HANDBOOK OF PEDIATRIC PSYCHOLOGY

The Society of Pediatric Psychology (Division 54 of the American Psychological Association) is pleased to sponsor the publication of this *Handbook*. Such sponsorship recognizes the scholarly significance of the volume and the care taken in the development of the chapters on scientific and professional issues. Topics were selected by experts in pediatric psychology, and recognized professionals in the field were solicited to contribute chapters. This was followed by an extensive peer review process for each chapter. This *Handbook* has not been considered by the Council of Representatives of the American Psychological Association, however, and does not represent official policy of the organization as a whole.

HANDBOOK OF PEDIATRIC PSYCHOLOGY

Third Edition

Edited by
MICHAEL C. ROBERTS

THE GUILFORD PRESS
New York London

A Division of Guilford Publications, Inc.
72 Spring Street, New York, NY 10012
www.guilford.com

Printed in the United States of America

This book is printed on acid-free paper.

Last digit is print number: 9 8 7 6 5 4 3 2 1

Library of Congress Cataloging-in-Publication Data

Handbook of pediatric psychology / edited by Michael C. Roberts.— 3rd ed.
p. cm.
Includes bibliographical references and index.
ISBN 1-57230-906-7 (alk. paper)
1. Pediatrics—Psychological aspects. 2. Sick children—Psychology.
I. Roberts, Michael C.
RJ47.5.H38 2003
618.92′0001′9—dc21

2003010143

Dedicated to the memory of
Lizette Peterson-Homer (1951–2002)
for her significant contributions to the
empirical foundations of pediatric psychology

And in recognition of Donald K. Routh
for his ongoing exceptional contributions
to the development of the field in numerous ways

About the Editor

Michael C. Roberts, PhD, ABPP, is Professor and Director of the Clinical Child Psychology Program at the University of Kansas. He formerly edited three journals—*Journal of Pediatric Psychology, Children's Health Care*, and *Children's Services: Social Policy, Research, and Practice*. In addition to conducting research in pediatric and clinical child psychology, Dr. Roberts has authored and coedited several books, including *Pediatric Psychology: Psychological Interventions and Strategies for Pediatric Problems, Casebook of Child and Pediatric Psychology, Handbook of Clinical Child Psychology, Readings in Pediatric Psychology, Helping Children Cope with Disasters and Terrorism, Beyond Appearances: A New Look at Adolescent Girls*, and *Managing Managed Care*. He has been President of the Society of Pediatric Psychology and the APA Section on Clinical Child Psychology, and is the current Chair of the Council of University Directors of Clinical Psychology and a member of the APA Council of Representatives on behalf of the Society of Pediatric Psychology.

Contributors

James D. Acton, MD, Cincinnati Children's Hospital Medical Center, University of Cincinnati College of Medicine, Cincinnati, Ohio

Ann Alriksson-Schmidt, MSPH, Civitan International Research Center and Department of Psychology, University of Alabama in Birmingham, Birmingham, Alabama

F. Daniel Armstrong, PhD, Mailman Center for Child Development, Department of Pediatrics, University of Miami School of Medicine, Miami, Florida

Glen P. Aylward, PhD, Division of Developmental and Behavioral Pediatrics, Southern Illinois University School of Medicine, Springfield, Illinois

Gerard A. Banez, PhD, Division of Pediatrics, Children's Hospital at The Cleveland Clinic, Cleveland, Ohio

Karen J. Bearman, MS, Department of Psychology, University of Miami, Coral Gables, Florida

Charmaine Biega, RN, NC, Columbus Children's Hospital, Columbus, Ohio

Maureen M. Black, PhD, Department of Pediatrics, University of Maryland School of Medicine, Baltimore, Maryland

Ronald L. Blount, PhD, Department of Psychology, University of Georgia, Athens, Georgia

Richard E. Boles, MS, Clinical Child Psychology Program, University of Kansas, Lawrence, Kansas

Barbara L. Bonner, PhD, Department of Pediatrics, Center on Child Abuse and Neglect, University of Oklahoma Health Sciences Center, Oklahoma City, Oklahoma

Anne Bradley, PhD, Department of Physical Medicine and Rehabilitation, University of Michigan, Ann Arbor, Michigan

Keri J. Brown, MA, Clinical Child Psychology Program, University of Kansas, Lawrence, Kansas

Ronald T. Brown, PhD, ABPP, College of Health Professions, Medical University of South Carolina, Charleston, South Carolina

Donald Brunnquell, PhD, Office of Ethics, Children's Hospitals and Clinics, Minneapolis and St. Paul, Minnesota

Lisa M. Buckloh, PhD, Department of Pediatric Medicine, Division of Psychology and Psychiatry, Nemours Children's Clinic, Jacksonville, Florida

Karen S. Budd, PhD, Department of Psychology, DePaul University, Chicago, Illinois
Catherine Butz, PhD, Department of Pediatrics, Columbus Children's Hospital and Ohio State University, Columbus, Ohio
Jonathan M. Campbell, PhD, Department of Educational Psychology, University of Georgia, Athens, Georgia
Edward R. Christophersen, PhD, Section of Developmental and Behavioral Sciences, Children's Mercy Hospital, Kansas City, Missouri
Lindsey L. Cohen, PhD, Department of Psychology, West Virginia University, Morgantown, West Virginia
Terry A. Crump, PhD, Division of Oncology, Children's Hospital of Philadelphia, Philadelphia, Pennsylvania
Carin Cunningham, PhD, Behavioral Pediatrics and Psychology, Department of Pediatrics, Rainbow Babies and Children's Hospital, Case Western Reserve University School of Medicine, Cleveland, Ohio
Lynnda M. Dahlquist, PhD, Department of Psychology, University of Maryland, Baltimore County, Baltimore, Maryland
Eugene J. D'Angelo, PhD, Department of Psychiatry, Children's Hospital, Harvard Medical School, Boston, Massachusetts
Melissa A. Davis, MHS, Department of Clinical and Health Psychology, University of Florida, Gainesville, Florida
Alan M. Delamater, PhD, Department of Pediatrics, University of Miami School of Medicine, Miami, Florida
Carrie A. Dittner, PhD, Department of Psychiatry and Psychology, Mayo Clinic, Rochester, Minnesota
Pamela Dixon, PhD, Department of Physical Medicine and Rehabilitation, University of Michigan, Ann Arbor, Michigan
Dennis Drotar, PhD, Behavioral Pediatrics and Psychology, Department of Pediatrics, Rainbow Babies and Children's Hospital, Case Western Reserve University School of Medicine, Cleveland, Ohio
George J. DuPaul, PhD, School Psychology Program, Lehigh University, Philadelphia, Pennsylvania
Lisa A. Efron, PhD, Departments of Psychiatry and Pediatrics, Children's National Medical Center and George Washington University, Washington, DC
Catherine C. Epkins, PhD, Department of Psychology, Texas Tech University, Lubbock, Texas
Alexandra E. Evans, PhD, Department of Health Promotion, Education, and Behavior, Norman J. Arnold School of Public Health, University of South Carolina, Columbia, South Carolina
Jennifer L. Fisher, PhD, Department of Psychiatry and Psychology, Mayo Clinic, Rochester, Minnesota
Esther Forti, PhD, Department of Health Professions, Medical University of South Carolina, Charleston, South Carolina
Bernard Fuemmeler, PhD, National Cancer Institute, Medical University of South Carolina, Charleston, South Carolina
Cynthia A. Gerhardt, PhD, Center for Biobehavioral Health, Columbus Children's Research Institute, Columbus, Ohio
Alan G. Glaros, PhD, Department of Dental Public Health and Behavioral Science, University of Missouri–Kansas City, Kansas City, Missouri

Peggy Greco, PhD, Department of Pediatric Medicine, Division of Psychology and Psychiatry, Nemours Children's Clinic, Jacksonville, Florida

Kelly Green, MSW, LISW, Columbus Children's Hospital, Columbus, Ohio

Cynthia Harbeck-Weber, PhD, Department of Psychiatry and Psychology, Mayo Clinic, Rochester, Minnesota

Dennis C. Harper, PhD, Department of Pediatrics, Division of Developmental Disabilities, Center for Disabilities and Development, University of Iowa, Iowa City, Iowa

Ahna Hoff, MS, Department of Psychology, Oklahoma State University, Stillwater, Oklahoma

E. Wayne Holden, PhD, ORC Macro, Atlanta, Georgia

Heather Huszti, PhD, Department of Health Psychology, Children's Hospital of Orange County, Orange, California

Jennie N. Jackson, BS, Department of Educational Psychology, University of Georgia, Athens, Georgia

Elissa Jelalian, PhD, Child and Family Psychiatry, Rhode Island Hospital and Brown University Medical School, Providence, Rhode Island

Christa Johnson, PhD, Department of Pediatrics, University of Oklahoma Health Sciences Center, Oklahoma City, Oklahoma

Anne E. Kazak, PhD, ABPP, Department of Psychology, Children's Hospital of Philadelphia and University of Pennsylvania, Philadelphia, Pennsylvania

Ambika Krishnakumar, PhD, Department of Family Studies, Syracuse University, Syracuse, New York

Michelle Kees, PhD, Department of Pediatrics, University of Oklahoma Health Sciences Center, Oklahoma City, Oklahoma

Donald G. Kewman, PhD, Department of Physical Medicine and Rehabilitation, University of Michigan, Ann Arbor, Michigan

Annette M. La Greca, PhD, Department of Psychology, University of Miami, Coral Gables, Florida

Kathleen L. Lemanek, PhD, Department of Psychology, Columbus Children's Hospital, Ohio State University College of Medicine, Columbus, Ohio

Carol B. Lindsley, MD, Department of Pediatrics, University of Kansas Medical Center, Kansas City, Kansas

Thomas R. Linscheid, PhD, Department of Pediatrics and Psychology, Columbus Children's Hospital, Ohio State University, Columbus, Ohio

Mary Beth Logue, PhD, Department of Pediatrics, University of Oklahoma Health Sciences Center, Oklahoma City, Oklahoma

Claudia Lupia, RN, BS, OCN, Columbus Children's Hospital, Columbus, Ohio

Laura M. Mackner, PhD, Columbus Children's Hospital, Ohio State University, Columbus, Ohio

Joanna O. Mashunkashey, BS, Clinical Child Psychology Program, University of Kansas, Lawrence, Kansas

Sunnye Mayes, BA, Clinical Child Psychology Program, University of Kansas, Lawrence, Kansas

Jennifer A. Mautone, MEd, School Psychology Program, Lehigh University, Philadelphia, Pennsylvania

Kara E. McGoey, PhD, School Psychology Program, Kent State University, Kent, Ohio

Ann M. McGrath, PhD, Department of Pediatrics, University of Kansas Medical Center, Kansas City, Kansas

Rodney McNeal, PhD, Department of Psychology, Central Missouri State University, Warrensburg, Missouri

Elizabeth L. McQuaid, PhD, Department of Psychiatry and Human Behavior, Brown University School of Medicine, Providence, Rhode Island

Robyn Mehlenbeck, PhD, Child and Family Psychiatry, Rhode Island Hospital and Brown University Medical School, Providence, Rhode Island

Montserrat C. Mitchell, BS, Clinical Child Psychology Program, University of Kansas, Lawrence, Kansas

Avani C. Modi, MS, Department of Clinical and Health Psychology, University of Florida, Gainesville, Florida

Sam B. Morgan, PhD, Department of Psychology, University of Memphis, Memphis, Tennessee

Susan L. Mortweet, PhD, Section of Developmental and Behavioral Sciences, Children's Mercy Hospital, Kansas City, Missouri

Robert B. Noll, PhD, Division of Hematology/Oncology, Children's Hospital Medical Center, Cincinnati, Ohio

Susana R. Patton, PhD, Division of Psychology, Cincinnati Children's Hospital Medical Center, University of Cincinnati College of Medicine, Cincinnati, Ohio

Tiina Piira, MPsych (Clinical), Pain Research Unit, Sydney Children's Hospital, Sydney, Australia

Alexandra L. Quittner, PhD, Department of Clinical and Health Psychology, University of Florida, Gainesville, Florida

William A. Rae, PhD, Department of Educational Psychology, Texas A&M University, College Station, Texas

Mark A. Ranalli, MD, Columbus Children's Hospital, Ohio State University College of Medicine, Columbus, Ohio

Michael A. Rapoff, PhD, Department of Pediatrics, University of Kansas Medical Center, Kansas City, Kansas

L. Kaye Rasnake, PhD, Department of Psychology, Denison University, Granville, Ohio

Jennifer Reiter-Purtill, MA, Division of Hematology/Oncology, Children's Hospital Medical Center, Cincinnati, Ohio

Michael C. Roberts, PhD, ABPP, Clinical Child Psychology Program, University of Kansas, Lawrence, Kansas

James R. Rodrigue, PhD, Center for Behavioral Health Research in Organ Transplantation and Donation, University of Florida Health Science Center, Gainesville, Florida

Mary T. Rourke, PhD, Department of Psychology, Children's Hospital of Philadelphia, Philadelphia, Pennsylvania

Terri L. Shelton, PhD, Center for the Study of Social Issues, University of North Carolina at Greensboro, Greensboro, North Carolina

Lawrence J. Siegel, PhD, Dean and Professor of Ferkauf Graduate School of Psychology, Yeshiva University, New York, New York

Amanda B. Sobel, PhD, Department of Pediatric Medicine, Division of Psychology and Psychiatry, Nemours Children's Clinic, Jacksonville, Florida

Karen Sorgen, PhD, Brooklyn Pediatric AIDS Network, Downstate Medical Center, Brooklyn, New York

Anthony Spirito, PhD, Department of Psychiatry and Human Behavior, Brown University Medical School, Providence, Rhode Island

Terry Stancin, PhD, Department of Pediatrics, MetroHealth Medical Center and Case Western Reserve University School of Medicine, Cleveland, Ohio

Lori J. Stark, PhD, Division of Psychology, Cincinnati Children's Hospital Medical Center, University of Cincinnati College of Medicine, Cincinnati, Ohio

Randi Streisand, PhD, Departments of Psychiatry and Pediatrics, Children's National Medical Center and George Washington University, Washington, DC

Jeremy R. Sullivan, BS, Department of Educational Psychology, Texas A&M University, College Station, Texas

Marni C. Switkin, MA, Department of Psychology, University of Maryland, Baltimore County, Baltimore, Maryland

Kenneth J. Tarnowski, PhD, ABPP, Psychology Program, Florida Gulf Coast University, Fort Myers, Florida

Kenneth P. Tercyak, PhD, Departments of Oncology and Pediatrics, Georgetown University School of Medicine and Lombardi Cancer Center, Georgetown University Medical Center, Washington, DC

Robert J. Thompson, Jr., PhD, Trinity College, Duke University, Durham, North Carolina

Kathryn Vannatta, PhD, Center for Biobehavioral Health, Columbus Children's Research Institute, Columbus, Ohio

Natalie Walders, PhD, Department of Psychiatry and Human Behavior, Brown University Medical School, Providence, Rhode Island

C. Eugene Walker, PhD, Department of Psychiatry and Behavioral Sciences, University of Oklahoma Medical School, Oklahoma City, Oklahoma

Jan L. Wallander, PhD, Civitan International Research Center and Department of Psychology, University of Alabama at Birmingham, Birmingham, Alabama

Seth Warschausky, PhD, Department of Physical Medicine and Rehabilitation, University of Michigan, Ann Arbor, Michigan

Dawn K. Wilson, PhD, Prevention Research Center, Department of Health Promotion, Education, and Behavior, Norman J. Arnold School of Public Health, University of South Carolina, Columbia, South Carolina

Elizabeth J. Willen, PhD, Department of Pediatrics, University of Miami School of Medicine, Miami, Florida

Tim Wysocki, PhD, ABPP, Department of Pediatric Medicine, Division of Psychology and Psychiatry, Nemours Children's Clinic, Jacksonville, Florida

Preface

The growth of pediatric psychology has been a remarkable phenomenon. The conceptualizations, research, and practice activities initially included in the field remain central to the daily lives of pediatric psychologists as scientist-practitioners. These original conceptualizations have been expanded daily with a multitude of activities in research and practice. This expansion is important for a vital and developing clinical profession built on empirical science. Notably, as a reflection of the field, this third edition builds on the foundations of the first two editions (Routh, 1988; Roberts, 1995), while adding some new concepts and topics. Thus this *Handbook* has continued to evolve to include newer aspects, as well as what may be understood as "traditional" pediatric psychology.

As with the second edition, I formed an advisory panel of experts in the field and solicited their ideas for topics and organization, including continuing or changing authors, and continuing, combining, expanding, or adding new topics, all while keeping the length similar to that of the previous edition. It is always interesting to see what professionals, scientists and clinicians, think is part of their field. Indeed, not all pediatric psychologists see the same things in the field as interesting and important (see, e.g., Brown & Roberts, 2000). Some panelists and authors commented that they would not have included certain topics in this volume because they personally have no interest in one or another topic, while wanting more space for their own interests. I valued their comments and perspectives, but ultimately I, as editor, had the final say in the contents and framework. In developing the book's outline and the topical coverage of the chapters, the advisory panel and I tried to take an open-minded perspective and include the diversity of activities and interests within pediatric psychology. The selection of topics and allocation of pages represents as much of the range of the field as we could put into the space available.

A handbook of this type can attempt to be comprehensive, but space limitations (and the need to keep the book's cost to a reasonable amount) inevitably constrain what could eventually be a multivolume set. All chapter authors suffered under these page constraints; each wanted much more space to cover essential topics. The reviewers and I tried to delete all such lamentations in the chapters because every author was under the same restrictions. Noting the page limits and remarking that there are other topics to cover takes up space, and it is simply a fact of life that we never get adequate space to cover all the things we ever want to include. I promised the authors that I would note here that severe space requirements were imposed and that they could not cover everything they would like to have included.

As noted in the imprimatur statement for this edition, this *Handbook* is a peer-reviewed publication of the Society of Pediatric Psychology. Each chapter was reviewed by at least two professional-level psychologists who are experts on the topics (the board of editors) and by a number of graduate students from several training programs (the student board of editors), in addition to my own reviewing and editing. The chapters were read with an eye to such considerations as content coverage and accuracy, readability, and references. This peer review process, although time-consuming and effortful, helped improve the overall quality and utility of the *Handbook* chapters for readers at all levels and with a range of clinical research interests. I thank the members of the advisory panel, the editorial board, and the student editorial board listed in the front of this book for their timely and substantive reviews of the chapters. Their contributions made this a stronger book than it would have been if only an editor had reviewed it.

I thank Tammie Zordel, the program secretary for the Clinical Child Psychology Program at the University of Kansas, for her assistance with this *Handbook* at all stages. Appreciation is also due to my wife, for putting up with the mess in the basement office while I devoted far too much attention to this "work of love," and to my children, for overlooking my heightened distractedness during the editing process.

The first edition of the *Handbook* was dedicated to Logan Wright, who passed away in 1999 and will be remembered for his contributions in founding the field of pediatric psychology and for early research and professional writings (Willis, 2000). The present volume is dedicated to two pediatric psychologists, each of whom has made significant contributions to the foundation, growth, and vitality of the field. While recognizing their professional accomplishments, this dedication honoring Lizette Peterson-Homer and Donald K. Routh is also a personal one for me. As I have noted,

> Lizette Peterson-Homer was an exceptional clinical researcher, dedicated teacher and mentor, and supportive colleague and friend to many in pediatric psychology. Her innovative applications were coupled with strong methodological standards in creating a superb portfolio of contributions to the field. Lizette's premature death on July 18, 2002, was a loss for the discipline of psychology and particularly for the field of pediatric psychology. . . . Among her strengths were the orientations she carried into her work, such as a critical founding in child development, behavior analysis, and cognitive behavior therapy, strong standards for research methodology, a practical reliance on theory, and a passion to make a better world for children. (Roberts, 2002, pp. 765–766)

Lizette wrote chapters in the two previous editions of this *Handbook*.

Don Routh, who edited the first edition of the *Handbook*, is honored here (as he was in the second edition) through a living dedication. In his many magnanimous ways, Don contributed and continues to contribute his knowledge, work ethic, and resources to vivify our field. Years ago, Don and his wife, Marion, established a fund within the Society of Pediatric Psychology for supporting research into injuries and injury prevention in memory of their daughter, who was tragically killed. After Lizette's unexpected death in the summer of 2002, Don generously requested that the Rebecca Routh Coon Injury Research Grant be renamed to honor Lizette as the Lizette Peterson-Homer Injury Prevention Research Grant administered by the Society of Pediatric Psychology with the American Psychological Foundation. The royalties from the sales of this *Handbook* will also fund this research award for students and faculty to support research related to the prevention of childhood injuries from a psychological perspective. Donations can also be made to American Psychological Foundation (750 First Street, NE, Washington, DC 20002) to honor both Don and Lizette and further the cause of reducing injury and death in childhood.

MICHAEL C. ROBERTS

REFERENCES

Brown, K. J., & Roberts, M. C. (2000). Future issues in pediatric psychology: Delphic survey. *Journal of Clinical Psychology in Medical Settings, 7*, 5–15.

Roberts, M. C. (Ed.). (1995). *Handbook of pediatric psychology* (2nd ed.). New York: Guilford Press.

Roberts, M. C. (2002). The legacy of Lizette Peterson-Homer in pediatric psychology (1951–2002). *Journal of Pediatric Psychology, 27*, 765–769.

Routh, D. K. (Ed.). (1988). *Handbook of pediatric psychology.* New York: Guilford Press.

Willis, D. J. (2000). In memoriam: Logan Wright, Jr., PhD (1933–1999). *Journal of Pediatric Psychology, 25*, 359–361.

Contents

HANDBOOK OF PEDIATRIC PSYCHOLOGY

Part I

PROFESSIONAL ISSUES

1

The Evolving Field of Pediatric Psychology

Critical Issues and Future Challenges

MICHAEL C. ROBERTS
MONTSERRAT C. MITCHELL
RODNEY McNEAL

Pediatric psychology as a field of science and clinical practice addresses the range of physical and psychological development, health, and illness issues affecting children, adolescents, and their families. As part of a multifaceted field, scientist/practitioners in pediatric psychology explore the relationship among psychological and physical health and the welfare of children and adolescents within a developmental perspective, considering the contexts of families, caregivers, health care systems, schools, peers, and community. Pediatric psychologists, in a variety of roles, seek to promote a better understanding of developmental disorders, emotional and behavioral problems, and the concomitants of disease, illness, and injuries. With this understanding, pediatric psychologists provide assessment and measurement, intervene preventively and therapeutically, promote health and psychosocial development, and prevent illness and injury (Roberts, La Greca, & Harper, 1988). Increasingly, pediatric psychologists are utilizing their clinical science for public policy and advocacy.

PEDIATRIC PSYCHOLOGY: CLINICAL AND RESEARCH ACTIVITIES

Clinical Services of Pediatric Psychology

At least five venues or settings can be identified for pediatric psychology services: (1) inpatient medical center units for disease and illness (e.g., consultation/liaison services for acute and chronic illness units such as neonatal/pediatric intensive care, oncology, and burns); (2) medical outpatient clinics (e.g., private pediatric practices, consultation/liaison services to general pediatrics, endocrinology, plastic surgery, gastrointestinal); (3) outpatient and primary care clinics for emotional and behavioral problems; (4) specialty facilities, clinics, and centers (e.g., physical rehabilitation centers, child study or developmental disabilities centers, university-affiliated facilities); and (5) camps or groups (e.g., summer or weekend camps for children with chronic illnesses such as asthma, diabetes, sickle cell disease, spina bifida; parenting groups for children with chronic illness). The range of clinical activities provided in these service settings includes the following:

1. Psychosocial services for problems related to pediatric health conditions (e.g., adjustment to disease, management of disease symptoms, adherence to treatment regimens, coping with procedural pain or invasive procedures, treatments for medical problems such as encopresis or tracheotomy addiction)
2. Psychological interventions for mental health problems and issues appearing in medical units, sometimes as a concomitant of a medical condition (e.g., negative behaviors resulting from extended hospitalization, grief and bereavement, reintegration into school and community)
3. General mental health services for behavior problems referred to and referred within pediatric settings but not necessarily related to a pediatric health condition
4. Programs for promotion of health and prevention of and early intervention for both physical and psychological problems
5. Assessment, training, and education for mental retardation and developmental disabilities
6. Education and consultation for pediatricians and family physicians in training
7. Public health and public policy domains (Roberts, Brown, & Puddy, 2002).

Research Activities in Pediatric Psychology

In addition to illustrating the clinical service activities of pediatric psychology, these aspects are also the focus of scientific research in the field. Indeed, much of pediatric psychology has been able to demonstrate an integration of applied clinical activities and scientific research, whereas other specialties of psychology have increasingly bifurcated into either practice or research as separate entities. Perhaps pediatric psychology has remained well integrated because research has been focused largely on applied problems. Instead of separating to conduct solely basic psychological research, pediatric psychology has asked research questions relevant to applications and interventions (Brown & Roberts, 2000; Elkins & Roberts, 1988).

Research in pediatric psychology may be found in a number of journals (e.g., *Pediatrics*, *Children's Health Care*, *Journal of Developmental and Behavioral Pediatrics*, and to lesser degree *Health Psychology*, *Journal of Clinical Psychology in Medical Settings*, and *Journal of Behavioral Medicine*). The *Journal of Pediatric Psychology* (*JPP*), the flagship publication of the Society of Pediatric Psychology (Division 54 of the American Psychological Association), constitutes the most concentrated scientific representation of this field. Therefore, the contents of *JPP* reflect the breadth and depth of the field's research activities. A large percentage of empirical studies have investigated the development and manifestation of children's physical conditions and their relationships to psychosocial problems (labeled "explicative research" by Roberts, 1992). Pediatric psychology research has also evaluated biopsychosocial interventions in order to improve functioning and prevent problem development, as well as to develop and improve assessment and clinical diagnoses. Much of pediatric psychology research has involved various chronic illnesses that affect children and adolescents, such as diabetes, asthma, and cancer. Conditions at the intersection of medicine and psychology are also frequently researched, such as failure to thrive, attention-deficit/hyperactivity disorder, feeding and eating disorders, enuresis, and encopresis. The scientific activities and the range of research methodologies have strengthened the clinical aspects of pediatric psychology (Roberts, McNeal, Randall, & Roberts, 1996). A multi- and interdisciplinary collaboration has also been at the core of much work in research and clinical services (Wertlieb, 1999).

Indeed, the rest of this *Handbook* relies on the empirical foundations established in the clinical research activities of pediatric psychologists. As noted by Roberts et al. (2002), several pragmatic reasons, both theoretical and clinical, contribute to the increased emphasis on evidence-based or empirically supported assessment and treatment. These include (1) intellectual curiosity for understanding of the development and manifestations of pediatric psychological problems; (2) a commitment to finding better ways to intervene and provide quality services that benefit children and families; (3) attempts to enhance accountability and honesty in providing worthwhile services; (4) improvements in measurement and assessment for evaluating the process and outcomes of pediatric psychology services; (5) new conceptualizations of basic and applied research and of evaluation of intervention models. Additionally, the field manifests a responsiveness and accountability to societal need. As a profession, pediatric psychology demonstrates a strong commitment to professional ethics and to providing competent services. To a large degree, these reasons have existed since the founding of the field known as pediatric psychology (Wright, 1967). More recently, managed care has affected the delivery of services and necessitated demonstrations of effective clinical work (Roberts & Hurley, 1997). Other disciplines, including medicine, nursing, and social work, have also moved toward an evidence-based orientation to treatment and organization of services. Thus, today, perhaps more than at any other time in the history of pediatric psychology, the reliance on integrating science and practice has its greatest value.

DEVELOPMENTS IN THE HISTORY OF PEDIATRIC PSYCHOLOGY

Conceptual Origins

The roots of pediatric psychology can be traced to the late 19th century, when Lightner Witmer established the first psychological clinic in the United States, at which he interacted with pediatricians and schools to help children with general and pediatric-related problems (Routh, 1975). Early in the 20th century, psychologists and pediatricians began to perceive the importance of recognizing the link between psychology and medicine. By 1919, Arnold Gesell, a psychologist and physician, had articulated the potential contributions of clinical psychology in the medical treatment of children (Gesell, 1919). This position was reiterated by J. E. Anderson (1938) in an address to the American Medical Association. In particular, he called for clinical psychologists to assist pediatricians through child assessments and parent training. However, little collaboration seems to have resulted from these presentations. Much later, Kagan (1965) called for a "new marriage" between psychology and pediatrics. As he envisioned it, this marriage of disciplines would be particularly beneficial for the purposes of prevention, early detection, and treatment.

The term "pediatric psychology" was first coined by Logan Wright (1967) in an article entitled "The Pediatric Psychologist: A Role Model." This work is considered pivotal in the conceptualization and vitalization of the field (Roberts, 1993). Wright defined pediatric psychology as "dealing primarily with children in a medical setting which is nonpsychiatric in nature" (1967, p. 323). Additionally, he outlined the need for pediatric psychologists to (1) establish a group identity through formal organization, (2) develop specialized professional training, and (3) construct a new body of applied research. As becomes evident in this chapter, these perceived needs led to concrete developments in the field of pediatric psychology.

Organizational Developments

One of these developments came in 1966, when George Albee, president of the Division of Clinical Psychology of the American Psychological Association (APA), requested that the division's Section on Clinical Child Psychology evaluate the potential for the organization of a group interested in pediatric issues. A committee was assembled, and, as part of its needs assessment, it sent letters to pediatric departments in every medical school in the United States, asking for names of psychologists on staff that might be interested in a society to meet the needs of pediatric psychologists. In response, they received the names of 250 interested professionals. Thus, in August 1968, the Society of Pediatric Psychology (SPP) was formed as an affiliate of the Section of Clinical Child Psychology, with 75 full members and 22 affiliate members. In 1980, the SPP became an independent section within the Division of Clinical Psychology.

Publications

Over time, one of SPP's methods of meeting the needs of pediatric psychologists has been through its publications. At the time of its initial formation, the society began publication of a newsletter entitled *Pediatric Psychology*. In 1975, this newsletter changed its format to that of a journal, and in 1976, the first issue of the *Journal of Pediatric Psychology* (*JPP*) was published. The publication of this journal solidified the foundation of SPP and established it as the organizational home for the field of pediatric psychology. As SPP has grown, it has also published professional texts, sponsored conferences, testified in front of the U.S. Senate, collaborated with other national organizations, and organized task forces on different issues important to children and families. Through these activities, SPP has fostered the development of professionals interested in the research and applications at the intersection of psychology and pediatric medicine. Roberts (1993) and Routh (1994) have provided a more detailed history of SPP. In order to document the historical foundations of pediatric psychology, the *JPP* has started publishing a series of articles on "Pioneers in Pediatric Psychology," in which early leaders reflect on the development of the field and their own contributions (Drotar, 2001; Routh, 2000; Walker, 2000). A brief history of the journal itself was also recently published (Kazak, 2000).

Early Clinical Activities

Surveys of pediatric psychologists have provided historical information about the differentiation of pediatric psychology from clinical child psychology. In a survey of pediatric psychologists and clinical child psychologists, Tuma and Grabert (1983) found that pediatric psychologists were different from clinical child psychologists not only in that they primarily dealt with medically related issues in children, collaborated with health care disciplines, and functioned more within the medical model, but also in that they spent more time in assessment than in treatment and were more likely to see clients of low socioeconomic status and with developmental delays. Other surveys have ascertained additional aspects of the field. For example, Stabler and Mesibov (1984) found that pediatric psychologists tended to practice in primary care facilities, in which a significant amount of their time was spent providing direct clinical services, including consultation and diagnostic testing. Compared with these earlier surveys, recent analyses show that the role and placements of pediatric psychologists are increasingly becoming more diverse (Drotar & Lemanek, 2001; see also Drotar, Spirito, & Stancin, Chapter 4, this volume).

In the beginning years of the field, the primary activities of pediatric psychologists involved clinical applications in service settings. Because this role was still under development, a great need existed for models and descriptions of the roles and functions of pediatric psychologists in clinical service. As a consequence, various practitioners published accounts of their settings, assessment and treatment activities, successes, and obstacles, as well as conceptual approaches. In the classic article noted earlier, Wright (1967) described a "model" role for the pediatric psychologist, which included psychological testing and diagnosis, training of child-rearing and behavioral skills, short-term psychotherapeutic methods, and applied research. In 1978, Lee Salk outlined the services then provided by the Division of Psychology in Pediatrics at the New York Hospital–Cornell Medical Center, which included "on the spot" consultations and case referrals from his pediatric department colleagues. Like Wright, Salk illustrated the role of pediatric psychologists in screening, diagnosis, and short-term therapy; however, he also emphasized the need for strong consultative relationships with the pediatric staff, particularly in regard to child emotional development, behavioral techniques, and the reduction of the traumatic nature of medical procedures and hospitalization. This aspect of pediatric psychology has been depicted in additional descriptions of clinical work. For example, Gerald Koocher and his colleagues outlined a model for pediatric oncology consultation in which children in treatment for cancer were routinely seen by a pediatric psychology team (Koocher, Sourkes, & Keane, 1979; O'Malley & Koocher, 1977). As in the previous examples, the team dealt with a wide range of issues, and referrals were also followed up for depression, developmental delay due to hospitalization, serious acting out, and behavioral management during medical events. Case examples provided specific illustrations of how pediatric psychology interventions were implemented. Also early in the descriptive phase of the field's development, service descriptions were published about other hospital units that required psychological consultation and intervention, such as intensive care nurseries (Magrab & Davitt, 1975), neurological units (Hartlage & Hartlage, 1978), and units specializing in renal dialysis and transplantation (Magrab, 1975). Over time, these narrative articles played an important role in defining the field.

As such services increased in number and sophistication, depictions of the nature of pediatric psychology began to move beyond case examples to descriptive data presentations. Publications portrayed the types of referrals, interventions, and other aspects of practice by including more empirical data. Roberts and Walker (1989) collated the types of cases typically seen in outpatient pediatric psychology practices by combining three analyses of case referrals by Walker (1979), Ottinger and Roberts (1980), and Kanoy and Schroeder (1985). The three analyses showed fairly consistent patterns of practice, with large numbers of referrals for what might be considered traditional child and family mental health concerns (e.g., negative behaviors, school-related problems, and personality disorders). However, the second most common set of problems represented those suited for the specialty of pediatric psychologists, such as physical complaints, adjustment to disease, developmental delays, toileting, and infant management problems. In another data-based examination, Olson et al. (1988) found that the most frequent referrals to inpatient psychological services at a children's hospital were for poor adjustment to a chronic illness, behavior problems, and depression or suicide attempts. These referrals were most frequently made from the pediatric, surgical, and adolescent units. Therapeutic contacts with the patient and his or her family were typically brief (fewer than four sessions); however, longer contacts were needed for problems such as decannulation of tracheostomy, pain management of burns, eating problems, and terminal illness. Evaluation of this unit found considerable satisfaction with the services provided. A similar examination of consultation/liaison services in another hospital also revealed positive findings (Rodrigue et al., 1995).

Descriptions of the types of services provided by pediatric psychologists and analyses of the variety of referrals they typically see help to define the field and convey the diverse and wide-ranging clinical applications of pediatric psychology (e.g., Armstrong et al., 1999; King, Cathers, King, & Rosenbaum, 2001; Singer & Drotar, 1989; Sobel, Roberts, Rapoff, & Barnard, 2001; Sobel, Roberts, Rayfield, Barnard, & Rapoff, 2001). The development of clinical practice has often been paralleled by changes in the research aspects of this field.

Development of Research Activities

Changes in the empirical basis of pediatric psychology can be traced by looking at analyses of the content of the field's primary journal, *JPP*. The first content analysis, done in 1979 by Routh and Mesibov, reported that in its first 3 years of official publication as a journal, *JPP* published mostly literature reviews and descriptions of clinical practice. These articles most frequently cited other articles published in *Pediatrics* and *Child Development*, illustrating the important merging of these two fields. Similarly, Routh (1980) later found that the authors most frequently cited in *JPP*'s first 4½ years included psychologists, child psychiatrists, and pediatricians, a variety that demonstrated the interdisciplinary nature of pediatric psychology.

In a further examination of the journal, Elkins and Roberts (1988) comprehensively analyzed the first 10 years of *JPP* articles (Volumes 1–10, 1976–1985). After categorizing the 351 articles according to participant population age groups, population types, article types, theoretical orientations, senior authors' affiliations, and gender of senior authors and editors, they found several interesting developments over time. For example, a trend emerged for an increasing number of articles to have female senior authors, and eventually female senior authors became the majority. Additionally, the more recent articles were more likely to have a senior author who was affiliated with a college or university rather than a medical setting, which had been the case for earlier articles. Over time, literature reviews and professional practice articles decreased, whereas the number of applied and basic research articles correspondingly increased. Consistent across time, the population ages for participants in research spanned two or more age groups, indicating a developmental focus; adolescents were the most underrepresented age group. Additionally, articles dealing with medically ill or developmentally delayed children accounted for 70.5% of the total. Roberts (1992) conducted a similar analysis of articles published from 1988 to 1992, the years of his editorship of the journal. Contrary to the Elkins and Roberts (1988) analysis, the majority of affiliations were with medical settings instead of universities. However, many results similar to the Elkins and Roberts (1988) analysis were obtained. A majority of the articles examined medical conditions, and most of the studied populations included several age groups. Only a few articles categorized in the Roberts (1992) study were literature reviews or dealt with professional practice; more than half of the articles were applied research reports, whereas one-third involved more basic research. He found that articles on intervention, prevention, and assessment constituted about 25% of *JPP*, whereas explicative research (i.e., investigating the connection between pediatric and psychological phenomena) made up about 75% of the articles. Roberts (1992) concluded that, although explicative research is necessary to increase understanding of the elements and processes of various pediatric and psychological phenomena, this improved understanding should also be translated into more effective interventions.

A similar article analysis by La Greca (1997), at the conclusion of her editorship, on *JPP* articles published between 1993 and 1997 illustrated that many of the trends evident in Roberts's (1992) analysis remained the same. For example, the majority of the empirical articles were still explicative (72%), although a slight increase occurred in articles on interventions and assessment. Additionally, as had been previously true, the majority of empirical articles published during this time period focused on pediatric chronic illnesses; however, La Greca commented that the research in this area appeared to be increasing in sophistication, offering, for instance, conceptual models to frame hypotheses. The most recent article analysis, done by Kazak (2002) on articles included in the *JPP* from 1998 to 2002 (conclusion of her editorship), supports some of the trends reported by Roberts (1992) and La Greca (1997). For example, the majority of empirical studies continued to be focused on chronic illnesses, and there continued to be an increasing number of female primary authors. Despite Roberts's call in 1992 for an increase in intervention research, this area still appeared to be lacking, because only 12 of 219 articles (5.4%) published during this time reported on intervention evaluations. This number is actually a decrease from the 1990–1994 period, which included 10.8% intervention/therapy reports (Roberts et al., 1996). This finding is of some concern because the future of pediatric psychology is perceived to rely on demonstrations of therapeutic utility (see later discussion of the Delphic survey by Brown & Roberts, 2000).

CONCEPTUALIZATIONS OF PEDIATRIC PSYCHOLOGY OVER TIME

The field of pediatric psychology was developed for a pragmatic reason. Pediatricians had been faced with a large number of problems in development, behavior, education, and child management (McClelland, Staples, Weisberg, & Berger, 1973). At the same time, psychologists discovered that the traditional office or outpatient practice did not meet the needs of clients and their families, especially those whose problems were related to medical phenomena. Therefore "pediatric and psychological practitioners found they could not meet the challenges of critical childhood problems from within the frameworks of either traditional pediatrics or traditional clinical child psychology" (Roberts, 1986, p. 2). The "new marriage" of psychology and pediatrics proposed by Kagan (1965) may have been fated. However, the interactions and collaborations between psychologists and pediatricians grew slowly and developed into institutionalized units only after individual interactions and relationships formed a foundation.

As this field has emerged, pediatric psychologists have generally elucidated some common characteristics of their practice. These commonalities include a clinical practice that is most likely done in a health care setting, either primary or tertiary, inpatient or outpatient. The patients are typically referred by colleagues in medically based fields, and clinical work is a balance between consultations with physicians and parents and direct interventions with children. The pediatric psychologist typically has a pragmatic orientation toward treatment techniques that are effective and time-efficient but flexible, while maintaining a problem-solving approach. Additionally, the practice of pediatric psychology demands a developmental perspective on diagnosis and intervention and an orientation to health promotion and problem prevention.

As the practice of pediatric psychology has evolved, so has its research. In particular, researchers have attempted to establish an empirical base for interventions and to gain a greater understanding of the interaction of psychology with pediatric problems and settings. The investigations have primarily focused on the problems that are most typically seen by pediatric psychologists, such as whether play therapy can ease the impact of hospitalization or what characteristics help a child adjust to a chronic illness. These types of studies illustrate the pragmatic nature of much of the practice-based research in pediatric psychology. As the field has developed this research base, more efforts have been made in the direction of model-based and theoretically driven studies. All of these research approaches have value; they help position pediatric psychology as an empirically based or scientifically applied field, and not just an intuitive, well-intentioned one.

Pediatric psychology has been conceptualized as a subspecialty of clinical child psychology, and therefore of clinical psychology (Roberts, Maddux, Wurtele, & Wright, 1982). However, this view may not be completely accurate. For example, many researchers and practitioners have obtained training in special education, developmental psychology, school psychology, and experimental psychology, but their interests have extended to children in medical settings. Pediatric psychology has become a multifaceted discipline, so its organizational home, the SPP, accommodates many diverse activities and backgrounds. This diversity has enriched the field.

CRITICAL RECENT DEVELOPMENTS IN THE HISTORY OF PEDIATRIC PSYCHOLOGY

Development as an APA Division

After years of sitting organizationally as a section of the Division of Clinical Psychology, in 2001 the Society of Pediatric Psychology (SPP) formally assumed greater status as Division 54 of the American Psychological Association. This increased visibility resulted from the efforts of its members to establish the knowledge base and applied practice dimensions of an area differentiated from other related areas (e.g., clinical psychology, health psychology, clinical child and adolescent psychology, and developmental psychology). By increasing its stature and recognition within the field of psychology, this historical event has enhanced the vitality of pediatric psychology as a concept and SPP as its organizational home. The SPP has also developed a strong liaison with the American Academy of Pediatrics through its Committee on Psychosocial Aspects of Child and Family Health (Armstrong, 1997; see also Spirito, 2002). As a result, pediatric psychologists' input has been included in the formulation of a number of position statements on such issues as psychosocial aspects of pediatric care; assessment and management of acute pain in infants, children, and adolescents; sexuality education; and insurance coverage of mental health and substance abuse services (e.g., American Academy of Pediatrics, 2000, 2001a, 2001b, 2001c).

New Challenges of Reimbursement

In another recent development affecting pediatric psychology (and all health care), the managed care model as a new form of financial reimbursement for services has negatively affected access and delivery of pediatric and psychological services (Brown & Roberts, 2000; Roberts & Hurley, 1997). The quality and quantity of care have been adversely influenced by lowered rates of reimbursement and restricted coverage of certain diagnoses and interventions for problems. Additionally, many pediatric psychology services for children—such as for managing pain, increasing adherence to medication regimens, enhancing adjustment to chronic disease, or working on multidisciplinary teams (for child abuse or feeding/eating disorders)—are not directly covered by many managed care organizations. Services for psychosocial problems that do not fit the psychiatrically based fourth edition of the *Diagnostic and Statistical Manual of Mental Disorders* (American Psychiatric Association, 1994) are also not covered. The American Academy of Pediatrics sponsored an interdisciplinary task force that developed a tool for diagnosing and managing psychosocial problems in pediatric primary care, titled the *Diagnostic and Statistical Manual for Primary Care* (DMS-PC; Wolraich, Felice, & Drotar, 1996). If adopted widely, DSM-PC could lead to greater reimbursement and access to psychosocial services (Drotar, 1999). The restrictive effects of managed care are likely to continue in some form, however, and the innovative contributions of pediatric psychologists will be needed. Drotar and Zagorski (2001) noted that one effect of the lowered reimbursement rate for mental health and medical services has been that professionals have to "work hard for less money" with greater potential for "burnout and disruption in quality of care" (p. 91). Further, Drotar and Zagorski (2001) also detailed the difficulties of pediatric psychology services within a managed care environment. These difficulties include a lack of support for challenges to collaboration and coordination of care with other professionals, to the detriment of effective, competent, and high-quality care of children and families.

The Promise of Primary Preventive Care

Drotar and Zagorski (2001) also observed an increasing trend for pediatric psychology services to be offered in satellite clinics, away from the typical hospital base but closer to where families live. The move to nonhospital clinics offers greater opportunity for participation in primary care interventions and prevention (Roberts & Brown, in press; Stancin, 1999; Wildman & Stancin, in press). Although some activities in treating psychosocial problems in primary care have long been a part of pediatric psychology (e.g., Schroeder, 1979, 1996), funding for consultation/liaison services in inpatient units was more prevalent. Thus interest in primary care services has not been as extensive as the apparent interest in inpatient services and care for patients with chronic illnesses. However, as with all health care services in managed care, proof of effectiveness and worth does not translate into adequate funding for providing psychosocial and early intervention services.

Challenges for Empirically Supported Treatments

The professional disciplines of medicine and psychology have recently moved toward empirically supported treatments and evidence-based practice, although both disciplines have long been engaged in establishing the scientific bases for assessment and practice. Within clinical psychology, criteria for listing a treatment as an empirically supported treatment (EST) required (1) details on the participants involved in treatment outcomes research, (2) randomized clinical trials and/or single case designs, (3) detailed descriptions of the therapeutic approach, usually in a treatment manual, and (4) replication by independent researchers. In clinical child psychology, the EST effort modified some criteria and produced excellent summaries of treatments in the literature (Chambless & Ollendick, 2001; Chorpita et al., 2002; Lonigan, Elbert, & Johnson, 1998). The Society of Pediatric Psychology commissioned a similar series of reviews that appeared in *JPP* (Spirito, 1999). Treatments covered in these EST reviews include regimen adherence, nocturnal enuresis, severe feeding problems, pain, and disease-related symptoms. More treatment summaries are planned, and a book is in the development stage. SPP recently appointed a task force to develop criteria and reviews of empirically supported assessments to parallel the treatment series.

The goals of the EST movement are to determine the most effective treatments for specific mental health and physical problems and to help pediatric psychologists select which interventions to use with particular patients. Although not without controversy, the EST activity has advanced the field, increased the quality and utility of clinical research, and exposed which treatments have been empirically established and which have not. A research agenda for pediatric psychology can be ascertained from these reviews. The future of pediatric psychology will include developments in refining EST criteria, as well as increasing the amount and nature of scientific evaluations of therapeutic outcomes. This work will establish the worth and position of pediatric psychologists as contributing to the health and development of pediatric patients. As Roberts noted in 1986, the field needed to move from the "intuitive" to the empirical; EST-related activities accelerate the momentum for the future.

FUTURE OF PEDIATRIC PSYCHOLOGY

Delphic Projections about the Future

As a formal assessment of projections for the future, Brown and Roberts (2000) conducted a Delphic poll of researchers and clinicians who were members of SPP. Participants were asked to identify the major issues that will affect the direction of pediatric psychology over the next 10 years. After three rounds of inquiry and Internet dialogue, the results of this Delphic survey indicated high consensus for the top ten issues identified. Table 1.1 depicts the issue domains viewed as most significant. As can be seen, the highest priority was assigned to the ability of the pediatric psychology field to demonstrate viability through empirical support for treatment interventions and improving health outcomes of pediatric conditions. Similarly, the integration of the psychologist into the pediatric primary care setting was also perceived as a high priority (second on the list), as were increased collaboration, prevention of problems, and promotion of physical and mental health. The effects of managed care may be evidenced in the third domain, which states that financial reimbursement policies need to be changed. Considerable linkages and overlaps exist across the domains.

As noted in several places in this chapter, the integration of research with clinical practice is taking a prominent position in the future of pediatric psychology. Indeed, much of the rest of this *Handbook* is a presentation of the empirical foundations for clinical applications. This integration has been stressed in each edition of the *Handbook*.

Efficacy–Effectiveness–Practice–Service System Research

As described by Roberts, Brown, and Puddy (2002), the goal of a Clinical Treatment and Services Research Workgroup of the National Institute of Mental Health (1998) was to narrow the gap between treatment research and practice. The work group provided four categories: (1) efficacy, (2) effectiveness, (3) practice, and (4) service system research. Efficacy research measures outcomes of very well specified interventions with specific disorders or problems (using careful screening of participants and random assignment, clinical trial methodology, and manualized treatments). Effectiveness research examines application of techniques that have been found efficacious to a broader population and in service delivery settings in the field rather than just in laboratory clinics. Effectiveness studies require methodological rigor and careful controls. These two domains of efficacy and effectiveness are most often invoked with EST descriptions (Chambless & Ollendick, 2001). The work group

TABLE 1.1. Top Issues for the Future of Pediatric Psychology

1. Demonstrating viability of pediatric psychology through
   a. empirical support for treatment interventions
   b. improved health outcomes of pediatric conditions due to psychological services
   c. evidence of medical cost offset
   d. evidence of efficacy of the integration of clinical research and practice
   e. evidence of effectiveness of psychological interventions in lowering societal costs
2. Integrating psychologists into pediatric primary care settings in which behavioral and developmental problems frequently first present by
   a. providing mental health services directly to patients in primary care
   b. providing consultation and collaboration with pediatricians and allied staff based on proximity to each other
   c. conducting clinically relevant research on issues related to primary care
3. Recognizing need for changes in reimbursement by
   a. creating non-DSM categories of reimbursable services
   b. eliminating behavioral health carve-outs
   c. paying for multidisciplinary teams providing services
   d. developing service systems that recognize the complexity of problems in children and families
4. Collaborating between pediatricians and psychologists in clinical research and practice activities by
   a. increasing at individual and local level
   b. creating more liaisons between major organizations such as the American Academy of Pediatrics and the Society of Pediatric Psychology, as well as the American Psychological Association
5. Emphasizing importance of prevention of problems in childhood and promotion of optimal physical and mental health by
   a. making practical applications in primary care (including injuries, smoking, obesity, and violence)
   b. conducting applications in prevention of behavioral and developmental problems
   c. developing conceptual models to guide prevention and promotion efforts
6. Responding to challenges to the professionalism of pediatric psychology by
   a. training pediatricians and other allied health personnel about psychological contributions to pediatric medicine, in order to promote an integration and acceptance of prevention and clinical intervention into pediatric care
   b. creating new models of training pediatric psychologists in the medical aspects of the care of children and the evolving aspects of health care system and reimbursement issues
   c. responding to new technology and medical/scientific advances that challenge professional ethics (e.g., telehealth, genetic testing, human–animal organ transplant, computerization of medical and psychological records)
7. Increasing awareness that pediatric psychology provides "value added" services to medical setting (e.g., better advertising or public relations), including education about its worth directed to the public, medical personnel, managed care companies, and psychologists
8. Facilitating collaborative research and evaluation efforts (e.g., multisite studies) for pediatric psychology investigations and interventions
9. Addressing changes in larger societal and socioeconomic conditions that affect child development, education, medical care, and psychological services
10. Changing direction of psychological research to problem prevention and primary care settings and away from issues of chronic illness

Note. Domains identified by panel members in final round of Delphic Survey conducted by Brown and Roberts (2000).

(1998) also described two additional domains of treatment research as "practice research" and "service system research." Practice research considers how various types of treatments or services are actually delivered to patients within settings and how this delivery in practice might be improved. Service system research investigates how different components and characteristics of health care service organization affect quality of care and therapeutic outcomes. Roberts et al. (2002) asserted:

> Pediatric psychology as a field has not engaged in enough of the first two, efficacy and effectiveness. The field has done even less work in the practice research domain and much less in the service system domain. What do practice research and service system research mean for pediatric psychology? The field needs to learn more about (a) who is being served, (b) what services are being provided, (c) how treatments are implemented, (d) how services are organized and staffed, (e) what are the outcomes of the services, (f) how do various consumers perceive services, (g) how services are reimbursed, and (h) what are alternatives and innovations? (p. 5)

Roberts et al. (2002) outlined a framework for evaluating outcomes in practice and services research with examples from the pediatric psychology literature. This framework overlapped with and yet was distinct from the efficacy and effectiveness research as examined in the EST summaries (Spirito, 1999). Relatedly, the EST activities will need to focus additionally on clinical relevance and costs–benefits of the clinical services provided. The future of this field must involve much more effort in all four domains in order to adequately demonstrate pediatric psychology's viability (as called for in the Delphic survey results of Brown & Roberts, 2000).

Medical Cost Offsets Research

The Delphic participants strongly endorse the issue of medical cost offsets as important to the future. That is, how can psychological services help diminish the patient's use of more expensive or unnecessary medical services? The cost of the pediatric psychology services would be "offset" by savings in medical expenditures (see Roberts & Hurley, 1997). The determination and importance of medical cost offsets is a complex issue, and the value of pediatric psychology services should not necessarily be predicated on such a demonstration. However, these considerations will be important overall as one component of evaluating outcomes in clinical practice (Roberts et al., 2002). Some research has indicated medical cost savings from pediatric psychology services (e.g., Finney, Lemanek, Cataldo, Katz, & Fuqua, 1989; Finney, Riley, & Cataldo, 1991; Rosen & Wiens, 1979). The SPP is currently establishing a task force to evaluate existing evidence and to develop a research agenda for future investigations of medical cost offsets.

Editorial Views of the Field

As noted in the content analyses of *JPP*, the last three editors of the journal authored *vale dictum* editorials in which they reviewed trends and progress reflected during their terms. Roberts (1992) offered three observations based on evidence from the journal articles published during his term:

> *Clinical Practice*: Pediatric psychologists are providing competent services well appreciated by referral sources and parents (p. 799).

Scientific Research: Pediatric psychologists are clarifying relationships of psychological and pediatric phenomena (p. 800).

Professional Issues: Pediatric psychologists are examining issues of ethics, training, and self-definition that articulate it as a profession (p. 801).

Roberts noted that these considerations would develop further as the field progresses. In her final editorial, La Greca (1997) predicted that the trends of the past will continue in the future, so that chronic pediatric conditions will continue as topics of primary interest, with a growing sophistication in the research methodology. She also noted two important areas of concern that were not well represented in the journal. First, she suggested that investigations focus on systems that affect children, such as peers, schools, and medical settings, in addition to the family. Second, she encouraged more research into the "cost–benefits" of interventions made by pediatric psychologists.

Kazak (2002), as the most recent retiring editor, observed several important issues for the field, including (1) the increasing reliance on grant funding for research in the field, (2) the increase of multisite investigations in which more than one setting or institution helped collect data in order to produce more representative samples of participants in sufficient numbers, (3) the necessity of attention to compliance with research regulations and ethics, and (4) the issues of increasing diversity in the clinical field and in research participants. Additionally, other commentators (often in presidential and award addresses for SPP) have articulated concerns and encouragement to help guide the future of pediatric psychology. For example, Wertlieb (1999) called for more effective collaborations; Seagull (2000) urged greater orientation to families in pediatric psychology research and practice; Clay, Modhorst, and Lehn (2002) pointed out the lack of diversity discussions in the EST reviews; Roberts et al. (1996) encouraged statements indicating the clinical relevance of research; Drotar (2002) outlined what needs to take place in order to advance the EST movement; Sifers, Puddy, Warren, and Roberts (2002) decried the lack of information in research about participant demographics, methodology, and ethical procedures. Although sometimes critical of the field, these commentaries help establish what pediatric psychology must do to retain its progress and enhance its stature as a profession of science and practice.

CONCLUDING REMARKS

The field of pediatric psychology remains vibrant and viable, from its founding throughout its evolution over time. No one topic or activity alone can capture the diversity and energy of pediatric psychology researchers and clinicians. The chapters in this *Handbook of Pediatric Psychology* (3rd edition) convey the findings and applications, as well as the excitement and challenges, of the integrative field of pediatric psychology.

REFERENCES

American Academy of Pediatrics. (2000). Policy statement: Insurance coverage of mental health and substance abuse services for children and adolescents: A consensus statement. *Pediatrics, 106*, 860–862.

American Academy of Pediatrics, Committee on Psychosocial Aspects of Child and Family Health. (2001a). Policy statement: Sexuality education for children and adolescents. *Pediatrics, 108*, 498–502.

American Academy of Pediatrics, Committee on Psychosocial Aspects of Child and Family Health. (2001b). Policy statement: The assessment and management of acute pain in infants, children, and adolescents. *Pediatrics, 108*, 793–797.

American Academy of Pediatrics, Committee on Psychosocial Aspects of Child and Family Health. (2001c). Policy statement: The New Morbidity revisited: A renewed commitment to the psychosocial aspects of pediatric care. *Pediatrics, 108*, 1227–1230.

American Psychiatric Association. (1994). *Diagnostic and statistical manual of mental disorders* (4th ed.). Washington, DC: Author.

Anderson, J. E. (1938). Pediatrics and child psychology. *Journal of the American Medical Association, 95*, 1015–1018.

Armstrong, F. D. (1997). Presidential column: Updates. *SPP Progress Notes, 21*(1), 13, 21.

Armstrong, F. D., Harris, L. L., Thompson, W., Semrad, J. L., Jensen, M. M., Lee, D. Y., et al. (1999). The outpatient developmental services project: Integration of pediatric psychology with primary medical care for children infected with HIV. *Journal of Pediatric Psychology, 24*, 381–391.

Brown, K. J., & Roberts, M. C. (2000). Future issues in pediatric psychology: Delphic survey. *Journal of Clinical Psychology in Medical Settings, 7*, 5–15.

Chambless, D. L., & Ollendick, T. H. (2001). Empirically supported psychological interventions: Controversies and evidence. *Annual Review of Psychology, 52*, 685–716.

Chorpita, B. F., Yim, L. M., Donkervoet, J. C., Arendorfer, A., Amundsen, M. J., McGee, C., et al. (2002). Toward large-scale implementation of empirically supported treatments for children: A review and observations by the Hawaii Empirical Basis to Services Task Force. *Clinical Psychology: Science and Practice, 9*, 165–190.

Clay, D., Modhorst, M., & Lehn, L. (2002). Empirically supported treatments in pediatric psychology: Where is the diversity? *Journal of Pediatric Psychology, 27*, 325–337.

Clinical Treatment and Services Research Workgroup, National Advisory Mental Health Council, National Institute of Mental Health. (1998). *Bridging science and service*. Retrieved December 22, 2000, from *http://nimh.nih.gov/research/bridge.htm*.

Drotar, D. (1999). *The Diagnostic and Statistical Manual for Primary Care (DSM-PC), Child and Adolescent Version*: What pediatric psychologists need to know. *Journal of Pediatric Psychology, 24*, 369–380.

Drotar, D. (2001). Pioneers in pediatric psychology: Between two professional worlds: Personal reflections on a career in a pediatric setting. *Journal of Pediatric Psychology, 26*, 185–192.

Drotar, D. (2002). Enhancing reviews of psychological treatments with pediatric populations: Thoughts on the next steps. *Journal of Pediatric Psychology, 27*, 167–176.

Drotar, D., & Lemanek, K. (2001). Steps toward a clinically relevant science of interventions in pediatric settings. *Journal of Pediatric Psychology, 26*, 385–394.

Drotar, D., & Zagorski, L. (2001). Providing psychological services in pediatric settings in an era of managed care: Challenges and opportunities. In J. N. Hughes, A. M. La Greca, & J. C. Conoley (Eds.), *Handbook of psychological services for children and adolescents* (pp. 89–104). New York: Oxford University Press.

Elkins, P. D., & Roberts, M. C. (1988). *Journal of Pediatric Psychology*: A content analysis of articles over its first 10 years. *Journal of Pediatric Psychology, 13*, 575–594.

Finney, J. C., Lemanek, K. L., Cataldo, M. F., Katz, H. P., & Fuqua, R. W. (1989). Pediatric psychology in primary health care: Brief targeted therapy for recurrent abdominal pain. *Behavior Therapy, 20*, 283–291.

Finney, J. W., Riley, A. W., & Cataldo, M. F. (1991). Psychology in primary health care: Effects of brief targeted therapy on children's medical care utilization. *Journal of Pediatric Psychology, 16*, 447–461.

Gesell, A. (1919). The field of clinical psychology as an applied science: A symposium. *Journal of Applied Psychology, 3*, 81–84.

Hartlage, L. C., & Hartlage, P. L. (1978). Clinical consultation to pediatric neurology and developmental pediatrics. *Journal of Clinical Child Psychology, 7*, 19–20.

Kagan, J. (1965). The new marriage: Pediatrics and psychology. *American Journal of Diseases of Children, 110*, 272–278.

Kanoy, K. W., & Schroeder, C. (1985). Suggestions to parents about common behavior problems in a pediatric primary care office: Five years of follow-up. *Journal of Pediatric Psychology, 10*, 15–30.

Kazak, A. E. (2000). *Journal of Pediatric Psychology*: A brief history (1969–1999). *Journal of Pediatric Psychology, 25*, 463–470.

Kazak, A. E. (2002). *Journal of Pediatric Psychology (JPP)*, 1998–2002: Editor's vale dictum. *Journal of Pediatric Psychology, 27*, 653–663.

King, G., Cathers, T., King, S., & Rosenbaum, P. (2001). Major elements of parents' satisfaction and dissatisfaction with pediatric rehabilitation services. *Children's Health Care, 30*, 111–134.

Koocher, G. P., Sourkes, B. M., & Keane, W. M. (1979). Pediatric oncology consultations: A generalizable model for medical settings. *Professional Psychology, 10*, 467–474.

La Greca, A. M. (1997). Reflections and perspectives on pediatric psychology: Editor's vale dictum. *Journal of Pediatric Psychology, 22*, 759–777.

Lonigan, C. J., Elbert, J. C., & Johnson, S. B. (1998). Empirically supported psychosocial treatments for children: An overview. *Journal of Clinical Child Psychology, 27*, 138–145.

Magrab, P. (1975). Psychological management and renal dialysis. *Pediatric Psychology, 3*, 3–6.

Magrab, P., & Davitt, M. K. (1975). The pediatric psychologist and the developmental follow-up of intensive care nursery infants. *Journal of Clinical Child Psychology, 4*, 16–18.

McClelland, C. Q., Staples, W. P., Weisberg, I., & Berger, M. E. (1973). The practitioner's role in behavioral pediatrics. *Journal of Pediatrics, 82*, 325–331.

Olson, R. A., Holden, E. W., Friedman, A., Faust, J., Kenning, M., & Mason, P. J. (1988). Psychological consultation in a children's hospital: An evaluation of services. *Journal of Pediatric Psychology, 13*, 479–492.

O'Malley, J. E., & Koocher, G. P. (1977). Psychological consultation to a pediatric oncology unit: Obstacles to effective intervention. *Journal of Pediatric Psychology, 2*, 256–260.

Ottinger, D. R., & Roberts, M. C. (1980). A university-based predoctoral practicum in pediatric psychology. *Professional Psychology, 11*, 707–713.

Roberts, M. C. (1986). *Pediatric psychology: Psychological interventions and strategies for pediatric problems.* New York: Pergamon.

Roberts, M. C. (1992). Vale dictum: The editor's view of the field of pediatric psychology. *Journal of Pediatric Psychology, 17*, 785–805.

Roberts, M. C. (1993). Introduction to pediatric psychology: An historical perspective. In M. C. Roberts, G. P. Koocher, D. K. Routh, & D. Willis (Eds.), *Readings in pediatric psychology* (pp. 1–21). New York: Plenum.

Roberts, M. C., & Brown, K. J. (in press). Primary care, prevention, and pediatric psychology: Challenges and opportunities. In B. Wildman & T. Stancin (Eds.), *Treating children's psychosocial problems in primary care.* Westport, CT: Greenwood.

Roberts, M. C., Brown, K. J., & Puddy, R. W. (2002). Service delivery issues and program evaluation in pediatric psychology. *Journal of Clinical Psychology in Medical Settings, 9*, 3–13.

Roberts, M. C., & Hurley, L. (1997). *Managing managed care.* New York: Plenum.

Roberts, M. C., La Greca, A. M., & Harper, D. C. (1988). *Journal of Pediatric Psychology*: Another stage of development [Editorial]. *Journal of Pediatric Psychology, 13*, 1–5.

Roberts, M. C., Maddux, J., Wurtele, S. K., & Wright, L. (1982). Pediatric psychology: Health care psychology for children. In T. Millon, C. J. Green, & R. B. Meagher (Eds.), *Handbook of clinical health care psychology* (pp. 191–226). New York: Plenum.

Roberts, M. C., McNeal, R., Randall, C., & Roberts, J. (1996). A necessary reemphasis on integrating explicative research with the pragmatics of pediatric psychology. *Journal of Pediatric Psychology, 21*, 107–114.

Roberts, M. C., & Walker, C. E. (1989). Clinical cases in child and pediatric psychology: Conceptualization and overview. In M. C. Roberts & C. E. Walker (Eds.), *Casebook of child and pediatric psychology*, (pp. 1–15). New York: Guilford Press.

Rodrigue, J. R., Hoffmann, R. G., Rayfield, A., Lescano, C., Kubar, W., & Streisand, R., et al. (1995). Evaluating pediatric psychology consultation services in a medical setting: An example. *Journal of Clinical Psychology in Medical Settings, 2*, 89–107.

Rosen, J. C., & Wiens, A. N. (1979). Changes in medical problems and use of medical services following psychological interventions. *American Psychologist, 34*, 420–431.

Routh, D. K. (1975). The short history of pediatric psychology. *Journal of Clinical Child Psychology, 4*, 6–8.

Routh, D. K. (1980). Research training in pediatric psychology. *Journal of Pediatric Psychology, 5*, 287–293.

Routh, D. K. (1994). *Clinical psychology since 1917: Science, practice, and organization.* New York: Plenum.

Routh, D. K. (2000). Growing older in pediatric psychology. *Journal of Pediatric Psychology, 25*, 47–52.

Routh, D. K., & Mesibov, G. B. (1979). The editorial policy of the *Journal of Pediatric Psychology. Journal of Pediatric Psychology, 4*, 1–3.

Salk, L. (1978). Psychologist in a pediatric setting. *Professional Psychology, 1*, 395–396.

Schroeder, C. S. (1979). Psychologists in a private pediatric practice. *Journal of Pediatric Psychology, 4*, 5–18.

Schroeder, C. S. (1996). Mental health services in pediatric primary care. In M. C. Roberts (Ed.), *Model programs in service delivery in child and family mental health* (pp. 265–284). Mahwah, NJ: Erlbaum.

Seagull, E. A. (2000). Beyond mothers and children: Finding the family in pediatric psychology. *Journal of Pediatric Psychology, 25*, 161–169.

Sifers, S., Puddy, R., Warren, J., & Roberts, M. C. (2002). Reporting of demographics, methodology, and ethical procedures in journals in pediatric and child psychology. *Journal of Pediatric Psychology, 27*, 19–25.

Singer, L., & Drotar, D. (1989). Psychological practice in a pediatric rehabilitation hospital. *Journal of Pediatric Psychology, 14*, 479–489.

Sobel, A. M., Roberts, M. C., Rapoff, M. A., & Barnard, M. U. (2001). Problems and interventions of a pediatric psychology clinic in a medical setting: A retrospective analysis. *Cognitive and Behavioral Practice, 8*, 11–17.

Sobel, A. M., Roberts, M. C., Rayfield, A. D., Barnard, M. U., & Rapoff, M. A. (2001). Evaluating outpatient pediatric psychology services in a primary care setting. *Journal of Pediatric Psychology, 26*, 395–405.

Spirito, A. (1999). Introduction: Special series on empirically supported treatments in pediatric psychology. *Journal of Pediatric Psychology, 24*, 87–90.

Spirito, A. (2002). The president's message: Strengthening our ties with pediatricians. *SPP Progress Notes, 26*(1), 1, 2, 4.

Stabler, B., & Mesibov, G. B. (1984). Role functioning of pediatric and health psychologists in health care settings. *Professional Psychology, 15*, 142–151.

Stancin, T. (1999). Introduction: Special issue on pediatric mental health services in primary care settings. *Journal of Pediatric Psychology, 24*, 367–368.

Tuma, J. M., & Grabert, J. (1983). Internship and postdoctoral training in pediatric and clinical child psychology: A survey. *Journal of Pediatric Psychology, 8*, 245–268.

Walker, C. E. (1979). Behavioral intervention in a pediatric setting. In J. R. McNamara (Ed.), *Behavioral approaches to medicine: Applications and analysis* (pp. 227–266). New York: Plenum.

Walker, C. E. (2000). Pioneers in pediatric psychology: A career in pediatric psychology. *Journal of Pediatric Psychology, 25*, 521–532.

Wertlieb, D. (1999). Society of Pediatric Psychology Presidential Address: Calling all collaborators, advancing pediatric psychology. *Journal of Pediatric Psychology, 24*, 77–83.

Wildman, B., & Stancin, T. (Eds.). (in press). *Treating children's psychosocial problems in primary care*. Westport, CT: Greenwood.

Wolraich, M. L., Felice, M. E., & Drotar, D. (Eds.). (1996). *The classification of child and adolescent mental diagnosis in primary care: Diagnosis and Statistical Manual for Primary Care (DSM-PC): Child and adolescent version*. Elk Grove, IL: American Academy of Pediatrics.

Wright, L. (1967). The pediatric psychologist: A role model. *American Psychologist, 22*, 323–325.

2

Training Pediatric Psychologists for the 21st Century

ANTHONY SPIRITO
RONALD T. BROWN
EUGENE J. D'ANGELO
ALAN M. DELAMATER
JAMES R. RODRIGUE
LAWRENCE J. SIEGEL

This chapter is designed to provide an overview of the types of training experiences considered important to the development of competencies in pediatric psychology. Although we review both general research and clinical skills, we place a particular emphasis on the special skills necessary to provide professional psychological services within primary care pediatric settings and tertiary health science centers that serve children and adolescents with health-related problems and chronic disease.

Pediatric psychologists must be prepared to provide general psychological services to children, adolescents, and families. As such, they need to receive training regarding "physical, cognitive, social, and emotional functioning and development as related to health and illness issues in children, adolescents, and families" (American Psychological Association, Division 54, Society of Pediatric Psychology, 1999, p. 1). Specific critical competencies that must also be included in training are (1) multicultural competencies; (2) delivery and evaluation of comprehensive and coordinated systems of care; (3) collaborative and interprofessional skills; (4) empirically supported assessment and treatments for promoting behavioral change in children, families, and other systems; and (5) entrepreneurial and supervisory skills (La Greca & Hughes, 1999).

Our premise is that clinical child psychology is the foundation for developing skills and expertise in pediatric psychology. Nonetheless, pediatric psychologists also share many aspects of their training and professional identity with health psychologists. Many of our recommendations reflect this close tie to health psychology.

The training opportunities described in this chapter are examples of specific experiences recommended for students in pediatric psychology. These are not to be construed as mandatory experiences necessary for competence in pediatric psychology, because similar training experiences specific to the many and varied training settings in pediatric psychology may serve the same training purpose. However, trainees are expected to have some familiarity, if only through readings, with each of these areas. The breadth of training in pediatric psychology described here will not be easily accomplished, nor is it mandatory. Psychologists in training will not participate intensively in all of these experiences across a typical graduate school, predoctoral, and postdoctoral training sequence.

BREADTH, DEPTH, AND SCOPE OF TRAINING AND PRACTICE

Different opportunities for implementing these training experiences are available at the graduate school, internship, and postdoctoral levels. At the graduate school level, the focus of training is typically on the acquisition of general child clinical skills. Where possible, the student may obtain additional experiences in pediatric psychology content through course work, directed readings, practicum experiences, student membership in relevant organizations, and research exposure. More intensive experience in health care settings will typically occur at the predoctoral internship level. Internships are available that provide programmatic focus in pediatric psychology. Subsequently, development of expertise within specialized areas of pediatric psychology practice is expected to occur at the postdoctoral level.

Pediatric psychology practice includes psychological applications to developmental issues in primary care, screening of psychopathology in primary care settings, chronic disease, acute illness, health promotion, and disease prevention, as well as contributions to the development of policy in psychosocial aspects of pediatric health care. Opportunities to practice pediatric psychology exist in tertiary care centers, ambulatory care clinics, community-based health clinics, private practice, primary care settings, and schools and through telehealth. Given the assumption that the careers of pediatric psychologists will involve multiple responsibilities and tasks, emphasis is placed on training in a variety of skills and the expansion of training beyond direct service to include research, consultation, program evaluation, and program development at the local, state, and national levels. New areas of practice will appear in the future, such as consultation on ethical issues that arise with biomedical advances (e.g., genetic testing; see Tercyak, Chapter 43, this volume), advocacy for children within the health care system, supervision of clinical programs staffed by masters-level providers, paraprofessionals and other treatment providers, as well as program development and public health policy, including prevention and intervention programs delivered via various media outlets. The training opportunities described in this document are sufficiently broad to provide students in pediatric psychology the training experiences necessary to participate in these new areas of practice.

In order to develop an area of expertise, training in one or two specific areas of interest is recommended, in addition to the emphasis on training in multiple skills. For example, primary career areas might include chronic illness, public policy, epidemiology, program evaluation, multicultural assessment and treatment, health disparities and health utilization, and preventive pediatric health psychology. The priority assigned to each training area will vary for every trainee according to his or her interests.

PRIMARY CARE

Although pediatric psychology practice in primary care has been advocated for many years (e.g., Routh, Schroeder, & Koocher, 1983), expansion of pediatric psychology efforts in such settings is nonetheless strongly recommended. In pediatrics, practice in primary care settings allows psychologists greater opportunities for the prevention of behavioral and health problems (including obesity and injuries), for managing children and adolescents and their families who are designated to be at risk, for educating primary care providers regarding the use of psychosocial treatments, as well as psychotropic medication, for managing "high utilizers" of health care services to reduce inappropriate medical utilization and promote better outcomes, and, finally, for identifying and referring patients in need of specialized mental health treatment. This model of integrating mental health and medical care requires a new training emphasis.

INTERDISCIPLINARY TRAINING

Pediatric psychologists should have opportunities to work in interdisciplinary settings with professionals and trainees from other health professions, including nursing, social work, occupational and physical therapy, and pediatrics. Joint training opportunities with pediatricians are particularly encouraged, because increased interdisciplinary training will result in productive interactions with pediatricians and other providers of child health services. Most particularly, we emphasize the importance of more systematic training in pediatric disease and medical management. Greater emphasis on the biological components of the biopsychosocial model to pediatric psychology training will enable pediatric psychologists to develop a greater understanding of important issues in comprehensive pediatric health care. Interdisciplinary training also is important as a means of developing skills for forging new partnerships in the health care system, including the training of pediatric residents and other health care professionals, enhancing pediatricians' understanding of the roles and skills of pediatric psychologists in the care of patients, and expanding future employment opportunities for pediatric psychologists.

DOMAINS OF TRAINING

The training domains described in this chapter correspond to those selected by the National Institute of Mental Health (NIMH) work group as training necessary to work with children (Roberts et al., 1998), with the exception of "consultant and liaison roles" and "disease process and medical management," both of which are specific to the training of health psychologists. We refer the reader to the model developed by Roberts et al. (1998) that carefully delineates and outlines the implementation goals for child clinical psychology training.

For each of the following topics, we first provide an overview of the content of the topic area and its importance in pediatric psychology training. Examples of the way in which the student may be trained in the knowledge and skills pertinent to a particular domain are included under sections labeled "Exposure" and "Experience." "Exposure" refers primarily to didactic materials (e.g., seminars, observation of a clinician), and "experience" denotes the actual practice of the activity (e.g., psychotherapy by means of a practicum experience).

Lifespan Developmental Psychology

Lifespan development includes the knowledge of typical development and behavior in infants, preschool-age children, school-age children, and adolescents within their ecological (family, school, community, and cultural) contexts. Developmental issues specific to the practice of pediatric psychology include the influence of the disease process and prescribed medical regimens on emotional, social, motor, and behavioral development, as well as physiological maturation.

Exposure

- Directed readings, seminars, and lectures on the effects of health-related issues on developmental processes.

Experience

- Opportunities to observe and conduct supervised clinical activities with children at various levels of development in health care settings.
- Supervised clinical cases, across age groups, in which developmental issues are exemplified, such as a case in which adherence to medical regimen affects typical developmental processes, including peer relations and autonomy from parents.

Lifespan Developmental Psychopathology

Pediatric psychologists need to be trained in models of developmental psychopathology that emphasize trajectories of adaptation and maladaptation under conditions of risk. Additionally, awareness of developmental psychopathology is necessary for pediatric psychologists whose tasks are to assist healthy children with behavioral or emotional problems who undergo diagnostic medical procedures (e.g., immunizations, computerized axial tomography scans, invasive treatments, surgical procedures). Knowledge of psychopathology is also necessary to make a differential diagnosis between psychological conditions and health-related symptoms. Through training in lifespan developmental psychopathology, pediatric psychologists may also identify children at risk for problems of adaptation in primary and other health care settings, thereby promoting positive psychological adaptation, emotional well-being, and optimal quality of life.

Exposure

- Directed readings, seminars, and lectures that highlight the influence of psychopathology on children with acute and chronic illness, as well as more general health-related issues.

Experience

- Opportunities to observe and conduct supervised clinical activities with children and adolescents who evidence varied types of psychopathology as they present in health care settings.

• Supervised experience in differentiating emotional distress within normal limits for children with acute and chronic medical conditions versus psychopathology independent of the health condition.

Child, Adolescent, and Family Assessment

Pediatric psychologists must be knowledgeable in the use of currently available health-related assessments, as well as measures that become available as this literature develops. Examples of such health-related topic areas include health beliefs, adherence (see La Greca and Bearman, Chapter 8, this volume), quality of life (see Quittner, Davis, and Modi, Chapter 41, this volume), and coping (see Harbeck-Weber, Fisher, and Dittner, Chapter 7, this volume); special topic areas in pediatric psychology (e.g., pediatric pain; see Blount, Piira, and Cohen, Chapter 13, this volume); as well as behavioral health assessments, including substance use, weight control, and exercise.

Pediatric psychologists should be well versed in the assessment of general family functioning given the impact of family functioning on health-related conditions (see Kazak, Rourke, and Crump, Chapter 10, this volume). For example, it is important to identify how family strengths and vulnerabilities may affect adaptation and treatment outcomes. When available, pediatric psychologists should use assessment tools with norms appropriate to children with chronic illness in order to differentiate symptoms associated with disease and treatment from those that are secondary to poor psychological adjustment (for a review of specific instruments available for children with chronic illness, see Rodrigue, Geffken, and Streisand, 2000). It is particularly important that pediatric psychologists be well versed in measures of coping and adaptation, in addition to those instruments that assess psychopathology. Expertise in screening instruments is a particularly important skill for pediatric psychologists working in a primary care setting.

Exposure

• Participate in seminars, lectures, and course work on (1) how individual and family processes affect child adaptation to health care and illness, (2) valid tools that assess individual and family functioning in health-related contexts, and (3) screening measures and how best to assess coping, adaptation, and behavioral health.

Experience

• Supervised training experiences should include application of standardized assessment instruments to specific pediatric populations in various settings, such as clinics and hospitals. Selection of instruments is important and includes generic and disease-specific measures and those measures used for screening and assessment of coping, adaptation, and behavioral health in both primary and tertiary health care settings.

• Supervised experience in family interview techniques that identify family strengths and problems, as well as problem-solving abilities, to assist the child in coping with a health-related stressor.

• Supervised experience in the preparation and writing of assessment reports, providing brief yet cogent case presentations, and communicating reliable feedback to pediatricians.

Intervention Strategies

Pediatric psychologists should receive training in theory-driven, empirically supported treatments for a variety of childhood problems. Because most of the empirically supported treatments to date are behavioral or cognitive–behavioral in nature, adequate training in individual and family-based behavioral intervention strategies should be provided at the graduate training level. However, it is equally important for trainees to be exposed to other treatment approaches, such as family systems therapy, that may show less demonstrated empirical support for chronically ill pediatric populations at this time but that are promising for the future because of their established efficacy with other populations.

Pediatric psychologists need to understand a child's disease status and to implement psychological interventions within the context of the child's medical condition and treatment. For example, if a child with congenital heart disease is referred for sleep-onset difficulties, the use of ignoring techniques (which may be appropriate for healthy toddlers) may not be appropriate given the possibility that prolonged crying episodes may be contraindicated due to the underlying medical condition. Alternatively, specific interventions developed for nonmedical problems (e.g., parent training for a child's disruptive behavior) must be modified when implemented within a medical system (e.g., a hospital) or when a psychological condition is comorbid with a medical condition (e.g., cancer). Similarly, pediatric psychologists need to have a basic working knowledge of pediatric psychopharmacology that includes an understanding of the differences in efficacy and side effects of specific psychotropic agents when administered to children with various health-related conditions and chronic diseases (see DuPaul, McGoey, and Mautone, Chapter 14, this volume). Finally, pediatric psychologists must be prepared for the unique challenges inherent in conducting psychotherapy with children and adolescents in medical settings (e.g., maintaining therapeutic confidentiality while collaborating with medical personnel who might be treating the child for medical problems).

Exposure

- Course work and directed readings on empirically supported treatments relevant to pediatric psychology, such as the empirically supported treatment series published in the 1999 and 2000 volumes of the *Journal of Pediatric Psychology.*
- Opportunities to observe clinical supervisors (*in vivo* or via videotape) conduct interventions for children with medical conditions.
- Course work, seminars, lectures, and readings on basic clinical psychopharmacology.

Experience

- Training in interventions unique to the pediatric setting via practica, internships, and fellowships, including (1) helping children prepare for and cope with stressful medical or surgical procedures (see Blount et al., Chapter 13, this volume); (2) management of pain and disease-related symptoms (see Dahlquist and Switkin, Chapter 12, this volume); (3) adherence to medical regimens as part of the treatment and recovery process (see La Greca and Bearman, Chapter 8, this volume); (4) management of anxiety symptoms that are secondary to receiving medical care; (5) medical crisis counseling, such as assisting in adaptation to a recent diagnosis of a medical condition; (6) family therapy to assist families in managing the impact of illness on child and family lifestyle (see Kazak et al., Chapter 10, this volume); (7) specific applications of biofeedback for certain biobehavioral conditions, such as dysfunctional voiding and headaches; (8) bereavement counseling on issues related to death of a patient or of a patient's family member and on making end-of-life decisions faced by both children and their family members; (9) assisting the children in families with a terminally ill adult; and (10) providing psychological support to health care providers who take care of children and their families in the terminal stages of illness.

Research Methods and Systems Evaluation

Pediatric psychologists conduct assessment, treatment, and epidemiological and prevention research. Training in the process and procedures necessary to conduct clinical research and treatment outcome studies is particularly important. Between-group design studies frequently require multisite collaborations, as the low incidence of certain diseases precludes sufficiently large sample sizes to adequately test empirical questions at a single site. Experimentally controlled single-subject research designs, such as reversal and multiple-baseline designs, allow empirically valid research at a single site with a small number of participants. Pediatric psychologists need to be cognizant of how cultural diversity and developmental issues affect research outcomes and to design studies accordingly. Pediatric psychologists should also gain familiarity with biomedical research concepts and terminology, as well as medical cost offset issues associated with access to care and health disparities (see Brown, Fuemmeler, and Forti, Chapter 40, this volume).

Exposure

- Course work and seminars in clinical trials, experimental design, and advanced statistics.
- Course work and seminars on health-related assessments, including health outcome measures, measures of disease severity, quality of life, medical cost offset, and indicators of functional status.
- Course work and seminars that provide information on health care service assessment, including patient and parent satisfaction, perception of treatment, access to care, health disparities, referral source satisfaction, and program evaluation.
- Observations of faculty collaboration on interdisciplinary research projects that involve the careful coordination of other disciplines, such as various pediatric subspecialties.

Experience

- Opportunities to conduct clinical research that includes analogue, observational, cross-sectional, prospective longitudinal and retrospective designs, as well as controlled treatment outcome research or clinical trials.
- Opportunities for students to design qualitative research and single-subject experimental methods that may be applied to low-incidence diseases.
- Opportunities to prepare grant applications in pediatric psychology for student awards, such as dissertation grants, hospital or university internal grants, local or national foundation grants, and federal grants.

Professional, Ethical, and Legal Issues Pertaining to Children, Adolescents, and Families

Pediatric psychologists need to be aware of professional, ethical, and legal issues pertinent to children and adolescents with specific physical challenges and those with chronic illnesses, their families, and the health care system (see Rae, Brunnquell, and Sullivan, Chapter 3, this volume). For example, it is important to understand the rights of caregivers and those of children in making decisions regarding medical care. Pediatric psychologists need to be cognizant of the complex issues involved in serving the best interests of children while at the same time attending to the needs of families in a variety of situations (e.g., end-stage care for terminal illness, use of sibling donors). Special ethical issues and problems may arise regarding situations of privileged communication, definition of the primary client (e.g., referring physician, child, caregiver, or family member), and delineation of the respective roles and boundaries of patient care among the providers. Many ethical and legal issues arise in communicating information to the patient, family members, and health care providers that need to be addressed during training.

Ethical and legal issues particularly important to pediatric psychologists also encompass health care delivery issues that include changes in the delivery of health care (e.g., telehealth; see Harper, Chapter 44, this volume), public policy, access to care, and health disparities (see Brown et al., Chapter 40, this volume). Pediatric psychologists also need to be aware of professional issues related to the training and practice of psychology in medical settings at state or provincial levels, as well as at the national level.

Exposure

- Seminars, lectures, and directed readings on the ethical and legal issues specific to pediatric psychology, such as those associated with the emerging fields of telehealth and genetic testing.
- Medical rounds that focus on ethical issues related to medical practice and hospital policies; presentations from hospital risk management teams that describe their roles and functions.

Experience

- Opportunities to provide clinical data and feedback to other health care professionals in team meetings and to prepare consultation reports and medical chart notes.
- Establishing the limits of confidentiality unique to health care settings and applying policies and regulations in a local health care setting.

Issues of Diversity. Pediatric psychology training should enhance clinicians' sensitivity to ethnic, cultural, and religious factors that affect health beliefs and medical treatment, as well as familial, health care, and professional relationships (see Brown et al., Chapter 40, this volume). In addition, pediatric psychologists should incorporate factors related to familial cultural backgrounds and religious beliefs into intervention programs that assist patients and families to cope with stressful medical situations, including terminal illness. Pediatric psychologists need to be cognizant of the problem of access to health care in certain minority and ethnic groups. Also important is an understanding of the nonmainstream health practices influenced by a family's cultural or religious beliefs, the association between spirituality and health, and how cultural beliefs affect recommendations to seek and comply with medical care.

Enhanced understanding of issues pertaining to gender is also essential in the training and practice of pediatric psychology. Gender differences in adult health outcomes have important ramifications for how pediatric psychologists approach health promotion and the modification of health-compromising behaviors and the medical utilization patterns of males and females during childhood and adolescence. Pediatric psychologists also must be sensitive to issues related to sexual orientation in the families with whom they work, particularly with adolescent clients. Pediatric psychologists often need to assist other pediatric health care providers in addressing issues of diversity in their patient care.

Exposure

- Course work and readings on diversity that include training about prejudice, cultural and religious beliefs relevant to health and illness, and issues of sexual orientation and the potential impact these issues have on adjustment and coping with health-related problems. Students should receive an understanding of community resources that are outside of the health care system, such as religious organizations, ethnic community centers, and the use of language translators that may facilitate or impede medical treatment with culturally and ethnically diverse client populations.

Experience

- Supervised clinical experience with patients of diverse ethnic and cultural backgrounds and different sexual orientations in a variety of health care settings.
- Evaluations in health care settings, with the assistance of an interpreter when providing services for non-English-speaking children and their families.

The Role of Multiple Disciplines in Service Delivery Systems

Children and adolescents served by health care systems often require evaluation by multiple disciplines. It is important for pediatric psychologists to understand the roles and hierarchy among the different disciplines and service systems in the delivery of health care (see Drotar, Spirito, and Stancin, Chapter 4, this volume).

Exposure

- Seminars, lectures, and readings on the roles of different disciplines in health care, as well as observation of various systems and settings, disciplines, and multidisciplinary teams.
- Observations of multidisciplinary services—for example, following a family through an entire evaluation in a multidisciplinary clinic and discussing the process with attending physicians and supervisors.
- Observation of examinations conducted by primary care pediatricians and subspecialists.
- Opportunities to participate in multidisciplinary staffings, team meetings, teaching rounds, and hospital administration and departmental meetings.

Experience

- Supervised experiences involving health delivery issues (e.g., documentation of information in chart, communicating with attending physicians prior to providing a specific intervention with a client).
- Supervised experience in conducting lectures to medical students and pediatric and psychiatric residents, as well as other health care professionals, on psychological factors during their various rotations.

Prevention, Family Support, and Health Promotion

An important role for pediatric psychologists is promoting healthy lifestyles (see Wilson and Evans, Chapter 5, this volume) and preventing the development of health-risk behaviors in children who are currently healthy (see Roberts, Brown, Boles, Mashunkashey, and Mayes, Chapter 6, this volume) and those with chronic illnesses. Particularly important in primary care is the promotion of exercise and a healthy diet to prevent childhood obesity and associated sequelae such as hypertension and Type 2 diabetes. For adolescents, other prevention efforts are geared toward health-risk behaviors such as unprotected sex (see Huszti, Hoff, and Johnson, Chapter 39, this volume), smoking, substance abuse and other high-risk health behaviors including behaviors, and lifestyles that may result in unintentional injuries.

For children with chronic illness, pediatric psychologists should employ primary, secondary, and tertiary preventive interventions when indicated to diminish the potential development of negative emotional sequelae in these children. Pediatric psychologists should work in conjunction with pediatric health care providers to identify and intervene with families at risk for domestic violence, child abuse, or neglect (see Bonner, Logue, and Kees, Chapter 39, this volume).

Exposure

- Course work, formal readings, or seminars on the science of prevention and principles of behavior change as pertinent to healthy development and prevention of disease in adulthood.
- Course work and lectures on healthy behavior and health-risk behavior, as well as seminars on screening and identifying children in primary care who experience or are at risk for abuse and neglect.

Experience

- Supervised experience in addressing multiple behavioral health issues that include the promotion of healthy lifestyles and disease prevention; safety, nutrition, weight management, stress management, and exercise; and how to address family risk factors, such as family violence, sexual and physical abuse, and individual risk factors, such as substance use (including nicotine).

Social Issues Affecting Children, Adolescents, and Families

Pediatric psychologists frequently are exposed to social issues as they present in health care settings. For example, pediatric psychologists often work with children who have been exposed to violence or have problems with access to health care resources. By identifying and providing early intervention for children at risk for behavioral and health disorders, pediatric psychologists can help to prevent more serious disorders. Advocacy for children, particularly as it relates to access to health care, should take place at the individual, local, state, and national levels.

Exposure

- Directed readings and seminars on advocacy in pediatric health care and social issues as these affect the development of children and health care delivery.

Experience

- Obtain experience in advocacy by becoming involved in local, state, and national professional associations.

Consultation and Liaison Roles

Pediatric psychologists often consult with providers from other disciplines, especially pediatricians, in a variety of settings. An understanding of consultation models and the ability to complete brief, focused consultations with patients, physicians, and medical and other health staff are particularly important skills for pediatric psychologists.

Pediatric psychologists also are in a unique position to educate and consult with nonmedical professionals, such as teachers, school psychologists, and counselors, regarding pediatric disease and its psychosocial sequelae. Pediatric psychologists provide support to other disciplines for issues related to the management of difficult families, stressful physician and family interactions, professional burnout, bereavement, and negotiating various stressful situations that present in medical settings.

Exposure

- Directed readings and seminars on consultation–liaison models as applied to pediatric psychology.
- Opportunities to observe supervisors providing consultation to pediatricians.
- Training in how best to teach the principles of learning, development, and behavioral health to other health care professionals.

Experience

- Supervised experiences in providing consultation with health care professionals via participation on a consultation–liaison service and preparing medical chart notes in both inpatient and outpatient settings.
- Supervised practica in consulting with community-based pediatricians on common childhood problems, as well as consultation regarding psychological sequelae of children with medical problems in nonmedical settings, and consultation with health care professionals regarding job-related stress.

• Supervised experience in consulting with parent groups on various issues related to child development and behavior and experience in communicating psychological knowledge to pediatricians, pediatric residents, and other health care professionals, as well as educating these professionals about the best practices in pediatric psychology.

Disease Process and Medical Management

As they routinely work with medical professionals, it is crucial that pediatric psychologists have a basic understanding of various diseases (see, for example, McQuaid and Walters, Chapter 16, this volume, and Stark, Mackner, Patton, and Acton, Chapter 17, this volume). It is equally important for the pediatric psychologist to keep informed of advances in current medical treatments for childhood diseases. Understanding of the illness better prepares pediatric psychologists to foresee areas in which psychological issues will be important and enables them to design interventions related to these factors. A sufficient working knowledge of the terminology relevant to various aspects of the disease process and treatment is necessary in order to communicate with physicians treating these patients and with their family caregivers, who rapidly can become knowledgeable about the specifics of the illness.

Exposure

• Course work, seminars, readings, and lectures on various diseases, disease processes and pathophysiology, and medical management and treatment of disease.

• Continuing education and medical rounds offered in most major medical centers on the advances in medical knowledge and care, as well as pediatric grand rounds and bedside rounds, medical procedures, and specific teaching rounds (e.g., walking rounds, tumor boards).

Experience

• Supervised rotations through primary care, community health clinics, and specialty clinics for firsthand knowledge of disease, management, and advances in treatment.

CLOSING COMMENTS

This chapter summarizes the recommendations of the Society of Pediatric Psychology Task Force on Training and suggests particular areas that are unique to the training of pediatric psychologists. These areas also further solidify an identity for pediatric psychology as a unique and separate discipline from clinical child psychology and extend this identity beyond the original conceptualizations of its founders (e.g., Wright, 1967). The training domains described here should allow pediatric psychologists to increase involvement of families in both disease prevention and adaptation to illness; should have a significant role in helping families manage complex medical systems; should allow a greater role for pediatric psychologists in health promotion and more frequent delivery of pediatric psychological services in the primary care setting than in previous years; and should improve knowledge of disease processes and innovative approaches to disease management among practicing pediatric psychologists. The broadening of these skills should allow pediatric psychologists greater opportunities for professional practice in the 21st century.

ACKNOWLEDGMENTS

This chapter is based on a task force report titled "Recommendations for the Training of Pediatric Psychologists," which was prepared at the request of the Executive Committee of the Society of Pediatric Psychology in 2000. The first author was chair of the task force, and the other authors volunteered to be members of the task force.

A copy of the full task force report is available from the Society of Pediatric Psychology. An expanded version of this chapter was published in the *Journal of Pediatric Psychology*, *28*(2), 2003. Spirito and Brown assumed final responsibility for preparing the task force document and this chapter. The other authors are listed in alphabetical order. The opinions and recommendations delineated in this document are those of the authors and the task force and have not been endorsed or recommended by the American Psychological Association.

REFERENCES

American Psychological Association, Division 54, Society of Pediatric Psychology. (1999). *The Society of Pediatric Psychology By-Laws*. Washington, DC: American Psychological Association.

La Greca, A., & Hughes, J. (1999). United we stand, divided we fall: The education and training needs of clinical child psychologists. *Journal of Clinical Child Psychology, 28*, 435–447.

Roberts, M., Carlson, C., Erickson, M., Friedman, R., La Greca, A., Lemanek, K., et al. (1998). A model for training psychologists to provide services for children and adolescents. *Professional Psychology: Research and Practice, 29*, 293–299.

Rodrigue, J., Geffken, G., & Streisand, R. (2000). *Child health assessment: A handbook of measurement techniques*. Boston: Allyn & Bacon.

Routh, D. K., Schroeder, C. S., & Koocher, G. P. (1983). Psychology and primary care for children. *American Psychologist, 38*, 95–98.

Wright, L. (1967). The pediatric psychologist: A role model. *American Psychologist, 22*, 323–325.

3

Ethical and Legal Issues in Pediatric Psychology

WILLIAM A. RAE
DONALD BRUNNQUELL
JEREMY R. SULLIVAN

Throughout their varied professional activities, pediatric psychologists must constantly acknowledge and apply general ethical principles, as well as more specific ethical guidelines, on behalf of their patients. The ethics code of the American Psychological Association (APA, 2002) includes several ethical principles of paramount importance to pediatric psychologists. The principles of beneficence and nonmaleficence imply that psychologists should always attempt to help their patients while also striving to cause no harm. The principles of fidelity and responsibility refer to the care psychologists take in establishing trustful relationships, maintaining awareness of their professional responsibilities, and upholding standards of conduct. Integrity refers to maintaining accuracy and honesty in all professional endeavors, and justice refers to psychologists treating all people equitably and recognizing the limitations of their professional competence. Finally, the principle of respect for people's rights and dignity entails recognition of patients' rights to confidentiality, autonomy, and self-determination. Within these general principles lies the importance of competence in all professional activities. Although these general principles underlie all of psychologists' work, this chapter focuses on more specific ethical guidelines and issues as applied to pediatric psychology.

The purpose of this chapter is to describe ethical and legal issues that may affect the pediatric psychologist in his or her multiple professional roles as a member of the health care team, as a mental health practitioner, and as a researcher. In the first section, bioethics is described within the context of real-world problems confronted by pediatric psychologists in hospital settings. The second section describes general mental health issues such as informed consent, confidentiality, and record keeping, all of which are important in the provision of psychological services. In the third section, research ethics for pediatric psychologists are described.

BIOETHICS FOR CHILDREN AND ADOLESCENTS

The growth of attention to ethical issues within the medical health care setting has been one of the most noticeable changes of the past decades. Coinciding with the patient autonomy movement and more recently with the cost containment movement in health care, discussions of ethical issues in medicine are taking place in numerous venues such as in hospital ethics committees, in courts over the right to refuse and obtain treatment, and in legislative bodies in the passage of federal and state mandates regarding certain aspects of decision making. The pediatric psychologist has a unique set of skills and viewpoints that can enhance both the patients' and care providers' approaches to ethical issues.

Bioethics, Ethics Committees, and Ethics Consultation

Although ethics have been a concern in ancient religious and philosophical traditions, explicit attention to bioethics increased during the last third of the 20th century. This increase occurred as the result of the advent of new technologies, the shift to a less paternalistic and more consumer-oriented health care system, an increase in resource allocation dilemmas, and the generally increasing pluralism of society (Evans, 2000; Pellegrino, 1993). Legal (*in re* Quinlan, 1976) and regulatory involvement in health care has further reinforced this growth. Current standards in health care organizations require specific notification of rights and mechanisms to address ethical dilemmas (Joint Commission on Accreditation of Healthcare Organizations [JCAHO], 2001).

In most hospital settings and many clinic settings, ethical issues are addressed by specific ethics committees that act to develop and implement polices in ethically troubling areas, as well as to provide consultation to staff and families in difficult cases. Most committees have adopted an approach based on defined principles of ethics such as those described in the work of Beauchamp and Childress (2001). This approach has been tempered in recent years by other approaches such as virtue ethics, feminist ethics, narrative ethics, and utilitarian approaches, but reliance on principles such as autonomy, justice, nonmaleficence, beneficence, truth telling, and respect for persons is still the dominant approach in health care (Benjamin, 2001).

Full committees, subcommittees, or individual consultants acting independently or as part of an ethics committee may carry out ethics consultations in individual cases. No standard format for consultation exists, although a task force of the American Society for Bioethics and Humanities (ASBH) attempted to outline core competencies for consultation (ASBH, 1998). This task force noted the assessments, processes, and interpersonal skills needed for consultation in ethical matters and emphasized the importance of core knowledge in the areas of bioethical issues and concepts (such as ethical theory, end-of-life decision making, and advance care planning). Other core knowledge areas included the health care system, the local institution and its policies, beliefs and perspectives of patients and staff, relevant professional ethics codes, and health care law. Although data on satisfaction with and effectiveness of ethics consultation are still quite limited, initial reports indicated that provider satisfaction is high (70–90%) but that family satisfaction was somewhat lower (50%; Orr, Morton, & de Leon, 1996; Yen & Schneiderman, 1999). An interview study

(Schneiderman, Gilmer, & Teetzel, 2000) suggested that, although consultation is seen by families as stressful, 75% found it helpful and would recommend it to others. In addition to clinical ethics, committees and consultants have become more involved with organizational ethics and the attempt to assess the effects of organizational decisions and policies on individuals and groups of patients (Potter, 1999).

Medical Decision Making for Children

Issues of informed consent and assent are discussed later in the chapter, but the discussion of who makes medical decisions for children is essential. Until 18 years of age, the legal guardian, usually the parent, is typically responsible for the consent to treatment. However, out of respect for autonomy and self-determination, the child or adolescent should be involved in medical decisions to the extent of his or her capacity, even when he or she not capable of understanding the entire situation or recognized as legally competent. Once the adolescent is no longer a minor and becomes his or her own legal guardian, the adolescent also becomes responsible for making his or her own medical decisions. Psychologists have a role in both assessing the child's capacity and advocating for the inclusion of the child's preferences to the extent possible.

Although there generally is no legal requirement for children's assent to medical treatment, as children enter adolescence, treatment without assent is difficult. The philosophical complexities of these decisions are manifold and include such variables as autonomy, consent, and competence, as well as practical issues of subrogation of rights and representation (Gaylin, 1982). Although parents are charged with the duty to act on their understanding of the child's best interests, it is still the rights and interests of the child that should determine the decision, not the interests or preferences of the parent. Although parents are presumed to have the legal authority to act on their child's behalf, this is not an unlimited authority.

One potential source of conflict over the medical consent to treatment is the religious view of the parents, which may affect the child's life and may have to be overridden by the court. In a fairly common situation, Jehovah's Witnesses may specifically request that blood products from one person not be given to another, a request based on religious and medical reasons (Watchtower Bible and Tract Society of New York, 1992). State laws and local judicial practices with regard to parents who are Jehovah's Witnesses differ. Thus courts may be used to override the parents' judgment in refusing blood transfusions for their children in life-threatening situations, while still recognizing the decision of legally competent patients (Layon, D'Amico, Caton, & Mollet, 1990). Debate is ongoing regarding the rights of parents who are Christian Scientists to refuse all medical treatment for their children and to provide spiritual healing (see American Academy of Pediatrics, Committee on Bioethics, 1988).

The ethical issues surrounding medical decision making become even more complex when adolescents, who are beginning to assert their own preferences, become involved. Blustein and Moreno (1997) address these issues by noting the combination of developmental and social factors that must be considered when determining whether an adolescent has the capacity to make decisions on his or her own, requires assisted decision making, or should be considered incapacitated. The laws of each state affect the definition of an emancipated minor. The basic principle of inclusion of the adolescent to the extent of his or her capacity should always drive decision making. Even in areas such as forgoing life-sustaining treatment, many ethicists argue that mature minors should have the right in most circumstances to refuse treatment (Derish & Vanden Heuvel, 2000).

Forgoing Life-Sustaining Treatment

Based on the right to autonomous decision making about health care, an almost absolute right to forgo treatments exists for the competent, adult patient. These rights include both refusing recommended treatments (i.e., withholding treatment) and withdrawing treatments already begun. Decisions to withhold or withdraw life-sustaining treatment have most often been discussed in the context of cardiopulmonary resuscitation (CPR) and so-called "do not resuscitate" (DNR) orders and also with regard to the issue of fluids and nutrition. General attempts to address these decisions (American Thoracic Society, 1991; Hastings Center, 1987; President's Commission, 1983; Stanley, 1992) indicated that there is no logical, philosophical distinction between withholding and withdrawing treatment. Those working in the situation confirm almost universally, however, that there is an emotional difference between the two situations. Exploration of this perceived difference is often helpful in discussions of particular cases. Work is beginning to emerge in which the description of forgoing life-sustaining treatment is being discussed in the context of "allowing natural death" rather than withholding or withdrawing a treatment.

The right to refuse resuscitation and other treatments is now among those guaranteed by the regulations of JCAHO (JCAHO, 2001) and the federal government's Centers for Medicare and Medicaid Services (CMS). The confusion of DNR, which refers specifically to withholding resuscitative services while continuing other life-sustaining treatment, continues. The right to refuse or have treatments withdrawn extends to all medical treatments. Variables such as the invasiveness of the treatment, the pain and suffering entailed in the treatment, the short- and long-term prognosis for the patient, and quality of life are all relevant during the decision-making process (Youngner, 1987). Issues such as the role of the family when patients are not competent (as is true of most children), patient's and family's fears of abandonment if a DNR order is instituted, and the use of DNR orders as a cost-containment method are also raised. These decisions are more complex for nonautonomous patients, for whom a surrogate (such as a parent) must make the decisions, even though the right to refuse treatment on behalf of someone else is recognized in law and ethics (Paris & Fletcher, 1987; Stanley, 1992; Weir & Gostin, 1990). As members of the health care team not directly involved in providing these services, pediatric psychologists can play an important advocacy role by assisting families in asking questions and carefully considering all of their options. Pediatric psychologists should also be aware of and discuss with families the various policies held by local schools, emergency medical technicians (EMTs), and first responders with regard to honoring DNR orders (Sabitino, 1999). The issue of withholding or withdrawing nutrition and hydration is even more contentious, especially when nonautonomous patients are involved. Ramer-Chrastek, Brunnquell, and Hasse (2002), Johnson and Mitchell (2000), and Nelson et al. (1995) provided discussions of the acceptable grounds for discontinuing medical nutrition and hydration in pediatrics.

Related to the discussion of forgoing life-sustaining treatment is the control of pain and suffering in end-of-life situations. There is general agreement that relief of pain and suffering in all medical care is an obligation. In fact, relief of pain is now required in hospitals (JCAHO, 2001), and practitioners are subject to malpractice claims if the problem is not properly addressed (Furrow, 2001). In end-of-life circumstances, however, medications used to control pain can also lead to diminished respiratory drive and other side effects that may hasten death; this quandary is often referred to as the "double effect." The unintended effects of the treatment are acceptable in certain limited circumstances in order to achieve the intended effect of pain management. Although no absolute consensus exists in American society, most people take the view in support of patient autonomy and quality of life and hold that the double effect is acceptable if (1) the patient is in a terminal phase; (2) there is no alternative method to control the pain and suffering; (3) the medications are used in response to symptoms; and (4) the patient or his or her proxy is fully informed of, and consents to, the course of treatment (Sulmasy, 2000). Wolfe (2000) presented a comprehensive argument for an affirmative duty to palliate pain in end-of-life situations with children and raises empirical questions about the existence of the double effect in most cases of aggressive pain palliation.

Issues in Neonatal Medicine

Neonatal medicine has remained a crucible for bioethics issues for the past 50 years. As the technology to save smaller and younger premature infants has emerged, battles have raged over the appropriate use of that technology, the duties owed helpless and dependent newborns, the long-term prognosis of survivors, and control over decision making. The well-known Baby Doe case and the subsequent federal guidelines regarding treatment of infants have dominated the discourse in neonatal ethics (see Caplan, Blank, & Merrick, 1992, for a complete discussion of this history from a wide variety of viewpoints). Recent views of these issues focus on the meaning of medically indicated treatment (King, 1992; Koppelman, Koppelman, & Irons, 1992; Paris, Ferranti, & Reardon, 2001). These views are discussed within the context of the debate in the general bioethics literature on the issue of obligatory treatment versus the right to refuse treatments (Miles, 1992; Schneiderman, Jecker, & Jonsen, 1990). In this view, the ethical task is to ask whether treatment is appropriate, given the understanding that (1) treatment decisions involve the probability that treatment will be effective, and (2) treatment serves the goals of the patient. Because in these cases those goals are defined by the surrogate decision makers (generally the parents), the issue of discrimination and unfair treatment of infants becomes salient.

The conundrum of the infant's individuation from the mother leads to numerous other issues. State requirements for prenatal and postnatal screening of infants and their mothers for illicit drug use vary widely, with differing emphases on the interests of the child and the parent. Due to this variability, familiarity with local law is essential. Informing mothers of drug testing, determining whether consent is necessary or desirable, and using objective standards for the decision to test are important issues that must be addressed. It is clearly preferable to obtain consent before implementing any procedure with significant social implications, but concerns about alienating families or causing families to remove their children from treatment against medical advice often influence this decision. Clear institutional protocols should be developed to address these questions. New reproductive technologies such as in vitro fertilization (IVF), preimplantation genetic screening, and selective reduction of embryos have a strong influence on the outcome for neonates and the psychological response of parents to neonatal crises (Cohen, 1996; White & Leuthner, 2001). These variables should be part of the pediatric psychologist's assessment of families facing ethical dilemmas in the newborn period.

Genetic Screening and Testing of Children

As genetic tests for specific diseases become available, the debate about use of those tests with children grows. Whereas adults are presumed to choose such tests based on their fully informed evaluation of their own interests, when tests are chosen by parents, the interests of the child may or may not be primary. Benefits to the child may include earlier understanding and treatment of disease conditions and therefore better life within the family. Harms may include labeling and self-fulfilling prophecies about development, overprotection of a child before symptoms occur, effects on self-image, future discrimination, or uninsurability. These claims remain largely unresearched on both sides. Interviews with 29 genetic counselors led Hall and Rich (2000) to claim that fears of effects on insurance are exaggerated, but news reports continue to emerge of insurance industry use of such information in spite of many state laws enacted ensuring privacy of genetic information. Cohen (1998) delineates four categories of factors that must be taken into account in assessing the decision to conduct genetic testing: (1) the disease and its characteristics (e.g., severity, onset); (2) the age and development of the child and effects on emotional development and possible future discrimination; (3) the effects of the knowledge on family dynamics; (4) the concerns and goals of the other family members. Emerging issues include the right of parents to prevent having children with disabilities (Parens & Asch, 1999), to have children with life conditions or "disabilities" the parents have (e.g., deafness; Davis, 1997), or to enhance their offspring (McGee, 1997).

Other Issues in Pediatric Bioethics

Pediatric patients with chronic illness often continue to be seen by their pediatric care providers, and these providers are required to implement certain procedures. The Patient Self-Determination Act (1990) requires that every hospital, nursing home, and home care agency have in place a mechanism to notify the adult patient of his or her right to have an advance directive in accordance with state law. An "advance directive" is a legal document that specifies a patient's wishes regarding health care that is to be used as a guide if the person becomes unable to communicate his or her own wishes. Pediatric psychologists should know the relevant requirements for documentation of advance directives in their organization and locale.

Growing attention to cultural competence has also emerged in the bioethics literature. Although aligned with the discussion of ethical analysis, this literature challenges the traditional medical model and academically based analysis of ethical issues. For example, Hern, Koening, Moore, and Marshall (1998) addressed culture in end-of-life decision making, and Levin and Schiller (1998) described social class as a cultural issue. In addition, it has become clear that racial and ethnic issues contribute to disparities in health care treatment in such diverse areas as access to transplantation (Alexander & Sehgal, 1998) and treatment of pain (Bonham, 2001). Cultural issues affect the child's and family's view of what is right and desirable. The pediatric psychologist can act as a powerful advocate for inclusion of those views into the discussion in a health care system that still attends to the medical model of disease and remains skeptical of other approaches. Carter and Klugman (2001) presented a comprehensive model for cultural engagement in ethics. Their approach involves interviewing the patient or family and practitioner about the nature of the health problem, the effects of quality of life, the causes of the problem, and discussion of past and proposed treatments with the patient and whoever advises them about their decision making.

Attention and debate has grown in the area of treatment of children with various genetic–anatomic–psychological conditions broadly categorized as intersexuality (previously labeled ambiguous genitalia). These are children with a variety of conditions, especially Turner and Klinefelter syndromes, congenital adrenal hypoplasia, and androgen insensitivity syndrome, who have external genitalia that do not conform to the societal dimorphic expectations, that is, either a boy or a girl. There is a wide variety of internal anatomy and underlying X–Y chromosome variants. In a comprehensive review of this topic, Fausto-Sterling (2000) estimated the total rate of nondimorphic sexual development as 1.78/100 live births. An early case report and subsequent publications by psychologist John Money (Money & Ehrhardt, 1972) led to frequent early definitive surgery to create an external genital appearance of a boy or girl on the theory that gender identity would then conform to this external anatomy and social stigma would be minimized. Recent reexamination of this approach by adults who experienced this treatment has led to a broad reassessment of the assumptions and approach. Dreger (1998), Howe (1998), and Beh and Diamond (2000) reviewed the complex elements of the area and concur with the calls of Kipnis and Diamond (1998) and the Intersex Society of North America (1994) to gather more information, to fully inform parents of children born with these conditions, and generally to postpone definitive surgeries. The pediatric psychologist must understand and assist children, families, and staff struggling to address these issues.

MENTAL HEALTH ETHICS FOR PEDIATRIC PSYCHOLOGISTS

Children and adolescents rarely request psychological services directly from pediatric psychologists. They are usually brought in for psychological services involuntarily by parents or guardians. Adolescents can be especially resistant to mental health assessment and treatment because of the stigma attached to receiving psychological services and their developmentally appropriate need to be independent of parental control. Special consideration by the pediatric psychologist must be given to informed consent, confidentiality, and record keeping.

Informed Consent

All pediatric psychologists should obtain informed assent from children and informed consent from parents when engaging in assessment, intervention, or consultation activities. The pediatric psychologist should use language that is understandable and developmentally appropriate for the patient and family. Any risks or benefits of the assessment, intervention, or consultation activity should be thoroughly explained. Most young children lack the cognitive ability and life experience to fully understand the potential risks and benefits of assessment, intervention, or consultation. In addition, children with chronic illnesses or other conditions (e.g., mental retardation) might have further diminished capacity to fully assent. For example, children who are medicated or who are in considerable pain may not be able to cognitively process information as well as unaffected children. In the same way, children and families who are undergoing the stress of hospitalization and/or treatment for a chronic illness are not always in the psychological state of mind to make the best decision about their care. In most cases children and adolescents are not legally able to provide informed consent for themselves. Thus pediatric psychologists should obtain permission from a legally authorized person (e.g., parent, guardian). Although the psychologist should always consider the minor child's preferences, the best interest of the child should be of paramount importance. Pediatric psychologists should always strive to benefit their patients and never do anything that would be harmful.

Children in hospital settings are often referred to a pediatric psychologist without their knowledge or consent. As part of the tacit consent in being hospitalized and certainly during the diagnostic phase, it is assumed that the child will receive appropriate care "as needed."

Although not required by the APA ethical guidelines (APA, 2002), the best practice would be to obtain a separate informed consent in writing for each activity of the pediatric psychologist, but this is often impractical during a hospitalization. When written consent is obtained, the consent form should include specific information about all aspects of psychological services, including the type of service (i.e., assessment, intervention, or consultation) and the recipient (e.g., child, parents, family). The limits of confidentiality should be specified, including circumstances under which confidentiality may be broken and what kinds of confidences will be kept between child, parents, and others.

Contexts of Consent

Different professional activities require different informed consent considerations. For assessment, informed consent is often implied because assessment is a routine hospital activity. Regardless of the child's capacity, the pediatric psychologist should always explain the nature and purpose of the assessment using language that is understandable to the child. Answering questions and being responsive to the concerns of the child or parents is helpful for avoiding misunderstandings. Even if a consent "form" has been signed, that form is not a substitute for a formal discussion of the nature and purpose of the assessment with the child and parents. Explaining the assessment process to the child and parents sometimes requires giving creative examples of assessment activities.

For intervention activities, pediatric psychologists should inform patients as early as possible about the nature and course of the treatment, involvement of third parties (e.g., family members, physicians), and confidentiality. Although fees should always be discussed prior to commencing outpatient psychotherapeutic intervention, fees may not be discussed during pediatric hospitalization. Pediatric psychologists should always inform children and their parents about potential risks and benefits of any intervention and whether the techniques being used are established, recognized therapeutic techniques or are emerging, less established techniques. Similarly, the child and parents should be informed of any alternative treatments that may be available and should be given the opportunity to withdraw from treatment at any time. Pediatric psychologists should also delineate the effect of managed care on the treatment process.

Confusion can exist about the nature of consultation in health care settings. Two types of consultation exist in pediatric health care settings, with particular requirements of informed consent for each context. First, consultation in a hospital can begin with a referral to the pediatric psychologist by a health care provider in order to answer a diagnostic question. A "consult" in this context usually involves the pediatric psychologist evaluating the pediatric patient and family in light of a specific referral question. Because the patient is evaluated, the pediatric psychologist should attempt to clarify his or her role at the onset of contact and indicate the probable use of the information obtained. Because within a health care setting information can be shared with other professionals, it is important to clarify who might be the intended recipients of information about the patient. Second, consultation for the pediatric psychologist may involve discussing general psychological issues surrounding the care and well-being of patients with other professionals without evaluating the patient directly. When consulting with professional colleagues, the pediatric psychologist does not disclose confidential information that might reveal the patient's identity and only discloses information necessary to achieve the purposes of the consultation (APA, 2002).

Informed consent can be problematic when working with families. The psychologist should delineate the nature of the relationship with the patient and the other family members at the onset of professional contact, clarifying who is being assessed and the way information will be used. If it becomes apparent that a conflicting role may exist (e.g., testifying for custody while acting as the family's therapist), the pediatric psychologist should modify or clarify his or her role accordingly and, if no resolution appears evident, should withdraw from providing care. Another dilemma for pediatric psychologists involves dealing with families in crisis or conflict; what may be therapeutically beneficial to one family member may not be beneficial to another.

Elements in Informed Decision Making

Four elements are essential in making an informed decision with regard to consent. The first element requires that the patient and parent be provided information that might affect his or her willingness to participate in the assessment, intervention, or consultation activity. The pediatric psychologist should provide an explanation that is clear and comprehensive; the explanation should be in language that is appropriate for the developmental understanding of the child, adolescent, or parent. Unfortunately, in harried hospital settings, there may not be adequate time to assess this understanding.

Second, the decision to participate in any assessment, intervention, or consultation activity must be made voluntarily, without undue influence or coercion (Corey, Corey, & Callanan, 2003; Koocher & Keith-Spiegel, 1998). It is important for the child, adolescent, or parent to feel that to decline participation will not result in a loss of benefit or respect. Children and their parents can be exposed to subtle coercion to participate when the referring physician strongly recommends psychological services. The pediatric psychologist must be careful not to exploit the power differential in his or her relationship with the child and family, because to do so might unfairly compel participation in psychological services. Because many children and parents can be intimidated in medical settings, they may not feel free to decline participation; they may believe that declining participation with the pediatric psychologist might affect the medical care that they receive. Children are also unaccustomed to making health care decisions for themselves, deferring instead to their parents. The pediatric psychologist should develop a cooperative relationship in which coercion is kept to a minimum.

Third, whether obtained orally or in written form, informed consent must be appropriately documented. Because of statutory or accrediting agency regulations in health care settings, pediatric psychologists usually have little trouble documenting informed consent. Pediatric psychologists should document that the child and parents were provided the opportunity to ask questions and receive answers about the psychological services proposed.

Finally, at the centerpiece of informed consent is the requirement of competence (Beauchamp & Childress, 2001). This principle states that the legally responsible person (e.g., parent) giving permission for a minor should have the capacity to competently assess the services being proposed. Each state mandates the age of majority for adult competence (Kitchener, 2000).

It is preferable to obtain permission from both parents for psychological services, not just the custodial parent. Because of their legally defined diminished competence, minors are not allowed to consent to services except in rare circumstances. At the same time, pediatric psychologists should inform children of the proposed interventions in a manner commensurate with their psychological capabilities, should seek their assent to those interventions, and should consider their preferences and best interests. The assessment of "competence" is poorly articulated in law (Melton, Ehrenreich, & Lyons, 2001) and often is not attempted by pediatric psychologists (Rae & Worchel, 1991). Therefore, although obtaining consent is legally required, once the parent has given permission for psychological services, the child's wishes become legally irrelevant.

Evaluation of Capacity to Consent

Because of their diminished capacity, children cannot always understand all the ramifications of making important health care decisions for themselves. Although there is no legal requirement that a minor assent to diagnostic or treatment services, a child who agrees to participate is generally more cooperative, which in turn should lead to a more effective therapeutic relationship and better outcomes. As noted by McCabe (1996), involving children in the decision-making process may have additional benefits, such as giving children a sense of autonomy and self-determination, facilitating communication, maximizing medical treatment compliance, and providing psychologists with an opportunity to demonstrate respect for children's abilities.

The evaluation of the child's capacity to consent or assent requires that the pediatric psychologist assess the child's cognitive development. Each child will need assistance in understanding the psychological services proposed. Thus the pediatric psychologist should use language and examples that are compatible with the child's own developmental abilities and life experiences. Koocher and Keith-Spiegel (1990) have summarized the child's abilities at each stage of Piagetian development. Each child or adolescent should be evaluated individually to determine the quality of his or her cognitive processing abilities, in addition to his or her social development and characteristics such as coping style, health beliefs, and relevant experiences (McCabe, 1996). Further, through clinical interviews the psychologist should also strive to understand the influence of additional factors on the child's decision, such as the complexity of the issues, clarity of communication, how the child perceives and processes consent information, environmental and situational factors, the child's emotional status, and the child's feelings about the treatment, thereby leading to a more comprehensive understanding of the child's capacity to consent or assent to services (Krener & Mancina, 1994; Reder & Fitzpatrick, 1998; Tymchuk, 1997). Unfortunately, as noted by Tymchuk (1997), psychometric methods with which to assess these constructs within the context of the informed consent situation and decision-making process have not been adequately examined.

Exceptions to Informed Consent

The past several decades have shown a trend for minors to be given the legal authority to both consent to and refuse psychological services under certain circumstances regardless of parental wishes. This change has come about because of an awareness that parents do not always act in the best interests of their children (Shields & Johnson, 1992). In many cases, exceptions are made to parental consent when it is believed that parental consent would discourage minors from seeking psychological services that would be beneficial to them (Brock, 1989). The legal regulations for consenting to treatment are made by individual states. As a result, what is permissible in one state may not be allowed in another state. Exceptions to informed consent fall into two categories. In the first category, the legal status of the minor can affect how informed consent is obtained. For example, most states have a category of "emancipated minor," which is usually defined as an individual younger than 18 years who is married, in the military, or living independently from parents while at the same time being financially self-supporting. In the same way, if a minor has been required by a court to obtain an assessment or treatment, informed consent is not necessary. In the second category, a minor has the legal right to consent to certain kinds of assessments (e.g., suicide) or interventions (e.g., drug abuse counseling) depending on the laws of the particular state in which the child or adolescent resides. For example, minors in the state of Texas can consent to assessment of drug addiction or suicide and treatment of physical, sexual, or emotional abuse and/or chemical addiction. In addition, in most states a minor can obtain emergency psychological services if the minor is a danger to self or others.

Confidentiality

Confidentiality is the cornerstone of the therapeutic relationship (Koocher & Keith-Spiegel, 1998) but also is at the center of one of the most frequent ethical dilemmas for psychologists (Pope & Vetter, 1992). Many patients and families might not divulge private information to the pediatric psychologist unless they were assured that private information would remain confidential, a situation that could lead to spurious assessments and interventions. Protecting confidentiality is a primary obligation for all psychologists. Pediatric psychologists should recognize that confidentiality practices are established not only legally but also within institutions and for professionals. Pediatric psychologists do not have confidentiality for themselves, but they may raise the privilege of confidentiality on behalf of their patients. A discussion of confidentiality issues should take place during the informed consent process at the initiation of the professional contact, although this discussion is not always feasible in the chaotic medical environment. During the informed consent procedure, the pediatric psychologist should discuss the limits to confidentiality and how confidential information will be used. In addition, if confidential information is transmitted electronically (e.g., e-mail or facsimile), the patient should be forewarned. Although the patient's understanding of confidentiality should always be assessed, many pediatric psychologists admit that they do not always assess it. In a study of ethical beliefs of pediatric psychologists, even though 97% of pediatric psychologists reported that it was ethical to assess the pediatric client's understanding of confidentiality, in practice 13% reported that they "never" or "rarely" assessed it (Rae & Worchel, 1991).

Confidentiality issues with children and adolescents are different from those with adults. Adults expect that private information obtained from a mental health professional will be kept confidential except when they give their written consent to have information released. Young children, in particular, do not expect broad confidentiality for private information as parents are knowledgeable about many of these details anyway. On the other hand, adolescents require more assurances of confidentiality, because they are often suspicious of parental motives and intentions. Many psychologists who treat adolescents require that confidentiality be maintained in regard to parents even though there is no legal basis for doing so. The pediatric psychologist must balance the *right* versus the *need* for the parents to obtain confidential information about their child.

Determining the limits of confidentiality can be problematic for pediatric psychologists. Conflicting expectations often exist for the patient, parent, referral agent (e.g., physician), and institution (e.g., hospital). In the same way, conflicting expectations may also occur for pediatric psychologists who work with families, because the patient, parents, siblings, and extended family members can all have different expectations about what information should be shared with whom. Before initiating professional services, the pediatric psychologist should attempt to clarify the confidentiality issues for all the stakeholders involved. Even after clarification, there may still be different expectations. For example, primary care pediatricians commonly expect to be privy to the most confidential information, but patients might not want certain private information divulged even to their physician. Ultimately, the parents and the child have to decide how information is shared with family members or health care providers.

Breaking confidentiality is legally mandated in most states under three circumstances. First, in all 50 states psychologists are required to break confidentiality if they suspect a child is being physically, emotionally, or sexually abused. In actual practice, the timing and manner of breaking this confidence can be influenced by circumstantial variables. In fact, there are times at which pediatric psychologists believe it is ethical not to report abusive situations, even though it is a legal requirement (Rae & Worchel, 1991). Second, psychologists must divulge confidential information if ordered by a court. Third, pediatric psychologists should always break confidentiality to report imminent danger to the patient or to others. The pediatric psychologist must evaluate the potential of danger and disclose that information only to appropriate public authorities, professional workers, potential victims, and/or parents as required by law. Pediatric psychologists appear to have little ambivalence about breaking confidentiality if a child or adolescent appears to be suicidal or homicidal (Rae & Worchel, 1991). In contrast to those unambiguous situations, pediatric psychologists often have to make judgments about risky behaviors before deciding to break confidentiality. Obviously, the psychologist's own values and biases affect these judgments. Pediatric psychologists have shown considerable variation when judging risky adolescent behaviors in such areas as sexual behavior, substance use, and suicidal behavior that are affected by intensity, frequency, and duration of the behavior (Rae, Sullivan, Razo, George, & Ramirez, 2002).

Record Keeping

The APA ethical principles state that psychologists must document the services they perform and maintain accurate, current, and pertinent records of services. In addition, they should maintain appropriate confidentiality in the creating, storing, accessing, transferring, and disposition of records (APA, 1993, 2002). This requirement would include written, recorded, or computerized records. The records should be sufficiently detailed to permit the continued provision of services by them or by other professionals. Any documentation of services should only include information germane to the purposes of that documentation. In actual practice, the pediatric psychologist's records can vary widely depending on the setting and institutional requirements. An ethical dilemma can occur for the hospital-based pediatric psychologist who must write chart notes in the hospital record. Although psychologists might want to have a private file in the psychologist's office, doing so could present some liability issues, because the private notes would not be part of the official medical record. More than half of pediatric psychologists do not think it is ethical to reveal personal psychological data in a hospital chart note (Rae & Worchel, 1991). The pediatric psychologist should strive to document thoroughly and accurately but also be sensitive to the potentially harmful effects to the child of revealing confidential information. In medical centers, other health care providers want access to information in order to provide comprehensive care, but the pediatric psychologist should continually assess the potential harm in revealing that information.

Another conflict can arise over confidential information about the patient being revealed to parents. Technically, parents have the legal rights to all medical records of their minor children. If a thorough pediatric psychologist documents potentially damaging information, parents could have access to it. For example, if information about substance abuse or sexual activity were revealed, it could destroy the cooperative relationship between the patient and the pediatric psychologist. In a similar way, when patients reach the age of legal majority, they can request copies of all records. Because of the trend toward increased patient access to records, written documentation should be maintained with the assumption that the child or family will eventually see the record (Koocher & Keith-Spiegel, 1998).

ETHICAL ISSUES IN RESEARCH WITH CHILDREN AND ADOLESCENTS

As with assessment, intervention, and consultation, conducting research in the area of pediatric psychology raises some special issues, largely because the populations in which pediatric psychologists are primarily interested include children and adolescents. Whereas the APA's ethical code (APA, 2002) provides some general ethical guidelines, the U.S. Department of Health and Human Services (DHHS) provides guidelines specifically related to conducting research with child participants (Protection of Human Services, 2001). Because of their minority status, children have fewer legal rights than adults, thereby making very clear the need for researchers to protect child research participants. This need for protection manifests itself in several ways: parental informed consent, child assent, and the risk-to-benefit ratio. This section briefly considers these ethical issues as applied to research with pediatric populations.

Obtaining Informed Consent

Researchers wishing to include children or adolescents as participants in research protocols are required to obtain written consent from the child's or adolescent's parents or legal guardians, unless the would-be participants are emancipated minors or adolescents 18 years of age or older. The consent form to be signed by parents should clarify the responsibilities of each party (i.e., researcher and participant) and should include detailed information about the nature and purpose of the research study and what participation would entail (APA, 2002; Protection, 2001; Fischman, 2000; Kitchener, 2000; Rae & Sullivan, 2003). This information must be conveyed in language that is understandable; professional jargon should be avoided. Further, researchers must be willing to respond to participants' questions and concerns. Drotar et al. (2000) suggested that researchers read consent forms aloud to parents and potential participants, in order to maximize the likelihood that everyone involved understands what participation in the research project will entail, especially with regard to potential risks and the opportunity for participants to withdraw from the study at any time. This process can be followed by a question-and-answer session in which the researcher addresses questions and clarifies any points of uncertainty.

Informed consent must be provided voluntarily and without coercion. In pediatric psychology research, the investigator should remember that parents may assume that the role of the researcher is identical to the role of the clinician, who is likely to be conceptualized as a helper of children and families. This assumption may lead parents to automatically consent to any research invitation under the assumption that the "doctor knows best" or that research participation will result in better medical or psychosocial care. Thus, in obtaining informed consent, researchers must clearly define their roles and assure children and their parents that consenting to or declining participation will have no bearing on the quality of treatment that they receive; that is, they will still receive appropriate treatment if they decline participation. Similarly, researchers are in positions of authority, and they must be careful to refrain from exerting subtle pressure on parents to provide consent for participation.

Parental Consent and Child Assent

As noted, in most circumstances written consent from parents or guardians is required before children and adolescents can be included in psychological research. Once parental consent has been obtained, it is desirable to obtain the child participant's assent as well, in the same way that assent is desirable for other activities such as assessment, intervention, and consultation. As with parental consent, child assent requires a description of what participation will entail in developmentally appropriate terms. Under certain circumstances, child assent for research participation may not be necessary. For example, the assent requirement may be waived if the child is too young or is incapable of making a reasonable decision regarding participation. Further, if the experimental procedures or interventions have the potential for direct benefit to the health or mental health of participants and if these procedures or interventions are available only through the research project, then assent is not necessary. The decision of whether child assent (and, for that matter, parental consent) is necessary is ultimately made by the institutional review board (IRB) upon review of the research proposal (Protection, 2001).

Risk versus Benefit

Risk may be defined as the potential for physical, psychological, emotional, or other harm to befall participants as the result of their involvement in a research project. Risk can be classified into three types. (1) A no-risk situation involves experimental procedures that constitute the routine care of the child, such as customer satisfaction questionnaires, and may not even require direct interaction between the researcher and child participants. (2) A minimal-risk situation involves procedures or interventions in which the potential for physical or psychological harm is no greater than that encountered in the daily lives of the children or in a normal medical or psychological examination. (3) A high-risk situation involves procedures or interventions that are not necessary for the treatment of the child and that may involve participation in emotionally stressful situations. In general, research that involves more than a minimal level of risk places participants in a situation that contains potential for emotional distress or psychological harm. Although the investigator should always minimize risk, the research participants (and their parents or guardians) must always be fully informed as to the nature and extent of any possible risk. Benefit, on the other hand, may be conceptualized as the potential for participation to result in positive effects. Thus the potential for benefit is always a desirable characteristic in research, and psychologists should always strive to make this potential a reality. An important task during the planning of a research project is to consider the risk-to-benefit ratio; doing so allows researchers to plan to conduct the study in a way that minimizes potential risk, maximizes potential benefit, and ultimately assesses whether the potential risks are proportionate to the potential benefits to the participants and to society as a whole.

In a research situation in which the potential exists for more than minimal risk, a strong potential must exist for direct benefit to individual research participants (Rae & Fournier, 1986). In psychological research, exposing a child to more than minimal risk can rarely be justified, as most psychological research does not hold promise of a degree of benefit commensurate with a high degree of risk. Thus, in pediatric psychology research, the potential benefits should always outweigh the potential risks. Research in pediatric psychology often entails minimal or no risk; it almost never involves any physical risk. Because of this comparatively lower risk, researchers might employ what McCormick (1976) calls an "accordion morality," in which they inadvertently stretch their ethical standards to fit the needs of a particular investigation. Similarly, the researcher's need to complete a research project might lead to taking ethical shortcuts with regard to participants' welfare. For example, a psychologist might feel work-related pressures (e.g., publish-or-perish, grant deadline) to complete a research project, which may lead to a less comprehensive evaluation of possible ethical conflicts. Therefore, it is critical that proposed research be evaluated carefully by external reviewers (e.g., IRBs) in order to ensure that an overzealous researcher has not biased the risk–benefit analysis. These outside committees can conduct an independent assessment of the risk-to-benefit ratio and determine whether the proposed research has sufficient promise of resulting in benefit while maintaining a minimal level of potential risk.

Although research represents a distinct professional activity of pediatric psychologists, the ethical responsibilities involved in research with children and adolescents in medical settings closely parallel the ethical responsibilities involved in other professional activities, such as assessment, intervention, and consultation. This situation means that the areas discussed here, including informed consent, confidentiality, and record keeping, also apply to research activities in pediatric psychology. For a more thorough consideration of the ethical issues involved in psychological research, see Drotar (2000), Kitchener (2000), Rae and Sullivan (2003), and Sales and Folkman (2000).

CONCLUSION

Applying ethical and legal standards to the care and treatment of children, adolescents, and families can be very complex for pediatric psychologists. In working with pediatric populations, it is critical for pediatric psychologists to recognize that children represent a vulnerable population and that, therefore, assessment, intervention, and research in pediatric psychology require special care and sensitivity to the participants' welfare. All psychologists must strive to be ethical, but pediatric psychologists should be held to a higher standard given their role as advocates for pediatric patients and their families.

REFERENCES

Alexander, G. C., & Sehgal, A. R (1998). Barriers to cadaveric renal transplantation among blacks, women and the poor. *Journal of the American Medical Association, 280*, 1148–1152.

American Academy of Pediatrics, Committee on Bioethics. (1988). Religious exemptions from child abuse statutes. *Pediatrics, 81*, 169–171.

American Psychological Association. (2002). Ethical principles of psychologists and code of conduct. *American Psychologist, 57,* 1060–1073.

American Psychological Association. (1993). Record keeping guidelines. *American Psychologist, 48*, 984–986.

American Society for Bioethics and Humanities, Task Force on Standards for Bioethics Consultation. (1998). *Core competencies for health care ethics consultation*. Glenview, IL: Author.

American Thoracic Society. (1991). Withholding and withdrawing life-sustaining therapy. *American Review of Respiratory Disease, 144*, 726–731.

Beauchamp, T. L., & Childress, J. F. (2001). *Principles of biomedical ethics* (5th ed.). New York: Oxford University Press.

Beh, H. G., & Diamond, M. (2000). An emerging ethical and medical dilemma: Should physicians perform sex assignment surgery on infants with ambiguous genitalia? *Michigan Journal of Gender and Law.* (WL, 7 Mich J. Gender and L. 1).

Benjamin, M. (2001). Between subway and spaceship: Practical ethics at the outset of the twenty-first century. *Hastings Center Report, 31,* 24–31.

Blustein, J., & Moreno, J. (1997). Valid consent to treatment and the unsupervised adolescent. In J. Blustein, C. Levine, & N. N. Dubler (Eds.), *The adolescent alone: Decision-making in health care in the United States* (pp. 100–110). New York: Cambridge University Press.

Bonham, V. L. (2001). Race, ethnicity and pain treatment: Striving to understand the causes and solutions to the disparities in pain treatment. *Journal of Law, Medicine, and Ethics, 29,* 52–68.

Brock, D. W. (1989). Children's competence for health care decision-making. In L. M. Koppelman & J. C. Moskop (Eds.), *Children and health care* (pp. 181–212). Boston, MA: Kluwer Academic.

Caplan, A. L., Blank, R. H., & Merrick, J. C. (Eds.). (1992). *Compelled compassion: Government intervention in the treatment of critically ill newborns.* Totowa, NJ: Humana Press.

Carter, M. A., & Klugman, C. M. (2001). Cultural engagement in clinical ethics: A model for ethics consultation. *Cambridge Quarterly of Healthcare Ethics, 10,* 16–33.

Cohen, C. B. (1996). "Give me children or I shall die!" New reproductive technologies and harm to children. *Hastings Center Report, 26,* 19–27.

Cohen, C. B. (1998). Wrestling with the future: Should we test children for adult-onset genetic conditions? *Kennedy Institute of Ethics Journal, 8,* 111–130.

Corey, G., Corey, M. S., & Callanan, P. (2003). *Issues and ethics in the helping professions* (6th ed.). Pacific Grove, CA: Brooks/Cole.

Davis, D. (1997). Genetic dilemmas and the child's right to an open future. *Hastings Center Report, 27,* 7–15.

Derish, M. T., & Vanden Heuvel, K. (2000). Mature minors should have the right to refuse life-sustaining medical treatment. *Journal of Law, Medicine, and Ethics, 28,* 109–124.

Dreger, A. D. (1998). The history of intersexuality: From the age of gonads to the age of consent. *Journal of Clinical Ethics, 9,* 345–355.

Drotar, D. (Ed.). (2000). *Handbook of research in pediatric and clinical child psychology: Practical strategies and methods.* New York: Kluwer Academic/Plenum.

Drotar, D., Overholser, J. C., Levi, R., Walders, N., Robinson, J. R., Palermo, T. M., & Riekert, K. A. (2000). Ethical issues in conducting research with pediatric and clinical child populations in applied settings. In D. Drotar (Ed.), *Handbook of research in pediatric and clinical child psychology: Practical strategies and methods* (pp. 305–326). New York: Kluwer Academic/Plenum.

Evans, J. H. (2000). A sociological account of the growth of principalism. *Hastings Center Report, 30,* 31–38.

Fausto-Sterling, A. (2000). *Sexing the body: Gender politics and the construction of sexuality.* New York: Basic Books.

Fischman, M. W. (2000). Informed consent. In B. D. Sales & S. Folkman (Eds.), *Ethics in research with human participants* (pp. 35–48). Washington, DC: American Psychological Association.

Furrow, B. R. (2001). Pain management and provider liability: No more excuses. *Journal of Law, Medicine, and Ethics, 29,* 28–51.

Gaylin, W. (1982). Who speaks for the child? In W. Gaylin & R. Macklin (Eds.), *Who speaks for the child? The problems of proxy consent* (pp. 3–26). New York: Plenum.

Hall, M. A., & Rich, S. S. (2000). Genetic privacy laws and patients' fears of discrimination by health insurers: A view from genetic counselors. *Journal of Law, Medicine, and Ethics, 28,* 245–257.

Hastings Center. (1987). *Guidelines on the termination of life-sustaining treatment and the care of the dying.* Briarcliff Manor, NY: Author.

Hern, H. E., Koening, B. A., Moore, L. J., & Marshall, P. A. (1998). The difference that culture can make in end-of-life decision-making. *Cambridge Quarterly of Healthcare Ethics, 7,* 27–40.

Howe, E. G. (1998). Intersexuality: What should care providers do now? *Journal of Clinical Ethics, 9,* 337–344.

In re Quinlan, 355 A.2d 647 (N.J. 1976).

Intersex Society of North America. (1994). *Recommendations for treatment.* Petaluma, CA: Author.

Johnson, J., & Mitchell, C. (2000). Responding to parental requests to forgo pediatric nutrition and hydration. *Journal of Clinical Ethics, 11,* 128–135.

Joint Commission on Accreditation of Healthcare Organizations. (2001). Patient rights and organizational ethics. In *Hospital accreditation standards* (pp. 69–81). Oakbrook Terrace, IL: Author.

King, N. M. P. (1992). Transparency in neonatal intensive care. *Hastings Center Report, 22,* 18–25.

Kipnis, K., & Diamond, M. (1998). Pediatric ethics and the surgical assignment of sex. *Journal of Clinical Ethics, 9,* 398–410.

Kitchener, K. S. (2000). *Foundations of ethical practice, research, and teaching in psychology.* Mahwah, NJ: Erlbaum.

Koocher, G. P., & Keith-Spiegel, P. C. (1990). *Children, ethics, and the law: Professional issues and cases.* Lincoln, NE: University of Nebraska.

Koocher, G. P., & Keith-Spiegel, P. (1998). *Ethics in psychology: Professional standards and cases* (2nd ed.). New York: Oxford University Press.

Koppelman, L. M., Koppelman, A. E., & Irons, T. G. (1992). Neonatalogists, pediatricians, and the Supreme Court criticize the "Baby Doe" regulations. In A. L. Caplan, R. H. Blank, & J. C. Merrick (Eds.), *Compelled compassion: Government intervention in the treatment of critically ill newborns* (pp. 237–266). Totowa, NJ: Humana Press.

Krener, P. K., & Mancina, R. A. (1994). Informed consent or informed coercion? Decision-making in pediatric psychopharmacology. *Journal of Child and Adolescent Psychopharmacology, 4,* 183–200.

Layon, A. J., D'Amico, R., Caton, D., & Mollet, C. J. (1990). And the patient chose: Medical ethics and the case of the Jehovah's Witness. *Anesthesiology, 73,* 1258–1262.

Levin, B. W., & Schiller, N. G. (1998) Social class and medical decision-making: A neglected topic in bioethics. *Cambridge Quarterly of Healthcare Ethics, 7,* 41–56.

McCabe, M. A. (1996). Involving children and adolescents in medical decision making: Developmental and clinical considerations. *Journal of Pediatric Psychology, 21,* 505–516.

McCormick, R. A. (1976). Experimentation in children: Sharing in sociality. *Hastings Center Reports, 6,* 41–46.

McGee, G. (1997). Parenting in an era of genetics. *Hastings Center Report, 27,* 16–22.

Melton, G. B., Ehrenreich, N. S., & Lyons, P. M., Jr. (2001). Ethical and legal issues in mental health services for children. In C. E. Walker & M. C. Roberts (Eds.), *Handbook of clinical child psychology* (3rd ed., pp. 1074–1093). New York: Wiley.

Miles, S. (1992). Medical futility. *Law, Medicine, and Health Care, 20,* 310–315.

Money, J., & Ehrhardt, A. A. (1972). *Man and woman/boy and girl: The differentiation and dimorphism of gender identity from conception to maturity.* Baltimore, MD: Johns Hopkins University Press.

Nelson, L., Rushton, C. H., Cranford, R. E., Nelson, R. M., Glover, J. J., & Truog, R. D. (1995). Forgoing medically provided nutrition and hydration in pediatric patients. *Journal of Law, Medicine, and Ethics, 23,* 33–46

Orr, R. D., Morton, K. R., & de Leon, D. M. (1996). Evaluation of an ethics consultation service: Patient and family perspective. *American Journal of Medicine, 101,* 135–141.

Parens, E., & Asch, A. (1999). The disabilities critique of prenatal testing. *Hastings Center Report, 29*(5, Special Suppl.), 1–22.

Paris, J. J., Ferranti, J., & Reardon, F. (2001). From the Johns Hopkins baby to Baby Miller: What have we learned from four decades of reflection on neonatal cases? *Journal of Clinical Ethics, 12,* 207–214.

Paris, J. J., & Fletcher, A. B. (1987). Withholding of nutrition and fluids in the hopelessly ill patient. *Clinics in Perinatology, 14,* 367–377.

Patient Self-Determination Act. Omnibus Budget Reconciliation Act of 1990, Pub. L. No. 101–508, §§4206, 4571 (1990).

Pellegrino, E. D. (1993). The metamorphosis of medical ethics: A 30–year retrospective. *Journal of the American Medical Association, 269,* 1158–1162.

Pope, K. S., & Vetter, V. A. (1992). Ethical dilemmas encountered by members of the American Psychological Association: A national survey. *American Psychologist, 47,* 397–411.

Potter, R. L. (1999). On our way to integrated bioethics: Clinical, organizational, communal. *Journal of Clinical Ethics, 10,* 171–177.

President's Commission for the Study of Ethical Problems in Medicine and Biomedical and Behavioral Research. (1983). *Deciding to forgo life-sustaining treatment: Ethical, medical, and legal issues in treatment decisions.* Washington, DC: US Government Printing Office.

Protection of Human Subjects, 45 C. F. R. 46 (2001).

Rae, W. A., & Fournier, C. J. (1986). Ethical issues in pediatric research: Preserving psychosocial care in scientific inquiry. *Children's Health Care, 14,* 242–248.

Rae, W. A., & Sullivan, J. R. (2003). Ethical considerations in clinical psychology research. In M. C. Roberts & S. S. Ilardi (Eds.), *Handbook of research methods in clinical psychology* (pp. 52–77). Malden, MA: Blackwell.

Rae, W. A., Sullivan, J. R., Razo, N. P., George, C. A., & Ramirez, E. (2002). Adolescent health risk behavior: When do pediatric psychologists break confidentiality? *Journal of Pediatric Psychology, 27,* 541–549.

Rae, W. A., & Worchel, F. F. (1991). Ethical beliefs and behaviors of pediatric psychologists: A survey. *Journal of Pediatric Psychology, 16,* 727–745.

Ramer-Chrastek, J., Brunnquell, D., & Hasse, S. (2002). Letting nature take its course. *American Journal of Nursing, 102,* 24CC–24JJ.

Reder, P., & Fitzpatrick, G. (1998). What is sufficient understanding? *Clinical Child Psychology and Psychiatry, 3,* 103–113.

Sabitino, C. P. (1999). Survey of state EMS-DNR laws and protocols. *Journal of Law, Medicine, and Ethics, 27,* 297–315.

Sales, B. D., & Folkman, S. (Eds.). (2000). *Ethics in research with human participants.* Washington, DC: American Psychological Association.

Schneiderman, L. J., Gilmer, T., & Teetzel, H. D. (2000). Impact of ethics consultation in the intensive care setting: A randomized, controlled trial. *Critical Care Medicine, 28,* 3920–3924.

Schneiderman, L. J., Jecker, N. S., & Jonsen, A. R. (1990). Medical futility: Its meaning and ethical implications. *Annals of Internal Medicine, 112,* 949–954.

Shields, J. M., & Johnson, A. (1992). Collision between law and ethics: Consent for treatment with adolescents. *Bulletin of the American Academy of Psychiatry and Law, 20,* 309–323.

Stanley, J. M. (1992). The Appleton International Conference: Developing guidelines for decisions to forgo life prolonging medical treatment. *Journal of Medical Ethics,* 18, 11–23.

Sulmasy, D. P. (2000). Commentary: Double effect-intention is the solution, not the problem. *Journal of Law, Medicine, and Ethics, 28,* 26–29.

Tymchuk, A. J. (1997). Informing for consent: Concepts and methods. *Canadian Psychology, 38,* 55–75.

Watchtower Bible and Tract Society of New York. (1992). *Family care and medical management for Jehovah's Witnesses.* Brooklyn, NY: Author.

Weir, R. F., & Gostin, L. (1990). Decisions to abate life-sustaining treatment for nonautonomous patients: Ethical standards and legal liability for physicians after Cruzan. *Journal of the American Medical Association, 264,* 1846–1853.

White, G. B., & Leuthner, S. R. (2001). Infertility treatments and neonatal care: The ethical obligation to transcend specialty practice in the interest of reducing multiple births. *Journal of Clinical Ethics, 12,* 223–230.

Wolfe, J. (2000). Suffering in children at the end of life: Recognizing an ethical duty to palliate. *Journal of Clinical Ethics, 11,* 157–163.

Yen, B., & Schneiderman, L. (1999). Impact of pediatric ethics consultations on patients, families, social workers, and physicians. *Journal of Perinatology, 19,* 373–378.

Youngner, S. J. (1987). Do-not-resuscitate orders: No longer secret, but still a problem. *Hastings Center Report, 17,* 24–33.

4

Professional Roles and Practice Patterns

DENNIS DROTAR
ANTHONY SPIRITO
TERRY STANCIN

Pediatric psychologists have made extraordinary inroads in developing services and advancing their professional roles over the past 30 years. They now provide services to children, adolescents, and their families in community, primary care, and inpatient hospital settings (Drotar, 1993, 1995; Drotar & Zagorski, 2001, Mullins, Gillman, & Harbeck, 1992; Olson et al., 1988; Schroeder & Mann, 1991). In recent years, the scope of practice, breadth of populations, and advent of managed care have expanded the professional roles of psychologists and changed practice patterns (Roberts & Hurley, 1997). Finally, recent advances in empirically supported treatments in the field of pediatric psychology (Spirito, 1999) have provided a sounder scientific foundation for interventions with a range of populations delivered in multiple settings (Drotar & Lemanek, 2001). To address these issues, this chapter describes current professional roles and practice patterns of psychologists in three settings—primary care, emergency departments, and inpatient settings—and considers relevant implications.

ROLES AND PRACTICE PATTERNS IN OUTPATIENT/PRIMARY CARE

The fact that the majority of child health services are provided in ambulatory care underscores the importance of pediatric psychology services in this context (Perrin, 1999; Stancin, 1999; Wildman & Stancin, in press). Ambulatory pediatric settings differ in *populations* served (rural vs. urban), *function* (community or public health clinics, medical education), *practice type* (private or public), and *scope* (primary vs. subspecialty care). In primary care, pediatricians, family practice physicians, and nurse practitioners provide a broad range of services, such as prevention (i.e., immunization) and early detection of disease, injury prevention, assessment of family health and safety, early identification and preventive interventions with developmental and behavioral problems, and comprehensive care of children with chronic health and developmental conditions (American Academy of Pediatrics [AAP], 1997; American Academy of Pediatrics Committee on Practice and Ambulatory Medicine [AAPCPAM], 2000; Green, 1994).

Pediatric Populations and Relevant Opportunities for Psychologists

The American Academy of Pediatrics Committee on Practice and Ambulatory Medicine (AAPCPAM, 2000) recommends eight preventive pediatric health care visits during the first year of life, three during the second year, and then once yearly until adulthood. In addition, younger children are seen for acute medical care more often than older children. This younger population provides important clinical opportunities for pediatric psychologists, such as monitoring the developmental progress of infants and children, screening for delays and dysfunction, providing follow-up assessments, and participating in prevention and early intervention strategies (Christophersen, 1982; Schroeder, in press).

School-age children in primary care present to pediatric psychologists with school-related problems, disruptive behavior disorders, internalizing conditions, adjustment to stresses, and attention-deficit/hyperactivity disorder (ADHD). Healthy adolescents are seen less frequently than younger children, but they seek services for sensitive concerns, such as reproductive health and sexuality issues (Rosenthal, 1995). Psychological services may be requested to address these issues, along with the more common adolescent mental health concerns such as depression, anxiety, and substance use problems or stress-related somatic complaints such as headaches, abdominal, or other pain concerns.

Identification and Management of Behavioral Problems in Primary Care

Behavior problems have been shown to be common in pediatric primary care settings (e.g., Costello & Shugart, 1992; Sharp, Pantell, Murphy, & Lewis, 1992; Starfield & Borkowf, 1969). Epidemiological studies have shown that between 10 and 20% of school-age children may have a diagnosable psychiatric disorder (Lavigne et al., 1993). Although the pediatrician is in a unique position to identify children's behavioral problems, studies have consistently shown underidentification and underreferral to mental health professionals for further evaluation and treatment (Costello, 1986). These findings have led to improved behavioral screening methods (Stancin & Palermo, 1997) and classification systems of children's behavior that are more oriented toward pediatric practice, such as the *Diagnostic and Statistical Manual for Primary Care (DSM-PC), Child and Adolescent Version* (Wolraich, Felice & Drotar, 1996) and have underscored the need to integrate pediatric and psychological services in primary care. For example, recent guidelines developed by the American Academy of Pediatrics' Committee on Quality Improvement and Subcommittee on ADHD for the assessment and treatment of Attention-Deficit/Hyperactivity Disorder (2000, 2001) highlight the need for pediatricians to conduct a comprehensive evaluation prior to diagnosing ADHD in children and emphasize the importance of integrating services with mental health professionals, including psychologists and other behavioral specialists (AAP, 2001). The fact that many pediatricians do not have the training or expertise to implement these guidelines, let alone have time within the standard 15-minute office visit to do so (Tynan, in press), creates important opportunities for psychologists in assessment and screening (Riekert, Stancin, Palermo, & Drotar, 1999) and in collaborative management of children with conditions such as ADHD (Tynan, Schuman, & Lampert, 1999), including comprehensive, integrated pediatric practice (AAP, 2001).

Psychologist Consultation Roles and Issues in Primary Care Settings

In primary care, pediatric psychology can be practiced at many levels, including consultation, direct clinical services, case management, forensics, and training and collaborating with school and community agencies (Schroeder, in press). In addition, pediatric psychologists who work as consultants in primary care settings are called on to respond to an extraordinary range of clinical problems that are detailed below.

Presenting Problems

Charlop, Parrish, Fenton, and Cataldo (1987) described the referral problems of 100 patients who received outpatient behavioral treatment during a 1-year period. Behavioral noncompliance (16.2%), tantrums (12.8%), and aggression (8.1%) were ranked as the three presenting problem behaviors of greatest concern to parents. Similarly, among Finney, Riley and Cataldo's (1991) analysis of 93 children referred for psychological treatment in a university-based health maintenance organization (HMO), the largest group (56%) were referred for behavioral problems such as aggression, sleep, and mealtime problems. Other frequent referral problems included toileting problems (e.g., enuresis and encopresis, 16%), and somatic problems (e.g., recurrent abdominal pain, headaches, tics, or obesity, 20%).

More recently, Sobel, Roberts, Rayfield, Barnard, and Rapoff (2001) described the most common referral problems in 100 children seen for psychological treatment at two primary care settings as school problems, behavior problems, anger, attention, depression, and temper tantrums. A total of 31 separate reasons for referral were summarized into the following six categories: externalizing problems (45%), internalizing problems (23%), education-related problems (15%), adjustment problems (7%), diagnosis for medical or psychological problems (4%), habit disorders (4%), and medical problems (3%). Taken together, these data consistently underscore the heterogeneity of the referral problems of children in primary pediatric care settings and suggest that psychologists in these settings need to be prepared to function (much as their pediatric counterparts) as generalists who can assess and manage a wide range of problems.

Evaluation of Psychological Services: Effectiveness Studies

Data from available research tend to support the effectiveness of interventions conducted by psychologists in primary care settings but have not as yet demonstrated efficacy in randomized trials (Drotar & Lemanek, 2001). Kanoy and Schroeder (1985) evaluated parental perceptions of the effectiveness of pediatric psychology services in a primary care setting. Between 2 months and 2 years after the original contact, at least 88% of parents rated the service as good in every area of concern except for developmental delays. Parents rated the suggestions concerning socialization and behavioral problems higher than those that were made for developmental problems.

Charlop et al. (1987) assessed the effectiveness of parent-based behavioral management of 100 children who were referred to a pediatric psychology service at a university-based center. Parents generally reported satisfaction with recommendations and improvement in their children's problem behaviors from intervention to termination, with most improvements maintained at a 12–month follow-up.

To address the question of whether outpatient pediatric psychology services reduced the level of pediatric health care utilization, Finney et al. (1991) evaluated a psychological consultation service that involved brief targeted therapy, including behavioral management. At 3–5 months following termination of treatment, the majority of parents (76%) reported that their children's problems were resolved (30%) or improved (40%). One of the most important findings was a significant decrease in the treated group's medical encounters, from a mean of 8.8 visits per person year before treatment to 6.3 visits after treatment. Use of medical services was unchanged during the same time period for a matched comparison group of children from the practice.

Finney, Lemanek, Cataldo, Katz, and Fuqua (1989) demonstrated a similar decrease in utilization of medical care, as well as an improvement of pain-related symptoms, among children with recurrent abdominal pain (N = 16) who received a multicomponent target therapy that included self-monitoring, limited parental attention to symptoms, relaxation training, and school attendance. In a recent evaluation of children contacted six weeks after outpatient treatment was terminated, Sobel et al. (2001) found that 48% (N = 44) of parents reported that their child's behavior was much improved after therapy began, 34% (N = 31) reported their child's behavior was a little better, and 16% (N = 15) reported that their child's behavior stayed the same. From pre- to posttreatment, children demonstrated a significant decrease in symptoms, and parents rated their children as functioning much better at home and at school compared with pretreatment. Finally, parent training in behavior management and child psychosocial skills training have also been shown to be effective and feasible treatment modalities for disruptive disorders, which commonly present in primary care settings (Tynan et al., 1999; Tynan, Chew, & Algermissen, in press).

Program Development and Systems Oriented Consultation in Primary Care Settings

Perhaps the most critical future challenge in primary care is to develop practices that carefully integrate the services of pediatricians and psychologists in order to enhance the professional development of each discipline and promote the quality of patient care. Schroeder's pediatric practice in Chapel Hill, North Carolina, has clearly been a model ahead of its time (Schroeder, 1979; Schroeder, in press; Schroeder, Goolsby, & Stangler, 1974; Schroeder & Mann, 1991). The Chapel Hill Pediatric Psychology Practice is a premier example of a "collaborative care model" in primary care, described as one that integrates biological and psychological domains of child health (Perrin, 1999). One of the first (and perhaps longest thriving) practices, it was initially established in response to growing demand for more developmental and behavioral services in a suburban pediatric practice. At first, services were provided during a biweekly "call-in hour" for general parenting advice, weekly parent groups, brief "come in" (or drop-in) opportunities for more in-depth discussions of child-related concerns, and developmental screening. One of a number of lessons from Schroeder's (in press) experience is the importance of systematic data collection concerning key practice and outcome variables in order to guide the development of the practice. A second important lesson in developing integrated practices in primary care settings involves the need to deal directly with economic issues that affect such practices (Hurley, 1995; Schroeder, in press). For example, Schroeder (in press) has underscored the need to obtain a variety of funding sources in order to provide for the array of services needed. Although fee-for-service is the usual payment arrangement, it may also be important to develop funded collaborations with community or granting agencies to augment or fund low-reimbursement services (Schroeder, in press).

Toward Promotion of a Public Health Pediatric Psychology Agenda in Primary Care

One of the most extraordinary and as yet underanswered questions concerning pediatric psychology services in primary care is how such services can best be used to develop and promote a public health agenda. Based on Schroeder's (in press) experience, successful collaborative experiences concerning individual cases can lead to public health initiatives, such as school or community agency interventions. Examples from the Chapel Hill practice included contracts for community training and expanded services for children who had been sexually abused (Schroeder & Mann, 1991).

To achieve the potential impact of a public health model in primary care, pediatric psychologists need to transcend individual practices to work within broad-based community initiatives to develop prevention-based program models. One such model is the integrated five-level ("Triple P": Positive Parenting Program) system of mental health care developed by Sanders (1999) in Australia, which is very well suited to a primary care practice. This model includes the following components:

1. Education and universal prevention (e.g., television-based promotional series on common child behavioral problems)
2. Brief problem-specific sessions conducted by medical providers in the office setting
3. Parent training series on common problems directed by medical staff over four sessions
4. Parent group sessions for more severe problems, conducted by mental health professionals or medical staff who have received additional training
5. Intensive group or individual interventions by mental health professionals (i.e., traditional mental health services)

The Triple P model, which emphasizes systematic training of medical providers in basic intervention strategies, may also be effective in the United States, where other primary care staff, including nurse practitioners and physician assistants, play key roles in delivering these services, allowing mental health professionals to focus on program development, evaluation, training, and interventions with more severe cases (Tynan, in press).

Future Directions in Research, Training, and Practice in Primary Care

Opportunities for Research and Practice in Preventive Intervention for Behavioral and Developmental Problems

Primary care is based on a longitudinal perspective that begins in infancy. Consequently, pediatric psychologists in these settings have a critical opportunity to provide prevention-focused and early-intervention services that target disruptive disorders and other common health issues. The development and empirical evaluation of such prevention strategies in primary care, along with an emphasis on training in such methods, are important next steps that should shape the direction of the field (Roberts & Brown, in press). In this regard, one interesting and potentially important opportunity for psychologists who work in primary care settings is to develop practice-based research networks to study relevant questions related to research on psychological practice. The Pediatric Research Office Settings (PROS) Network is a model for such work (Kelleher, McInerny, Gardner, Childs, & Wasserman, 2000).

Opportunities for Training Pediatricians

Primary care pediatricians who practice in primary care carry a heavy burden of patient management in that they must respond to multiple tasks involving health supervision, as well as the identification and management of behavioral and developmental problems. Given such demands, it is not surprising that it is difficult for pediatricians to receive sufficient training to help them identify and manage psychosocial and behavioral problems. Consequently, psychologists who work in academic medical settings have important opportunities to assume critical roles in training pediatricians to identify, manage, and refer children with behavioral and developmental problems. Due in no small measure to the influence of psychologists and their colleagues in behavioral and developmental pediatrics, pediatricians are now receiving more training in psychosocial issues (Coury, Berger, Stancin, & Tanner, 1999). Indeed, Yerkey, Stancin, and Wildman (2000) found that at an urban teaching clinic, pediatricians detected behavior problems in school-age children at rates approaching 20%, suggesting that pediatricians, at least in some settings, may be more adept at recognizing behavior problems than they were in the past. But there is still a long way to go in developing and promoting adequate training opportunities for pediatricians to learn to identify and manage behavioral and developmental problems.

Training Opportunities for Psychologists in Primary Care

Given the relevance of primary care to the field of pediatric psychology, it is important that trainees have opportunity for formal, supervised experiences in such settings. One such training model involves pediatric residents at MetroHealth Medical Center in Cleveland and pediatric psychology graduate students from Case Western Reserve University who participate in the resident Continuity Care Clinic (Drotar, 1995). Psychology trainees assigned to a clinic afternoon for the year have the following opportunities: (1) to observe pediatric providers and all aspects of well-child care (e.g., appointments, immunizations, medical procedures, precepting from the attending pediatrician or team psychologist), (2) to participate in team meetings used for case discussion or topical presentations, (3) to provide direct consultation and service under the supervision of the psychologist, and (4) to learn a range of clinical management strategies that are appropriate to the primary care setting. These experiences provide an opportunity for psychology trainees to become familiar with the applications of the DSM-PC in teaching and practice (Drotar, 1999), as well as to participate in research that is relevant to clinical care in the primary care setting (e.g., research on the feasibility and impact of a behavioral screening service; Riekert et al., 1999).

ROLES AND PRACTICE PATTERNS IN EMERGENCY DEPARTMENT SETTINGS

Setting Characteristics and Patient Populations

Emergency department (ED) settings are an integral part of pediatric hospitals, although they have not traditionally been a setting in which pediatric psychologists have been visible. In recent years, such services have continued to expand, and they now provide important opportunities for intervention by mental health professionals, including pediatric psychologists (Horowitz, Kassam-Adams, & Bergstein, 2001). Unfortunately, only about one-fourth of all U.S. hospitals offer any comprehensive mental health services for children (U.S. Consumer Product Safety Commission, 1997). Consequently, even pediatric psychology referral and service patterns in ED settings have not been extensively described.

Presenting Problems

Presenting problems in ED settings include depression and suicidal behavior; acute psychological and psychiatric emergencies, such as psychosis, violent or aggressive behavior, and fire setting; being exposed to violence or experiencing violence; and pediatric medical emergencies, such as traumatic injury or acute illness exacerbations, which have significant psychological sequelae. Peterson, Zhang, Santa-Lucia, King, and Lewis (1996) examined more than 1,400 consecutive consultations to a pediatric psychiatric emergency service composed of psychologists, psychiatrists, and mental health professionals. The most common reasons for consultation were suicidal behavior (47%), followed by oppositional behavior (24%) and physical aggression or threats of violence or homicide (17%). Repeat visits accounted for 330 of the cases, with about half of the repeat visits occurring within 1 month of the original visit. Although the incidence of suicide attempts seen in the ED is difficult to determine precisely, suicidal ideation and suicide attempts are the most common reasons for a psychiatric consultation in the ED. Injuries are also common, although psychological and psychiatric consultations for such violence-related injuries are relatively rare (Centers for Disease Control, 1995).

Kharasch, Yuknek, Vinci, Herbert, and Zuckerman (1997), conducting a 6–month retrospective chart review, found that 3% of the admissions during this time period were for violence-related injuries; most were the result of an interpersonal conflict. In addition, the incidence of pediatric gunshot wounds presenting to EDs increased almost twofold from 1987 to 1993 (Ary, Waldrop, & Harper, 1996).

Psychological Consultation Roles and Issues in ED Settings

The primary role of the psychologist in the ED is to provide consultation to families and health care professionals regarding the mental health needs of their pediatric patients in the ED. Consultation in the ED generally follows a traditional medical model, with a premium on arriving at a disposition as quickly as possible (Drotar, 1995). Irrespective of the specific referral problem, the basic steps in psychological consultation in the ED are as follows: (1) discuss referral questions with ED personnel and solicit their observations; (2) observe the patient and take a history from parent or guardian or other adults accompanying the child; (3) conduct a mental status exam; and (4) make a diagnosis, disposition, and appropriate referral, if necessary (Kalogerakis, 1992). The services provided by psychologists and/or psychiatrists in the ED, who ideally operate as members of a team, can be divided into those involving (1) suicidal behavior; (2) assaultive behavior; and (3) medical crises and/or unintentional injury.

Consultation for Suicidal Behavior

In such a case, which is a very common presenting problem, the primary referral question is whether the adolescent is at risk for continued suicidal behavior following discharge. To accomplish this task, the clinician must evaluate the intent of the suicide attempt, whether or not the adolescent remains suicidal, his or her support network, ability of parents to monitor his or her behavior following discharge, and his or her problem-solving and coping skills. If an outpatient disposition is indicated, the psychologist or psychiatrist in the ED must arrange referral to the outpatient clinician. Referral to a mental health practitioner within 24 hours is the preferred disposition, whenever possible. In addition, the ED psychologist or psychiatrist must also be prepared to arrange for emergency services if the adolescent becomes suicidal prior to receiving outpatient care.

For those adolescents discharged to outpatient care, the base rates for a repeat suicide attempt following discharge from an ED are low (one study documented rates of 2% in the month following discharge and 9% at 3 months after discharge; Spirito et al., 1992). Consequently, predicting which adolescent suicide attempters are at highest risk for repeat attempts 3 months after their attempts is very difficult, particularly if sociodemographic and attempt characteristics are the only available data concerning predictors (Spirito, Lewander, Levy, Kurkjian, & Fritz, 1994). Level of depression at the time of evaluation in the hospital predicted repeat attempts at 3–month follow-up for suicide attempters seen in an ED (Spirito, Valeri, Boergers, & Donaldson, 2003).

In general, studies have demonstrated a very poor rate of adherence to recommendations for psychological treatment in patients who have attempted suicide. These findings need to be considered in disposition planning across a range of settings. For example, Spirito et al. (1992) found that one-third of families who were referred from the ED to a variety of agencies and private practitioners in the community attended fewer than three treatment sessions. Trautman, Stewart, and Morishima (1993) found that among minority female adolescents, suicide attempters dropped out of treatment much more quickly (median number of sessions = 3) than nonsuicidal adolescents.

Consultation for Victims or Witnesses to Assault

Child abuse and violence-related problems are common reasons for psychological consultation in the ED (Fontana & Besharov, 1996) and are managed by well-established child abuse teams (see Deblinger, Heflin, & Fishet, 2000; Gordon & Jaudes, 1996). Adolescents who are assaulted or who witness violence present special problems and are at risk for developing a wide variety of symptoms, including posttraumatic stress disorder (PTSD; Arroyo & Eth, 1995). Unfortunately, in current practice patterns, psychological consultation in the ED for child and adolescent victims who were violently injured following an assault is not common, and these individuals are much less likely to be referred for outpatient services than those who are evaluated for suicidal behavior (Schuchman, Silbernagel, Chesney, & Villarreal, 1996).

The pediatric psychologist who evaluates assault victims needs to assess the child or adolescent's emotional functioning pre- and postassault, to provide psychological support, and to assist the family with discharge planning, which can include changing schools (if the assailant attends school with the victim) and facilitating legal action by attending court appearances (AAP Task Force on Adolescent Assault Victim Needs, 1996). Because psychological symptoms may develop or escalate in the weeks following traumatic violence, psychologists consulting to the ED need to help arrange adequate mental health follow-up for child and adolescent victims of violence and to make contact with the child's primary care physician (PCP) to help ensure that a mental health referral is kept following the ED visit.

In some instances, psychologists and other mental health professionals may also be called on to evaluate adolescents who present in the ED with assaultive behavior that is triggered by alcohol and substance use, agitated depression, environmental factors, and/or a psychotic episode. Finally, in some EDs that routinely encounter children and adolescents who have experienced violence, psychologists may be called on to assist in the development of violence prevention programs that are managed from EDs (e.g., Smith, 1997).

Consultation for Medical Crises and/or Intentional Injury

Psychological interventions for children and adolescents who are treated for medical crises and/or unintentional injury include providing support for children and families during emergency medical treatment, identifying traumatic emotional responses in these children, and educating health care professionals regarding the emotional needs of these patients. Such interventions are best incorporated into a team that treats children in the ED (Cardona, 1994; Williams, 1995).

Psychologists who consult in the ED also have an important opportunity to educate parents and others who care for children on how to identify and assess the emotional reactions and respond to emotional needs of children who have experienced physical trauma (Brunnquell & Kohen, 1991). For example, psychologists can inform parents or guardians about the increased risk for behavioral difficulties (e.g., the signs of potential PTSD that occur after a child experiences a traumatic injury; Basson et al., 1991) so that an appropriate referral for treatment can be made (Aaron, Zaglul, & Emery, 1999; DeVries et al., 1999).

Whenever a child is ill or injured and being treated in the ED, families are under a great deal of stress, are removed from their support systems, and are often asked to make very difficult decisions on short notice. In such circumstances, strong emotions are aroused, and anger at health care professionals is not uncommon. For this reason, an important potential role for psychologists and others, such as social workers in the ED, is to serve as an intermediary who facilitates communication between families and ED staff (Athey, O'Malley, Henderson, & Ball, 1997).

Program or Systems-Oriented Consultation in the ED

Pediatric psychologists and other mental health professionals have an important role in educating health care professionals about the critical psychological issues that are involved in the management of emergencies, as well as about the development of policies involving the aspects of care in this setting (e.g., whether or not parents should be allowed in the treatment room during procedures; Sacchetti, Lichenstein, Carraccio, & Harris, 1996). Psychologists also can educate medical and nursing staff regarding how to best respond to the emotional needs of pediatric patients who require potentially traumatic procedures (Brunnquell & Kohen, 1991; Raikow, 1998; Thomas, 1991) and to individualize the management of families' psychological and psychiatric crises based on their culture and ethnicity (Wright, 1998; Zayas, Evans, Mejia, & Rodriguez, 1997).

Other services in the ED in which psychologists may play a pivotal role include routine screening for mental health problems such as depression (Porter, Fein, & Ginsburg, 1997). For example, psychologists may help ED staff establish procedures for screening and then consult to ED staff when a patient is identified. Psychologists can also be involved in developing bereavement protocols for use in the ED, as well as in direct support to families who are coping with the loss of a child or adolescents who are coping with the loss of a fellow teenage occupant in a fatal car crash (AAP Committee on Pediatric Emergency Medicine, 1994). Finally, psychologists also play an important role in supporting ED staff as they cope with their considerable work-related stressors (Raikow, 1998; Zayas et al., 1997).

Future Directions in Research, Training, and Practice in ED Settings

Teaching Opportunities

Staff education regarding the psychological factors that affect the emotional responses of patients in the ED, such as guilt, preexisting stressors, and family history can facilitate patient care. Moreover, ED staff can benefit from knowledge on the effects of stress, such as that encountered in the ED, on attention and memory and the implications for parents (Grover, Berkowitz, & Lewis, 1994).

Research Opportunities in the ED

The ED provides important opportunities and challenges for conducting research. Basic descriptive research, such as description of the mental health consultation questions typically encountered in the EDs and the mental health needs of these children, is both necessary and feasible. Such record reviews do not typically require obtaining individual consent from patients and families. In fact, expanding the description of the incidence of psychological symptoms following a medical emergency, as well as the effects of psychological distress on care and recovery, is an important research need (Horowitz et al., 2001). Other important future research should address the development of screening tools to identify children who are at elevated risk for continued emotional distress following ED visits for evaluation of medical and psychological crises and the evaluation of brief intervention protocols designed to prevent the emotional sequelae that result from a medical emergency (Horowitz et al., 2001).

Approaching parents to obtain informed consent presents obstacles to more intensive research protocols, including intervention research, owing to the distress experienced by families when being treated in an ED. Nonetheless, the ED is an ideal setting in which to reach populations such as adolescents who are desperately in need of psychological intervention owing to a range of risk factors but who do not have access to other resources (Glynn, Anderson, & Schwartz, 1991). For example, alcohol-positive adolescents seen in the ED for an injury have been shown to have significantly higher alcohol use, alcohol problems, prior alcohol-related injuries, and episodes of driving after drinking and riding with a drinking driver than alcohol-negative adolescents (Spirito et al., 2001).

A compelling reason to conduct interventions in medical settings such as EDs is to capitalize on the "window of opportunity" for behavior changes that is framed by the child's and adolescent's visit to the ED. For example, a brief motivational interview designed to enhance adolescents' recognition of behavioral risk that might result from alcohol use resulted in significantly fewer incidents of drinking and driving, alcohol-related problems, and alcohol-related injuries compared with a standard care group at follow-up (Monti et al., 1999).

ROLES AND PRACTICE PATTERNS IN THE INPATIENT SETTING

The inpatient service remains the cornerstone of pediatric care for children who are hospitalized for intensive medical treatment for a wide range of medical crises due to acute and chronic illnesses. Owing to advances in medical treatment and changes in reimbursement related to managed care, the average length of stay for hospitalized children has been significantly reduced, heightening the need for very rapid medical and/or psychological management in this setting.

Setting Characteristics and Patient Populations

Pediatric inpatient settings include extraordinarily heterogeneous patient populations. Variation in patients seen in different settings reflect the population served by individual hospitals, as well as the structure and availability of psychological services, especially in collaboration with child psychiatry. In a survey of 528 hospitalized children and adolescents, Drotar (1977) identified several common referral problems, including children with presumed developmental delay (*N* = 243), psychological adaptation to chronic disease and handicap (*N* = 104), the role of psychological factors in physical symptoms (*N* = 92), evaluation of behavioral problems (*N* = 48), and management of psychological crises (*N* = 41). In Olson and colleagues' (1988) evaluation (*N* = 740), the largest number of referral problems (*N* = 145) were related to depression and/or suicide attempts. Relatively large numbers of children were also seen for adjustment to chronic illness (*N* = 92), behavioral problems (*N* = 69), psychosomatic problems (*N* = 61), and pain management (*N* = 57).

Carter et al. (2001) recently conducted what is to our knowledge the only controlled study of hospitalized children referred for psychological consultation who were compared with non-referred hospitalized children matched on age, gender, and illness. The diverse reasons for referral included: coping/adjustment (*N* = 30); depression (*N* = 24); anxiety (*N* = 13); acute evaluation (*N* = 12); illness exacerbation (*N* = 12); parental coping (*N* = 12); new diagnosis (*N* = 12); ongoing treatment (*N* = 10); treatment compliance (*N* = 10), acting-out behaviors (*N* = 8); and pain management (*N* = 6). Pediatric inpatients who were referred for consultation demonstrated significantly more behavioral and adjustment difficulties than nonreferred children. On the other hand, a significant proportion (up to 40%) of the nonreferred patients showed levels of distress within the clinical range.

Consultation Process

Psychological consultation for hospitalized children follows a medical model in which the consultant's primary responsibilities involve assessment and communication to the physician about findings and advice concerning management. (See Drotar, 1995, for a comprehensive description.) Some of these consultation requests are straightforward and discrete (e.g., a request to assess the developmental status of a young child with a history of prematurity). Others are much more complex (e.g., a request to determine whether an adolescent with sickle cell anemia is "faking" his pain in order to manipulate the staff). Such complex consultations may require comprehensive, time-consuming assessment procedures, such as multiple interviews with the child and family or repeated behavioral observations (Drotar, 1995).

Communication of findings to hospital staff, which is a critical component of consultation, is accomplished by face-to-face contact and through notes in the medical chart and/or on a consultation sheet. Referring physicians appreciate the following areas of feedback: (1) a brief description of presenting problems, history, and procedures; (2) a brief appraisal of the child's problem; and (3) recommendations for management (Drotar, 1995). In some cases, the consultant's communication of the results of the evaluation will be sufficient to allow the physician to conduct appropriate management. In other cases, the consultation may involve comanagement with the physician to signal the beginning of intensive contact with the child for support and behavioral management during the hospitalization and after the child returns home (Olson et al., 1988).

Program- or Systems-Oriented Consultation

Although a timely, individualized approach is a critical ingredient of psychological consultation in inpatient settings, it does not address the complex, systems-related issues that can influence the staff's appraisals of referral problems and management (Mullins et al., 1992). Consequently, depending on resources, psychologists and other professionals can utilize other methods, such as multidisciplinary case reviews, in working with medical and nursing staff in inpatient settings. Multidisciplinary case reviews and planning for psychosocial services have the following advantages over an individual, more traditional case-centered consultation: (1) comprehensive assessment based on observations from multiple staff, (2) promotion of more effective interdisciplinary problem solving concerning patient care, and (3) opportunity for teaching about psychosocial management issues (Mullins et al., 1992).

Teaching Opportunities in Inpatient Settings

Psychological consultations with hospitalized children provide useful opportunities for psychological training. Psychologists at graduate, intern, or postdoctoral levels can benefit significantly from experience in observing, supervising, or managing inpatient consultations (Rodrigue et al., 1995). These consultations can provide important opportunities for trainees to learn skills in rapid assessment and treatment planning, integrating information from sources (e.g., chart notes, conversation with pediatric and nursing staff, observations and interviews with children and families), and written and oral communication with staff (Drotar, 1995).

In general, the demand for a rapid response and some inpatient consultations limits the potential for certain kinds of teaching (e.g., formal lectures) for both psychologists and pediatric residents. On the other hand, specialized teaching conferences can also be developed to address the management problems that are typically presented by children on different inpatient units (e.g., "live" demonstrations of developmental assessments on a 25–bed acute-care division for infants up to age 2 years; Drotar & Malone, 1982). Moreover, collaborative case reviews also can be a very effective means of coordinating interdisciplinary planning, as well as teaching residents concerning difficult problems (Mullins et al., 1992).

Research Opportunities in Inpatient Settings

Research opportunities with hospitalized children include documentation of the efficacy of interventions that are designed to improve the outcomes of severe problems (e.g., feeding, compliance with medical treatment, chronic pain) in research studies, as well as case studies and reports (Drotar, La Greca, Lemanek, & Kazak, 1995). In one recent example, Palermo and Scher (2001) described the results of an inpatient intervention that successfully improved the functioning of a child who was severely incapacitated by pain.

The need for rapid, objective psychological evaluation of hospitalized children also provides a clinical context in which to develop or extend methods of assessment. An excellent example is the development of the Pediatric Inpatient Behavior Scale, which is suitable for observational assessment of hospitalized children who present with a wide range of clinical problems (Kronenberger, Carter, & Thomas, 1997).

FUTURE CHALLENGES IN DEVELOPING PEDIATRIC PSYCHOLOGICAL SERVICES IN MULTIPLE SETTINGS

The development of the professional roles and careers of psychologists who provide multifaceted services in the range of settings described in this chapter presents a number of significant challenges involving administrative organization of services and programs, proactive planning for service delivery, and research concerning the effectiveness of pediatric psychology services in applied settings (Drotar & Zagorski, 2001).

Administrative Organization of Services and Programs

The development and continued growth of pediatric psychology services in multiple settings raises a great many practical and administrative challenges. Settings vary considerably as a function of resources, collaborators, and level of program development involving services in ambulatory care, inpatient care, or the ED. Nonetheless, it should be recognized that successful administration of multifaceted pediatric psychology programs, as defined by their longevity, growth, and comprehensiveness of educational, research, and clinical care programs in a range of settings (Drotar, 1995), have the following characteristics: (1) multiple funding sources (patient care, research and service, grants, hospital and department) for their programs, (2) energetic leaders who advocate for psychologists and who also collaborate closely with pediatric leadership in program development, and (3) core administration in a division of psychology, along with very close administrative ties to a department of pediatrics (Drotar, 1995; Drotar & Zagorski, 2001).

Proactive Planning for Service Delivery

Psychologists and others who are engaged in service provision in medical settings are continually challenged to develop innovative, cost-effective, and consumer-friendly services in a managed care environment that continues to limit the payment for such services (Drotar & Zagorski, 2001). For this reason, psychologists in pediatric settings need to engage in proactive planning for psychological services in collaboration with departmental faculty and leadership that may include such issues as enhancing community pediatricians' awareness of available psychological and psychiatric services, facilitating family access to psychological services, and improving coordination of care among psychologists and pediatricians.

One new frontier in managing and planning for psychological services in pediatric settings is the need to develop proactive strategies of dialogue and advocacy with managed care companies, including informing companies about the efficacy of psychological services and advocacy for reimbursement (Roberts & Hurley, 1997). To remain competitive in a managed care environment, pediatric psychologists also need to work closely with their hospital administrators and planners at the level of contracting with managed care companies. Consequently, advocacy with managed care companies is also needed to address limits in reimbursement by educating them concerning the efficacy of psychological services (Foxhall, 2001) and encouraging patients' families to advocate with employers who hold managed care contracts to include pediatric psychologists in their health plans (Drotar & Zagorski, 2001).

Research Concerning the Efficacy and Effectiveness of Pediatric Psychology Services in Applied Settings

Pediatric psychologists have developed an extraordinary array of services in a wide range of settings. The continued development of services and professional roles in pediatric psychology in the next millenium will depend on our collective ability to meet a number of significant challenges in service delivery. One of the most important of these is the generation of data concerning the efficacy in randomized controlled trials and effectiveness of clinical services as they are delivered in practice settings (Drotar & Lemanek, 2001). Such information will be critical to planning the pediatric psychological service programs of the future.

REFERENCES

Aaron, J., Zaglul, H., & Emery, R. E. (1999). Posttraumatic stress in children following acute physical injury. *Journal of Pediatric Psychology, 24*, 335–343.

American Academy of Pediatrics. (1997). *Guidelines for health supervision: III*. Elk Grove Village, IL: Author.

American Academy of Pediatrics, Committee on Pediatric Emergency Medicine. (1994). Death of a child in the emergency department. *Pediatrics, 93*, 861–862.

American Academy of Pediatrics, Committee on Practice and Ambulatory Medicine. (2000). Recommendations for preventive pediatric health care. *Pediatrics, 105*, 645.

American Academy of Pediatrics, Committee on Quality Improvement and Subcommittee on Attention-Deficit/Hyperactivity Disorder. (2000). Diagnosis and evaluation of the child with attention-deficit/hyperactivity disorder. *Pediatrics, 105*, 1158–1170.

American Academy of Pediatrics, Subcommittee on Attention-Deficit/Hyperactivity Disorder and Committee on Quality Improvement. (2001). Clinical practice guidelines: Treatment of the school-aged child with attention-deficit/hyperactivity disorder. *Pediatrics, 108*, 1033–1044.

American Academy of Pediatrics Task Force on Adolescent Assault Victim Needs. (1996). Adolescent assault victim needs: A review of issues and a model protocol. *Pediatrics, 98*, 991–1001.

Arroyo, W., & Eth, S. (1995). Assessment following violence-witnessing trauma. In W. Arroyo & S. Eth (Eds.), *Ending the cycle of violence: Community responses to children of battered women* (pp. 27–42). Thousand Oaks, CA: Sage.

Ary, R., Waldrop, R., & Harper, D. (1996). The increasing burden of pediatric firearm injuries in the emergency department. *Pediatric Emergency Care, 12*, 391–393.

Athey, J., O'Malley, P., Henderson, D., & Ball, J. (1997). Emergency medical services for Children: Beyond lights and sirens. *Professional Psychology: Research and Practice, 28*, 464–470.

Basson, M., Guinn, J., McElligott, J., Vitale, R., Brown, W., & Fielding, L. (1991). Behavioral disturbances in children after trauma. *Journal of Trauma, 31*, 1363–1368.

Brunnquell, D., & Kohen, D. (1991). Emotions in pediatric emergencies: What we know, what we can do. *Children's Health Care, 20*, 240–247.

Cardona, L. (1994). Behavioral approaches to pain and anxiety in the pediatric patient. *Child and Adolescent Psychiatric Clinics of North America, 3*, 449–464.

Carter, B. D., Baker, J., Grimes, L., Smith, C., Crabtree, V., & McGraw, K. (2001, April). *A case-controlled study of pediatric consultations in a tertiary care children's hospital setting: Parent-report, self-report and nursing-*

report of psychological symptoms and adjustment. Paper presented at Florida Conference on Child Health Psychology, Gainesville, FL.

Centers for Disease Control. (1995). Fatal and non-fatal suicide attempts among adolescents: Oregon, 1988–1993. *Morbidity and Mortality Weekly Report*, *44*, 312–323.

Charlop, M. H., Parrish, J. M., Fenton, L. R., & Cataldo, M. J. (1987). Evaluation of hospital-based pediatric psychology services. *Journal of Pediatric Psychology*, *12*, 485–503.

Christophersen, E. R. (1982). Incorporating behavioral pediatrics into primary care. *Pediatric Clinics of North America*, *29*, 261–296.

Costello, E. J. (1986). Primary care pediatrics and child psychopathology: A review of diagnostic, treatment, and referral practices. *Pediatrics*, *78*, 1044–1051.

Costello, E. J., & Shugart, M. A. (1992). Above and below the threshold: Severity of psychiatric symptoms and functional impairment in a pediatric sample. *Pediatrics, 90*, 359–368.

Coury, D., Berger, S., Stancin, T., & Tanner, L. (1999). Curricular guidelines for residency training in developmental and behavioral pediatrics. *Journal of Developmental and Behavioral Pediatrics*, *20*, S1–S38.

Deblinger, E., Heflin, A., & Fisher, C. (2000). Child sexual abuse. In F. M. Dattilio & A. Freeman (Eds.), *Cognitive-behavioral strategies in crisis intervention* (2nd ed., pp. 166–195). New York: Guilford Press.

DeVries, A., Kassam-Adams, N., Canaan, A., Sherman Slate, E., Gallagher, P., & Winston, F. K. (1999). Looking beyond the physical injury: Post-traumatic stress disorder in children and parents after pediatric traffic injury. *Pediatrics*, *104*, 1293–1299.

Drotar, D. (1977). Clinical psychological practice in the pediatric hospital. *Professional Psychology*, *8*, 72–80.

Drotar, D. (1993). Influences on collaborative activities among psychologists and physicians: Implications for practice, research, and training. *Journal of Pediatric Psychology*, *18*, 159–172.

Drotar, D. (1995). *Consulting with pediatricians: Psychological perspectives for research and practice*. New York: Plenum Press.

Drotar, D. (1999). *The Diagnostic and Statistical Manual for Primary Care (DSM-PC), Child and Adolescent Version*: What pediatric psychologists need to know. *Journal of Pediatric Psychology*, *24*, 369–380.

Drotar, D., La Greca, A. M., Lemanek, K. L., & Kazak, A. E. (1995). Case reports in pediatric psychology: Uses and guidelines for authors and reviewers. *Journal of Pediatric Psychology*, *20*, 549–565.

Drotar, D., & Lemanek, K. (2001). Steps toward a clinically relevant science of interventions in pediatric settings. *Journal of Pediatric Psychology*, *26*, 385–394.

Drotar, D., & Malone, C. A. (1982). The developmental case conference as a method of teaching pediatricians about child development on an inpatient service. *Clinical Pediatrics*, *19*, 261–262.

Drotar, D., & Zagorski, L. (2001). Providing psychological services in pediatric settings in an era of managed care: Challenges and opportunities. In J. N. Hughes, A. M. La Greca, & J. C. Conoley (Eds.), *Handbook of psychological services for children and adolescents* (pp. 89–104). New York: Oxford University Press.

Finney, J. W., Lemanek, K. L., Cataldo, M. F., Katz, H. P., & Fuqua, R. W. (1989). Pediatric psychology in primary health care: Brief target therapy for recurrent abdominal pain. *Behavior Therapy*, *29*, 283–291.

Finney, J. W., Riley, A. W., & Cataldo, M. F. (1991). Psychology in primary care: Effects of brief targeted therapy on children's medical care utilization. *Journal of Pediatric Psychology*, *16*, 447–461.

Fontana, V., & Besharov, D. (1996). *The maltreated child: The maltreatment syndrome in children: A medical, legal, and social guide* (5th ed.). Springfield, IL: Thomas.

Foxhall, K. (2001). Winning one with Medicare. *American Psychological Association Monitor on Psychology*, *32*, 64–65.

Glynn, T., Anderson, M., & Schwartz, L. (1991). Tobacco-use reduction among high-risk youth: Recommendations of a National Cancer Institute expert advisory panel. *Preventive Medicine*, *20*, 279–291.

Gordon, S., & Jaudes, P. (1996). Sexual abuse evaluations in the emergency department: Is the history reliable? *Child Abuse and Neglect*, *20*, 315–322.

Green, M. (Editor). (1994). *Bright futures: Guidelines for health supervision of infants, children and adolescents*. Arlington VA: National Center for Education in Maternal and Child Health.

Grover, G., Berkowitz, C., & Lewis, R. (1994). Parental recall after a visit to the emergency department. *Clinical Pediatrics*, *33*, 194–201.

Horowitz, L., Kassam-Adams, N., & Bergstein, J. (2001). Mental health aspects of emergency medical services for children: Summary of a consensus conference. *Journal of Pediatric Psychology*, *26*, 491–502.

Hurley, L. K. (1995). Developing a collaborative pediatric psychology practice in a pediatric primary care setting. In D. Drotar (Ed.), *Consulting with pediatricians: Psychological perspectives* (pp. 159–184). New York: Plenum Press.

Kalogerakis, M. (1992). Emergency evaluation of adolescents. *Hospital and Community Psychiatry*, *43*, 617–621.

Kanoy, K. W., & Schroeder, C. S. (1985). Suggestions to parents about common behavior problems in a pediatric primary care office: Five years of follow-up. *Journal of Pediatric Psychology*, *10*, 15–30.

Kelleher, K. J., McInerny, E. K., Gardner, W. P., Childs, G. P., & Wasserman, R.C. (2000). Increasing identification of psychosocial problems. *Pediatrics, 105*, 1313–1321.

Kharasch, S., Yuknek, J., Vinci, R., Herbert, B., & Zuckerman, B. (1997). Violence-related injuries in a pediatric emergency department. *Pediatric Emergency Care, 13*, 95–97.

Kronenberger, W. G., Carter, B. D., & Thomas, D. (1997). Assessment of behavior problems in pediatric inpatient settings: Development of the Pediatric Inpatient Behavior Scale (PIBS). *Children's Health Care, 26*, 211–232.

Lavigne, J. V., Binns, H. J., Christoffel, K. K., Rosenbaum, D., Arend, R., Smith, K,, et al. (1993). Behavioral and emotional problems among preschool children in pediatric primary care: Prevalence and pediatricians' recognition. *Pediatrics, 91*, 649–655.

Monti, P. M., Colby, S. M., Barnett, N. P., Spirito, A., Rohsenow, D. J., Myers, M., Woolard, R., & Lewander, W. (1999). Brief intervention for harm reduction with alcohol positive older adolescents in a hospital emergency department. *Journal of Consulting and Clinical Psychology, 67*, 989–994.

Mullins, L. D., Gillman, J., & Harbeck, C. (1992). Multiple-level interventions in pediatric psychology setting: A behavioral systems perspective. In A. M. La Greca, L. J. Siegel, J. L. Wallander, & C. E. Walker (Eds.), *Stress and coping in child health* (pp. 371–399). New York: Guilford Press.

Olson, R. A., Holden, E. W., Friedman, A., Faust, J., Kenning, M., & Mason, P. J. (1988). Psychological consultation in a children's hospital: An evaluation of services. *Journal of Pediatric Psychology, 13*, 479–492.

Palermo, T. M., & Scher, M. (2001). Treatment of functional impairment in severe somatoform pain disorder. *Journal of Pediatric Psychology, 26*, 429–434.

Perrin, E. C. (1999). The promise of collaborative care. *Journal of Developmental and Behavioral Pediatrics, 20*, 57–62.

Peterson, B., Zhang, H., Santa-Lucia, R., King, R., & Lewis, M. (1996). Risk factors for presenting problems in child psychiatric emergencies. *Journal of the American Academy of Child and Adolescent Psychiatry, 35*, 1162–1173.

Porter, S., Fein, J., & Ginsburg, K. (1997). Depression screening in adolescents with somatic complaints presenting to the emergency department. *Annals of Emergency Medicine, 29*, 141–145.

Raikow, S. (1998). Meeting the emotional needs of the pediatric patient. *Emergency Medical Services, 27*, 28–32.

Riekert, K. A., Stancin, T., Palermo, T. M., & Drotar, D. (1999). A psychological behavioral screening service: Use, feasibility, and impact in a primary care setting. *Journal of Pediatric Psychology, 24*, 405–414.

Roberts, M. C., & Brown, K. J. (in press). Primary care, prevention and pediatric psychology: Challenges and opportunities. In B. W. Wildman & T. Stancin (Eds.), *New directions for research and treatment of pediatric psychosocial problems in primary care*. Westport CT: Greenwood.

Roberts, M. S., & Hurley, L. K. (1997). *Managing managed care*. New York: Plenum Press.

Rodrigue, J. R., Hoffmann, R. G., Rayfield, A., Lescano, C., Kubar, W., Streisand, R., & Banko, C. G. (1995). Evaluating pediatric psychology consultation services in a medical setting: An example. *Journal of Clinical Psychology in Medical Settings, 2*, 89–107.

Rosenthal, S. R. (1995). Consultation in an adolescent medicine clinic. In D. Drotar (Ed.), *Consulting with pediatricians* (pp. 185–194). New York: Plenum Press.

Sacchetti, A., Lichenstein, R., Carraccio, C., & Harris, R. (1996). Family member presence during pediatric emergency department procedures. *Pediatric Emergency Care, 12*, 268–271.

Sanders, M. R. (1999). The Triple P positive parenting program: Towards an empirically validated multilevel parenting and family support strategy for the prevention of behavior and emotional problems in children. *Clinical Child and Family Psychology, 2*, 71–90.

Schroeder, C. S. (1979). Psychologists in a private pediatric practice. *Journal of Pediatric Psychology, 4*, 5–18.

Schroeder, C. S. (in press). Reaching beyond the guild. In B. W. Wildman & T. Stancin (Eds.), *New directions for research and treatment of pediatric psychosocial problems in primary care*. Westport, CT: Greenwood.

Schroeder, C. S., Goolsby, E., & Stangler, S. (1974). Preventive services in a private pediatric practice. *Journal of Clinical Child Psychology, 4*, 32–33.

Schroeder, C. S., & Mann, J. (1991). A model for clinical child practice. In C. S. Schroeder & B. N. Gordon (Eds.), *Assessment and treatment of childhood problems: A clinician's guide* (pp. 375–398). New York: Guilford Press.

Schuchman, M., Silbernagel, K., Chesney, M., & Villarreal, S. (1996). Interventions among adolescents who were violently injured and those who attempted suicide. *Psychiatric Service, 47*, 755–757.

Sharp, L., Pantell, R. H., Murphy, L. O., & Lewis, C. C. (1992). Psychosocial problems during child health supervision visits: Eliciting, then what? *Pediatrics, 89*, 619–623.

Smith, T. (1997). Chicago hospital tries to save money and lives through violence prevention. *Health Care Strategic Management, 15*, 18–20.

Sobel, A. B., Roberts, M. C., Rayfield, A. D., Barnard, M. U., & Rapoff, M. D. (2001). Evaluating outpatient pediatric psychology services in a primary care setting. *Journal of Pediatric Psychology, 26*, 395–405.

Spirito, A. (1999). Introduction to special series on empirically supported treatments in pediatric psychology. *Journal of Pediatric Psychology, 24*, 87–90.

Spirito, A., Barnett, N. P., Lewander, W., Colby, S. M., Rohsenow, D. J., Eaton, C. A., & Monti, P. M. (2002). Risks associated with alcohol-positive status among adolescents in the ED. *Journal of Pediatrics, 139*, 694–699.

Spirito, A., Lewander, W., Levy, S., Kurkjian, J., & Fritz, G. (1994). Emergency department assessment of adolescent suicide attempters: Factors related to short-term follow-up outcome. *Pediatric Emergency Care, 10*, 6–12.

Spirito, A., Plummer, B., Gispert, M., Levy, S., Kurkjian, J., Lewander, W., et al. (1992). Follow-up outcome of adolescent suicide attempters. *American Journal of Orthopsychiatry, 62*, 464–468.

Spirito, A., Valeri, S., Boergers, J., & Donaldson, D. (2003). Predictors of continued suicidal behavior in adolescents following a suicide attempt. *Journal of Clinical Child and Adolescent Psychology, 32*, 284–289.

Stancin, T. (1999). Special issue on pediatric mental health services in primary care settings [Introduction]. *Journal of Pediatric Psychology, 24*, 367–368.

Stancin, T., & Palermo, T. M. (1997). A review of behavioral screening practices in pediatric settings: Do they pass the test? *Journal of Developmental Behavioral Pediatrics, 18*, 183–194.

Starfield, B., & Borkowf, S. (1969). Physicians' recognition of complaints made by parents about their children's health. *Pediatrics, 43*, 168–172.

Thomas, D. (1991). How to deal with children in the emergency department. *Journal of Emergency Nursing, 17*, 49–50.

Trautman, P., Stewart, M., & Morishima, A. (1993). Are adolescent suicide attempters noncompliant with outpatient care? *Journal of the American Academy of Child and Adolescent Psychiatry, 32*, 89–94.

Tynan, W. D. (in press). Interventions in primary care: Psychology privileges for pediatricians. In B. W. Wildman & T. Stancin (Eds.), *New directions for research and treatment of pediatric psychosocial problems in primary care*. Westport, CT: Greenwood.

Tynan, W. D., Chew, C., & Algermissen, M. (in press). Concurrent parent and child therapy groups for externalizing disorders: The rural replication. *Cognitive & Behavioral Practice.*

Tynan, W. D., Schuman, W., & Lampert, N. (1999). Concurrent parent and child therapy groups for externalizing disorders: From the laboratory to the world of managed care. *Cognitive & Behavioral Practice, 6*, 3–9.

U.S. Consumer Product Safety Commission, Division of Hazard and Injury Data Systems. (1997). *Hospital-based pediatric emergency resource survey*. Bethesda, MD: Author.

Wildman, B. W. & Stancin, T. (Eds.). (in press). *New directions for research and treatment of pediatric psychosocial problems in primary care*. Westport, CT: Greenwood.

Williams, C. (1995). Children's understanding of treatment in the A&E department. *British Journal of Nursing, 4*, 385–387.

Wolraich, M. L., Felice, M. E., & Drotar, D. (Eds.). (1996). *The classification of child and adolescent mental diagnoses in primary care: Diagnostic & Statistical Manual for Primary Care (DSM-PC), Child and Adolescent Version*. Elk Grove, IL: American Academy of Pediatrics.

Wright, J. (1998). Effective communication and cultural competencies in emergency care of the adolescent: A curriculum for emerging medical service providers. In *U.S. Department of Health and Human Services, Emergency Medical Services for Children: Abstracts of active projects, 1998–1999* (pp. 15–16). Washington, DC: EMSC National Resource Center

Yerkey, T. M., Stancin T., & Wildman, B. G. (April, 2000). *Identification of maternal distress and child psychosocial problems by primary care pediatricians*. Poster presented at the Millennium Conference of the Great Lakes Society of Pediatric Psychology, Cleveland, OH.

Zayas, L., Evans, M., Mejia, L., & Rodriguez, D. (1997). Cultural-competency training for staff serving Hispanic families with a child psychiatric emergency. *Families in Society, 78*, 405–412.

Part II

CROSS-CUTTING ISSUES IN PEDIATRIC PSYCHOLOGY

5

Health Promotion in Children and Adolescents

An Integration of Psychosocial and Environmental Approaches

DAWN K. WILSON
ALEXANDRA E. EVANS

Clinicians and health care providers are particularly interested in understanding the unique health problems that children and adolescents face. For example, the increasing prevalence of obesity in U.S. children and adolescents is a major health threat to our society. Over the past decade the rate of obesity has increased in youth by 64% (Kumanyika, 2001) and is directly associated with an increased prevalence of Type 2 diabetes, high blood pressure, and high cholesterol (Dietz & Gortmaker, 2001; Solomon & Manson, 1997). Previous research indicates a 50% decline in physical activity in youths between the ages of 6 and 16 years old (Taylor, Beech, & Cummings, 1997) and inadequate fruit and vegetable intake among adolescents (Neumark-Sztainer, Story, Resnick, & Blum, 1998). National studies also indicate a rise in cigarette and drug use (e.g., marijuana, stimulants) in adolescents (Johnston, O'Malley, & Bachman, 1994). Although the national birth rate among girls ages 15–19 years is currently decreasing (Klerman, 2002), youth continue to engage in risky sexual behaviors, and teen pregnancy is still a significant public health problem (Kahn et al., 2000).

Previous research suggests that efforts to improve health habits among children, such as increasing physical activity and healthy dietary habits, can lead to positive health benefits. For example, physical activity and healthy diets in youth have been positively associated with improvements in aerobic fitness, blood lipids, blood pressure, body composition, glucose, and insulin, as well as in psychological variables, such as self-efficacy and outcome expectations (Baranowski et al., 1992; Sallis & Patrick, 1994). Furthermore, increasing evidence suggests that engaging in health-promoting behaviors such as physical activity is associated with a reduction in health-compromising behaviors such as cigarette smoking (Winnail, Valois, McKeown, Saunders, & Pate, 1995).

The purpose of this chapter is to provide an overview of the literature on health promotion among children and adolescents, with a primary emphasis on improving physical activity and dietary intake and decreasing drug use (e.g., cigarette, drug, alcohol use) and unsafe sexual behaviors. An ecological model is provided that illustrates the importance of integrating the child's perspective with environmental influences and public health policy (Bronfenbrenner, 1979, 1992). This approach is consistent with the perspective that health and lifestyle behaviors are multifaceted and dynamic and are developed in a social context through personal, interpersonal, and environmental interactions. In this chapter, we highlight the promotion of positive lifestyle behaviors in youth within the context of an ecological framework.

AN INTEGRATED MODEL OF HEALTH PROMOTION IN YOUTH

Figure 5.1 presents an integrated model for understanding factors that affect health-promoting and health-compromising behaviors in children and adolescents. This integrated model is derived from ecologically based models (Bronfenbrenner, 1979, 1992; McLeroy, Bibeau, Steckler, & Glanz, 1988). Ecological models consider the interactions between individuals and their environments. According to the ecological model, health behavior is affected by intrapersonal, social, cultural, and physical environmental variables. For example, restrictions or bans on cigarette smoking in a public setting restrict smokers' behaviors and change the distribution of smoking over a day and the ways other people, such as children and adolescents, are affected by the smoke. A basic tenet of the ecological perspective and social cognitive theory (SCT) is reciprocal determinism (Bandura 1986, 1989; Glanz, Lewis, & Rimer, 1997), which suggests that behavior and the environment influence each other.

The integrated model in Figure 5.1 emphasizes the need to consider multiple levels of variables. These variables include the child's individual perspective, family and peer influences, school, community, worksite, mass media, and public policy. In this model, child and adolescent health-promoting behaviors are conceptualized as a function of individual and environmental influences. The environmental influences may be divided into proximal and distal contexts. The proximal ones are embedded within the distal ones (Bronfenbrenner, 1979, 1992). Consistent with McLeroy et al. (1988) model, we specify five levels of influence that include: (1) intrapersonal influences (e.g., biological and psychosocial), (2) interpersonal influences (e.g., family, peers), (3) institutional factors (e.g., school, worksites), (4) community factors (e.g., relationship among organizations, institutions, and social networks in a defined area), and (5) public policy (e.g., laws and policies at the local, state, national, and international levels).

The child's perspective (intrapersonal influences) includes cognitive factors such as self-efficacy, self-identity, outcome expectancies, attitudes, intention, and motivation for change. These variables may be age-, gender-, or cultural-dependent. For example, younger children, such as preschoolers, may not have the cognitive capacity to consider outcome expectancies and the relevance to changing health behaviors (Dweck & Leggett, 1988). In contrast, adolescents may be able to process information about outcome expectancies but may not have the intentions or motivation to make desirable changes (Iannotti & Bush, 1993). Thus health care providers must consider the relevance of these cognitive and motivational factors

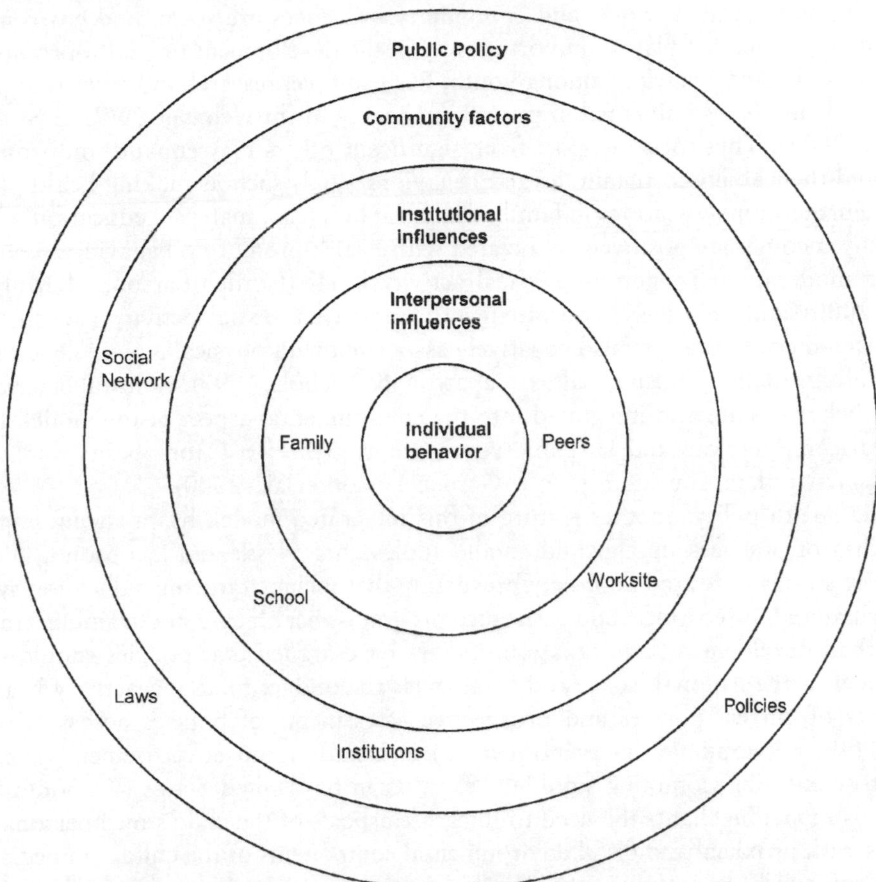

FIGURE 5.1. The model shown in this figure emphasizes the need to consider multiple levels of variables that integrate both psychosocial and environmental variables. These variables include the child's individual perspective, family and peer influences, school, community, worksite, mass media, and public policy. In this model, child and adolescent health-promoting behaviors are conceptualized as a function of individual and environmental influences.

within the context of the child's developmental stage. The child's perspective will also be influenced by the surrounding social and environmental factors.

An increasingly popular approach to youth risk prevention involves the identification of protective factors. Protective factors include positive characteristics, predispositions, and influences in adolescents' lives that can buffer negative influences (Benard, 1991). Examples of protective factors include involvement in structured activities (both in and outside schools), parental boundary setting, religious commitment, and adult mentors (Greene, 1998; Jessor, Van Den Bos, Vanderryn, Costa, & Turbin, 1995). Over time, protective factors help adolescents to become more resilient and to resist negative influences effectively (Benson, Leffert, Scales, & Blythe, 1998; Rak & Patterson, 1996). Previous research (Jessor et al., 1995) indicates an inverse relationship between protective and risk factors in the prediction of problem behavior. Greater numbers of protective factors present in the lives of adolescents predict lower engagement in problem behavior (e.g., violence, drug use, sexual activity).

Family, peers, school, work, and community influences are social and environmental aspects of the model that play an important role in the development of health-promoting or health-compromising behaviors among youth. For example, research indicates that positive family social support is influential in promoting healthy dietary change (Wilson & Ampey-Thornhill, 2001). Thus social support from significant others may enhance individuals' resources and their ability to obtain desired behavioral goals such as making healthy dietary changes. Furthermore, variations in family demographics (e.g., maternal education level, annual family income) are positively associated with health-promoting behaviors such as engaging in moderate and vigorous physical activity levels (Gorden-Larson, McMurray, & Popkin, 2000) and negatively associated with adolescent sexual activity (Lynch, 2001). Neighborhood crime rates are also negatively associated with physical activity levels in children and adults (Sallis, Johnson, Calfas, Caparosa, & Nichols, 1997). Cultural determinants of health behaviors are also integrated into the environmental aspect of the model. For example, African American and Hispanic youth are at greater risk for obesity and are less physically active than Caucasian youth (Gorden-Larson et al., 2000).

Public health policy, another feature of this integrated model, has a strong impact on health behavior practices among children and adolescents. Nestle and Jacobson (2000) outlined policy strategies related to obesity prevention that include targeting education systems, food labeling and advertising, food assistance programs, health care and training, transportation, urban development, and taxation. Others have argued that policies should involve commitment at the national, state, and local levels to conduct food and activity health impact audits of current policies and prospective assessments of policies across all sectors (Lock, 2000). For example, interventions such as taxation and advertisement regulations were instrumental in promoting smoking cessation in the United States (Economos et al., 2001). This model highlights the need to integrate aspects of the child's intrapersonal characteristics with proximal and distal environmental components of the child's immediate and extended surroundings, including the development of public health policies. We argue that this integrated approach to improving health behaviors in youth will be more effective than approaches that focus on simply one aspect of the model.

INDIVIDUAL AND PSYCHOSOCIAL INFLUENCES ON HEALTH BEHAVIORS

During the past decade a number of psychosocial approaches have been implemented as a means for changing health behaviors in youth. These theoretical approaches examine specific aspects of SCT such as self-efficacy theory, behavioral control theory, and outcome expectancy models (Bandura, 1986, 1989; Karoly & Kanfer, 1982). Other theoretical approaches include the transtheoretical model (Prochaska & DiClemente, 1984), the health belief model (Becker, 1974), motivational approaches (Resnicow, Jackson, Wang, Dudley, & Baranowski, 2001; Wilson et al., 2002), and theory of planned behavior (Ajzen & Fishbein, 1980; Fishbein, 1980). We provide a brief review and highlight the need to expand on these theoretical models by incorporating environmental and public health policy.

Social Cognitive Theory–Based Interventions

One of the most utilized models for explaining health promotion behavior change has been Bandura's SCT (1986). The theory assumes that cognitive factors, environmental events, and behavior function as interacting and reciprocal determinants of each other. With respect to cognitive factors, behavioral control is composed of expectancies about outcomes and confidence in personal ability (self-efficacy) to make the desired behavior change. According to Bandura (1986), individuals who adopt challenging goals and are confident (have high self-efficacy) attain their goals more effectively than individuals who have little confidence in their ability to perform the desired behaviors. Thus, if a child feels confident about his or her ability to be physically active, then he or she may be more likely to reach the goal of exercising 30 to 60 minutes a day.

Several intervention studies provide evidence for the role of self-efficacy as a determinant of health behaviors. In these studies, self-efficacy increased as a function of teaching the youth behavioral skills relevant to promoting healthy diets and physical activity. For example, the Child and Adolescent Trial on Cardiovascular Health (CATCH) is one of the largest clinical trials to examine the effects of an SCT intervention on lowering saturated fat, cholesterol, and sodium intake and increasing physical activity in children (Edmundson et al., 1996; Nader et al., 1999). Ninety-six elementary schools were randomized to either an SCT treatment or a control condition. The findings indicated sustained significant effects for improved knowledge, intentions, self-efficacy, dietary behavior, and perceived social reinforcement for healthy food choices 3 years later for children in the elementary schools that had received the intervention. Intermittent effects for self-efficacy were also observed for increasing physical activity. Similar results have also been demonstrated by Parcel, Simons-Morton, O'Hara, Baranowski, and Wilson (1989), who examined the effects of a school-based SCT dietary intervention on changing early adolescents' dietary self-efficacy beliefs. In summary, SCT has been successfully used as a theoretical framework for understanding the relationship between self-efficacy and physical activity; however, the mediational influence of self-efficacy on behavioral change has not been demonstrated.

Motivational Theory–Based Interventions

Motivational theory is an extension of SCT that involves increasing motivation by creating cognitive dissonance (inconsistency between attitudinal beliefs and behavior) and inducing shifts in the self-concept through increasing public commitment (Eitel & Friend, 1999; Leake, Friend, & Wadhwa, 1999). Motivational theory is based on a large body of research on role play and commitment (Lewin, 1958; Schlenker, Dlugolecki & Doherty, 1994), cognitive dissonance theory (Aronson, Fried, & Stone, 1991; Bem, 1972; Brehm & Cohen, 1962), and self-perception theory (Bem, 1972). The underlying premise of this approach is that how individuals present themselves to others has a powerful influence on how they perceive themselves and subsequently behave (Rhodewalt, 1998). Thus individuals who freely choose to commit themselves publicly to a particular identity ("I eat healthy") and a course of action (e.g., eating 6–8 servings of fruit and vegetables a day) should be more likely to do so than individuals who only hold such beliefs privately. Findings from several decades of experimental research have demonstrated that public self-presentation has a strong influence on private self-appraisal that in turn influences behavior (Bem, 1972; Fazio, Zanna, & Cooper, 1977; Schlenker, 1986).

Research has also provided evidence for the contingent role of commitment when implementing motivational theory–based interventions to produce health behavior change (Brehm & Cohen, 1962; Schlenker et al., 1994). Lewin (1958) was the first to demonstrate the importance of commitment and decisional processes in translating motivation into action. For example, Lewin (1958) showed that groups of housewives and students who publicly agreed to change their dietary habits were more likely to do so (immediately and long term) than those who were individually lectured and who made no commitment or decision to change. In a recent study by Wilson et al. (2002), adolescents who were randomized to a motivational + SCT intervention participated either in a strategic self-presentation videotape session in which they discussed their positive coping strategies for increasing fruit and vegetable intake or in a standard SCT session. Although both treatment groups showed greater increases in fruit and vegetable intake from pre- to posttreatment than the control group, only the motivational + SCT intervention group showed that self-concept (r .58, $r = .67$, $p < .05$) and self-efficacy for behavioral skills (r .65, $r = .85$, $p < .05$) were significantly correlated with posttreatment fruit and vegetable intake and change in intake, respectively. Although few studies have been conducted in young children, motivational approaches to changing health behaviors may be promising. These approaches may be developmentally appropriate for adolescents who are trying to gain autonomy and may easily be incorporated into environmental approaches such as school and community settings.

Other theoretical perspectives can be compared and contrasted to motivational theory, specifically with the strategic self-presentation approach. For example, motivational interviewing is another theoretical approach that involves the use of a therapeutic method for assisting individuals to work through their ambivalence about behavior change (Miller & Rollnick, 2002). In contrast to motivational interviewing, the strategic self-presentation approach is a directive approach that engages individuals in presenting themselves within the context of positive change regardless of their ambivalence. Motivational interviewing and strategic self-presentation may appear similar in that both models' ultimate goal is to get the individual to see the importance and relevance of taking on a more positive lifestyle after overcoming barriers.

Transtheoretical Model

The transtheoretical model (Prochaska & DiClemente, 1984) is based on stages of behavioral change, including precontemplation, contemplation, preparation, action, and maintenance. This model proposes that tailoring an intervention to an individual's stage of readiness may be most effective in promoting behavior change. Research indicates that children and adolescents are not capable of staging themselves according to the five different stages (Domel et al., 1996). Instead, for these age groups, two different stages may be more appropriate. In a study by Domel et al. (1996), a measure of stages of change in fruit and vegetable intake was developed among fourth and fifth graders. Principal components analysis from the study indicated that two subscales (precontemplation and beyond precontemplation) accounted for almost 40% of the variance. Students in the "beyond precontemplation" stage had higher levels of self-efficacy and outcome expectancies regarding eating fruit and vegetables. Further research is needed to better understand the role of stage-tailoring health promotion interventions in youth.

Theory of Reasoned Action

Ajzen and Fishbein's (1980) theory of reasoned action has been applied in several studies evaluating health promotion interventions for physical activity in children. The theory focuses on identifying personal intentions as immediate determinants of behavior. Intentions are directly influenced by attitudes and subject norms (social influence about what a person thinks significant others want them to do and the motivation to conform). Attitudes and beliefs about the behavior and consequences of performing a desired behavior are evaluated as either positive or negative in the context of social norms. In a study by Woodward et al. (1996), students (12–15 years old) provided self-report data concerning their perceptions of the qualities of food (enjoyable, healthy) and their descriptive social norms for the food (its usage by parents and friends). The results indicated that liking and parental usage were both strong predictors of food selection and that parental usage was a stronger predictor than friend usage. In the area of health-compromising behaviors, peer influences have been shown to be a factor in cigarette smoking and drug use (Pentz et al., 1989; Sussman, Dent, Stacy, & Sun, 1993). Further research is needed to better understand the role of social norms in child and adolescent health promotion.

Health Belief Model

The health belief model, developed by Becker (1974), suggests that attitudes and beliefs are important determinants of health behavior change. For example, if a student has a positive attitude about eating healthy and exercising, he or she should be more likely to engage in such behaviors. A large literature exists that has evaluated the role of health beliefs in understanding health behaviors; however, the results of these studies show mixed support for the model. In a recent study focusing on youth, Resnicow et al. (1997) found no relationship between health beliefs and students' preferences for healthy food choices. In general, the health belief model has an important heuristic appeal that may not directly translate into health behavior change; thus in recent years fewer researchers have made these factors the focus of their work.

CRITIQUE OF INTERPERSONAL INTERVENTIONS

Some evidence suggests that psychosocial factors have not been associated with change in actual health behaviors. For example, in a recent review of the literature, psychosocial variables demonstrated low predictiveness of dietary fat and fruit and vegetable intake (Baranowski, Cullen, & Baranowski, 1999). However, as these authors point out, only a few studies have examined theoretical mediators of health behavior change in children and adolescents. In another review by Baranowski, Anderson, and Carmack (1998), psychosocial theoretical interventions were found to account for only 30% or less of the variability in physical activity behaviors across both adult and child populations. Thus these authors argue for an approach that takes into consideration a broader environmental context than did past studies.

ENVIRONMENTAL INFLUENCES ON HEALTH BEHAVIORS

Researchers are extending the field of health promotion to include ecological or social-ecological perspectives (McLeroy et al., 1988; Sallis, Bauman, & Pratt, 1998). The following review focuses on the interactions between individual and collective behaviors and the health resources and constraints that exist in specific environmental settings.

Family Environment and Structure

The immediate family environment influences adolescents' behavior significantly. For example, parents' modeling of certain behaviors can influence their children's behavior. Through modeling, family members can encourage or discourage certain lifestyle patterns such as overeating, cigarette smoking, and exercise habits (Patterson, Rupp, Sallis, Atkins, & Nader, 1988; Sallis, Patterson, Buono, Atkins, & Nader, 1988). In addition, research indicates that siblings can have a significant influence on adolescents' sexual behavior (Brooks-Gunn & Furstenberg, 1989).

The structure of families in the United States has changed over the past 40 years. Compared with 1960, more adolescents today live in single-parent households (27%; Bowers, 2000; U.S. Department of Health & Human Services, 2002), and more adolescents live in households in which the mother is employed outside the home (74%; U.S. Department of Health & Human Services, 1999). Consequently, because of this lack of adult supervision, adolescents spend more time with peers. Unsupervised time can also provide more opportunities for adolescents to engage in behaviors of which adults may disapprove. Behaviors such as alcohol and drug use may also be appealing to adolescents because of their desire to achieve maturity and independence at this developmental stage (Perry & Jessor, 1985). A second concern about the increase of unsupervised time available to adolescents is the lessening of quality time that is available for communication and intimacy with parents or other supportive adults. Research indicates that adolescents who feel close to their parents or other adults show more positive psychosocial development, behavioral competence, and psychological well-being (Jessor et al., 1995). Additionally, adolescents with less parental supervision are more susceptible to peer influences. However, this association seems to be mediated by the extent of parental monitoring of and communication about the adolescent's activities during the parent's absence (Kandel, 1973).

In addition to the resulting increase in available unsupervised time, family structure affects adolescents' health behaviors in other ways. For example, in terms of dietary intake, single parents and parents in two-earner households have less time available to prepare meals (Bowers, 2000), which may lead to fewer family meals and an increase in the consumption of snacks (Siega-Riz, Carson, & Popkins, 1998). Family meals are associated with more healthful dietary intake patterns, including more fruits and vegetables, less fried food and soft drinks (Gillman et al., 2000), fewer meals eaten outside the home, and less consumption of convenience and prepared foods. Foods eaten away from home are also higher in energy and fat than foods made at home (Biing-Hwan, Guthrie, & Frazao, 1999), and among single-parent households, adolescents eat more high-energy, high-fat snacks and fewer meals (Siega-Riz et al., 1998). In terms of physical activity, family structure may also mean that parents from single-parent households are less available to provide transportation to locations at which adolescents can be physically active.

Peer Groups and Behavioral Practices

During adolescence, peer bonding with concurrent distancing from the family constitutes a central task (Erickson, 1988). At this time, adolescents spend a significant amount of their free time with peers. During this time, peer norms become very salient, especially to adolescents in the 13- to 14-year age group, in which peak conformity occurs (Berndt, 1979). Because adolescents seek peer approval and social identity, those behaviors found acceptable by their peer group will be the ones they tend to engage in. Peer influence can have both positive and negative effects. Adolescents who associate with peers who smoke and abuse drugs are more likely to smoke and abuse drugs than teens who do not have friends who engage in those behaviors (Mosbach & Leventhal, 1988; Sussman et al., 1990). Peers also influence whether or not adolescents will engage in sexual activity (Brooks-Gunn & Firstenberg, 1989). In contrast, previous research on health-promoting behaviors has shown mixed results. Results from one study indicate that for habitual fat and food intake, parental influence is stronger than peer influence (Feunekes, de Graaf, Meyboom, & van Staveren, 1998).

School Environments

The school environment has significant proximal influences on adolescent health behaviors because the educational system is the main formal community institution that is responsible for the socialization of adolescents. More than 95% of youth ages 5–17 years attend school for approximately 8 hours daily; no other institution has as much continuous and intense contact with children during their first two decades of life (Resnicow, 1993). Consequently, the school environment can have a significant effect on the behaviors of large numbers of adolescents. For example, almost 33% of all adolescent eating occurs outside of the home, and approximately 52% of out-of-home eating takes place in the school setting (Lin, Guthrie, & Frazao, 1999). Foods eaten at school lunch make up 35–40% of students' total daily energy intake (U.S. Department of Health & Human Services, 2002). Thus the accessibility and availability of certain foods at the school cafeteria or from vending machines directly influence the specific foods that adolescents consume. When low-nutritional-density foods are highly available, adolescents will be more likely to purchase and consume these types of foods.

Current evidence suggests that modeling by both peers and teachers may be influential in promoting healthy behavioral practices in youths. Previous research indicates a positive relationship between the numbers of teachers who smoke and adolescent smoking rates (Murray, Kiryluk, & Swan, 1984). In addition, lower rates of student smoking have also been associated with policies that restrict teacher smoking to certain areas (e.g., staff room), thereby precluding direct modeling (Cooreman & Perdrizet, 1980). Similar teacher modeling effects have been demonstrated for dietary change among youths (Cullen et al., 1999).

Worksite Environments

The worksite environment also has significant proximal environmental influences on adolescent health behaviors. Many adolescents spend a significant number of hours at work; more than 75% of high school students will have been employed before high school graduation (Barton, 1989). Working during after-school hours limits the time teens have available to participate in certain behaviors. For example, after-school employment will make it less likely that teens can participate in after-school sport activities. It may also limit the time they have available to engage in health-compromising behaviors, such as smoking, because after-school hours include the time period during which adolescents most frequently engage in unhealthy behaviors. Nearly 60% of those teens who work are employed in restaurants (mainly fast-food restaurants) and retail businesses (Mortimer, Finch, Shanahan, & Ryu, 1992). Because many fast-food establishments have policies that provide their employees with food discounts and free sodas, they directly influence adolescents' food intake. In addition, friends may visit their peers at work and "hang out," which often times coincides with eating unhealthy foods.

Community Factors

Researchers have shown that community resources such as churches, supermarkets, and restaurants can also influence children's and adolescents' eating behaviors. Church-led dietary interventions have been effective, especially among minority populations, because of the important role of the church in providing communication and social networks (Hatch & Lovelace, 1980). Supermarkets are another important community resource that can be instrumental in changing children's and adolescents' food intake. In one study (Mayer, Dubbert, & Elder, 1989), supermarkets used a point-of-choice strategy to influence youths' food choices. Mayer et al. (1989) concluded that many of the foods used in these strategies were of low nutritional value and recommended that supermarkets implement specific nutritional targets to promote healthier food selections among children and adolescents. Based on census tracts, some investigators have reported that the availability of foods in local grocery stores is positively associated with the consumption of foods. For example, Edmonds, Baranowski, Baranowski, Cullen, and Myres (2001) examined whether median family income and the availability of fruit, juice, and vegetables in grocery stores, restaurants, and homes were associated with consumption of these foods in African American Boy Scouts. Results indicated that median household income was significantly correlated with restaurant fruit availability, and significant correlations were demonstrated between restaurant availability and Boy Scout consumption of juice and vegetables. Safety, gang involvement, community norms, availability and accessibility of certain stores and recreation facilities, and police presence are other community factors that influence adolescent's engagement in health-compromising and health-promoting behaviors.

Mass Media Influences

The meanings that are communicated through the mass media may be particularly salient in adolescence, as decisions about adult values and lifestyles are being made and responsibility assumed. Although radio, movies, and magazines all play a major role, the major mass communication system is television. Televisions are present in over 98% of American households (Res, 2000), and two-thirds of children and adolescents ages 8–18 years old have their own televisions in their bedrooms (Roberts, Foehr, Rideont, & Brodie, 1999). Children 8–13 years old watch approximately 3.5 hours of television per day, and adolescents ages 14–18 years old watch almost 3 hours per day (Roberts et al., 1999). Television watching affects adolescents' diet and physical activity directly. Time that could be spent being physically active is replaced by inactivity. Additionally, television has been cited as a contributing factor to unhealthy dietary intake (Hill & Peters, 1998; Jefferey & French, 1998). Exposure to advertising, such as commercials for convenience or fast foods, can influence adolescents' food choices toward high-fat or high-energy foods (DuRant, Baranowski, Johnson, & Thompson, 1994; Jefferey & French, 1998).

Public Policy

The field of health promotion has long endorsed the value of policy interventions. Green and Kreuter (1999) define health promotion as the combination of educational and environmental supports for behaviors and living conditions that are central to healthy lifestyles. Environmental and policy interventions can play a large role in health promotion, such as the enactment of legislation ensuring food safety and wearing seatbelts. However, the study of how policies affect adolescent health behaviors is relatively new, and much more work is needed to conceptualize the relevant policy variables for individual behaviors among this population group. Policies are organizational statements or rules that are meant to influence behavior. They may be explicit or implicit, and their effects may be intentional or unintentional. Policies are considered sociocultural influences because people often create policies to respond to the perceived needs or desires of their constituents (Sallis, Bauman, & Pratt, 1998). Thus policies can affect health behaviors in that they can restrict or encourage certain behaviors. For example, a no-smoking policy at school that prohibits adolescents from smoking during school time may decrease the number of adolescents who smoke or the number of cigarettes they consume on a daily basis. Policies that promote physical activity during school time could increase the number of adolescents who are physically active and the level of physical activity for those who are already active. However, at this time, few efficacy studies have been conducted (French, Story, & Jeffery, 2001; Sallis et al., 1998).

An Example of Integrated Interventions

The CATCH study (Edmundson et al., 1996) is a good example of a multilevel intervention. The CATCH study was designed to reduce young children's (3rd to 5th grade) risk factors for cardiovascular disease by specifically targeting dietary (decreasing fat and sodium intake), physical activity (increasing moderate and vigorous activity), and smoking (abstaining from tobacco use) behaviors. CATCH intervened at the individual, the family, and the institutional levels. CATCH focused on individual behavior change through changes in the school health education and physical education curricula. Behaviors supportive of cardiovascular health were reinforced by features of the school environment. For example, meals with lower fat and sodium content were served in the cafeterias of the intervention schools; moderate and vigorous physical activities were offered through the physical education classes; and school policies supporting these behaviors were put in place. CATCH intervened at the family level by including family members at Family Fun Nights and by implementing home-based curricula focusing on healthier eating and increased physical activity at the intervention schools.

Three-year follow-up results (Nader et al., 1999; Luepker et al., 1996) indicated that CATCH positively affected the school environment and students' eating and physical activity behaviors. After 3 years, the amount of fat and saturated fat in foods served in the intervention schools was decreased significantly compared with the lunches served at the control schools. In addition, compared with the 5th-grade students in the control schools, the students in the intervention schools decreased their fat intake and reported being more physically active. The family component increased students' knowledge and attitudes but did not create additional behavior change (Luepker et al., 1996). CATCH students were followed (without further intervention) and measured again in the 8th grade. Results indicated that the significant difference in fat intake between the students at the intervention schools and the control schools remained (30.6% vs. 31.6%, $p = .01$). Lastly, intervention students maintained significantly higher self-reported daily vigorous activity (Luepker et al., 1996).

Brondino et al.'s (1997) work using multisystemic interventions to treat adolescent substance abuse provides another good example of a multilevel intervention. In one study, 120 youths who were referred by the South Carolina Department of Juvenile Justice and who had been diagnosed with substance abuse and dependence participated in a 5-year intervention program (Pickrel & Henggeler, 1996). The multisystemic intervention program focuses on close evaluation of the cultural context, counselor characteristics, socioecological pressures, social isolation, provision of services that address the juvenile and family needs, and overcoming mistrust of people and systems providing services. The results showed that only 1 of 60 families in the multisystemic condition left treatment prematurely. Similar findings have also been reported by other studies using this approach (Henggeler et al., 1991; Henggeler, Melton, & Smith, 1992).

SUMMARY AND CONCLUSIONS

In this chapter we have proposed a model that integrates both psychosocial and environmental approaches to health promotion in youth. Although many of the psychosocial theoretical approaches have not been shown to mediate the actual change in health behaviors, their use in combination with environmental approaches may be most promising. More comprehensive or environmental approaches that include policy making and coalition building have yet to be tested. Because of the increasing environmental threats to children's health, it will be an ongoing challenge to develop and implement programs that target change at the level of policy. The most effective approach for promoting healthy lifestyle changes in youth may be one that takes into account the multiple levels of factors, including the child's perspective, social, and environmental contexts.

ACKNOWLEDGMENTS

The research projects reported in this chapter were supported by a National Kidney Foundation Grant to the first author and by a GCRC grant (No. M01RR00065) at Virginia Commonwealth University.

REFERENCES

Ajzen, I., & Fishbein, M. (1980). *Understanding attitudes and predicting social behavior.* Englewood Cliffs, NJ: Prentice-Hall.

Aronson, E., Fried, C. B., & Stone, J. (1991). Overcoming denial and increasing the intention to use condoms through the induction of hypocrisy. *American Journal of Public Health, 81,* 1636–1638.

Bandura, A. (1986). *Social foundations of thought and action.* Englewood Cliffs, NJ, Prentice-Hall.

Bandura, A. (1989). Perceived self-efficacy in the exercise of personal agency. *The Psychologist: Bulletin of the British Psychological Society, 10,* 411–424.

Baranowski, T., Anderson, C., & Carmack, C. (1998). Mediating variable framework in physical activity interventions: How are we doing? How might we do better? *American Journal of Preventive Medicine, 15,* 266–297.

Baranowski, T., Bouchard, C., Bar-Or, O., Bricker, T., Heath, G., Kimm, S. Y., et al. (1992). Assessment, prevalence, and cardiovascular benefits of physical activity and fitness in youth. *Medicine and Science in Sports and Exercise, 24*(Suppl.), S237–S247.

Baranowski, T., Cullen, K. W., & Baranowski, J. (1999). Psychosocial correlates of dietary intake: Advancing dietary intervention. *Annual Review of Nutrition, 19,* 17–40.

Barton, P. (1989). *Earning and learning.* Princeton, NJ: Educational Testing Services, National Assessment of Educational Progress.

Becker, M. H. (1974). The health belief model and personal health behavior. *Health Education Monographs, 2,* 324–508.

Bem, D. J. (1972). Self-perception theory. In L. Berkowitz (Ed.), *Advances in experimental social psychology* (Vol. 6, pp. 1–62). New York: Academic Press.

Benson, P. L., Leffert, N., Scales, P. C., & Blythe, D. A. (1998). Beyond the village rhetoric: Creating healthy communities for children and adolescents. *Applied Developmental Science, 2,* 138–159.

Berndt, T. (1979). Developmental changes in conformity to peers and parents. *Developmental Psychology, 15,* 608–616.

Biing-Hwan, L., Guthrie, J., & Frazao, E. (1999). *America's eating habits: Changes and consequences.* Washington, DC: USDA/Economic Research Service.

Bowers, D. (2000). Cooking trends echo changing roles of women. *Food Review, 23*, 23–29.

Brehm, J. W., & Cohen, A. R. (1962). *Explorations on cognitive dissonance*. New York: Wiley.

Brondino, M. J., Henggeler, S. W., Rowland, S. G., Pickrel, S. G., Cunningham, P. B., & Schoenwald, S. K. (1997). Multisystemic therapy and the ethnic minority client: Culturally responsive and clinically effective. In D. K. Wilson, J. R. Rodrigue, & W. C. Taylor (Eds.), *Health-promoting and health-compromising behaviors among minority adolescents* (pp. 229–250). Washington, DC: American Psychological Association.

Bronfenbrenner, U. (1979). *The ecology of human development: Experiments by nature and design*. Cambridge, MA: Harvard University Press.

Bronfenbrenner, U. (1992). Ecological systems theory. In R. Vasta (Ed.), *Six theories of child development* (pp. 187–250). London: Jessica Kingsley.

Brooks-Gunn, J., & Furstenberg, F. (1989). Adolescent sexual behavior. *American Psychologist, 44*, 249–257.

Cooreman, J., & Perdrizet, S. (1980). Smoking in teenagers: Some psychological aspects. *Adolescence, 15*, 581–588.

Cullen, K. W., Baranowski, T., Baranowski, J., Hebert, D., deMoor, C., Hearn, M. D., & Resnicow, K. (1999). Influence of school organization characteristics on the outcomes of a school health promotion program. *Journal of School Health, 69*, 376–380.

Dietz, W. D., & Gortmaker, S. L. (2001). Preventing obesity in children and adolescents. *Annual Review of Public Health, 22*, 337–353.

Domel, S. B., Baranowski, T., Davis, H. C., Thompson, W. O., Leonard, S. B., & Baranowski, J. (1996). A measure of stages of change in fruit and vegetable consumption among fourth- and fifth-grade school children: Reliability and validity. *Journal of the American College of Nutrition, 15*, 56–64.

DuRant, R. H., Baranowski, T., Johnson, M., & Thompson, W. O. (1994). The relationship among television watching, physical activity, and body composition of young children. *Pediatrics, 94*, 449–455.

Dweck, C. S., & Leggett, E. L. (1988). Goals: An approach to motivation and achievement. *Journal of Personality and Social Psychology, 54*, 5–12.

Economos, C., Brownson, R. C., DeAngelis, M. A., Novelli, P., Foerster, S. B., Foreman, C. T., et al. (2001). What lessons have been learned from other attempts to guide social change? *Nutrition Review, 59*, S40–S56.

Edmonds, J., Baranowski, T., Baranowski, J., Cullen, K. W., & Myres, D. (2001). Ecological and socioeconomic correlates of fruit, juice, and vegetable consumption among African-American boys. *Preventive Medicine, 2*, 476–481.

Edmundson, E., Parcel, G. S., Perry, C. L,. Feldman H. A., Smyth, M., Johnson, C. C., et al. (1996). The effects of the child and adolescent trial for cardiovascular health upon psychosocial determinants of diet and physical activity behavior. *Preventive Medicine, 25*, 442–454.

Erickson, J. (1988). Real American children: The challenge for after school programs. *Child and Youth Care Quarterly, 17*, 86–103.

Eitel, P., & Friend, R. (1999). Reducing denial of STD and HIV risk in college students: A comparison of a cognitive and motivational approach. *Annals of Behavioral Medicine, 21*, 12–19.

Fazio, R. H., Zanna, M. P., & Cooper, J. (1977). Dissonance and self-perception: An integrated view of each theory's proper domain of application. *Journal of Experimental Social Psychology, 13*, 464–479.

Feunekes, G., de Graaf, C., Meyboom, S., & van Staveren, W. (1998). Food choice and fat intake of adolescents and adults: Associations of intakes within social networks. *Preventive Medicine, 27*, 645–656.

Fishbein, M. (1980). A theory of reasoned action: Some applications and implications. In H. Howe & M. Page (Eds.), *Nebraska Symposium on Motivation* (pp. 65–116). Lincoln: University of Nebraska Press.

French, S. A., Story, M., & Jeffery, R. W. (2001). Environmental influences on eating and physical activity. *Annual Reviews of Public Health, 22*, 309–335.

Gillman, M., Rifas-Shiman, S., Frazier, L., Rockett, H., Camargo, C. A., Fulce, A., et al. (2000). Family dinner and diet quality among older children and adolescents. *Archives of Family Medicine, 9*, 235–240.

Glanz, K., Lewis, F. M., & Rimer, B. (1997). *Health behavior and health education*. San Francisco: Jossey-Bass.

Gorden-Larson, P., McMurray, R. G., & Popkin, B. M. (2000). Determinants of physical activity and inactivity patterns. *Pediatrics, 105*, 70–83.

Green, L. W., & Kreuter, M. W. (1999). *Health promotion planning: An educational and environmental approach*. Mountain View, CA: Mayfield.

Greene, M. B. (1998). Youth violence in the city: The role of educational interventions. *Health Education and Behavior, 25*, 175–193.

Hatch, J. W., & Lovelace, K. A. (1980). Involving the southern rural church and students of the health professions in health education. *Public Health Reports, 95*, 23–25.

Henggeler, S. W., Borduin, C. M., Melton, G. B., Mann, B. J., Smith, L., Hall, J. A., et. al. (1991). Effects of multisystemic therapy on drug use and abuse in serious juvenile offenders: A progress report from two outcome studies. *Family Dynamics of Addiction Quarterly, 1*, 40–51.

Henggeler, S. W., Melton, G. B., & Smith, L. A. (1992). Family prevention using multisystemic therapy: An effective alternative to incarcerating serious juvenile offenders. *Journal of Counsulting and Clinical Psychology, 60*, 953–961.

Hill, J. O., & Peters, J. C. (1998). Environmental contributions of the obesity epidemic. *Science, 280*, 1371–1374.

Iannotti, R. J., & Bush, P. J. (1993). Toward a developmental theory of compliance. In N. A. Krasnegor, L. Epstein, S. Bennett-Johnson, & S. J. Yaffe (Eds.), *Developemental aspects of health compliance behavior* (pp. 59–76). Hillsdale, NJ: Erlbaum.

Jeffery, R., & French, S. (1998). Epidemic obesity in the United States: Are fast foods and television contributing? *American Journal of Public Health, 88*, 277–280.

Jessor, R., Van Den Bos, J., Vanderryn, J., Costa, F. M., & Turbin, M. S. (1995). Protective factors in adolescent problem behavior: Moderator effects and developmental change. *Developmental Psychology, 31*, 923–933.

Johnston, L. D., O'Malley, P. M., & Bachman, J. G. (1994). *National survey results on drug use from the Monitoring the Future Study, 1975–1993: Secondary school students* (Vol. 1). Rockville, MD: U. S. Department of Health and Human Services.

Kahn, L., Kinchen, S. A., Williams, B. I., Ross, J. G., Lowry, R., Grunbaum, J. A., et al. (2000). Youth Risk Behavior Surveillance, 1999—United States. *Morbidity and Mortality Weekly Report, 48* (SS-7), 1–44.

Kandel, D. B. (1973). Adolescent marijuana use: Roles of parents and peers. *Science, 181*, 1067–1070.

Karoly, P., & Kanfer, F. H. (Eds.) (1982). *Self management and behavior change: From theory to practice*. New York: Pergamon Press.

Klerman, L. V. (2002). Adolescent pregnancy in the United States. *International Journal of Adolescent Medical Health, 14*(2), 91–96.

Kumanyika, S. K. (2001). Minisymposium on obesity: Overview and some strategic considerations. *Annual Review of Public Health, 22*, 293–308.

Leake, R., Friend, R., & Wadhwa, N. (1999). Improving adjustment to chronic illness through strategic self-presentation: An experimental study on a renal dialysis unit. *Health Psychology, 18*, 54–62.

Lewin, K. (1958). Group decision and social change. In E. E. Maccoby, T. M. Newcomb, & E. L. Hartley (Eds.), *Readings in social psychology* (pp. 197–212), New York: Holt.

Lin, B. H., Guthrie, J., & Frazao, E. (1999). *Nutrient contribution of food away from home: America's eating habits: Changes and consequences* (pp. 213–242). Washington, DC: USDA/Economic Research Service.

Lock, K. (2000). Health impact assessment. *British Medical Journal, 320*, 1395–1398.

Luepker, R. V., Perry, C. L., McKinlay, S. M., Nader, P. R., Parcel, G. S., Stone, E. J., et al. (1996). Outcomes of a field trial to improve children's dietary patterns and physical activity: Child and Adolescent Trial for Cardiovascular Health (CATCH). *Journal of the American Medical Association, 257*, 768–776.

Lynch, C. O. (2001). Risk and protective factors associated with adolescent sexual activity. *Adolescent and Family Health, 2*, 99–107.

Mayer, J. A., Dubbert, P. M., & Elder, J. P. (1989). Promoting nutrition at the point of choice: A review. *Health Education Quarterly, 16*, 31–43.

McLeroy, K. R., Bibeau, D., Steckler, A., & Glanz, K. (1988). An ecological perspective on health promotion programs. *Health Education Quarterly, 15*, 351–378.

Miller, W., & Rollnick, S. (2002). *Motivational interviewing: Preparing people to change addictive behavior* (2nd ed.). New York: Guilford Press.

Mortimer, J., Finch, M., Shanahan, M., & Ryu, S. (1992). Adolescent work history and behavioral adjustment. *Journal of Research on Adolescence, 2*, 59–80.

Mosbach, P., & Leventhal, H. (1988). Peer group identification and smoking: Implications for intervention. *Journal of Abnormal Psychology, 97*, 238–245.

Murray, M., Kiryluk, S., & Swan, A. (1984). School characteristics and adolescent smoking: Results from the MRC Derbyshore Smoking Study of 1974–8 and from a follow-up in 1981. *Journal of Epidemiology and Community Health, 38*, 167–172.

Nader, P. R., Stone, E. J., Lytle, L. A., Perry, C. L., Osganian, S. K., Kelder, S., et al. (1999). Three-year maintenance of improved diet and physical activity: The CATCH Cohort. *Archives of Pediatric Adolescent Medicine, 153*, 695–704.

Nestle, M., & Jacobson, M. F. (2000). Halting the obesity epidemic: A public health policy approach. *Public Health Reports, 115*, 12–24.

Neumark-Sztainer, D., Story, M., Resnick, M. D., & Blum, R. W. (1998). Lessons learned about adolescent nutrition from the Minnesota Adolescent Health Survey. *Journal of the American Dietetic Association, 98*, 1449–1456.

Parcel, G. S., Simons-Morton, B., O'Hara, N. M., Baranowski, T., & Wilson, B. (1989). School promotion of healthful diet and physical activity: Impact on learning outcomes and self-reported behavior. *Health Education Quarterly, 16*, 181–199.

Patterson, T., Rupp, J., Sallis, J. F., Atkins, C., & Nader, P. (1988). Aggregation of dietary calories, fats and sodium in Mexican American and Anglo families. *American Journal of Preventive Medicine, 4*, 75–82.

Pentz, M. A., Dwyer, J. H., MacKinnon, D. P., Flay, B. R., Hansen, W. B., Wang, E. Y.. et al. (1989). A multicommunity trial for primary prevention in adolescent drug abuse: Effects on drug prevalence. *Journal of the American Medical Association, 261*, 3259–3266.

Perry, C. L., & Jessor, R. (1985). The concept of health promotion and the prevention of adolescent drug abuse. *Health Education Quarterly, 12*, 169–184.

Pickrel, S. G., & Henggeler, S. W. (1996). Multisystemic therapy for adolescent substance abuse and dependence. *Child and Adolescent Psychiatric Clinics of North America, 5*, 201–211.

Prochaska, J. O., & DiClemente, C. C. (1984). *The transtheoretical approach: Crossing traditional boundaries of change*. Homewood, IL: Dow Jones-Irwin.

Rak, C. F., & Patterson, L. E. (1996). Promoting resilience in at-risk children. *Journal of Counseling and Development, 74*, 368–373.

Res, N. M. (2000). *2000 report on television: The first 50 years*. New York: A.C. Nielsen.

Resnicow, K. (1993). School-based obesity prevention population versus high-risk interventions. *Annals of the New York Academy of Sciences, 7*, 154–166.

Resnicow, K., Davis-Hearn, M., Smith, M., Baranowski, T., Lin, L. S., Baranowski, J., et al. (1997). Social-cognitive predictors of fruit and vegetable intake in children. *Health Psychology, 16*, 272–276.

Resnicow, K., Jackson, A., Wang, T., Dudley, W., & Baranowski, T. (2001). A motivational interviewing intervention to increase fruit and vegetable intake through Black churches: Results of the Eat for Life Trial. *American Journal of Public Health, 9*, 1686–1693.

Rhodewalt, F. (1998). Self-presentation and the phenomenal self: The "carryover effect" revisited. In J. Cooper, J. M. Darley (Eds.), *Attributional processes, person perception, and social interaction: The legacy of Edward E. Jones* (pp. 373–421). Washington, DC: American Psychological Association.

Roberts, D. F., Foehr, U. G., Rideont, V. T., & Brodie, M. (1999). *Kids and media: A Kaiser Family Foundation report*. Menlo Park, CA: J. Kaiser Family Foundation.

Sallis, J. F., & Patrick, K. (1994). Physical activity guidelines for adolescents: Consensus statement. *Pediatric Exercise Science, 6*, 302–314.

Sallis, J. F., Bauman, A., & Pratt, M. (1998). Environmental and policy interventions to promote physical activity. *American Journal of Preventive Medicine, 15*, 379–397.

Sallis, J. F., Johnson, M. F., Calfas, K. J., Caparosa, S., & Nichols, J. F. (1997). Assessing perceived physical environmental variables that may influence physical activity. *Research Quarterly for Exercise and Sport, 68*, 345–351.

Sallis, J. F., Patterson, T., Buono, M., Atkins, C., & Nader, P. (1988). Aggregation of physical activity habits in Mexican American and Anglo families. *Journal of Behavioral Medicine, 11*, 31–41.

Schlenker, B. R. (1986). *Self-identification: Toward an integration of the public and private self*. In R. F. Baumeister (Ed.), *Public self and private self* (pp. 21–62). New York: Springer-Verlag.

Schlenker, B. R., Dlugolecki, D. W, & Doherty, K. (1994). The impact of self-presentations on self-appraisals and behavior: The power of public commitment. *Journal of Personality and Social Psychology, 66*, 20–33.

Siega-Riz, A., Carson, T., & Popkins, B. (1998). Three square meals or mostly snacks: What do teens really eat? A sociodemographic study of meal patterns. *Journal of Adolescent Health, 22*, 29–36.

Solomon, C. G., & Manson, J. E. (1997). Obesity and mortality: A review of the epidemiologic data. *American Journal of Clinical Nutrition, 66*, 1044S–1050S.

Sussman, S., Dent, C., Stacy, A., Burciaaga, C., Raynor, A., Turner, C., et al. (1990). Peer-group association and adolescent tobacco use. *Journal of Abnormal Psychology, 99*, 349–352.

Sussman, S., Dent, C. W., Stacy, A. W, & Sun, P. (1993). Project Towards No Tobacco Use: One-year behavior outcomes. *American Journal of Public Health, 83*, 1245–1250.

Taylor, W. C., Beech, B. M., & Cummings, S. S. (1997). Increasing physical activity levels among youth: A public health challenge. In D. K. Wilson, J. R. Rodrigue, & W. C. Taylor (Eds.), *Health-promoting and health-compromising behaviors among minority adolescents* (pp. 107–128). Washington, DC: American Psychological Association.

U.S. Department of Health and Human Services. (1999). *Child Health USA, 1999*. Rockville, MD, Maternal and Child Health Bureau.

U.S. Department of Health and Human Services. (2002). *America's children: Key national indicators of well-being*. Washington, DC: Author.

Wilson, D. K., & Ampey-Thornhill, G. (2001). Gender differences in social support and dietary compliance in African-American adolescents. *Annals of Behavioral Medicine, 23*, 59–67.

Wilson, D. K., Friend, R., Teasley, N., Green, S., Reeves, L., & Sica, D. A. (2002). Motivational versus social cognitive interventions for promoting fruit and vegetable intake and physical activity in African-American adolescents. *Annals of Behavioral Medicine, 24*, 310–319.

Winnail, S. D., Valois, R. F., McKeown, R. E., Saunders, R. P., & Pate, R. R. (1995). Relationship between physical activity level and cigarette, smokeless tobacco, and marijuana use among public high school adolescents. *Journal of School Health, 65*, 438–442.

Woodward, D. R., Boon, J. A., Cumming, F. J., Ball, P. J., Williams, H. M., & Hornsby, H. (1996). Adolescents' reported usage of selected foods in relation to their perceptions and social norms for those foods. *Appetite, 27*, 109–117.

6

Prevention of Disease and Injury in Pediatric Psychology

MICHAEL C. ROBERTS
KERI J. BROWN
RICHARD E. BOLES
JOANNA O. MASHUNKASHEY
SUNNYE MAYES

At the beginning of each of the past three decades, the United States government has issued a comprehensive report on the status of the nation's health. These *Healthy People* reports present an agenda for the improvement of citizens' health by establishing health objectives for the United States through identifying preventable threats to health and setting up goals for the nation to reduce these threats (*Centers for Disease Control and Prevention, 2000*). In the current report, *Healthy People 2010*, there are two overriding goals: (1) to improve quality of life and increase years of healthy life, and (2) to eliminate health disparities. Focus area chapters within this report provide detail on existing knowledge and outline specific goals for such health threats as physical activity, overweight and obesity, tobacco and substance use, sexual behavior, environmental quality, immunization and access to care, injury and violence, and mental health. Significant portions of such health threats are behaviorally based or preventable through behavioral actions. This observation places the *Healthy People* goals well within the bailiwick of pediatric psychologists, whose field has long recognized the need for health promotion, prevention, and early interventions to improve the health and development of children and adolescents (Roberts, 1986, 1994). Whereas the chapter by Wilson and Evans (Chapter 5, this volume) covers health promotion topics, in the present chapter we examine research and interventions to prevent disease and injury in pediatric populations.

Prevention involves taking action to stop the occurrence of a negative outcome before adverse effects develop. Prevention may also include the early identification of problems and intervening to diminish negative effects. In an historical overview, Caplan (1964) outlined three types of prevention. *Primary prevention* includes actions taken *before* any problems have occurred. *Secondary prevention* is done when problems are considered likely to occur (a person or group is at risk) or in the early stages of a problem or disorder. These actions may include screening, early detection, and treatment. *Tertiary prevention* attempts to reduce impairment resulting from an existing problem or disorder and to avoid development of further difficulties. Frequently conceptualized as prevention-oriented, the essential goal of these interventions is rehabilitative or therapeutic.

More recently, a new terminology has been advanced to conceptualize prevention in the mental health areas of application, but it has relevance to the prevention of physical health threats as well (Greenberg, Domitrovich, & Bumbarger, 2001; Mrazek & Haggerty, 1994). *Universal* prevention refers to preventive interventions applied to everybody, not necessarily only to those who are at risk for development of a disorder. Adding fluoride to the drinking water, removing lead from gasoline and paint, requiring childhood immunizations for school enrollment, and installing air bags in motor vehicles are examples of universal prevention. *Selective* prevention interventions target those who are at higher risk for developing a negative outcome. Installing smoke detectors into older homes and establishing regulations or providing incentives for bicycle or motorcycle helmet use illustrate selective prevention. *Indicated* preventive interventions are those provided to individuals with early signs of problems, and these programs are intended to forestall further development. For example, a program may be designed to identify individuals with risk factors, such as failing in school and consuming alcohol, aiming to prevent the development or severity of a drug abuse problem. As can be seen, the newer terminology parallels the older concepts to some degree.

Other conceptualizations have also been applied to prevention activities. Researchers frequently differentiate between *passive* and *active* prevention. Passive prevention requires no or minimal effort or behavior on an individual's part to gain prevention benefit. For example, passive modalities include air bags and automatic seat belts in cars, firewalls in apartment buildings, improved water and sewage treatment, and fluoride added to drinking water. Thus passive prevention often requires structural changes to environmental elements to build in safety. Active prevention, in contrast, requires an individual to take frequent action to achieve safety benefits each time. Exemplars include buckling into a seat belt each time a person rides in a car, washing hands to remove bacteria, and putting on a helmet every time an individual rides a bicycle. Safety professionals advocate for passive prevention whenever possible in order to overcome the limitations of active prevention models. However, not all situations are amenable to passive or structural approaches, and, for optimal effect, many may require interventions that actively involve behavior change in taking safety action.

In another conceptualization, Roberts, Elkins, and Royal (1984) outlined preventive interventions targeted to (1) the individual child, (2) the environment and institutions in which the child is engaged, and (3) the child's caregivers to change their own and their child's safety. This framework was later elaborated in a matrix that also included (4) tactics for presenting prevention to these targets, (5) methods of reducing injury risk, and (6) contingencies or consequences for engaging in preventive action (Peterson & Mori, 1985; Tremblay & Peterson, 1999). Other psychological models for conceptualizing injury development and prevention have been articulated and reviewed by Roberts, Brown, Boles, and Mashunkashey (2003).

In a frequently cited model, the interdisciplinary approach to prevention and health promotion derives from the integrative traditions of public health. The epidemiological model of considering the host, agent, and environmental vector or vehicle applies to prevention of both diseases and injuries. The *host* refers to the person (child or adult) who is at risk for disease or injury. The *agent* includes the causative force (energy transfer in injuries; germs or virus in disease contagion). The *vector* or *vehicle* involves the elements in the environment that convey or allow the agent to produce negative effects, such as injury or disease. Elaborations on this basic model have been applied to injuries (Haddon, 1972; Rivara & Mueller, 1987; Wilson & Baker, 1987).

These models provide the framework for scientific research. If a scientific approach is taken to understanding the development of and preventively intervening with disease and injury in childhood, then the view of injury and disease as due to chance factors or fate becomes untenable. Scientific investigations into how disease and injury occur demonstrate clearly that these are not "accidents" or chance occurrences that are somehow unpredictable and unavoidable. Prevention to avoid or mitigate the effects of negative conditions can be taken through behavioral and environmental actions. In the following sections, we describe the characteristics of disease and injury separately as health threats to children and adolescents and then present prevention approaches for both.

DISEASE

Since the field's initial inception, pediatric psychologists have been concerned about the medical, developmental, and psychological difficulties faced by children who have contagious diseases or chronic illnesses. Although still a concern today, contagious diseases prevalent in childhood have decreased due to medical advances such as antibiotics and immunizations and therefore are no longer the leading killer of children over the age of 1 year in the United States.

The primary way to prevent the spread of childhood contagious diseases remains regularly scheduled immunizations. Immunizations protect children against major diseases, including polio, measles, mumps, rubella, pertussis, diphtheria, and *hemophilus influenzae* Type B. The decrease in morbidity as a result of immunizations has been remarkable, with reductions of 96% for deaths from pertussis and elimination of polio, measles, and rubella (Centers for Disease Control and Prevention, [CDC], 1999b, 2002). Childhood immunization has also been effective toward the reduction of various diseases (e.g., measles and smallpox), yet many families identified as being at risk remain underimmunized, particularly preschool children. In general, three primary components exist as major barriers: (1) difficulty complying with immunization schedules, (2) access to medical services, and (3) family factors, such as low socioeconomic status.

Ironically, the decrease in incidence of contagious diseases may give parents a false sense of security, and in turn parents may be less vigilant with scheduled immunizations. Continued parental action, however, is necessary to protect children from disease. Only smallpox has been eradicated globally due to immunization efforts; other contagious diseases still claim lives in other parts of the world. It has been estimated that 22% of children in the United States do not receive all of their scheduled vaccinations, with minority children and children from impoverished families being less likely to receive the recommended vaccinations. Decreases in immunization may be due, in part, to unsubstantiated parental fears regarding vaccinations. These parental misperceptions include the belief that varicella (i.e., chicken pox) is a harmless illness; however, in 1999 an average of one child per week died from complications of chicken pox in the United States ("ABCs of Childhood Vaccines," 2002). Another parental concern is the unsubstantiated claim that the MMR vaccine (measles, mumps, rubella) causes autism in children. Current research does not support this link. Because of these types of misconceptions and barriers, several infectious diseases have shown increased prevalence resulting from decreased immunizations. For example, reports of pertussis increased 81% from 1992 to 1993 in the United States, with the communities of Cincinnati and Chicago being particularly affected (CDC, 1993). Pediatric psychologists can play instrumental roles in preventing the spread of contagious diseases by developing empirically supported parental education and implementation of interventions to increase immunizations.

INJURY

Injuries are damages to the physical body of a child, incurring pain and trauma, as well as potential psychological impact for the child and caregivers. Injuries may result from intentional (e.g., violence: assaults, child abuse) or unintentional (e.g., what the public calls "accidents") actions. The codes for the International Classification of Diseases recognize the importance of considering the presumed intent of the commission of injury-producing actions or the omission of injury-preventive actions when presenting the categories of unintentional, homicidal, and suicidal (World Health Organization, 1992). Although some have argued that the distinctions based on intentionality are not useful (Peterson & Gable, 1998), research and preventive intervention programming have predominantly tended to differentiate on this basis. This chapter section is focused on *unintentional* injuries. Nonetheless, the *Healthy People 2010* report combined injury and violence prevention in the same section because the "outcomes and extent of the injury are similar" (CDC, 2000, ch. 15, para. 4), even though the events leading up to the injuries are dissimilar in many ways.

Unintentional injuries are the leading causes of death and disability in children and adolescents from ages 1 to 19 years (Guyer et al., 1999) and represent the single largest threat to the health and well-being of humans (Finney et al., 1993). Each year, approximately one-fourth of all children are brought to medical attention due to an injury (Kogan, Overpeck, & Fingerhut, 1995; Scheidt et al., 1995). Danseco, Miller, and Spicer (2000) estimated that injuries in childhood involved a projected loss of $347 billion annually (including medical costs, future lost wages, and diminished quality of life). Thus unintentional injuries and deaths due to injury significantly affect the lives of children and their families in a multitude of ways. Injuries occur "neither randomly nor capriciously but rather in predictable patterns" (Widome, 1991, p. v). The involvement of behavior places the scientific study of unintentional injuries in childhood well within psychology's purview.

PREVENTION APPROACHES FOR DISEASE AND INJURY

The interaction of human behavior with the environment has the potential of resulting in injury and disease. The prevention approaches are consequently directed at making those interactions safer and healthier. We have categorized these prevention interventions as modifications to the environment (structural changes), modifications in human behavior (behavior change), and legislative regulations. Although made distinctive here, it should be recognized that these two approaches overlap to some degree, and certainly interact and combine to effectively prevent disease and injury.

Environmental Modifications

Environmental changes or structural modifications that either remove potential hazards or separate humans from hazards create safer conditions. Such structural changes range from abating lead paint in housing to mandated crib construction (in which slats are close enough to prevent infant asphyxiation) to legislation requiring that children's sleepwear meet flammability standards. Once implemented, structural changes have been empirically shown to be effective toward the reduction of disease and injury (National Committee for Injury Prevention and Control, 1989).

Lead Exposure

Lead poisoning in children is completely preventable with a decrease in lead exposure. Although lead toxicity has been recognized for several centuries, only within recent decades have countries identified and controlled sources of lead in the environment, such as in the air, water, soil, and food (Silbergeld, 1997). Moreover, the very definition of lead poisoning has evolved to reflect the recognition that neurotoxicity can be linked with even small doses of lead and few observable symptoms. The reduction of lead in gasoline, house paint, and drinking water has been largely effective toward the decline in elevated blood levels in children (Silbergeld, 1997). Unfortunately, with a 5% prevalence rate of lead poisoning remaining across the United States and greater than 5 times that amount within disadvantaged areas, a continued commitment by communities and professionals remains necessarily high to enhance the development of successful preventive interventions for childhood lead toxicity.

Dental Caries

The fluoridation of drinking water is a classic example of a structural change by which childhood dental caries (i.e., tooth decay) has been dramatically reduced (CDC, 1999a). Although other modalities of fluoridation exist (e.g., toothpastes, mouth rinses, and gels), water fluoridation continues to be "the most equitable and cost-effective method of delivering fluoride to all members of most communities, regardless of age, educational attainment, or income level" (CDC, 1999a, p. 939). With fluoridation, the average number of decayed, missing, or filled teeth (DMFT) for children at age 12 years was reduced by 68% (CDC, 1999a). Low socioeconomic status populations are even more benefited by water fluoridation, given that children in such populations often have more limited access to adequate dental care. The proportion of children drinking fluoridated water increased rapidly from the 1940s into the 1970s and is holding steady. Resistance to fluoridation has come from individuals and groups who argue that fluoride is a health hazard (e.g., causing cancer), although no credible evidence presently exists.

Automobile Transportation Injuries

Many examples of structural changes are associated with automobile transportation, including the implementation of daytime running lights to increase visibility to pedestrians and other drivers, strengthening of side door beams in motor vehicles, and equipping automobiles with front-seat air bags (Graham, Corso, Morris, Segui-Gomez, & Weinstein, 1998). In particular, air bags have been empirically shown to reduce deaths among automobile passengers, although recent child deaths in front passenger seats caused a reevaluation of present designs and continued development of "smart" air bag systems that can detect the presence of children (National Highway Traffic Safety Administration [NHTSA], 1999). Additionally, behavior changes have been required, such as placing children in back seats. Other transportation strategies include efforts to "calm" traffic via lowered speed limits within residential areas, directing busy traffic away from neighborhoods, and installing speed bumps (Deal, Gomby, Zippiroli, & Behrman, 2000).

Home Injuries

High rates of childhood injuries in and around the home have illustrated numerous vectors for safety interventions. For instance, Blum and Shield (2000) noted that more than half of toddler drowning deaths occurred at in-ground home swimming pools around which no or inadequate fencing was used. Within the home, medicines and household cleaning products often cause childhood poisoning. Consequently, legislation mandating manufacturers to produce childproof containers for poisons and medications resulted in an effective reduction of previous rates of childhood poisoning (Walton, 1982).

Fire-Related Injuries

Childhood burns have also been reduced using structural changes. Burns as a result of fire to children's clothing are often severe and result in extensive tissue damage and often death. The Flammable Fabrics Act of 1971 was passed to require children's bedtime clothing to be flame retardant (Deal et al., 2000). Thus childhood burns due to flammable sleepwear have been substantially reduced (McLoughlin, Clarke, Stahl, & Crawford, 1977). Similarly, scalding burns have been circumvented when manufacturers produce water heaters that are preset at lower, safe temperatures. Housing codes requiring safer construction, electrical wiring standards, and fire and smoke detectors also have positive effects in reducing fire-related injuries through structural changes.

Modification in Human Behavior

Psychological principles of behavioral change have been recognized as key components in persuading individuals to make environments safer or their behaviors less risky (Roberts, Fanurik, & Layfield, 1987). Past efforts toward injury prevention based on behavioral change have relied on education as a possible strategy. Primarily, it was thought that families would alter their behavior based on provided information that detailed how to prevent common injuries. Unfortunately, linking increased injury prevention knowledge to behavioral changes has not been very successful (Deal et al., 2000).

Community Information Campaigns

Project Burn Prevention is one example of a community-based program designed to specifically reduce burn injuries using public education (McLoughlin, Vince, Lee, & Crawford, 1982). The program was based on three components: (1) media promotion, (2) community-initiated interventions, and (3) school-initiated interventions (MacKay & Rothman 1982). The program, however, showed no significant effect on burn prevention knowledge. Furthermore, the program showed no overall reduction of incidence or severity of burn-related injuries. In contrast, a notably successful combination of a structural and educational program designed to reduce residential fire-related injuries was the Oklahoma City Smoke Alarm Project (Mallonee, 2000). The chief program component was the distribution of smoke alarms to an area within the city known for high rates of fire injuries and deaths. The educational material provided families with knowledge of typical fire causes, how to make emergency calls, installing and maintaining smoke alarms, and escaping fires. Over a 6-year period following the study, the targeted population showed an 81% decrease in fire-related rates of injury compared with only 7% of the rest of the city population.

Successful behavior change was found by DiGuiseppi, Rivara, Koepsell, and Polissar (1989) when a community-wide campaign in Seattle was instituted to raise childhood rates of bicycle helmet use. Specifically, the campaign employed public service announcements, stickers, brochures, electronic and print media articles, motivational activities, and coupons for helmets. Across a 5-year period, helmet use increased significantly, due in part to the intensive and comprehensive nature of the behavior change program.

Physician Counseling

Health care providers have multiple opportunities to employ interventions with families in order to promote the prevention of disease and injury. Such individual-level tactics can be delivered within clinics, emergency rooms, hospitals, or physicians' offices (DiGuiseppi & Roberts, 2000). Recently, a systematic review of 22 randomized controlled trials investigated: (1) the effects of child-based prevention interventions delivered in a clinic on safety behaviors and (2) the effects of these interventions on injuries. Measured outcomes included motor vehicle restraint use, bicycle helmet use, safe water temperatures, smoke alarm possession, and various behaviors designed to childproof the home. Known causes of unintentional injuries, such as firearms, drowning, car–pedestrian collisions, and motorcycles, and their interventions were not included in the review due to a lack of relevant trials. In general, clinical setting interventions, which emphasized reinforcement or resources, were significantly effective toward increasing motor vehicle restraint use, although long-term effects were limited. Interventions that utilized education alone revealed only modest effects toward restraint use and no increase of bicycle helmet ownership and use or effect on injury rates after individual counseling.

In contrast, when families were counseled, not only were they more likely to assess and lower their water temperature, but they also increased their smoke alarm ownership by nearly twofold. The effects of physician counseling on childproofing homes (e.g., against burns, smoke inhalation, drowning, cuts, falls, poisoning, suffocation, and choking) revealed very small effects toward home-based safety practices. There are also physician-related barriers within injury prevention counseling. For instance, a recent survey of 160 physicians in pediatric training showed that, although most physicians felt that discussing injury prevention during family visits was important, they also felt that they had more important agenda items, lacked time, or simply did not think to bring up the topic (Cohen & Runyan, 1999).

The Injury Prevention Project (TIPP) was initiated by the American Academy of Pediatrics (AAP) in 1983 to provide parents with information on how to keep their children safe. This program is implemented by pediatricians and other physicians who provide parents of infants through 12-year-olds with education on how to prevent the occurrence of unintentional injuries. Although various research projects have reported results of differing effectiveness, reviews have concluded that injury prevention counseling can be cost-effective (Bass et al., 1993; Miller & Galbraith, 1995). Gielen and colleagues (2001) found that the effectiveness of this program can be enhanced when it is paired with additional safety and counseling instruction. Families involved in the program reported greater levels of satisfaction when the additional instruction was given.

Rewards and Incentive Programs

Interventions designed to reward parents and children for decreasing risky behavior have been shown to have positive effects. For instance, Roberts and Fanurik (1986) utilized rewards contingent on children's use of seat belts when arriving at school. When all passengers arrived each morning at school wearing seat belts properly, various prizes were awarded that included stickers, coloring books, and bumper stickers. A significant increase in seat belt use occurred—from 18% to 63%—in the participating schools. Roberts, Fanurik, and Wilson (1988) later implemented a community-wide intervention with 25 elementary schools. Both adult and child seat belt use increased significantly. Children colored winning posters, which were featured on nightly news broadcasts, along with other novel rewards. (See summary by Roberts, Layfield, and Fanurik, 1992.)

A playground safety program developed by Heck, Collins, and Peterson (2001) rewarded lower-grade elementary school children for safe playground behavior. Specifically, children were taught safe and unsafe play on climbing apparatus and slides during a 5-day intervention that used large photos of safe and unsafe behavior and class discussions. When the class as a whole decreased risky slide and climbing behavior, each individual student received a small reward. Using a multiple baseline design with more than 300 children, these researchers found a decrease in unsafe behaviors on the slide for the kindergarten, second-, and third-grade classes after the skills training. Insignificant reductions in unsafe play behavior for the slide (first grade) and climber (all grades) were attributed to low-base-rate risk behaviors.

Individual/Small Group Training for Skills Building

Individual and group skill building is another behavior change method implemented by pediatric psychologists to reduce the incidence of injuries in children and adolescents. Jones and McDonald (1986) developed a prevention model to guide these skill-building interventions. This model outlined the following steps in designing a successful program: (1) identify the area of need for intervention, (2) determine and validate skills to be taught, (3) determine how, when, and by whom these skills will be taught, and (4) decide to what extent the community will be involved. These steps are exemplified by training programs to improve safety behaviors.

Jones and Kazdin (1980) developed a primary prevention program to train children to respond appropriately to fire emergencies at home. In this school-based intervention, children were taught proper evacuation procedures in a simulated bedroom. The program included the behavioral techniques of shaping, feedback, modeling, and reinforcement of appropriate evacuation behaviors. The results showed that the behavioral intervention was effective in teaching preschoolers the skills necessary to make emergency phone calls. Other studies have found that behavioral interventions have also been effective in teaching young children to discriminate between nonemergency and emergency situations (Jones & Kazdin, 1980; Rosenbaum, Creedon, & Drabman, 1981)

Peterson developed a program for latchkey children to increase their safety skills while home alone (e.g., Peterson, 1984a, 1984b). The Safe at Home program included modeling, external reinforcement (verbal praise, small incentives), group discussions, rehearsal, and successive approximations. It focused on teaching children safety behaviors in nine modules, including what to do when confronted with an emergency (e.g., fire), stranger confrontation, bicycle and pedestrian safety, and general daily activities at home (e.g., selecting safe things to do). Compared with a control group, the trained children demonstrated significantly more home-safety knowledge. This series of studies also identified ineffective means of increasing safety knowledge, including self-help texts and 1-day workshops, and the limitations associated with having a parent who is unmotivated to participate fully in the program.

Another home-safety program was developed to enhance parenting skills in parents who have been referred by the courts for alleged abuse and neglect. Project SafeCare is an ecobehavioral and multicomponent treatment package for children under 5 and their families and includes family training in the health and physical care of the child, injury prevention and home safety, and parent–child bonding. This 15-week program proved to be effective in decreasing the number of home hazards and maintained reductions over time (see Lutzker & Bigelow, 2002, for a complete program description).

Another area of concentration for skill-building instruction for behavior change is the prevention of child sexual abuse. The majority of the many programs implemented in the United States target elementary-school-age children in an effort to decrease their vulnerability to sexual abuse. These programs use a variety of formats (e.g., role playing, videos) to teach children the following skills: recognizing and exiting situations that are potentially abusive, saying no, and telling a trusted adult about abuse (and to keep telling until someone believes the child). Interactive teaching techniques have reportedly been most effective in gaining skills. Wurtele, Marrs, and Miller-Perrin (1987) indicated that modeling, role playing, and behavioral rehearsal were most useful. Skill building may also lead to disclosure of current abuse and contribute to halting ongoing abuse (Finkelhor & Daro, 1997). Although many programs report increased knowledge gain, it is more difficult to determine whether this knowledge translates into greater safety for those program participants and whether the programs decrease overall rates of child sexual abuse. Overall, there is no direct evidence that sexual abuse education decreases the incidence of child abuse. Renk, Liljequist, Bosco, and Phares (2002) argued that

> Placing the burden of preventing abuse squarely on the children, who should have only to worry about growing and learning, has not been effective in reducing rates of sexual abuse. Although these types of interventions may help potential victims lower their risk of victimization, they should be supplemented with interventions focused on potential perpetrators as it is these individuals who are truly responsible for sexual abuse. (p. 70)

Another targeted group for skills training is adolescent drivers. Improving teenage driving skills and safety through driver education programs is the primary intervention approach. The basic tenet of driver education is to teach teenagers responsible and defensive driving tactics in both classroom and vehicle settings. A comprehensive program might cover vehicle control skills, environmental factors, driver impairments, emergency situations, and personal readiness. Evaluation of these programs often found no differences in the mean number of crashes or driver convictions. Although driver's education alone does not provide solid evidence of its efficacy, it may be more effective combined with graduated driver licensing regulations. In addition to the basic elements of driver's education, the program typically includes a three-level licensure system. In Michigan, for example, inexperienced drivers are limited to low-risk situations (e.g., only daytime driving) and must "clock" a sufficient number of hours before moving to more advanced driving situations. A comprehensive evaluation of the Michigan program found a 25% reduction of crash involvement for 16-year-olds between 1996 and 1999 (Shope, Molnar, Elliott, & Waller, 2001).

Comprehensive Combined Community Programs

Numerous community-based initiatives as behavior change strategies have been implemented to prevent children and adolescents from sustaining injuries and developing illnesses. These interventions have met with varying levels of success. For example, the Safe Kids/Healthy Neighborhoods injury prevention program was implemented in central Harlem in New York (Davidson et al., 1994). This program involved renovating playgrounds, implementing organized activities for youth, informing children about injury and violence prevention, and providing safety equipment (e.g., bicycle helmets) at reduced costs. Surveillance of injuries and deaths that occurred to children in this area determined that the program decreased the number of injuries to children and adolescents in the targeted age group (5–16 years old) from the targeted injury causes (traffic accidents, assaults, firearms, and outdoor falls; Davidson et al., 1994).

Another program in New York, "Children Can't Fly," was a community initiative aimed at preventing the death or injury of young children due to falling from windows (Spiegel & Lindaman, 1977). This program provided education on the prevention of falls from windows and provided families with installed window guards. Concurrently, legislation was passed to hold landlords accountable for equipping windows with proper safety guards. This program reduced the number of children's deaths caused by window falls by 35%.

Other community initiatives have been less effective. Drug Abuse Resistance Education (D.A.R.E.) is the most widely implemented community-based prevention program in the United States. Lynam and colleagues (1999) evaluated the long-term effectiveness of the D.A.R.E. program 10 years after its initial presentation to the children. They found that there was no relationship between D.A.R.E. education and behavior or attitudes regarding the use of cigarettes, alcohol, marijuana, and illicit drug use. These findings are consistent with other evaluations of the D.A.R.E. program (e.g., Clayton, Cattarello, & Johnstone, 1996) that found few, if any, beneficial results of this intervention. These results underscore the need for continuing evaluations of community intervention programs, as well as for the revision or elimination of ineffective programs.

Violence prevention programs conducted in the schools are another comprehensive intervention for changing behavior that many communities are implementing to promote the health of their children. For example, Grossman et al. (1997) conducted an evaluation of an intervention called Second Step: A Violence Prevention Curriculum, designed to teach second and third graders social skills through the use of role playing, discussion, and group activities. Results from the evaluation found no differences in parent- and teacher-reported violence-related behavior between the control and intervention schools. However, observers rated the children's behavior as significantly less aggressive and more prosocial after the intervention. These changes were maintained 6 months following the intervention. Another community intervention, the Piscataway Project, was designed to decrease violent and aggressive behavior and to increase social competence and interethnic contact in children from fourth to sixth grade (Hunter, Elias, & Norris, 2001). The evaluation of this project indicated that some benefits were achieved on measures of social competence and violent and aggressive behaviors; however, these effects were not maintained over time.

Several community interventions have been implemented with the goal of increasing immunization compliance. Stille, Christison-Lagay, Bernstein, and Dworkin (2001) found that an educational intervention presented at a child's first well-care visit and rewards given at subsequent visits improved immunization rates. Infants whose parents were given this intervention, compared with infants whose parents received routine information, did not have greater 7-month immunization rates but did miss fewer of their appointments. In another intervention for immunization compliance, Dini, Linkins, and Sigafoos (2000) found that children whose families received any of the interventions were 21% more likely to have completed the immunizations by the time the child was 24 months of age than were children in the control group. These results demonstrate that even relatively inexpensive interventions, such as telephone reminders, can have a beneficial effect on children's health.

Legislative Interventions

Legislative interventions have been implemented in an effort to reduce the amount of childhood injuries, often with success in promoting desired safety behaviors. Legislation may be aimed at creating or compelling environmental changes or behavioral changes, thus overlapping with the other approaches. There are many other legislative acts that have affected injury prevention efforts, such as immunization, seat belt use, water safety, and prevention of sexual abuse. Of course, legislative interventions for safety may be only as effective as the enforcement of these regulations.

Immunizations

Although child immunization rates have improved, fewer numbers of immunizations are being given to children under 2 years of age (Centers for Disease Control and Prevention, 1999b). Immunization rates increased dramatically in school-age children, most likely because of immunization requirements for school entry. Although laws differ from state to state regarding the immunization requirements for children before beginning school, the majority of states require a minimum of doses of vaccines for tetanus, diphtheria, polio, measles, mumps, and rubella ("Is Your Child," n.d.).

Transportation

Automobile collisions are one of the leading causes of childhood mortality. Children are at higher risk of injury in automobiles than are adults and are less able to take safety precautions for themselves. Many of the childhood injuries and deaths that result from motor vehicle crashes could be prevented with the proper use of child safety seats. One of the main problems with increasing the use of child safety seats is motivating parents to use them (Faber, 1986). However, with implementation of child restraint laws, beginning with Tennessee in 1978, there has been an increase in the use of safety seats for children. By 1985, all states had passed similar laws regarding child safety seat use in automobiles. The laws and enforcement thereof vary in each state, but they usually apply to children from birth through age 4 (Faber, 1986). Faber (1986) reported that from 1978 to 1983 the number of child deaths in Tennessee decreased by 50%. Additionally, California reported a 35% reduction in injuries, and Michigan announced a 25% decrease after implementation of child restraint laws.

Consumer Product Safety Commission

The U.S. Consumer Product Safety Commission (CPSC) was established in 1972 at the federal level to improve safety in manufactured goods marketed to the public. The CPSC is authorized to "ban hazardous consumer products, to initiate recalls for products which pose imminent or substantial hazards to the public, and to establish mandatory performance standards and warning and instruction requirements for consumer products" (Christoffel & Christoffel, 1989, p. 336). According to data collected by the CPSC, children suffer from a significant number of fireworks-related injuries (CPSC, 1999a). A large number of fireworks regulations overseen by the CPSC have decreased the amount of fireworks-related injuries. The CPSC (1999b) mandated a safety standard for all bicycle helmets sold in the United States. A number of legislative acts are enforced by this agency, with considerable evidence of their effectiveness in reducing childhood injury (e.g., the Poison Prevention Packaging Act of 1970; the Flammable Fabric Act of 1967; the Refrigerator Safety Act of 1982). However, the CPSC has relatively limited powers and is restricted in its reach; not all consumer products are reviewed, although the public perceives that marketed products have been deemed safe (Christoffel & Christoffel, 1989). Nonetheless, regulations and legislative action can be demonstrated as effective and useful in injury prevention.

Over 275 children have drowned in household buckets containing liquid since 1984 (Consumer Product Safety Commission, 2002). Therefore, warning signs are placed on most buckets as voluntary and mandatory actions by manufacturers that encourage parents not to leave buckets unattended around children. The CPSC has encouraged the implementation of these types of warnings as education interventions (with limited evidence of effectiveness). Several approaches have been used to decrease the amount of tap water scalds and burns. The Gas Appliance Manufacturers' Association set up voluntary self-regulations, and several states have adopted the regulatory approach on reducing thermostat settings on hot water heaters. A study by Webne and Kaplan (1993) reported that, whereas some families increased their hot water heater settings after installation, over 50% of the families reduced or did not change the thermostat settings. To contravene these actions, statewide legislation for using regulatory approaches on hot water heaters seems to be effective in decreasing the risk of tap water scalds.

As another example of legislative approaches to improving safety, the Child Abuse Prevention and Enforcement Act of 2000 enhances the ability of different agencies to report information to each other. For example, the act gives the criminal justice system the authority to report to child welfare services and organizations the criminal history of people who will be in contact with the children. The purpose of this act is to reduce the amount of child abuse and neglect and to ensure the safety of children.

CONCLUSIONS

In order to effectively decrease the occurrence of disease and injury in childhood, comprehensive approaches are needed, involving structural, behavioral, and legislative change:

> Because it is rare that a single intervention will significantly reduce a complex injury problem, program designers should carefully consider a mix of legislation/enforcement, education/behavior change, and engineering/technology interventions that complement each other and increase the likelihood of success. (National Committee for Injury Prevention and Control, 1989, p. 72)

Multifaceted interventions, as applicable to disease prevention as to injury prevention, are needed from numerous disciplines, agencies, and orientations.

The concepts and methods of psychology are clearly applicable to the prevention of injury and disease in terms of improving the understanding of etiological causes, developmental sequences and risk factors, and situational characteristics. Psychologists have designed interventions to prevent unintentional injuries and disease, as well as to ameliorate the effects of disease and injury. Psychological techniques are also useful in evaluating these preventive intervention activities. Pediatric psychology as a field with fundamental interests in improving the healthy development of children has a significant role to play in formulating, implementing, and evaluating prevention activities (Roberts, 1986, 1994). Unfortunately, the involvement of pediatric psychologists in these areas has not been commensurate with the enormity of the problems. The approaches and applications discussed here provide a glimpse at the potential contributions that can result if efforts are enhanced by researchers and practitioners in the field.

REFERENCES

ABCs of childhood vaccines. (2002). Retrieved February 4, 2003, from Centers for Disease Control website: *http://www.cdc.gov/nip/vaccine/ABCs/5-ABCS-primary.txt*

Bass, J. C., Christoffel, K. K., Widome, M., Boyle, W., Scheidt, P., Stanwick, R., & Roberts, K. (1993). Childhood injury prevention counseling in primary care settings: A critical review of the literature. *Pediatrics, 92*, 544–550.

Blum, C., & Shield, J. (2000). Toddler drowning in domestic swimming pools. *Injury Prevention, 6*, 288–290.

Caplan, G. (1964). *The principles of preventive psychiatry*. New York: Basic Books.

Centers for Disease Control and Prevention. (1993). Resurgence of pertussis: United States, 1993 and editorial note. *Morbidity and Mortality Weekly Review, 42*, 952–960.

Centers for Disease Control and Prevention. (1999a). Achievements in public health, 1900–1999: Fluoridation of drinking water to prevent dental caries. *Morbidity and Mortality Weekly Report, 41*, 939–940.

Centers for Disease Control and Prevention. (1999b). Impact of vaccines universally recommended for children—United States, 1900–1998. *Morbidity and Mortality Weekly Review, 48*, 243–248.

Centers for Disease Control and Prevention. (2000). *Healthy People 2010*. Retrieved February 12, 2001, from *http://web.health.gov/healthypeople/document*

Centers for Disease Control and Prevention. (2002). Provisional cases of selected notifiable diseases preventable by vaccination, United States, weeks ending December 29, 2001, and December 30, 2000 (52nd week). *Morbidity and Mortality Weekly Review, 50*, 1174–1175.

Christoffel, T., & Christoffel, K. K. (1989). The Consumer Product Safety Commission's opposition to consumer product safety: Lessons for public health advocates. *American Journal of Public Heath, 79*, 336–339.

Clayton, R. R., Cattarello, A. M., & Johnstone, B. M. (1996). The effectiveness of Drug Abuse Resistance Education (Project D.A.R.E.): 5-year follow-up results. *Preventive Medicine, 25*, 307–318.

Cohen, L. R., & Runyan, C. W. (1999). Barriers to pediatric injury prevention counseling. *Injury Prevention, 5*, 36–40.

Consumer Product Safety Commission. (1999a). Fireworks safety. *Consumer Product Safety Review, 3*(4).

Consumer Product Safety Commission. (1999b). Bike helmets. *Consumer Product Safety Review, 4*(1).

Consumer Product Safety Commission. (2002). *Infants and toddlers can drown in 5-gallon buckets*. Retrieved August 4, 2002, from http://www.cpsc.gov/CPSCPUB/PUBS/5006.html

Danseco, E. R., Miller, T. R., & Spicer, R. S. (2000). Incidence and costs of 1987–1994 injuries: Demographic breakdowns. *Pediatrics, 105*, e27.

Davidson, L. L., Durkin, M. S., Kuhn, L., O'Connor, P., Barlow, B., & Heagarty, M. C. (1994). The impact of the Safe Kids/Healthy Neighborhoods injury prevention program in Harlem, 1988 through 1991. *American Journal of Public Health, 84*, 580–586.

Deal, L. W., Gomby, D. S., Zippiroli, L., & Behrman, R. E. (2000). Unintentional injuries in childhood: Analysis and recommendations. *The Future of Children, 10*, 4–22.

DiGuiseppi, C. G., Rivara, F. P., Koepsell, T. D., & Polissar, L. (1989). Bicycle helmet use by children: Evaluation of a community-wide helmet campaign. *Journal of the American Medical Association, 262*, 2256–2261.

DiGuiseppi, C., & Roberts, I. G. (2000). Individual-level injury prevention strategies in the clinical setting. *The Future of Children, 10*, 53–82.

Dini, E. F., Linkins, R. W., & Sigafoos, J. (2000). The impact of computer-generated messages on childhood immunization coverage. *American Journal of Preventive Medicine, 18*, 132–139.

Faber, M. M. (1986). A review of efforts to protect children from injury in car crashes. *Family and Community Health, 9*, 25–41.

Finkelhor, D., & Daro, D. (1997). Prevention of child sexual abuse. In M. E. Helfer & R. S. Kempe (Eds.), *The battered child* (5th ed., pp. 615–626). Chicago: University of Chicago Press.

Finney, J. W., Christophersen, E. R., Friman, P. C., Kalnins, I. V., Maddux, J. E., Peterson, L., Roberts, M. C., & Wolraich, M. (1993). Society of Pediatric Psychology Task Force Report: Pediatric psychology and injury control. *Journal of Pediatric Psychology, 18*, 499–526.

Gielen, A. C., Wilson, M. E., McDonald, E. M., Servint, J. R., Andrews, J. S., Hwang, W., & Wang, M. (2001). Randomized trial of enhanced anticipatory guidance for injury prevention. *Archives of Pediatric and Adolescent Medicine, 155*, 42–49.

Graham, J. D., Corso, P. S., Morris, J. M., Segui-Gomez, M., & Weinstein, M. C. (1998). Evaluating the cost-effectiveness of clinical and public health measures. *Annual Review of Public Health, 19*, 125–152.

Greenberg, M. T., Domitrovich, C., & Bumbarger, B. (2001, March 30). The prevention of mental disorders in school-aged children: A current state of the field. *Prevention and Treatment, 4*, Article 1. Retrieved May 27, 2002, from *http://journals.apa.org/prevention/volume4/pre0040001a.html*

Grossman, D. C., Neckerman, H. J., Koepsell, T. D., Liu, P. Y., Asher, K. N., Beland, K., et al. (1997). Effectiveness of a violence prevention curriculum among children in elementary school: A randomized controlled trial. *Journal of the American Medical Association, 277*, 1605–1611.

Guyer, B., Hoyert, D. L., Martin, J. A., Ventura, M. A., MacDorman, M. F., & Stobino, D. M. (1999). Annual summary of vital statistics 1998. *Pediatrics, 104*, 1229–1246.

Haddon, W. (1972). A logical framework for categorizing highway safety phenomena and activity. *Journal of Trauma, 12*, 193–207.

Heck, A., Collins, J., & Peterson, L. (2001). Decreasing children's risk taking on the playground. *Journal of Applied Behavior Analysis, 34*, 349–352.

Hunter, L., Elias, M. J., & Norris, J. (2001). School-based violence prevention: Challenges and lessons learned from an action research project. *Journal of School Psychology, 39*, 161–175.

Is your child adequately immunized to begin school? (n.d.). Retrieved May 2, 2002, from *http://www.healthatoz.com/atoz/Lifestyles/BackSchool/Bsimmunized.html*

Jones, R. T., & Kazdin, A. (1980). Teaching children how and when to make emergency telephone calls. *Behavior Therapy, 11*, 509–521.

Jones, R. T., & McDonald, D. W. (1986). Childhood injury: A prevention model for intervention. *Education and Treatment of Children, 9*, 307–319.

Kogan, M. D., Overpeck, M. D., & Fingerhut, L. A. (1995). Medically attended nonfatal injuries among preschool-age children: National estimates. *American Journal of Preventive Medicine, 11*, 99–104.

Lutzker, J. R., & Bigelow, K. M. (2002). *Reducing child maltreatment: A guidebook for parent services.* New York: Guilford Press.

Lynam, D. R., Milich, R., Zimmerman, R., Novak, S. P., Logan, T. K., Martin, C., et al. (1999). Project D.A.R.E.: No effects at 10-year follow-up. *Journal of Consulting and Clinical Psychology, 67*, 590–593.

MacKay, A. M., & Rothman, K. J. (1982). The incidence and severity of burn injuries following Project Burn Prevention. *American Journal of Public Health, 72*, 248–252.

McLoughlin, E., Clarke, N., Stahl, K., & Crawford, J. D. (1977). One pediatric burn unit's experience with sleepwear-related injuries. *Pediatrics, 60*, 405–409.

McLoughlin, E., Vince, C. J., Lee, A. M., & Crawford, J. D. (1982). Project Burn Prevention: Outcome and implications. *American Journal of Public Health, 72*, 241–247.

Mallonee, S. (2000). Evaluating injury prevention programs: The Oklahoma City Smoke Alarm Project. *The Future of Children, 10*, 164–174.

Miller, T. R., & Galbraith, M. (1995). Injury prevention counseling by pediatricians: A benefit-cost comparison. *Pediatrics, 96*, 1–4.

Mrazek, P. J., & Haggerty, R. J. (1994). *Reducing risks for mental disorders: Frontiers for preventive intervention research.* Washington, DC: National Academy Press.

National Committee for Injury Prevention and Control. (1989). *Injury prevention: Meeting the challenge.* New York: Oxford University Press.

National Highway Traffic Safety Administration. (1999, October 1). *Special crash investigation report.* Retrieved February 4, 2003, from *http://www-nrd.nhtsa.dot.gov/departments/nrd-30/mcsa/SCI.html.*

Peterson, L. (1984a). The "Safe-at-Home" game: Training comprehensive safety skills in latchkey children. *Behavior Modification, 8*, 474–494.

Peterson, L. (1984b). Teaching home safety and survival skills to latchkey children: A comparison of two manuals and methods. *Journal of Applied Behavior Analysis, 17*, 279–293.

Peterson, L., & Gable, S. (1998). Holistic injury prevention. In J. Lutzker (Ed.), *Handbook of child abuse research and treatment* (pp. 291–318). New York: Plenum.

Peterson, L., & Mori, L. (1985). Prevention of child injury: An overview of targets, methods, and tactics for psychologists. *Journal of Consulting and Clinical Psychology, 53*, 586–595.

Renk, K., Liljequist, L., Bosco, G., & Phares, V. (2002). Prevention of child sexual abuse: Are we doing enough? *Trauma, Violence, & Abuse, 3*, 68–84.

Rivara, F. P., & Mueller, B. A. (1987). The epidemiology and causes of childhood injuries. *Journal of Social Issues, 43*, 13–31.

Roberts, M. C. (1986). Health promotion and problem prevention in pediatric psychology: An overview. *Journal of Pediatric Psychology, 11*, 147–161.

Roberts, M. C. (1994). Prevention/promotion in America: Still spitting on the sidewalk. *Journal of Pediatric Psychology, 19*, 267–281.

Roberts, M. C., Brown, K. J., Boles, R. E., & Mashunkashey, J. O. (2003). Prevention of injuries: Concepts and interventions for pediatric psychology in the schools. In R. Brown (Ed.), *Handbook of pediatric psychology in school settings* (pp. 65–80). New York: Erlbaum.

Roberts, M. C., Elkins, P. D., & Royal, G. P. (1984). Psychological applications to the prevention of accidents and illness. In M. C. Roberts & L. Peterson (Eds.), *Prevention of problems in childhood: Psychological research and applications* (pp. 173–199). New York: Wiley.

Roberts, M. C., & Fanurik, D. (1986). Rewarding elementary schoolchildren for their use of safety belts. *Health Psychology, 5*, 185–196.

Roberts, M. C., Fanurik, D., & Layfield, D. (1987). Behavioral approaches to prevention of childhood injuries. *Journal of Social Issues, 43*, 105–118.

Roberts, M. C., Fanurik, D., & Wilson, D. R. (1988). A community program to reward children's use of seat belts. *American Journal of Community Psychology, 16*, 395–407.

Roberts, M. C., Layfield, D. A., & Fanurik, D. (1992). Motivating children's use of car safety devices. In M. Wolraich & D. Routh (Eds.), *Advances in developmental and behavioral pediatrics* (Vol. 10, pp. 61–87). London: Jessica Kingsley.

Rosenbaum, M. S., Creedon, D. I., & Drabman, R. S. (1981). Training preschool children to identify emergency situations and make emergency phone calls. *Behavior Therapy, 12*, 425–435.

Shope, J. T., Molnar, L. J., Elliott, M. R., & Waller, P. F. (2001). Graduated driver licensing in Michigan: Early impact on motor vehicle crashes among 16-year-old drivers. *Journal of the American Medical Association, 286*, 1593–1598.

Silbergeld, E. K. (1997). Preventing lead poisoning in children. *Annual Review of Public Health, 18*, 187–210.

Spiegel, C. N., & Lindaman, F. C. (1977). Children's can't fly: A program to prevent childhood morbidity and mortality from window falls. *American Journal of Public Health, 67*, 1143–1147.

Stille, C. J., Christison-Lagay, J., Bernstein, B. A., & Dworkin, P. H. (2001). A simple provider-based educational intervention to boost infant immunization rates: A controlled trial. *Clinical Pediatrics, 40*, 365–373.

Tremblay, G. C., & Peterson, L. (1999). Prevention of childhood injury: Clinical and public policy challenges. *Clinical Psychology Review, 19*, 415–434.

Walton, W. W. (1982). An evaluation of the Poison Prevention Packaging Act. *Pediatrics, 69*, 363–370.

Webne, S. L., & Kaplan, B. J. (1993). Preventing tap water scalds: Do consumers change their preset thermostats? *American Journal of Public Health, 83*, 1469–1470.

Widome, M. D. (1991). Foreword. In M. H. Wilson, S. P. Baker, S. P. Teret, S. Shock, & J. Garbarino (Eds.), *Saving children: A guide to injury prevention* (pp. v–vii). New York: Oxford University Press.

Wilson, M. H., & Baker, S. (1987). Structural approach to injury control. *Journal of Social Issues, 43*, 73–86.

World Heath Organization. (1992). *International statistical classification of diseases and related health problems* (10th rev.). Geneva, Switzerland: Author.

Wurtele, S., Marrs, S., & Miller-Perrin, C. (1987). Practice makes perfect? The role of participant modeling in sexual abuse prevention programs. *Journal of Consulting and Clinical Psychology, 55*, 599–602.

7

Promoting Coping and Enhancing Adaptation to Illness

CYNTHIA HARBECK-WEBER
JENNIFER L. FISHER
CARRIE A. DITTNER

Almost all children will need to cope with medical stressors during their childhood. Most children receive at least 10 preventive injections by 5 years of age. In addition, 5 million children undergo diagnostic or treatment-oriented medical procedures yearly (Bush, Melamed, Sheras, & Greenbaum, 1986), with more than 2 million children below age 15 hospitalized each year (Popovic & Hall, 2001). Even more children (approximately 12.6 million) will experience chronic illnesses or conditions (Newacheck et al., 1998), which often involve multiple symptoms and exposures to medical events. The importance of helping these children adapt to medical stressors is important to their childhoods but also to their adult functioning, as childhood experiences with medical events may influence future anxiety, pain, and coping with medical encounters (Pate, Blount, Cohen, & Smith, 1996; Steward, 1993).

Studies describing children's coping and adaptation to medical stressors have been a hallmark of the field of pediatric psychology. The stressors examined have ranged from brief, acute procedures, such as injections and venipunctures, to lengthy procedures, such as hospitalization, to lifelong chronic illnesses, such as cystic fibrosis and diabetes. Numerous factors affecting adaptation to illness have been described, including demographic variables, illness variables, individual variables (e.g., temperament, coping), marital and family factors, and aspects of the health care system. This chapter takes a broad look at factors that promote a child's coping with various aspects of illness. We begin by reviewing two general concepts related to children's coping with medical stressors that provide a context for the remainder of the chapter. Next, we examine interventions that promote children's coping with a relatively brief but intense stressor—surgery. We then examine interventions that have helped children and their families cope with more chronic medical conditions. After considering these family and peer interventions, we briefly explore aspects of the health care system that can affect coping. Rather than focusing on the numerous descriptive studies that elucidate children's coping attempts, we have tried to emphasize current research on interventions that promote coping with chronic conditions.

DEVELOPMENTAL FACTORS

Numerous developmental factors affect a child's ability to cope with medical stressors. For example, as children grow, they become more independent in their coping efforts. Infants and toddlers will primarily depend on caregivers to provide coping resources during medical events (e.g., distraction during preparation and encounter, soothing during recovery); preschool and young elementary children are able to utilize internal coping resources (e.g., positive self-talk, imagery) but need cueing or coaching from caregivers. Adolescents are often able to cope with brief medical stressors quite independently, while requiring family and peer support to successfully cope with chronic medical stressors.

Young children may not have the linguistic skills to understand a medical event or to accurately encode it in memory, thus affecting their experience of future medical encounters. Research suggests that knowledge regarding an upcoming medical stressor or completion of a complex medical regimen can facilitate coping and adherence. Studies have demonstrated a positive correlation between children's knowledge of health concepts and general cognitive development (for review, see Harbeck-Weber & Peterson, 1993). Thus younger children may be most at risk for difficulty coping with medical stressors. Indeed, research suggests that younger children are more likely than older children to have misconceptions regarding hospitalization and surgery (Redpath & Rogers, 1984) and are less able to ask questions about what will happen during a medical procedure (Pidgeon, 1981). In addition to cognitive differences, young children also have less experience with coping, a fact that may affect their coping attempts.

COPING STYLE

Coping has been described as "constantly changing cognitive and behavioral efforts to manage specific external and/or internal demands that are appraised as taxing or exceeding the resources of the person" (Lazarus & Folkman, 1984, p. 141). Peterson, Oliver, and Saldana (1997) argued that studies of children's coping should be divided into studies of coping during the anticipation and preparation phase versus coping during the encounter. It is easy to understand how a coping strategy such as asking questions may be adaptive during preparation but less helpful during the encounter phase if the questions serve to delay or lengthen the procedure. Studies of coping during the anticipation phase have characterized children as "sensitizers" or "repressors" by diverse methods such as interviews (Peterson & Toler, 1986), play behaviors (Burstein & Meichenbaum, 1979), and Rorschach protocols (Knight et al., 1979). Sensitizers cope with a stressor by attempting to gather information and familiarize themselves with their upcoming medical encounter. Repressors may turn away from the stressor and use denial or distraction as a preferred coping mechanism. Sensitizers have more adaptive responses to hospitalization and surgery, including less anxiety and more cooperation before and after surgery, and lower rates of cortisol production. They also require less monitoring in the intensive care unit (Field, Alpert, Vega-Lahr, Goldstein, & Perry, 1988; Knight et al., 1979; Peterson & Toler, 1986).

Some studies of coping during the encounter phase have examined a different coping construct, that of primary–secondary control (Rothbaum, Weisz & Snyder, 1982). Primary control refers to coping that attempts to modify objective conditions, and secondary control attempts to modify oneself to adapt to the stressor. In a study of children with leukemia, Weisz, McCabe, and Dennig (1994) found that children using secondary control coping exhibited less distress during painful procedures and had lower internalizing and externalizing problem scores on the Child Behavior Checklist (CBCL) than children using primary control coping. Some researchers suggested that secondary control coping strategies are most effective with uncontrollable stressors (e.g., necessary medical procedures) while primary control strategies may be most effective with controllable stressors (Blount, Landolf-Fritsche, Powers, & Sturges, 1991; Compas, Malcarne, & Banez, 1992).

Children's coping attempts also change over time. Research suggests that children's use of emotion-focused coping strategies generally increases with age (Band & Weisz, 1988; Compas, Malcarne, & Fondacaro, 1988). Older children are more likely than younger children to utilize a greater number and variety of coping responses, as well as to focus on positive factors related to the stressor (Brown, O'Keeffe, Sanders, & Baker, 1986). Older children are also better able to differentiate between situations in which they can exert some control and those in which they cannot (Band & Weisz, 1988; Harris & Lipian, 1989), perhaps increasing their ability to match their coping strategy to the stressor involved. In addition to controllability, medical situations vary in severity and chronicity. The next section reviews interventions that promote adaptation to acute medical stressors, using the examples of surgery and hospitalization.

COPING WITH ACUTE MEDICAL STRESSORS

The rich history of studies assessing the effectiveness of preparation programs for decreasing children's distress during surgery and hospitalization followed research suggesting that hospitalization and medical procedures were significant stressors for children. More recent reports suggested that as many as 54% of children exhibit behavioral changes following outpatient surgery (Kain, Mayes, O'Connor, & Cicchetti, 1994) and that 11% of children experience relatively severe behavior problems within 2 weeks of surgery (Lumley, Melamed, & Abeles, 1993), suggesting that although hospital environments have changed dramatically over the last four to five decades, medical procedures continue to be distressing for children. Melamed (1998) lists three primary goals for preparing children for hospitalization and medical procedures: (1) encouraging trusting relationships, (2) providing emotional support, and (3) giving age-appropriate information that will help children develop coping strategies before and during a medical procedure. The three following primary modalities have been developed to achieve these important goals, and each has received significant empirical support.

Preventive Interventions

Education

One of the earliest studies to evaluate an educational intervention with presurgery patients utilized a nurse to prepare children by using a doll as a model and telling a story to the child about what would happen next (Wolfer & Visintainer, 1975). These sessions occurred at defined stress points (e.g., admission to the hospital, before a blood test, preceding the first night's stay, prior to any preoperative medication, and immediately after returning from the recovery room). Mothers were also given information and a chance to ask questions. The children participating in the educational program were rated by an independent observer as showing fewer distress behaviors at all of the identified stress points. These children also displayed less resistance to anesthesia induction, greater fluid intake, and earlier voiding after surgery. Mothers also reported being more satisfied with their child's nursing care and appeared less anxious. Other authors have confirmed the efficacy of educational interventions with children and adolescents undergoing gastrointestinal endoscopy (Mahajan et al., 1998), acute appendectomy (Edwinson, Arnbjornsson, & Ekman, 1988), ENT surgery (Hatava, Olsson, & Lagerkranser, 2000), and emergency surgery (Mansson, Fredrikzon, & Rosberg, 1992).

For educational interventions to be optimal, they must provide developmentally appropriate information to children and adolescents. Rasnake and Linscheid (1989) clearly demonstrated the importance of providing developmentally congruent information in their study of 48 children undergoing a proctoscopy. They designed three separate educational videotapes for the children. The developmentally appropriate videotape for preschoolers focused on external, observable events (e.g., the noise the machine would make and the light on the instruments) and utilized a simple linguistic pattern. The videotape for the children in the concrete operational stage included a description of previous experiences related to the upcoming medical procedure, the relationship between symptoms and the examination, approximate time of the procedure, and analogies such as comparing the external part of the proctoscope to a microscope. Children were randomly assigned to three conditions: (1) standard preparation, (2) developmentally appropriate information, or (3) developmentally advanced information. Observers uninformed about the children's group status rated the children given developmentally appropriate information as less distressed than children given either the control information or the developmentally advanced information.

Modeling

Modeling interventions are based on Bandura's social learning theory. They include an educational component that exposes the child to the sights, sounds, equipment, and techniques used in the child's upcoming medical procedure. In addition, they provide a peer model who experiences the upcoming event and demonstrates positive coping skills. In one of the first studies to evaluate the effectiveness of a modeling intervention, Melamed and Siegel (1975) randomly assigned 60 children undergoing elective surgery to view either the film *Ethan Has an Operation* or a control film. *Ethan Has an Operation* depicts a boy's adaptive responses to a blood test, presurgical injection, IV insertion, anesthesia induction, surgery recovery, and discharge from the hospital. They found that children viewing the *Ethan* film had lower palmar sweating before and after surgery, reported fewer medical concerns, and exhibited less behavioral distress as rated by objective observers both before and after surgery than did children who viewed the control film.

Peterson and colleagues later confirmed the importance of a modeling intervention (Peterson, Ridley-Johnson, Tracy, & Mullins, 1984) and demonstrated that modeling interventions presented by a puppet or a locally produced videotape are also effective (Peterson, Schultheis, Ridley-Johnson, Miller, & Tracy, 1984). Klingman, Melamed, Cuthbert, and Hermecz (1984) also found that participant modeling (i.e., the child is cued to imitate the model during the preparation program) is more effective than symbolic modeling (i.e., child observes the model).

Coping Skills

A third type of preparation program typically includes education and modeling components but emphasizes teaching the child coping techniques for the upcoming medical stressor. In one of the earliest studies, Peterson and Shigetomi (1981) randomly assigned children to one of the following four groups: basic preparation using a puppet model; basic preparation plus the *Ethan Has an Operation* film; basic preparation plus coping skills training (i.e., deep muscle relaxation, imagery, and self-instruction); or all three components. Parents, observers, and nurses who were not informed about the children's treatment group rated the children receiving the coping skills training as less upset and more cooperative both before and after surgery than children who did not receive the coping skills training. In addition, children who received all three components of the preparation program were rated by the lab technician as less upset and more cooperative than children in the other groups. Zastowny, Kirschenbaum, and Meng (1986) later confirmed the importance of teaching coping skills in presurgery preparation programs.

Techniques for Children Undergoing Repeated Procedures

Research indicates that children who have previously experienced hospitalization or surgery may not respond as well to traditional preparations as naïve children do (Melamed, Dearborn, & Hermecz, 1983). Perhaps children with prior experience need to be evaluated to determine the quality of their experience before receiving preparation (Melamed, 1992). Children who report positive prior experiences and successful coping during previous hospital experience may benefit from a "refresher course" style of preparation. Children who report a negative prior experience may require a more extensive preparation tailored to their needs. Alternatively, novel techniques may be useful in preparing children expected to receive multiple procedures or hospitalizations. In a recent study, Chen, Zeltzer, Craske, and Katz (1999) evaluated a memory intervention with 50 children diagnosed with leukemia who were undergoing repeated lumbar punctures (LPs). After their initial LP, children in the treatment group were interviewed by a therapist, who helped the children and adolescents reevaluate their reaction to the recent LP by enhancing their beliefs about the efficacy of their coping attempts, helping them to realistically appraise their actual responses to the LP and to increase the accuracy of their subjective memories. In comparison with children and adolescents in the attention control group, children in the treatment group reported greater decreases in pain during a subsequent LP and showed greater decreases in observable distress in the postprocedure phase and greater decreases in pre-LP cortisol levels. No differences in heart rate or blood pressure emerged. Although conducted with children receiving repeat LPs, this methodology may have important implications for children receiving other repeated procedures and surgeries.

Additional Behavior Therapy Techniques

Although many children will benefit from the approaches outlined here, a few particularly anxious children or children who have had previous negative experiences may have difficulty coping with hospitalization or repeated medical procedures, difficulty severe enough to interfere with their treatment. For those children, the addition of traditional behavioral therapy techniques may be needed. For example, operant techniques such as tangible rewards (e.g., praise, points to be exchanged for preferred activities) may be useful to increase a child's cooperation with repeated medical procedures such as dialysis or growth hormone injections. Systematic desensitization can also be helpful to reduce the fear associated with some procedures, such as diagnostic studies (e.g., MRI, CT) and medical interventions (e.g., radiation, chemotherapy).

Parental Participation

Research regarding parental presence during medical procedures has been mixed. Some studies have found that parental presence during anesthesia reduces child distress (Glazebrook, Lim, Sheard, & Standen, 1994), whereas other studies have found that parental presence did not reduce child distress and may even increase it in children with an anxious parent (Beven et al., 1990). However, most studies have found that parental presence during presurgery preparation programs is helpful. For example, Pinto and Hollandsworth (1989) contrasted two viewer conditions (parent present and parent absent) and three treatments (adult-narrated videotape, peer-narrated videotape, and a no-videotape control). They randomly assigned 60 children to one of the six interventions. Patients who viewed one of the tapes with a parent present exhibited less preoperative arousal than did children who did not have a parent present. Although they did not compare parental presence with parental absence during a preparation program, both Peterson and Shigetomi (1981) and Zastowny et al. (1986) utilized parents as coaches during the surgery preparation process and instructed the parents to cue their children to utilize their coping skills. The parents who received the coping skills training reported less anxiety and increased feelings of competence. Instead of including parents in the preparation program, Campbell et al. (1992) directly prepared the mothers of preschoolers undergoing cardiac catheterization. Mothers who received the stress management training reported a more favorable posthospital adjustment for their children than did mothers in the other preparation groups. Children whose mothers received the stress management training were significantly less upset and more cooperative with venipuncture and catheterization than were children in the other groups.

Although several studies have suggested that parental inclusion in preparation and medical procedures is beneficial, not all children benefit from parental presence. In a study of same-day surgery patients, Faust, Olson, and Rodriguez (1991) reported that parental presence during preparation did not result in less distress than children receiving preparation alone. Whether the contrasting results are due to the limited amount of time parents and children had to practice their newly learned skills remains a question for further research.

Same-Day Surgery

With few exceptions (e.g., Faust et al., 1991), the majority of the studies reviewed here were conducted with children undergoing hospitalization and surgery. In a recent review, Palermo, Drotar, and Tripi (1999) suggested that current research regarding interventions for children undergoing same-day surgery are not as positive. Three randomized studies utilizing a pain education booklet (Chambers, Reid, McGrath, Finley, & Ellerton, 1997), an interactive teaching book (Margolis et al., 1998), or a distraction intervention by written instructions or parent training (Palermo & Drotar, 1999) did not yield differences between prepared and unprepared children. In contrast, three quasi-experimental design studies utilizing an education and modeling intervention (Atkins, 1987), videotape, tour, and play intervention (Ellerton & Merriam, 1994), or participant modeling (Faust et al., 1991) found mixed results, with prepared children exhibiting less distress and lower anxiety before surgery, as well as more accurate knowledge concerning hospitalization. These same patients generally did not differ in terms of parent or child postoperative behavior. Whether the difference in findings is due to the increased methodological rigor of the first three studies or the difference in preparation programs remains for future research to discover.

Implications for Health Promotion Policy

An extensive literature has shown that preparing children for the experience of hospitalization and surgery through education, modeling, and teaching effective coping strategies can improve children's cooperation with surgery procedures, reduce their distress, and lower health care costs. However, O'Byrne, Peterson, and Saldana (1997), found that only 50% of hospitals serving children taught coping skills for surgery, 43% taught relaxation, and 48% utilized films. Instead, hospitals preferred narrative preparation (89%), tours (87%), play therapy (86%), and printed material (84%), all techniques that do not have sufficient empirical support. Of equal concern, O'Byrne and colleagues discovered that only 10% of hospitals had empirically evaluated their own preparation programs. When discussing reasons for the discrepancy between scientific findings and practice, the authors report that health care personnel who choose preparation programs rarely read psychology research journals but instead rely on information from informal teaching settings and discussions, pediatric research and nursing journals, and commercially available materials.

Future Research

O'Byrne et al.'s (1997) work highlights a critical need for research in this area. At this point, the research has clearly delineated effective interventions that help most children adapt to the stressors of surgery and hospitalization. Programs that utilize modeling and teach coping skills, that include parents, and that promote active participation are generally the most effective. Unfortunately, the most effective interventions are not the most widely utilized. How can this be changed? O'Byrne and colleagues suggest that researchers interested in helping children cope with hospitalization and medical procedures should also focus on effective methods of disseminating research findings to health care personnel who choose preventive interventions (O'Byrne et al., 1997). Further research on the cost-effectiveness of programs designed to promote adaptation to hospitalization and surgery is also needed. Particularly in the current health care culture, rapid preparation programs are likely to be the most accepted; however, very brief interventions (i.e., written instructions provided to parents) have not been found to be effective. Therefore, determining the essential components of programs and time needed may help keep preparation programs from being minimized below their level of effectiveness. Further research continues to be needed on the best preparation programs for special populations, including very young children, children with previous negative experiences, and children with anxious parents. Continued research on preparation for same-day surgery also appears warranted. Finally, ensuring that programs are developmentally appropriate and evaluating the impact of coping style on children's responses to preparation programs would also be beneficial.

This section has focused on methods that may help a child or adolescent cope with an acute stressor such as hospitalization or surgery. However, many children with medical illnesses need to adapt to a series of hospitalizations and procedures rather than to an acute event. Whether children and adolescents are experiencing one or numerous medical stressors, they also are spending more time with their families and peers than children with illnesses have in the past. Hospitalizations have grown much shorter, and the complexity of medical regimens has increased. Thus identifying family and peer variables that may help a child or adolescent adjust to his or her illness becomes very important.

FAMILY VARIABLES THAT PROMOTE ADJUSTMENT TO CHRONIC ILLNESS

The importance of parent and family variables in the adjustment of children with chronic illnesses has been highlighted in a number of conceptual models (Kliewer, 1997; Kliewer, Sandler, & Wolchik, 1994; Thompson & Gustafson, 1996; Wallander, Varni, Babani, Banis, & Wilcox, 1989). For example, Wallander et al. (1989) included parental mental health, marital satisfaction, family cohesion, and utilitarian resources under "social-ecological factors" that influence children's coping with and adjustment to chronic illness. Thompson and Gustafson (1996) speculated that maternal adaptation processes are important for determining children's adjustment. In their model, patient and family processes are felt to be more important in mediating the illness–outcome relationship than illness-related or demographic factors. Kliewer et al. (1994) based their conceptual model on the hypothesis that parents influence their children's coping through several mechanisms: coaching their children to use various coping strategies, modeling their own coping strategies and emotional reactions, and creating a home environment that is characterized either by conflict or by cohesion and communication. Unfortunately, although multiple conceptual models have been developed to explain children's adjustment to chronic illness, only a limited number of empirical studies of these models have been conducted. In fact, the impact of children's chronic illnesses on parental mental health and family functioning has received more empirical attention than has the impact of these family mediators on children's coping and adjustment. In the following sections, we review studies that assess the relationship between parent and family mediators and children's coping and adjustment in families with a chronically ill child.

Family Environment

The social-ecological variable that has received the most attention is the family environment (Wallander & Thompson, 1995), including the relationship between variables such as adaptability, cohesion, communication, and conflict on the coping of children with chronic illnesses. These studies generally find strong support for the role of family functioning in determining children's coping with and adjustment to chronic illness.

For example, in families of children with diabetes, family flexibility was related to dietary adherence (Hanson, DeGuire, Schinkel, Henggeler, & Burghen, 1992); high family cohesion was related to good metabolic control, particularly in children who had diabetes for a brief time (Hanson, Henggeler, Harris, Burghen, & Moore, 1989); and low family cohesion was related to higher levels of avoidant coping (Hanson, Cigrang, et al., 1989). Seiffge-Krenke (1998) proposed three hypothetical links between family environments and metabolic control in diabetes patients: (1) a structure hypothesis that suggests that control and organization within the family are important for metabolic control in an adolescent; (2) a cohesion hypothesis that supports the relation of family warmth and cohesion to good metabolic control; and (3) the flexibility hypothesis, in which family adaptability is important for determining metabolic control.

More recently, family environment variables have received attention in determining the adjustment of sickle cell patients. Kell, Kliewer, Erickson, and Ohene-Frempong (1998) showed that parent reports of family competence, as defined by the family's ability to work together to solve problems and respect one another, were negatively related to somatic complaints by children with sickle cell disease. In addition, they found that high family competence was associated with fewer internalizing and externalizing behaviors by adolescent girls with sickle cell disease. Burlew, Telfair, Colagelo, and Wright (2000) also identified a significant negative relationship between family relations (cohesion and expression) and internalizing symptoms in children with sickle cell disease. Finally, Thompson and colleagues demonstrated a positive relationship between family conflict and maternal reports of child behavior problems in sickle cell patients (Thompson et al., 1999).

Parental Mental Health

Numerous studies have shown a relationship between parental mental health and children's coping and adjustment. Not surprisingly, this relationship also appears to exist in families that include children with chronic illnesses. This association is important to understand because it may be bidirectional. For example, the experience of children's chronic illnesses within a family appears to contribute to parental mental health challenges. In a major epidemiological study assessing the psychological adjustment of parents of children with chronic illnesses (Cadman, Rosenbaum, Boyle, & Offord, 1991), the number of parents receiving mental health treatment was significantly (2 to 3 times) higher for parents of children with chronic illnesses than for parents of well children. This finding has been supported in other studies of families with chronically ill children (Dahlquist et al., 1993; Wallander, Varni, Babani, Banis, DeHaan, & Wilcox, 1989). Kazak and her colleagues have conducted research showing that children with cancer and their family members, especially mothers, often experience symptoms of posttraumatic stress disorder after children's cancer diagnosis and treatment (Best, Streisand, Catania, & Kazak, 2001; Kazak et al., 1998).

Several studies have shown a positive association between parental mental health challenges and problems in children with chronic illnesses. For example, Thompson, Gustafson, Hamlett, and Spock (1992) found that, in families of children with cystic fibrosis, maternal anxiety was positively related to children's internalizing and externalizing symptoms, even after controlling for demographic factors and disease severity. In a study of children with juvenile rheumatoid arthritis, Ross et al. (1993) found that maternal distress was one of several variables positively correlated with self-reported pain levels. In other words, children with parents who have emotional challenges may show higher levels of somatic symptomatology. Unfortunately, it is not possible to determine the direction of the relationship from these studies; children's challenges, psychological or medical, may also be contributing to parents' mental health problems.

Variables that influence parental mental health may also influence children's coping and adjustment to chronic illness. For example, social support has long been identified as an important stress-buffering resource, and studies have found that parents who show better psychological adjustment to their children's illness have more social support (Hoekstra-Weebers, Jaspers, Kamps, & Klip, 2001). Similarly, the parents of children with cancer who reported high levels of family cohesion, as defined by close, supportive relationships between family members, typically reported less emotional distress than those with low levels of family cohesion (Sloper, 2000). Yet these studies rarely investigated the relationship of mental health–enhancing resources available to parents to the coping and adjustment of the children. Thus the strength of this relationship has yet to be established.

Family Interventions

Interventions to enhance parent and family functioning are routinely conducted in mental health clinics and health care centers, with the implicit goal of improving children's adjustment to chronic illness. Unfortunately, because of the difficulty of undertaking randomized, controlled intervention trials, few of these interventions have published empirical support. Three notable exceptions, each of which used random assignment to treatment and control groups, are described next. Satin, La Greca, Zigo, and Skyler (1989) were the first to report on a family-oriented group intervention for adolescents with diabetes. They randomly assigned families to one of three groups: a multifamily group, a multifamily group including parent simulation of diabetes, and a wait-list control group. Although group effects were found such that the children in the multifamily-plus-simulation group improved their diabetic control, no differences in family environment variables were observed, suggesting that group content did not effectively target these mediators and that group differences were observed for other reasons.

Sanders, Shepherd, Cleghorn, and Woolford (1994) randomly assigned families with children who have chronic abdominal pain to a cognitive–behavioral family intervention or to standard pediatric care. The cognitive–behavioral group involved training parents in contingency management (e.g., reinforcing well behaviors, ignoring pain behaviors) and self-management training for children (e.g., deep breathing and relaxation). Standard pediatric treatment included the same number of sessions, but families received only reassurance and support, not any specific training in pain management. Results showed that children in both groups had reduced levels of pain at postintervention. However, children in the cognitive–behavioral family group also showed lower levels of long-term relapse, better functional abilities, and higher rates of complete pain elimination.

Finally, Wysocki and colleagues investigated the efficacy of behavior therapy for families in improving the diabetic control of adolescents (Wysocki et al., 2000). They randomized 119 families with diabetes to one of three groups: a behavior family therapy group, a diabetes education and support group, or the standard treatment group. Unfortunately, no group differences were observed for diabetic adherence. However, the behavior family therapy group resulted in improved parent–child relations and reduced diabetes-related conflict. Also, some adolescents in this group showed improvements in adjustment to diabetes and diabetic control.

Future Research

The preceding review clearly suggests that characteristics of parents and families, such as good maternal mental health, high family flexibility, competence and cohesion, and low family and parental conflict, can promote children's adjustment to chronic illness. Unfortunately, most of this descriptive research includes mothers and children, neglecting the important perspectives and influence of other family members (Seagull, 2000). Clearly, the current models explaining children's adjustment to chronic illness support the inclusion of fathers, siblings, other relatives, and friends in future studies. Future intervention studies are also warranted. Existing family intervention studies appear useful in facilitating the adjustment of children with chronic illnesses. However, the varied results of these interventions highlight the challenges of conducting well-controlled clinical trials with families of chronically ill patients. These challenges include recruitment of participants, many of whom are already overburdened by daily cares and responsibilities; attrition of participants, resulting in low power to detect significant group differences; and implementation of complex interventions that target multiple individuals and variables within each family. Despite these challenges, more intervention research is needed to fully appreciate the value of family interventions in determining children's adjustment to chronic illness. As with family variables, research on peers of children with a chronic illness has been primarily descriptive, with limited randomized intervention studies.

PROMOTING ADAPTATION TO CHRONIC ILLNESS THROUGH PEER INTERVENTIONS

Children with chronic illness often face disruptions in their achievement of social development tasks and the formation of friendships. Chronic illness may result in decreased school attendance and limited participation in play or sports activities, as well as adherence to medical regimens that make a child or adolescent seem "different" (Kliewer, 1997). Autonomy may also be difficult to achieve for children and adolescents who require parental involvement in the management of their disease. Side effects of treatment can also reduce children's confidence about and willingness to engage in social activities (Novakovic et al., 1996). For example, they may fear being teased because of their appearance or worry about keeping up with healthy peers. This anxiety has implications for the development of a maladaptive cycle characterized by less social initiation, increased peer perceptions of withdrawal, and fewer opportunities to learn and practice skills related to making and keeping friends. All of these issues place youth with chronic illness at greater risk for the maladaptive outcomes associated with the absence of peer support. Indeed, the risk of significant psychological or social problems for chronically ill children may be 1.3 to 3 times greater than for healthy children (Thompson, Zeman, Fanurik, & Sirotkin-Roses, 1992).

Research with healthy children suggests that an absence of social support can lead to maladaptive outcomes such as loneliness and social dissatisfaction (Asher, Parkhurst, Hymel, & Williams, 1990) and to increased likelihood of school dropout, criminal activity, and mental health problems (Kupersmidt, Coie, & Dodge, 1990; Parker & Asher, 1987). Moreover, without the establishment of positive peer relations, children's sense of competence and identity formation may be challenged (Garrison & McQuiston, 1989). Therefore, helping children with chronic illness maximize their social support seems beneficial.

Peer relationships have been found to both help and hinder treatment adherence in children and adolescents with chronic illness. For example, Skinner, John, and Hampson (2000) found that support from family and friends was predictive of better dietary self-care in adolescents with Type I diabetes. Research also has shown that adolescents perceive greater support from their friends with regard to "feeling good about diabetes" (La Greca et al., 1995), as well as adhering to exercise and diet regimens. This finding is consistent with general developmental research that shows that friends, particularly during adolescence, are a primary means of emotional support.

In contrast, adolescents with cystic fibrosis (CF) have been found to skip medications because they do not want to be perceived as different or risk interfering with romantic possibilities (Christian & D'Auria, 1997). This same study, however, found that friendships that were characterized by acceptance and validation reduced the need to hide differences among CF youth.

In a review of the literature, Thompson and Gustafson (1996) noted several shortcomings of studies on social adaptation of children with chronic illness, including: emphasis on global constructs (i.e., psychological adjustment), use of between-group and cross-sectional methodological designs, failure to use multiple informants, and limits in the use of direct and multiple assessment measures. Fortunately, research is also moving beyond an examination of the relationship between social relationships and chronic illness to interventions that may foster both positive social relationships and successful coping with a chronic disease.

Interventions

Intervention efforts geared toward improving social adjustment have typically focused on helping children to form friendships with other children who are experiencing similar medical difficulties and to establish healthy relationships outside of the disease context. Such programs include group therapy, social skills programs, school reintegration services, and computer-based interventions (i.e., STARBRIGHT).

Group Therapy

Given the critical role of peers in the adjustment to and management of illness in pediatric populations, group interventions may be particularly beneficial to patients. Plante, Lobato, and Engel (2001) recently completed an excellent review of group interventions for pediatric chronic illness. Groups were classified as providing emotional support, psychoeducation, adaptation and skill development, or symptom reduction. The Society of Pediatric Psychology Task Force modification of the Chambless criteria for efficacious interventions was used to evaluate the literature. In brief, emotional support and psychoeducation groups did not meet minimal Chambless criteria, given the lack of well-controlled studies. Adaptation and skill development groups were deemed a well-established intervention for physical symptoms and a probably efficacious intervention for psychosocial outcomes for children with diabetes and asthma. Finally, for symptom-reduction groups, efficacy was demonstrated, from the level of a promising intervention (e.g., relaxation for headaches) to a well-established treatment (e.g., pediatric obesity groups).

Unfortunately, many studies involving group interventions have included children diagnosed with chronic illnesses, rather than typical peers who are encountered on a daily basis and who often play a role in adjustment. The research examining social interactions of adolescents with diabetes have found that peers can be negative influences (Thomas, Peterson, & Goldstein, 1997), as well as providers of companionship and emotional support (La Greca et al., 1995). In a rather informal, unstructured peer group intervention with typical peers and adolescents with cancer and hematological diagnoses, Clark and colleagues (1992) found that the interaction helped patients cope with their illness and improve quality of life. Greco, Pendley, McDonnell, and Reeves (2001) developed a structured intervention for integrating peers into diabetes care regimens. Adolescents with diabetes and their best friends participated in a group aimed at increasing knowledge about diabetes and social support in diabetes care. Some of the sessions included reflective listening and problem solving, as well as general stress management. The intervention proved to be effective at improving peers' knowledge about diabetes and ways to offer support. Peers also evidenced improved self-perception following the intervention.

Social Skills Training

Research has clearly shown the influences of social support and social competence on a child's ability to cope with stress associated with illness, such as cancer (Varni & Katz, 1997). It follows that maximizing the social competence of children would therefore place them at lower risk for the adjustment difficulties typically associated with peer problems. Indeed, the effectiveness of social skills training programs has been well documented in general developmental literature. Varni and colleagues have developed a successful social skills training program aimed at meeting these needs in pediatric cancer patients (Varni, Katz, Colegrove, & Dolgin, 1993). Results show that children who participated in treatment showed significantly fewer behavior problems and greater social support at 9-month follow-up compared with pretreatment levels of adjustment.

School Re-Entry

School adjustment issues can be the result of direct effects of the illness (i.e., central nervous system impairment) or of indirect effects such as fatigue, absenteeism, or psychological stress (Thompson & Gustafson, 1996). Many children and adolescents with chronic illness require some type of special consideration from school. Public policy has produced several laws to develop educational plans for children with medical conditions (i.e., "Other Health Impaired" classification of the Individuals with Disabilities Education Act, 1990, amended in 1997). In addition, school reintegration programs have been developed to assist with the goals of enhancing academic and peer support. Although various school re-entry programs have been proposed (e.g., Farmer & Peterson, 1995; Worchel-Prevatt et al., 1998), the empirical literature describing the school re-entry process and impact of such programs is scant. Madan-Swain, Fredrick, and Wallander (1999) identify three major phases of school re-entry: educational planning while the child is in the hospital, preparing teachers and peers for the classmate's return, and ensuring follow-up contact with school personnel and parents to continue to monitor school progress. This model, though comprehensive in nature, has yet to be validated by empirical research.

Summer Camps

Summer camp programs are considered a popular means of addressing the social needs of children with chronic illness. Although the programmatic basis of such camps may vary, almost all share the common goal of improving children's attitudes toward their medical or physical condition. In a recent review of summer camp programs, Plante and colleagues (2001) reported that pre- and postevaluations of summer camp programs reveal that campers gain disease-related knowledge and may show improvements in self-esteem, anxiety, attitudes toward illness, and management of the disease. Treatment moderator variables may include gender, age, family functioning, and experience with camp. Unfortunately, most studies that focus on summer camps have not utilized standardized empirical measures to assess effectiveness and usually lack a controlled comparison group. In a recent study, Briery and Rabian (1999) attempted to address some of these limits by quantifying children's attitudes toward illness (Child Attitude Toward Illness scale), as well as their overall trait anxiety (State–Trait Anxiety Inventory for Children). Their data suggest that specialized camping experiences can improve attitudes toward illness and decrease anxiety.

Support via Computer Network

Another means of facilitating social adjustment in pediatric chronically ill patients involves the development of a private computer network for hospitalized children that enables them to interact with other hospitalized children in an online community (i.e., STARBRIGHT World at www.starbright.org). Holden and colleagues have evaluated the impact of STARBRIGHT on two occasions (Holden, Bearison, Rode, Kapliloff, & Rosenberg, 2000; Holden, Bearison, Rode, Rosenberg, & Fishman, 1999). Hospitalized children ages 9 to 19 years reported less pain intensity, pain aversiveness, and anxiety in the STARBRIGHT condition than in normal pediatric care.

Future Research

Continued research in promoting positive peer adjustment among chronically ill youth is clearly needed. It is evident that social skills training programs are effective in children with social difficulties. The challenge is to tailor these programs to suit children with chronic illness. To begin, it would be helpful for future investigations to focus on assessing perceptions of the unique social challenges and degree of social satisfaction of chronically ill children across different developmental levels. Within-group design studies to determine what differentiates chronically ill children with good social adjustment and positive peer relations from those with social difficulties would also yield helpful information. Finally, given that social acceptance has often been associated with long-term, positive psychosocial adjustment, interventions that include same-age, healthy peers may also facilitate acceptance, as well as disease adaptation.

HEALTH CARE SYSTEM FACTORS THAT PROMOTE ADJUSTMENT

In addition to individual, family, and peer factors that may promote adjustment to illness, pediatric psychology has become increasingly aware of how the medical system affects a child's and family's adaptation. Early efforts of the health care system to promote adjustment focused on helping children adapt to hospitalization. For example, when the literature suggested that separation from parents was perhaps the most traumatic aspect of hospitalization for many children, policies regarding parental rooming-in changed. In the 1950s, most New York hospitals limited parental visiting to 2 hours per week. By the 1970s, 83% of children's hospitals and 54% of general hospitals allowed the parent to be with the child day and night (Hardgrove, 1980). Currently, most hospitals also encourage parents to be present at presurgical preparation programs, and some hospitals allow parents to be present during medical procedures, including anesthesia induction. Hospitals have also provided child life therapists and school tutors to give children developmentally appropriate experiences during hospitalization. Unfortunately, in some areas, these important services are being reduced due to budget constraints.

Recent efforts to investigate and improve health system variables have focused more closely on outpatient services. Some studies have suggested that primary care physicians may underestimate parental needs for information about children's diagnosis, treatments, and prognosis (Liptak & Revell, 1989) and overestimate the opportunities available for parents to discuss their concerns (Bradford, 1991). Recent efforts have also focused on helping children and their parents adhere to complex medical regiments. Studies suggest that adherence may be directly linked to knowledge about the medical regimen (Ievers et al., 1999). However, the knowledge may not come easily without health system interventions. For example, an early study noted significant discrepancies between what information providers told their patients and the information patients recalled after a clinic visit. Page, Verstraete, Robb, and Etzwiler (1981) found that providers typically gave seven recommendations per patient. Patients (and parents of younger children) recalled an average of two recommendations. Perhaps even more concerning is the finding that 40% of the patient-recalled recommendations were not recorded by the provider. Patients fared even worse in a high-stress medical encounter (visit to the emergency room). Grover, Berkowitz, and Lewis (1994) found that only half of parents given a follow-up appointment knew the date and place of their child's follow-up, 30% of parents knew the name of the medication their child was prescribed, and 51% knew how to administer it. Only 13% of parents given multiple medications recalled the names of the medications and only 10% could recall how to administer the medications.

Providing written recommendations during outpatient and emergency department (ED) visits is likely to be helpful, and this has been highlighted in the area of asthma care. National guidelines issued in 1991 recommend providing a written management plan to patients with asthma (National Asthma Education Program, 1991). This relatively simple procedure has been associated with decreased hospitalization and emergency department visits (Lieu et al., 1997). Drotar et al. (2000) recommended several further health care system efforts, including further study of physician influences to treatment adherence, development and design of programs to improve communication with patients and physicians, and utilization of a multidisciplinary approach to improving adherence and self-care for children with chronic illness. Using technology (i.e., e-mail, Web sites, teleconferencing) to improve adherence and other aspects of adaptation is another area deserving further attention.

FUTURE DIRECTIONS

As can be seen from this review, much is known about factors that promote children's adjustment to acute and chronic medical stressors. Research has effectively demonstrated that modeling and coping skills preparation programs help children cope with hospitalization and surgery. Several family and peer interventions show promise in helping children and adolescents cope with chronic illness, and the profession is beginning to delineate some health care system variables that affect adaptation to illness. This important literature has already had a significant impact on children and adolescents, as pediatric psychologists and other health care professionals use this information on a daily basis to help children involved in the medical system. However, as seen in the surgery preparation literature, effective research approaches do not always translate easily to practice. Clearly, further research on interventions that promote adaptation to chronic illness is warranted, and finding effective ways to translate these programs to daily practice is equally important. Numerous challenges impede easy transfer of methods from researchers to clinicians, including clinician variables (e.g., increased productivity demands, varied caseload, patients with multiple complex issues), health care system variables (e.g., reimbursement issues), and patient factors (e.g., motivation, distance from health care setting). Finding methods to help clinicians use the most effective interventions is clearly an area for further research and policy development. Keeping a developmental focus for all research and clinical programs appears critical.

The health care culture is changing, creating further challenges for patients, clinicians, and researchers. An emphasis on cost-effectiveness is present throughout the health care system, and psychologists need to respond to this reality. Throughout our review, only one study was found that documented the cost-effectiveness of a preventive intervention (Pinto & Hollandsworth, 1989). This study deserves replication and extension in the area of surgery preparation. It may be more difficult to document cost-effectiveness with peer and family interventions. Currently, many of these studies document factors related to the intervention (i.e., family communication, peer support) that are clearly important. However, expanding those measures to include disease-specific symptoms, measures of emotional well-being, and health care costs (e.g., specialty health care, primary health care, and mental health care visits) may be helpful.

Finally, research suggests that hospitalization and chronic illness may be conceptualized as stressors. Many children and adolescents cope successfully with these stressors, whereas other children and their families clearly struggle with the additional demands. Future research aimed at predicting which children and families will benefit from preventive interventions would be helpful. For children experiencing acute stressors, brief measures of anxiety or a short interview may help predict which children and families will require additional or different preparation. For children with chronic illnesses, using a more global measure, such as health-related quality of life, may be most useful (e.g., Varni, La Greca, & Spirito, 2000). Using measures as screening tools to determine which children would benefit from intervention *before* significant problems develop clearly deserves further attention.

REFERENCES

Asher, S., Parkhurst, J., Hymel, S., & Williams, G. (1990). Peer rejection and loneliness in childhood. In S. Asher & J. Coie (Eds.), *Peer rejection in childhood* (pp. 252–273). Cambridge, UK: Cambridge University Press.

Atkins, D. (1987). Evaluation of pediatric preparation program for short-stay surgical patients. *Journal of Pediatric Psychology, 12*, 285–290.

Band, E., & Weisz, J. (1988). How to feel better when it feels bad: Children's perspectives of coping with everyday stress. *Developmental Psychology, 24*, 247–253.

Best, M., Streisand, R., Catania, L., & Kazak, A. (2001). Parental distress during pediatric leukemia and Posttraumatic Stress Symptoms (PTSS) after treatment ends. *Journal of Pediatric Psychology, 26*, 299–307.

Beven, J., Johnston, C., Haig, M., Tounsignant, G., Lucy, S., Kirnon, V., et al. (1990). Pre-operative parental anxiety predicts behavioral and emotional responses to induction of anesthesia in children. *Canadian Journal of Anesthesia, 37*, 177–182.

Blount, R., Landolf-Fritsche, B., Powers, S., & Sturges, J. (1991). Differences between high and low coping children and between parent and staff behaviors during painful medical procedures. *Journal of Pediatric Psychology, 16*, 795–809.

Bradford, R. (1991). Staff accuracy in predicting the concerns of parents of chronically ill children. *Child: Care, Health and Development, 17*, 39–47.

Briery, B., & Rabian, B. (1999). Psychosocial changes associated with participation in a pediatric summer camp. *Journal of Pediatric Psychology, 24*, 183–190.

Brown, J., O'Keeffe, J., Sanders, S., & Baker, B. (1986). Developmental changes in children's cognition to stressful and painful situations. *Journal of Pediatric Psychology, 11*, 343–357.

Burlew, K., Telfair, J., Colagelo, L., & Wright, E. (2000). Factors that influence adolescent adaptation to sickle cell disease. *Journal of Pediatric Psychology, 25*, 287–299.

Burstein, S., & Meichenbaum, D. (1979). The work of worrying in children undergoing surgery. *Journal of Abnormal Child Psychology, 7*, 121–132.

Bush, J., Melamed, B., Sheras, P., & Greenbaum, P. (1986). Mother–child patterns of coping with anticipatory medical stress. *Health Psychology, 5*, 137–157.

Cadman, D., Rosenbaum, P., Boyle, M., & Offord, D. (1991). Children with chronic illness: Family and parent demographic characteristics and psychological adjustment. *Pediatrics, 87*, 884–889.

Campbell, L., Kirkpatrick, S., Berry, C., Penn, N., Waldman, J., & Mathewson, J. (1992). Psychological preparation of mothers of preschool children undergoing cardiac catheterization. *Psychology and Health, 7*, 175–185.

Chambers, C., Reid, G., McGrath, P., Finley, G., & Ellerton, M. (1997). A randomized trial of a pain education booklet: Effects on parents' attitudes and postoperative pain management. *Children's Health Care, 26*, 1–13.

Chen, E., Zeltzer, L., Craske, M., & Katz, E. (1999). Alteration of memory in the reduction of children's distress during repeated aversive medical procedures. *Journal of Consulting and Clinical Psychology, 67*, 481–490.

Christian, B., & D'Auria, J. (1997). The child's eye: Memories of growing up with cystic fibrosis. *Journal of Pediatric Nursing, 12*, 3–12.

Clark, H., Ichinose, C., Meseck-Bushey, S., Perez, K., Hall, M., Gibertini, M., & Crowe, T. (1992). Peer support group for adolescents with chronic illness. *Children's Health Care, 21*, 233–238.

Compas, B., Malcarne, V., & Banez, G. (1992). Coping with psychological stress: A developmental perspective. In B. Carpenter (Ed.), *Personal coping: Theory, research, and application* (pp. 47–64). Westport, CT: Praeger.

Compas, B., Malcarne, V., & Fondacaro, K. (1988). Coping with stressful events in older children and young adolescents. *Journal of Consulting and Clinical Psychology, 56*, 405–411.

Dahlquist, L., Czyzewski, K., Copeland, K., Jones, C., Taub, E., & Vaughan, J. (1993). Parents of children newly diagnosed with cancer: Anxiety, coping, and marital distress. *Journal of Pediatric Psychology, 18*, 365–376.

Drotar, D., Riekert, K., Burgess, E., Levi, R., Nobile, C., Kaugars, A., & Walders, N. (2000). Treatment adherence in childhood chronic illness: Issues and recommendations to enhance practice, research, and training. In D. Drotar (Ed.), *Promoting adherence to medical treatment in chronic childhood illness* (pp. 455–476). Mahwah, NJ: Erlbaum.

Edwinson, M., Arnbjornsson, E., & Ekman, R. (1988). Psychologic preparation program for children undergoing acute appendectomy. *Pediatrics, 82*, 30–36.

Ellerton, M., & Merriam, C. (1994). Preparing children and families psychologically for day surgery: An evaluation. *Journal of Advanced Nursing, 19*, 1057–1062.

Farmer, J., & Peterson, L. (1995). Pediatric traumatic brain injury: Promoting successful school re-entry. *School Psychology Review, 24*, 230–243.

Faust, J., Olson, R., & Rodriguez, H. (1991). Same-day surgery preparation: Reduction of pediatric patient arousal and distress through participant modeling. *Journal of Consulting and Clinical Psychology, 59*, 475–478.

Field, T., Alpert, B., Vega-Lahr, N., Goldstein, S., & Perry, S. (1988). Hospitalization stress in children: Sensitizer and repressor coping styles. *Health Psychology, 7*, 433–445.

Garrison, W., & McQuiston, S. (1989). *Chronic illness during childhood and adolescence: Psychological aspects.* Newbury Park, CA: Sage.

Glazebrook, C., Lim, E., Sheard, C., & Standen, P. (1994). Child temperament and reaction to induction of anesthesia: Implications for maternal presence in the anaesthetic room. *Psychology and Health, 10*, 55–67.

Greco, P., Pendley, J., McDonnell, K., & Reeves, G. (2001). A peer group intervention for adolescents with type I diabetes and their best friends. *Journal of Pediatric Psychology, 26*, 485–490.

Grover, G., Berkowitz, C., & Lewis, R. (1994). Parental recall after a visit to the emergency room. *Clinical Pediatrics, 33*, 194–201.

Hanson, C., Cigrang, J., Harris, M., Carle, D., Relyea, G., & Burghen, G. (1989). Coping styles in youths with insulin-dependent diabetes mellitus. *Journal of Consulting and Clinical Psychology, 57*, 644–651.

Hanson, C., DeGuire, M., Schinkel, A., Henggeler, S., & Burghen, G. (1992). Comparing social learning and family systems correlates of adaptation in youths with IDDM. *Journal of Pediatric Psychology, 17*, 555–572.

Hanson, C., Henggeler, S., Harris, M., Burghen, G., & Moore, M. (1989). Family system variables and the health status of adolescents with insulin-dependent diabetes mellitus. *Health Psychology, 8*, 239–253.

Harbeck-Weber, C., & Peterson, L. (1993). Children's conceptions of illness and pain. In R. Vasta (Ed.), *Annals of child development* (pp. 133–162). Bristol, PA: Jessica Kingsley.

Hardgrove, C. (1980). Helping parents on the pediatric ward: A report on a survey of hospitals with "Living-In" programs. *Paediatrician, 9*, 220–223.

Harris, P., & Lipian, M. (1989). Understanding emotion and experiencing emotion. In C. Saarni & P. Harris (Eds.), *Children's understanding of emotion* (pp. 241–258). New York: Cambridge University Press.

Hatava, P., Olsson, G., & Lagerkranser, M. (2000). Preoperative psychological preparation for children undergoing ENT operations: A comparison of two methods. *Paediatric Anaesthesia, 10*, 477–486.

Hoekstra-Weebers, J., Jaspers, J., Kamps, W., & Klip, E. (2001). Psychological adaptation and social support of parents of pediatric cancer patients: A prospective longitudinal study. *Journal of Pediatric Psychology, 26*, 225–235.

Holden, G., Bearison, D., Rode, D., Kapliloff, M., & Rosenberg, G. (2000). The effects of a computer network on pediatric pain and anxiety. *Journal of Technology in Human Services, 17*, 27–47.

Holden, G., Bearison, D., Rode, D., Rosenberg, G., & Fishman, M. (1999). Evaluating the effects of a virtual environment (STARBRIGHT World) with hospitalized children. *Research on Social Work Practice, 9*, 365–382.

Ievers, C., Brown, R., Drotar, D., Caplan, D., Pishevar, B., & Lambert, R. (1999). Knowledge of physician prescriptions and adherence to treatment among children with cystic fibrosis and their mothers. *Developmental and Behavioral Pediatrics, 20*, 335–343.

Individuals with Disabilities Education Act Amendments of 1997, H.R. 5, 105th Congress (1997).

Kain, Z., Mayes, L., O'Connor, T., & Cicchetti, D. (1994). Preoperative anxiety in children: Predictors and outcomes. *Archives of Pediatrics and Adolescent Medicine, 150*, 1238–1245.

Kazak, A., Stuber, M., Barakat, L., Meeske, K., Guthrie, D., & Meadows, A. (1998). Predicting posttraumatic stress symptoms in mothers and fathers of survivors of childhood cancers. *Journal of the American Academy of Child and Adolescent Psychiatry, 37*, 823–831.

Kell, R., Kliewer, W., Erickson, M., & Ohene-Frempong, K. (1998). Psychological adjustment of adolescents with sickle cell disease: Relations with demographic, medical, and family competence variables. *Journal of Pediatric Psychology, 23*, 301–312.

Kliewer, W. (1997). Children's coping with chronic illness. In S. Wolchik & I. Sandler (Eds.), *Handbook of children's coping: Linking theory and intervention* (pp. 275–300). New York: Plenum Press.

Kliewer, W., Sandler, I., & Wolchik, S. (1994). Family socialization of threat appraisal and coping: Coaching, modeling, and family context. In K. Hurrelmann & F. Festmann (Eds.), *Social networks and social support in childhood and adolescence* (pp. 271–291). Berlin, Germany: de Gruyter.

Klingman, A., Melamed, B., Cuthbert, M., & Hermecz, D. (1984). Effects of participant modeling on information acquisition and skill utilization. *Journal of Consulting and Clinical Psychology, 52*, 414–422.

Knight, R., Atkins, A., Eagle, C., Evans, N., Finkelstein, J., Fukushima, D., et al. (1979). Psychological stress, ego defenses, and cortisol production in children hospitalized for elective surgery. *Psychosomatic Medicine, 41*, 40–49.

Kupersmidt, J., Coie, J., & Dodge, K. (1990). The role of poor peer relationships in the development of disorder. In S. Asher & J. Coie (Eds.), *Peer rejection in childhood* (pp. 274–305). Cambridge, UK: Cambridge University Press.

La Greca, A. M., Auslander, W. F., Greco, P., Spetter, D., Fisher, E. B., Jr., & Santiago, J. V. (1995). I get by with a little help from my family and friends: Adolescents' support for diabetes care. *Journal of Pediatric Psychology, 20*, 449–476.

Lazarus, R., & Folkman, S. (1984). *Stress, appraisal, and coping*. New York: Springer.

Lieu, T., Quesenberry, C., Capra, A., Sorel, M., Martin, K., & Mendoza, G. (1997). Outpatient management practices associated with reduced risk of pediatric asthma hospitalization and emergency department visits. *Pediatrics, 100*, 334–341.

Liptak, G., & Revell, G. (1989). Community physicians' role in case management of children with chronic illnesses. *Pediatrics, 84*, 465–471.

Lumley, M., Melamed, B., & Abeles, L. (1993). Predicting children's presurgical anxiety and subsequent behavior changes. *Journal of Pediatric Psychology, 18*, 481–497.

Madan-Swain, A., Fredrick, L., & Wallander, J. (1999). Returning to school after a serious illness or injury. In R. Brown (Ed.), *Cognitive aspects of chronic illness in children* (pp. 312–332). New York: Guilford Press.

Mahajan, L., Wyllie, R., Steffen, R., Kay, M., Kitaoka, G., Dettorre, J., et al. (1998). The effects of a psychological preparation program on anxiety in children and adolescents undergoing gastrointestinal endoscopy. *Journal of Pediatric Gastroenterology and Nutrition, 27*, 161–165.

Mansson, M., Fredrikzon, B., & Rosberg, B. (1992). Comparison of preparation and narcotic-sedative premedication in children undergoing surgery. *Pediatric Nursing, 18*, 337–342.

Margolis, J., Ginsberg, B., Dear, G., Ross, A., Goral, J., & Bailey, A. (1998). Paediatric preoperative teaching: Effects at induction and postoperatively. *Paediatric Anaesthesia, 8*, 17–23.

Melamed, B. (1992). Family factors predicting children's reaction to anesthesia induction. In A. M. La Greca, L. J. Siegel, J. L. Wallander, & C. E. Walker (Eds.), *Stress and coping in child health* (pp. 140–156). New York: Guilford Press.

Melamed, B. (1998). Preparation for medical procedures. In R. Ammerman & J. Campo (Eds.), *Handbook of pediatric psychology and psychiatry: Disease, injury and illness* (Vol. 2, pp. 16–30). Boston: Allyn & Bacon.

Melamed, B., Dearborn, M., & Hermecz, D. (1983). Necessary considerations for surgery preparation: Age and previous experience. *Psychosomatic Medicine, 45*, 517–525.

Melamed, B., & Siegel, L. (1975). Reduction of anxiety in children facing hospitalization and surgery by use of filmed modeling. *Journal of Consulting and Clinical Psychology, 43*, 511–521.

National Asthma Education Program. (1991). *Guidelines for the diagnosis and management of asthma*. Bethesda, MD: U.S. Department of Health and Human Services, National Institutes of Health.

Newacheck, P., Strickland, B., Shonkoff, J., Perrin, J., McPherson, M., McManus, M., et al. (1998). An epidemiologic profile of children with special health care needs. *Pediatrics, 102*(1, Pt. 1), 117–123.

Novakovic, B., Fears, T., Wexler, L., McClure, L., Wilson, D., McCalla, J., & Tucker, M. (1996). Experiences of cancer in children and adolescents. *Cancer Nursing, 19,* 54–59.

O'Byrne, K., Peterson, L., & Saldana, L. (1997). Survey of pediatric hospitals' preparation programs: Evidence of the impact of health psychology research. *Health Psychology, 16,* 147–154.

Page, P., Verstraete, D., Robb, J., & Etzwiler, D. (1981). Patient recall of self-care recommendations in diabetes. *Diabetes Care, 4,* 96–98.

Palermo, T., & Drotar, D. (1999). Coping with pediatric ambulatory surgery: Effectiveness of parent-implemented behavioral distraction strategies. *Behavior Therapy, 30,* 657–671.

Palermo, T., Drotar, D., & Tripi, P. (1999). Current status of psychosocial intervention research for pediatric outpatient surgery. *Journal of Clinical Psychology in Medical Settings, 6,* 405–426.

Parker, J., & Asher, S. (1987). Peer relations and later personal adjustment: Are low-accepted children at risk? *Psychological Bulletin, 102,* 357–389.

Pate, J., Blount, R., Cohen, L., & Smith, A. (1996). Childhood medical experience and temperament as predictors of adult functioning in medical situations. *Children's Health Care, 25,* 281–298.

Peterson, L., Oliver, K., & Saldana, L. (1997). Children's coping with stressful medical procedures. In S. Wolchik & I. Sandler (Eds.), *Handbook of children's coping: Linking theory and intervention* (pp. 333–360). New York: Plenum Press.

Peterson, L., Ridley-Johnson, R., Tracy, K., & Mullins, L. (1984). Developing cost-effective presurgical preparation: A comparative analysis. *Journal of Pediatric Psychology, 9,* 439–455.

Peterson, L., Schultheis, K., Ridley-Johnson, R., Miller, D., & Tracy, K. (1984). Comparison of three modeling procedures on the presurgical and postsurgical reactions of children. *Behavior Therapy, 15,* 197–203.

Peterson, L., & Shigetomi, C. (1981). The use of coping techniques to minimize anxiety in hospitalized children. *Behavior Therapy, 12,* 1–14.

Peterson, L., & Toler, S. (1986). An information seeking disposition in child surgery patients. *Health Psychology, 5,* 343–358.

Pidgeon, V. (1981). Children's concepts of illness: Implications for health teaching. *Maternal–Child Nursing Journal, 14,* 23–35.

Pinto, R., & Hollandsworth, J., Jr. (1989). Using videotape modeling to prepare children psychologically for surgery: Influence of parents and costs versus benefits of providing preparation services. *Health Psychology, 8,* 79–95.

Plante, W., Lobato, D., & Engel, R. (2001). Review of group interventions for pediatric chronic conditions. *Journal of Pediatric Psychology, 26,* 435–453.

Popovic, J., & Hall, M. (2001). *1999 National Hospital Discharge Survey.* Hyattsville, MD: National Center for Health Statistics.

Rasnake, L., & Linscheid, T. (1989). Anxiety reduction in children receiving medical care: Developmental considerations. *Journal of Developmental and Behavioral Pediatrics, 10,* 169–175.

Redpath, C., & Rogers, C. (1984). Healthy young children's concepts of hospitals, medical personnel, operations, and illness. *Journal of Pediatric Psychology, 9,* 29–40.

Ross, C., Lavigne, J., Hayford, J., Berry, S., Sinacore, J., & Packman, L. (1993). Psychological factors affecting reported pain in juvenile rheumatoid arthritis. *Journal of Pediatric Psychology, 18,* 561–573.

Rothbaum, F., Weisz, J. R., & Snyder, S. S. (1982). Changing the world and changing the self: A two-process model of perceived control. *Journal of Personality and Social Psychology, 42,* 5–37.

Sanders, M., Shepherd, R., Cleghorn, G., & Woolford, H. (1994). The treatment of recurrent abdominal pain in children: A controlled comparison of cognitive-behavioral family intervention and standard pediatric care. *Journal of Consulting and Clinical Psychology, 62,* 306–314.

Satin, W., La Greca, A., Zigo, M., & Skyler, J. (1989). Diabetes in adolescence: Effects of multifamily group intervention and parent simulation of diabetes. *Journal of Pediatric Psychology, 14,* 259–275.

Seagull, E. (2000). Beyond mothers and children: Finding the family in pediatric psychology. *Journal of Pediatric Psychology, 25,* 161–169.

Seiffge-Krenke, I. (1998). The highly structured climate in families of adolescents with diabetes: Functional or dysfunctional for metabolic control? *Journal of Pediatric Psychology, 23,* 313–322.

Skinner, T., John, M., & Hampson, S. (2000). Social support and personal models of diabetes as predictors of self-care and well-being: A longitudinal study of adolescents with diabetes. *Journal of Pediatric Psychology, 25,* 257–267.

Sloper, P. (2000). Predictors of distress in parents of children with cancer: A prospective study. *Journal of Pediatric Psychology, 25,* 79–91.

Steward, M. (1993). Understanding children's memories of medical procedures: "He didn't touch me and it didn't hurt." In C. A. Nelson (Ed.), *The Minnesota Symposia on Child Psychology* (Vol. 26, pp. 171–225). Hillsdale, NJ: Erlbaum.

Thomas, A., Peterson, L., & Goldstein, D. (1997). Problem solving and diabetes regimen adherence by children and adolescents with IDDM in social pressure situations: A reflection of normal development. *Journal of Pediatric Psychology, 22,* 541–561.

Thompson, R., Jr., Armstrong, F., Kronenberger, W., Scott, D., McCabe, M., Smith, B., et al. (1999). Family functioning, neurocognitive functioning, and behavior problems in children with sickle cell disease. *Journal of Pediatric Psychology, 24,* 491–498.

Thompson, R. J., Jr., & Gustafson, K. (1996). *Adaptation to chronic childhood illness.* Washington, DC: American Psychological Association.

Thompson, R., Jr., Gustafson, K., Hamlett, K., & Spock, A. (1992). Psychological adjustment of children with cystic fibrosis: The role of child cognitive processes and maternal adjustment. *Journal of Pediatric Psychology, 17,* 741–755.

Thompson R., Jr., Zeman, J., Fanurik, D., & Sirotkin-Roses, M. (1992). The role of parent stress and coping and family functioning in parent and child adjustment to Duchenne muscular dystrophy. *Journal of Clinical Psychology, 48,* 11–19.

Varni, J., & Katz, E. (1997). Stress, social support and negative affectivity in children with newly diagnosed cancer: A prospective transactional analysis. *Psycho-Oncology, 6,* 267–278.

Varni, J., Katz, E., Colegrove, R., Jr., & Dolgin, M. (1993). The impact of social skills training on the adjustment of children with newly diagnosed cancer. *Journal of Pediatric Psychology, 18,* 751–767.

Varni, J., La Greca, A., & Spirito, A. (2000). Cognitive-behavioral interventions for children with chronic health conditions. In P. C. Kendall (Ed.), *Child and adolescent therapy: Cognitive-behavioral procedures* (2nd ed., pp. 291–333). New York: Guilford Press.

Wallander, J., & Thompson, R., Jr. (1995). Psychosocial adjustment of children with chronic physical conditions. In M. C. Roberts (Ed.), *Handbook of pediatric psychology* (2nd ed., pp. 124–141). New York: Guilford Press.

Wallander, J., Varni, J., Babani, L., Banis, H., DeHaan, C., & Wilcox, K. (1989). Disability parameters, chronic strain, and adaptation of physically handicapped children and their mothers. *Journal of Pediatric Psychology, 14,* 23–42.

Wallander, J., Varni, J., Babani, L., Banis, H., & Wilcox, K. (1989). Family resources as resistance factors for psychological maladjustment in chronically ill and handicapped children. *Journal of Pediatric Psychology, 14,* 157–173.

Weisz, J., McCabe, M., & Dennig, M. (1994). Primary and secondary control among children undergoing medical procedures: Adjustment as a function of coping style. *Journal of Consulting and Clinical Psychology, 62,* 324–332.

Wolfer, J., & Visintainer, M. (1975). Pediatric surgery patients' and parents' stress responses and adjustment. *Nursing Research, 24,* 244–255.

Worchel-Prevatt, F., Heffer, R., Prevatt, B., Miner, J., Young-Saleme, T., Horgan, D., et al. (1998). A school re-entry program for chronically ill children. *Journal of School Psychology, 36,* 261–279.

Wysocki, T., Harris, M., Greco, P., Bubb, J., Danda, C., Harvey, L., et al. (2000). Randomized, controlled trial of behavior therapy for families of adolescents with insulin-dependent diabetes mellitus. *Journal of Pediatric Psychology, 25,* 23–33.

Zastowny, T., Kirschenbaum, D., & Meng, A. (1986). Coping skills training for children: Effects on distress before, during, and after hospitalization for surgery. *Health Psychology, 5,* 231–247.

8

Adherence to Pediatric Treatment Regimens

ANNETTE M. LA GRECA
KAREN J. BEARMAN

Adherence to pediatric treatment regimens is a major health concern. Estimates suggest that the overall treatment adherence rate for pediatric populations is about 50% (Litt & Cuskey, 1980), although rates of noncompliance may be substantially higher for chronic conditions (Rapoff, 1999).

Adherence is a complex issue, and several considerations are important. First, although health providers may view complete adherence as desirable, it is important to adopt a realistic family perspective in trying to understand youngsters' health behaviors. This means giving up the notion that the "doctor knows best" and that adaptive patient behavior means complying fully with medical recommendations, regardless of their effectiveness, cost, inconvenience, or discomfort. In many cases, complete adherence does not guarantee symptom relief or illness recovery, even for acute illnesses (Mattar, Markello, & Yaffe, 1975). For chronic illnesses requiring complex management skills, the relationship between adherence and disease control is modest at best (e.g., Johnson, 1994). Faced with an inexact medical science, families must decide how to balance health care needs with efforts to achieve normal social and emotional functioning for their child. When viewed from this perspective, problems with adherence may represent reasoned decision making (Donovan & Blake, 1992) or "adaptive noncompliance" (Deaton, 1985). Thus, to understand adherence, it is critical to view the child and family as active participants in the medical decision-making process.

A second consideration is that, with few exceptions, studies have examined adherence at one time point in the context of an ongoing disease. Little attention has been devoted to the *process* of disease management, despite the fact that adherence declines over time for those with acute or chronic conditions (Rapoff, 1999). A child's and family's history of adherence and the effects of their behaviors on health status are likely to be important determinants of disease management.

A final consideration is the complexity of understanding and predicting adherence behavior. Although several models for conceptualizing health care behaviors are discussed briefly in this chapter, most of the research on pediatric adherence has been atheoretical. Further attention to model development will be essential for further progress in the field. Even though the complexity of managing various diseases and the varied challenges faced by youngsters at different developmental stages may preclude the establishment of one all-encompassing model, conceptual frameworks are needed to guide research and intervention efforts.

This chapter addresses some of the complexities of pediatric adherence. Specifically, it reviews the definition and measurement of adherence, the variables associated with adherence, conceptual models of adherence, and interventions to improve pediatric treatment adherence.

DEFINITION AND MEASUREMENT ISSUES

Definitions of Adherence

Investigators have used widely divergent definitions of adherence, even for the same illness or regimen. In addition, the terms "adherence" and "compliance" have been used interchangeably.

Most measures of adherence do not measure a person's behavior *in relation to a prescribed medical regimen* (La Greca, 1990a), and, in fact, different regimens may be prescribed for the same disease. Because of these complications, some investigators have examined adherence in relation to an *ideal* regimen (e.g., Johnson, Silverstein, Rosenbloom, Carter, & Cunningham, 1986), or have measured the frequency of health behaviors without making comparisons to standards or prescriptions (e.g., Davis et al., 2001). In the latter case, the term "self-care behavior" has been used in lieu of "adherence" (see Rapoff, 1999).

Operational definitions tend to view adherence as: (1) categorical versus continuous and (2) unitary versus multidimensional. Using a *categorical* approach, researchers may specify criteria for successful adherence and then use the criteria to define groups of "adherent" and "nonadherent" patients (e.g., Phipps & DeCuir-Whalley, 1990) or to define patients with "good," "moderate," and "poor" adherence (e.g., Dolgin, Katz, Doctors, & Siegel, 1986). The categorical approach often has been used for initial investigations of adherence in pediatric populations; however, a limitation of this approach is the arbitrary nature of the cutoff criteria. It is not known what constitutes adequate adherence for most medical problems. A further drawback is that the nonstandard use of cutoff scores makes it difficult to compare adherence levels across studies, across different aspects of a regimen, or across different diseases (La Greca, 1990a).

For chronic regimens with multiple treatment tasks, a related approach has involved *combining multiple indicators* (e.g., taking medication, completing self-monitoring forms) into an index of overall adherence (e.g., Becker, Drachman, & Kirscht, 1972). Although this takes into account the multiple aspects of a treatment regimen, such decision rules lack scientific rigor and mask the significance of individual adherence behaviors. The behaviors selected for inclusion in the "index" may vary tremendously in therapeutic importance.

More recent studies have examined adherence on a *continuum* and also consider adherence to be *multidimensional*. For example, adherence rates have been computed by dividing the number of adherence behaviors completed by the number prescribed, doing this for multiple tasks (e.g., Carney, Schechter, & Davis, 1983). Interviews or self-reports have also been used to obtain an index of adherence for multiple aspects of a regimen (e.g., Hanson, DeGuire, Schinkel, & Kolterman, 1995; Johnson et al., 1992). This approach allows a comparison of adherence levels across different behaviors and pediatric conditions but does not address the *relative* importance of some health behaviors compared with others.

Methods for Measuring Adherence

Perhaps the single most difficult question confronting pediatric researchers is how to measure adherence (La Greca, 1990a), as measures are diverse and each has its advantages and limitations. In addition, most methods overestimate adherence, although some do so more than others. In fact, it is difficult to obtain *any* assessment of adherence from the most nonadherent youngsters, as they may refuse to comply with the requirements of the assessment method (e.g., completing diaries).

Several considerations are important in selecting a measure. First, measures that are appropriate for short-term regimens (e.g., pill counts) may not be appropriate for chronic diseases with complex regimens. Regimens that involve multiple, complex behaviors may need a variety of strategies for comprehensive assessment. Second, many measures focus on self-care behaviors without regard for how well the behaviors match the prescribed treatment. In such cases, an assessment of the prescribed regimen may be useful (both from patients' and providers' perspectives) to determine the extent to which patients' behaviors correspond to medical recommendations. What appears to be "nonadherent behavior" may reflect the patient's inaccurate knowledge of the regimen or the provider's inexact specification of the desired behaviors. Finally, it is important to recognize that adherence behaviors and *health outcomes* are not synonymous. Although health outcomes are important for evaluating the impact of adherence on health, medical treatments are largely based on patients' *typical* response to a regimen and do not take into account individual variability and responsiveness to treatment (Dunbar, 1983). Furthermore, in most cases, a high correspondence between adherence and health outcome is lacking. For example, Johnson (1994) found that more than one-third of the youngsters with "good" adherence to a diabetes regimen had poor metabolic control (a measure of health status) and that about one-third of those with "poor" adherence had good disease control. This underscores the point that health status and adherence are not interchangeable. Nevertheless, health outcome measures are important to evaluate a treatment's efficacy. Negative outcomes, in the presence of good adherence, may help to detect ineffective regimens.

Drug Assays

Assays are one of the most direct, objective, reliable, and easily quantifiable methods for assessing adherence. Assays typically involve obtaining blood, urine, or saliva samples to determine the presence or concentration of a particular drug that has been prescribed. Drug assays are best for evaluating adherence to short-term medication regimens, provided that the medication can be traced via an assay and that the cost of the assay is not prohibitive. Unfortunately, many regimens cannot be monitored by an assay. Another problem is that, even when assays are financially feasible, they generally assess adherence over relatively short time periods and thus can be misleading. For instance, assays may overestimate adherence in youngsters who are generally nonadherent but who take their medications just prior to testing. The results obtained from drug assays also may be affected by individual variability in drug absorption rates (see Lemanek, 1990).

Self-Reports

Child, adolescent, and parent reports are frequently used for assessing adherence, as they are easy and inexpensive to obtain and can assess a complex array of behaviors (e.g., amount and timing of meals, frequency and duration of exercise). As a result, self-reports have been widely used for evaluating adherence to complex regimens (e.g., Davis et al., 2001; Kovacs, Goldston, Obrosky, & Iyengar, 1992). Self-reports are more accurate when recall periods are kept to a minimum and detailed objective questions are asked. As an example, patients' recall over the previous 24 hours will be more accurate than for extended, retrospective time periods. In fact, researchers have developed a 24-hour recall interview for assessing adherence to chronic disease regimens, such as for diabetes (e.g., Freund, Johnson, Silverstein, & Thomas, 1991; Johnson et al., 1986). Typically, children and parents are separately interviewed, often by phone, regarding daily regimen tasks; two to three assessments may be averaged to estimate adherence over an extended time period. The 24-hour recall method has good reliability and good correspondence with observations of heath behaviors and self-reports (Johnson et al., 1986). The main drawback is the labor-intensive nature of data collection and scoring. Although self-reports have been useful for detecting nonadherent children and families (e.g., Gordis, Markowitz, & Lilienfeld, 1969), they may be influenced by social desirability and tend to overestimate adherence (Rapoff, 1999).

Ratings by Health Professionals

Ratings by health care providers have been used to assess adherence (e.g., Dolgin et al., 1986; La Greca, Follansbee, & Skyler, 1990). Because physician estimates are based, in part, on information provided by children and families, they are subject to the same biases and limitations as self-reports. Additional concerns with provider ratings include the influence of or confusion with other information (e.g., history of disease, cooperation with medical staff) or with health status as indicators of adherence (La Greca, 1990a). Nonetheless, health care providers see a wide range of patients and may detect extremes in adherence. In addition, providers' impressions of adherence are of interest, as they may lead to adjustments in youngsters' regimens.

Behavioral Observations

Observations, typically in the form of self-monitoring of adherence tasks via daily diaries, appear to be an improvement over verbal reports. Observations have been used to assess adherence with medications and with multicomponent regimens (e.g., Baum & Creer, 1986). In some studies (e.g., Wilson & Endres, 1986) children were asked to keep daily records that were checked for accuracy by family members or metering devices. Although self-monitoring is an improvement over verbal reports, parents and children have been found to misrepresent adherence behaviors. For example, some youngsters fabricate records or test results (Wilson & Endres, 1986) or complete daily records just prior to bringing them into the medical setting. Another drawback is the intensive effort self-monitoring requires. Children who do not comply with medical recommendations often do not provide *any* monitoring information (Chaney & Peterson, 1989).

Pill Counts

Pill counts are useful for assessing medication regimens. Pill counts compare the amount of medication remaining in a container with the amount that would be left if the patient consumed all that was prescribed. Pill counts are more accurate and reliable than verbal self-reports (Epstein & Cluss, 1982), although they may overestimate adherence (e.g., youngsters may remove some pills but not ingest them). Moreover, pill counts cannot track other behaviors related to medication usage, such as the time of ingestion or the administration of the proper dose.

Monitoring Devices

Recent advances in technology have improved the accuracy and reliability of the data obtained from daily monitoring activities or pill counts. For instance, glucose reflectance meters for evaluating daily blood samples in youngsters with diabetes can be equipped with memory chips to record the date, time, and results of glucose testing (Wilson & Endres, 1986). In addition, the Medication Event Monitor System embeds a microprocessor in a standard medication vial cap to record the date and time of vial openings and closings (Cramer, 1995). The main drawback to such devices is their cost; however, further advances in monitoring devices, with accompanying reductions in cost, will likely make such devices commonplace in the near future.

VARIABLES THAT AFFECT ADHERENCE

Multiple variables affect medical adherence. This section reviews four major areas related to pediatric adherence: (1) developmental issues, (2) characteristics of the child and family, (3) characteristics of the health care system, and (4) characteristics of the disease or regimen. In addition, conceptual models of adherence are discussed.

Developmental Issues

In general, demographic variables, such as race, gender, religion, and educational level, have not been consistent predictors of adherence in pediatric populations (Cromer & Tarnowski, 1989; Lemanek, 1990). However, developmental variables (e.g., cognitive, motor, social, emotional, and physiological functioning) have been consistently linked to adherence. Developmental status, as indexed by chronological age, is critical for understanding children's reactions to physical illness, their involvement in disease management, and the types of interventions that may be most effective. Despite its importance, a developmental perspective has been neglected in adherence research.

Age

Adolescents usually have more difficulties with adherence than children do (Brownbridge & Fielding, 1994; Kovacs et al., 1992). Specifically, adolescents have difficulty managing regimens that require major lifestyle adjustments (e.g., dietary restrictions, exercise) or have cosmetic side effects or that interfere with social interactions (La Greca, 1990b). However, adolescents may be *more* adherent than younger children with invasive and aversive treatments such as bone marrow aspirations (Phipps & DeCuir-Whalley, 1990). In general, little is known about the mechanisms that link age and adherence. When adolescents show poor adherence, a common interpretation is that the turmoil of this developmental period contributes to teens' rebellion and problems with parental and medical authority (La Greca, 1990a), although studies have not documented that poorly adhering teens are in fact high on measures of rebellion or have "authority" issues. Furthermore, other competing factors, such as decreased levels of parental support and treatment involvement (La Greca et al., 1995), might contribute to the adherence problems observed during adolescence. However, alternative mechanisms such as these have not been well studied.

Social and Emotional Development

Children's social and emotional development is another important consideration (La Greca, 1990b). Generally, children progress from a state of dependent, close attachment to parents during infancy and the preschool years to an expanding awareness of and desire for friendships during the elementary school years to a preoccupation with peer acceptance and personal independence during adolescence. These varying social and emotional needs can have a dramatic effect on disease management. Some adolescents neglect their medical care to avoid appearing different from peers, and this may be particularly true for treatments that produce undesirable cosmetic effects (e.g., Korsch, Fine, & Negrete, 1978). Efforts to improve adolescents' adherence may need to address ways of coping with peer pressure and social demands while adhering to the regimen (e.g., Gross, Johnson, Wildman, & Mullett, 1981).

Responsibility

Responsibility for disease management varies greatly as a function of youngsters' age and developmental level. Family members assume the major responsibility for implementing the medical regimen for young children and preadolescents (e.g., Anderson, Auslander, Jung, Miller, & Santiago, 1990; La Greca et al., 1990); however, even for adolescents, parental involvement may remain high for certain aspects of treatment, such as meal planning (e.g., La Greca et al., 1990). To understand adherence, one needs to know *who* assumes responsibility for various aspects of medical care or *how* that responsibility is shared within the family (e.g., Anderson et al., 1990).

When family members are involved in treatment, it is usually the mother (or primary caretaker) who assumes substantial responsibility for implementing the regimen. More information on the ways that other family members support or hinder these efforts would be of interest.

Biological Development

Developmental variables also influence disease management from a biological perspective. Certain diseases are more difficult to control during periods of rapid growth and metabolic fluctuation (Bennett & Ward, 1977). For example, puberty is associated with a marked decrease in insulin sensitivity; thus adolescents with diabetes need to have their insulin needs reevaluated and appropriate changes made to their treatment regimens. Puberty also changes the distribution of body fat and muscle mass, which in turn can affect drug absorption rates (Brooks-Gunn & Graber, 1994). These biological variables are important to consider in prescribing regimens; if the regimen is ineffective, adolescents may disengage entirely from self-care efforts.

Child and Family Characteristics

Characteristics of the child and family (e.g., disease knowledge, adjustment) are important for understanding adherence. Efforts to improve adherence behaviors have often focused on ways to change or improve these characteristics (e.g., increasing knowledge or enhancing social support).

Knowledge and Problem Solving

Youngsters' and families' understanding of a disease and their active knowledge of how to manage the disease are important for adherence. Active knowledge of a disease goes beyond basic understanding of the illness process and includes an accurate understanding of the tasks that constitute successful treatment management and the ability to execute such tasks accurately and to make adjustments when problems arise. Disease knowledge and skills are especially important for complex disease regimens. For young children, *parents'* disease knowledge and management skills may be important because of their active involvement in their youngsters' treatment regimens. For instance, among children with PKU, Fehrenbach and Peterson (1989) found that parents' problem-solving skills were positively related to their child's adherence. On the other hand, *children's* disease knowledge and skills are critical when they are responsible for disease management. Lorenz, Christensen, and Pichert (1985) found that diet-related knowledge and skill predicted dietary adherence among youngsters with diabetes.

Relationships among knowledge, problem solving, and adherence may change over time. La Greca and colleagues (1990) found that *maternal* knowledge was a significant predictor of diabetes adherence for preadolescent children, but not for adolescents; however, *adolescents'* knowledge significantly predicted their own level of adherence with diabetes care. Based on these findings, further consideration of children's and parents' knowledge and problem-solving skills is of interest.

Psychosocial Adjustment

Most pediatric problems affect heterogeneous groups of youngsters, with tremendous variability in their coping styles and adjustment. Because of this, numerous studies have examined linkages between youngsters' emotional functioning and their adherence and disease adaptation. This body of work is primarily cross-sectional in nature, highlighting linkages between youngsters' adaptation and adherence without clarifying causal relationships. A common *assumption* is that youngsters' psychosocial functioning influences their disease management.

In general, positive psychosocial adaptation has been associated with good treatment adherence, particularly for youngsters with chronic disease. For example, more highly adherent youngsters have been found to have better self-esteem (Littlefield et al., 1992), less anxiety and depression (Brownbridge & Fielding, 1994), and more adaptive coping styles (Jacobson et al., 1990). In contrast, youngsters with serious emotional difficulties often have problems with treatment adherence. Kovacs et al. (1992) followed children and adolescents for 9 years after their initial diagnosis of diabetes, finding that serious noncompliance was associated with having a major psychiatric disorder. Others have found behavioral and emotional problems to be related to poor disease control for youngsters with diabetes (see Rubin & Peyrot, 1992) or asthma (Rubin, Bauman, & Lauby, 1989).

Family Support and Conflict

Families play a critical role in the medical management of children and adolescents. Furthermore, the degree to which family members cope with and adjust to children's or adolescents' illness may influence adherence. In particular, research has highlighted the importance of social support for successful adaptation and disease management (Burroughs, Harris, Pontious, & Santiago, 1997). Parents represent a primary source of support for children (Cauce, Reid, Landesman, & Gonzales, 1990), and the types of parental support youngsters receive are predominantly instrumental (e.g., tangible assistance and resources) and emotional (e.g., acceptance, praise). Parents and family members who provide more support for diabetes care have been found to have adolescents who are more adherent with their regimens (La Greca et al., 1995; La Greca & Bearman, 2002). One of the challenges facing parents is finding ways to remain supportive and involved in their youngsters' treatment, while also encouraging adolescents' increased self-responsibility for health care (La Greca et al., 1995).

Although family support may be beneficial, adherence problems are likely to arise in families affected by stress and conflict. Management of pediatric conditions can be challenging, and a child's medical treatment may disrupt the entire family's routine and lifestyle (La Greca, 1998). Regimens requiring dietary modifications, such as those for hypertension, PKU, diabetes, and obesity, can alter family eating habits. Other medical protocols may require frequent hospital-based treatments, as is the case with renal dialysis or chemotherapy, or unexpected emergency room visits, as can occur with asthma, sickle cell disease, or seizure disorders. Such treatments interfere with the family's routine and may be barriers to adherence. Because the family is always critical for pediatric health care, problems with adherence are almost certain to emerge when a child develops an illness within the context of a dysfunctional family. Numerous studies have found an inverse relationship between family conflict and youngsters' adherence (e.g., Hauser et al., 1990).

Individual Differences in Biological Functioning

Although they are understudied, individual variability in physiological functioning and responsiveness to medical interventions are also important for adherence. For example, the therapeutic dose for chemotherapy treatment is determined by its *typical* effect, yet marked variability in the frequency and magnitude of aversive side effects, such as nausea and vomiting, have been observed (Barofsky, 1984). Variable response to treatment may affect children and adolescents' motivation to follow through with a prescribed regimen.

The Health Care System

In comparison with research on the child and family, relatively little attention has been devoted to the influence of the health care system on adherence. Yet, with recent, major changes in health care delivery, it becomes critical to understand how the health care system can affect children's and families' participation and cooperation in their medical treatment.

Personal and Contextual Aspects of the Health Care Setting

Certain aspects of the doctor–patient relationship have been linked with adherence. Parents are more likely to adhere to medical recommendations for their youngsters when they are satisfied with the medical care provided (e.g., Cromer & Tarnowski, 1989; Litt & Cuskey, 1984). Other personal variables important for adherence include doctor–patient rapport and perceptions of the medical provider as friendly, warm, empathic, and supportive (e.g., Francis, Korsch, & Morris, 1969; Litt & Cuskey, 1980). A survey of mothers' and professionals' ratings of strategies to enhance families' participation in an intervention program for special-needs infants highlighted several effective strategies for health care providers (Saylor, Elksnin, Farah, & Pope, 1990), including verbal support and encouragement, phone reminders for appointments, and staff support. In addition, continued contact with the *same* provider has been linked with better adherence (e.g., Litt & Cuskey, 1980). Unfortunately, "managed care" and other changes in the health care delivery system that emphasize cost containment and profitability make it difficult to provide "personal" care. One consequence of cost containment has been reductions in the length of time available for direct patient contact (Walders, Nobile, & Drotar, 2000). Shortened visits may lead to communication problems and ultimately contribute to deterioration in patients' quality of care (Emanuel & Dubler, 1995; Probst, Greenhouse, & Selassie, 1997).

In addition to the patient–provider relationship, other aspects of the medical setting may promote or hinder adherence. Specifically, the convenience of medical care (e.g., closeness to home; accessible location; short waiting-room time) has been related to better adherence (e.g., Hazzard, Hutchinson, & Krawiecki, 1990). Providing transportation and babysitters may also enhance families' participation in their youngsters' treatment (Saylor et al., 1990).

Communication of Regimen Requirements

In many cases, medical advice may be inconsistent or unclear. One index of the quality of doctor–patient communication is the parents' or patients' ability to recall the specific regimen (Ievers-Landis & Drotar, 2000), which has been associated with better adherence. For instance, among families of children with asthma, reasons for nonadherence have included incorrect and insufficient information regarding asthma management, unclear instructions provided in technical terms, and failure to repeat and rephrase instructions (Alexander, 1983; Schraa & Dirks, 1992). A study by Page, Verstraete, Robb, and Etzwiler (1981) compared providers' recommendations for diabetes care with patients' and families' recall of the recommendations. Providers made *seven* recommendations on average, although children and families recalled only *two*. Moreover, families recalled recommendations that were not made by the health care providers. Such communication gaps may lead to inadvertent nonadherence.

Disease and Regimen Considerations

Diseases differ markedly in the demands placed on youngsters and families. Several aspects of diseases and regimens are described in this section, along with their implications for adherence.

Chronicity

Pediatric conditions vary from acute problems requiring a few days of treatment to chronic conditions involving lifelong management. Although acute and chronic conditions are often dichotomized, marked variability within these broad categories can be observed. Asthma, for instance, is considered to be a chronic condition, yet about 50% of youngsters with asthma become asymptomatic as adolescents (Lemanek, 1990). In contrast, diabetes is a chronic disease with no available cure, and youngsters with diabetes are confronted with a lifelong effort to control their disease. Disease chronicity has been linked with poorer treatment adherence. Even with acute conditions, adherence rates for medication fall off dramatically over time, as many patients discontinue some or all medications once symptoms have abated (see Rapoff, 1999). Adherence difficulties abound with long-term regimens. Youngsters with diabetes (Jacobson et al., 1990) and renal disease (Brownbridge & Fielding, 1994) display significant declines in adherence over the length of treatment. Such findings suggest that it is unrealistic to expect consistently good adherence with a chronic disease regimen. Periodic nonadherence should be viewed *as the rule,* rather than the *exception.* Health care providers might focus on supporting adherence before problems arise and providing encouragement when inevitable difficulties occur. In fact, incentives for health behaviors are a component of several adherence interventions (e.g., Wysocki, Green, & Huxtable, 1989).

Complexity

Treatment complexity increases the likelihood of adherence problems. For medication regimens, prescriptions of more than one medication are associated with lower adherence rates (Francis et al., 1969), as are prescriptions of multiple medications on different administration schedules (Mattar et al., 1975). Treatments for HIV are especially challenging in that they require multidrug regimens and that the medications have varied side effects (Johnson, 2000).

Problems with adherence also arise with regimens that involve activity limitations or changes in lifestyle and personal habits (e.g., diet, exercise), which are much more difficult to comply with than medication prescriptions. For example, youths with diabetes have higher rates of adherence to taking insulin injections than to the meal-related aspects of their regimen (La Greca et al., 1990).

Variables that influence adherence to complex regimens include the parents' or youngsters' disease knowledge and their skills in implementing self-care tasks. As discussed previously, disease knowledge and problem solving have been linked with better adherence for complex, chronic diseases (Alexander, 1983; La Greca et al., 1990). Good family communication also has been linked to better adherence for adolescents with diabetes (e.g., Bobrow, Avruskin, & Siller, 1985).

Immediate and Future Consequences

Fewer problems arise when adherence brings immediate, positive results, as in the case of pain relief or symptom reduction (e.g., Arnhold et al., 1970). In contrast, regimens with no immediate consequences for adherence, of uncertain efficacy, or that produce aversive side effects are problematic (Litt & Cuskey, 1980; Tamaroff, Festa, Adesman, & Walco, 1992).

Regimens such as chemotherapy or steroid medication, that produce immediate negative physical side effects, have proven to be especially difficult for adherence, even in the face of the life-threatening consequences of nonadherence (Blowey et al., 1997; Korsch et al.,

1978). Regimens that interfere with children's normal development or daily activities may also lead to problems with adherence (Fotheringham & Sawyer, 1995; Matsui, 2000).

For diseases that are largely asymptomatic (e.g., diabetes), the benefits of adherence are associated with *future* outcomes. However, future-oriented goals are often insufficient motivators for daily adherence behaviors and are outweighed by the immediate and ongoing efforts needed to comply (Litt & Cuskey, 1980). Such regimens may require the use of incentives to promote compliance. An additional problem with asymptomatic diseases is that there may not be any consequences for *nonadherence*. Dunbar (1983) noted that youngsters who experienced an episode of nonadherence without any adverse consequences were more likely to repeat the nonadherence.

Models of Medical Adherence

Because adherence is a complex problem, it is important to consider the multiple contexts that influence youngsters' self-care behaviors. Several multivariate models have been offered for conceptualizing and understanding health care behaviors, and they are reviewed briefly here.

Health Belief Model (HBM)

Perhaps the most well-known model of health behavior developed from the work of Becker and colleagues (1972, 1978), who consolidated available knowledge on health care behavior into a model for predicting individuals' adherence to ongoing and preventive regimens. The key elements of the HBM that predict good adherence include the individual's perceptions of *susceptibility* to a particular illness or illness complications, *severity* or *seriousness* of the disease or its complications, and the *benefits* of prescribed health care actions (i.e., how likely the regimen is to produce positive results). Perceived *barriers* to health care (e.g., cost, risk level of the treatment, limitations on daily activities) serve as negative predictors of adherence. In theory, the most adherent individuals are those who perceive themselves as vulnerable to disease, view the disease as serious, believe the regimen will produce positive results, and are not hindered by obstacles to treatment. The relationship between these perceptions and adherence may be further moderated by other variables, including the quality of the doctor–patient relationship, the presence of cues to action, the availability of social support, the person's age, and personality variables.

Tests of the HBM have been conducted primarily with low-income mothers whose children were seen in outpatient clinics for a variety of health problems (e.g., Becker et al., 1972; Becker et al., 1978). In general, this research supports the utility of the HBM. A few studies have examined the links between adolescents' health beliefs and their adherence with chronic regimens. Consistent with the HBM, higher perceived *barriers* to treatment have been linked with poorer compliance; however, contrary to the HBM, *perceived threat* (e.g., susceptibility, disease severity) has been linked with *poorer* adherence among teens (Bond, Aiken, & Somerville, 1992; Brownlee-Duffeck et al., 1987).

A major criticism of the HBM has been its questionable relevance for health care interventions. Other strengths and limitations of the HBM have been discussed at length by Rapoff (1999).

Disease-Specific Models

Several investigators have developed disease-specific, cross-sectional models of disease adaptation that include adherence as a component of the model. For instance, models of associations between psychosocial factors and health outcomes have been developed for youths with diabetes (e.g., Hanson, 1992; La Greca & Skyler, 1991). These models reveal several common factors predictive of adherence, including: *knowledge* about the disease and its management, parental and family *support* of treatment, youngsters' levels of *stress*, youngsters' *coping* strategies, and current *disease status* (i.e., how well or poorly the disease is controlled). Extending these disease-specific models to other pediatric populations may be an important future goal. However, in addition to cross-sectional models, longitudinal perspectives will be necessary for understanding how adherence changes over time and how and when to intervene.

Longitudinal Models

A longitudinal approach is reflected in the work of Prochaska and DiClemente (1984), who developed a transtheoretical model (TTM) of behavior change to identify the best fit between an individual's characteristics and health care interventions. Applications of TTM have focused on reducing high-risk behaviors (e.g., smoking, alcohol abuse) or promoting health-enhancing behaviors (e.g., exercise, reducing dietary fat) in adolescents and adults. However, this model has not been applied to pediatric conditions.

The TTM model postulates five *stages of change* in the acquisition of health-enhancing behaviors (or cessation of risk behaviors): (1) *precontemplation* (i.e., not thinking about making changes), (2) *contemplation* (i.e., considering change in the future), (3) *preparation* (i.e., considering change in the immediate future), (4) *action* (i.e., changing behavior), and (5) *maintenance* (i.e., continued change over time). Two intervening variables, *decisional balance* and *self-efficacy*, may influence when and how a person progresses through the five stages. Decisional balance refers to the process of weighing the benefits against the costs of the desired behavior; self-efficacy refers to the person's confidence in his or her ability to make the desired behavior change. Progression through the stages is not linear, as individuals may relapse and recycle back through previous stages (Ruggiero & Prochaska, 1993); moreover, individuals could be at different stages for different health care tasks.

An important feature of TTM is that it matches different types of intervention strategies with different stages in the model. For instance, an adolescent with diabetes who has not been monitoring glucose levels but has good future intentions (i.e., contemplation stage) might respond well to efforts from health care providers that emphasize the benefits of monitoring. Not until the action stage, however, will this adolescent be ready for specific instructions on monitoring. In contrast, youngsters with good monitoring skills (maintenance stage) may need support and reinforcement to prevent relapse to less desirable monitoring levels. TTM may also be helpful in predicting which individuals are likely to withdraw from intervention, as individuals in the precontemplation or contemplation stages are not likely to follow through with intensive efforts to improve behaviors. (See Rapoff, 1999, for a further discussion of TTM.)

INTERVENTIONS FOR PEDIATRIC ADHERENCE

Relative to the number of studies on correlates of adherence, substantially less attention has been devoted to methods for improving adherence. This section briefly reviews common strategies for facilitating adherence and self-care behaviors in children, adolescents, and families.

Interventions That Emphasize Learning New Skills and Behaviors

Educational Approaches

Children's and families' knowledge of the disease and its regimen are important for adherence. Education has been stressed for regimens that involve complex skills (e.g., factor replacement therapy for hemophilia), that require major lifestyle modifications (e.g., obesity and eating-related problems), or that demand a high degree of self-regulation (e.g., diabetes).

Education alone may be appropriate for short-term medication regimens. For example, Colcher and Bass (1972) examined the effects of an educational intervention for parents of youngsters with streptococcal pharyngitis. The parents who were given information on how to administer medication plus written instructions were more adherent (80%) than those receiving usual care (50%).

Educational approaches are also important for children and families at the time of initial disease diagnosis (e.g., Delamater et al., 1990) or for adolescents with a chronic disease who are beginning to assume increased responsibility for their treatment regimens (La Greca & Skyler, 1995). In such cases, it is important to ensure that youngsters and families have the knowledge and skills necessary to effectively carry out the treatment regimen. However, knowledge alone is insufficient for successful adherence with complex, chronic, or aversive regimens (La Greca & Skyler, 1991). In such cases, additional procedures (e.g., support, supervision, or reinforcement) are necessary.

Modeling

Several studies used modeling to improve children's or parents' skills in executing difficult regimen tasks. Although these studies have not directly investigated the impact of improved skills on adherence, they are of interest because anxiety about how to administer complex tasks could serve as a deterrent to adherence. Sergis-Deavenport and Varni (1982) taught parents of children with hemophilia to administer factor replacement therapy (FRT) at home. FRT consists of administering a factor concentrate via venipuncture whenever a sudden bleeding episode occurs. FRT was modeled by a nurse practitioner, and parents were given instructions and behavioral rehearsal with corrective feedback. Parents increased their skill levels from 15% correct during baseline to over 90% correct during treatment and follow-up. These findings suggest that further investigation of modeling for improving skills on difficult management tasks would be desirable.

Interventions That Emphasize Supervision, Feedback, or Reminders

Medical Supervision

Supervision by health care providers has shown promise as a method for enhancing adherence. Supervision might take the form of more frequent medical visits or of monitoring medications through assays of drug levels or inactive markers in body fluids. Specifically, medical supervision appears to enhance adherence to short-term regimens. In a study of children with acute medical problems, Fink, Malloy, Cohen, Greycloud, and Martin (1969) assigned families randomly to a usual-care group or a nurse follow-up condition that provided increased supervision of medications. The adherence rate in the nurse follow-up condition was 59%, as compared with an 18% adherence rate for the control patients. Increased medical supervision has also been a part of multicomponent interventions (e.g., Delamater et al., 1990).

Visual Cues or Reminders

Reminders or cues, such as signs in key places (e.g., refrigerator or bathroom mirror), calendars, postcards, and phone calls, may prompt the performance of regimen tasks. This approach might be considered (1) for appointment keeping, (2) for acute, short-term regimens, (3) during the initial phases of more complex, chronic treatment protocols; and (4) in situations in which parents are trying to increase children's involvement in their own medical management. In such cases, new health behaviors must be acquired and integrated into the individual's daily routine, and visual cues and reminders might facilitate this process.

Reminders, such as phone calls or postcards, are often used to assist appointment keeping. Casey, Rosen, Glowasky, and Ludwig (1985) investigated the use of phone reminders, with or without an educational session, to increase appointment adherence in 183 children with otitis media. The "telephone reminder" group had the highest percentage of children who kept their follow-up appointments (56%), compared with the "education" (39%) and control groups (25%). Thus phone reminders can increase adherence with medical appointments, although the highest level of adherence demonstrated in this study still fell well below the ideal (100%). Reminders alone may be insufficient to improve adherence for some patients and families.

Visual cues also may prompt performance of regimen tasks, such as taking medication. Lima, Nazarian, Charney, and Lahti (1976) studied the impact of two visual cues (a printed clock with the times for medication circled and a bright sticker for posting at home) on adherence to a 10-day antibiotic regimen. The low-income sample included 158 children and adults with a variety of acute problems. Children and parents were helped considerably more by the visual cues than were adult patients. Moreover, children in the "reminder" group had adherence levels that were more than twice as high as the controls. These and other findings suggest that reminders can improve adherence, although additional procedures (e.g., incentives) may be needed for difficult tasks.

Self-Monitoring

Self-monitoring of disease symptoms or regimen behaviors may be useful for acute illnesses with short-term medication regimens, although few well-controlled investigations are available and most studies that included self-monitoring also used other strategies. For example, Mattar et al. (1975) provided parents with calendars to monitor a 10-day regimen of oral antibiotics for their children; parents also were given written instructions on medication use and a measuring device for the medication. The rate of adherence in the intervention group was 51%, as compared with an 8.5% rate in control cases. In contrast, for complex regimens, self-monitoring interventions have been less promising. Wysocki and colleagues (1989) taught adolescents with diabetes to self-monitor blood glucose levels using reflectance meters with memory chips that recorded the results of each blood test. Adolescents were randomly assigned to a "meter-alone" (i.e., self-monitoring) or "meter-plus-contract" (i.e., self-monitoring plus monetary incentive) condition; additional patients served as controls. Findings revealed that blood testing frequency declined sharply during the 16-week intervention for the meter-alone group but remained at or above baseline levels for the meter-plus-contract group. Thus, self-monitoring alone had no positive effect on adolescents' adherence; incentives were necessary to achieve adequate levels of testing. In general, self-monitoring *alone* is of limited utility for diabetes or illnesses with complex regimens. Moreover, unless the information obtained from monitoring can be used to improve disease management, the benefits of self-monitoring are likely to be limited (Wysocki et al., 1989).

Providing Incentives for Adherence Behaviors

Reinforcement contingencies for improving adherence have been very successful with medication regimens, with complex, chronic treatments, with challenging lifestyle behaviors (e.g., diet, exercise), and with children's or parents' treatment participation. As one example, Lowe and Lutzker (1979) combined written instructions, parental home monitoring, and a token reward system to increase adherence to foot care, urine glucose testing, and diet in a 9-year-old girl with diabetes. Similarly, for youngsters with hemophilia, Greenan-Fowler, Powell, and Varni (1987) used a contingency contract and token exchange system for improving adherence to prescribed exercises, completing self-monitoring forms, and attending group exercise sessions. Six-month follow-up revealed average adherence rates ranging from 81% to 90%.

Although promising, reinforcement procedures have limitations. Variable responsiveness (Killam, Apodaca, Manella, & Varni, 1983) and treatment failures (e.g., Carney et al., 1983; Finney, Lemanek, Brophy, & Cataldo, 1990) have been evident. Furthermore, adherence levels may not be maintained when reinforcement procedures are discontinued. Future investigations might explore methods for modifying effective reinforcement systems over time to maintain long-term adherence gains. More immediate and frequent reinforcement may be needed for complex or demanding tasks or for younger or less motivated youngsters (Friedman & Litt, 1987). Over time, reinforcement might be contingent on longer periods of adherence and greater self-management.

Interventions That Emphasize Social Support or Problem Solving

Family interventions are extremely important. In fact, many of the studies cited in this chapter included parents in the treatment program, primarily to dispense reinforcement or to provide supervision for youngsters' self-care (e.g., Lowe & Lutzker, 1979). Few studies, however, have directly tried to improve family support, communication, and problem solving.

A study by Satin, La Greca, Zigo, and Skyler (1989) examined a 6-week multifamily intervention for adolescents with diabetes. Adolescents and their parents were randomly assigned either to one of two multifamily conditions or to a control group. Multifamily sessions stressed effective communication concerning diabetes-specific situations, problem solving for diabetes management, and family support for adolescents' self-care. In one of the multifamily conditions, parents simulated diabetes for a week (e.g., daily injections, glucose tests, dietary plan, exercise prescription) to heighten their awareness of the difficulties of daily management. Adolescents who participated in the multifamily groups demonstrated significant improvements in self-care and metabolic control 6 months posttreatment relative to controls. In contrast to these findings, however, Wysocki and colleagues (2000) conducted a randomized, controlled trial of behavioral family systems therapy (BFST) with families of adolescents with diabetes and found minimal effects on adherence, diabetes control, or health care utilization. The authors proposed several explanations, including that BFST may be more appropriate as a preventive intervention for younger adolescents than as an adolescent intervention and that treatment barriers may need to be targeted directly in treatment.

In addition to family involvement, youngsters' adherence may benefit from peer support. Recent studies suggest that peers with the *same* medical condition can improve youngsters' health behaviors (e.g., Anderson, Wolf, Burkhart, Cornell, & Bacon, 1989). However, support from *healthy* peers (especially close friends) may also determine the extent to which a youngster will carry out health care tasks, such as following prescribed dietary guidelines or testing glucose following a meal at school. Along these lines, Greco, Pendley, McDonell, and Reeves (2001) developed a group intervention for adolescents with diabetes and their best friends. The sessions were structured to encourage friends to become involved with diabetes care in order to improve adolescents' adherence and disease control. The four sessions covered information about diabetes, reflective listening skills and problem solving, and ways that friends could assist with diabetes care. After the intervention, adolescents and their friends reported greater diabetes knowledge and support and a higher ratio of friend-to-family support. Although parents rated their adolescents as having less diabetes-related conflict, no direct effects on adolescents' treatment adherence were observed.

Reducing Barriers to Adherence

Children and adolescents report many different obstacles to treatment management (e.g., La Greca & Hanna, 1983), yet few investigators have matched their intervention to the types of problems that interfere with youngsters' medical management. One exception is the work of Schafer, Glasgow, and McCaul (1982), who helped three children with diabetes reduce their barriers to daily glucose testing, insulin administration, and exercise. Based on the children's and parents' reports of barriers to daily management, individualized programs were designed and specific goals for adherence were determined. For glucose testing and exercise adherence, the combination of barrier reduction and goal setting was effective for two children. However, a combination of barrier reduction, goal setting, and contingent reinforcement was needed to achieve a satisfactory level of adherence for one child who had difficulty administering injections on time.

Multicomponent Interventions

Given the complexity of chronic pediatric conditions and the multiple variables and barriers that contribute to adherence, it may be unrealistic to expect that any single intervention strategy will lead to successful adherence. Thus several multicomponent intervention programs have been developed to improve adherence and/or health outcomes; a few key examples are described here. In general, these studies have examined health outcomes rather than adherence behaviors, although better adherence was *presumed* to underlie improvements in health outcomes.

Delamater and colleagues (1990) taught self-management training (SMT) to newly diagnosed youngsters with diabetes and their parents; SMT combined education, problem solving, social support, and reinforcement. Children and parents who received SMT met for nine sessions that stressed the use of self-monitoring of blood glucose, parental reinforcement of children's monitoring and recording behaviors, and the use of self-monitoring data for making adjustments in the regimen. Children in the SMT group achieved significantly better metabolic control (a key health outcome) 1 and 2 years postdiagnosis than those who received only conventional treatment.

Baum and Creer (1986) used multiple treatment strategies, including SMT, to improve adherence among children with asthma. Youngsters receiving SMT did not show gains in medication adherence relative to those in the self-monitoring group; however, they were more likely to avoid the cause of an asthma attack, to manage an asthma attack by themselves without immediately seeking adult attention, and to institute other measures before resorting to medication. In short, the combination of self-monitoring, incentives, and education led to better *management*.

In contrast to interventions that focus on children and families, Anderson and colleagues (1989) worked with adolescents and parents. Adolescents with diabetes were randomly assigned to either an intervention or a standard-care condition and were seen in clinic every 3 to 4 months over an 18-month period. Adolescents and parents receiving the intervention met in concurrent but separate groups. Adolescent sessions focused on the use of self-monitoring of blood glucose (SMBG) as a tool for solving diabetes management problems. The adolescents also ate, exercised, and monitored blood glucose together, creating an atmosphere of peer support. Clinic nurses provided increased medical supervision by routinely contacting adolescents. Parent sessions focused on ways to negotiate appropriate levels of parental involvement and adolescent responsibility for diet, exercise, and monitoring. Results indicated that postintervention metabolic control (a key health outcome) deteriorated in 50% of the adolescents in the standard-care condition but in only 23% of the intervention group. Although adherence was not measured directly, more teens in the intervention group reported changing their exercise patterns based on information from SMBG. This is an example of an intervention that combined education, self-monitoring, medical supervision, and family and peer support to prevent deterioration in metabolic control and to improve self-care.

In summary, multicomponent programs for improving health outcomes appear to be promising, although the effects on adherence have been less clear. Nevertheless, given the multiple demands of many regimens, multicomponent interventions will continue to be important for research and practice.

Summary of Adherence Interventions

Relatively few systematic investigations have been done of interventions to improve treatment adherence in children, adolescents, and families. In general, effective strategies for acute illnesses with short-term medication regimens include providing verbal and written instructions, providing visual cues or reminders, and increasing medical supervision. However, treatments for complex regimens remain a challenge. The most success has been associated with programs that combine treatment strategies, such as intensive education, parental involvement, self-monitoring, and reinforcement procedures, or that reflect a high degree of family involvement and problem solving.

Studies have been limited by a variety of methodological difficulties, including a reliance on small samples, focus on short-term interventions with limited follow-up periods, or use of participant selection procedures that may exclude resistant or nonadherent patients. Even with well-controlled studies, the active ingredients of the treatment packages are not well understood. These caveats are not limited to interventions for nonadherence but, in fact, are similar to concerns regarding the status of intervention research in pediatric psychology (La Greca & Varni, 1993).

In future research, it will be important to examine child and family characteristics that *moderate* treatment responsiveness, such as: the severity and duration of the pediatric condition; youngsters' developmental level; comorbidity with other problems; children's and families' experience of distress; and the degree of parental involvement in treatment (La Greca & Varni, 1993). In addition, attention to the cost-effectiveness of the interventions will be essential if they are to be of practical use in today's managed care environment (Greineder, Loane, & Parks, 1999; Walders et al., 2000).

CONCLUDING COMMENTS

Adherence to prescribed medical regimens is a complex and challenging problem. Although substantial progress has been made, considerably more remains to be accomplished. Understanding the parameters *underlying* adherence to pediatric regimens will be advanced by greater attention to the conceptual, practical, and methodological issues described in this chapter. Returning to several themes noted earlier, the importance of considering developmental, child, and family variables in future investigations, in addition to key aspects of the health care environment (e.g., physician communication and support, characteristics of the health care setting), cannot be overemphasized. Systematic analysis of these and other variables may enable clinicians and researchers to tailor interventions to the specific needs of children, adolescents, and families. Finally, future investigations might focus on factors conducive to successful health care. A positive approach may broaden professionals' understanding of adherence, suggest new avenues for intervention, and shift the emphasis away from the current negative approach of searching out causes for nonadherence. With a fresh perspective, future efforts may go a long way toward improving the health outlook and quality of life for youngsters affected by disease.

ACKNOWLEDGMENTS

Preparation of this chapter was supported, in part, by a grant from the National Institute of Child Health and Development (No. T32 HD07510).

REFERENCES

Alexander, A. B. (1983). The nature of asthma. In P. J. McGrath & P. Firestone (Eds.), *Pediatric and adolescent behavioral medicine: Issues in treatment* (pp. 28–66). New York: Springer.

Anderson, B. J., Auslander, W. F., Jung, K. C., Miller, J. P., & Santiago, J. V. (1990). Assessing family sharing of diabetes responsibilities. *Journal of Pediatric Psychology, 15,* 477–492.

Anderson, B. J., Wolf, F. M., Burkhart, M. T., Cornell, R. G., & Bacon, G. E. (1989). Effects of peer-group intervention on metabolic control of adolescents with IDDM: Randomized outpatient study. *Diabetes Care, 3,* 179–183.

Arnhold, R. G., Adebonojo, F. O., Callas, E. R., Callas, J., Carte, E., & Stein, R. C. (1970). Patients and prescriptions: Comprehension and compliance with medical instructions in a suburban pediatric practice. *Clinical Pediatrics, 9,* 648–651.

Barofsky, I. (1984). Therapeutic compliance and the cancer patient. *Health Education Quarterly, 10,* 43–56.

Baum, D., & Creer, T. (1986). Medication compliance in children with asthma. *Journal of Asthma, 23,* 49–59.

Becker, M. H., Drachman, R. H., & Kirscht, J. P. (1972). Predicting mothers' compliance with pediatric medical regimens. *Journal of Pediatrics, 81,* 843–854.

Becker, M. H., Radius, S. M., Rosenstock, I. M., Drachman, R. H., Shuberth, K. C., & Teets, K. C. (1978). Compliance with a medical regimen for asthma: A test of the Health Belief Model. *Public Health Reports, 93*, 268–277.

Bennett, D. L., & Ward, M. S. (1977). Diabetes mellitus in adolescents: A comprehensive approach to outpatient care. *Southern Medical Journal, 70*, 705–708.

Blowey, D. L., Hebert, D., Arbus, G. S., Pool, R., Korus, M., & Koren, G. (1997). Compliance with cyclosporine in adolescent renal transplant recipients. *Pediatric Nephrology, 11*, 547–551.

Bobrow, E. S., Avruskin, T. W., & Siller, J. (1985). Mother–daughter interaction and adherence to diabetes regimens. *Diabetes Care, 8*, 146–151.

Bond, G. G., Aiken, L. S., & Somerville, S. C. (1992). The health belief model and adolescents with insulin-dependent diabetes mellitus. *Health Psychology, 11*, 190–198.

Brooks-Gunn, J., & Graber, J. A. (1994). Puberty as a biological and social event: Implications for research on pharmacology. *Journal of Adolescent Health, 15*, 663–671.

Brownbridge, G., & Fielding, D. M. (1994). Psychosocial adjustment and adherence to dialysis treatment regimens. *Pediatric Nephrology, 8*, 744–749.

Brownlee-Duffeck, M., Peterson, L., Simonds, J. F., Goldstein, D., Kilo, C., & Hoette, S. (1987). The role of health beliefs in the regimen adherence and metabolic control of adolescents and adults with diabetes mellitus. *Journal of Consulting and Clinical Psychology, 55*, 139–144.

Burroughs, T. E., Harris, M. A., Pontious, S. L., & Santiago, J. V. (1997). Research on social support in adolescents with IDDM: A critical review. *The Diabetes Educator, 23*, 438–448.

Carney, R. M., Schechter, K., & Davis, T. (1983). Improving adherence to blood glucose testing in insulin dependent diabetic children. *Behavior Therapy, 14*, 247–254.

Casey, R., Rosen, B., Glowasky, A., & Ludwig, S. (1985). An intervention to improve follow-up of patients with otitis media. *Clinical Pediatrics, 24*, 149–152.

Cauce, A. M., Reid, M., Landesman, S., & Gonzales, N. (1990). Social support in young children: Measurement, structure, and behavioral impact. In B. R. Sarason, I. G. Sarason, & G. R. Pierce (Eds.), *Social support: An interactional view* (pp. 64–94). New York: Wiley.

Chaney, J. M., & Peterson, L. (1989). Family variables and disease management in juvenile rheumatoid arthritis. *Journal of Pediatric Psychology, 14*, 389–403.

Colcher, I. S., & Bass, J. W. (1972). Penicillin treatment of streptococcal pharyngitis: A comparison of schedules and the role of specific counseling. *Journal of the American Medical Association, 222*, 657–659.

Cramer, J. A. (1995). Microelectric systems for monitoring and enhancing patient compliance with medication regimens. *Drugs, 49*, 321–327.

Cromer, B. A., & Tarnowski, K. J. (1989). Noncompliance in adolescents: A review. *Developmental and Behavioral Pediatrics, 10*, 207–215.

Davis, C. L., Delamater, A. M., Shaw, K. H., La Greca, A. M., Eidson, M. S., Perez-Rodriguez, J. E., & Nemery, R. (2001). Parenting styles, regimen adherence, and glycemic control in 4– to 10–year-old children with diabetes. *Journal of Pediatric Psychology, 26*, 123–129.

Deaton, A. V. (1985). Adaptive noncompliance in pediatric asthma: The parent as expert. *Journal of Pediatric Psychology, 10*, 1–14.

Delamater, A. M., Bubb, J., Davis, S. G., Smith, J. A., Schmidt, L., White, N. H., & Santiago, J. V. (1990). Randomized prospective study of self-management training with newly diagnosed diabetic children. *Diabetes Care, 13*, 492–498.

Dolgin, M. J., Katz, E. R., Doctors, S. R., & Siegel, S. E. (1986). Caregivers' perceptions of medical compliance in adolescents with cancer. *Journal of Adolescent Health Care, 7*, 22–27.

Donovan, J. L., & Blake, D. R. (1992). Patient noncompliance: Deviance or reasoned decision making? *Social Science and Medicine, 34*, 507–513.

Dunbar, J. (1983). Compliance in pediatric populations: A review. In P. J. McGrath & P. Firestone (Eds.), *Pediatric and adolescent behavioral medicine: Issues in treatment* (pp. 210–230). New York: Springer.

Emanuel, E. J., & Dubler, N. N. (1995). Preserving the physician–patient relationship in the era of managed care. *Journal of the American Medical Association, 273*, 323–329.

Epstein, L. H., & Cluss, P. A. (1982). A behavioral medicine perspective on adherence to long-term medical regimens. *Journal of Consulting and Clinical Psychology, 50*, 950–971.

Fehrenbach, A. M. B., & Peterson, L. (1989). Parental problem-solving skills, stress, and dietary compliance in phenylketonuria. *Journal of Consulting and Clinical Psychology, 57*, 237–241.

Fink, D., Malloy, M. J., Cohen, M., Greycloud, M. A., & Martin, F. (1969). Effective patient care in the pediatric ambulatory setting: A study of the acute care clinic. *Pediatrics, 43*, 927–935.

Finney, J. W., Lemanek, K. L., Brophy, C. J., & Cataldo, M. F. (1990). Pediatric appointment keeping: Improving adherence in a primary care allergy clinic. *Journal of Pediatric Psychology, 15*, 571–579.

Fotheringham, M. J., & Sawyer, M. G. (1995). Adherence to recommended medical regimens in childhood and adolescence. *Journal of Pediatrics and Child Health, 31*, 72–78.

Francis, V., Korsch, B. M., & Morris, M. J. (1969). Gaps in doctor–patient communication: Patients' response to medical advice. *New England Journal of Medicine, 280,* 535–540.

Freund, A., Johnson, S. B., Silverstein, J., & Thomas, J. (1991). Assessing daily management of childhood diabetes using 24–hour recall interviews: Reliability and stability. *Health Psychology, 10,* 200–208.

Friedman, I. M., & Litt, I. F. (1987). Adolescents' compliance with therapeutic regimens: Psycho-logical and social aspects and intervention. *Journal of Adolescent Health Care, 8,* 52–65.

Gordis, L., Markowitz, M., & Lilienfeld, A. M. (1969). The inaccuracy in using interviews to estimate patient reliability in taking medications at home. *Medical Care, 1,* 49–54.

Greco, P., Pendley, J. S., McDonell, K., & Reeves, G. (2001). A peer group intervention for adolescents with type 1 diabetes and their best friends. *Journal of Pediatric Psychology, 26,* 485–490.

Greenan-Fowler, E., Powell, C., & Varni, J. W. (1987). Behavioral treatment of adherence to therapeutic exercise by children with hemophilia. *Archives of Physical Medicine and Rehabilitation, 68,* 846–849.

Greineder, D. K., Loane, K. C., & Parks, P. (1999). A randomized controlled trial of a pediatric asthma outreach program. *Journal of Allergy and Clinical Immunology, 103,* 436–440.

Gross, A. M., Johnson, W. G., Wildman, H. E., & Mullett, M. (1981). Coping skills training with insulin dependent preadolescent diabetics. *Child Behavior Therapy, 3,* 141–153.

Hanson, C. L. (1992). Developing systemic models of the adaptation of youths with diabetes. In A. M. La Greca, L. J. Siegel, J. L. Wallander, & C. E. Walker (Eds.), *Stress and coping in child health* (pp. 212–241). New York: Guilford Press.

Hanson, C. L., De Guire, M. J., Schinkel, A. M., & Kolterman, O. G. (1995). Empirical validation for a family-centered model of care. *Diabetes Care, 18,* 1347–1356.

Hauser, S. T., Jacobson, A. M., Lavori, P., Wolfsdorf, J. I., Herskowitz, R. D., Milley, J. E., et al. (1990). Adherence among children and adolescents with insulin-dependent diabetes mellitus over a four-year longitudinal follow-up: II. Immediate and long-term linkages with the family milieu. *Journal of Pediatric Psychology, 15,* 527–542.

Hazzard, A., Hutchinson, S. J., & Krawiecki, N. (1990). Factors related to adherence to medication regimens in pediatric seizure patients. *Journal of Pediatric Psychology, 15,* 543–555.

Ievers-Landis, C. E., & Drotar, D. (2000). Parental and child knowledge of the treatment regimen for childhood chronic illnesses: Related factors and adherence to treatment. In D. Drotar (Ed.), *Promoting adherence to medical treatment in chronic childhood illness: Concepts, methods, and interventions* (pp. 259–282). Mahwah, NJ: Erlbaum.

Jacobson, A. M., Hauser, S. T., Lavori, P., Wolfsdorf, J. I., Herskowitz, R. D., Milley, J. E., et al. (1990). Adherence among children and adolescents with insulin-dependent diabetes mellitus over a four-year longitudinal follow-up: I. The influence of patient coping and adjustment. *Journal of Pediatric Psychology, 15,* 511–526.

Johnson, S. B. (1994). Health behavior and health status: Concepts, methods, and applications. *Journal of Pediatric Psychology, 19,* 129–141.

Johnson, S. B. (2000). Compliance behavior in clinical trials: Error or opportunity? In D. Drotar (Ed.), *Promoting adherence to medical treatment in chronic childhood illness: Concepts, methods, and interventions* (pp. 307–321). Mahwah, NJ: Erlbaum.

Johnson, S. B., Kelly, M., Henretta, J. C., Cunningham, W. R., Tomer, A., & Silverstein, J. H. (1992). A longitudinal analysis of adherence and health status in childhood diabetes. *Journal of Pediatric Psychology, 17,* 537–553.

Johnson, S. B., Silverstein, J., Rosenbloom, A., Carter, R., & Cunningham, W. (1986). Assessing daily management of childhood diabetes. *Health Psychology, 5,* 545–564.

Killam, P. E., Apodaca, L., Manella, K. J., & Varni, J. W. (1983). Behavioral pediatric weight rehabilitation for children with myelomeningocele. *American Journal of Maternal Child Nursing, 8,* 280–286.

Korsch, B. M., Fine, R. N., & Negrete, V. F. (1978). Noncompliance in children with renal transplants. *Pediatrics, 61,* 872–876.

Kovacs, M., Goldston, D., Obrosky, D. S., & Iyengar, S. (1992). Prevalence and predictors of pervasive noncompliance with medical treatment among youths with insulin-dependent diabetes mellitus. *Journal of the American Academy of Child and Adolescent Psychiatry, 31,* 1112–1119.

La Greca, A. M. (1990a). Issues in adherence with pediatric regimens. *Journal of Pediatric Psychology, 15,* 423–436.

La Greca, A. M. (1990b). Social consequences of pediatric conditions: Fertile area for future investigation and intervention? *Journal of Pediatric Psychology, 15,* 285–308.

La Greca, A. M. (1998). It's "all in the family": Responsibility for diabetes care. *Journal of Pediatric Endocrinology and Metabolism, 11*(Suppl. 2), 379–385.

La Greca, A. M., Auslander, W. F., Greco, P., Spetter, D., Fisher, E. B., Jr., & Santiago, J. V. (1995). I get by with a little help from my family and friends: Adolescents' support for diabetes care. *Journal of Pediatric Psychology, 20,* 449–476.

La Greca, A. M., & Bearman, K. J. (2002). The Diabetes Social Support Questionnaire—Family Version: Evaluating adolescents' diabetes-specific support from family members. *Journal of Pediatric Psychology, 27*, 665–676.

La Greca, A. M., Follansbee, D., & Skyler, J. S. (1990). Developmental and behavioral aspects of diabetes management in youngsters. *Children's Health Care, 19*, 132–137.

La Greca, A. M., & Hanna, N. C. (1983). Health beliefs of children and their mothers: Implications for treatment [Abstract]. *Diabetes, 32*(Suppl. 1), 66.

La Greca, A. M., & Skyler, J. S. (1991). Psychosocial issues in IDDM: A multivariate framework. In P. McCabe, N. Schneiderman, T. Field, & J. S. Skyler (Eds.), *Stress, coping and disease* (pp. 169–190). Hillsdale, NJ: Erlbaum.

La Greca, A. M., & Skyler, J. S. (1995). Psychological management of diabetes. In C. J. H. Kelnar (Ed.), *Childhood diabetes* (pp. 295–310). London: Chapman & Hall.

La Greca, A. M., & Varni, J. W. (1993). Intervention in pediatric psychology: A look to the future. *Journal of Pediatric Psychology, 18*, 667–679.

Lemanek, K. (1990). Adherence issues in the medical management of asthma. *Journal of Pediatric Psychology, 15*, 437–458.

Lima, J., Nazarian, L., Charney, E., & Lahti, C. (1976). Compliance with short-term antimicrobial therapy: Some techniques that help. *Pediatrics, 57*, 383–386.

Litt, I. F., & Cuskey, W. R. (1980). Compliance with medical regimens during adolescence. *Pediatric Clinics of North America, 27*, 1–15.

Litt, I. F., & Cuskey, W. R. (1984). Satisfaction with health care: A predictor of adolescents' appointment keeping. *Journal of Adolescent Health Care, 5*, 196–200.

Littlefield, C. H., Craven, J. L., Rodin, G. M., Daneman, D., Murray, M. A., & Rydall, A. C. (1992). Relationship of self-efficacy and binging to adherence to diabetes regimen among adolescents. *Diabetes Care, 15*, 90–94.

Lorenz, R. A., Christensen, N. K., & Pichert, J. W. (1985). Diet-related knowledge, skill, and adherence among children with insulin-dependent diabetes mellitus. *Pediatrics, 75*, 872–876.

Lowe, K., & Lutzker, J. R. (1979). Increasing compliance to a medical regimen with a juvenile diabetic. *Behavior Therapy, 10*, 57–64.

Matsui, D. M. (2000). Children's adherence to medication treatment. In D. Drotar (Ed.), *Promoting adherence to medical treatment in chronic childhood illness: Concepts, methods, and interventions* (pp. 135–152). Mahwah, NJ: Erlbaum.

Mattar, M. F., Markello, J., & Yaffe, S. J. (1975). Pharmaceutic factors affecting pediatric compliance. *Pediatrics, 55*, 101–108.

Page, P., Verstraete, D. G., Robb, J. R., & Etzwiler, D. D. (1981). Patient recall of self-care recommendations in diabetes. *Diabetes Care, 4*, 96–98.

Phipps, S., & DeCuir-Whalley, S. (1990). Adherence issues in pediatric bone marrow transplantation. *Journal of Pediatric Psychology, 15*, 459–475.

Probst, J. C., Greenhouse, D. L., & Selassie, A. W. (1997). Patient and physician satisfaction with an outpatient care visit. *Journal of Family Practice, 45*, 419–425.

Prochaska, J. O., & DiClemente, C. C. (1984). *The transtheoretical approach: Crossing traditional boundaries of change*. Homewood, IL: Dorsey Press.

Rapoff, M. A. (1999). *Adherence to pediatric medical regimens*. New York: Kluwer Academic,

Rubin, D. H., Bauman, L. J., & Lauby, J. L. (1989). The relationship between knowledge and reported behavior in childhood asthma. *Journal of Behavioral and Developmental Pediatrics,10*, 307–312.

Rubin, R. R., & Peyrot, M. (1992). Psychosocial problems and intervention in diabetes: A review of the literature. *Diabetes Care, 15*, 1640–1657.

Ruggiero, L., & Prochaska, J. (1993). Introduction: Application of the transtheoretical model to diabetes. *Diabetes Spectrum, 6*, 22–24.

Satin, W., La Greca, A. M., Zigo, M. A., & Skyler, J. S. (1989). Diabetes in adolescence: Effects of multifamily group intervention and parent simulation of diabetes. *Journal of Pediatric Psychology, 14*, 259–275.

Saylor, C. F., Elksnin, N., Farah, B. A., & Pope, J. A. (1990). Depends on who you ask: What maximizes participation of families in early intervention programs. *Journal of Pediatric Psychology, 15*, 557–569.

Schafer, L. C., Glasgow, R. E., & McCaul, K. D. (1982). Adherence to IDDM regimens: Relationship to psychosocial variables and metabolic control. *Diabetes Care, 6*, 493–498.

Schraa, J. C., & Dirks, J. F. (1992). Improving patient recall and comprehension of the treatment regimen. *Journal of Asthma, 19*, 159–162.

Sergis-Deavenport, E., & Varni, J. (1982). Behavioral techniques in teaching hemophilia factor replacement procedures to families. *Pediatric Nursing, 8*, 416–419.

Tamaroff, M. H., Festa, R. S., Adesman, A. R., & Walco, G. A. (1992). Therapeutic adherence to oral medication regimens by adolescents with cancer. *Journal of Pediatrics, 120*, 812–817.

Walders, N., Nobile, C., & Drotar, D. (2000). Promoting treatment adherence in childhood chronic illness: Challenges in a managed care environment. In D. Drotar (Ed.), *Promoting adherence to medical treatment in chronic childhood illness: Concepts, methods, and interventions* (pp. 201–236). Mahwah, NJ: Erlbaum.

Wilson, D. P., & Endres, R. K. (1986). Compliance with blood glucose monitoring in children with type 1 diabetes mellitus. *Journal of Pediatrics, 108,* 1022–1024.

Wysocki, T., Green, L., & Huxtable, K. (1989). Blood glucose monitoring by diabetic adolescents: Compliance and metabolic control. *Health Psychology, 8,* 267–284.

Wysocki, T., Harris, M. A., Greco, P., Bubb, J., Danda, C. E., Harvey, L. M., et al. (2000). Randomized, controlled trial behavior therapy for families of adolescents with insulin-dependent diabetes mellitus. *Journal of Pediatric Psychology, 25,* 23–33.

9

Psychosocial Adjustment of Children with Chronic Physical Conditions

JAN L. WALLANDER
ROBERT J. THOMPSON, JR.
ANN ALRIKSSON-SCHMIDT

Nowadays children with serious physical conditions that used to cause premature death often live well into adulthood. This outcome follows enormous advances in medical treatment (e.g., insulin, antibiotics, radiation, antileukemic drugs, surgical procedures). Previously lethal threats to life therefore became *chronic* physical conditions to be managed throughout life. However, it was not sufficient only to survive these conditions. Issues of quality of life and the psychosocial functioning of children with chronic physical conditions rightly become of concern. In this chapter, we first provide an overview of the topic, and then discuss findings on the adjustment of children with chronic physical conditions. This discussion is followed by a review of correlates of psychosocial adjustment and of the most salient theoretical models used to study these. We conclude with a critique and suggestions for future research. Since the previous edition of this chapter (Wallander & Thompson, 1995), several other reviews have been published of this literature (e.g., Thompson & Gustafsson, 1996; Wallander & Varni, 1997).

OVERVIEW

Definition of a Chronic Physical Condition

A "chronic physical condition" is defined as one that (1) interferes with daily functioning for more than 3 months a year; or (2) causes hospitalization lasting more than 1 month a year; or (3) is thought at the time of diagnosis to be likely to do either of the preceding (Pless & Pinkerton, 1975). These conditions affect children for extended periods of times, typically for life. Although many conditions appear at birth or soon thereafter, they can appear at varying ages up to adulthood. They can be managed to the extent that a degree of pain control, fewer exacerbations, or reduction of symptoms can generally be achieved, but they typically cannot be cured. Some examples of chronic physical conditions are asthma, cerebral palsy, congenital heart disease, cystic fibrosis, diabetes, hemophilia, leukemia, sickle cell diseases, and spina bifida.

Diagnosis-Specific and Noncategorical Approaches

Each chronic physical condition has a distinct biological process and can result in diverse and often demanding treatment regimens. Most treatment is conducted in condition-specific contexts, such as a specialty clinic by specialists focusing on one illness. Most research also tends to focus on a single diagnostic category, despite considerable commonality in the psychosocial ramifications of chronic physical conditions. For example, the burden of daily care falls on the family; treatment necessitates the involvement of a variety of health care professions, often in a fragmented fashion; specific conditions are rare; pain and discomfort are common; there can be considerable uncertainty; and the child can be stigmatized among peers, lose time from school, and experience other negative influences on development. Because of these commonalities, Pless and Pinkerton (1975) argued that psychosocial study and treatment of children with chronic physical conditions would benefit from a *noncategorical* approach. Along with others, they suggest that such conditions can be placed on common dimensions, with differing implications for psychosocial functioning (Stein & Jessop, 1982; Rolland, 1994). These dimensions include nature of onset and course, life-threat potential, intrusiveness or pain of treatment, visibility and social stigma, stability versus crises, and secondary functional and cognitive disability. They suggest that it is the variability within each of these dimensions that has implications for adjustment rather than the different diagnoses. In corollary, there is often more variation on some of these dimensions within a diagnosis than between diagnoses (Gartstein, Short, Vannatta, & Noll, 1999). A broader conceptual framework—one that is not condition specific but that focuses on these common issues—will enhance our understanding of the impact of chronic physical conditions on psychological adjustment and will improve quality of care.

Size of Population

Children with chronic physical conditions constitute 10–20% of the general population (e.g., Aron, Loprest, & Steuerie, 1996; Newacheck et al., 1998). This range includes all degrees of chronic conditions; however, most are biologically rather benign, creating few ongoing problems for the children. Only about 10% of the children with chronic physical conditions, or 1–2% of the total child population, have severe conditions (Gortmaker & Sappenfield, 1984). With the exception of allergies, which affect 10–15% of the total childhood population, most conditions affect fewer than 1 child in 1,000. Nonetheless, when all severe chronic conditions are taken together, approximately 1–2 children out of every 100—or more than 1 million children in the United States—have such conditions.

PSYCHOSOCIAL ADJUSTMENT

Concerns about the psychosocial adjustment of children with chronic physical conditions thus apply to a sizable population. "Adjustment," "adaptation," and "mental health" are closely related terms, but the term "adjustment" is mainly used in this chapter because it implies a broad range of levels of functioning, can incorporate a clinical range in terms of maladjustment, and inherently suggests temporal and situational variability. Because the predominant task for children is to develop into autonomous, healthy, and well-functioning adults, as defined by their social and historical context, adjustment should be defined in developmental-normative terms. Good adjustment is reflected as age-appropriate, normative, and healthy behavior that follows a trajectory toward positive adult functioning. Maladjustment is evidenced in behavior that is age inappropriate, especially when it is qualitatively pathological or clinical in nature. Applying this definition necessitates norms for behaviors at different ages. An advantage of this definition is its general applicability across age, contexts, and multiple dimensions of behavior. A common alternative is using psychiatric diagnoses based on explicit criteria. However, there are limitations to applying diagnoses to children whose behavioral symptomatology, although perhaps uncommon in a healthy population, may be adaptive to their experience (Drotar & Bush, 1985).

Measurement of Adjustment

There is no inherently preferred way of measuring developmental-normative adjustment. Parent- or teacher-completed paper-and-pencil instruments can be used, as well as self-report procedures, clinical interviews, or observations. However, the Child Behavior Checklist (CBCL; Achenbach, 2002), and related scales, is by far the most commonly used measure of psychosocial adjustment of children with chronic physical conditions. At the same time, the following potential problems must be considered when the scales are used for this purpose (Perrin, Stein, & Drotar, 1991): the CBCL may have limited sensitivity for the identification of less serious adjustment problems; assessment of social competence can be grossly misleading in this population; and longitudinal research, especially with small heterogeneous samples, may be limited. However, the concern that adjustment scores may be confounded by physical symptomatology is not supported by data. Indeed, Holmes, Respess, Greer, and Frentz (1998) reported that when physical symptom items or other items deemed to be directly affected by diabetes are excluded, children with diabetes still obtained elevated CBCL scores.

Compelling evidence now exists that the adequate assessment of children's adjustment requires multiple methods and informants. This need is exemplified in recent research on chronic conditions (Holmes et al., 1998; Klinnert, McQuaid, McCormick, Adinoff, & Bryant, 2000; Radcliffe, Bennett, Kazak, Foley, & Phillips, 1996). Parent and teacher checklists and child interview methods show differential sensitivity to types of adjustment problems, and the concordance among reporters is relatively low.

An emerging concept in considering the adjustment of children with chronic physical disorders is *quality of life* (QL; Drotar, 1998; Koot & Wallander, 2001a). Wallander (2001) defines QL as "the combination of objectively and subjectively indicated well being in multiple domains of life considered salient in one's culture and time, while adhering to universal standards of human rights" (p. 34). Progress is being made in measuring QL, both for children with specific physical disorders (Koot & Wallander, 2001a) and in general (Spieth, 2001; Varni, Seid, & Rode, 2000). Two QL constructions can be discerned, the narrower health-related QL and generic QL (Koot & Wallander 2001b). The former focuses on the functional implications and disease- and treatment-related symptoms specific to a particular disease, as well as how the disease is influencing psychological and social well-being. Generic QL metaphorically asks the child the question of "How are you?" (Koot, 2001) without constraining the answer to the impact of the disease. The latter approach is important for children with chronic physical conditions, because they need to be considered as whole children and not merely as children with a disease. Koot and Wallander also point to the methodological problems inherent in asking a child to sort out what is and is not disease-related.

Is There an Increased Risk for Adjustment Problems?

By now, several hundred studies have provided data on the adjustment of children with chronic physical conditions. When these are examined individually, the results are often contradictory and confusing. This is a consequence of the different definitions, measures, and samples used across studies. Encompassing this literature as a whole, we continue to conclude that a simple or direct universal relationship between chronic physical condition and psychosocial adjustment does not exist. Rather, a wide range of responses to this source of life stress is evidenced. Although major psychiatric disturbance is not common among children with chronic conditions, nonetheless this population is at *increased risk* for psychological adjustment problems. Cadman, Boyle, Szatmari, and Offord (1987), for example, interviewed 1,869 randomly sampled families during home visits, which included an oral administration of the CBCL parent and youth self-report forms. The 20% of the children and adolescents who had various chronic physical conditions were at 2 to 3 times greater risk for psychiatric disorder than were healthy children. About 33% of the children with a chronic physical condition were diagnosed with at least one DSM-III disorder.

Lavigne and Faier-Routman (1992) conducted a meta-analysis of 87 articles selected from over 700 published between 1928 and 1990 that included some form of comparison group and a quantifiable outcome measure of overall adjustment. Children with a chronic physical disorder, on the average, reported or were reported as having more adjustment problems than those in comparison groups. This result was found regardless of whether comparisons were made against within-study controls or normative samples representing the child population. Irrespective of how adjustment was operationalized, on the average the body of literature reported twice the number of children with chronic physical conditions to have maladjustment than children in comparison groups. Although the prevalence was higher, only a minority of children with chronic physical conditions appeared maladjusted. These findings reinforce the conclusions that children with chronic physical conditions constitute a group vulnerable for maladjustment but indicate that this is not the most common outcome. Because the literature on psychosocial adjustment in children with chronic physical conditions continues to expand, this meta-analysis needs to be updated. Some recent studies indeed have reported no increased risk (Bachanas et al., 2001; Noll, Vannatta, Koontz, & Kalinyak, 1996).

What Types of Adjustment Problems Are Experienced?

Few efforts have been made to identify the specific types of problems these children tend to develop when difficulties occur. However, Thompson and colleagues used a clinical diagnostic interview with children with cystic fibrosis (Thompson, Hodges, & Hamlett, 1990) and sickle cell disease (Thompson, Gil, Burbach, Keith, & Kinney, 1993). Specifically, for cystic fibrosis, 58% received a major diagnosis; of these, 37% were diagnosed with an anxiety disorder, 23% with oppositional disorder, 14% with enuresis, 12% with conduct disorder, and

2% with a depressive disorder. For sickle cell disease, 50% received a major diagnosis, of which 34% were diagnosed with an anxiety disorder, 12% with phobia, 8% with enuresis, 8% with obsessive-compulsive disorder, 4% with conduct disorder, and 3% with encopresis. It would be beneficial if future studies of children with chronic physical conditions added to these findings by identifying what specific types of problems they develop. This research can aid in the development of intervention programs.

Does Adjustment Change over Time?

Longitudinal studies of children with chronic physical conditions can provide information about the psychosocial prognosis, as well as how psychosocial adjustment can affect physical health. For example, Bryden et al. (2001) reported that adjustment problems in adolescence predicted poorer metabolic control during the subsequent 8 years and into early adulthood (ages 20–28). A potential complication in studying children with chronic physical conditions is that their physical health can change. Orr, Weller, Satterwhite, and Pless (1984) found that 40% of those who had chronic physical conditions when their study commenced were well 8 years later (at ages 13–22). Furthermore, 47% of the originally healthy controls had acquired chronic conditions in this time span, although these were largely mild allergic and dermatological conditions. Initially rare, longitudinal studies are becoming more common in this area. Few studies follow patients prospectively from diagnosis, but they report improvements once the child is past the initial phases of adjusting to the disease and treatment (Northam, Anderson, Adler, Werther, & Warne, 1996). Others constitute samples for a follow-up assessment only to address the long-term "survival" of children with chronic physical disorders (Noll et al., 1997; Sullivan, 2001), finding generally good adjustment later in life.

In contrast, Thompson and colleagues reported that the rates of poor psychological adjustment remained fairly constant over 10 and 12 months in children with cystic fibrosis and sickle cell disease (Thompson, Gil, Keith, Gustafson, George, & Kinney, 1994; Thompson, Gustafson, George, & Spock, 1994). Breslau and Marshall (1985) examined the 5-year stability of behavioral problems among children with cystic fibrosis, cerebral palsy, spina bifida, or multiple physical disabilities. The rate of psychiatric impairment among children with conditions involving the brain (cerebral palsy, spina bifida, multiple physical disabilities) did not change with passage of time, whereas it did decline in those with cystic fibrosis, which is not considered to affect the brain. Almost two-thirds of the children initially considered severely psychiatrically impaired were still impaired 5 years later. Consequently, divergence appears as more findings emerge on the time course of adjustment in children with chronic conditions. It is likely that differences in samples, conditions, developmental periods covered, and length of follow-up, among others, contribute to this situation. Clearly, much more research into the psychosocial development of these children using longer term longitudinal designs, is needed.

CORRELATES OF PSYCHOSOCIAL ADJUSTMENT

Given the considerable variability in the psychosocial adjustment of children with chronic conditions, research has attempted to identify correlates of adjustment. These efforts are motivated not only to acquire a better understanding of adjustment but also to guide intervention efforts. Integration of findings on correlates and factors that mediate or moderate the psychosocial adjustment of children to the stress of chronic conditions was facilitated by another meta-analysis by Lavigne and Faier-Routman (1993), although only 38 studies could be incorporated. Their findings and those of other representative studies are reviewed here in terms of three broad dimensions that form an organizational framework: condition parameters, child parameters, and social-ecological parameters. Because of the volume of work, however, only representative studies are noted.

Condition Parameters

The findings of the meta-analysis (Lavigne & Faier-Routman, 1993) support a significant contribution of condition parameters, in general, to adjustment. In fact, significant correlations with adjustment were obtained for severity, functional status, and prognosis. In addition to these variables, studies have also addressed the contribution of type of condition and duration. However, it is not clear that condition parameters are stronger correlates of adjustment than psychosocial factors. For example, Burlew, Telfair, Colangelo, and Wright (2000) reported that intrapersonal, stress-processing, and social-ecological factors predicted adjustment in children with sickle cell disease, whereas condition parameters did not.

Condition Type

Contrasts among conditions that do not involve the brain, such as heart defects and types of cancer, have generally yielded no significant differences in behavioral problems or social functioning. Studies that contrast multiple conditions have not produced a consistent pattern of psychological adjustment as a function of condition type (Perrin, Ayoub, & Willett, 1993; Wallander, Varni, Babani, Banis, & Wilcox, 1988). However, children with conditions involving the brain have more behavior problems and poorer social functioning than children with conditions not involving the brain (Breslau, 1985; Walker, Ortiz-Valdes, & Newbrough, 1989). Furthermore, across conditions, levels of intellectual functioning have been shown to make independent contributions to psychological adjustment (DeMaso, Beardslee, Silbert, & Fyler, 1990; Perrin et al., 1993).

Condition Severity

Lavigne and Faier-Routman's (1993) meta-analysis supports a contribution of condition severity to adjustment. It is possible, however, that severity was confounded with condition type, because numerous studies show no relationship of severity to behavioral problems, for example, studies of children with sickle cell disease (Hurtig, Koepke, & Park, 1989) and diabetes (Kovacs et al., 1990). In terms of self-esteem or self-worth, the evidence is inconclusive. Similarly, severity and self-esteem were not significantly related in studies of children with sickle cell disease (Hurtig et al., 1989) and limb deficiencies (Varni & Setoguchi, 1991), but they were significantly related in a study of children with epilepsy (Westbrook, Bauman, & Shinnas, 1992). In terms of social functioning, the findings are also mixed. Increased severity was associated with poorer social functioning in children with asthma (Perrin, MacLean, & Perrin, 1989). Across studies of children with spina bifida, the findings have been inconsistent (Wallander, Feldman, & Varni, 1989; Wallander, Varni, Babani, Banis, DeHaan, & Wilcox, 1989).

Functional Status

Rather than assessing medical severity per se, we can examine the relationship of children's functional status to psychosocial adjustment. For example, in children with physical disabilities, poor social functioning was related to teachers' assessment of children's functional abilities (Wallander, Varni, Babani, Banis, DeHaan, & Wilcox, 1989). Motor skills were found to be associated with behavior problems in children with hydrocephalus, even when considered together with treatment, sex, and family variables (Fletcher et al., 1995). Measuring condition-related impairment in terms of functional status is potentially a useful way to operationalize severity, particularly as a common unit to be used across different conditions. It is important that these measures be based on biomedical parameters (such as degree of ambulation, pulmonary functioning, or metabolic control) or on objective measures of competency in relation to age expectations. This approach is necessary to keep this dimension distinct from psychological adjustment and other potentially mediating or moderating variables, such as *perceived* severity.

Duration

Few studies have explicitly examined the relationship between disease duration and adjustment. The previously noted longitudinal studies on prognosis addressed this issue indirectly. However, among the more direct studies, Daniels, Moos, Billings, and Miller (1987) found that longer disease duration was related to more psychological adjustment problems in children with juvenile rheumatoid arthritis. In a longitudinal study of the first 6 years subsequent to diagnosis, children appraised their diabetes as increasingly stressful and management as increasingly difficult over time (Kovacs et al., 1990). Over time, both boys and girls exhibited a mild increase in depressive symptoms; girls exhibited an increase in anxiety, and boys exhibited a decrease. If the field is to incorporate a developmental perspective, it is essential that investigations include duration as one of the factors that can mediate or moderate adjustment. To complicate matters, duration is usually confounded with age. What is most needed are longitudinal studies to determine how condition parameters interact over time with child characteristics and social-ecological parameters to influence psychological adjustment. Also, more sophisticated models of how condition parameters may be related to psychosocial adjustment need to be tested, as nicely illustrated by Hommeyer, Holmbeck, Wills, and Coers (1999).

Child Parameters

Lavigne and Faier-Routman (1993) included as child characteristics such variables as temperament, distractibility, coping methods, self-concept, and IQ. Child characteristics were found to be more significantly associated with child adjustment than were the condition variables. In addition, studies have addressed the contributions to adjustment of age, sex, social support, and an array of cognitive processes.

Gender

The contribution of gender to children's psychological adjustment has received mixed support, dependent on who is the reporting source. Most studies have found no significant differences in parent- and/or teacher-reported behavior problems as a function of gender. When adjustment was assessed through child self-report, girls reported more symptoms of distress than boys (e.g., Ryan & Morrow, 1986). However, it may be that girls are more willing than boys to report distress.

Age/Age of Onset

Studies consistently report a lack of an age effect on behavior problems or self-esteem. In contrast, the findings regarding age of onset are mixed. For example, boys who developed diabetes after age 4 had more behavior problems than boys with early-onset and girls with both early and late onset (Rovet, Ehrlich, & Hoppe, 1987). However, age of onset was not related to self-reported symptoms of psychological distress (Kovacs et al., 1990). There was no age-of-onset effect in terms of self-esteem in two studies (Rovet et al., 1987; Hanson et al., 1990); however, in another study, girls with early onset reported poorer self-concept than boys with early onset (Ryan & Morrow, 1986). These interactions warrant further examination. As with duration, the influences of age and age of onset on adjustment of children with chronic conditions need to be investigated developmentally. Such investigation requires longitudinal assessment of psychological adjustment as a function of developmental tasks associated with specific periods, such as school entry, movement to middle school or junior high, and graduation from high school.

Temperament

Given the centrality of biologically determined temperament in explanations of psychosocial functioning, it is surprising that so few studies have examined this relationship in children with chronic physical conditions. Existing studies, however, consistently show that difficult temperament is associated with poorer adjustment (e.g., Gartstein, Noll, & Vannatta, 2000; Weissberg-Benchell & Glasgow, 1997). For example, child activity level and child reactivity were related to reported behavior problems in children with spina bifida and cerebral palsy (Wallander, Hubert, & Varni, 1988). Research needs to apply more sophisticated theories of temperament and also to consider the influence of chronic conditions on temperament.

Child Coping Methods

An increasing number of studies examine the relationship of children's coping methods to their adjustment. Some have confirmed this relationship (Bachanas et al., 2001), especially the positive relationship between use of avoidance coping and psychosocial problems (Frank, Blount, & Brown, 1997; Lewis & Kliewer, 1996). In a more sophisticated test, Lewis and Kliewer (1996) also found that active, as well as support, coping moderated the negative relationship between a sense of hope and anxiety in children with sickle cell disease. Earlier studies found no relationship between coping and adjustment (Kovacs, Brent, Steinberg, Paulauskas, & Reid, 1986; Thompson et al., 1993). This area of investigation has been hampered by the lack of agreed-upon measures of children's coping, reflecting the need for conceptual clarity regarding what constitutes coping and how coping changes developmentally.

Cognitive Processes

The contribution of an array of cognitive processes to children's adjustment has been demonstrated. Perceived stress (in terms of negative life events or daily hassles) has been related to adjustment problems in multiple studies with different conditions (Kovacs et al., 1990;

Thompson, Gustafson, Gil, Godfrey, & Murphy, 1998). Additionally, perception of physical appearance and stigma has been related to self-esteem in children with epilepsy (Westbrook et al., 1992) and to self-worth (Varni, Rubenfeld, Talbot, & Setoguchi, 1989), depressive symptoms, and trait anxiety (Varni & Setoguchi, 1991) in children with limb deficiencies. A depressive attributional style was related to poorer psychological adjustment overall in older adolescents and young adults with asthma (Mullins, Chaney, Pace, & Hartman, 1997) and to depressive, anxiety, and externalizing behavior problems in children with cancer (Frank et al., 1997). However, the findings regarding perceptions of health locus of control have been mixed. No significant relationship was found in terms of behavior problems in children with cystic fibrosis (Thompson, Gustafson, Hamlett, & Spock, 1992), but "powerful other" health locus of control perceptions in children with sickle cell disease contributed to internalizing behavior problems (Thompson et al., 1993). Although few studies have been done of each cognitive factor, the evidence across factors attests to some role for cognitive processes in children's adjustment. A challenge will be to find the most salient, common dimensions of cognitive style that influence adjustment. Once accomplished, those cognitive processes could be important intervention targets.

Social-Ecological Parameters

The meta-analysis conducted by Lavigne and Faier-Routman (1993) examined social-ecological variables. Maternal adjustment, marital and family adjustment or conflict, and family support or cohesiveness, but not paternal adjustment, were significantly correlated with child adjustment. In addition, parent ratings of life stressors were significantly related to child adjustment, but socioeconomic status (SES) was not.

Family Functioning

Family functioning has been the most frequently investigated social-ecological correlate of adjustment. Conceptually, the role of the family has been reflected in terms of the dimensions of cohesion, expressiveness, organization, independence, and control identified by Moos and Moos (1981) and of the adaptability and cohesion dimensions identified by the circumplex model (Olson, Sprenkle, & Russell, 1979). There is strong, consistent support for the role of family functioning in child psychological adjustment across different conditions. Some studies investigate a single dimension of family functioning. For example, cohesion was related to the adjustment of children with spina bifida (Lavigne, Nolan, & McLone, 1988). It is possible that this association stems from the positive effect of family cohesion over time on children's use of problem-focused coping strategies, demonstrated in a longitudinal study (McKernon et al., 2001). In contrast, Wallander, Varni, Babani, Banis, and Wilcox (1989) formulated a multidimensional measure of family psychological resources, which accounted for a significant increment in variance in children's behavior problems and social functioning above the contribution of family income and maternal education. Family cohesion made a particularly significant contribution to social functioning. Other studies have confirmed that family conflict is correlated with adjustment problems (Manne & Miller, 1998; Thompson et al., 1999).

Not only have dimensions of family functioning been shown to have direct associations with adjustment, but also interaction effects with other potential correlates of adjustment have been demonstrated. Murch and Cohen (1989) demonstrated that low conflict, low control, and high cohesion in the family served to buffer depression in children with spina bifida in the situation of uncontrollable life stress, whereas high independence exacerbated depression and anxiety in the context of controllable life stress. This study illustrates a sophisticated examination of ways in which sets of correlates may act together on adjustment. The contribution of family functioning may vary not only in relation to perceptions of stress but also in terms of SES, coping methods, and child characteristics. In particular, patterns of family functioning conducive to adjustment may vary with the child's developmental level.

Parental Stress and Adjustment

The mental health literature also supports a relationship between children's adjustment and parental stress and distress (Banez & Compas, 1990). Several studies have found a relationship between maternal distress and mother-reported child adjustment. For example, Thompson and colleagues have reported such findings for children with cystic fibrosis and sickle cell disease, both concurrently and longitudinally (Thompson et al., 1992; Thompson, Gustafson, et al., 1994; Thompson, Gil, et al., 1993, 1994). Although there is a possibility that this relationship reflects maternal report bias, other studies indicate that mothers' reports of their children's behavior are influenced by child behavior, as well as by their own mood (Walker et al., 1989). Child adjustment needs to be assessed through both child and maternal reports to differentiate the association between parental adjustment and child adjustment from that between maternal adjustment and maternal perceptions of their children's behavior.

Of course, the relationship between maternal and child adjustment is likely transactional, but this possibility is rarely considered empirically. Utilizing both interview and self-report methods, Chaney et al. (1997) examined such patterns longitudinally among child, mother, and father in families in which the child has diabetes. Interestingly, increases in fathers' but not mothers' distress over time predicted poorer subsequent adjustment in the children. Child adjustment in this case was not associated with mothers' adjustment. This study illustrates the transactional nature of other relationships that exist in families and exemplifies how families can be studied as a system.

Peer Relationships

Research on the peer relationships of children with chronic conditions was largely absent at the time of Lavigne and Faier-Routman's (1993) meta-analysis. Although the number of studies exploring peer relationships has increased, their role in the adjustment of children with chronic conditions has rarely been examined. However, Wallander and Varni (1989) found that for children with chronic conditions, those who had high levels of social support from both family and peers showed significantly better adjustment than those with social support from only one of those sources. This finding is of concern because reports on the quality of these children's peer relationships conflict (Graetz & Shute, 1995; Vannatta, Zeller, Noll, & Koontz, 1998), even though peers are considered to be important sources of emotional support for children (La Greca & Thompson, 1998). Much more research is needed into this important area of children's lives.

Conclusions

The search for correlates of psychological adjustment of children with chronic conditions has involved many variables and various measures of children's adjustment. Overwhelmingly, specific variables have too often been investigated in only one study. When correlates have been addressed in more than one study, findings are often inconsistent across studies, whether they use the same or different measures of children's adjustment. Thus, in spite of the efforts to date, the knowledge base is limited. At this point, there is relatively stronger support for brain involvement, child reports of high levels of stress and low levels of self esteem, family functioning characterized as low in cohesion and supportiveness or high in conflict, and maternal distress as correlates of poor adjustment in children with chronic conditions. In particular, the role of child parameters and the interrelationship among condition, child, and social-ecological parameters are ripe for investigation, especially in longitudinal studies. Currently, there is a need to determine whether positive and negative findings can be replicated. To provide a sound basis for the pattern of variables investigated and to integrate findings across studies, these efforts need to be theoretically driven. To this end, we now review prominent conceptual models.

INTEGRATIVE THEORETICAL MODELS

Several researchers have attempted to make sense of the multiple purported influences on adjustment in children with chronic physical conditions. Beginning with Pless and Pinkerton's (1975) groundbreaking effort, more complex but integrative models have been proposed to attempt to explain this phenomenon. Two of these models are discussed briefly here.

Wallander and Varni's Model

Wallander and Varni's disability–stress–coping model (Wallander & Varni, 1992, 1997; Wallander, Varni, Babani, Banis, & Wilcox, 1989; see Figure 9.1) builds on notions put forth for the understanding of adjustment more generally in both children (Rutter, 1990) and adults (Lazarus & Folkman, 1984; Moos & Schaefer, 1984), as well as notions of disease processes advanced in epidemiology. The various variables hypothesized in this model to play a role in adjustment are organized into a risk-and-resilience framework. The variable thought to be primarily responsible for elevating the risk for psychosocial problems is stress. That is, children with chronic physical conditions display adjustment problems because they are exposed to negative life events. Some of this stress emanates from their physical condition (i.e., disease/disability parameters) and closely associated behavioral and environmental circumstances (i.e., functional limitations, disability-related stress). However, added to this must be the more general stress occurring in their lives, which may be indirectly or not at all related to their condition. For example, stressors experienced by most children (e.g., the start of middle school) may be harder to deal with for a child with a chronic physical condition, possibly because condition-related limitations or disability-related stressors are already present. Adjustment is also influenced by intrapersonal, social-ecological, and stress-processing factors. In addition, the impact of the risk factors on adjustment is hypothesized to be moderated by resilience factors. This conceptual model has guided Wallander's and Varni's research programs (cf. Wallander & Varni, 1997) and is also frequently referenced by others. However, because of its complexity, only portions of this model are evaluated in any given study.

Thompson's Model

Thompson has proposed a transactional stress and coping model (Thompson et al., 1992) (see Figure 9.2), set within ecological-systems theory. A chronic physical condition is a

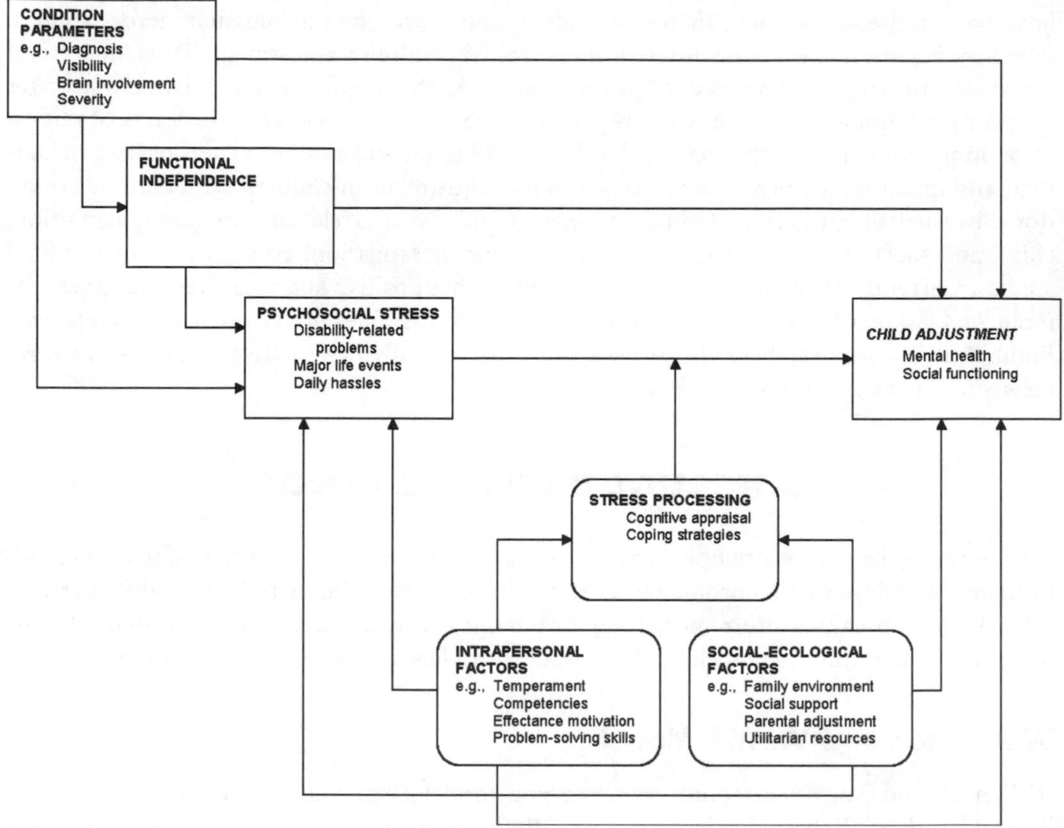

FIGURE 9.1. Wallander and Varni's disability–stress–coping model of adjustment. Square corner boxes indicate risk factors; round-corner boxes indicate resilience factors. Adapted from Wallander and Varni (1992). Copyright 1992 by The Guilford Press. Adapted by permission.

potential stressor to which the child and family system endeavor to adapt. The relationship between the chronic physical condition and adjustment is a function of the transactions of biomedical, developmental, and psychosocial processes. However, the focus is on the contribution of child and family adaptation that is hypothesized to influence the psychological adjustment of children, above the contribution of biomedical and demographic parameters. In terms of child adjustment, hypothesized adaptational processes currently include expectations of self-esteem and health locus of control. It is also hypothesized that child adjustment affects and is affected by maternal adjustment. Hypotheses based on this model have now been tested in studies of children with different chronic physical conditions (Thompson & Gustafson, 1996).

CRITIQUE AND RECOMMENDATIONS

Developmental Perspective

Children with chronic physical disorders are developing beings. Their families also experience development. Models and concepts within theories, as well as the research methods, need to reflect these basic tenets. General developmental processes should become more salient features of the conceptualizations of adjustment in this special group. Prospective longitudinal designs need to become the norm. The course of the disorder and its treatment need to be taken into account, as well as the interactions of these with individual and family development. The study of the effects of chronic disorders should in many ways become a specific case of the study of the effects of challenging circumstances on child development.

Theory

Although conceptually driven research has increased considerably during the recent past, more varied models need to be proposed. These models should incorporate richer perspectives, novel concepts, and more explicit causal processes. More attention should be paid to intrapersonal correlates of adjustment, including the range of traditional personality traits and biologically linked temperament to situation-specific cognitive–affective processes. The study of the family context must reflect advances in family research more generally. We need to move beyond considering just the mother in this context. Additional social contexts also need to be considered, such as the peer, school, and treatment environments. Future studies will need to begin to test the multivariate models being proposed *in toto*. These theoretical advancements, as well as adopting a more explicit developmental perspective, will require

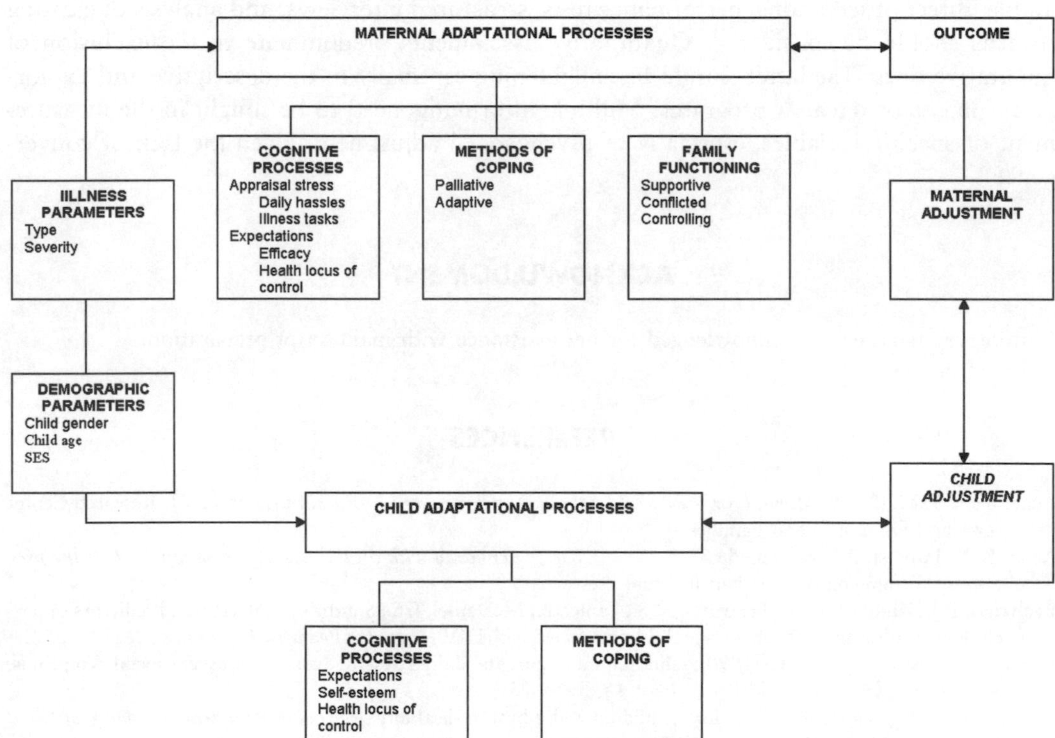

FIGURE 9.2. Thompson's stress and coping model of adjustment. From Roberts (1998). Copyright 1998 by the Guilford Press.

analytical procedures better suited to these challenges (e.g., structural equations analysis, hierarchical growth modeling).

Methods

Population-based studies will be required to test these multivariate models with sufficient power. Furthermore, the generalizability of results will be substantially enhanced when study samples are drawn from defined populations. Although clinic samples will continue to be studied, they will need to be constituted from multiple sites. As well, multiple disorders should be studied, whether based on a noncategorical perspective or for purposes of comparing different biomedical or psychosocial processes that they may represent. Understudied populations, such as ethnic groups, the economically disadvantaged, and those without access to specialty care, need to be targeted. Cross-cultural comparisons can illuminate the role of behaviors of the children and their families, as well as the health care models employed in different cultures.

Measurement

Measurement of variables should employ the whole range of methods available. Researchers tend to overrely on paper-and-pencil self-reports, especially from mothers. Whereas this method and source obviously remain important, additional ones will be informative. For example, direct observations, performance tests, structured interviews, and analysis of existing records should be considered. Quantitative assessments predominate to the exclusion of qualitative ones. The latter should be enlightening especially in the descriptive and exploratory phases of research programs. Multiple informants need to be sought in the measurement of specific variables, especially of psychosocial adjustment, given the lack of convergence.

ACKNOWLEDGMENT

Kym Storey is gratefully acknowledged for her assistance with manuscript preparation.

REFERENCES

Achenbach, T. M. (2002). *Manual for the ASEBA School-Age Forms and Profiles*. Burlington, VT: Research Center for Children, Youth, and Families.

Aron, L. Y., Loprest, P. J., & Steuerie, C. E. (1996). *Serving children with disabilities: A systematic look at the programs*. Washington, DC: Urban Institute Press.

Bachanas, P. J., Kullgren, K. A., Schwarts, K. S., Lanier, B., McDaniel, J. S., Smith, J., et al. (2001). Predictors of psychological adjustment in school-age children infected with HIV. *Journal of Pediatric Psychology, 26*, 343–352.

Banez, G. A., & Compas, B. E. (1990). Children's and parents' daily stressful events and psychosocial symptoms. *Journal of Abnormal Child Psychology, 18*, 591–605.

Breslau, N. (1985). Psychiatric disorder in children with physical disability. *Journal of American Academy of Child Psychiatry, 24*, 87–94.

Breslau, N., & Marshall, I. A. (1985). Psychological disturbance in children with physical disabilities: Continuity and change in a 5-year follow-up. *Journal of Abnormal Child Psychology, 13*, 199–216.

Bryden, K. S., Peveler, R. C., Stein, A., Neil, A., Mayou, R. A., & Dunger, D. B. (2001). Clinical and psychological course of diabetes from adolescence to young adulthood: A longitudinal cohort study. *Diabetes Care, 24*, 1536–1540.

Burlew, K., Telfair, J., Colangelo, L., & Wright, E. C. (2000). Factors that influence adolescent adaptation to sickle cell disease. *Journal of Pediatric Psychology, 25*, 287–299.

Cadman, D., Boyle, M., Szatmari, P., & Offord, D. R. (1987). Chronic illness, disability, and mental and social well-being: Findings of the Ontario Child Health Study. *Pediatrics, 79*, 805–813.

Chaney, J. M., Mullins, L. L., Frank, R. G., Peterson, L., Mace, L. D., Kashani, J. H., et al. (1997). Transactional patterns of child, mother, and father adjustment in insulin-dependent diabetes mellitus: A prospective study. *Journal of Pediatric Psychology, 22*, 229–244.

Daniels, D., Moos, R. H., Billings, A. G., & Miller, J. J. (1987). Psychosocial risks and resistance factors among children with chronic illness, healthy siblings, and healthy controls. *Journal of Abnormal Child Psychology, 15*, 295–308.

DeMaso, D. R., Beardslee, W. R., Silbert, A. R., & Fyler, D. C. (1990). Psychological functioning in children with cyanotic heart defects. *Journal of Developmental and Behavioral Pediatrics, 11*, 289–294.

Drotar, D. (1998). *Measuring health-related quality of life in children and adolescents: Implications for research and practice.* Mahway, NJ: Erlbaum.

Drotar, D., & Bush, M. (1985). Mental health issues and services. In N. Hobbs & J. M. Perrin (Eds.), *Issues in the care of children with chronic illness* (pp. 514–550). San Francisco: Jossey-Bass.

Fletcher, J. M., Brookshire, B. L., Landry, S. H., Bohan, T. P., Davidson, K. C., Francis, D. J., et al. (1995). Behavioral adjustment of children with hydrocephalus: Relationships with etiology, neurological and family status. *Journal of Pediatric Psychology, 20*, 109–125.

Frank, N. C., Blount, R. L., & Brown, R. T. (1997). Attributions, coping, and adjustment in children with cancer. *Journal of Pediatric Psychology, 22*, 563–576.

Gartstein, M. A., Noll, R. B., & Vannatta, K. (2000). Childhood aggression and chronic illness: Possible protective mechanisms. *Journal of Applied Developmental Psychology, 21*, 315–333.

Gartstein, M. A., Short, A. D., Vannatta, K., & Noll, R. B. (1999). Psychosocial adjustment of children with chronic illness: An evaluation of three models. *Journal of Developmental and Behavioral Pediatrics, 20*, 157–163.

Gortmaker, S. L., & Sappenfield, W. (1984). Chronic childhood disorders: Prevalence and impact. *Pediatric Clinics of North America, 31*, 3–18.

Graetz, B., & Shute, R. (1995). Assessment of peer relationships in children with asthma. *Journal of Pediatric Psychology, 20*, 205–216.

Hanson, C. L., Rodrigue, J. R., Henggeler, S. W., Harris, M. A., Klesges, R. C., & Carle, D. L. (1990). The perceived self-competence of adolescents with insulin-dependent diabetes mellitus: Deficit or strength? *Journal of Pediatric Psychology, 10*, 605–618.

Holmes, C. S., Respess, D., Greer, T., & Frentz, J. (1998). Behavior problems in children with diabetes: Disentangling possible scoring confounds on the Child Behavior Checklist. *Journal of Pediatric Psychology, 23*, 179–185.

Hommeyer, J. S., Holmbeck, G. N., Wills, K. E., & Coers, S. (1999). Condition severity and psychosocial functioning in preadolescents with spina bifida: Disentangling proximal functional status and distal adjustment outcomes. *Journal of Pediatric Psychology, 24*, 499–509.

Hurtig, A. L., Koepke, D., & Park, K. B. (1989). Relation between severity of chronic illness and adjustment in children and adolescents with sickle cell disease. *Journal of Pediatric Psychology, 14*, 117–132.

Klinnert, M. D., McQuaid, E. L., McCormick, D., Adinoff, A. D., & Bryant, N. E. (2000). A multimethod assessment of behavioral and emotional adjustment in children with asthma. *Journal of Pediatric Psychology, 25*, 35–46.

Koot, H. (2001). The study of quality of life: Concepts and methods. In H. Koot & J. L. Wallander (Eds.), *Quality of life in child and adolescent illness: Concepts, methods, and findings* (pp. 3–20). Hove, East Sussex, UK: Brunner-Routledge.

Koot, H. M., & Wallander, J. L. (Eds.). (2001a). *Quality of life in child and adolescent illness: Concepts, methods, and findings.* Hove, East Sussex, UK: Brunner-Routledge.

Koot, H. M., & Wallander, J. L. (2001b). Challenges in child and adolescent quality of life research. In H. M. Koot & J. L. Wallander (Eds.), *Quality of life in child and adolescent illness: Concepts, methods, and findings* (pp. 431–456). Hove, East Sussex, UK: Brunner-Routledge.

Kovacs, M., Brent, D., Steinberg, T. F., Paulauskas, S., & Reid, J. (1986). Children's self-reports of psychological adjustment and coping strategies during first year of insulin-dependent diabetes mellitus. *Diabetes Care, 9*, 472–479.

Kovacs, M., Iyengar, S., Goldston, D., Obrosky, D. S., Stewart, J., & Marsh, J. (1990). Psychological functioning among mothers of children with insulin-dependent diabetes mellitus: A longitudinal study. *Journal of Consulting and Clinical Psychology, 58*, 189–195.

La Greca, A. M., & Thompson, K. (1998). Family and friend support for adolescents with diabetes. *Analise Psicologica, 1*, 101–113.

Lavigne, J. V., & Faier-Routman, J. (1992). Psychological adjustment to pediatric physical disorders: A meta-analytic review. *Journal of Pediatric Psychology, 17*, 133–157.

Lavigne, J. V., & Faier-Routman, J. (1993). Correlates of psychological adjustment to pediatric physical disorders: A meta-analytic review and comparison with existing models. *Journals of Developmental and Behavioral Pediatrics, 14*, 117–123.

Lavigne, J. V., Nolan, P., & McLone, P. G. (1988). Temperament, coping, and psychological adjustment in young children with myelomeningocele. *Journal of Pediatric Psychology, 13*, 363–378.

Lazarus, R. S., & Folkman, S. (Eds.). (1984). *Stress, appraisal, and coping*. New York: Springer.

Lewis, H. A., & Kliewer, W. (1996). Hope, coping, and adjustment among children with sickle cell disease: Tests of mediator and moderator models. *Journal of Pediatric Psychology, 21*, 25–41.

Manne, S., & Miller, D. (1998). Social support, social conflict, and adjustment among adolescents with cancer. *Journal of Pediatric Psychology, 23*, 121–130.

McKernon, W. L., Holmbeck, G. N., Grayson, N., Colder, C. R., Hommeyer, J. S., Shapera, W., et al. (2001). Longitudinal study of observed and perceived family influences on problem-focused coping behaviors of preadolescents with spina bifida. *Journal of Pediatric Psychology, 26*, 41–54.

Moos, R. H., & Moos, B. S. (Eds.). (1981). *Family Environment Scale Manual*. Palo Alto, CA: Consulting Psychologists Press.

Moos, R. H., & Schaefer, J. (1984). The crisis of physical illness: An overview and conceptual approach. In R. H. Moos (Ed.), *Coping with physical illness: New perspectives* (pp. 3–25). New York: Plenum.

Mullins, L. L., Chaney, J. M., Pace, T. M., & Hartman, V. L. (1997). Illness uncertainty, attributional style, and psychological adjustment in older adolescents and young adults with asthma. *Journal of Pediatric Psychology, 22*, 871–880.

Murch, R. L., & Cohen, L. H. (1989). Relationships among life stress, perceived family environment, and the psychological distress of spina bifida adolescents. *Journal of Pediatric Psychology, 14*, 193–214.

Newacheck, P. W., Strickland, B., Shonkoff, J. P., Perrin, J. M., McPherson, M., McManus, M., et al. (1998). An epidemiologic profile of children with special health care needs. *Pediatrics, 102*, 117–123.

Noll, R. B., MacLean, W. E., Jr., Whitt, J. K., Kaleita, T. A., Stehbens, J. A., Waskerwitz, M. J., et al. (1997). Behavioral adjustment and social functioning of long-term survivors of childhood leukemia: Parent and teacher reports. *Journal of Pediatric Psychology, 22*, 827–841.

Noll, R. B., Vannatta, K., Koontz, K., & Kalinyak, K. (1996). Peer relationships and emotional well-being of youngsters with sickle cell disease. *Child Development, 67*, 423–436.

Northam, E., Anderson, P., Adler, R., Werther, G., & Warne, G. (1996). Psychosocial and family functioning in children with insulin-dependent diabetes at diagnosis and one year later. *Journal of Pediatric Psychology, 21*, 699–717.

Olson, D. H., Sprenkle, D., & Russell, C. (1979). Circumplex model of marital and family systems: I. Cohesion and adaptability dimensions, family types, and clinical applications. *Family Process, 18*, 3–28.

Orr, D. P., Weller, S. C., Satterwhite, B., & Pless, I. B. (1984). Psychosocial implications of chronic illness in adolescence. *Journal of Pediatrics, 194*, 152–157.

Perrin, E. C., Ayoub, C. C., & Willett, J. B. (1993). In the eyes of the beholder: Family and maternal influences on perceptions of adjustment of children with a chronic illness. *Journal of Developmental and Behavioral Pediatrics, 14*, 94–105.

Perrin, E. C., Stein, R. E. K., & Drotar, D. (1991). Cautions on using the Child Behavior Checklist: Observations based on research about children with a chronic illness. *Journal of Pediatric Psychology, 16*, 411–421.

Perrin, J. M., MacLean, W. E., Jr., & Perrin, E. C. (1989). Parents' perception of health status and psychological adjustment of children with asthma. *Pediatrics, 83*, 26–30.

Pless, I. B., & Pinkerton, P. (Eds.). (1975). *Chronic childhood disorder: Promoting patterns of adjustment*. Chicago: Year Book Medical Publishers.

Radcliffe, J., Bennett, D., Kazak, A. E., Foley, B., & Phillips, P. C. (1996). Adjustment in childhood brain tumor survival: Child, mother, and teacher report. *Journal of Pediatric Psychology, 21*, 529–539.

Rolland, J. S. (1994). *Families, illness, and disability: An integrative treatment model*. New York: Basic Books.

Rovet, J. F., Ehrlich, R. M., & Hoppe, M. (1987). Behavior problems in children with diabetes as a function of sex and age of onset of disease. *Journal of Child Psychology and Psychiatry, 28*, 477–491.

Rutter, M. (1990). Psychosocial resilience and protective mechanisms. In J. Rolf, A. S. Masten, D. Cicchetti, K. Nuechterlein, & S. Weintraub (Eds.), *Risk and protective factors in the development of psychopathology* (pp. 181–214). New York: Cambridge University Press.

Ryan, C. M., & Morrow, L. A. (1986). Self-esteem in diabetic adolescents: Relationship between age at onset and gender. *Journal of Consulting and Clinical Psychology, 54*, 730–731.

Speith, L. (2001). Generic health-related quality of life measures for children and adolescents. In H. Koot & J. L. Wallander (Eds.), *Quality of life in child and adolescent illness: Concepts, methods, and findings* (pp. 49–88). Hove, East Sussex, UK: Brunner-Routledge.

Stein, R. E. K., & Jessop, D. J. (1982). A noncategorical approach to chronic childhood illness. *Public Health Reports, 97*, 354–362.

Sullivan, J. E. (2001). Emotional outcomes of adolescents and young adults with early and continuously treated phenylketonuria. *Journal of Pediatric Psychology, 26*, 477–484.

Thompson, R. J., Jr., Armstrong, F. D., Kronenberger, W. G., Scott, D., McCabe, M. A., Smith, B., et al. (1999). Family functioning, neurocognitive functioning, and behavior problems in children with sickle cell disease. *Journal of Pediatric Psychology, 24*, 491–498.

Thompson, R. J., Jr., Gil, K. M., Burbach, D. J., Keith, B. R., & Kinney, T. R. (1993). Role of child and maternal processes in the psychological adjustment of children with sickle cell disease. *Journal of Consulting and Clinical Psychology, 61*, 468–474.

Thompson, R. J., Jr., Gil, K. M., Keith, B. R., Gustafson, K. E., George, L. K., & Kinney, T. R. (1994). Psychological adjustment of children with sickle cell disease: Stability and change over a 10-month period. *Journal of Consulting and Clinical Psychology, 62*, 856–860.

Thompson, R. J., Jr., & Gustafson, K. E. (1996). *Adaptation to chronic childhood illness.* Washington, DC: American Psychological Association.

Thompson, R. J., Jr., Gustafson, K. E., George, L. K., & Spock, A. (1994). Change over a 12-month period in the psychological adjustment of children and adolescents with cystic fibrosis. *Journal of Pediatric Psychology, 19*, 189–203.

Thompson, R. J., Jr., Gustafson, K. E., Gil, K. M., Godfrey, J., & Murphy, L. M. (1998). Illness specific patterns of psychological adjustment and cognitive adaptational processes in children with cystic fibrosis and sickle cell disease. *Journal of Clinical Psychology, 54*, 121–128.

Thompson, R. J., Jr., Gustafson, K. E., Hamlett, K. W., & Spock, A. (1992). Stress, coping, and family functioning in the psychological adjustment of mothers of children with cystic fibrosis. *Journal of Pediatric Psychology, 17*, 573–585.

Thompson, R. J., Jr., Hodges, K., & Hamlett, K. W. (1990). A matched comparison of adjustment in children with cystic fibrosis and psychiatrically referred and non-referred children. *Journal of Pediatric Psychology, 15*, 745–759.

Vannatta, K., Zeller, M., Noll, R. B., & Koontz, K. (1998). Social functioning of children surviving bone marrow transplantation. *Journal of Pediatric Psychology, 23*, 169–178.

Varni, J. W., Rubenfeld, L. A., Talbot, D., & Setoguchi, Y. (1989). Determinants of self-esteem in children with congenital/acquired limb deficiencies. *Journal of Developmental and Behavioral Pediatrics, 10*, 13–16.

Varni, J. W., Seid, M., & Rode, C. A. (2000). The PedsQL^{TM}: Measurement Model for the Pediatric Quality of Life Inventory. *Medical Care, 37*, 126–139.

Varni, J. W., & Setoguchi, Y. (1991). Correlates of perceived physical appearance in children with congenital/acquired limb deficiencies. *Journal of Developmental and Behavioral Pediatrics, 12*, 171–176.

Walker, L. S., Ortiz-Valdes, J. A., & Newbrough, J. R. (1989). The role of maternal employment and depression in the psychological adjustment of chronically ill, mentally retarded, and well children. *Journal of Pediatric Psychology, 14*, 357–370.

Wallander, J. L. (2001). Theoretical and developmental issues in quality of life for children and adolescents. In H. M. Koot & J. L. Wallander (Eds.), *Quality of life in child and adolescent illness: Concepts, methods and findings* (pp. 23–48). Hove, East Sussex, UK: Brunner-Routledge.

Wallander, J. L., Feldman, W. S., & Varni, J. W. (1989). Physical status and psychosocial adjustment in children with spina bifida. *Journal of Pediatric Psychology, 14*, 89–102.

Wallander, J. L., Hubert, N. C., & Varni, J. W. (1988). Child and maternal temperament characteristics, goodness of fit, and adjustment in physically handicapped children. *Journal of Clinical Child Psychology, 17*, 336–344.

Wallander, J. L., & Thompson, R. J., Jr. (1995). Psychosocial adjustment of children with chronic physical conditions. In M. C. Roberts (Ed.), *Handbook of pediatric psychology* (2nd ed., pp. 124–141). New York: Guilford Press.

Wallander, J. L., & Varni, J. W. (1992). Adjustment in children with chronic physical disorders: Programmatic research on a disability-stress-coping model. In A. M. La Greca, L. Siegel, J. L. Wallander, & C. E. Walker (Eds.), *Stress and coping in child health* (pp. 279–298). New York: Guilford Press.

Wallander, J. L., & Varni, J. W. (1997). Effects of pediatric chronic physical disorders on child and family adjustment. *Journal of Child Psychology and Psychiatry, 39*, 29–46.

Wallander, J. L., & Varni, J. W. (1989). Social support and adjustment in chronically ill and handicapped children. *American Journal of Community Psychology, 17*, 185–201.

Wallander, J. L., Varni, J. W., Babani, L., Banis, H. T., DeHaan, C. B., & Wilcox, K. T. (1989). Disability parameters: Chronic strain and adaptation of physically handicapped children and their mothers. *Journal of Pediatric Psychology, 14*, 23–42.

Wallander, J. L., Varni, J. W., Babani, L., Banis, H. T., & Wilcox, K. T. (1988). Children with chronic physical disorders: Maternal reports of their psychological adjustment. *Journal of Pediatric Psychology, 13*, 197–212.

Wallander, J. L., Varni, J. W., Babani, L., Banis, H. T., & Wilcox, K. T. (1989). Family resources as resistance factors for psychological maladjustment in chronically ill and handicapped children. *Journal of Pediatric Psychology, 14*, 157–173.

Weissberg-Benchell, J., & Glasgow, A. (1997). The role of temperament in children with insulin-dependent diabetes mellitus. *Journal of Pediatric Psychology, 22*, 795–809.

Westbrook, L. E., Bauman, L. J., & Shinnas, S. (1992). Applying stigma theory to epilepsy: A test of a conceptual model. *Journal of Pediatric Psychology, 17*, 633–658.

10

Families and Other Systems in Pediatric Psychology

ANNE E. KAZAK
MARY T. ROURKE
TERRY A. CRUMP

A FAMILY/SYSTEMS APPROACH IN PEDIATRIC PSYCHOLOGY

Child health-related concerns, both chronic and acute, inherently and unquestionably affect not only the child but also parents, siblings, extended family, classmates, school personnel, and the health care team. Likewise, issues related to each of these groups, or subsystems, reciprocally influence the child. In pediatric psychology, this is most clearly evident in childhood chronic illnesses. Children and their families must balance the complicated tasks of growing up with the symptoms of their disease and implications of their treatment. The course of the child's life and the family's development may be profoundly affected by a shortened lifespan, a lifetime of unpredictable medical problems, cognitive impairments, and/or the financial impact of long-term illness. Also relevant, although less developed, is the importance of family in acute illnesses, which are often treated in primary care settings, and in the field of primary prevention.

There is much to be learned from a broader inclusion of families in our conceptualization of children and health. Historically, families of ill children tended to be viewed as disrupted, complicated, or sometimes even pathological. Despite a substantial literature refuting these views, the idea of competence in families is only now beginning to be appreciated more fully. When the family is viewed as essential and inseparable from patients in understanding illness and adaptation, the complexity of family systems in pediatric psychology becomes evident.

Where does the family fit in pediatric psychology? Family research, family therapy, and family policy are multidisciplinary fields, with psychologists often contributing less than might be expected, perhaps based on a traditional focus on individuals. Indeed, most pediatric psychologists are not trained to work with whole families and may not appreciate the conceptual and clinical arguments for doing so. A relatively small amount of family therapy coursework and supervised practice is provided in clinical child and pediatric training programs. Nonetheless, several models use a systemic framework to organize family and disease factors (Wallander & Varni, 1992; Thompson & Gustafson, 1999; Wood, 1995; Fiese & Sameroff, 1989).

The role of families in pediatric psychology remains relatively underdeveloped (Mullins, Gillman, & Harbeck, 1991; Seagull, 2000). Indeed, the majority of research published in the *Journal of Pediatric Psychology* (JPP) rests heavily on data from and about children. Although data from other family members are frequently included, the data are generally parent reports on child behavior, not differentiating mothers and fathers. However, there is evidence of a shift over the 1990s, with more papers reporting data from multiple members of the family system (Kazak, Simms, & Rourke, 2002) and advancing methodologies for multiinformant, multimethod research relevant to families (Holmbeck, Li, Schurman, Friedman, & Coakley, 2002).

Our family–systems approach to pediatric illness presents the family and contextual factors as *foreground*. That is, rather than considering linear relationships between family variables and child outcome, we focus on those studies that take a family orientation and clarify family issues relevant to pediatric psychology. Our approach also emphasizes family strength or competence in the face of childhood illness. With this in mind, we focus less on studies documenting psychopathology and more on studies that focus on the presumably adaptive processes that families demonstrate when confronted with illness.

A SOCIAL-ECOLOGICAL FRAMEWORK APPLIED TO PEDIATRIC PSYCHOLOGY

Social ecology (Figure 10.1) is a useful model for conceptualizing the many systems relevant to pediatric patients and their families (Kazak, 1989). Based on the work of developmental psychologist Bronfenbrenner (1979), social ecology provides a context for understanding the many interactions among childhood illnesses and the individuals and systems affected, and it can help to organize systemically oriented interventions. Social ecology emphasizes the importance of individual development within an ecological context and the implications of developmental processes for coping and adaptation.

The most proximal levels of influence on the developing child within a social ecological model are *microsystems*, or the "patterns of activities, roles, and interpersonal relations experienced by the developing person" (Bronfenbrenner, 1979, p. 22). The microsystem includes the immediate settings in which the child functions, such as schools, or in the case of children with health-related concerns, health care settings. Other important microsystems include the family (the most frequently addressed microsystem) and subsystems of the family (e.g., siblings, marital relationships, parent–child interactions). In our work, we view the disease and its treatment—including members of the health care team—as a critical microsystem. Diseases and their treatments place many demands on children and families and remain an important part of the lives of affected families for many years.

Mesosystems are interrelated microsystems, or the overlap of two or more microsystems. It is misleading that mesosystems are sometimes oversimplified, with emphasis on their more distal relationship to the child rather than on systemic interactions. Mesosystems allow us to ask, for example, how interactions among families, health care teams, and

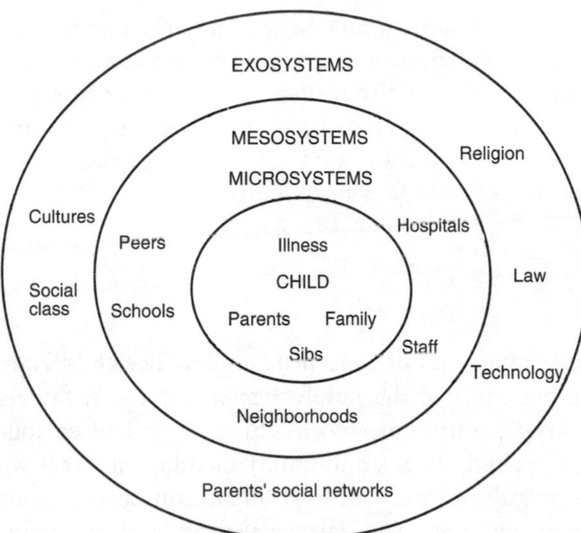

FIGURE 10.1. The social ecology of pediatric illness. From Power, DuPaul, Shapiro, and Kazak (2003). Copyright 2003 by The Guilford Press. Reprinted by permission.

school personnel affect children with chronic illness and their families. The *exosystem* includes aspects of the social ecology that do not have direct effects on the child but that rather may have profound indirect effects. Relevant research in this area includes the impact of parental social networks and employment on children. Given the importance of caregiving for ill children and the fact that the majority of care is provided by parents, it is crucial to include an appreciation of parental social ecologies in order to (indirectly) affect the care of children.

Finally, at the outermost level of social ecology is the *macrosystem,* which refers to the impact of subculture, culture, and general belief patterns throughout the ecology. Although broader systems issues are frequently not considered within the realm of psychological theory or intervention, neglect of these issues can result in a dangerously myopic view of families. For example, local, state, and federal laws and policies have direct implications for the types of care and services available to children and families. Over the past decade, the United States has witnessed the impact of dramatic changes in health care on families and have seen the passage of legislation (e.g., Family Medical Leave Act) that assists families by providing more options for balancing their family and work demands. Understanding ways in which broader systems constrain or support family adaptation during the course of an illness is critical to designing more effective interventions.

Representative Work Related to Microsystems

In the following section, we present empirical work related to the primary microsystems for children. In doing so, we inevitably cover the interaction of some of these microsystems with each other—that is, mesosystems (e.g., child-illness, family-illness, and family-health care teams). Where possible, we aim to integrate exo- and macrosystem influences. Readers can find more about specific macrosystem influences (culture, health care organization, technology, legal) elsewhere in this volume. When including studies about *families*, we sought: (1)

studies that included data from more than one person in the family (e.g., patient, mother, father) and/or more than one person from multiple systems (e.g., mother–nurse, child–peer); and (2) study questions that were either conceptualized or interpreted from a family–systems perspective. We generally excluded parent self-report questionnaire data reporting on child behavior. These criteria yielded a narrow band of research. Occasionally, research that did not fully meet the criteria was included because it offered an important systemic perspective.

The Child

The child is at the center of a series of concentric circles. The child's circle is nested within a larger circle including members of the family system (mothers, fathers, siblings, extended family) and the illness (type, course, prognosis, chronicity). This ecological context is highly interactional. That is, the child, illness, and family members interact with one another, continuously refining the overall context and its influence on development. For example, children must have parental consent to initiate treatment, and, even for adolescents, family members assume substantial responsibility for assuring adherence to treatment recommendations. Despite the family's broad and powerful impact throughout the course of treatment, however, most of what is known about child adjustment to illness focuses on the individual child.

The substantial literature on child adjustment demonstrates that children with chronic illness are at some elevated risk for psychological difficulties. There is a discernable need for methodologically rigorous research that identifies the variables that place a chronically ill child and family at risk. In addition, consistent with medicine's organization by organ systems and specific diseases, much of the existing literature focuses on specific illnesses. An ecological perspective, considering the concurrent interaction of many systems, provides an opportunity to identify common parameters of illness, treatment, and family responses across conditions.

A key social ecology concept involves understanding how reciprocal interactions provide a context for development. Children with illnesses continue to grow and develop like their healthy counterparts as they adjust to and cope with their health-related concerns. Developmental issues may be evident in at least three ways when a child has a chronic illness. First, there is risk of developmental arrest. As families cope and adjust to the realities of their child's health concerns, they may initially (and perhaps appropriately) treat the child differently. For example, a child who is not feeling well physically may behave like a younger child, may be excused temporarily from some developmentally appropriate expectations, and may seek comfort and emotional support in a way similar to a younger child. As treatment progresses, the child is expected to participate in a developmentally appropriate manner. The child and family reorganize around the illness, perhaps in a new configuration (e.g., people in the family may shift roles), with a common goal of achieving successful treatment.

Second, because many childhood illnesses are chronic, illness-specific developmental issues may need to be frequently renegotiated, requiring reconfigurations of the family. For example, as adolescence unfolds, parents and children need to recognize the increasing independence of the child, and anticipate how that independence changes their roles. For instance, when can the adolescent with diabetes check blood sugars and administer insulin without supervision? When and how can a kidney transplant recipient track complex medication regimens correctly? As prognoses improve for many serious childhood conditions (e.g., premature birth, HIV/AIDS, cancer, cystic fibrosis, muscular dystrophy), increasing numbers of children are surviving into adulthood. Long-term survivorship is another developmental phase of the illness, for the patient and family. Over time, the long-term medical effects of intense treatments, complicated but potentially disruptive medical regimens that are necessary for health maintenance, and real or perceived functional impairment become more apparent.

Research has begun to explore the psychological sequelae that may accompany these medical issues for survivors and family members. Survivors of heart, heart and lung, and liver transplantation experience higher than average levels of anxiety, depression, and other behavioral concerns (Shemesh et al., 2000). Posttraumatic stress has provided a helpful model for understanding long-term psychological adjustment for survivors and family members for cancer and organ transplantation patients (Kazak et al., 1997; Shemesh et al., 2000). Further, pilot data indicate that posttraumatic stress in adolescents after organ transplant may affect adherence to medical regimens, linking psychosocial sequelae and physical health (Shemesh et al., 2000). The meaning of survivorship is also likely to change over time, perhaps resulting in an associated change in psychosocial sequelae. Although no research currently examines this developmental change directly, young adult survivors of childhood cancer reported higher levels of posttraumatic stress than was reported in younger groups of survivors (Hobbie et al., 2000).

The Illness and Treatment

The illness and its treatment are located within the innermost circle of the social ecology framework. Diseases and treatment differ vastly and can assume different roles within the family context. Even within each diagnosis (e.g., cancer, diabetes, epilepsy), there may be variability in psychosocial parameters. As discussed previously, illnesses also have their own developmental trajectories. Particularly in childhood, with the changes characteristic of development, the nature of the illness and its impact may also shift over time.

Illnesses also vary in their severity, although it is more difficult than might be expected to characterize severity. Some conditions are highly visible (e.g., cerebral palsy, amputation), whereas others cannot be discerned visually unless the child is acutely ill (e.g., diabetes, epilepsy). In general illness severity is not associated with adjustment, although it may affect the demands placed on the child and family for treatment. There are also potential indirect effects; for example, disease severity may influence parental behavior but not be directly associated with health care utilization (Logan, Radcliffe, & Smith-Whitley, 2002).

An exception is the case in which the child's illness affects the central nervous system (CNS). For example, the severity of neurological impairment has been shown to predict adaptive functioning (Max et al., 1998). This impact of illness severity is consistent with the added complexity of caring for children with neurocognitive impairments and may reflect the difficulty of modifying sequelae of CNS insults (Wade et al., 2001).

In illnesses other than those involving CNS injury, however, subjective factors (e.g., what the patient and family believe about the illness and its treatment) are generally more powerful predictors of outcome than typical "objective" measures of illness severity (e.g., physician ratings). For example, for childhood cancer survivors and their parents, physician ratings of degree of medical complications due to treatment and treatment intensity were unrelated to posttraumatic stress, but perceptions of life threat and perceived treatment intensity predicted posttraumatic stress (Kazak et al., 1998). Similarly, for congenital heart disease, mothers' perceptions, but not physician ratings, of illness severity correlated with psychological distress postdischarge (Van Horn, DeMaso, Gonzalez-Heydrich, & Erickson, 2001). Similarly, sibling adjustment was not associated with severity of the illness (as measured by mortality rates), although a more negative adjustment was evident with conditions in which daily functioning was more heavily affected (Sharpe & Rossiter, 2002).

The lack of association between distress and more objective measures of illness severity emphasizes the importance of focusing on the subjective illness experience of children and their caregivers. Even in diseases with more positive prognoses, family members must confront the losses associated with the illness and treatments (Kazak & Simms, 1996). How families balance the psychological issues of grief, fear, and uncertainty with the practical issues of family and illness management depends not simply on the medical facts of the disease but also on issues including pre-illness family adjustment and risk and other family resources that may constrain flexibility and adaptation. The combination of factors makes a child's illness more than just a set of medical facts that can be summed up by a physician's rating of illness severity. To date, little research has explored this important issue.

Siblings

Pediatric illnesses and their treatments have many direct and indirect effects on siblings. Although parents frequently worry about the impact of a child's illness on other children, siblings have received relatively little attention. A meta-analysis of research on siblings of children with chronic illness published between 1976 and 2000 concluded that having a sibling with a chronic illness was associated with psychological distress, most often in the form of internalizing disorders (Sharpe & Rossiter, 2002). These elevated rates of distress, however, are accompanied by positive outcomes associated with having an ill sibling (cf. Cadman, Boyle & Offord, 1988; Lobato, Faust, & Spirito, 1988). Positive outcomes have also been reported in siblings who donate bone marrow relative to nondonor siblings (Packman, 1999).

Studies have begun to examine the correlates of risk and resilience for siblings and to identify distal and proximal influences on sibling adjustment. Family cohesion, maternal social support, and maternal mood or psychological distress are associated with the adaptive functioning of siblings. Williams and colleagues (1999) found that the relationship between maternal mood and sibling mood was mediated by family cohesion. Individual characteristics have also been associated with sibling functioning. Younger siblings at the time of diagnosis are more likely to experience externalizing problems (Cohen et al., 1994); gender and birth order effects have also been reported (Silver & Frohlinger-Graham, 2000). Illness characteristics have been linked to sibling adjustment. Specifically, a negative association between time since diagnosis and number of internalizing and externalizing problems has been reported in the literature (Cohen et al., 1994). The relationships among contextual variables (family, parent, individual, illness) and sibling functioning provide a good illustration of the social-ecological model. Our understanding could be further enhanced through an examination of the relationships among related psychosocial risk and protective factors. Although support and psychoeducational groups for siblings have been developed and evaluated (Lobato & Kao, 2002; Houtzager, Grootenhuis, & Last, 2001) more intervention research is needed.

Parents

Across family models, parents are central to effective family functioning. Parents are the usual informants about the child's health, developmental history, and emotional and social functioning. When parents have been the focus of pediatric investigations, the main aim has been to describe parental adaptation to the child's illness and related demands. Mothers are frequently the only parents included in research and are often asked to be the sole informants of family functioning. Psychological knowledge about the bidirectional interaction between parenting and the child's illness has been limited by the failure to empirically examine the role of both fathers and mothers. Although this bias reflects the focus of services toward mothers and children in pediatric health care, its persistence is remarkable and limits professionals' understanding of how families function, maintaining a view of fathers as peripheral to the well being of children. Seagull (2000, p., 164) bluntly asks, "are we just avoiding the extra work involved in making a place for them [fathers] in our treatment? . . . We need to be more flexible in adjusting to the family's needs for realistic appointment times that respect the work schedules. . . . We must develop skills in making the family members feel not only invited, but vitally important." Although the recruitment of fathers into studies can be more difficult, it is possible and has been standard practice among several research groups for many years. Research documenting paternal distress in a pediatric sample (Wiener, Vasquez, & Battles, 2001) highlights the importance of including both parents.

Marital Relationships

One of the most frequently heard comments about the impact of serious childhood illness on families suggested that marital separation and divorce is inevitable, despite compelling evidence from the 1980s arguing against differences between families with and without a chronically ill child in terms of marital satisfaction (Sabbeth & Leventhal, 1984). More recent research on the impact of chronic illness on the marital relationship has begun to disentangle the individual and family factors that predict marital outcomes for pediatric parents (Gaither, Bingen, & Hopkins, 2000). For example, laboratory research with parents of children with asthma, when compared with families without an ill child, found that they expressed less disagreement, more frequently detoured potentially conflictual conversations, and more often drew the child into parental disputes (Northey, Griffin, & Krainz, 1998). Interestingly, marital quality was not related to these behavioral patterns. Quittner and colleagues have described the importance of role strain in marital satisfaction for parents with children with cystic fibrosis (CF; Quittner et al., 1998). Role strain refers to stressors associated with the parenting role, frustration about role expectations or the division of labor, role conflict, and affective exchanges. Compared with those without an ill child, parents of children in pediatric care reported greater role strain, with specific stressors that varied according to gender. The work of Holmbeck and colleagues has also identified gender differences in how coping relates to marital adjustment (Holmbeck et al., 1997). Specifically, parents of children with spina bifida and parents of healthy children reported similar levels of marital satisfaction. For women, marital satisfaction was negatively associated with the tendency to use behavioral disengagement (i.e., avoidance strategies) as a means of coping with their child's illness. For men, marital satisfaction was significantly associated with positive reinterpretation and growth.

In a study of the longitudinal impact of chronic illness on marriages, Dahlquist, Czyzewski, and Jones (1996) examined emotional distress, coping style, and marital adjustment in 42 couples who had children with cancer at 2 and at 20 months postdiagnosis. Both individual (affective functioning) and relational variables (spouse's marital satisfaction) predicted marital adjustment. In general, to the extent that parents perceived their partners as very committed and assessed that the marital relationship was relatively free of conflict, they reported greater overall satisfaction. Additionally, the marital relationship changed over time; for a subset there were significant changes in marital distress, in both positive and negative directions.

Research on the marital relationship of pediatric parents has been limited by various methodological flaws, including sampling biases, lack of control groups, omission of child and family developmental stages, use of unstandardized measures, and a preponderance of retrospective, cross-sectional studies rather than prospective research (Gaither et al., 2000). Despite these constraints, evidence shows that the relationship between pediatric illness and marital functioning is a complex one mediated by several factors. The factors that contribute to marital satisfaction appear to be gender specific, dependent on the types of coping styles or strategies employed, and are transactional (i.e., affect and influence others). Parenting stress, specifically conflict over role negotiation, coupled with limited time for social activities, bodes poorly for marital satisfaction.

Families

It is important to think broadly about family composition and function. Although it is important to ask, "Who is in your family?" and to include people who may not have blood ties to the child, the definition of family must be even more inclusive. There are many different types of families, with single-parent families, remarried families, gay and lesbian families, adoptive families, and foster care families among the most commonly encountered. There are literatures on each that provide cogent summaries based on empirical studies and clinical experience. In most cases, however, illness-specific issues that confront more diverse families have not been addressed. This is a serious shortcoming because different types of families may respond differently to childhood illness. For example, the family members that mobilize in a crisis, the family members that help assure that the family functions as routinely as possible, or the family as defined by ethnic, religious, or other cultural parameters may vary.

A large body of research on families and childhood illness exists and may be summarized by examining some of the consistent predictors of well-being. These include, for example, family flexibility, integration into a supportive social network, ability to balance the demands of the illness with other family needs and responsibilities, clear family boundaries, effective communication, positive attributions, active coping, and the encouragement of development of individuals within the family (Kazak, 2001). Our research on families, as an example, has contributed to emphasizing the competencies of families as they cope with childhood disabilities and illnesses. Across a series of studies (Kazak, 2001), we found that families with an affected child were more like other, nonaffected families than they were different, with only a subset of families demonstrating psychosocial difficulties at a clinical level. This is not meant to imply that families do not "need" or benefit from additional assistance but rather underscores the many possibilities for including parents and families as partners in the development and delivery of interventions in child health. We have shown, for example, the positive outcomes of interventions for procedural pain that incorporate parents in helping to reduce the distress of their child with leukemia (Kazak, Penati, Brophy, & Himelstein, 1998) and the feasibility and helpfulness of an intervention that combines cognitive–behavioral and family therapy approaches for reducing symptoms of posttraumatic stress in survivors of childhood cancer (Kazak et al., 1999).

Research focusing on family-level variables can refine our understanding of the complex process of adaptation to a child's chronic illness. For example, lower levels of cohesion were observed in families with a child with spina bifida, compared with a matched sample, although there were no group differences in family conflict (Holmbeck, Coakley, Hommeyer, Shapera, & Westhoven, 2002). Although illness may disrupt family cohesion, these families are resilient and adapt to these illness-related issues, which may avert higher levels of family conflict. Interestingly, socioeconomic status (SES) was an important determinant across groups, with lower SES families evidencing less cohesion, more conflict, and more stressful life events than higher SES families. This same line of research highlights how normative developmental experiences may differ for the child and family managing chronic illness. Early puberty was associated with higher levels of family conflict and lower levels of family cohesion for well children but not for those with spina bifida, suggesting that the impact of puberty on the family may be different when a child is ill (Coakley, Holmbeck, Friedman, Greenley, & Thill, 2002). These kinds of developmental differences, their meanings for individuals and for families, and similarities and differences across illnesses remain to be explored.

Some research suggests the potential for dysfunction or pathology, at either an individual or family level, to influence diseases, their course, and even their outcome. For example, Wood et al. (1989) found disease activity for gastrointestinal disorders to be related to specific family patterns, with evidence that patterns differ by disease. Patterns of family interaction have also been linked to disease activity in families of children with diabetes (Martin, Miller-Johnson, Kitzmann, & Emery, 1998). Families may also play an indirect role in illness management. Using the example of childhood asthma, Fiese and Wamboldt (2000) describe family rituals as a potentially mediating factor in treatment adherence. Family rituals describe a broad range of family behavior, from highly structured religious activities to daily household routines. Rituals may help families in maintaining disease-related treatment regimens indirectly by reducing anxiety in family members, increasing predictability, or helping families adapt and apply effective problem solving to new demands.

Other potentially important family characteristics are parenting style and parent–child relatedness. Davis and colleagues reported that authoritative parenting, characterized by warmth, support and control, was associated with better adherence in preschool and school-age children with diabetes (Davis et al., 2001). These data are quite intriguing given the associations among parent–child conflict and adherence difficulties in adolescents with diabetes (e.g., Jacobson et al., 1994). Parenting variables have also been implicated in the development of coping skills in children with spina bifida. Specifically, parental responsiveness predicted 8- and 9-year-old children's use of problem-focused coping concurrently and 2 years later (McKernon et al., 2001). Evidence also exists that attachment styles between mothers and children mediate the relationship between functional health status and depressive symptoms in children with asthma (Bleil, Ramesh, Miller, & Wood, 2000).

Schools

For children, schools are essential ecologies that interact with other systems (e.g., families, hospitals, communities). It is these interactions that are central to the social-ecological model. Integrated interventions across the child, family, and school remains the exception rather than the rule. Most hospital-based health care providers do not explicitly consider how treatment recommendations will be communicated to the child's school. These communications usually happen between families and schools, perhaps including the child, but generally without considering approaches that would build on the strengths of all three systems in pursuing a common goal (i.e., the child's health).

Most literature on family–school relationships has not focused specifically on health-related issues. However, it is readily transferable to these issues. For example, Power and Bartholomew (1987) describe five types of interaction styles between schools and families (avoidant, competitive, merged, one-way, and collaborative). These patterns might also be applied to relationships between schools and hospitals and between hospitals and families. The addition of a third component amplifies the complications (and underscores why three-way collaboration can be so challenging). For example, a family–school relationship may be avoidant, and the hospital–school relationship might be one-way. In this case, the school might look to the hospital for guidance on an asthma treatment plan, but the school and family do not have a solid, collaborative relationship (e.g., the family fails to attend meetings or indicates that there are no problems with the current plan). Or, in the case of a competitive school–family relationship, the school may feel that they have better ways of controlling the asthma than the family (e.g., if there is smoking in the home). This situation is ripe for misunderstanding, conflict, and adverse outcomes.

At a broader level, collaborations among families, schools, and health care systems necessitate thoughtful consideration of the resources and challenges associated with meeting the health care needs of children in each system and in terms of their active collaborations among systems. Identifying and developing these approaches is particularly important, given changes in health care delivery and the increasing responsibility placed on communities for caring for children with health care needs (Power, DuPaul, Shapiro, & Kazak, 2003). Alternatively, schools are an optimal environment for health promotion, providing community-based settings that are accessible to families.

Peers

Another essential system that interacts with the child, family, and health care setting and that directly overlaps, in part, with the school is the peer system. Peers are critical in the process of socialization and are recognized within the pediatric psychology literature as influencing the behavior of children, adolescents in particular (see Reiter-Purtill & Noll, Chapter 11, this volume). Peers are generally invisible in health care settings, but they are central in educational environments and thus provide an optimal area in which to link the health care and school ecologies across both chronic disease and health promotion and prevention.

The Health Care System

Given the prominence of the health care system in pediatric psychology, it is surprising how little has been written describing models of hospital–family collaboration. Family-centered care is perhaps the most widely described (e.g., Johnson, 2000), with its clearly articulated principles affirming the importance and role of families in pediatric health care. This model is also widely accepted, with many of its recommendations (e.g., expanded roles for families with hospitals, "consumers" (parents) employed by health care facilities, on-site family resource centers) implemented in children's hospitals nationwide.

Another movement advocating for consideration of families and health care teams in patient care is the Collaborative Family Healthcare Association (CFHA). With its mission highlighting collaboration, "The . . . model envisions seamless collaboration between psychosocial, biomedical, nursing and other health care providers. It views patient, family, community and provider systems as equally important participants in the health care process" (CFHA, 2002). In addition, the CFHA emphasizes the potential for this care model to affect fiscal resources. That is, a coordinated, collaborative approach, viewing clinical medicine from a biopsychosocial framework, may be translated into economic outcomes by reducing duplicative care, by treating "medical" issues in isolation from "psychosocial" ones, and by building on the adaptive competencies of patients and families.

Most literature on parent–physician interaction has focused on the conflicts in the relationship and has typically proposed approaches to prevent escalation of these tensions. There are data that show, for example, that pediatricians view verbal, cooperative, and compliant mothers more positively than those who demonstrate fewer of these attributes (Tellerman & Medio, 1988). This type of interaction is often viewed as a training issue in that pediatricians often do not have the skills or training necessary to deal with families whom they find difficult and may not utilize some of the relatively simple steps that can facilitate these relationships (Sunde, Mabe, & Josephson, 1993). Cohen and Wamboldt (2000) analyzed speech samples of parents of children with asthma and their asthma specialists talking about their perceptions of one another and their relationships. They found relationship difficulties in 15–40% of these interactions.

Waters (2001) describes the lack of attention to the relationship aspects of the doctor–patient–family interaction as "medicine's dirty secret." Noting that the lack of attention to the relational aspects of medicine are widely known (but not discussed), Waters (2001) notes that collaborative models of health care are "revolutionary" in offering a solution. In advocating the practice of a family systems model in pediatric health care, tasks that are common to families and to staff can be identified. These include soothing oneself in the face of stress, developing trust (in the relationships one must form to ensure optimal health care), and managing the inevitable conflicts that arise in modern health care (Kazak et al., 2002). Using this framework, a clinical protocol is proposed that guides the consultant to help the health care team address situations in which relationships between families and health care providers become strained.

FAMILY/SYSTEMS INTERVENTIONS IN PEDIATRIC PSYCHOLOGY

Most interventions for ill children have either focused on the child (e.g., cognitive–behavioral interventions) or included members of the family system (e.g., in parent education), but without an explicit family framework. Few have included family members in interventions that focus on changing disease management or family outcome. This lack of research reflects the developmental stage of the field. Only recently has more basic research focused on outlining family risk and protective factors, as well as family processes relevant to disease management. This "preintervention" research is a necessary precursor to intervention studies that can take a family-level focus (Weihs, Fisher, & Baird, 2002).

In order to promote family intervention research in child health, difficult conceptual and methodological challenges must be addressed (Kazak, 2002). For example, family research must measure changes not simply in one individual but in several family members and must conceptualize how change in related individuals can be interpreted and measured. Indeed, existing measures of family functioning are insufficiently specific to pediatric illness experience and limit the ability to accurately assess change (Kazak, 2002). Although family interventions are often discussed as if they were one type of intervention, it is important to distinguish among the various types, including therapy, psychoeducation, information and support, and direct service (Campbell & Patterson, 1995). Each differs in its goals, approaches, and outcomes. Several pediatric family interventions focus primarily on psychoeducation while another group addresses family interactions and change at the level of the family or system.

Behavioral group treatment for children with cystic fibrosis and their families has been effective in increasing adherence to a high-energy, high-fat diet to treat pancreatic insufficiency (Stark, 2001). The treatment protocols provide interventions for parents and patients separately, in each case emphasizing nutritional information, calorie goals, and developmentally appropriate behavioral approaches for encouraging intake of targeted foods. Comparatively, family-based behavioral treatment for childhood obesity that focuses on eating and exercise behaviors in both parents and children has been shown to be effective in long-term child weight reduction (i.e., 2 years) and diminished child behavior problems. Further, when this treatment is expanded to incorporate problem-solving training, improvements in parents' distress have been observed over time (Epstein, Paluch, Gordy, Saelens & Ernst, 2000). A family psychoeducational approach integrating biological (e.g., knowledge about sickle cell disease), psychological (e.g., psychological symptoms, cognitive functioning) and sociocultural (e.g., racial identity, family resources) issues related to disease management has been piloted with families of children with sickle cell disease (Kaslow et al., 2000). Relative to standard treatment, this intervention has been associated with increased knowledge about sickle cell disease for both children and parents; for child participants, enhanced disease knowledge was maintained over time (6 months). Although findings about the efficacy of this treatment in addressing psychological adjustment and family functioning are equivocal, there is evidence that an intervention of this kind might be beneficial for children and families with sickle cell disease.

Interventions that promote adherence in children with diabetes are among the most advanced in their incorporation of families. Although most approaches to adherence involve family members, the involvement is often based on necessity (i.e., that children need to have adults oversee their behavior) rather than on viewing the family as the unit of intervention. Satin conducted a randomized clinical trial of a 6-week multifamily intervention for adolescents with diabetes (compared with a wait-list control condition; Satin, La Greca, Zigo, & Skyler, 1989). The intervention covered major topics associated with adherence (e.g., communication skills, problem solving, support for self-care). The intervention also included creative elements in which other family members "simulated" diabetes for a week in order to experience the demands of the treatment regimen. The study results were interpreted as showing the importance of family support in improving self-care outcomes.

Because adherence regimens can create or accentuate naturally occurring conflict in families (particularly for adolescents), interventions that address family conflict are particularly compelling. Wysocki and his colleagues (Wysocki et al., 2000) have compared behavioral family systems therapy (BFST) to a standard treatment and to an education and support condition in adolescents with diabetes. BFST targeted family conflict by emphasizing problem solving and negotiation, communication skills, cognitive restructuring of beliefs that may maintain conflicts, and intervening in family patterns that were contradictory to adaptive functioning. The BFST condition was associated with improvements in family relationships and reduced diabetes-specific conflict but was not strongly associated with diabetes control and adherence. The data reflect both the advantages and disadvantages of taking a broader perspective on adherence. That is, improvements in conflict are important and may relate indirectly to variables relevant to adherence, although they may not show direct and clear relationships. BFST is currently being evaluated in cystic fibrosis (Quittner et al., 2001).

Anderson and her team developed a brief teamwork intervention protocol directed toward preventing the increase in conflict related to diabetes care that is typically seen over the early adolescent years (Anderson, Brackett, Ho, & Laffel, 2000). This 20–30 minute intervention appeared to reduce the expected increase in parent–adolescent conflict that was seen in the comparison group. Similar to the BFST outcomes, additional research is necessary in order to determine possible indirect pathways among family variables (including conflict, among others), disease characteristics, and outcomes (including multiple measures of adherence).

Building on research that documented symptoms of posttraumatic stress at the family level (e.g., mothers, fathers) in childhood cancer survival, our team has developed and is evaluating an intervention that integrates cognitive–behavioral therapy and family therapy. The goals of the intervention are to decrease symptoms of posttraumatic stress and to enhance family functioning for survivors and their families during adolescence. Adolescent cancer survivors (*N* = 151) and their mothers, fathers, and siblings participated in the Surviving Cancer Competently Intervention Program (SCCIP). Although results from the randomized clinical trial are not yet available, SCCIP pilot data were promising (Kazak et al., 1999).

Family and systems interventions can also be integrated into other areas of pediatric psychology practice. In the area of procedural pain, for example, parents can be active and effective interventionists with their children (Kazak et al., 1998). It is possible to conceptualize change at the level of the health care team and to anticipate systemic forces that can help or hinder the introduction of procedural pain interventions (Kazak, Blackall, Himelstein, Brophy, & Daller, 1995). Our empirical work in this regard was helpful in showing how medical and nursing staff are accepting of approaches to procedural pain intervention that require shifting their practice patterns (Kazak et al., 1996). Additionally, emotionally focused therapy (EFT) has strong empirical support for addressing family adjustment to chronic illness. This marital intervention, which targets the couple's negative patterns of interaction and attachment bond, has been shown to reduce marital distress; improvements have been reported to be stable over a 2-year period (Walker, Johnson, Manion & Cloutier, 1996). The EFT model offers an opportunity not only to examine how the marital relationship is affected by the illness but also how the disease course and the child's functioning is influenced by the marital relationship.

The examples of family intervention research provided share some commonalities, despite differences in patient groups and theoretical orientations. That is, these findings represent work that has evolved from more basic research in pediatric psychology. These researchers are all also applying family interventions to problems that are central to pediatric health care and that are concerns shared by families and health care teams (e.g., adherence, knowledge about disease and treatment, long-term sequelae of treatment). They are responding to the challenges of conducting research in "real world" settings, including difficulties with small sample sizes and recruitment and attrition concerns. These are important challenges and ones that will hopefully continue to be refined and evaluated empirically.

Some of what is lost in pediatric family research are the rich clinical perspectives from family therapy models, such as structural family therapy, which were among the earliest applied to pediatric samples (Minuchin et al., 1975) and others that are highly applicable, such as medical family therapy (McDaniel, Hepworth, & Doherty, 1992). Although this is unlikely to be changed in the near future, with the current and important focus on empirically supported treatments, these family therapy frameworks provide important perspectives for treating ill children and their families. The medical family therapist, for example, will supplement behavioral strategies with an awareness of family systems issues such as perceived closeness in the family, interactional patterns, and generational boundaries. Similarly, therapy goals are likely to include a consideration of individual and family developmental tasks that are affected by or that change in the presence of illness. Opportunities exist for the development of family therapy–based interventions that could be manualized and tested in pediatric practice.

As family interventions in pediatric psychology develop, it will be important for researchers to creatively address some challenges that have impeded the development of this field. These include, for example, utilizing the descriptive and explicative research on family variables to identify malleable risk and protective factors associated with disease management and to develop family assessment strategies that provide focused information to gauge the type and target of intervention.

SUMMARY

Perhaps the single most important "take home" message with respect to families and other systems in pediatric psychology is to encourage pediatric psychologists to incorporate broader perspectives in their work. Clinically, children facing health challenges live in the context of social systems, the most prominent of which are families, schools, and hospital systems. Interventions that focus on interpersonal relationships have the potential to change not only the specific individuals but also the broader contexts in which children grow and develop.

One of the most obvious steps is to ask research questions that incorporate the perspective of other important individuals in the child's life and to view these questions from an interactional perspective. For example, how does the behavior among and between parents and staff affect the child's coping ability in the procedural context? How do family patterns and the family's relationships with schools and community support systems affect an adolescent's diabetes management? Should we only be changing the behavior of a disruptive pediatric inpatient or also be asking that parents and staff shift their perceptions and behaviors to understand the family and systemic factors contributing to the behavior? These are questions that are easier asked than answered. Indeed, the relatively small body of research in this area speaks to the difficulty of conducting these studies.

However, a few general recommendations can be made. First, assuring that multidisciplinary family and systems perspectives are integrated into curricula, in terms of both didactics and supervised clinical experience, will expose more pediatric psychologists to these approaches. Second, pediatric psychologists can and should assume an optimistic and energetic approach to including other members of the family in our studies. At a minimum, psychologists should no longer tolerate generalizations made from mother-only data to represent the perspective of parents more broadly, but rather should consider how exclusion of family members limits the knowledge contributed. Third, children do not seek health care in isolation from the broader contexts in which they live. Pediatric psychologists must identify ways to better account for not just family influences but also the broader impact of health care systems and factors that affect access to care. This is relevant at many levels, from clinical work with an individual family that takes into account socioeconomic status and ethnicity to consulting with medical teams about family-focused treatment approaches to advocating for the needs of children and families more broadly to influence health care policy.

REFERENCES

Anderson, B., Brackett, J., Ho, J., & Laffel, L. (2000). An intervention to promote family teamwork in diabetes management tasks. In D. Drotar (Ed.), *Promoting adherence to medical treatment and chronic childhood illness* (pp. 71–93). Mahwah, NJ: Erlbaum.

Bleil, M., Ramesh, S., Miller, B., & Wood, B. (2000). The influence of parent–child relatedness on depressive symptoms in children with asthma: Tests of moderator and mediator models. *Journal of Pediatric Psychology, 25*, 481–491.

Bronfenbrenner, U. (1979). *The ecology of human development.* Cambridge, MA. Harvard University Press.

Cadman, D., Boyle, M. H., & Offord, D. R. (1988). The Ontario Child Health Study; Social adjustment and mental health of siblings of children with chronic health problems. *Journal of Developmental and Behavioral Pediatrics, 9*, 117–121.

Campbell, T., & Patterson, J. (1995). The effectiveness of family interventions in the treatment of physical illness. *Journal of Marital and Family Therapy, 21*, 545–583.

Coakley, R., Holmbeck, G., Friedman, D., Greenley, R., & Thill, A. (2002). A longitudinal study of pubertal timing, parent–child conflict, and cohesion in families of young adolescents with spina bifida. *Journal of Pediatric Psychology, 27*, 461–473.

Cohen, D. S., Friedrich, W. N., Jaworski, T. M., Copeland, D., & Pendergrass, T. (1994). Pediatric cancer: Predicting sibling adjustment. *Journal of Clinical Psychology, 50*, 303–319.

Cohen, S., & Wamboldt, F. (2000). The parent-physician relationship in pediatric asthma care. *Journal of Pediatric Psychology, 25*, 69–77.

Collaborative Family Healthcare Association. (2002). *The collaborative family healthcare model.* Retrieved June 23, 2002 from *http://www.cfha.net/model.asp*

Dahlquist, L. M., Czyzewski, D. I., & Jones, C. L. (1996). Parents of children with cancer: A longitudinal study of emotional distress, coping style, and marital adjustment two and twenty months after diagnosis. *Journal of Pediatric Psychology, 21*(4), 541–554.

Davis, C., Delamater, A., Shaw, K., La Greca, A., Eidson, M., Perez-Rodriques, J., & Nemery, R. (2001). Brief report: Parenting styles, regimen adherence and glycemic control in 4–10-year-old children with diabetes. *Journal of Pediatric Psychology, 26*, 123–129.

Epstein, L., Paluch, R., Gordy, C., Saelens, B., & Ernst, M. (2000). Problem solving in the treatment of childhood obesity. *Journal of Consulting and Clinical Psychology, 68*, 717–721.

Fiese, B., & Sameroff, A. (1989). Family context in pediatric psychology: A transactional perspective. *Journal of Pediatric Psychology, 14*, 293–314.

Fiese, B., & Wamboldt, F. (2000). Family routines, rituals and asthma management: A proposal for family-based strategies to increase treatment adherence. *Families, Systems, and Health, 18*, 405–418.

Gaither, R., Bingen, K., & Hopkins, J. (2000). When the bough breaks: The relationship between chronic illness in children and couple functioning. In K. B. Schmaling & T. G. Sher (Eds.), *The psychology of couples and illness* (pp. 337–365). Washington, DC: American Psychological Association.

Hobbie, W., Stuber, M., Meeske, K., Wissler, K., Rourke, M., Ruccione, K., et al. (2000). Symptoms of posttraumatic stress in young adult survivors of childhood cancer. *Journal of Clinical Oncology, 18*, 4060–4066.

Holmbeck, G., Coakley, R., Hommeyer, J., Shapera, W., & Westhoven, V. (2002). Observed and perceived dyadic and systemic functioning in families of preadolescents with spina bifida. *Journal of Pediatric Psychology, 27*, 177–189.

Holmbeck, G., Gorey-Ferguson, L., Hudson, T., Seefeldt, T., Shapera, W., Turner, T., & Uhler, J. (1997). Maternal, paternal and marital functioning in families of preadolescents with spina bifida. *Journal of Pediatric Psychology, 22*, 167–181.

Holmbeck, G., Li, S., Schurman, J., Friedman, D., & Coakley, R. (2002). Collecting and managing multisource and multimethod data in studies of pediatric populations. *Journal of Pediatric Psychology, 27*, 5–18.

Houtzager, B. A., Grootenhuis, M. A., & Last, B. F. (2001). Supportive groups for sibs of pediatric oncology patients: Impact on anxiety. *Psycho-Oncology, 10*, 315–324.

Jacobson, A., Hauser, S., Lavori, P., Willett, J., Cole, C., Wolfsdorf, J., et al. (1994). Family environment and glycemic control: A four-year prospective study of children and adolescents with insulin-dependent diabetes mellitus. *Psychosomatic Medicine, 56*, 401–409.

Johnson, B. (2000). Family-centered care: Four decades of progress. *Families, Systems, and Health, 18*, 137–156.

Kaslow, N., Collins, M., Rashid, F., Baskin, M., Griffith, J., Hollins, L., & Eckman, J. (2000). The efficacy of a pilot family psychoeducational intervention for pediatric sickle cell disease. *Families, Systems and Health, 18*, 381–404.

Kazak, A. (1989). Families of chronically ill children: A systems and social ecological model of adaptation and challenge. *Journal of Consulting and Clinical Psychology, 57*, 25–30.

Kazak, A. (2001). Comprehensive care for children with cancer and their families: A social ecological framework guiding research, practice and policy. *Children's Services: Social Policy, Research and Practice, 4*, 217–233.

Kazak, A. (2002). Challenges in family health intervention research. *Families, Systems and Health, 20*, 51–59.

Kazak, A., Barakat, L., Meeske, K., Christakis, D., Meadows, A., Casey, R., et al. (1997). Posttraumatic stress, family functioning, and social support in survivors of childhood leukemia and their mothers and fathers. *Journal of Consulting and Clinical Psychology, 65*, 120–129.

Kazak, A., Blackall, G., Boyer, B., Brophy, P., Buzaglo, J., Penati, B., & Himelstein, B. (1996). Implementing a pediatric leukemia intervention for procedural pain: The impact on staff. *Families, Systems and Health, 14*, 43–56.

Kazak, A., Blackall, G., Himelstein, B., Brophy, P., & Daller, R. (1995). Producing systemic change in pediatric practice: An intervention protocol for reducing distress during painful procedures. *Family Systems Medicine, 13*, 173–185.

Kazak, A., Penati, B., Brophy, P., & Himelstein, B. (1998). Pharmacologic and psychologic interventions for procedural pain. *Pediatrics, 102, 59–66.*

Kazak, A., & Simms, S. (1996). Family systems interventions in pediatric neuropsychiatric disorders. In C. E. Coffee & R. Brumback (Eds.), *Textbook of pediatric neuropsychiatry* (pp 1449–1464) Washington, DC: American Psychiatric Press.

Kazak, A., Simms, S., Barakat, L., Hobbie, W., Foley, B., Golomb, B., & Best, M. (1999). Surviving Cancer Competently Intervention Program (SCCIP): A cognitive-behavioral and family therapy intervention for adolescent survivors of childhood cancer and their families. *Family Process, 38*, 175–192.

Kazak, A., Simms, S., & Rourke, M. (2002). Family systems practice in pediatric psychology. *Journal of Pediatric Psychology, 27*, 133–143.

Kazak, A., Stuber, M., Barakat, L., Meeske, K., Guthrie, D., & Meadows, A. (1998). Predicting postttraumatic stress symptoms in mothers and fathers of survivors of childhood cancer. *Journal of the American Academy of Child and Adolescent Psychiatry, 37*, 823–831.

Lobato, D., Faust, D., & Spirito, A. (1988). Examining the effects of chronic disease and disability on children's relationships. *Journal of Pediatric Psychology, 13*, 389–407.

Lobato, D. & Kao, B. (2002). Sibling-parent group intervention to improve sibling knowledge and adjustment to chronic illness and disability. *Journal of Pediatric Psychology, 27*, 711–716,

Logan, D., Radcliffe, J., & Smith-Whitley, K. (2002). Parent factors and adolescent sickle cell disease: Associations with patterns of health service use. *Journal of Pediatric Psychology, 27*, 475–484.

Martin, M., Miller-Johnson, S., Kitzmann, K., & Emery, R. (1998). Parent–child relationships and insulin-dependent diabetes mellitus: Observational ratings of clinically relevant dimensions. *Journal of Family Psychology, 12*, 102–111.

Max, J. E., Castillo, C. S., Robin, D. A., Lindgren, S. D., Smith, W. L., Sata, Y., et al. (1998). Predictors of family functioning following traumatic brain injury in children and adolescents. *Journal of the American Academy of Child and Adolescent Psychiatry, 37*, 83–90.

McDaniel, S., Hepworth, J., & Doherty, W. (1992). *Medical family therapy.* New York: Basic Books.

McKernon, W., Holmbeck, G., Colder, C., Hommeyer, J., Shapera, W., & Westhoeven, V. (2001). Longitudinal study of observed and perceived family influences on problem-focused coping behaviors of preadolescents with spina bifida. *Journal of Pediatric Psychology, 26*, 41–54.

Minuchin, S., Baker, L., Rosman, B., Liebman, R., Millman, L., & Todd, T. (1975). A conceptual model of psychosomatic illness in children: Family organization and family therapy. *Archives of General Psychiatry, 32*, 1031–1038.

Mullins, L., Gillman, J., & Harbeck, C. (1992). Multiple level interventions in pediatric psychology settings: A behavioral systems perspective. In A. M. La Greca, L. J. Siegel, J. L. Wallander & C. E. Walker (Eds.), *Stress and coping in child health* (pp. 377–399). New York: Guilford Press.

Northey, S., Griffin, W., & Krainz, S. (1998). A partial test of the psychosomatic family model: Marital interaction patterns in asthma and nonasthma families. *Journal of Family Psychology, 12*, 220–223.

Packman, W. L. (1999). Psychosocial impact of pediatric BMT on siblings. *Bone Marrow Transplantation, 24*, 701–706.

Power, T., & Bartholomew, K. (1987). Family–school relationship patterns: An ecological perspective. *School Psychology Review, 16*, 498–512.

Power, T., DuPaul, G., Shapiro, E., & Kazak, A. (2003). *Promoting children's health: Integrating school, family, and community.* New York: Guilford.

Quittner, A., Drotar, D., Ievers-Landis, C., Slocom, N., Seidner, D. & Jacobsen, J. (2001). Adherence to medical treatments in adolescents with cystic fibrosis. In D. Drotar (Ed.). *Promoting adherence to medical treatment and chronic childhood illness* (pp. 383–407). Mahwah, NJ: Erlbaum.

Quittner, A., Espelage, D., Opipari, L., Carter, B., Eid, N., & Eigen, H. (1998). Role strain in couples with and without a child with a chronic illness: Associations with marital satisfaction, intimacy, and daily mood. *Health Psychology, 17*, 112–124.

Sabbeth, B., & Leventhal, J. (1984). Marital adjustment to chronic childhood illness. *Pediatrics, 73*, 762–768.

Satin, W., La Greca, A., Zigo, M., & Skyler, J. (1989). Diabetes in adolescence: Effects of multifamily group intervention and parent simulation of diabetes. *Journal of Pediatric Psychology, 14*, 259–275.

Seagull, E. (2000). Beyond mothers and children: Finding the family in pediatric psychology. *Journal of Pediatric Psychology, 25*, 161–169.

Sharpe, D., & Rossiter, L. (2002). Siblings of children with a chronic illness: A meta-analysis. *Journal of Pediatric Psychology, 27*, 699–710.

Shemesh, E., Lurie, S., Stuber, M., Emre, S., Patel, Y., Vohra, P., et al. (2000). A pilot study of posttraumatic stress and nonadherence in pediatric liver transplant recipients. *Pediatrics, 105*, e29.

Silver, E. J., & Frohlinger-Graham, M. J. (2000). Brief report: Psychological symptoms in healthy female siblings of adolescents with and without chronic conditions. *Journal of Pediatric Psychology, 25*, 279–284.

Stark, L. (2001). Adherence to diet in chronic conditions. In D. Drotar (Ed.), *Promoting adherence to medical treatment and chronic childhood illness* (pp. 409–427). Mahwah, NJ: Erlbaum.

Sunde, E., Mabe, P., & Josephson, A. (1993). Difficult parents: From adversaries to partners. *Clinical Pediatrics, 32*, 213–219.

Tellerman, K., & Medio, F. (1988). Pediatricians' opinions of mothers. *Pediatrics, 81*, 186–189.

Thompson, R., & Gustafson, K. (1999). *Adaptation to chronic childhood illness*. Washington, DC: American Psychological Association.

Van Horn, M., DeMaso, D., Gonzalez-Heydrich, J., & Erickson, J. (2001). Illness-related concerns of mothers of children with congential heart disease. *Journal of the American Academy of Child and Adolescent Psychiatry, 40*, 847–854.

Wade, S. L., Borawski, E. A., Taylor, H. G., Drotar, D., Yeates, K. O., & Stancin, T. (2001). The relationship of caregiver coping to family outcomes during the initial year following pediatric traumatic injury. *Journal of Consulting and Clinical Psychology, 69*(3), 406–415.

Walker, J., Johnson, S., Manion, I., & Cloutier, P. (1996). Emotionally focused marital intervention for couples with chronically ill children. *Journal of Consulting and Clinical Psychology, 64*, 1029–1036.

Wallander, J., & Varni, J. (1992). Adjustment in children with chronic physical disorders: Programmatic research on a disability-stress-coping model. In A. M. La Greca, L. J. Siegel, J. L. Wallander, & C. E. Walker (Eds.), *Stress and coping in child health*, (pp. 279–298). New York: Guilford Press.

Waters, D. (2001). Commentary: The revolutionary subtext of collaborative care. *Families, Systems and Health, 19*, 59–63.

Weihs, K., Fisher, L., & Baird, M. (2002). Families, health and behavior. *Families, Systems and Health, 20*, 7–46.

Wiener, L., Vasquez, M. J., & Battles, H. (2001). Brief report: Fathering a child living with HIV/AIDS: Psychosocial adjustment and parenting stress. *Journal of Pediatric Psychology, 26*, 353–358.

Williams, P. D., Williams, A. R., Hanson, S., Graff, C., Redder, C., Ridder, L., et al. (1999). Maternal mood, family functioning, and perceptions of social support, self-esteem, and mood among siblings of chronically ill children. *Children's Health Care, 28*, 297–310.

Wood, B. (1995). A developmental biopsychosocial approach to the treatment of chronic illness in children and adolescents. In R. H. Mikesell, D. D. Lusterman, & S. H. McDaniel (Eds.), *Integrating Family Therapy* (pp. 437–455). Washington, DC: American Psychological Association.

Wood, B., Watkins, J., Boyle, J., Nogueira, J., Zimand, E., & Carroll, L. (1989). The psychosomatic family model: An empirical and theoretical analysis. *Family Process, 28*, 399–417.

Wysocki, T., Harris, M., Greco, P., Bubb, J., Danda, C., Harvey, L., et al. (2000). Randomized controlled trial of behavioral therapy for families of adolescents with insulin-dependent diabetes mellitus. *Journal of Pediatric Psychology, 25*, 23–33.

11

Peer Relationships of Children with Chronic Illness

JENNIFER REITER-PURTILL
ROBERT B. NOLL

Considerable research during the past 30 years has examined the role of peer relationships in the social and emotional development of children. This work has suggested that relationships with peers are stable and predictive of future functioning. Children who get along well with peers feel better about themselves and perform better academically. Conversely, children who do not get along well with peers do not perform as well in school and experience behavioral difficulties. Because children with chronic illness may experience school absences, changes in appearance, restrictions on activities, physical complaints, or cognitive impairments, they seem to be at risk for problems with peers that could be the harbingers of future trouble.

Estimates of the numbers of youths under age 18 who experience a chronic health condition range from 10 to 30% and are rising due, in part, to significant advances in medical care that reduce mortality (e.g., Cadman, Boyle, Szatmari, & Offord, 1987; Newacheck & Taylor, 1992; Stein & Silver, 1999). Approximately 5% of these children are affected by conditions that are sufficiently severe to limit normative activities, and these children account for 24% of all school absences, 19% of physician visits, and 33% of hospital days (Newacheck & Taylor, 1992). With improved treatments and better mortality rates, concerns have been voiced about quality of life, particularly for those children with more severe conditions. This chapter reviews some of the most recent empirical literature on the peer relationships of children with chronic conditions and discusses some of the methodological limitations that serve as challenges to future research in this area.

CATEGORICAL AND NONCATEGORICAL APPROACHES

Research examining the impact of pediatric chronic illness on children's psychosocial adjustment has followed two conceptually distinct approaches. Some researchers have used a biological model to study the impact of different chronic illnesses on the psychosocial functioning of affected children. This categorical model suggests that each chronic illness or condition is associated with a unique set of challenges. In contrast, the noncategorical approach contends that children with different chronic conditions experience many common stressors (Rolland, 1988; Stein & Jessop, 1982). These stressors can include illness chronicity and severity, whether or not the condition is life threatening, the number of hospitalizations, and treatment side effects. A noncategorical approach has been slowly gaining acceptance in research (e.g., Gartstein, Short, Vannatta, & Noll, 1999; Wallander & Varni, 1998) and for planning services (Stein & Silver, 1999). Empirical studies from a noncategorical approach have found few differences between disease groups (Apter et al., 1991; Meijer, Sinnema, Bijstra, Mellenbergh, & Wolters, 2000a; Nassau & Drotar, 1995; Westbrook, Silver, Coupey, & Shinnar, 1991). When differences have been identified, they most often occur in the domain of restrictions on activities (Eiser, Havermans, Pancer, & Eiser, 1992; Meijer, Sinnema, Bijstra, Mellenbergh, & Wolters, 2000b; Padur et al., 1995) or when diseases affect central nervous system (CNS) functioning (Noll, Ris, Davies, Bukowski, & Koontz, 1992; Wallander, Varni, Babani, Banis, & Wilcox, 1989).

CHRONIC ILLNESS AND PEER RELATIONSHIPS

Within a noncategorical paradigm, chronic illness may be considered a potentially stressful life event. A considerable amount of research has examined the impact of severe stressors (e.g., natural disasters, child maltreatment, exposure to violence, and persistent poverty) on the emotional and behavioral functioning of children. Experiences with these stressors have been associated with both internalizing and externalizing problems such as depression, anxiety, and aggression (e.g., Durkin, Khan, Davidson, Zaman, & Stein, 1993; Margolin & Gordis, 2000). Fewer studies have addressed the peer relationships of these children. Research in this area has primarily focused on children exposed to violence or abuse who have been reported to be at risk for social difficulties (for a review, see Margolin & Gordis, 2000).

Chronic illness involves both acute stressors (e.g., invasive/painful medical procedures, pain episodes) and chronic stressors (e.g., repeated hospitalizations and doctor's appointments, long-term management of illness). Similar to the literature regarding other severe stressors, multiple studies have suggested that youth with chronic illnesses are at risk for experiencing difficulties with emotional well-being, particularly internalizing difficulties (Cadman et al., 1987; Lavigne & Faier-Routman, 1992). Unfortunately, less attention has been given to their peer relationships. The literature concerning peer relationships is listed in Table 11.1.

Peer relationships have been described as both excellent measures of current social competence and predictive of subsequent adjustment (Morison & Masten, 1991; Parker & Asher, 1987). Friendships in childhood are considered developmentally significant because they provide both cognitive and social resources, especially during times of stress (Hartup, 1996). In contrast, poor peer adjustment is a risk for later life difficulties (Parker & Asher, 1987). Low acceptance and aggressiveness are predictive of academic difficulties, exter-

TABLE 11.1. Peer Relationships and Children with Chronic Illness

Reference	Sample/age	Control	Measure of social functioning	Findings
Aasland, Flato, & Vandvik (1997)	JRA (N = 52) R = 9–25 at 9-year follow-up	No	Parent: CBCL-SCS Child: Interview, Global Assessment Scale, YSR	7 of 23 children < 18 had CBCL-SCS scores in the clinical range; 1 adolescent of 20 had a YSR-SCS score in clinical range; most impairment in the activities domain; in children < 18, psychosocial functioning negatively correlated with parent-rated physical disability but was unrelated to other disease severity measures.
Apter et al. (1991)	Temporal lobe epilepsy (N = 26) R = 13–16	Yes (asthma N = 26; nonchronically ill N = 90)	Parent: CBCL-SCS	Both groups with chronic illness had lower CBCL-SCS scores on the Activities and Social subscales than nonchronically ill controls but were not different from each other.
Barbarin, Whitten, & Bonds (1994)	SCD (N = 327) R = 4–17	No	Parent and child (older than 8 years of age): interview-social adjustment domain	Social adjustment (e.g., shyness, loneliness, and a lack of a close friend) was a problem for one child in five; those with serious pain episodes were more likely to experience activity disruption and teasing.
Boni, Brown, Davis, Hsu, & Hopkins (2001)	SCD with a cerebral vascular accident (HbSS; CVA) (N = 21) R = 6–16	Yes (HbSS without CVA N = 20; milder SCD N = 11)	Parent and teacher: SSRS Child: Diagnostic Analysis of Nonverbal Accuracy, CDI	Controlled for IQ; children with CVA exhibited more errors on tasks involving adult–child vocal emotional recognition (low intensity) and facial emotional recognition (low intensity) for African American adults than both control groups; no differences in terms of social–emotional functioning according to parent, teacher, and self-report.
Casey, Sykes, Craig, Power, & Mulholland (1996)	CHD (N = 26) R = 4–16	Yes (innocent heart murmur N = 26)	Parent and teacher: CBCL (Withdrawn and Social Problems subscales)	According to teachers, children with CHD had higher scores on Withdrawn scale relative to controls; parents report children with CHD had higher scores on Withdrawn and Social Problems scales than controls; when somatic items removed from Withdrawn scale, differences no longer significant for both teacher and parent report; parents report children with CHD participate in fewer activities.
Colegrove & Huntzinger (1994)	Hemophilia (56% with HIV) (N = 37) R = 8–19	No	Parent: CBCL, SSRS Teacher: teacher versions of CBCL, SSRS, and SPPC Child: SSRS	All parent, child, and teacher ratings of social competency and teacher-reported SPPC scores were within normative range; more absences from school associated with lower teacher ratings of scholastic, social, and athletic competence, physical attractiveness, and social activities; no differences between children with HIV and those without.

Daltroy, Larson, et al. (1992)	JRA ($N = 102$) R = 4–16	No	Parent: CBCL-SCS, Profile of Mood States	Older children, particularly older males, children with recent disease onset, and those with more parent-reported severe disease, showed the poorest social competence relative to norms; parental distress not associated with children's social competence.
Eiser, Havermans, Pancer, & Eiser (1992)	Diabetes ($N = 144$), Asthma ($N = 53$), Epilepsy ($N = 35$), Leukemia ($N = 17$), SB ($N = 19$), Cardiac ($N = 16$) R = 4–14	No	Parent: Modified Child and Adolescent Adjustment Profile Scale (Peer Relations and Withdrawal subscales)	Children with epilepsy rated by mothers as having more problems in peer relations compared with children with diabetes, leukemia, or cardiac problems; girls were better adjusted than boys on peer relations scale; children with epilepsy or leukemia had the most restrictions on activities. Fathers reported that children with epilepsy had most restrictions on activities but no other differences. According to both parents, children were rated as having more difficulties in peer relations as disease restrictions increased.
Graetz & Shute (1995)	Asthma ($N = 21$) R = 8–13	Yes (nonchronically ill $N = 21$)	Peer: Revised Class Play (RCP), Three Best Friends, Like Rating Scale Child: The Loneliness Scale	No differences between groups on most measures; children with asthma were perceived by peers as sicker and missing more school; children who experienced more hospitalizations were less popular, more lonely, and exhibited more sensitive-isolated behavior, according to peers.
Harris, Newcomb, & Gewanter (1991)	JRA ($N = 12$) R = 6–11	Yes (nonchronically ill $N = 12$)	Observation in the classroom	No differences in classroom observations of social functioning.
Hoffman, Rodrigue, Andres, & Novak (1995)	Liver disease ($N = 30$) R = 4–13	No	Parent: CBCL-SCS Child: PCSC–Social Subscale	Parents reported lower social competence than norms but no differences in social functioning according to child report; after controlling for IQ and disease severity, parent reported family functioning was significantly associated with social competence as reported by parent but not child.
Johnson, Saal, Lovell, & Schorry (1999)	Neurofibromatosis ($N = 43$) R = 5–18	Yes (unaffected siblings $N = 22$)	Parent and teacher: CBCL	Parents and teachers reported a higher score on Social Problems scale compared with norms and controls; parents also reported a higher score on Withdrawn scale compared with norms and controls, as well as lower scores than controls on Activities and Social Competence scales.
Kapp-Simon & McGuire (1997)	CFC ($N = 13$) R = 12–14	Yes (nonchronically ill $N = 12$)	Observation at school	Relative to controls, adolescents with CFC were less likely to start conversations with peers, to respond if approached, and to have an extended conversation; peers addressed them less frequently and responded less often if the adolescent with CFC approached them.

(*continued*)

TABLE 11.1. *(continued)*

Reference	Sample/age	Control	Measure of social functioning	Findings
Kapp-Simon, Simon, & Kristovich (1992)	CFC (N = 45) R = 10–16	No	Parent: PIC-Adjustment and Social Skills scales, RBPC (Anxiety/ Withdrawal subscale) Child: SPPC	Mean scores of self-perception, social skills, and withdrawal were within normative levels; mean score on adjustment scale of PIC was below normative levels; parent reported social skills and self-reported athletic competence accounted for 73.5% of variance in parent-reported adjustment; according to parents, more poorly adjusted adolescents exhibited greater social inhibition; no gender differences.
Manne & Miller (1998)	Cancer (N = 50) R = 12–20	No	Child: Network of Relationships Inventory; Psychological Distress scale of the Mental Health Inventory	No difference from norms in levels of perceived support/conflict with friends; physical impairment accounted for the most variance in psychological distress; maternal conflict significantly associated with distress after controlling for physical impairment but support/conflict with friends did not account for significant amounts of variance.
Meijer, Sinnema, Bijstra, Mellenbergh, & Wolters (2000a)	Asthma (N = 44), CF (N = 23), Diabetes (N = 7), JRA (N = 11), Osteogenesis imperfecta (N = 7), Eczema (N = 11) R = 8–12	No	Parent: CBCL-SCS, Children's Assertive Behavior Scale Child: MESSY, SPPC (Social Acceptance), SASK	Number of hospitalizations negatively correlated with social activities; no differences between chronic illness groups on measures of social functioning; children with chronic illness self-reported less aggressive behavior and less prosocial behavior than norms; no differences from norms for CBCL-SCS or SPPC; physical restrictions and pain were associated with less participation in social activities but not with any other measures.
Meijer, Sinnema, Bijstra, Mellenbergh, & Wolters (2000b)	Asthma (N = 31), CF (N = 23), Diabetes (N = 6), JRA (N = 15), Osteogenesis imperfecta (N = 5), Eczema (N = 15) R = 13–16	No	Parent: CBCL-SCS Child: SPPA (Social Acceptance, Close Friendships, and Romantic Appeal), Scale of Interpersonal Behavior for Adolescents, MESSY	Diagnosis was associated with social activities such that adolescents with asthma had the highest level of social activities and adolescents with OI or diabetes had the lowest; age positively associated with social self-esteem and social skills; compared with norms, girls participated in fewer social activities and displayed more assertive behavior; boys report less inadequate social skills; functional limitations not associated with social functioning but illness duration positively correlated with social skills and assertive behavior; pain was associated with restricted social activities for boys only.
Moss, Bose, Wolters, & Brouwers (1998)	HIV (N = 24) R = 8–15	No	Parent: CBCL-SCS, Life Events Scale-R, Conner's Parent Rating Scales Child: CDI, PCSC	Two-year longitudinal study; social self-concept decreased over time; more negative life events at Time 1 associated with more psychosocial difficulties at both times, including lower CBCL-SCS scores at Time 1 and lower social self-concept at both times.

Moss, Wolters, Brouwers, Hendricks, & Pizzo (1996)	HIV, Encephalopathic (N = 45) Infants, M age = 1.08 and Children, M age = 5.15	Yes (HIV, nonencephalopathic (N = 38)	Observation	Nonencephalopathic infants had higher activity levels, better motor and verbal skills, and more social and emotional responsiveness than encephalopathic infants; older children with encephalopathy were less able to act purposefully, were emotionally and socially unresponsive, were inactive, and had impaired motor and verbal functioning.
Nassau & Drotar (1995)	IDDM (N = 25) Asthma (N = 19) R = 8–10	Yes (nonchronically ill N = 24)	Parent: PARS, TOPS Child: PCSC-SCS, Children's Self-Efficacy for Peer Interaction Scale, Friendship Questionnaire Teacher: PARS, TOPS	No significant differences between groups on any of the measures.
Newby, Brown, Pawletko, Gold, & Whitt (2000)	Survivors of cancer (N = 42) R = 6–18	No	Parent: CBCL-SCS, SSRS Teacher: SSRS	Survivors show mean social skills within normative levels; academic functioning was positively associated with parent and teacher rated social skills; age/age at diagnosis and time off therapy not associated with social skills.
Noll, Bukowski, Davies, Koontz, & Kulkarni (1993)	Off treatment for cancer (N = 19) R = 11–18	Yes (nonchronically ill N = 19)	Peer: RCP, Three Best Friends, Like Rating Scale Teacher: RCP Child: RCP, LSDQ	Two-year longitudinal study of adolescents primarily off treatment for cancer; relative to controls, these adolescents were more socially isolated and withdrawn according to peer and self-report; no other significant differences identified on measures of social reputation, acceptance, or self-reported feelings.
Noll, Bukowski, Rogosch, LeRoy, & Kulkarni (1990)	Cancer (N = 24) R = 8–18	Yes (nonchronically ill N = 24)	Teacher: RCP	Relative to controls, children with cancer were perceived by teachers as less sociable and more socially isolated and withdrawn; children with cancer were perceived as being sick a lot, missing more school, and more tired than controls; no effects for gender, age, or whether child had received cranial radiation.
Noll et al. (1999)	Cancer (N = 76) R = 8–15	Yes (nonchronically ill N = 76)	Peer: RCP, Three Best Friends, Like Rating Scale Teacher: RCP Child: LSDQ, SPPC Parent: CBCL-SCS	Relative to controls, children were perceived by teachers as more sociable; by teachers and peers as being less aggressive; and by peers as having greater social acceptance; no differences in parent-reported social functioning nor on loneliness and self-concept measures except that children with cancer reported lower athletic competence; children receiving more intense treatment were perceived by peers as less aggressive and more well liked and by teachers as more withdrawn.
Noll et al. (2000)	JRA (N = 74) R = 8–14	Yes (nonchronically ill N = 74)	Peer: RCP, Three Best Friends, Like Rating Scale Teacher: RCP Child: LSDQ, SPPC Parent: CBCL-SCS	Relative to controls, children with JRA were similar on all measures of social functioning; no differences in social functioning between children with mild disease and children with moderate/severe disease; mothers reported children with disease in remission as more socially competent on the CBCL than children with active disease.

(*continued*)

TABLE 11.1. *(continued)*

Reference	Sample/age	Control	Measure of social functioning	Findings
Noll, LeRoy, Bukowski, Rogosch, & Kulkarni (1991)	Cancer (*N* = 24) R = 8–18	Yes (nonchronically ill *N* = 24)	Peer: RCP, Three Best Friends, Like Rating Scale Child: RCP, LSDQ, SPPC/A	Relative to controls, children with cancer were perceived by peers as more socially withdrawn and more tired, and by peers and self-report as more sick and missing more school; no other significant differences identified on measures of social reputation, acceptance, or self-reported feelings; no effects for gender, age, or whether child had received cranial radiation.
Noll, Ris, Davies, Bukowski, & Koontz (1992)	Cancer (nonprimary brain tumors *N* = 26) Brain tumor survivors (*N* = 15) SCD (*N* = 33) R = 8–18	Yes (nonchronically ill *N* = 74)	Teacher: RCP	Relative to controls, children with cancer were perceived as more sociable and less aggressive; survivors of brain tumors were perceived as more socially isolated and withdrawn; children with SCD were not significantly different from controls; children receiving treatment for cancer and children with SCD were perceived as being more sick, tired, and missing more school than controls.
Noll et al. (1996)	SCD (*N* = 34) R = 8–14	Yes (nonchronically ill *N* = 34)	Peer: RCP, Three Best Friends, Like Rating Scale Teacher: RCP Child: LSDQ	Relative to controls, girls with SCD were perceived by peers as less sociable and less well accepted; males with SCD were perceived by peers as less aggressive; no other differences in social functioning were identified; disease severity was not related to measures of social functioning.
Padur et al. (1995)	Asthma (*N* = 25) R = 8–16	Yes (Cancer *N* = 25; diabetes *N* = 25; nonchronically ill *N* = 25)	Parent: CBCL-SCS, CDI Child: CDI, PHCSC	No differences between groups on CBCL-SCS; children with asthma had most restrictions on activities (i.e., functional impairment); children with asthma had more parent-reported internalizing symptoms and lower self-concept than other groups; internalizing symptoms were no longer significant after functional impairment was controlled.
Pendley, Dahlquist, & Dreyer (1997)	Survivors of cancer (*N* = 21) R = 11–21	Yes (nonchronically ill *N* = 21)	Child: SPPA, Loneliness Questionnaire, SASC-Revised, body image questionnaires, and Peer Interaction Record	Survivors participate in fewer activities than controls; no significant differences on measures of loneliness, social anxiety, or body image; negative body image correlated with social anxiety, loneliness, and low global self-worth but not with peer activities or peer network.

Pope & Ward (1997a)	CFC (N = 24) R = 11–14	No	Parent: Parental Involvement Checklist, CBCL (Social Problems and Withdrawn) Child: NRI, Loneliness Questionnaire, SPPC	All means for social functioning were within normative levels; no gender differences; children with less social competence reported more social anxiety and loneliness, and less companionship with peers; parents rated them as having more internalizing problems; positive self-perceptions of academics, athletics, and physical appearance were associated with good social competence; parents with more socially competent children provided more encouragement and opportunities for their children to be with peers.
Pope & Ward (1997b)	CFC (N = 24) R = 11–14	No	Parent: Parental Involvement Checklist, CBCL (Social Problems and Withdrawn) Child: NRI, Loneliness Questionnaire, SPPC, Social Anxiety and Social Avoidance Questionnaire	Loneliness and parent-reported social problems (e.g., withdrawal and being disliked by peers) were negatively correlated with facial appearance (altered physical appearance scale of SPPC); self-reported number of close friends, as well as perceived social acceptance and global self-worth, were positively correlated with facial appearance; dissatisfaction with facial appearance was not associated with other aspects of self-concept or adjustment problems.
Reiter-Purtill, Gerhardt, Vannatta, Passo, & Noll (2003)	JRA (N = 57) R = 10–17	Yes (nonchronically ill N = 63)	Peer: RCP, Three Best Friends, Like Rating Scale Teacher: RCP Child: RCP	Cross-sectional analyses indicated no significant differences between children with JRA and controls on measures of behavioral reputation and social acceptance; longitudinal assessments indicated that for children with more severe disease, like ratings declined over a 2-year period relative to children with mild disease; children with active disease were chosen fewer times over the 2-year period as best friends relative to children in remission.
Rodrigue, Streisand, Banko, Kedar, & Pitel (1996)	SCD (N = 85) R = 4–18	Yes (nonchronically ill N = 46)	Parent, teacher, child (10 years and older): CBCL and Missouri Peer Relations Inventory	Compared with controls, children with SCD report more social problems; no differences identified between groups on parent and teacher reports of social competence, social problems, emotional bonding, aggression, and emotional maturity; disease severity not associated with any of the measures.
Sanger, Copeland, & Davidson (1991)	Cancer (N = 48) R = 4–17	No	Parent: PIC Teacher: Health Resources Inventory	33% experienced difficulties in cognitive functioning and academic performance; mean scores were above clinical cutoff on Withdrawal scale but not different from norms for Social Skills scale; children with two or more clinically significant PIC scale elevations (52% of sample) were seen as less socially competent by teachers.

(*continued*)

TABLE 11.1. *(continued)*

Reference	Sample/age	Control	Measure of social functioning	Findings
Shelby, Nagle, Barnett-Queen, Quattlebaum, & Wuori (1998)	Survivors of acute lymphocytic leukemia (N = 34) R = 6–17	No	Parent: CBCL-SCS, Behavior Assessment for Children (BASC)	All means within normative levels; more scores in clinically significant range for CBCL-Social Problems and for the Social Competence subscales relative to norms; on BASC, more children, particularly adolescents, had social skills and leadership difficulties than normative sample; children receiving special education had more problem behaviors and lower levels of social competence than those who did not; no differences between children who received cranial irradiation and those who had not; age at diagnosis not associated with functioning.
Spirito et al. (1990)	Survivors of cancer (N = 56) R = 5–12	Yes (nonchronically ill N = 52)	Parent: Interview, TOPS, questions from CBCL-SCS Child: SPPC, Social Skills Questionnaire, YSR-SCS Teacher: TOPS, Deasy-Spinetta Behavioral Questionnaire	Children with cancer spent more time with adults than controls but few other differences in social functioning according to parent report; teachers rated children with cancer as higher than controls in eagerness to attend school and in school attendance and lower than controls in their anxiety about school, restlessness, getting teased and arguing; children with cancer reported significantly fewer friends their own age.
Timko, Stovel, Moos, & Miller (1992)	JRA (N = 165) M=(9.8)	Yes (nonchronically ill siblings N = 126)	Parent: Health and Daily Living Form (peer problems) Child: Health and Daily Living Form (School Activities and Activities with Friends), PHCSC, Feelings About Illness	Few problems according to parent report at both times; self-report at Time 1: Relative to controls, children with JRA participated less in social activities; children with severe disease had fewer friends than mild group or controls. Time 2: Relative to controls, children with JRA participated in fewer activities with friends and perceived themselves as less popular; children with more severe disease reported fewer friends than mild group or controls; children with mild disease perceived themselves as less attractive than controls.
Van Hasselt, Ammerman, Hersen, Reigel, & Rowley (1991)	SB (N = 26) R = 7–9	Yes (nonchronically ill N = 29)	Observation: Role Play Tests Parent: CBCL-SCS Teacher: CBCL	Controlling for IQ, groups did not differ on tasks of conversational skill and negative assertion on the Role Play Tests; groups did not differ on CBCL according to teachers and mothers, although children with SB had lower father-rated School Social Competence scores.

Vannatta, Gartstein, Short, & Noll (1998)	Brain tumor survivors (*N* = 28) R = 8–18	Yes (nonchronically ill *N* = 28)	Peer: RCP, Three Best Friends, Like Rating Scale Teacher: RCP Child: RCP	Relative to controls, children diagnosed with brain tumors received fewer friendship nominations from peers and were described by peer, teacher, and self-report as socially isolated; peers perceived survivors as being more sick, more fatigued, and more often absent from school.
Vannatta, Zeller, Noll, & Koontz (1998)	Bone marrow transplant (BMT) survivors (*N* = 48) R = 8–16	Yes (nonchronically ill *N* = 48)	Peer: RCP, Three Best Friends, Like Rating Scale Teacher: RCP Child: RCP	Relative to controls, survivors were described by teachers as less aggressive and by peers as more socially isolated; survivors had fewer friends; peers described survivors as sick a lot, missing school, less physically attractive, and less athletically skilled than controls; physical appearance, athletic ability and whether cranial radiation was received mediated the social difficulties of survivors.
Westbrook, Silver, Coupey, & Shinnar (1991)	Epilepsy (mild) (*N* = 34) R = 13–19	Yes (chronically ill, *N* = 32; nonchronically ill, *N* = 50)	Child: Interview	Few differences between groups in social functioning (e.g., time spent in social/solitary activities); children with epilepsy were more likely to attend learning disabled classes than both control groups; children with epilepsy were less likely than controls with chronic illness to discuss disorder and to make all of their friends aware of their illness.
Zbikowski & Cohen (1998)	Asthma (*N* = 22) R = 6–12	Yes (nonchronically ill *N* = 84)	Parent: CBCL-SCS Peer: Three Peers They Like Best, Like Rating Scale, Friendship Nominations	Young children with asthma had lower parent-rated social competence than older children with asthma or controls and fewer close friends than young controls; according to peers, young children with asthma had fewer reciprocated friends compared with controls, but all children with asthma were as well liked as controls.

Note. BRP, Behavior Rating Profile; CBCL-SCS, Child Behavior Checklist—Social Competence Scale; CBP, Child Behavior Profile; CDI, Children's Depression Inventory; CHD, congenital heart disease; CF, cystic fibrosis; CFC, craniofacial conditions; CP, cerebral palsy; CVA, cerebral vascular accidents; HbSS, homozygous form of sickle cell disease; HDLF, Health and Daily Living Form; IDDM, insulin-dependent diabetes mellitus; JRA, juvenile rheumatoid arthritis; LSDQ, Loneliness and Social Dissatisfaction Questionnaire; MESSY, Matson Evaluation of Social Skills with Youngsters; NRI, Network of Relationships Inventory; PARS, Personal Adjustment and Role Skills Scale; PCSC, Perceived Competence Scale for Children; PHCSC, Piers–Harris Children's Self-Concept Scale; PIC, Personality Inventory for Children; R, age range (in years); RBPC, Revised Behavior Problem Checklist; RCP, Revised Class Play; SB, spina bifida; SPPA, Self-Perception Profile for Adolescents; SPPC, Self-Perception Profile for Children; SCD, sickle cell disease; SASK, Social Anxiety Scale for Children; SSRS, Social Skills Rating System; TOPS, Taxonomy of Problematic Situations; YSR-SCS, Youth Self-Report—Social Competence Scale.

nalizing symptoms, delinquency, and leaving school early (Hymel, Rubin, Rowden, & LeMare, 1990; Morison & Masten, 1991; Parker & Asher, 1987). Similarly, socially isolated behavior is a risk factor predictive of future problems with social acceptance by peers, negative self-perceptions, anxiety, and depression (Hymel et al., 1990; Rubin & Mills, 1988).

Two distinct aspects of peer relationships can be characterized broadly as peer acceptance and behavioral reputation. Measures of peer acceptance and friendships address the question, Is the child liked? whereas reports of a child's behavioral reputation are concerned with, What is the child like? (Parker & Asher, 1987). Although peer acceptance and behavioral reputation are interrelated, they are not redundant. "Knowledge of a child's behavioral style can only suggest that child's level of acceptance and findings from studies identifying children by one type of measure may not generalize to children identified by the other type of measure" (Parker & Asher, 1987, p. 359). In addition, some data suggest that the associations between social behaviors and peer acceptance vary across cultural groups (Chen, Rubin, & Li, 1995).

THEORETICAL APPROACHES

Several theories concerning the impact of pediatric chronic illness on the psychosocial adjustment of children have been proposed. Wallander and Varni's (1998) disability–stress–coping model suggests that chronic illness creates ongoing strain for children and their families, which may result in the disruption of a child's psychosocial functioning and development. This model contains a number of risk (e.g., disease severity) and resistance (e.g., cognitive abilities, family environment) factors that determine how well a child with a chronic illness adapts. Similarly, Thompson's (Thompson et al., 1994; Wallander & Thompson, 1995) transactional stress and coping model describes chronic physical conditions as possible stressors to which children and their families must adapt. Adjustment or lack of adjustment is a consequence of the transactions of illness factors (e.g., disease severity), demographic factors (e.g., age, gender), and adaptational processes (e.g., child coping, maternal adjustment).

Other theoretical literature has suggested that children are resilient in the face of adversity. Resilience has been defined as "good outcomes in spite of serious threats to adaptation or development" (Masten, 2001, p. 228). Masten has suggested that resilience results from the working of basic human adaptational systems and is a common phenomenon, consisting of "ordinary, rather than extraordinary, processes" (2001, p. 227). Severe, persistent adversity creates few significant effects on adjustment unless two important adaptive systems, neurocognitive functioning or parenting, are seriously impaired (Masten, 2001).

PEER OUTCOMES FOR CHILDREN WITH CHRONIC ILLNESS

La Greca (1990) has suggested several characteristics of diseases and/or treatments that might be expected to affect children's peer relationships. First, chronic conditions or treatments for them may cause restrictions in physical activities or interfere with daily activities, resulting in a child being less able or less available to participate in peer-oriented activities. Second, some conditions may affect physical appearance (e.g., growth and pubertal delays), leading to negative self-perceptions or negative reactions from peers. Finally, children who have cognitive impairment as a result of their illness or treatment may be particularly susceptible to experiencing difficulties in peer relationships (Nassau & Drotar, 1997; Schuman & La Greca, 1999).

Physical Restrictions and Interruptions in Daily Activity

A number of studies have reported that chronically ill children participate in fewer social activities than healthy children (Aasland, Flato, & Vandvik, 1997; Casey, Sykes, Craig, Power, & Mulholland, 1996; Daltroy et al., 1992; Johnson, Saal, Lovell, & Schorry, 1999; Timko, Stovel, Moos, & Miller, 1992). Participation in fewer activities has been attributed to pain, fatigue, disability, or other physical restrictions or to the ongoing disruptions created by treatment demands, visits to the doctor, and hospitalizations (e.g., Meijer et al., 2000a, 2000b). For instance, children with sickle cell disease (SCD) who experienced serious pain episodes were more likely to have also experienced activity disruption and teasing (Barbarin, Whitten, & Bonds, 1994).

Although limitations in activities are not necessarily an indication of poor social functioning, participation in fewer activities and diminished peer contact could lead to fewer opportunities to develop the social skills necessary to make and keep friends. For instance, Eiser et al. (1992) found that children with chronic illness were rated by both parents as having more problems with peer relations as disease restrictions increased. Similarly, Graetz and Shute (1995) reported that children with asthma who experienced more hospitalizations were less popular and more lonely and exhibited more sensitive-isolated behavior, according to peers.

Impairment that leads to serious limitations of normal functional abilities (e.g., walking, eating, playing) has been shown to be a particularly important factor in psychosocial adjustment of youth with chronic illness. In an epidemiological study of over 3,000 children 4–16 years of age, children with both chronic illness and disability were at greater risk for psychiatric disorders and social adjustment problems than were children with chronic illness alone (Cadman et al., 1987). However, most illness-related variables indicative of severity (e.g., number of hospitalizations, complications, frequency of pain) have not consistently been found to be associated with peer difficulties (Noll et al., 1996, 1999, 2000; Rodrigue, Streisand, Banko, Kedar, & Pitel, 1996; Zbikowski & Cohen, 1998). When differences between severity groups have been identified, greater disease severity has been primarily associated with more school absences and participation in fewer social activities (Daltroy et al., 1992; Meijer et al., 2000a; Timko et al., 1992). Although objective measures of disease severity have generally failed to be indicative of peer difficulties, we agree with the suggestion of Wallander and Thompson (1995). They emphasize that it is important that measures of disease severity or impairment continue to be defined by biomedical parameters (e.g., pulmonary functioning, hemoglobin levels) in order to keep them distinct from psychosocial factors.

Few studies have examined the role of parental interest and involvement in the social adjustment of children with chronic illness. Pope and Ward (1997a) reported that parents of more socially competent children with craniofacial conditions offered more encouragement and greater opportunities for their children to participate in activities with peers than did parents of children low on social competence. Pope and Ward concluded that parental encouragement might prevent some children from withdrawing from peer-oriented activities. Similarly, Wallander et al. (1989) reported that both utilitarian family resources (e.g., income and maternal education) and psychological family resources (e.g., levels of family cohesion, conflict, and control) accounted for a significant proportion of variance in the social adjustment of children with chronic illness. Social adjustment was assessed using the Child Behavior Checklist Social Competence Scale (CBCL-SCS), which focuses on parent report of participation in activities, sports, and organizations. Wallander et al. (1989) suggest that taking part in some of these activities requires financial resources and cooperation among family members and that it may be especially challenging for parents to sustain a child with physical impairment in these activities. Thus, children from families with limited resources or from families experiencing conflict may have fewer opportunities to interact with peers.

Physical Appearance

Physical attractiveness is highly valued by peers and has been reported to be a strong predictor of friendship and peer acceptance (Hanna, 1998; Lerner et al., 1991; Vannatta, Gartstein, Zeller, & Noll, 2003). Differences in appearance experienced due to a chronic condition or treatment may negatively affect a child's peer relationships. Some of these differences may be temporary, but others are permanent consequences of the illness and its treatment. These differences in appearance might create negative self-perceptions of attractiveness and body image concerns in the child, leading to self-consciousness and more withdrawn behaviors (Spirito, DeLawyer, & Stark, 1991). Some research has indicated that children who are dissatisfied with their appearance are perceived by peers as displaying more passive withdrawal behaviors, suggesting that they may choose to limit their interactions with peers (Cobb, Cohen, Houston, & Rubin, 1998). Youth with chronic illness who report less satisfaction with their appearance than those from comparison groups have also been reported to experience difficulties in peer relations (e.g., Timko et al., 1992). Pendley, Dahlquist, and Dreyer (1997) found that negative body image in adolescent survivors of cancer was correlated with greater social anxiety, loneliness, and lower global self-worth, although not with the number of peer activities or size of the peer network.

Changes in appearance may also affect how peers perceive children with chronic conditions, particularly those conditions that are highly visible to peers and to which peers may react negatively. In a study using naturalistic observation, Kapp-Simon and McGuire (1997) reported that not only were adolescents with craniofacial conditions less likely than controls to initiate a conversation with a peer and to respond if approached, but also that peers spoke to these adolescents less frequently than to controls and responded less often if the adolescent spoke to them (also see Pope & Ward, 1997a,1997b). Vannatta, Zeller, Noll, and Koontz (1998) assessed the peer relationships of a group of children who had survived bone marrow transplantation (BMT). Many of these children experience permanent alterations in appearance. Vannatta, Zeller, et al. (1998) reported that peers perceived these children as less physically attractive and less athletically skilled than healthy comparison peers. These physical attributes mediated the social difficulties of the survivors such that survivors who were perceived as less attractive and less athletically skilled had more peer difficulties, including having fewer best friends and being more actively isolated by peers.

In some instances, the treatment regimens rather than physical appearance per se may be experienced as stigmatizing (La Greca, 1990). For example, children with diabetes may need to use insulin and may be required to follow strict dietary and exercise programs. Despite the potentially stigmatizing aspects of this treatment, some evidence demonstrates the importance to children of receiving the support of friends and peers during treatment. La Greca et al. (1995) evaluated the support provided by family and friends for the care of adolescents with diabetes. They concluded that the support provided by the adolescents' friends, compared with that provided by family, was unique, and they further suggested that adolescents who do not have friends with whom they can discuss their condition may be lacking an important source of emotional support.

Cognitive Impairment

A number of chronic illnesses may negatively affect CNS functioning (see Nassau & Drotar, 1997). Some of these illnesses are primarily distinguished by their CNS involvement (e.g., brain tumors, epilepsy, spina bifida, cerebral palsy), whereas others may have a more subtle impact (e.g., leukemia, SCD). Nassau and Drotar's (1997) recent review of the social competence of children with CNS-related chronic health conditions indicated that these children are at considerable risk for difficulties in social functioning. They suggested several reasons why social functioning may be a particular problem for these children, including visible appearance changes, restrictions on activities, or cognitive impairments that affect social understanding.

Some CNS conditions may be experienced by children as stigmatizing because of their high visibility. For example, Vannatta, Gartstein, et al. (1998) reported that children who had survived brain tumors were perceived by peers as being sick, more fatigued, and missing more school relative to comparison peers, suggesting that the physical sequelae of their therapy was still apparent to peers even though they were no longer receiving treatment for their disease. These survivors received fewer friendship nominations from classmates than nonchronically-ill comparison peers and were described by peer, teacher, and self-report as socially isolated.

Children with CNS conditions may participate in fewer activities than peers because of physical limitations or because they must attend special education classes (Nassau & Drotar, 1997; Schuman & La Greca, 1999). Kazak and Meadows (1989) reported that cancer survivors receiving educational assistance were rated by mothers as having lower levels of social competence than survivors not receiving such assistance. However, those survivors receiving assistance also reported getting more help and support from friends than other survivors.

Finally, Nassau and Drotar (1997) suggested that cognitive limitations (e.g., intelligence, memory, or attention) experienced by some children may have a negative impact on peer relationships through their effect on social understanding (Dodge & Price, 1994). Subtle neurocognitive impairments such as nonverbal learning difficulties have been suggested to be associated with social problems (Gresham, 1992; Rourke, 1995). Indeed, children with cognitive impairments have been reported to experience difficulty in expressing social behavior, as well as in understanding social information. In a comparison of expressive behavior in infants and young children with HIV who were classified as either encephalopathic or nonencephalopathic, children with CNS disease were less responsive socially and emotionally and displayed difficulties in motor functioning and verbal behavior (Moss, Wolters, Brouwers, Hendricks, & Pizzo, 1996). Boni, Brown, Davis, Hsu, and Hopkins (2001) investigated social information processing in school-aged children with SCD with a cerebral vascular accident (CVA) compared with children with SCD without CVA. Children with SCD with CVA demonstrated more errors on tasks involving recognition of subtle facial and vocal expression of emotion compared with children without CVA. The authors concluded that children with CVA might have particular difficulty understanding complex or ambiguous social situations. Vannatta, Zeller, et al. (1998) reported that BMT survivors who had received cranial radiation, which has been associated with neurocognitive morbidity, were perceived as more passive, anxious, and socially withdrawn than BMT survivors who had not received cranial radiation.

Gender and Age

In general, when gender differences in social functioning are found, boys with chronic illness appear to be at greater risk for difficulties than girls (Daltroy et al., 1992; Eiser et al., 1992; Sanger, Copeland, & Davidson, 1991). La Greca (1990) suggested that conditions that restrict physical activities or create increased fatigue or growth and pubertal delays have a greater social impact on boys. This finding may be attributed to the nature of boys' play, which often involves more group-oriented and athletic activities in comparison to the activities preferred by girls, making athletic ability of particular importance for the social behavior of males (Adler, Kless, & Adler, 1992; Maccoby, 1988; Vannatta et al., 2003).

When age differences in adjustment have been examined, older children with chronic illness appear to be at greater risk for social difficulties than younger children (Daltroy et al., 1992; Shelby, Nagle, Barnett-Queen, Quattlebaum, & Wuori, 1998). Adolescence is a time during which identification with and acceptance by the peer group are particularly important. Decreased time with peers, potentially stigmatizing differences in appearance and treatment regimens, and a dependence on adults to manage their illness may disrupt normal developmental tasks of adolescence, such as establishing a comfortable body image or gaining a sense of autonomy (Fritz & McQuaid, 2000). However, longitudinal studies need to be conducted to follow children with chronic illnesses and healthy comparison children through such developmental transitions (Wallander & Thompson, 1995).

Conclusions

In general, the majority of studies concerning the peer relationships of children with chronic illness have found few problems (Table 11.1). When difficulties have been reported, they most often involve restrictions on activities, but not problems getting along with peers. The exception is children who experience cognitive impairment as a consequence of their illness or its treatment. In addition, children who appear physically different from their peers may also encounter peer difficulties (Kapp-Simon & McGuire, 1997; Pope & Ward, 1997b; Vannatta, Zeller, et al., 1998), although these findings are less consistent. Finally, the experience of chronic illness may serve a protective function. For example, several studies have reported that children with chronic illness were less aggressive than controls or normative samples (Meijer et al., 2000a; Noll et al., 1999; Noll et al., 1996; Spirito et al., 1990). The physical limitations and fatigue that accompany many illnesses may make some children less likely to be contentious with peers, thereby disrupting developmental pathways to future externalizing behaviors or conduct problems.

METHODOLOGY

A number of methodological shortcomings in the literature on the peer relationships of children with chronic illness limit the conclusions and generalizability of the results.

Participants

One of the major concerns with this literature is determining the representativeness of the samples of participants with chronic illness. Common problems have included a failure to report recruitment rates, ascertainment bias, and small sample sizes (Eiser, Hill, & Vance, 2000; Miller, 1993). For example, a frequent practice is to recruit participants from the children who come for treatment at specialty clinics. Thus samples tend to include those who most often attend these clinics, potentially excluding children of families who are less compliant or with less severe disease. We strongly recommend recruitment from clinic rosters that include all children who have been diagnosed with a chronic illness at a particular center. In addition, information needs to be provided concerning what percentage of available children were located and refusal rates (Lavigne & Faier-Routman, 1992).

The recruitment of controls also warrants careful attention and can be accomplished in a number of ways. Controls matched on race, gender, and age may be recruited from the same classrooms as the children with chronic illness. Door-to-door canvassing techniques or "snowball" techniques, in which the child with a chronic illness is asked for the names of several same-race, same-gender, similar-aged peers, can be utilized to recruit neighborhood controls (Noll et al., 1992). Although sibling controls may be useful for some questions (e.g., neurocognitive functioning), nonaffected siblings are typically a different age and gender. Recruitment of volunteers through advertisements or from other clinics results in numerous potential confounds. The use of random digit dialing may also be biased because some communities have a high percentage of households with unlisted numbers or without phones.

Measures

Much of the reviewed work has utilized measures that do not primarily assess social functioning. Such measures may assess peer relations in a cursory way, as they often have only a few questions or one scale regarding social functioning (Nassau & Drotar, 1997; Spirito et al., 1991). In particular, many studies have described the global social functioning of children with chronic illness in terms of parent-reported social competence. One of the most widely used instruments in the literature concerning the adjustment of children with a chronic illness is the Child Behavior Checklist (CBCL; Achenbach, 1991). Drotar, Stein, and Perrin (1995) pointed out that some of the competencies assessed by the CBCL-SCS are not social but rather concern general activities such as skills at jobs (Schneider & Byrne, 1989). Other items focus on achievements at school, such as grades, that have little to do with social competence. More recently, studies have begun to include measures to assess other aspects of social functioning, including behavioral reputation, social acceptance, social skills, social self-concept, social anxiety, and loneliness.

There is also some question as to whether some of these instruments can validly measure the social functioning of children with a chronic illness. In particular, it is important to know whether items on measures normed on healthy children are confounded by illness factors (Spirito et al., 1991). Drotar et al. (1995) have suggested that caution must be exercised when using the CBCL as a measure of social functioning for children with chronic illness. The CBCL contains items that reflect physical symptoms, and they may be particularly difficult to interpret when used with children with chronic illness (Drotar et al., 1995; Perrin, Stein, & Drotar, 1991). For instance, in an investigation of children with congenital heart disease, Casey et al. (1996) found that these children had higher scores on the Withdrawn subscale of the CBCL relative to controls, according to parents and teachers. However, this difference was no longer significant when the item "underactive," which may be a symptom of the child's medical condition, was removed from the subscale.

Source of Information

The majority of studies assessing social functioning of children with a chronic illness use parent report alone or in combination with teacher report or self-report. Reliance on parent report when assessing peer relations may be particularly problematic, because parents primarily observe their children at home rather than during direct interactions with peers. For instance, the activities and social subscales of the CBCL-SCS have shown a lack of convergent validity with children's self-ratings and with peer nominations (Schneider & Byrne, 1989). Adults such as teachers are often biased by other knowledge about the child (e.g., academic success), and they primarily interact with children in classrooms, in which peer interactions are limited (Parker & Asher, 1987; Newcomb, Bukowski, & Pattee, 1993). For instance, when Colegrove and Huntzinger (1994) evaluated the social skills and competence of 37 boys with hemophilia, 56% of whom were HIV positive, all parent, child, and teacher ratings fell within the normal range according to instrument norms. However, more absences from school were associated with lower teacher ratings not only of scholastic competence but of social and athletic competence, physical attractiveness, and social activities. Parent ratings of behavior and social activities and self-ratings of social activities were not associated with the number of days absent.

Peers may be the best judges of a child's social functioning, as they have the most daily interactions with the child. In addition, peer report often consists of multiple raters (e.g., a child's classmates) of each child, thereby providing a more stable measure of social functioning in contrast to single-rater sources (e.g., teachers). Unfortunately, few studies have obtained data from peers.

Design

Only about half of the studies reviewed used a control group, whereas the rest relied on normative comparisons. Reliance on instrument norms may be limited by cohort (Achenbach & Howell, 1993) or regional effects (Sandburg, Meyer-Bahlburg, & Yager, 1991), even for measures that have national norms with periodic updates. Moreover, without appropriate comparison groups, it is difficult to determine whether findings are specific to youths with a chronic illness or due to confounds with demographic characteristics such as SES or family background variables. For instance, Lemanek and colleagues (Lemanek, Moore, Gresham, Williamson, & Kelley, 1986) assessed the psychosocial functioning of children with SCD and healthy controls and found no group differences. However, when compared with measure norms, both groups of children reported greater problems in school and with peers. The authors concluded that these differences were likely due to the low SES of black children in their sample rather than a result of the experience of SCD.

Another problem with study designs in this literature is the lack of long-term longitudinal studies that follow children and controls prospectively. The overwhelming majority of studies have utilized cross-sectional or short-term longitudinal designs that prevent researchers from identifying whether changes in adjustment occur over time, as well as potential mechanisms to explain why differences in adjustment may be present in subgroups of children. New analytic methods such as individual growth modeling may be particularly advantageous in understanding how adjustment to chronic illness changes over time for individuals (e.g., Frank et al., 1998). More traditional methods tend to analyze change over time as a characteristic of groups by examining the mean response of all participants across groups between arbitrary time points. Growth curve modeling represents change as a continuous process and focuses on defining trajectories of change in adjustment for individuals over time (Francis, Fletcher, Stuebing, Davidson, & Thompson, 1991). Such techniques can be employed to identify different trajectories among children with chronic illness and perhaps identify potential disease-related (e.g., severity, prognosis), nonsocial (e.g., appearance, athletic competence), psychological (e.g., coping skills, temperament), and environmental (e.g., family variables, social support) mediators that might aid in understanding why some children with chronic illness do well socially, whereas others experience difficulties (e.g., Frank et al., 1998). Unfortunately, few studies have given consideration to directly testing potential mechanisms that might affect continuing transactions between the child with a chronic illness and his or her social relationships.

Finally, a significant limitation of work in this area involves conducting studies at single sites, with small samples of children with chronic illness. This practice may introduce bias because sites may differ from each other in terms of the SES, age, gender, race, or disease characteristics of the patient population treated there (Lavigne & Faier-Routman, 1992). A multisite approach would mitigate some of these biases, increase sample size, and reduce methodological differences in how data are obtained (Lavigne & Faier-Routman, 1992). In addition, the effects of differing levels of services available at various health care facilities could also be evaluated. For instance, Noll et al. (1999) found that children with cancer were perceived as more sociable by teachers and as having greater social acceptance by peers relative to controls. One explanation offered for these positive outcomes is the basic supportive care activities at the center at which the participants received treatment. These positive results may not be representative of children in other areas of the country for whom extensive psychosocial services are not available.

Conclusions

There are a number of methodological challenges to future research concerning the peer relationships of children with chronic illness that must be met in order to advance understanding in this area and better serve intervention efforts. First, longitudinal studies must be completed that follow children prospectively through different developmental periods, as well as through different stages of the illness. Second, multisite studies are necessary to minimize bias and increase sample size. Recruitment of participants with chronic illness from clinic rosters or through the use of epidemiological methods would also reduce biases and improve the generalizability of studies. Measures should assess the different aspects of peer relations and social functioning and have sound psychometric properties. Third and finally, multiple informants, especially peers, should be included.

ACKNOWLEDGMENTS

We wish to acknowledge Kathryn Vannatta and Cynthia A. Gerhardt for their help and support on this project.

REFERENCES

Aasland, A., Flato, B., & Vandvik, I. (1997). Psychosocial outcome in juvenile chronic arthritis: A nine-year follow-up. *Clinical and Experimental Rheumatology, 15,* 561–568.

Achenbach, T. M. (1991). *Manual for the Child Behavior Checklist/4–18 and 1991 Profile.* Burlington, VT: University of Vermont, Department of Psychiatry.

Achenbach, T. M., & Howell, C. T. (1993). Are American children's problems getting worse?: A 13-year comparison. *Journal of American Academy of Child and Adolescent Psychiatry, 32,* 1145–1154.

Adler, P. A., Kless, S. J., & Adler, P. (1992). Socialization to gender roles: Popularity among elementary school boys and girls. *Sociology of Education, 30,* 887–892.

Apter, A., Aviv, A., Kaminer, Y., Weizman, A., Lerman, P., & Tyano, S. (1991). Behavioral profile and social competence in temporal lobe epilepsy of adolescence. *Journal of the American Academy of Child and Adolescent Psychiatry, 30,* 887–892.

Barbarin, O. A., Whitten, C. F., & Bonds, S. M. (1994). Estimating rates of psychosocial problems in urban and poor children with sickle cell anemia. *Health and Social Work, 19,* 112–119.

Boni, L. C., Brown, R. T., Davis, P. C., Hsu, L., & Hopkins, K. (2001). Social information processing and magnetic resonance imaging in children with sickle cell disease. *Journal of Pediatric Psychology, 26,* 309–319.

Cadman, D., Boyle, M., Szatmari, P., & Offord, D. R. (1987). Chronic illness, disability, and mental and social well-being: Findings of the Ontario Child Health Study. *Pediatrics, 79,* 805–813.

Casey, F., Sykes, D. H., Craig, B. G., Power, R., & Mulholland, H. C. (1996). Behavioral adjustment of children with surgically palliated complex congenital heart disease. *Journal of Pediatric Psychology, 21,* 335–352.

Chen, X., Rubin, K. H., & Li, Z. (1995). Social functioning and adjustment in Chinese children: A longitudinal study. *Developmental Psychology, 31,* 531–539.

Cobb, J. C., Cohen, R., Houston, D. A., & Rubin, E. C. (1998). Children's self-concepts and peer relationships: Relating appearance self-discrepancies and peer perceptions of social behaviors. *Child Study Journal, 28,* 291–308.

Colegrove, R. W., & Huntzinger, R. M. (1994). Academic, behavioral, and social adaptation of boys with hemophilia/HIV disease. *Journal of Pediatric Psychology, 19,* 457–473.

Daltroy, L. H., Larson, M. G., Eaton, H. M., Partridge, A. J., Pless, I. B., Rogers, M. P., & Liang, M. H. (1992). Psychosocial adjustment in juvenile arthritis. *Journal of Pediatric Psychology, 17,* 277–289.

Dodge, K. A., & Price, J. M. (1994). On the relations between social information processing and socially competent behavior in early school-aged children. *Child Development, 65,* 1385–1397.

Drotar, D., Stein, R. E. K., & Perrin, E. (1995). Methodological issues in using the child behavior checklist and its related instruments in clinical child psychology research. *Journal of Clinical Child Psychology, 24,* 184–192.

Durkin, M. S., Khan, N., Davidson, L. L., Zaman, S. S., & Stein, Z. A. (1993). The effects of a natural disaster on child behavior: Evidence for posttraumatic stress. *American Journal of Public Health, 83,* 1549–1553.

Eiser, C., Havermans, T., Pancer, M., & Eiser, R. (1992). Adjustment to chronic disease in relation to age and gender: Mothers' and fathers' reports of their children's behavior. *Journal of Pediatric Psychology, 17,* 261–275.

Eiser, C., Hill, J. J., & Vance, Y. H. (2000). Examining the psychological consequences of surviving childhood cancer: Systematic review as a research method in pediatric psychology. *Journal of Pediatric Psychology, 25,* 449–460.

Francis, D. J., Fletcher, J. M., Stuebing, K. K., Davidson, K. C., & Thompson, N. M. (1991). Analysis of change: Modeling individual growth. *Journal of Consulting and Clinical Psychology, 59,* 27–37.

Frank, R., Thayer, J., Hagglund, K., Vieth, A., Schopp, L., Niels, C., et al. (1998). Trajectories of adaptation in pediatric chronic illness: The importance of the individual. *Journal of Consulting and Clinical Psychology, 66,* 521–532.

Fritz, G. K., & McQuaid, E. L. (2000). Chronic medical conditions: Impact on development. In A. J. Sameroff, M. Lewis, & S. M. Miller (Eds.), *Handbook of developmental psychopathology* (2nd ed., pp. 277–289). New York: Kluwer Academic/Plenum.

Gartstein, M., Short, A., Vannatta, K., & Noll, R. (1999). Psychosocial adjustment of children with chronic illness: An evaluation of three models. *Developmental and Behavioral Pediatrics, 20,* 157–163.

Graetz, B., & Shute, R. (1995). Assessment of peer relationships in children with asthma. *Journal of Pediatric Psychology, 20,* 205–216.

Gresham, F. M. (1992). Social skills and learning disabilities: Causal, concomitant, or correlational? *School Psychology Review, 21,* 348–360.

Hanna, N. A. (1998). Predictors of friendship quality and peer group acceptance at summer camp. *Journal of Early Adolescence, 18,* 291–318.

Harris, J. A., Newcomb, A. F., & Gewanter, H. L. (1991). Psychosocial effects of juvenile rheumatic disease: The family and peer systems as a context for coping. *Arthritis Care and Research, 4,* 123–130.

Hartup, W. W. (1996). The company they keep: Friendships and their developmental significance. *Child Development, 67,* 1–13.

Hoffman, R. G., Rodrigue, J. R., Andres, J., & Novak, D. A. (1995). Moderating effects of family functioning on the social adjustment of children with liver disease. *Children's Health Care, 24,* 107–117.

Hymel, S., Rubin, K. H., Rowden, L., & Lemare, L. (1990). Children's peer relationships: Longitudinal prediction of internalizing and externalizing problems from middle childhood. *Child Development, 61,* 2004–2021.

Johnson, N. S., Saal, H. M., Lovell, A. M., & Schorry, E. K. (1999). Social and emotional problems in children with neurofibromatosis type 1: Evidence and proposed interventions. *Journal of Pediatrics, 134,* 767–772.

Kapp-Simon, K. A., & McGuire, D. (1997). Observed social interaction patterns in adolescents with and without craniofacial conditions. *Cleft Palate–Craniofacial Journal, 34,* 380–384.

Kapp-Simon, K. A., Simon, D., & Kristovich, S. (1992). Self-perception, social skills, adjustment, and inhibition in young adolescents with craniofacial anomalies. *Cleft Palate–Craniofacial Journal, 29,* 352–356.

Kazak, A. E., & Meadows, A. T. (1989). Families of young adolescents who have survived cancer: Social-emotional adjustment, adaptability, and social support. *Journal of Pediatric Psychology, 14,* 175–191.

La Greca, A. M. (1990). Social consequences of pediatric conditions: Fertile area for future investigation and intervention? *Journal of Pediatric Psychology, 15,* 285–307.

La Greca, A. M., Auslander, W. F., Greco, P., Spetter, D., Fisher, E. B., & Santiago, J. V. (1995). I get by with a little help from my family and friends: Adolescents' support for diabetes care. *Journal of Pediatric Psychology, 20,* 449–476.

Lavigne, J. V., & Faier-Routman, J. (1992). Psychological adjustment to pediatric physical disorders: A meta-analytic review. *Journal of Pediatric Psychology, 17,* 133–157.

Lemanek, K. L., Moore, S. L., Gresham, D. A., Williamson, D. A., & Kelley, M. L. (1986). Psychological adjustment of children with sickle cell anemia. *Journal of Pediatric Psychology, 11,* 397–410.

Lerner, R. M., Lerner, J. V., Hess, L. E., Schwab, J., Jovanovic, J., Talwar, R., & Kucher, J. S. (1991). Physical attractiveness and psychosocial functioning among early adolescents. *Journal of Early Adolescence, 11,* 300–320.

Maccoby, E. E. (1988). Gender as a social category. *Developmental Psychology, 24,* 755–765.

Manne, S., & Miller, D. (1998). Social support, social conflict, and adjustment among adolescents with cancer. *Journal of Pediatric Psychology, 23,* 121–130.

Margolin, G., & Gordis, E. B. (2000). The effects of family and community violence on children. *Annual Review of Psychology, 51,* 445–479.

Masten, A. S. (2001). Ordinary magic: Resilience processes in development. *American Psychologist, 56,* 227–238.

Meijer, S. A., Sinnema, G., Bijstra, J. O., Mellenbergh, G. J., & Wolters, W. (2000a). Social functioning in children with a chronic illness. *Journal of Child Psychology and Psychiatry, 41,* 309–317.

Meijer, S. A., Sinnema, G., Bijstra, J. O., Mellenbergh, G. J., & Wolters, W. (2000b). Peer interaction in adolescents with a chronic illness. *Personality and Individual Differences, 29,* 799–813.

Miller, J. J. (1993). Psychosocial factors related to rheumatic diseases in childhood. *Journal of Rheumatology, 20,* 1–11.

Morison, P., & Masten, A. S. (1991). Peer reputation in middle childhood as a predictor of adaptation in adolescence: A seven-year follow-up. *Child Development, 62,* 991–1007.

Moss, H., Bose, S., Wolters, P., & Brouwers, P. (1998). A preliminary study of factors associated with psychological adjustment and disease course in school-age children infected with the Human Immunodeficiency Virus. *Developmental and Behavioral Pediatrics, 19,* 18–25.

Moss, H. A., Wolters, P. L., Brouwers, P., Hendricks, M. L., & Pizzo, P. A. (1996). Impairment of expressive behavior in pediatric HIV-infected patients with evidence of CNS disease. *Journal of Pediatric Psychology, 21,* 379–400.

Nassau, J. H., & Drotar, D. (1995). Social competence in children with IDDM and asthma: Child, teacher, and parent reports of children's social adjustment, social performance, and social skills. *Journal of Pediatric Psychology, 20,* 187–204.

Nassau, J. H., & Drotar, D. (1997). Social competence among children with central nervous system–related chronic health conditions: A review. *Journal of Pediatric Psychology, 22,* 771–793

Newacheck, P. W., & Taylor, W. R. (1992). Childhood chronic illness: Prevalence, severity, and impact. *American Journal of Public Health, 82,* 364–371.

Newby, W. L., Brown, R. T., Pawletko, T. M., Gold, S., & Whitt, K. (2000). Social skills and psychological adjustment of child and adolescent cancer survivors. *Psycho-oncology, 9,* 113–126.

Newcomb, A. F., Bukowski, W. M., & Pattee, L. (1993). Children's peer relations: A meta-analytic review of popular, rejected, neglected, controversial, and average sociometric status. *Psychological Bulletin, 113,* 99–128.

Noll, R. B., Bukowski, W. M., Davies, W. H., Koontz, K., & Kulkarni, R. (1993). Adjustment in the peer system of children with cancer: A two-year follow up study. *Journal of Pediatric Psychology, 18,* 351–364.

Noll, R. B., Bukowski, W. M., Rogosch, F. A., LeRoy, S. S., & Kulkarni, R. (1990). Social interactions between children with cancer and their peers: Teacher ratings. *Journal of Pediatric Psychology, 15,* 43–56.

Noll, R. B., Gartstein, M. A., Vannatta, K., Correll, J., Bukowski, W. M., & Davies, W. H. (1999). Social, emotional, and behavioral functioning of children with cancer. *Pediatrics, 103,* 71–78.

Noll, R. B., Kozlowski, M. A., Gerhardt, C. A., Vannatta, K., Taylor, J., & Passo, M. H. (2000). Social, emotional, and behavioral functioning of children with juvenile rheumatoid arthritis. *Arthritis and Rheumatism, 43,* 1387–1396.

Noll, R. B., LeRoy, S. S., Bukowski, W., Rogosch, F. A., & Kulkarni, R. (1991). Peer relationships and adjustment of children with cancer. *Journal of Pediatric Psychology, 16,* 307–326.

Noll, R. B., Ris, M. D., Davies, W. H., Bukowski, W. M., & Koontz, K. (1992). Social interactions between children with cancer or sickle cell disease and their peers: Teacher ratings. *Journal of Developmental and Behavioral Pediatrics, 13,* 187–193.

Noll, R. B., Vannatta, K., Koontz, K., Kaylinyak, K., Bukowski, W. M., & Davies, W. H. (1996). Peer relationships and emotional well-being of youngsters with sickle cell disease. *Child Development, 67,* 423–436.

Padur, J. S., Rapoff, M. A., Houston, B. K., Barnard, M., Danovsky, M., Olson, N. Y., et al. (1995). Psychosocial adjustment and the role of functional status for children with asthma. *Journal of Asthma, 32,* 345–353.

Parker, J. G., & Asher, S. R. (1987). Peer relations and later personal adjustment: Are low-accepted children at risk? *Psychological Bulletin, 102,* 357–389.

Pendley, J. P., Dahlquist, L. M., & Dreyer, Z. (1997). Body image and psychosocial adjustment in adolescent cancer survivors. *Journal of Pediatric Psychology, 22,* 29–43.

Perrin, E. C., Stein, R. E. K., & Drotar, D. (1991). Cautions in using the Child Behavior Checklist: Observations based on research with children with a chronic illness. *Journal of Pediatric Psychology, 16,* 411–421.

Pope, A., & Ward, J. (1997a). Factors associated with peer social competence in preadolescents with craniofacial anomalies. *Journal of Pediatric Psychology, 22,* 455–469.

Pope, A., & Ward, J. (1997b). Self-perceived facial appearance and psychosocial adjustment in preadolescents with craniofacial anomalies. *Cleft Palate–Craniofacial Journal, 34,* 396–401.

Reiter-Purtill, J., Gerhardt, C. A., Vannatta, K., Passo, M. H., & Noll, R. B. (2003). A controlled longitudinal study of the social functioning of children with juvenile rheumatoid arthritis. *Journal of Pediatric Psychology, 28,* 17–28.

Rodrigue, J. R., Streisand, R., Banko, C., Kedar, A., & Pitel, P. (1996). Social functioning, peer relations, and internalizing and externalizing problems among youths with sickle cell disease. *Children's Health Care, 25,* 37–52.

Rolland, J. S. (1988). Family systems and chronic illness: A typological model. In F. Walsh & C. Anderson (Eds.), *Chronic disorders and the family* (pp. 143–168). New York: Haworth Press.

Rourke, B. P. (Ed.). (1995). *Syndrome of nonverbal learning disabilities: Neurodevelopmental manifestations.* New York: Guilford Press.

Rubin, K. H., & Mills, R. S. (1988). The many faces of social isolation in childhood. *Journal of Consulting and Clinical Psychology, 56,* 916–924.

Sandburg, D. E., Meyer-Bahlburg, H. F. L., & Yager, T. J. (1991). The Child Behavior Checklist nonclinical standardization samples: Should they be utilized as norms? *Journal of American Academy of Child and Adolescent Psychiatry, 30,* 124–134.

Sanger, M. S., Copeland, D. R., & Davidson, E. R. (1991). Psychosocial adjustment among pediatric cancer patients: A multidimensional assessment. *Journal of Pediatric Psychology, 16,* 463–474.

Schneider, B. H., & Byrne, B. M. (1989). Parents rating children's social behavior: How focused the lens? *Journal of Clinical Child Psychology, 18,* 237–241.

Schuman, W. B., & La Greca, A. M. (1999). Social correlates of chronic illness. In R. T. Brown (Ed.), *Cognitive aspects of chronic illness in children* (pp. 289–311). New York: Guilford Press.

Shelby, M. D., Nagle, R. J., Barnett-Queen, L. L., Quattlebaum, P. D., & Wuori, D. F. (1998). Parental reports of psychosocial adjustment and social competence in child survivors of acute lymphocytic leukemia. *Children's Health Care, 27,* 113–129.

Spirito, A., DeLawyer, D. D., & Stark, L. J. (1991). Peer relations and social adjustment of chronically ill children and adolescents. *Clinical Psychology Review, 11,* 539–564.

Spirito, A., Stark, L. J., Cobiella, C., Drigan, R., Androkites, A., & Hewett, K. (1990). Social adjustment of children successfully treated for cancer. *Journal of Pediatric Psychology, 15,* 359–371.

Stein, R., & Jessop, D. (1982). A noncategorical approach to chronic childhood illness. *Public Health Reports, 97,* 354–362.

Stein, R. E. K., & Silver, E. J. (1999). Operationalizing a conceptually based noncategorical definition. *Archives of Pediatric Adolescent Medicine, 153,* 68–74.

Thompson, R. J., Gil, K. M., Keith, B. R., Gustafson, K. E., George, L. K., & Kinney, T. R. (1994). Psychological adjustment of children with sickle cell disease: Stability and change over a 10–month period. *Journal of Consulting and Clinical Psychology, 62,* 856–860.

Timko, C., Stovel, K. W., Moos, R. H., & Miller J. J. (1992). Adaptation to juvenile rheumatic disease with a one-year follow-up. *Health Psychology, 11,* 67–76.

Van Hasselt, V. B., Ammerman, R. T., Hersen, M., Reigel, D. H., & Rowley, F. L. (1991). Assessment of social skills and problem behaviors in young children with spina bifida. *Journal of Developmental and Physical Disabilities, 3,* 69–80.

Vannatta, K., Gartstein, M. A., Short, A., & Noll, R. B. (1998). A controlled study of peer relationships of children surviving brain tumors: Teacher, peer, and self ratings. *Journal of Pediatric Psychology, 23,* 279–288.

Vannatta, K., Gartstein, M. A., Zeller, M., & Noll, R. B. (2003). *Appearance, athletic ability and academic competence: Contributions to peer acceptance and behavioral reputation.* Manuscript submitted for publication.

Vannatta, K., Zeller, M., Noll, R. B., & Koontz, K. (1998). Social functioning of children surviving bone marrow transplantation. *Journal of Pediatric Psychology, 23,* 169–178.

Wallander, J. L., & Thompson, R. J. (1995). Psychosocial adjustment of children with chronic physical conditions. In M. C. Roberts (Ed.), *Handbook of pediatric psychology* (2nd ed., pp. 124–141). New York: Guilford Press.

Wallander, J. L., & Varni, J. W. (1998). Effects of pediatric chronic physical disorders on child and family adjustment. *Journal of Child Psychology and Psychiatry, 39,* 29–46.

Wallander, J. L., Varni, J. W., Babani, L., Banis, H. T., & Wilcox, K. T. (1989). Family resources as resistance factors for psychological maladjustment in chronically ill and handicapped children. *Journal of Pediatric Psychology, 14,* 157–173.

Westbrook, L. E., Silver, E. J., Coupey, S. M., & Shinnar, S. (1991). Social characteristics of adolescents with idiopathic epilepsy: A comparison to chronically ill and nonchronically ill peers. *Journal of Epilepsy, 4,* 87–94.

Zbikowski, S., & Cohen, R. (1998). Parent and peer evaluations of the social competence of children with mild asthma. *Journal of Applied Developmental Psychology, 19,* 249–265.

12

Chronic and Recurrent Pain

LYNNDA M. DAHLQUIST
MARNI C. SWITKIN

Few psychologists or pediatricians today would dispute the idea that children experience pain. However, the widespread appreciation of the need to understand and to effectively manage children's pain actually developed relatively recently. Prior to 1987, major pediatric textbooks did not even discuss pain management (McGrath & Finley, 1999; Schechter & Zeltzer, 1999). Children were thought to have a limited capacity to experience pain because of their immature neurological systems. As a result, pain medications were considered unnecessary for children undergoing invasive medical procedures; chronic pain was viewed as an adult rather than a pediatric problem. In contrast, today's professionals are much more sensitive to the pain experiences of children and infants and to the impact that pain can have on their developing nervous systems (Schechter & Zeltzer, 1999; Taddio, 1999). Most pediatric medical settings now routinely offer some sort of analgesia or anesthetic for invasive medical procedures. Pain management strategies typically are integrated into the specialty care of children with chronic or recurrent pain conditions, such as arthritis and headaches.

Despite the tremendous progress in the empirical and professional pediatric pain literature over the past decade, the attitudes of the lay public and practitioners who are not pain experts often lag far behind. Dualistic views of pain (i.e., either it is "real" or it is all in the child's head) are still common. Such misperceptions, unfortunately, often lead professionals to discount or ignore children's pain complaints that are not clearly tied to physical pathology or to label children as psychologically disturbed if their pain appears excessive (McGrath & Finley, 1999). These problems are evident with both chronic and acute pain in children; they are especially pronounced in pain conditions in which the source of the child's pain is less easily identified—such as chronic, recurrent pain conditions that fluctuate in unpredictable ways or that are difficult to tie to underlying disease activity.

The purpose of this chapter is to provide an overview of the variables that influence the experience of pain in children and to summarize the primary approaches to the evaluation and the treatment of chronic and recurrent pain in children. Our review is selective rather than comprehensive. We have highlighted studies that are good illustrations of certain techniques, examples of tests of theory, or critical reviews of existing literature.

BIOLOGICAL BASES OF PAIN

The human experience of pain is one that conjures up unpleasant images and negative connotations. It is an experience that both children and adults attempt to avoid altogether or terminate as quickly as possible. In fact, it is the most common reason for seeking medical care (Covington, 2000). However, the experience of pain also serves adaptive functions and is one of several biological safety mechanisms.

Pain sensation initially results from the partial destruction of or injury to tissue adjacent to specific nerve fibers (Rosenzweig, Breedlove, & Leiman, 2002). At the site of tissue damage, chemical substances (e.g., neuropeptides, serotonin, and histamines) are released, which then activate pain fibers during the process of inflammation. These pain fibers are called nociceptors—specialized receptors that respond to noxious stimulation (Covington, 2000; Rosenzweig et al., 2002). The quality of pain sensation is directly related to the type of nociceptor activated. Stimulation of cutaneous Aδ nociceptors (large-diameter, mylenated, high-threshold receptors) results in a pricking pain, stimulation of cutaneous C nociceptors (thin, unmyelinated fibers) results in burning or dull pain, and stimulation of nociceptors in muscle nerves results in aching pain (Rosenzweig et al., 2002; Willis & Westlund, 1997).

Based on physiological characteristics, pain can be classified as nociceptive (either superficial or deep) or neuropathic (Ness & Gebhart, 1990). Wilkie, Huang, Reilly, and Cain (2001) define nociceptive pain as the activation of primary afferent nociceptors located in the peripheral nervous system in somatic (skin, muscle, or bone) or visceral tissues. Superficial pain is the product of stimulation of cutaneous structures, whereas deep pain is caused by muscle, fascia, joints, bone, vascular structures, and viscera stimulation (Ness & Gebhart, 1990). In contrast, neuropathic pain is initiated or caused by a primary lesion or transitory functional disturbance in the peripheral or central nervous system (Wilkie et al., 2001).

Neuropathic pain processes differ from nociceptic pain processes (Wilkie et al., 2001). For example, neuropathic pain tends to be resistant to pharmacological therapies that typically relieve nociceptive pain (e.g., opioid therapy). Furthermore, patients tend to describe neuropathic pain differently. Adult patients with pain at the site of injury (nociceptive pain) describe their pain experience as beating, crushing, heavy, dull, tiring, exhausting, nauseating, fearful, frightful, obsessive, and wretched, whereas patients with neuropathic pain utilize descriptors such as burning, electric shock, tingling, pricking, itching, and cold (Wilkie et al., 2001).

Pain sensation in neuropathic pain often does not correspond to the injury or tissue stimulation. For example, innocuous stimulation of normal tissue with a soft brush can evoke pain (allodynia), noxious stimulation can yield greater than usual or greater than expected pain (hyperalgesia), and transient stimulation can result in persistent pain or hyperalgesia affecting uninjured tissue (referred pain; Covington, 2000). Pain perception also can linger at the injury site (primary hyperalgia) or at a remote site (secondary hyperalgia) long after the injury has healed (Willis & Westlund, 1997).

Type I complex regional pain syndrome (formerly called reflex sympathetic dystrophy or neurovascular dystrophy) is the most common type of neuropathic pain in children

(Olsson, 1999). This disorder usually involves pain in the distal portion of an arm or leg, which may begin after an injury but persists long after the injury appears to have healed. Children experience spontaneous pain and allodynia or hyperalgesia. They also show signs of autonomic dysfunction; for example, the affected foot may be significantly colder or warmer than the other foot. Muscle weakness and other motor impairments also can develop as a result of inactivity or attempts to guard the limb.

VARIABLES THAT MODULATE PAIN PERCEPTION: GATE CONTROL THEORY

According to Melzack and Wall's now-classic papers on the "gate control theory" of pain, both peripheral efferent impulses and central afferent impulses influence whether or not noxious stimulation reaches the cortex and is interpreted as pain (Melzack & Wall, 1965, 1982). They proposed the existence of a "gating" mechanism, a complex receiving and relay system, in the dorsal horn of the spinal cord, through which both sensory and pain fibers relay signals. If the "gate" is open, pain sensations are transmitted to the cortex, where they are recognized as pain. If the "gate" is closed, no signal is sent to the brain and no pain is perceived. Melzack and Wall argued that, if an impulse from a large-diameter, fast-transmitting myelinated sensory A-fiber reaches the "gate" before a pain fiber impulse, the connecting neuron would be activated by the sensory fiber and thereby be unresponsive to the pain impulse. In other words, the sensory stimulation closes the "gate." Perhaps even more important, however, they proposed that descending messages from central cognitive variables also could open or close the "gate," thus introducing the important role of cognition and emotion in all pain experiences.

Today, the importance of cognition and emotion in pain perception is widely acknowledged in pain research. In fact, the International Association for the Study of Pain (IASP) defines pain as "an unpleasant sensory and emotional experience associated with actual or potential tissue damage, or described in terms of such damage" (Mersky & Bogduk, 1994; Pain Terms, paragraph 1). In this respect, all pain is to some degree "psychogenic."

PSYCHOLOGICAL VARIABLES THAT INFLUENCE PAIN

Stress and Negative Emotions

Stress, depression, and anxiety are among the most commonly reported precipitants of chronic, recurrent pain syndromes in adults (e.g., Flor & Turk, 1989; Martin, 1993) and in children (Martin-Herz, Smith, & McMahon, 1999). For example, recurrent abdominal pain symptoms have been reported to correlate with mothers' reports of stressful life events (e.g., Walker, Garber, & Greene, 1994) and with children's reports of daily stressors (Varni et al., 1996; Walker, Garber, Smith, Van Slyke, & Claar, 2001). Experimental manipulation of stress in the laboratory also has been shown to increase headache intensity in adult headache patients (Martin & Seneviratne, 1997). Such studies support the notion that some chronic pain conditions are caused, at least in part, by physiological vulnerability to stress (Davis, Zautra, & Reich, 2001) or problems with recovery from stress (Compas, 1999). Stress also may exacerbate the impact of pain on the child's quality of life (Langeveld, Koot, & Passchier, 1999). Finally, the experience of pain itself may serve as an important stressor

(Compas, 1999). Thus stress can be conceptualized to cause or influence pain, as well as to be caused by pain.

Although the results are not consistently positive, higher levels of depression and anxiety also have been reported in children and adolescents with various chronic pain conditions, such as headache (e.g., Andrasik et al., 1988; Carlsson, Larsson, & Mark, 1996). Studies of adults suggest that the effects of stress on pain may be greatest during negative mood states (Burns, Wiegner, Derleth, Kiselica, & Pawl, 1997; Davis et al., 2001). Although fewer studies have been conducted with children, similar findings were reported by Walker et al. (2001). Children with higher trait levels of negative affect showed the strongest relations between stress and physiological symptoms.

Cognitive Coping Strategies

Both laboratory studies of pain and clinical studies of chronic pain suggest that cognitive variables affect pain experiences. For example, individuals who demonstrate negative thinking or catastrophize when faced with pain report more intense pain (Jacobsen & Butler, 1996; Thomsen et al., 2002) and psychological distress (Gil, Williams, Thompson, & Kinney, 1991; Gil et al., 2001), utilize more postsurgical pain medications (Jacobsen & Butler, 1996), and experience greater activity reduction (Gil et al., 1991). Coping styles have been found to relate to pain in children without a history of pain, as well as in children with current pain, and to predict which children recovered from recurrent abdominal pain (Walker, Smith, Garber, & Van Slyke, 1997).

Predictability/Controllability

In laboratory studies, predictability and perceived controllability have been shown to affect pain perception. For example, adults rated electric shock that was signaled by a light as less painful than did adults who received the same shock without a signal. Adults who were told that they could adjust the intensity of the shock if it became too painful (even though they never did adjust the intensity) rated the pain as less aversive and habituated more rapidly to the stimulus than did adults who were not given the perception of control (Staub, Tursky, & Schwartz, 1971). Similarly, children who were given ongoing information about the time that a cold presser trial would end reported less pain than children who underwent the same duration cold pressor trial without any temporal information (Coldwell et al., 2002).

PAIN ASSESSMENT

Because of the subjective nature of pain and the important roles of cognitive appraisal and emotions in the experience of pain, it is challenging to measure validly and reliably. Nevertheless, the assessment of pain in children is crucial in order to aid in medical diagnosis and determine treatment efficacy (McGrath, 1987). A number of developmental issues must be taken into consideration. For example, young children may not possess the vocabulary necessary to adequately describe their pain in ways that adults can interpret. Moreover, pain scales may require young children to discriminate constructs (e.g., intensity and duration) that are too sophisticated for their cognitive development (Dahlquist, 1990).

Child Self-Report

Visual analogue scales (VAS) are among the most common forms of child pain intensity assessment. These scales involve graphic representations of pain intensity by marking a point on a line or thermometer and appear valid for children as young as 5 years old (Dahlquist, 1990). Older children (over 9 years old) may be able to use Likert-type 5- or 10-point ratings of pain frequency, duration, and intensity (e.g., Walker, Smith, Garber, & Van Slyke, 1997). Simpler pain intensity scales include the poker chip tool (Hester, Foster, & Kristensen, 1990), which consists of four red chips that represent "pieces of hurt" (with one chip indicating a "little hurt" and all four chips indicating "the most hurt a child could have"), and the Tactile Analog Scale (Westerling, 1999), which consists of nine red wooden balls of increasing size on a metal pole and does not require sight to use. In some studies, body outlines have been used in conjunction with intensity ratings to identify the location of the child's pain (e.g., the Adolescent Pediatric Pain Tool, Savedra, Tesler, Holzemer, Wilkie, & Ward, 1990, and the Pediatric Pain Questionnaire [PPQ], Varni & Thompson, 1987).

Faces scales consist of a set of line drawings or photographs of faces that depict pain states (Chambers, Giesbrecht, Craig, Bennett, & Huntsman, 1999). They are argued to be appropriate for children because they do not employ sophisticated words or abstract numerical values. To our knowledge, only the Oucher Scale (Beyer, 2000; Beyer & Knott, 1998) provides different photographs for Caucasian, Hispanic, and African American children. For the most part, faces scales have been shown to correlate highly with other self-report and behavioral measures of pain, to be sensitive to analgesic interventions, and to correlate somewhat with pain ratings by other individuals (e.g., parents and nurses; Chambers et al., 1999). However, faces scales have been criticized for using different endpoint stimuli (children tend to report higher pain ratings when a scale begins with a smiling rather than neutral "no pain" face) and for validation studies that merely ask healthy children to rate hypothetical pain (Chambers et al., 1999). McGrath (1987) also raised the concern that faces with numerical scales alongside them may confound the affective component of pain (presumably captured in the faces) and pain intensity (reflected in the numbers). Finally, it cannot be assumed that faces scales yield interval or ratio data, even if each face is labeled with an integer. At best, the data should be considered ordinal; the intervals between stimuli might well be unequal from the child's perspective (McGrath, deVeber, & Hearn, 1985).

Structured interviews with children and their parents are the main vehicles for assessing historical and contextual variables contributing to pain experiences (Allen & Matthews, 1998). For example, the Pediatric Pain Questionnaire (PPQ) developed by Varni and Thompson (1985) taps a variety of aspects of the child's pain experience through individual structured interviews with patients and their parents. The PPQ measures pain intensity and location (through VAS ratings and coloring in body diagrams), sensory and affective aspects of the child's pain (through a list of pain descriptors), and the child and family's pain histories. Although originally designed for children with arthritis, the scale has been used with a number of illness populations. (For other disease-specific examples of structured interviews or multicomponent questionnaires, see Budd, Workman, Lemsky, and Quick, 1994; McGrath, 1990; McGrath et al., 2000; and Mikkelsson, Salminen, and Kautiainen, 1997.)

Because of the error that often accompanies retrospective recall, prospective monitoring of pain symptoms through daily pain diaries often is recommended. The use of pain diaries varies widely, from noting the occurrence of pain only when it happens to recording the presence or absence of pain at regular, fixed intervals. Some diaries require intensity ratings and calculation of duration, in addition to frequency. Pain diaries also may include functional disability (e.g., withdrawal from typical activities or social interactions or number of school absences), as well as pain triggers, coping strategies employed, and medication taken (Allen & Matthews, 1998; Gil et al., 2001; Holden, Levy, Deichmann, & Gladstein, 1998). In a recent study of the quality of life of adolescents with chronic pain (Hunfeld et al., 2001), participants reported significantly lower average pain intensities in 3-week daily diaries than they did on a retrospective questionnaire assessing pain intensity over the previous month. Hunfeld et al. argued that retrospective evaluations are more likely to overestimate pain intensity, because more severe pain is recalled more easily. Thus diary data are more valid.

Studies of the reliability and validity of child pain reports often compare the child's ratings with estimates of the child's pain by other adults. However, the results of such studies are mixed. Some have obtained good adult–child agreement (e.g., Sanders, Cleghorn, Shepherd & Patrick, 1996). Other studies have found evidence of nurses underestimating children's pain (Romsing, Moller-Sonnergaard, Hertel, & Rasmussen, 1996) and parents both underestimating (Chambers, Reid, Craig, McGrath, & Finley, 1998) and overreporting (Graumlich et al., 2001) pain. However, as Gragg and colleagues (1996) argued, these discrepancies should not be surprising given that there is a subjective component of pain perception that may not be adequately assessed by anyone other than the individual in pain. Thus there may be a ceiling on the degree of child–adult agreement that can be obtained.

Observational Assessment

Some researchers argue that behavioral observations are more reliable and valid than self-report measures because they are objective in nature, recording the presence or absence of discrete pain behaviors (McGrath, 1987). However, behavioral observations can capture only one aspect of the pain experience—the overt expression of pain. One must infer the subjective experience of pain severity from the frequency and duration of distress behaviors. Moreover, expressions of fear, anxiety, noncompliance, and pain may look identical in children, thus further complicating the measurement of pain (Chambers & Craig, 1998). Although behavioral observations should not be used in isolation if self-report also can be obtained, they may be the only pain measurement available for preverbal children. The Children's Hospital of Eastern Ontario Pain Scale (CHEOPS; McGrath et al., 1985) is one of the most widely studied and clinically utilized behavioral observational coding systems for children (Stein, 1995; Tyler, Tu, Douthit, & Chapman, 1993). The CHEOPS includes six behavioral subscales—crying, facial expression, verbal expression, torso position, touch behavior, and leg position—that are each rated on a 5-point scale (no pain to severe pain).

Behavioral observational coding systems specifically for infant pain usually rely on facial movements, crying, and gross body movements (van Dijk et al., 2000). The Postoperative Pain Score (POPS; Barrier, Attia, Mayer, Amiel-Tison, & Shnider, 1989), the Nursing Assessment of Pain Intensity (NAPI; Stevens, 1990), and the Riley Infant Pain Scale (RIPS; Joyce, Schade, & Keck, 1994) rate from 4 to 10 categories of infant behavior (Schade, Joyce, Gerkensmeyer, & Keck, 1996). The Neonatal Facial Coding System (NFCS; Grunau & Craig, 1987) and the Baby Facial Action Coding System (Baby FACS; Oster & Rosenstein, 1993) are even more detailed scales—coding the presence or absence of 10 facial expressions during five consecutive 2-second intervals. However, these scales have had limited applications in medical settings because of the cumbersome, time-intensive nature of the assessment (Schade et al., 1996). The COMFORT Scale (Ambuel, Hamlett, Marx, & Blumer, 1992) is a less complicated observational system designed for children from birth to

3 years of age. The six behavioral ratings (alertness, calmness, muscle tone, movement, facial tension, and respiratory response) can be obtained in 3 minutes and require only about 2 hours of nurse training (van Dijk et al., 2000).

PHARMACOLOGICAL INTERVENTIONS

Non-Narcotic Agents

Non-narcotic analgesics are used for mild to moderate pain. They are thought to reduce pain by affecting the peripheral nervous system and inhibiting the metabolism of pain-producing substances in body tissues and also may affect the central nervous system. For example, aspirin is thought to affect prostaglandin synthesis and to reduce inflammation at the site of an injury. Its use is discouraged in children, however, because of the increased risk of Reye syndrome (McGrath, 1990). Acetaminophen (e.g., Tylenol) appears to have less anti-inflammatory effect than does aspirin (McGrath, 1990), but it is prescribed more often because it does not interfere with platelet function and has fewer gastrointestinal side effects (Meyer et al., 1997). Nonsteroidal anti-inflammatory drugs (NSAIDS; e.g., ibuprofen, Motrin) inhibit prostaglandin synthesis and exert peripheral anti-inflammatory and analgesic effects. However, they also are associated with gastrointestinal, kidney, liver, and blood system (platelet) side effects (McGrath, 1990).

Narcotic Agents

Narcotic pain medications (sometimes referred to as "opioids" because they are derived from opium) include drugs such as codeine and morphine. These drugs relieve pain by affecting the central nervous system rather than the peripheral nervous system. They are most often used for moderate to severe pain. Although the mechanisms of action are only beginning to be understood, narcotics appear to inhibit the release of pain neurotransmitters, as well as activate descending neural pathways involved in pain control (McGrath, 1990). Dizziness, sedation, and nausea are common side effects. Higher doses of morphine can cause respiratory depression (Meyer et al., 1997). Over time, tolerance can develop, such that the child will require higher doses of the drug in order to obtain the same level of pain control. Drugs such as morphine also can cause physical dependence, meaning that the child's body will react with withdrawal symptoms if the medications are discontinued abruptly.

Because it is more difficult to titrate doses of any drug for children's small bodies, health professionals are particularly cautious about narcotic dosing with children. However, these realistic concerns often interact with misconceptions about the risks of psychological addiction, resulting in the underutilization of appropriate pain medications in many children. A dangerous cycle can then develop, with patients becoming more dramatic or manipulative in efforts to obtain pain relief and providers interpreting their behaviors as drug seeking (Schechter, 1999).

Combinations

In some instances, it is possible to achieve better pain control by combining pharmacological agents than by using any one agent alone. For example, codeine often is manufactured in combination with acetaminophen or aspirin and is used for moderate pain (such as after tooth extraction). Burn patients often are given acetaminophen on a regular schedule to control the constant background pain they experience. Opioids are then added if the acetaminophen does not sufficiently reduce the pain or to help children tolerate acutely painful procedures, such as dressing changes and wound treatments (Meyer et al., 1997).

Antidepressants also are commonly used in conjunction with other pain medications (McGrath, 1990). For the patients who are both depressed and experiencing chronic pain, there is evidence that their pain improves when their depression remits. However, tricyclic antidepressants also have been shown to have benefits for children with neuropathic pain who do not demonstrate depression (Sethna, 1999). Tricyclic antidepressants also appear to potentiate the effectiveness of opioids when used in combination—thus enabling better pain control to be achieved at lower doses of narcotics. Finally, tricyclic antidepressants can improve sleep in patients whose sleep cycles have been disrupted by pain (McGrath, 1990; Sethna, 1999).

Medication Schedules

Pain medications are most effective when administered around the clock (i.e., at regular intervals) rather than on a p.r.n (*pro re nata* or "as needed") basis (World Health Organization, 1990). Regular schedules maintain a constant level of medication in the body and help prevent the recurrence of pain. In contrast, p.r.n. schedules require the child to communicate the presence of pain before receiving medication. This is a problem for children who may be unwilling or unable to indicate when they are in pain. Moreover, p.r.n schedules delay the administration of pain medications, thus ensuring that the child will experience intervals of potentially preventable pain. Occasional breakthrough pain (pain that emerges despite regularly scheduled pain medication) can be treated by additional "as needed" dosing of oral medication. For children on intravenous pain medications, patient-controlled analgesia (PCA) allows the child to self-administer an additional dose of intravenous drugs at predetermined intervals, thus ameliorating breakthrough pain in a quick, efficient manner. (See McGrath, 1990, and McGrath and Finley, 1999, for more on the biological bases of pain pharmacology and Dahlquist, 1999b, for a more extensive discussion of medication schedules and family and medical system variables.)

PHYSICAL INTERVENTIONS

Transcutaneous electrical nerve stimulation (TENS) therapy is based on gate control theory (Melzack & Wall, 1965). TENS therapy involves electrical stimulation of large afferent nerve fibers (A fibers) near the site of the child's pain in such a way that nociceptive C fiber input is inhibited (Merkel, Gutstein, & Malviya, 1999). Thus the child feels a tingling or vibration sensation rather than an aching pain sensation. TENS also may relieve pain by activating endogenous opioids. Although there has been little research on the effectiveness of TENS for chronic pain in children, available data suggest that it can help reduce postoperative pain, wound care pain, and the pain associated with reflex sympathetic dystrophy, sickle cell crises, and skin ulcers (Merkel et al., 1999). In cases of severe neuropathic pain, surgical procedures or nerve blocks are sometimes used to prevent the transmission of pain impulses (Olsson, 1999).

Although sleep deprivation is widely acknowledged as one of many variables contributing to the suffering of chronic pain patients, Lewin and Dahl (1999) argued that sleep also affects pain perception and coping skills. By causing irritability, emotional lability, and impaired attention and behavioral control, Lewin and Dahl proposed that sleep deprivation interferes with children's efforts to divert their attention away from pain sensations. Improving children's sleep should facilitate pain control. Sleep also facilitates the healing process.

BIOFEEDBACK

Biofeedback training involves the monitoring and quantifying of a physiological response and conveying this information to the patient in such a way that the child perceives minute changes in his or her physiological status. Muscle tension (typically measured in the frontalis muscle or at the site of the child's pain) and skin temperature are the most common physical functions monitored for pain relief. Children as young as 7 years old appear to be able to learn to increase finger skin temperature (Labbe, Delaney, Olson, & Hickman, 1993) and to reduce muscle tension (Holden, Deichmann, & Levy, 1999).

The nature of the actual feedback provided to children varies considerably across studies. Simple auditory feedback involves a tone that increases or decreases in pitch and/or beeps. Simple visual feedback methods include digital finger temperature readings, temperature strips that change color, or lights that turn on or off to signal changes in temperature or muscle tension. More complex computer game-like feedback systems involve animals or race cars that change speed or spaceships that descend in response to changes in the child's muscle tension; these may be particularly appealing to children (Culbert, Kajander, & Reaney, 1996).

Depending on the pain application, biofeedback is used either as a means to achieve a heightened state of relaxation (Holden et al., 1999; Lavigne, Ross, Berry, Hayford, & Pachman, 1992) or to alter a physiological process thought to cause the pain sensations (e.g., Hermann, Kim, & Blanchard, 1995). For example, tension headaches are thought to be caused, in part, by sustained tension in pericranial muscles. Consequently, electromyographic (EMG) biofeedback is used to teach patients to relax the frontalis muscle (Gauthier, Ivers, & Carrier, 1996). Migraine headaches, on the other hand, are thought to be caused by constriction of intra- and extracranial arteries (Gauthier et al., 1996). Therefore, biofeedback procedures for migraines typically target vascular activity. Patients are taught to warm the index finger, which is thought to cause a decrease in sympathetic vascular activity and a concomitant vascular dilation of the arteries that would constrict in the event of a migraine headache (Gauthier et al., 1996). More recent headache models have proposed that vascular and muscular systems may have roles in both migraine and tension headaches; thus thermal biofeedback relieves tension headaches, as well as migraines (e.g., Arndorfer & Allen, 2001).

The variables that moderate biofeedback treatment effectiveness, such as age or baseline symptom severity, remain unclear. There is some indication in the literature that children with more severe headaches may benefit the most from biofeedback (Hermann, Blanchard, & Flor, 1997). However, this observation may merely reflect regression to the mean or floor effects in the less severely affected children (Hermann et al., 1997). With respect to age effects, the data are mixed. Hermann et al. (1997) obtained better outcomes with younger, elementary school–age migraine patients than with adolescents. In contrast, Osterhaus et al. (1993) reported better outcomes in older adolescents than in younger adolescents. Other researchers have found no age effects (e.g., Labbe et al., 1993).

COGNITIVE–BEHAVIORAL PAIN MANAGEMENT STRATEGIES

Because cognitive–behavioral interventions for chronic pain conditions are most often provided in a package format—teaching children several different pain management skills as part of a comprehensive pain management intervention—there are no outcome data for the individual components of intervention. Consequently, except where otherwise noted, the following sections describe the different components of treatment programs that, as part of a package, have been found to be effective.

Relaxation

Progressive muscle relaxation training has been conceptualized as both a distraction from pain sensations and a way to reduce subjective pain intensity (Walco, Varni, & Ilowite, 1992). Children typically are taught to tense and then relax specific groups of muscles. Most researchers use an abridged version of Jacobson's 16-muscle groups, but they usually do not report the specific number of muscle groups used. If more than one session of relaxation training is conducted, the number of muscle groups is gradually reduced until a more rapid, cue-controlled strategy is taught, in which the entire body is relaxed at once while the child subvocalizes a relaxation cue word (e.g., Dahlquist, 1999b; Larsson & Carlsson, 1996). Children are expected to practice relaxation at home and may be offered an audiotape of a relaxation session to assist with home practice (e.g., Walco et al. 1992). Some investigators also include deep breathing exercises as part of the relaxation exercise. More recently, relaxation via massage has been associated with lower reported pain in children with arthritis (Field et al., 1997).

Imagery

In some instances imagery is used as distraction. For example, Walco et al. (1992) used guided imagery in conjunction with progressive muscle relaxation and meditative breathing for pain management for children with arthritis. In the distracting-imagery component of their intervention, children were taught to imagine themselves in a setting in which they had been pain free. In other instances, children are instructed to use imagery to imagine the pain diminishing. For example, Walco et al. (1992) taught children to imagine turning off "pain switches" throughout their bodies or imagine joint pain as a blowtorch being extinguished. Imagery strategies that acknowledge pain but then transform it in some way to make it less noxious may be particularly useful for high-intensity pain, which may be too difficult to ignore.

Self-Statements

Gil and colleagues (Gil et al., 1997; Gil et al., 2001) developed a coping skills intervention that specifically targeted negative and catastrophizing cognitions. They taught children with sickle cell disease to use calming self-statements, deep breathing and counting relaxation, and pleasant imagery. The children then practiced using positive self-statements and the other coping strategies while undergoing two laboratory-induced pressure pain trials. Children who received the coping training demonstrated less negative thinking and lower pain during the laboratory pain task; however, the improvements were not maintained over a 1-month follow-up period. The authors speculated that an intervention more intensive than the two sessions and weekly follow-up phone calls they provided may be needed to achieve longer lasting changes in pain cognitions.

Sanders and colleagues (Sanders et al., 1989; Sanders, Shepherd, Cleghorn, & Woolford, 1994) included coping statements as part of a two-session cognitive–behavioral treatment program for children with recurrent abdominal pain. Children were taught to make encouraging self-statements (e.g., "be brave, hang in there") when experiencing pain and to then engage in relaxation and divert their attention from the pain (Sanders et al., 1989, p. 297). If their pain diminished, they were told to reward themselves with a positive self-statement. If the pain persisted, they were instructed to imagine a cartoon character "eating the pain away." Parents also received training in contingency management. A greater proportion of the children who received the cognitive–behavioral treatment program were pain free after treatment, compared with wait-list controls (Sanders et al., 1989) and children receiving standard pediatric care (Sanders et al., 1994).

OPERANT INTERVENTIONS

The types of interventions described so far focus primarily on decreasing the child's subjective experience of pain. In contrast, operant interventions focus on modifying the child's overt manifestations of pain. Common pain behaviors include crying, whimpering, groaning, verbal complaints, grimacing, protective postures or guarding, breath holding, limping, lying down, rubbing, pulling or holding part of the body, and gagging or vomiting (Allen & Matthews, 1998; Dahlquist, 1999b).

Many pain behaviors may be maintained by intermittent positive or negative reinforcement. Parents may comfort or spend extra time with the child when he or she is in pain. Friends and family may visit or send gifts or provide access to other positive consequences during pain episodes. Teachers and peers also may pay more attention to the child whose pain causes a limp or requires the use of a wheelchair. Pain behaviors also may enable the child to escape or avoid chores, a difficult class, or stressful peer or family interactions. Walker (1999) proposed that children who are having difficulty accomplishing normal developmental tasks, who experience or anticipate failure, and who perceive themselves to be incompetent are especially at risk for activity restriction and social withdrawal in response to pain. This tendency is likely to be exacerbated in highly competitive academic environments or in highly critical home environments.

An often-ignored negative reinforcement contingency is the fact that many pain behaviors actually do reduce pain sensations. For example, lying down, keeping a part of the body still, or restricting activities often reduce pain intensity in the short term (Allen & Matthews, 1998). However, in chronic or recurrent pain syndromes, these palliative measures have little impact on long-term pain frequency (Allen & Matthews, 1998) and can seriously interfere with the child's long-term adaptive functioning (Dahlquist, 1999b).

In a study of 7- to 18-year-olds with migraine headaches, Allen and Shriver (1998) compared biofeedback alone with an intervention consisting of biofeedback plus training of parents in ways to avoid reinforcing inappropriate pain behaviors and to provide positive reinforcement for adaptive coping strategies and for maintaining daily activities. Although both groups showed reductions in headache frequency, children in the group receiving parent training made greater gains and were more likely to be headache free at the end of treatment and at 3-month follow-up. At 1-year follow-up, however, the groups no longer differed. It is not clear whether the parents failed to maintain their behavior management skills or whether the behavior management skills of the parents of children who received only biofeedback spontaneously improved as their children assumed greater responsibility for managing their pain.

Competing contingencies also may interfere with parents' management of their children's pain behavior. Providing comfort and pain relief may make some parents feel closer to their children or may allow them to avoid aversive situations, such as work or marital conflict (Dahlquist, 1999b; Walker, 1999). In such cases, the contingencies that maintain the parent's behavior also should be targeted in the pain management intervention. Moreover, when parents who are ill or in pain themselves decrease their activity levels or do not fulfill their work or home responsibilities, children are likely to demonstrate similar behaviors when they are in pain (Allen & Matthews, 1998; Dahlquist, 1999b; Walker, 1999). However, only a few researchers (e.g., Sanders et al., 1994) have specifically targeted parental modeling of sick-role behaviors as part of their behavior management program.

SOCIOCULTURAL CONSIDERATIONS IN PAIN MANAGEMENT

Gender

Unruh and Campbell (1999) conducted a comprehensive review of the literature examining gender differences in children's pain across a variety of medical disorders. Although the findings are mixed, in general, the existing literatures on both adult and child pain suggest that females are at greater risk for pain, report lower pain thresholds and lower pain tolerance, and tend to report higher pain intensity. Although few gender differences emerged in infancy and young childhood, school-age and adolescent girls reported greater frequencies, longer duration, and higher pain intensity ratings for headaches, migraines, facial pain, upper back pain, and sickle cell disease. Unruh and Campbell (1999) also cited evidence that girls required more pain medication for dental procedures and tended to visit school and camp infirmaries more often. In a more recent experimental investigation (Chambers, Craig, & Bennett, 2002), mothers' behavior was found to affect the pain reports of girls but not boys who were undergoing cold pressor pain, suggesting that girls may be particularly sensitive to pain-reinforcing social contingencies.

Culture

There is very little empirical research documenting the role of cultural variables in the evaluation and management of pain. Research that does exist historically has been housed in other disciplines, such as sociology and anthropology (Lasch, 2000). Past research in child health and pain has almost exclusively used a Western approach, regardless of the child's ethnic background (Banoub-Baddour & Laryea, 1991). Only recently have psychologists recognized the importance of including cultural dimensions in pain research.

In a recent review of the literature, Lasch (2000) found evidence to suggest that pain reactions do vary according to cultural affiliations. Certain cultural groups tend to demonstrate higher pain tolerance, requiring less analgesia for pain management. Culture also appears to influence how children are expected to respond to painful stimuli, to whom they should report pain, what words to use to describe pain, and under what circumstances, if any, one should admit to feelings of pain (Banoub-Baddour & Laryea, 1991).

Current research suggests that minorities not only experience disproportionately high incidence and mortality rates for cancer but also report more ineffective treatment of cancer pain (Lasch, 2000). These trends may reflect the differential access to and utilization of health care services for minorities. Culture or bias also may affect health care providers' perceptions of patients' pain, thus leading to ineffective pain control (Schechter, 1999). For example, Calvillo and Flaskerud (1993) found that nurses estimated more pain in Anglo-American patients than in Mexican patients, despite no differences in patients' self-reports of pain.

A culturally sensitive health care provider assessing and treating pain must consider such variables as degree of acculturation; immigration status; language preferences; cultural attitudes and beliefs toward illness, health care, and mental health; and the education and resources of family members, as well as the individual child. Furthermore, practitioners must be aware of common cultural values and practices while remaining careful not to overgeneralize and stereotype individual cases.

FUTURE DIRECTIONS

Although there is considerable evidence that cognitive–behavioral, operant, and biofeedback pain management programs are effective, there is a pressing need for component analyses of these intervention programs. Multifaceted treatment package approaches have clinical utility in that they may maximize the chances of offering the child and family an intervention that will fit their needs. However, multicomponent interventions do not allow for the study of important questions that might help refine pain management techniques, develop more cost-effective strategies, or provide more effective treatment matching. In addition, as Holden et al. (1999) argued, pharmacological treatments for chronic and recurrent pain need to be integrated into psychosocial intervention packages. Future studies could then assess whether psychological intervention potentiates pharmacological treatment and vice versa, as well as identify which patients or families benefit from which combinations of treatment modalities.

Future studies also should pay greater attention to treatment failures, as well as treatment successes. A better understanding of which children and families respond best to which types of intervention has important theoretical and clinical implications (Dahlquist, 1999a). For example, Sanders et al. (1996) found that their combination of cognitive–behavioral pain management techniques and parent training in behavior management was most effective with children with recurrent abdominal pain whose parents believed their pain to be stress- rather than illness-related and were already encouraging independent pain management at baseline. These findings suggest that parental variables may mediate or moderate pain management outcomes. A certain cognitive set (i.e., that stress influences pain) or certain fundamental behavior management skills may be required before parents can benefit from instruction in pain management strategies. If so, future research should address the problem of what to offer families with poorer behavior management skills or more medical views of their child's pain. It also may be important to consider the messages the child and family receive from the medical care providers. It may not be feasible to conduct a pain management intervention based on an integrative biopsychosocial conceptualization of pain while medical personnel are conducting diagnostic studies to find a purely medical explanation for the child's pain. Other potential moderators of treatment effectiveness include developmental level and contextual variables such as culture, ethnicity, and the community and home environment. Medical variables such as severity or frequency of the child's pain also may affect treatment outcome or necessitate different treatment strategies.

Janicke and Finney (1999) argued that many intervention research protocols require such intensive time commitments from participants, both for treatment and for data collection, that the research findings may not be representative of the actual population of children with chronic pain. More data on treatment refusers and treatment dropouts would help determine the extent of this potential problem and determine whether protocols need to be modified to make them easier to follow or better suited to the unique needs of certain children and families. For example, innovations in service delivery, such as Larsson and Carlsson's (1996) school-based intervention for headache, may enable psychologists to provide pain management care for children who might otherwise be unable to participate.

More consistency in outcome evaluation would be helpful in evaluating pain management programs across studies and across disorders. Clearer standards for clinically significant pain reductions also are needed. It may not be reasonable to expect complete elimination of pain, especially in conditions with high base-rate pain frequency in the normal population (i.e., headaches and abdominal pain). Instead, it may be more useful to identify the magnitude of change in pain that is clinically significant, such as the 50% reduction in pain criterion used in the headache literature (Hermann et al., 1995).

More research also is needed to demonstrate changes in adaptive functioning, such as school attendance and achievement, social activities, sleep, burden on the family, and utilization of medical services as they relate to reductions in pain. As Palermo (2000) illustrated in her review of the impact of chronic pain on children and families, the limited data available suggest that all of these domains of functioning can be affected by chronic pain. However, there is little research designed to clarify *why* these functional outcomes occur. For example, do children with chronic pain interact less often with peers because they are too uncomfortable to play, or do they behave in ways that cause others to avoid them? By addressing the functional impact of chronic pain, as well as the experience of pain, health care providers will be better able to improve the quality of life of children and their families.

Finally, effective pain interventions for chronic, persistent pain conditions must, by definition, be long lasting. However, in several studies, treatment gains that were evident immediately after intervention were not maintained over time. More research on the long-term effectiveness of pain interventions is needed. In particular, future research should attempt to identify the variables that predict the maintenance of pain reduction and the intervention strategies needed for children whose initial improvements are not maintained.

REFERENCES

Allen, K. D., & Matthews, J. R. (1998). Behavior management of recurrent pain in children. In T. S. Watson & F. M. Gresham (Eds.), *Handbook of child behavior therapy* (pp. 263–285). New York: Plenum.

Allen, K. D., & Shriver, M. D. (1998). Role of parent-mediated pain behavior management strategies in biofeedback treatment of childhood migraines. *Behavior Therapy, 29*, 477–490.

Ambuel, B., Hamlett, K. W., Marx, C. M., & Blumer, J. L. (1992). Assessing distress in pediatric intensive care environments: The COMFORT Scale. *Journal of Pediatric Psychology, 17*, 95–109.

Andrasik, F., Kabela, E., Quinn, S., Attanasio, V., Blanchard, E. B., & Rosenblum, E. L. (1988). Psychological functioning of children who have recurrent migraine. *Pain, 34*, 43–52.

Arndorfer, R. E., & Allen, K. D. (2001). Extending the efficacy of a thermal biofeedback treatment package to the management of tension-type headaches in children. *Headache, 41*, 183–192.

Banoub-Baddour, S., & Laryea, M. (1991). Children in pain: A culturally sensitive perspective for child care professionals. *Journal of Child and Youth Care, 6*, 19–24.

Barrier, G., Attia, J., Mayer, M. N., Amiel-Tison, C., & Shnider, S. M. (1989). Measurement of post-operative pain and narcotic administration in infants using a new clinical scoring system. *Intensive Care Medicine, 15*, S37–S39.

Beyer, J. E. (2000). Judging the effectiveness of analgesia for children and adolescents during vaso-occlusive events of sickle cell disease. *Journal of Pain and Symptom Management, 19*, 63–72.

Beyer, J. E., & Knott, C. (1998). Construct validity estimation for the African-American and Hispanic Oucher Scale. *Journal of Pediatric Nursing, 13*, 20–31.

Budd, K. S., Workman, D. E., Lemsky, C. M., & Quick, D. M. (1994). The Children's Headache Assessment Scale (CHAAS): Factor structure and psychometric properties. *Headache, 17*, 159–179.

Burns, J. W., Wiegner, S., Derleth, M., Kiselica, K., & Pawl, R. (1997). Linking symptom-specific physiological reactivity to pain severity on chronic low back pain patients: A test of mediation and moderation models. *Health Psychology, 16*, 319–326.

Calvillo, E. R., & Flaskerud, J. H. (1993). Evaluation of the pain response by Mexican American and Anglo American women and their nurses. *Journal of Advanced Nursing, 18*, 451–459.

Carlsson, J., Larsson, B., & Mark, A. (1996). Psychosocial functioning in school children with recurrent headaches. *Headache, 36*, 77–82.

Chambers, C. T., & Craig, K. D. (1998). An intrusive impact of anchors in children's faces pain scales. *Pain, 78*, 27–37.

Chambers, C. T., Craig, K. D., & Bennett, S. M. (2002). The impact of maternal behavior on children's pain experiences: An experimental analysis. *Journal of Pediatric Psychology, 27*, 293–301.

Chambers, C. T., Giesbrecht, K., Craig, K. D., Bennett, S. M., & Huntsman, E. (1999). A comparison of faces scales for the measurement of pediatric pain: Children's and parents' ratings. *Pain, 83*, 25–35.

Chambers, C. T., Reid, G. J., Craig, K. D., McGrath, P. J., & Finley, G. A. (1998). Agreement between child and parent reports of pain. *Clinical Journal of Pain, 14*, 336–342.

Coldwell, S. E., Kaakko, T., Gaertner-Makihara, A. B., Williams, T., Milgrom, P., Weinstein, P., & Ramsay, D. S. (2002). Temporal information reduces children's pain reports during a multiple-trial cold pressor procedure. *Behavior Therapy, 33*, 45–63.

Compas, B. E. (1999). Coping and responses to stress among children with recurrent abdominal pain. *Developmental and Behavioral Pediatrics, 20*, 323–324.

Covington, E. C. (2000). The biological basis of pain. *International Review of Psychiatry, 12*, 128–147.

Culbert, T., P., Kajander, R. L., & Reaney, J. B. (1996). Biofeedback with children and adolescents: Clinical observations and patient perspectives. *Developmental and Behavioral Pediatrics, 17*, 342–350.

Dahlquist, L. M. (1990). Obtaining child reports in health care settings. In A. La Greca (Ed.), *Through the eyes of the child: Obtaining self-reports from children and adolescents* (pp. 395–439). Boston: Allyn & Bacon.

Dahlquist, L. M. (1999a). Commentary on treatments that work in pediatric psychology: Procedure-related pain. *Journal of Pediatric Psychology, 24*, 153–154.

Dahlquist, L. M. (1999b). *Pediatric pain management*. New York: Kluwer.

Davis, M. C., Zautra, A. J., & Reich, J. W. (2001). Vulnerability to stress among women in chronic pain from fibromyalgia and osteoarthritis. *Annals of Behavioral Medicine, 23*, 215–226.

Field, T., Hernandez-Reif, M., Seligman, S., Krasnegor, J., Sunshine, W., Rivas-Chacon, R., et al. (1997). Juvenile rheumatoid arthritis: Benefits from massage therapy. *Journal of Pediatric Psychology, 22*, 607–617.

Flor, H., & Turk, D. C. (1989). Psychophysiology of chronic pain: Do chronic pain patients exhibit symptom-specific psychophysiological responses? *Psychological Bulletin, 105*, 215–259.

Gauthier, J. G., Ivers, H., & Carrier, S. (1996). Nonpharmacological approaches in the management of recurrent headache disorders and their comparison and combination with pharmacotherapy. *Clinical Psychology Review, 16*, 543–571.

Gil, K. M., Anthony, K. K., Carson, J. W., Redding-Lallinger, R., Daeschner, C. W., & Ware, R. E. (2001). Daily coping practice predicts treatment effects in children with sickle cell disease. *Journal of Pediatric Psychology, 26*, 163–173.

Gil, K. M., Williams, D. A., Thompson, R. J., & Kinney, T. R. (1991). Sickle cell disease in children and adolescents: The relation of child and parent pain coping strategies to adjustment. *Journal of Pediatric Psychology, 16*, 643–663.

Gil, K. M., Wilson, J. J., Edens, J. L., Workman, E., Ready, J., Sedway, J., et al. (1997). Cognitive coping skills training in children with sickle cell disease pain. *International Journal of Behavioral Medicine, 4*, 364–377.

Gragg, R. A., Rapoff, M. A., Danovsky, M. B., Lindsley, C. B., Varni, J. W., Waldron, S. A., & Bernstein, B. H. (1996). Assessing chronic musculoskeletal pain associated with rheumatic disease: Further validation of the Pediatric Pain Questionnaire. *Journal of Pediatric Psychology, 21*, 237–250.

Graumlich, S. E., Powers, S. W., Byars, K. C., Schwarber, L. A., Mitchell, M. J., & Kalinyak, K. A. (2001). Multidimensional assessment of pain in pediatric sickle cell disease. *Journal of Pediatric Psychology, 26*, 203–214.

Grunau, R. V. E., & Craig, K. D. (1987). Pain expression in neonates: Facial action and cry. *Pain, 28*, 395–410.

Hermann, C., Blanchard, E. B., & Flor, H. (1997). Biofeedback for pediatric migraine: Prediction of treatment outcome. *Journal of Consulting and Clinical Psychology, 65*, 611–616.

Hermann, C., Kim, M., & Blanchard, E. B. (1995). Behavioral and prophylactic pharmacological intervention studies of pediatric migraine: An exploratory meta-analysis. *Pain, 60*, 239–256.

Hester, N. O., Foster, R., & Kristensen, K. (1990). Measurement of pain in children: Generalizability and validity of the pain ladder and the poker chip tool. In D. C. Tyler & E. J. Krane (Eds.), *Advances in pain research and therapy* (Vol. 15, pp. 79–84). New York: Raven Press.

Holden, E. W., Deichmann, M. M., & Levy, J. D. (1999). Empirically supported treatments in pediatric psychology: Recurrent pediatric headache. *Journal of Pediatric Psychology, 24*, 91–109.

Holden, E. W., Levy, J. D., Deichmann, M. M., & Gladstein, J. (1998). Recurrent pediatric headaches: Assessment and intervention. *Developmental and Behavioral Pediatrics, 19*, 109–116.

Hunfeld, J. A. M., Perquin, C. W., Duivenvoorden, H. J., Hazebroek-Kampschreur, A. A. J. M., Passchier, J., van Suijlekom-Smit, L. W. A., & van der Wouden, J. C. (2001). Chronic pain and its impact on quality of life in adolescents and their families. *Journal of Pediatric Psychology, 26*, 145–153.

Jacobsen, P. B., & Butler, R. W. (1996). Relation of cognitive coping and catastrophizing to acute pain and analgesic use following breast cancer surgery. *Journal of Behavioral Medicine, 19*, 17–29.

Janicke, D. M., & Finney, J. W. (1999). Empirically supported treatments in pediatric psychology: Recurrent abdominal pain. *Journal of Pediatric Psychology, 24*, 115–127.

Joyce, B. A., Schade, J. G., & Keck, J. F. (1994). Reliability and validity of preverbal pain assessment tools. *Issues in Comprehensive Pediatric Nursing, 17*, 121–134.

Labbe, E. E., Delaney, D., Olson, K., & Hickman, H. (1993). Skin-temperature biofeedback training: Cognitive and developmental variables in a nonclinical child population. *Perceptual and Motor Skills, 76*, 955–962.

Langeveld, J. H., Koot, H. M., & Passchier, J. (1999). Do experienced stress and trait negative affectivity moderate the relationship between headache and quality of life in adolescents? *Journal of Pediatric Psychology, 24*, 1–11.

Larsson, B., & Carlsson, J. (1996). A school-based, nurse-administered relaxation training for children with chronic tension-type headache. *Journal of Pediatric Psychology, 21*, 603–614.

Lasch, K. E. (2000). Culture, pain, and culturally sensitive pain care. *Pain Management Nursing, 1*, 16–22.

Lavigne, J. V., Ross, C. K., Berry, S. L., Hayford, J. R., & Pachman, L. M. (1992). Evaluation of a psychological treatment package for treating pain in juvenile rheumatoid arthritis. *Arthritis Care and Research, 5*, 101–110.

Lewin, D. S., & Dahl, R. E. (1999). The importance of sleep in the management of pediatric pain. *Developmental and Behavioral Pediatrics, 20*, 244–252.

Martin, P. R. (1993). *Psychological management of chronic headaches*. New York: Guilford Press.

Martin, P. R., & Seneviratne, H. M. (1997). Effects of food deprivation and a stressor on head pain. *Health Psychology, 16*, 310–318.

Martin-Herz, S. P., Smith, M. S., & McMahon, R. J. (1999). Psychosocial variables associated with headache in junior high school students. *Journal of Pediatric Psychology, 24*, 13–23.

McGrath, P. A. (1987). An assessment of children's pain: A review of behavioral, physiological, and direct scaling techniques. *Pain, 31*, 147–176.

McGrath, P. A. (1990). *Pain in children: Nature, assessment and treatment*. New York: Guilford Press.

McGrath, P. A., deVeber, L. L., & Hearn, M. T. (1985). Multidimensional pain assessment in children. In H. L. Fields, R. Dubner, & F. Cervero (Eds.), *Advances in pain research and therapy* (Vol. 9, pp. 387–393). New York: Raven Press.

McGrath, P. A., Speechley, K. N., Siefert, C. E., Biehn, J. T., Cairney, A. E. L., Gorodzinsky, F. P., et al. (2000). A survey of children's acute, recurrent, and chronic pain: Validation of the pain experience interview. *Pain, 87*, 59–73.

McGrath, P. J., & Finley, G. A. (Eds.). (1999). *Progress in pain research and management: Vol. 13. Chronic and recurrent pain in children and adolescents*. Seattle, WA: International Association for the Study of Pain (IASP) Press.

McGrath, P. J., Johnson, G., Goodman, J., Schillinger, J., Dunn, J., & Chapman, J. (1985). CHEOPS: A behavioral scale for rating postoperative pain in children. *Advanced Pain Research Theory, 9*, 395–402.

Melzack, R., & Wall, P. D. (1965). Pain mechanisms: A new theory. *Science, 150*, 971–979.

Melzack, R., & Wall, P. D. (1982). *The challenge of pain*. New York: Basic Books.

Merkel, S. I., Gutstein, H. B., & Malviya, S. (1999). Use of transcutaneous electrical nerve stimulation in a young child with pain from open perineal lesions. *Journal of Pain and Symptom Management, 18*(5), 376–381.

Merskey, H., & Bogduk, N. (Eds.). (1994). *Classification of chronic pain, Second Edition, IASP Task Force on Taxonomy* (pp. 209–214). Retrieved February 19, 2003, from IASP website: *http://www.iasp-pain.org/terms-p.html*

Meyer, W. J., Nichols, R. J., Cortiella, J., Villarreal, C., Marvin, J. A., Blakeney, P. E., & Herndon, D. N. (1997). Acetaminophen in the management of background pain in children post-burn. *Journal of Pain and Symptom Management, 13*, 50–55.

Mikkelsson, M., Salminen, J. J., & Kautiainen, H. (1997). Non-specific musculoskeletal pain in preadolescents: Prevalence and 1–year persistence. *Pain, 73*, 29–35.

Ness, T. J., & Gebhart, G. F. (1990). Visceral pain: A review of experimental studies. *Pain, 41*, 167–234.

Olsson, G. L. (1999). Neuropathic pain in children. In P. J. McGrath & G. A Finley (Eds.), *Progress in pain research and management: Vol. 13. Chronic and recurrent pain in children and adolescents* (pp. 75–98). Seattle, WA: IASP Press.

Oster, H., & Rosenstein, L. (1993). *Baby-FACS: Analyzing facial movement in infants*. Unpublished manuscript.

Osterhaus, S. O. L., Passchier, J., Van der Helm-Hylkema, H., deJong, K. T., Orlebke, J. F., deGrauw, A. J. C., & Dekker, P. H. (1993). Effects of behavioral psychophysiological treatment of schoolchildren with migraine in a nonclinical setting: Predictors and process variables. *Journal of Pediatric Psychology, 18*, 697–715.

Palermo, T. M. (2000). Impact of recurrent and chronic pain on child and family daily functioning: A critical review of the literature. *Developmental and Behavioral Pediatrics, 21*, 58–69.

Romsing, J., Moller-Sonnergaard, J., Hertel, S., & Rasmussen, M. (1996). Postoperative pain in children: Comparison between ratings of children and nurses. *Journal of Pain and Symptom Management, 11*, 42–46.

Rosenzweig, M. R., Breedlove, S. M., & Leiman, A. L. (2002). General principles of sensory processing, touch, and pain. In *Biological Psychology: An introduction to behavioral, cognitive, and clinical neuroscience* (3rd ed., pp. 213–245). Sunderland, MA: Sinauer.

Sanders, M. R., Cleghorn, G., Shepherd, R., & Patrick, M. (1996). Predictors of clinical improvement in children with recurrent abdominal pain. *Behavioural and Cognitive Psychotherapy, 24*, 27–38.

Sanders, M. R., Rebgetz, M., Morrison, M., Bor, W., Gordon, A., Dadds, M., & Shepherd, R. (1989). Cognitive-behavioral treatment of recurrent nonspecific abdominal pain in children: An analysis of generalization, maintenance and side effects. *Journal of Consulting and Clinical Psychology, 57*, 294–300.

Sanders, M. R., Shepherd, R. W., Cleghorn, G., & Woolford, H. (1994). The treatment of recurrent abdominal pain in children: A controlled comparison of cognitive–behavioral family intervention and standard pediatric care. *Journal of Consulting and Clinical Psychology, 62*, 306–314.

Savedra, M., Tesler, M., Holzemer, W., Wilkie, D., & Ward, J. (1990). Testing a tool to assess postoperative pediatric and adolescent pain. In D. C. Tyler & E. J. Krane (Eds.), *Advances in pain research and therapy* (Vol. 15, pp. 85–94). New York: Raven Press.

Schade, J. G., Joyce, B. A., Gerkensmeyer, J., & Keck, J. F. (1996). Comparison of three preverbal scales for postoperative pain assessment in a diverse pediatric sample. *Journal of Pain and Symptom Management, 12*, 348–359.

Schechter, N. L. (1999). Management of pain in sickle cell disease. In P. J. McGrath & G. A. Finley (Eds.), *Progress in pain research and management: Vol. 13. Chronic and recurrent pain in children and adolescents* (pp. 99–114). Seattle, WA: IASP Press.

Schechter, N. L. & Zeltzer, L. K. (1999). Pediatric pain: New directions from a developmental perspective. *Developmental and Behavioral Pediatrics, 20*, 209–210.

Sethna, N. F. (1999). Pharmacotherapy in long-term pain. In P. J. McGrath & G. A. Finley (Eds.), *Progress in pain research and management: Vol. 13. Chronic and recurrent pain in children and adolescents* (pp. 243–266). Seattle, WA: IASP Press.

Staub, E., Tursky, B., & Schwartz, G. E. (1971). Self-control and predictability: Their effects on reactions to aversive stimulation. *Journal of Personality and Social Psychology, 18*, 157–162.

Stein, P. R. (1995). Indices of pain intensity: Construct validity among preschoolers. *Pediatric Nursing, 21*, 119–123.

Stevens, B. (1990). Development and testing of a pediatric pain management sheet. *Pediatric Nursing, 16*, 543–548.

Taddio, A. (1999). Effects of early pain experience: The human literature. In P. J. McGrath & G. A. Finley (Eds.), *Progress in pain research and management: Vol. 13. Chronic and recurrent pain in children and adolescents* (pp. 57–74). Seattle, WA: IASP Press.

Thomsen, A. H., Compas, B. E., Colletti, R. B., Stanger, C., Boyer, M. C., & Konik, B. S. (2002). Parent reports of coping and stress responses in children with recurrent abdominal pain. *Journal of Pediatric Psychology, 27*, 215–226.

Tyler, D. C., Tu, A., Douthit, J., & Chapman, C. R. (1993). Toward validation of pain measurement tools for children: A pilot study. *Pain, 52*, 301–309.

Unruh, A. M., & Campbell, M. A. (1999). Gender differences in children's pain experiences. In P. J. McGrath & G. A. Finley (Eds.), *Progress in pain research and management: Vol. 13. Chronic and recurrent pain in children and adolescents* (pp. 199–241). Seattle, WA: IASP Press.

van Dijk, M., de Boer, J. B., Koot, H. M., Tibboel, D., Passchier, J., & Duivenvoorden, H. J. (2000). The reliability and validity of the COMFORT scale as a postoperative pain instrument in 0- to 3-year-old infants. *Pain, 84*, 367–377.

Varni, J. W., Rapoff, M. A., Waldron, S. A., Gragg, R. A., Bernstein, B. H., & Lindsley, C. B. (1996). Effects of perceived stress on pediatric chronic pain. *Journal of Behavioral Medicine, 19*, 515–528.

Varni, J. W., Thompson, K. L., & Hanson, V. (1987). The Varni/Thompson pediatric pain questionnaire: I. Chronic musculoskeletal pain in juvenile rheumatoid arthritis. *Pain, 28,* 27–38.

Walco, G. A., Varni, J. W., & Ilowite, N. T. (1992). Cognitive–behavioral pain management in children with juvenile rheumatoid arthritis. *Pediatrics, 89,* 1075–1079.

Walker, L. (1999). The evolution of research on recurrent abdominal pain: History, assumptions, and a conceptual model. In P. J. McGrath & G. A. Finley (Eds.), *Progress in pain research and management: Vol. 13. Chronic and recurrent pain in children and adolescents* (pp. 141–172). Seattle, WA: IASP Press.

Walker, L. S., Garber, J., & Greene, J. W. (1994). Somatic complaints in pediatric patients: A prospective study of the role of negative life events, child social and academic competence, and parental somatic symptoms. *Journal of Consulting and Clinical Psychology, 62,* 1213–1221.

Walker, L. S., Garber, J., Smith, C. A., Van Slyke, D. A., & Claar, R. L. (2001). The relation of daily stressors to somatic and emotional symptoms in children with and without recurrent abdominal pain. *Journal of Consulting and Clinical Psychology, 69,* 85–91.

Walker, L. S., Smith, C. A., Garber, J., & Van Slyke, D. A. (1997). Development and validation of the Pain Response Inventory for Children (PRI). *Psychological Assessment, 9,* 392–405.

Westerling, D. (1999). Postoperative recovery evaluated with a new, tactile scale (TaS) in children undergoing ophthalmic surgery. *Pain, 83,* 297–301.

Wilkie, D. J., Huang, H. Y., Reilly, N., & Cain, K. C. (2001). Nociceptive and neuropathic pain in patients with lung cancer: A comparison of pain quality descriptors. *Journal of Pain and Symptom Management, 22,* 899–910.

Willis, W. D., & Westlund, K. N. (1997). Neuroanatomy of the pain system and of the pathways that modulate pain. *Journal of Clinical Neurophysiology, 14,* 2–31.

World Health Organization. (1990). Cancer pain relief and palliative care. Report of a WHO expert committee (WHO Technical Report Series No. 804, pp. 1–75). Geneva, Switzerland: World Health Organization.

13

Management of Pediatric Pain and Distress Due to Medical Procedures

RONALD L. BLOUNT
TIINA PIIRA
LINDSEY L. COHEN

All children, regardless of their health status, gender, race, or socioeconomic class, may experience medical procedures that can cause fear, anxiety, and pain for them and for the adults who accompany them. In addition to this immediate distress, there may be long-term physiological (e.g., Ruda, Ling, Hohmann, Peng, & Tachibana, 2000; Taddio, Katz, Ilersich, & Koren, 1997) and psychological (e.g., Pate, Blount, Cohen, & Smith, 1996) effects.

Inadequately managed pediatric pain can have detrimental consequences, which can in turn lead to higher levels of pain during future medical treatments. For example, evidence suggests that early painful stimuli might permanently alter the neuronal circuits that process pain in the spinal cord (Ruda et al., 2000). Compared with babies receiving topical anesthesia for circumcision or with those uncircumcised, babies exposed to unanesthetized circumcision shortly after birth demonstrated an accentuated behavioral response to immunization injections at 4 to 6 months of age (Taddio et al., 1997). Emotional factors, such as elevated anxiety, distress, anger, and low mood, can increase children's pain perception (McGrath, 1994) and render subsequent medical procedures and pain management more difficult (e.g., Frank, Blount, Smith, Manimala, & Martin, 1995). Diagnosable posttraumatic stress disorder (PTSD) has also been found in one-fifth of a young adult sample of survivors of childhood cancer (Hobbie et al., 2000). The intensity of cancer treatment was one of the medical variables that was most highly correlated with PTSD symptoms. Further, reports of fear and pain experienced during medical procedures in childhood are predictive of fear and pain during medical procedures and even avoidance of medical care during young adulthood

(Pate et al., 1996). Thus acute procedural pain has both short- and long-term consequences. In this chapter we review some of the medical contexts in which children experience procedural pain, factors correlated with pain perception, methods of assessment, and medical and psychological treatments for pain. We propose a theoretical position and suggest future research.

ACUTE PROCEDURAL PAIN IN PEDIATRIC PATIENTS

Procedural pain comes in many forms. For example, infants experience painful heel sticks, immunizations, and circumcision. Premature and low-birthweight infants are likely to require additional invasive procedures (e.g., venous or arterial catheter insertion, chest tube placement, tracheal intubation, lumbar puncture, and subcutaneous or intramuscular injections). It has been reported that 2 to 10 invasive procedures are conducted per day on the average newborn under 32 weeks gestational age and weighing less than 1,500 grams at birth (Johnston, Collinge, Henderson, & Anand, 1997). In light of the considerable number of medical procedures conducted with neonates, it is important for clinicians to recognize that pain responses develop as early as 23 weeks after conception (Lagercrantz & Ringstedt, 2001). Further, neonates may have an increased sensitivity to pain (Anand, 1998).

Children experience painful procedures due to disease, injury, and routine health care. For example, children with cancer endure a variety of invasive procedures, including bone marrow aspirations, lumbar punctures, finger sticks, and injections. These children and their parents have reported that pain due to medical procedures was a greater problem than pain due to cancer itself (Ljungman, Gordh, Sorensen, & Kreuger, 1999). Children with severe burns typically require daily painful wound-care procedures. Without adequate pain management, highly aversive procedures are likely to result in a cycle of pain, distress, conditioned anticipatory anxiety, and more pain (Choinière, 2001). The intensive care unit also involves frequent painful procedures. In a study of a pediatric intensive care unit in Staffordshire, United Kingdom, it was reported that 55 patients between the ages of 1 month and 12½ years endured a total of 181 invasive procedures, with a median duration of 5 minutes per procedure (Southall, Cronin, Hartmann, Harrison-Sewell, & Samuels, 1993). Of these procedures, 50 (28%) were conducted without additional analgesia or sedation.

Needle pain is the most common source of procedural pain. Healthy children typically experience two to four immunization injections on five separate occasions between 2 and 15 months of age and again prior to entering school (e.g., Blount et al., 1992; Cohen, 2002). This is problematic because younger children typically report greater pain intensity from needles than older children (e.g., Goodenough et al., 1997). More than 50% of children and adolescents who undergo venipuncture for routine blood sampling experience moderate to severe distress or pain (Fradet, McGrath, Kay, Adams, & Luke, 1990). Some children with cancer undergo as many as 300 venipunctures during the course of their treatment (Jacobsen et al., 1990). Frequent needles may also be needed for children with chronic conditions such as insulin-dependent diabetes mellitus, renal failure, and growth hormone deficiency. Although needle pain can be significantly reduced with the use of topical anesthetics such as EMLA (eutectic mixture of local anesthetics), there is considerable variability among health professionals in the use of topical anesthetics for venipuncture or venous cannulation (Schechter, Blankson, Pachter, Sullivan, & Costa, 1997), and anesthetics are rarely used for immunization procedures.

CHILDREN'S INDIVIDUAL DIFFERENCES

Age, Gender, and Experience

Younger children tend to give higher pain intensity ratings than older children for the same procedures (Goodenough et al., 1997) and exhibit more overt distress (e.g., Rudolph, Denning, & Weisz, 1995). Even though data on differences in distress associated with gender are somewhat equivocal, when differences have been found they tend to indicate greater distress in females (see Rudolph et al., 1995). Distress during prior medical procedures is predictive of distress during future procedures (e.g., Dahlquist et al., 1986; Frank et al., 1995; Rudolph et al., 1995). Although the impact of painful prior experiences is thought to be primarily mediated by cognitive/psychological mechanisms, experiencing pain in infancy may also result in physiological changes to the neuronal circuits that process pain in the spinal cord, thus influencing the way subsequent nociceptive stimuli are experienced (Ruda et al., 2000).

Temperament

Difficult temperaments may render individuals more vulnerable to experiencing higher levels of pain and somatization problems (e.g., Grunau, Whitfield, Petrie, & Fryer, 1994). In a prospective study, Grunau et al. (1994) found that high emotionality assessed at 3 years was related to somatization at 4½ years of age. Also, children with low levels of adaptability and rhythmicity responded to injections at 5 years of age with greater distress (Schechter, Bernstein, Beck, Hart, & Scherzer, 1991). In addition, children who were rated as more adaptable, less intense, and more positive in mood were more likely to be better prepared for their medical procedures (Lee & White-Traut, 1996).

Coping Style

Coping style has been classified along many dimensions (e.g., information-seeking/information-avoiding, active/passive, approach/avoidance, problem-focused/emotion-focused, primary/secondary, behavioral/cognitive). For a review of the association between children's coping and their reactions to medical stressors, see Rudolph et al. (1995). The various terminologies used have both contributed nuances to researchers' understanding and created confusion. In one of the more popular typologies, information-seeking/information-avoiding (also called approach/avoidance, sensitizer/repressor), research is consistent in showing that children who endorse an information-seeking coping style have better outcomes when confronting medical stressors (see Blount, Davis, Powers, & Roberts, 1991; Rudolph et al., 1995). A closer examination of behavioral coping strategy, as opposed to overall coping style, yields additional findings. In the period *prior to* a procedure, seeking information is a preferable behavioral strategy to information avoiding. However, *during* the medical procedure, information seeking has been shown to be a distress behavior in at least two popular inventories, the Observational Scale of Behavioral Distress (OSBD; Elliott, Jay, & Woody, 1987) and the Child–Adult Medical Procedure Interaction Scale (CAMPIS; Blount et al., 1989; Blount et al., 1997). On these scales, information seeking correlates +.30 or higher with the children's total distress (Elliott et al., 1987) and shows the same unique pattern of antecedents and consequences as other distress behaviors (Blount et al., 1991; Blount et al., 1989).

As a further example of the complexities in this area of research, the coping style of information avoiding has some features in common with the coping strategy of distraction. However, distraction typically involves a purposeful refocusing of attention from the threatening aspects of the situation to more pleasant thoughts, objects, or events, while still remaining in the situation. In contrast, information avoiding prior to and during medical procedures could be active or passive and represents a cognitive or physical avoiding of, or fleeing or escaping from, an aversive situation. Although children's use of distraction during a stressful medical procedure is inversely related to their distress (e.g., Blount et al., 1997; Blount, Powers, Cotter, Swan, & Free, 1994; Blount, Sturges, & Powers, 1990), an avoidance coping style is not generally considered to be beneficial (e.g., Blount et al., 1991).

It is an appealing concept to attempt to match a psychological intervention to the child's coping style. However, empirical studies that have evaluated this proposal have produced conflicting results (see Blount et al., 1991). In an effort to evaluate the utility of matching versus mismatching psychological intervention to children's existing coping styles, Fanurik, Zeltzer, Roberts, and Blount (1993) provided children who were classified as either "distractors" or "attenders" with sensory information or imagery-based distraction interventions. When exposed to the cold pressor task, distractors who were given the imagery intervention could tolerate the cold water 3 times longer than distractors who were given the sensory-focusing intervention or no intervention, and at least twice as long as the attenders in any condition. There were no significant differences in tolerance across conditions for the attenders. Distractors in the imagery condition had lower self-reported pain intensity ratings than those in the sensory focusing condition or attenders in the imagery condition. The inference from these findings is that if any given child walked into a clinic for an acute painful medical procedure, the preferred intervention immediately prior to and during the procedure would be distraction based. At this point it seems best to consider coping style as one of many markers for determining those children who may be at greater risk during medical procedures and those who may do reasonably well without much additional help. Currently, knowledge of a child's coping style does not inform the clinician about how to train the child.

ASSESSMENT METHODS

Assessment of children's procedural pain and distress may be accomplished by use of self-report, reports by adults who are with the children, physiological monitoring, and observational methods. Researchers generally advocate including a range of assessment instruments to attain a comprehensive evaluation (e.g., McGrath, 1990). However, it is not unusual for there to be low correlations among the measures, which complicates the issue.

Children's Self-Report and Ratings by Adults

Because pain and distress are personal and subjective events, self-report has been referred to as the 'gold standard' of assessment (Finley & McGrath, 1998). However, the use of self-report measures with young children, particularly those age 5–6 years and below, has a number of limitations. Compared with adults, young children might be less accurate in their estimates of pain; more susceptible to situational demands; less able to separate pain from other emotions, such as fear; and have fewer painful experiences with which to compare the current event.

Nevertheless, there is a significant body of literature on various pediatric self-report instruments (for a review, see Champion, Goodenough, von Baeyer, & Thomas, 1998). The most widely used child self-report scales are pictorial ones, usually with photographed or cartoon faces ranging in expression from positive (e.g., smiling) or neutral to negative (e.g., crying, frowning), and are most often used with preschool and older children. For example, the Oucher Scale (Beyer, Denyes, & Villarruel, 1992) depicts six photographs of children's faces ranging from a neutral expression to one of distress, with a corresponding number scale from 0 to 100 for older children. The scale is available in versions for Caucasian, African American, and Hispanic populations. Other scales, such as the Faces Pain Scale—Revised (FPS-R; Hicks, von Baeyer, Spafford, van Korlaar, & Goodenough, 2001), utilize six drawn faces depicting varying degrees of pain severity. In addition to these faces scales, researchers have used other pictorial measures for young children, such as pain thermometers (e.g., Bush & Holmbeck, 1987). Older children and adolescents can use measures similar to those used with adults, such as visual analogue line scales (VASs) or Likert-type ratings (Champion et al., 1998). An advantage of the VAS is that there is less clustering of scores than with categorical scales (Goodenough et al., 1997).

In addition to self-report, or when working with children who are unable to provide self-report (e.g., infants), parents and medical staff can rate children's pain, anxiety, and cooperation (e.g., Blount et al., 1997), as well as their own distress and their ability to help the child (e.g., Blount et al., 1992; Cohen, Blount, & Panopoulos, 1997).

Physiological Monitoring

There are a number of physiological measures of pediatric procedural pain. For example, studies have been conducted evaluating a number of different supraspinal processing measurement techniques (e.g., EEG, fMRI), vagal tone (e.g., Gunnar, Porter, Wolf, Rigatuso, & Larson, 1995), heart rate (e.g., Cohen, Blount, Cohen, Schaen, & Zaff, 1999), blood pressure, and cortisol (e.g., Chen, Zeltzer, Craske, & Katz, 1999). Despite the lack of response bias and apparent objectivity, no single physiological index has been shown to be ideal. In fact, many physical measures vary not just according to pain but also to emotional states, room temperature, movement, and other extraneous factors. Further, some of the measures are invasive and introduce other factors (e.g., discomfort) that might influence distress. Lastly, physiological instruments can be impractical in terms of time and cost.

Observational Measures

Another method for assessing pediatric distress is via children's overt behavior. Observational measures are generally applicable to various painful medical procedures. Among the first observational measures was the Procedural Behavior Rating Scale (PBRS; Katz, Kellerman, & Siegel, 1980). With the PBRS, the occurrence or nonoccurrence of 11 behaviors indicative of behavioral distress were recorded during the anticipatory, encounter, and recovery phases of medical procedures. Based in part on the PBRS, the Observational Scale of Behavioral Distress (OSBD) was developed (Elliott et al., 1987). With the OSBD, distress behaviors are coded as occurring or not occurring during 15-second intervals. Distress behaviors are weighted for severity on a 1.0 to 4.0 scale. Weighted scores are added to provide phase or whole session distress scores. The OSBD has been reliably scored and widely used.

In addition to child distress, other important variables are children's coping behaviors and the behaviors of parents and medical staff that promote children's coping, and distress (for reviews, see Blount, Bunke, & Zaff, 2000a, 2000b; Varni, Blount, Waldron, & Smith,

1995). To address this need, the Child–Adult Medical Procedure Interaction Scale (CAMPIS; Blount et al., 1989) was developed and has been applied to various acute medical procedures. The CAMPIS includes 35 child and adult behaviors. These 35 codes were later grouped into the 6-code CAMPIS-R (Blount et al., 1990; Blount et al., 1997) based on conceptual and empirical factors. The CAMPIS-R includes adults' coping promoting, distress promoting, and neutral behaviors and children's coping, distress, and neutral behaviors. Reliability and validity are high for both the CAMPIS and CAMPIS-R. However, as with most direct observation scales, their use can be labor intensive. To help address this practical issue, the CAMPIS-Short Form was developed (CAMPIS-SF; Blount, Bunke, Cohen, & Forbes, 2001). It is used to monitor the same important categories as the CAMPIS-R and it requires much less time, but it gives less detailed data. Initial reliability and validity data are promising (Blount et al., 2001).

Observational scales are critical for a thorough evaluation of infants' procedural distress. The Modified Behavioral Pain Scale (MBPS; Taddio, Nulman, Goldbach, & Ipp, 1994) is a rating scale of facial expression, cry, and body movement indicators of infant pain. Using an alternative approach, the Neonatal Facial Coding System (NFCS; Grunau & Craig, 1987) examines 10 facial movements indicative of infant pain expression (e.g., eyes squeezed, taut cupped tongue). Crying is probably the most recognized infant distress reaction and has been examined in terms of latency, duration, intensity, and frequency of cry (Gunnar et al., 1995). The limitations of an examination of crying are that not all infants cry when distressed and that it is difficult to distinguish among different reasons for crying (e.g., hunger, anger, pain).

Summary and Recommendations for Assessment

The choice of specific measures should be determined by the child's developmental level, the setting, and whether assessment is for research or clinical purposes. Self-report and reports by adults have the advantages of being easily collected and of providing unique perspectives on children's reactions to painful procedures. Self-report is a more valid method for older children. Physiological monitoring offers the possibility of objective assessment, but the measures may be influenced by factors other than pain, and they can be invasive and expensive.

Observational methods offer a wealth of information about children's distress and coping and about the behaviors of adults in the treatment room. However, comprehensive observational scales can be time-consuming. To help extend their utility, rating scales, such as the CAMPIS-SF (Blount et al., 2001), or use of particular individual coping and coping-promoting codes from the CAMPIS (Blount et al., 1997) are recommended. Children's coping behaviors and adults' coping-promoting behaviors have a direct impact on children's distress and are too important for researchers and clinicians to ignore.

TREATMENTS TO REDUCE PAIN AND DISTRESS

Procedural pain has been treated using medical, psychological, and combined interventions. Medical interventions include pharmacological agents and improvements in medical equipment and procedures. With less pain, children should be less likely to develop conditioned anticipatory anxiety for subsequent procedures. Psychological interventions also can reduce fear and anxiety prior to and during procedures and distress and pain during procedures, and can increase children's and parents' sense of mastery over challenging medical procedures.

Medical Approaches

Pharmacological interventions for pediatric pain include anti-inflammatory and antipyretic drugs such as aspirin and acetaminophen; opiate analgesics such as morphine and codeine; psychotropic drugs such as tranquilizers, antidepressants, and psychostimulants; nitrous oxide; midazolam (Versed); and combinations of medications (Anand & McGrath, 1993). Despite the efficacy of these approaches for children's surgery, chronic pain, and highly invasive procedures (e.g., bone marrow aspiration), they would not be recommended for brief outpatient procedures such as venipuncture (McGrath, 1991). Pharmacological interventions for more common procedures such as immunizations and venipuncture include lidocaine, benzocaine, ketocaine, and mixtures of anesthetics. However, these have not been widely accepted due to inadequate pain reduction, the requirement of a painful needle injection to anesthetize the skin, dermal irritation, or toxicity (Hallén, Carlsson, & Uppfeldt, 1985). The topical anesthetic EMLA, available in cream or patch form, inhibits ionic fluxes that initiate and conduct pain impulses. EMLA requires approximately 1 hour to provide sufficient epidermal and dermal anesthesia.

To help reduce the sensory aspects of pain, many pediatric hospitals have taken initiatives to ensure that children receive fewer injections, such as through the use of a central line. There are also less painful methods of injection, such as the use of automatic needle insertion (Main, Jorgensen, Hertel, Jensen, & Jakobsen, 1995), microfabricated microneedles (Kaushik et al., 2001), and needle-free injectors (Murray et al., 2000). Compared with needle injections, needle-free injectors have resulted in better ratings for convenience, nervousness, pain, and overall performance (e.g., Murray et al., 2000). However, needle-free injectors are more typically used for children who require repeated injections, such as children with diabetes or growth hormone problems. Despite these medical advancements, acute procedures remain a source of considerable anxiety, pain, and distress for many children.

Cognitive-Behavioral Approaches

Psychological approaches to managing children's procedural pain and distress are divided into *preparation*, which occurs in advance of a medical procedure, and *treatment*, which has focused on the phases immediately prior to, during, and after a medical procedure. Preparation has usually focused on more complex, multicomponent stressors, such as hospitalization. In contrast, treatment research has focused on more discrete procedures, such as injections. Preparation and treatment programs can be combined, although that is rare.

Preparation

Preparation of children prior to a painful procedure may prevent or minimize potential problems. Preparation programs typically incorporate one or more of three main approaches: information provision, modeling, and teaching coping strategies. The timing of preparation appears to be critical. One study found that children older than 6 years were least anxious if they received preparatory information 5 or more days prior to surgery and most anxious if prepared 1 day prior to the surgery (Kain, Mayes, & Caramico, 1996). Similarly, children 7 years or older who watched a modeling film 1 week prior to hospitalization displayed fewer posthospital behavioral problems than those who viewed the film during hospital admission (Melamed, Meyer, Gee, & Soule, 1976).

The content of information provided is also central to the efficacy of a preparatory intervention. In a meta-analytic review of the child and adult pain coping literature, Suls and Wan (1989) concluded that preparatory information is most effective if it includes sensory information, which describes the sensations a patient is likely to experience, as well as procedural information, which emphasizes the sequence of medical events and procedures. The same conclusion was also reached in a recent study in which parents provided information to their children prior to the children undergoing ear piercing (Spafford, von Baeyer, & Hicks, 2002). Information promotes the development of accurate expectations that may help the patient focus on specific sensations and experiences in concrete, nonemotional ways and that allow them to use more adaptive coping strategies. This is especially important for children who have negatively distorted expectations prior to the medical procedures (Cohen et al., 2001). Habituation may also be facilitated through informational exposure.

Modeling provides an opportunity to observe a peer, usually by way of a video, using successful coping behaviors during a medical procedure while demonstrating successful coping behaviors. The effectiveness of film modeling seems to be enhanced when the model is of a similar age and race to the patient (Melamed et al., 1976).

The effectiveness of preparation programs is supported by a meta-analysis (Vernon & Thompson, 1993) indicating that for the stressor of hospitalization, beneficial effects seem to endure for at least 1 month. Further, children 7 years or older benefited more from preparation than younger children. Perhaps most instructive, stress-point preparation was found to be superior to modeling or information alone. Stress-point procedures provide individualized intervention prior to or after typical hospital stressors (e.g., admission, blood drawing, and return from surgery). Training sessions are tailored to the demands of the stressor. Stress-point interventions contrast to the usual single preparation session for multiple hospital stressors.

O'Byrne, Peterson, and Saldana (1997) surveyed hospitals in the United States and found that 75% had increased their use of filmed modeling and coping skills instruction during the last two decades. Medical professionals at the hospitals rated different preparation programs in terms of their perceived effectiveness during acute painful procedures. Coping skills training was ranked most effective, followed by relaxation training or videotape modeling, puppet shows, play therapy, narrative preparation, printed materials, and tours (stress-point intervention was not included in the survey). However, coping skills training and relaxation were used by about 50% of the hospitals, whereas narrative presentation, play therapy, tours, and printed materials were used in up to 89% of hospitals. Therefore, overall, the less expensive and less effective preparation programs were used most often. Evaluation of effectiveness of the preparation programs was seldom conducted.

Treatment

In a review of the literature, Powers (1999) determined that cognitive-behavioral therapy is a well-established and "empirically supported treatment" for acute procedural pain in children and adolescents. Some of the particular cognitive-behavioral approaches that have been utilized include relaxation (e.g., Jay, Elliott, Woody, & Siegel, 1991), desensitization and *in vivo* exposure (e.g., Blount et al., 1994), breathing exercises or using a distracting party blower (e.g., Blount et al., 1994; Kazak et al., 1996), counting (e.g., Powers, Blount, Bachanas, Cotter, & Swan, 1993), behavioral rehearsal (e.g., Blount et al., 1992; Powers et al., 1993), reinforcement (e.g., Jay, Elliott, Katz, & Siegel, 1987), modeling (e.g., Jay et al., 1987), imagery (e.g., Jay et al., 1987), distraction (e.g., Cohen et al., 1997), making coping statements, and parental and/or nurse coaching of the child to use coping behaviors (e.g., Cohen et al., 1997; Manimala, Blount, & Cohen, 2000). All of the approaches noted have been found to be useful. However, it should be noted that there are considerable differences in the specific procedures used in these programs, even though they could all be classified as cognitive behavioral. For detailed reviews of the treatment programs, see Powers (1999), Dahlquist (1999), and Blount et al. (2000a, 2000b). It should also be noted that nonpharmacological treatments for procedural distress with infants have begun to emerge. For example, there is some support for infant pain reduction using sucrose (Stevens, Taddio, Ohlsson, & Einarson, 1997), pacifiers (Field, 1999), rocking (Campos, 1994), and distraction (Cohen, 2002).

Common ingredients in the treatment interventions include the use of various methods to promote distraction and the use of other specific coping behaviors. Distraction involves refocusing attention *from* threatening, anxiety-provoking aspects of medical treatments *to* nonthreatening, and ideally pleasant and engaging, objects or situations. The threatening stimuli include the sights, smells, and sounds accompanying and predicting the medical procedure and the children's own sensations of fear, distress, and pain. Cognitive refocusing should be seen as engaging in behaviors that are incompatible with anxiety, distress, and pain. It is generally better to use observable distracting activities in order to ensure that the child is engaging in the activity, rather than utilizing unobservable coping behaviors (e.g., telling them to "relax"). Focusing concentration away from the noxious and toward positive stimuli may modify cognitive pain perceptions by altering nociceptive responses and triggering an internal pain-suppressing system (McGrath, 1991). It should be noted that even distraction-based programs include some information about the upcoming medical procedure, particularly if behavioral rehearsal is used. As with preparation programs, information and rehearsal may facilitate habituation of distress.

Numerous other psychological interventions for the management of children's pain exist, some of which have shown beneficial results in some studies. However, these approaches have insufficient empirical support or otherwise do not meet criteria (e.g., no manual or explicit procedure section) to be classified as an empirically supported treatment (Powers, 1999). For example, there are no child-hypnosis interventions that currently qualify as well-established, efficacious interventions (Milling & Constantino, 2000), even though this approach has been used to treat acute procedural pain for a number of years (Varni et al., 1995).

Only a few studies have compared or combined pharmacological and cognitive-behavioral interventions. In a comparison between EMLA and music distraction (Arts et al., 1994), EMLA was found to be superior to the music distraction for the 4- to 6-year-old children, but not for the 7- to 11- or the 12- to 16-year-olds. It is possible that music distraction was not sufficiently engaging of the younger children's attention. Later, Cohen et al. (1999) compared EMLA to a more potent, nurse-prompted, child-selected videotaped cartoon distraction for reducing distress in fourth-grade African American males undergoing a series of three immunization injections. Nurses prompted the children to attend to the videotape at critical procedural events, such as just prior to the injection, and at signs of distress. Nurse-prompted distraction resulted in better child coping and less behavioral distress than either EMLA or standard medical care. Children preferred both EMLA and the cartoon distraction to standard care. The distraction intervention was more cost-effective than EMLA. Further, in a 6-month follow-up (Cohen et al., 2001), children recalled no differences in pain relief between EMLA and distraction, and both were superior to standard medical care. For anxiety relief, EMLA was recalled to be superior to distraction, which was remembered to be superior to standard care.

Susan Jay and her colleagues compared their cognitive-behavioral therapy (CBT) treatment package to pharmacological alternatives (e.g., Jay et al., 1987). This package included filmed modeling, instruction, behavioral rehearsal, emotive imagery, and reinforcement for lying still. CBT treatment was found to be superior to diazepam (Valium) for reducing distress, pain, and pulse rates for children undergoing bone marrow aspirations (BMAs; Jay et al., 1987). Adding diazepam to CBT did not improve children's responses during BMAs beyond CBT alone (Jay et al., 1991). This group then compared CBT with general anesthesia (halothane delivered using a face mask). They found less distress for the anesthesia condition during the painful phase but fewer negative adjustment symptoms in the 24 hours following the BMA for CBT. There were no differences in the children's preferences for the two treatments (Jay, Elliott, Fitzgibbons, Woody, & Siegel, 1995). As was found by Cohen et al. (1999), CBT was more cost-effective than general anesthesia. Kazak et al. (1996) compared conscious sedation using midazolam and morphine with conscious sedation plus distraction during BMAs and lumbar punctures (LPs). Conscious sedation plus distraction resulted in less child distress than conscious sedation alone.

There are several new approaches for reducing procedural distress, including the modification of children's memories of past distress and coping, virtual reality interventions, and the use of interactive CDs. Chen et al. (1999) intervened with 3- to 18-year-old children with cancer shortly following one LP and again just prior to the next LP. The therapist encouraged reevaluations and remembering of greater efficacy of their efforts to cope and reevaluation of their distress during the procedure. Prior to the next LP, the children were given a fluorescent card depicting a child thinking about his or her LP and listing coping and other memories. Results indicated that during the posttreatment LP, only parental report of children's expected pain was lower for the intervention versus the control group. Other data were equivocal or not significant. However, during the third LP, children in the memory condition reported less pain, had lower cortisol levels, and displayed less observable distress. Results were interpreted in terms of unconditioned stimulus (US) reevaluation theory (Davey, 1992), in which making memory for the painful stimulus (the US) less aversive leads to decreases in unconditioned (UR) and conditioned (CR) responses. Memory manipulation offers a promising new approach, and replication in other laboratories is needed.

New technological approaches to this area have also been developed. Virtual–reality based distraction proved beneficial during range of motion exercises for two adolescents who had suffered burns (e.g., Hoffman, Patterson, Carrougher, & Sharar, 2001). The STARBRIGHT Foundation (www.starbright.org), chaired by Steven Speilberg and General Norman Schwarzkopf, have produced virtual reality, interactive CD-ROM, and videotapes intended to reduce anxiety and pain in children undergoing medical treatments. As indicated at the Web site, the initial results evaluating the STARBRIGHT techniques are encouraging.

Role of Parents and Nurses during Painful Procedures

Studies evaluating the impact of parental presence or absence during children's medical procedures have yielded equivocal results (see Blount et al., 1991). The characteristics and behaviors of parents with the child in the treatment room have also been considered. Children accompanied by anxious parents displayed more distress than those with less anxious parents (e.g., Jacobsen et al., 1990). Parent behavior in the treatment room accounts for 53%

of the variance in child distress behavior (Frank et al., 1995). Parent behaviors likely to facilitate better child coping include nonprocedural talk, humor, and other distraction methods (such as facilitating play with toys, bubble blowing, party blowers, and watching of cartoons), commands to engage in coping, and encouraging deep-breathing techniques (e.g., Blount et al., 1992; Cohen et al., 1997; Manimala et al., 2000).

In contrast, parental behaviors likely to promote child distress include making reassuring or empathetic statements, apologizing, criticizing, bargaining with the child, providing explanations during the procedure, giving the child control over when to start the procedure, catastrophizing, and becoming agitated (e.g., Blount et al., 1989; Manimala et al., 2000; Piira & von Baeyer, 2001). Maternal reassurance is also associated with higher distress in infants undergoing immunization (Sweet & McGrath, 1998). Deleterious effects of parental reassurance have been confirmed in experimental treatment studies of children undergoing immunizations (Manimala et al., 2000) and the analogue cold pressor task (Chambers, Craig, & Bennett, 2002), but not in another study examining injections (Gonzalez, Routh, & Armstrong, 1993). We speculate that reassurance prompts children to focus on their own pain and fear and on the threatening medical procedure, leading to heightened distress. Similar adult behaviors, including apologizing and making empathic comments, that focus the child's attention on his or her own distress and how difficult the procedure is, could be expected to have a similar distress-producing effect. Nurses' and parents' behaviors have been found to have similar effects on children's coping and distress (e.g., Blount et al., 1992; Blount et al., 1997; Cohen et al., 1997).

In the social environment of the medical treatment room, parents and nurses cue each other about how to interact with each other and with the child (Blount et al., 1989, 1992). This finding was used to develop a cost-effective training program in which the nurse modeled coping-promoting behaviors and the untrained mother also engaged in high rates of coping-promoting behaviors, resulting in less child distress (Cohen et al., 1997). Parents who have been trained in the use of coping promoting behaviors report that they experience less distress than they had during their child's previous injections, whereas untrained parents reported experiencing more distress than during previous injections (Blount et al., 1992). Nurse and parent distress are both lower when the adults effectively coach the child to use coping behaviors, leading to less child distress (Blount et al., 1997; Cohen et al., 1997). Our experience is that the best way to reduce the distress of parents and medical staff during children's medical procedures is to equip them with better ways to help the children (e.g., Powers et al., 1993).

Summary of Treatment Efficacy and Recommendations for Clinical Practice

Both medical and cognitive-behavioral approaches can help reduce children's fear, anxiety, distress, and pain. The use of smaller needles, less frequent medical procedures, conscious sedation, and topical anesthesia are some of the medical alternatives to reduce procedural pain. Preparation programs that use information provision, modeling, stress-point procedures, and training children in use of coping skills can be conducted prior to medical procedures. Regarding treatment, cognitive-behavioral treatment programs are empirically supported treatments for the reduction of acute procedural anxiety, pain, and distress (Powers, 1999). We further emphasize the key importance of high levels of distraction, that is, refocusing of the child's attention from threatening to pleasant stimuli, in order to produce therapeutic benefit during the medical procedure (e.g., Varni et al., 1995). Information provision should predominate during preparation, whereas distraction should predominate just before and during the medical procedure. The method of distraction should be salient and appealing to the child and should involve observable behavior. Training adults to prompt children to use coping behaviors should be included in treatment programs. Children, parents, and medical staff working together to ensure that children cope should be a feature of most therapeutic interventions. Combinations of cognitive-behavioral and medical approaches should be used whenever possible. The interventions described in this chapter and the phase-specific recommendations for their use are summarized in Table 13.1. We believe this prescriptive model reflects the literature and that it can be used to help guide clinical and research activities.

Cost-effectiveness is an additional important consideration in medical care. Cost factors include (1) the time and personnel required to promote the effective use of coping and coping-promoting behaviors; (2) costs of medications and other medical approaches used to reduce pain; (3) the length of medical stay and care associated with different treatments; and (4) other health-related dependent variables. Additional clinically relevant dependent variables are consumer satisfaction and preference for particular pain reduction approaches. Documentation of cost-effectiveness and consumer preference and satisfaction (e.g., Cohen et al., 1997, 1999, 2001; Jay et al., 1987) could go far toward the justification, enhancement, and dissemination of pain management services, as well as toward helping to ensure reimbursement of such services.

THEORETICAL FRAMEWORK

Few well-developed theories have been applied to the area of acute pediatric pain. For this reason, even though it is necessarily brief, we present a behavior analytic conceptualization as being representative of the empirical literature. We believe it could have heuristic value for guiding future research and clinical work in this area. The proposed framework is based on a variation of O. H. Mower's two-factor theory of anxiety disorders (Mower, 1939). The two factors, classical conditioning and negative reinforcement, help explain the acquisition, maintenance, and generalization of children's fear, pain, distress, and avoidance during medical procedures, as well as some of the mechanisms of therapeutic effect. In this framework, the unconditioned stimulus (US), the painful medical procedure, elicits the unconditioned response (UR), namely the pain, distress, and associated emotional and physical arousal. The conditioned stimulus (CS) also comes to elicit distress through close temporal pairing with the US, through imagining or being told of the pain of the procedure, or through observing another person experiencing high levels of procedural distress. Thus the circumstances, people, places, sights, sounds, smells, the child's arousal, and other stimuli associated with the painful procedure may become CSs.

The CS comes to predict the US and to take on some of the power of the US, thereby eliciting the conditioned response (CR). The CR is the anticipatory distress, fear, and anxiety prior to the medical procedure. Preprocedural distress correlates +.86 with distress and pain during the medical treatment, and higher levels seem to facilitate the experience of more procedural distress (Blount et al., 1990). Once classical conditioning has taken place, generalization can occur. In practical terms, this means that a child may experience anxiety going to the school health clinic because it has features in common with the clinic at which the

TABLE 13.1. Prescriptive Model of Medical and Coping Interventions by Phase of Medical Procedure

	Phase 1	Phase 2	Phase 3	Phase 4	Phase 5	Phase 6	Phase 7
Temporal proximity to procedure	Scheduling of the procedure	Approach of the procedure	Preprocedure (immediately before procedure)	Procedure (during the procedure)	Postprocedure (immediately after the procedure)	Completion (hours to longer after the procedure)	Next procedure scheduled
Child experiences	Recollection of distant past experiences	Preparation for upcoming event	Anticipation of imminent event	Encounter with the stimulus and stress	Recovery from pain and distress	Recollection of procedure and resumption of life	Remembering, and preparing for the future
			Goals and interventions for each phase				
Information provision and distraction	• Provide information to child in a calm, nonemotional manner. Answer questions and instill confidence.	• Offer age appropriate information about the procedures and sensations to expect. Provide opportunities to ask questions.	• Decrease both information provision and the child's focus on the upcoming procedure. • Increase distraction.	• Provide distraction and minimal information. Distraction is greatest and information provision lowest in this phase.	• Focus child's attention on positive coping efforts and continue distraction. • Allow child time to recover. Be sensitive to child's lead.	• Prompt memory encoding of successful coping and nonexaggerated distress. • Minimize focus on upcoming procedures, if any.	• Avoid focusing excessively on upcoming event until nearer to the time.
Coping	• Age, temperament and coping style may influence current coping. • Consider prior effective or ineffective coping and child's expectations. • Provide adequate social support for child and parents.	• Train child and adults in specific coping and coping-promoting behaviors and when to use them. • Anxiety reduction via exposure to aspects of the stressor. • Increase sense of mastery and hope.	• Parents/staff prompt child's use of coping strategies. • Use problem-focused, not emotion-focused coping. • Supportive, skilled parents and staff instill confidence.	• Coach/prompt child to use coping behaviors and praise attempts. • Minimize avoidance behaviors. • Low distress/pain should lead to less classical conditioning.	• Focus on successful coping and instill sense of achievement. • Encourage resumption of normal pleasant conversation and activities as appropriate.	• Engender a sense of mastery and hope in the face of challenge. • Begin resumption of adaptive, normal life activities. • Encourage general healthy adjustment.	• Practice and refine coping skills (only as needed) in light of previous experiences. • Encourage child's sense of confidence.
Medical factors	• Consider the child's previous experiences with medical procedures. • Consider the child's physical condition.		• Consider using medications for anesthesia and to lower arousal. • Use less threatening instruments.	• Use less painful medical equipment and topical anesthesia. • Keep unexpected events to a minimum.	• Use pain-reducing medications as needed.		

child received painful treatments. Children and adults tend to avoid upcoming aversive situations or try to escape once in them. Cognitive and motoric avoidance bring about an immediate and short-term reduction of fear, pain, and distress. Because of this reduction, the avoidant behaviors are negatively reinforced, as are the fears and anxieties that preceded them. For the child who may be trapped in this cycle, avoidance and escape result in short-term gain but long-term pain and distress.

Pharmacological interventions and technical improvements, such as the use of EMLA and needle-free injectors, may help prevent or attenuate this cycle by reducing the physical sensation of pain, thus reducing the potency of the US. To the extent this is accomplished, classical conditioning, as well as avoidance and escape, would be less likely. It should be noted that this is the main way in which improved medical interventions can assist the child. Psychological approaches are more far reaching and include alternatives for assisting the child before, during, and after the procedure. Preparation programs, as well as behavioral rehearsal of coping skills, allows for exposure to the CS without the US/UR following. Thus extinction of avoidant and other distress behaviors may occur. In our clinical research we have seen children flinch repeatedly, but gradually less often, when touched on their backs during coping skills rehearsal under simulated conditions prior to LPs (e.g., Blount et al., 1994).

Coping skills are incompatible behaviors with the distress children might otherwise experience prior to and during medical treatments. Like any behavioral skills, they require effort to train and to prompt their occurrence. Techniques that promote generalization, such as parents' and nurses' prompts, cue the desired behaviors when children move from training situations to the actual medical procedures. Equipped with effective coping skills, the child who previously was overwhelmed may develop a sense of mastery, or at least knowledge that he or she will survive, during the medical procedure. This sense of mastery can generalize to other life challenges as well. After the procedures the child can be helped to consolidate memories of what worked and what did not which can help to ensure that pain and distress are not encoded in greater proportion than was experienced (Chen et al., 1999). The memory manipulation approach has also been conceptualized in terms of unconditioned stimulus reevaluation theory (Davey, 1992) and is harmonious with the theoretical framework being presented. Following from the theory we are presenting, each of the therapeutic approaches we have described contribute to the US becoming less potent due to technological, pharmacological, or cognitive coping interventions; to the CSs either failing to develop or decreasing in potency; and to the CRs failing to develop or diminishing. In this situation, avoidance and escape are unnecessary. Further, the child develops an accurate sense of mastery by successfully confronting challenging medical situations.

The Proximal–Distal Model of Children's Coping and Distress During Painful Medical Procedures is described elsewhere (Blount, Bunke, & Zaff, 2000a, 2000b; Varni et al., 1995). In this model, the distal variables tend to be trait-like, temporally removed from the medical procedure, and assessed by paper-and-pencil measures, and they may serve as markers for which children are more likely to show distress. Examples include temperament, coping style, age, gender, history of distress, and the child's psychological characteristics. Distal variables are often difficult or impossible to modify. In contrast, proximal variables occur close in time to the medical procedure, tend to be behavioral as opposed to trait-like, are often assessed by observation of the child and others in the medical setting, and are more easily modified. The proximal variables are the ones that are most likely to be functional, in that they may develop into CSs and also serve as the antecedents and consequences for children's coping and distress.

FUTURE DIRECTIONS

Much of the correlational research in this area has examined the associations among distal variables of the Proximal–Distal model and children's distress and coping (Blount et al., 2000a, 2000b; Varni et al., 1995). Although useful for the development of theories, years of research on coping style and other distal, trait-like variables have thus far provided little in the way of direct treatment implications for reducing child distress. In contrast, correlational studies of proximal variables have yielded findings that have directly informed both theory and the design of effective treatment interventions. Future research that emphasizes modifiable proximal variables—such as the behaviors of adults; children's knowledge, thoughts, memories, and coping behaviors; and less painful and frightening medical technology and procedures—has the greatest potential to reduce the suffering and improve the lives of those we serve.

Cost-effectiveness and consumer satisfaction should also be features of future research in this area. In this regard, we note that there is a push in this and other areas of pediatric psychology for easier-to-use, economical, and briefer assessment instruments and interventions. This is largely due to the financial constraints in medical settings. However, in responding to this issue, effectiveness is primary and should not be sacrificed for ease and economy, or both science and clinical work will eventually suffer. The scientist/practitioner model is the guiding principle, with good clinical practice flowing from sound research, and, in turn, clinical practice informing the science so that the research that is conducted is clinically meaningful (Blount et al., 2000a, 2000b).

Although much progress has been made in this area over the past couple of decades, many intriguing questions remain. Among these issues are determining the effective components of treatment packages; determining other long-term effects of pain, as well as additional benefits of effective coping; promoting cross-situational generalization of the use of effective coping behaviors; further study of the effect of parent and staff behaviors on infants and other pediatric groups during various medical procedures; research on the dissemination of effective treatments; matching treatment to particular child and/or stressor characteristics; and further refinement and development of theoretical models to help guide future clinical research.

REFERENCES

Anand, K. J. (1998). Clinical importance of pain and stress in preterm neonates. *Biology of the Neonate, 73,* 1–9.

Anand, K. J., & McGrath, P. J. (1993). *Pain in neonates.* Amsterdam: Elsevier.

Arts, S. E., Abu-Saad, H. H., Champion, G. D., Crawford, M. R., Fisher, R. J., Juniper, K. H., et al. (1994). Age-related response to lidocaine-prilocaine (EMLA) emulsion and effect of music distraction on the pain of intravenous cannulation. *Pediatrics, 93,* 797–801.

Beyer, J. E., Denyes, M. J., & Villarruel, A. M. (1992). The creation, validation, and continuing development of the Oucher: A measure of pain intensity in children. *Journal of Pediatric Nursing, 7,* 335–346.

Blount, R. L., Bachanas, P .J., Powers, S. W., Cotter, M., Franklin, A., Chaplin, W., et al. (1992). Training children to cope and parents to coach them during routine immunizations: Effects on child, parent and staff behaviors. *Behavior Therapy, 23,* 689–705.

Blount, R. L., Bunke, V. L., Cohen, L. L., & Forbes, C. J. (2001). The Child–Adult Medical Procedure Interaction Scale—Short Form (CAMPIS-SF): Validation of a rating scale for children's and adults' behaviors during painful medical procedures. *Journal of Pain and Symptom Management, 22,* 591–599.

Blount, R. L., Bunke, V. L., & Zaff, J. F. (2000a). The integration of basic research, treatment research, and clinical practice in pediatric psychology. In D. Drotar (Ed.), *Handbook of research in pediatric and child clinical psychology: Practical strategies and methods* (pp. 491–510). New York: Kluwer Academic/Plenum.

Blount, R. L., Bunke, V. L., & Zaff, J. F. (2000b). Bridging the gap between explicative and treatment research: A model and practical implications. *Journal of Clinical Psychology in Medical Settings, 7,* 79–90.

Blount, R. L., Cohen, L. L., Frank, N. C., Bachanas, P. J., Smith, A. J., Manimala, M. R., et al. (1997). The Child–Adult Medical Procedure Interaction Scale—Revised: An assessment of validity. *Journal of Pediatric Psychology, 22,* 73–88.

Blount, R. L., Corbin, S. M., Sturges, J. W., Wolfe, V. V., Prater, J. M., & James, L. D. (1989). The relationship between adults' behavior and child coping and distress during BMA/LP procedures: A sequential analysis. *Behavior Therapy, 20,* 585–601.

Blount, R. L., Davis, N., Powers, S. W., & Roberts, M. C. (1991). The influence of environmental factors and coping style on children's coping and distress. *Clinical Psychology Review, 11,* 93–116.

Blount, R. L., Powers, S. W., Cotter, M. W., Swan S. C., & Free, K. (1994). Making the system work: Training pediatric oncology patients to cope and their parents to coach them during BMA/LP procedures. *Behavior Modification, 18,* 6–31.

Blount, R. L., Sturges, J. W., & Powers, S. W. (1990). Analysis of child and adult behavioral variations by phase of medical procedure. *Behavior Therapy, 21,* 33–48.

Bush, J. P., & Holmbeck, G. N. (1987). Children's attitudes about health care: Initial development of a questionnaire. *Journal of Pediatric Psychology, 12,* 429–443.

Campos, R. G. (1994). Rocking and pacificiers: Two comforting interventions for heel stick pain. *Research in Nursing and Health, 17,* 321–331.

Chambers, C. T., Craig, K. D., & Bennett, S. M. (2002). The impact of maternal behavior on children's pain experiences: An experimental analysis. *Journal of Pediatric Psychology, 3,* 293–301.

Champion, G. D., Goodenough, B., von Baeyer, C. L., & Thomas, W. (1998). Measurement of pain by self-report. In G. A. Finley & P. J. McGrath (Eds.), *Progress in pain research and management: Vol. 10. Measurement of pain in infants and children* (pp. 123–160). Seattle, WA: IASP Press.

Chen, E., Zeltzer, L. K., Craske, M. G., & Katz, E. R. (1999). Alternation of memory in the reduction of children's distress during repeated aversive medical procedures. *Journal of Consulting and Clinical Psychology, 67,* 481–490.

Choinière, M. (2001). Burn pain: A unique challenge. *Pain: Clinical Updates, 7,* 1–4.

Cohen, L. L. (2002). Reducing infant immunization distress through distraction. *Health Psychology, 21,* 207–211.

Cohen, L. L., Blount, R. L., Cohen, R. J., McClellan, C. B., Bernard, R. S., & Ball, C. M. (2001). Children's expectations and memories of acute distress: The short and long-term efficacy of pain management interventions. *Journal of Pediatric Psychology, 26,* 367–374.

Cohen, L. L., Blount, R. L., Cohen, R. J., Schaen, E. R., & Zaff, J. (1999). Comparative study of distraction versus topical anesthesia for pediatric pain management during immunizations. *Health Psychology, 18,* 591–598.

Cohen, L. L., Blount, R. L., & Panopoulos, G. (1997). Nurse coaching and cartoon distraction: An effective and practical intervention to reduce child, parent, and nurse distress during immunizations. *Journal of Pediatric Psychology, 22,* 355–370.

Dahlquist, L. M. (1999). *Pediatric pain management.* New York: Kluwer Academic / Plenum.

Dahlquist, L. M., Gil, K., Armstrong, D., DeLawyer, D., Greene, P., & Wouri, D. (1986). Preparing children for medical examinations: The importance of previous medical experience. *Health Psychology, 5,* 249–259.

Davey, G. (1992). Classical conditioning and the acquisition of human fears and phobias: A review and synthesis of the literature. *Advances in Behaviour Research and Therapy, 14,* 29–66.

Elliott, C. H., Jay, S. M., & Woody, P. (1987). An observational scale for measuring children's distress during medical procedures. *Journal of Pediatric Psychology, 12,* 543–551.

Fanurik, D., Zeltzer, L. K., Roberts, M. C., & Blount, R. L. (1993). The relationship between children's coping styles and psychological interventions for cold pressor pain. *Pain, 53,* 213–222.

Field, T. (1999). Sucking and massage therapy reduce stress during infancy. In M. Lewis & D. Ramsay (Eds.), *Soothing and stress* (pp. 157–169). Mahway, NJ: Erlbaum.

Finley, G. A., & McGrath, P. J. (1998). The roles of measurement in pain management and research. In G. A. Finley & P. J. McGrath (Eds.), *Progress in pain research and management: Vol. 10. Measurement of pain in infants and children* (pp. 1–4). Seattle, WA: IASP.

Fradet, C., McGrath, P. J., Kay, J., Adams, S., & Luke, B. (1990). A prospective survey of reactions to blood tests by children and adolescents. *Pain, 40,* 53–60.

Frank, N. C., Blount, R. L., Smith, A. J., Manimala, M. R., & Martin, J. K. (1995). Parent and staff behavior, previous child medical experience, and maternal anxiety as they relate to child procedural distress and coping. *Journal of Pediatric Psychology, 20,* 277–289.

Gonzalez, J. C., Routh, D. K., & Armstrong, F. D. (1993). Effects of maternal distraction versus reassurance on children's reactions to injections. *Journal of Pediatric Psychology, 18,* 593–604.

Goodenough, B., Kampel, L., Champion, G. D., Laubreaux, L., Nicholas, M. K., Ziegler, J. B., & McInerney, M.

(1997). An investigation of the placebo effect and age-related factors in the report of needle pain from venipuncture in children. *Pain, 72,* 383–391.

Grunau, R. V., & Craig, K. D. (1987). Pain expression in neonates: Facial action and cry. *Pain, 28,* 395–410.

Grunau, R. V. E., Whitfield, M. F., Petrie, J. H., & Fryer, E. L. (1994). Early pain experience, child and family factors, as precursors of somatization: A prospective study of extremely premature and fullterm children. *Pain, 56,* 353–359.

Gunnar, M. R., Porter, F. L., Wolf, C. N., Rigatuso, J., & Larson, M. C. (1995). Neonatal stress reactivity: Predictions to later emotional temperament. *Child Development, 66,* 1–13.

Hallén, B., Carlsson, P., & Uppfeldt, A. (1985). Clinical study of a lignocaine-prilocaine cream to relieve the pain of venipuncture. *British Journal of Anaesthesia, 57,* 326–328.

Hicks, C. L., von Baeyer, C. L., Spafford, P. A., van Korlaar, I., & Goodenough, B. (2001). The Faces Pain Scale—Revised: Toward a common metric in pediatric pain measurement. *Pain, 93,* 173–183.

Hobbie, W. L., Stubler, M., Meeske, K., Wissler, M., Rourke, M. T., Ruccione, K., et al. (2000). Symptoms of posttraumatic stress in survivors of childhood cancer. *Journal of Clinical Oncology, 18,* 4060–4066.

Hoffman, H. G., Patterson, D. R., Carrougher, G., & Sharar, S. (2001). Effectiveness of virtual reality–based pain control with multiple treatments. *Clinical Journal of Pain, 17,* 229–235.

Jacobsen, P., Manne, S., Gorfinkle, K., Schorr, O., Rapkin, B., & Redd, W. (1990). Analysis of child and parent activity during painful medical procedures. *Health Psychology, 9,* 559–576.

Jay, S., Elliott, C. H., Fitzgibbons, I., Woody, P., & Siegel, S. (1995). A comparative study of cognitive behavior therapy versus general anesthesia for painful medical procedures in children. *Pain, 62,* 3–9.

Jay, S. M., Elliott, C. E., Katz, E., & Siegel, S. E. (1987). Cognitive–behavioral and pharmacologic interventions for children's distress during painful medical procedures. *Journal of Consulting and Clinical Psychology, 55,* 860–865.

Jay, S. M., Elliott, C. E., Woody, P. D., & Siegel, S. (1991). An investigation of cognitive–behavior therapy combined with oral Valium for children undergoing medical procedures. *Health Psychology, 10,* 317–322.

Johnston, C. C., Collinge, J. M., Henderson, S. J., & Anand, K. J. (1997). A cross-sectional survey of pain and pharmacological analgesia in Canadian neonatal intensive care units. *Clinical Journal of Pain, 13,* 308–312.

Kain, Z. N., Mayes, L. C., & Caramico, L. A. (1996). Preoperative preparation in children: A cross sectional study. *Journal of Clinical Anesthesia, 8,* 508–514.

Katz, E. R., Kellerman, J., & Siegel, S. E. (1980). Distress behavior in children with cancer undergoing medical procedures: Developmental considerations. *Journal of Consulting and Clinical Psychology, 48,* 356–365.

Kaushik, S., Hord, A. H., Denson, D. D., McAllister, D. V., Smitra, S., Allen, M. G., & Prausnitz, M. R. (2001). Lack of pain associated with microfabricated microneedles. *Anesthesia and Analgesia, 92,* 502–504.

Kazak, A. E., Penati, B., Boyer, B. A., Himelstein, B., Brophy, P., Waibel, M. K., et al. (1996). A randomized controlled prospective outcome study of a psychological and pharmacological intervention protocol for procedural distress in pediatric leukemia. *Journal of Pediatric Psychology, 21,* 615–631.

Lagercrantz, H., & Ringstedt, T. (2001). Organization of the neuronal circuits in the central nervous system during development. *Acta Paediatrica, 90,* 707–715.

Lee, L. W., & White-Traut, R. C. (1996). The role of temperament in pediatric pain response. *Comprehensive Issues in Pediatric Nursing, 19,* 49–63.

Ljungman, G., Gordh, T., Sorensen, S., & Kreuger, A. (1999). Pain in paediatric oncology: Interviews with children, adolescents and their parents. *Acta Paediatrica, 88,* 623–630.

Main, K., Jorgensen, J., Hertel, N., Jensen, S., & Jakobsen, L. (1995). Automatic needle insertion diminishes pain during growth hormone injection. *Acta Paediatrica, 84,* 331–334.

Manimala, R., Blount, R. L., & Cohen, L. L. (2000). The effects of parental reassurance versus distraction on child distress and coping during immunizations. *Children's Health Care, 29,* 161–177.

McGrath, P. A. (1990). *Pain in children: Nature, assessment and treatment.* New York: Guilford Press.

McGrath, P. A. (1991). Intervention and management. In J. P. Bush & S. W. Harkins (Eds.), *Children in pain: Clinical and research issues from a developmental perspective* (pp. 83–115). New York: Springer-Verlag.

McGrath, P. A. (1994). Psychological aspects of pain perception. *Archives of Oral Biology, 39,* 55–62.

Melamed, B. G., Meyer, R., Gee, C., & Soule, L. (1976). The influence of time and type of preparation on children's adjustment to hospitalization. *Journal of Pediatric Psychology, 1,* 31–37.

Milling, L. S., & Constantino, C. A. (2000). Clinical hypnosis with children: First steps toward empirical support. *International Journal of Clinical and Experimental Hypnosis, 48,* 113–137.

Mower, O. H. (1939). A stimulus–response analysis of anxiety and its role as a reinforcing agent. *Psychological Review, 46,* 553–565.

Murray, F. T., Silverstein, J., Johnson, S. B., Gertner, J. H., Frye, K., Gironda, G., et al. (2000). Bioequivalence and patient satisfaction with a growth hormone (Siazen) needle-free device: Results of clinical and laboratory studies. *Today's Therapeutic Trends, 18,* 71–86.

O'Byrne, K. K., Peterson, L., & Saldana, L. (1997). Survey of pediatric hospitals' preparation programs: Evidence of the impact of health psychology research. *Health Psychology, 16,* 147–154.

Pate, J. T., Blount, R. L., Cohen, L. L., & Smith, A. J. (1996). Childhood medical experience and temperament as predictors of adult functioning in medical situations. *Children's Health Care, 25,* 281–296.

Piira, T., & von Baeyer, C. L. (2001). Commentary: Parents' role in helping children to cope with painful procedures. *Pediatric Pain Letter, 5*(2), 13–15.

Powers, S. W. (1999). Empirically supported treatments in pediatric psychology: Procedure-related pain. *Journal of Pediatric Psychology, 24,* 131–145.

Powers, S. W., Blount, R. L., Bachanas, P. J., Cotter, M. C., & Swan, S. C. (1993). Helping preschool leukemia patients and their patents cope during injections. *Journal of Pediatric Psychology, 18,* 681–695.

Ruda, M. A., Ling, Q., Hohmann, A., Peng, Y. B., & Tachibana, T. (2000). Altered nocioceptive neuronal circuits after neonatal peripheral inflammation. *Science, 289,* 628–631.

Rudolph, K. D., Dennig, M. D., & Weisz, J. R. (1995). Determinants and consequences of children's coping in the medical setting: Conceptualization, review, and critique. *Psychological Bulletin, 118,* 328–357.

Schechter, N. L., Bernstein, B. A., Beck, A., Hart, L., & Scherzer, L. (1991). Individual differences in children's response to pain: Role of temperament and parental characteristics. *Pediatrics, 87,* 171–177.

Schechter, N. L., Blankson, V., Pachter, L. M., Sullivan, C. M., & Costa, L. (1997). The ouchless place: No pain, children's gain. *Pediatrics, 99,* 890–894.

Southall, D. P., Cronin, B., Hartmann, H., Harrison-Sewell, C., & Samuels, M. (1993). Invasive procedures in children receiving intensive care. *British Medical Journal, 306,* 1512–1513.

Spafford, P. A., von Baeyer, C. L., & Hicks, C. L. (2002). Expected and reported pain in children undergoing ear piercing: A randomized trial of preparation by parents. *Behaviour Research and Therapy, 40,* 37–50.

Stevens, B., Taddio, A., Ohlsson, A., & Einarson, T. (1997). The efficacy of sucrose for relieving procedural pain in neonates: A systematic review and meta-analysis. *Acta Paediatrica, 86,* 837–842.

Suls, J., & Wan, C. K. (1989). Effects of sensory and procedural information on coping with stressful medical procedures and pain: A meta-analysis. *Journal of Consulting and Clinical Psychology, 57,* 372–379.

Sweet, S. D., & McGrath, P. J. (1998). Relative importance of mothers' versus medical staffs' behavior in the prediction of infant immunization pain behavior. *Journal of Pediatric Psychology, 23,* 249–256.

Taddio, A., Katz, J., Ilersich, A. L., & Koren, G. (1997). Effect of neonatal circumcision on pain response during subsequent routine vaccination. *Lancet, 349,* 599–603.

Taddio, A., Nulman, I., Goldbach, M., & Ipp, M. (1994). Use of lidocaine-prilocaine cream for vaccination pain in infants. *Journal of Pediatrics, 124,* 643–648.

Varni, J. W., Blount, R. L., Waldron, S. A., & Smith, A. J. (1995). Management of pain and distress. In M. C. Roberts (Ed.), *Handbook of pediatric psychology* (2nd ed., pp. 105–123). New York: Guilford Press.

Vernon, D. T. A., & Thompson, R. H. (1993). Research on the effects of experimental interventions on children's behavior after hospitalizations: A review and synthesis. *Developmental and Behavioral Pediatrics, 14,* 36–44.

14

Pediatric Pharmacology and Psychopharmacology

GEORGE J. DuPAUL
KARA E. McGOEY
JENNIFER A. MAUTONE

Pharmacotherapy is an integral component of treatment for most disorders of childhood and adolescence. This is true not only for physical illnesses (e.g., asthma), but for psychopathological conditions (e.g., attention-deficit/hyperactivity disorder [ADHD]) as well. Medications that have been found effective for the treatment of adult disorders are assumed to achieve similar outcomes in children; however, this assumption has not necessarily been supported by empirical data (e.g., antidepressant medications; Gadow, 1999). Nevertheless, practitioners are increasingly relying on drugs as a primary treatment approach for most of the disorders encountered in pediatric settings. For several compelling reasons, pediatric psychologists should be cognizant of the behavioral and physiological effects of medications used in the treatment of childhood mental and physical disorders. First, as mentioned, pharmacotherapy is a common intervention for many childhood conditions. In fact, for some disorders, medication may be the treatment of choice. For example, approximately 2–5% of children in the United States are treated with psychostimulant medication (e.g., methylphenidate) for ADHD (Safer & Zito, 2000). Although few research data exist on the extent to which medications are used for other childhood disorders, it is clear that psychologists are being asked to evaluate and treat many children who are receiving some form of medication.

The importance of pharmacological knowledge is underscored by the current debate in psychology concerning the relative merits of pursuing prescription privileges for psychologists (Gutierrez & Silk, 1998). If, as is argued here, behavioral assessment strategies are an essential component of evaluating the efficacy of medication therapy, particularly when psychotropic medications are used, then psychologists who are knowledgeable about assessment methodology *and* pharmacological principles would be in a better position to prescribe and monitor medication than others without such training. Another impetus for pediatric psychologists to gain expertise in pharmacotherapy is the dearth of empirical data underlying child psychopharmacology relative to the available research on psychotropic medications in adult populations. Given their expertise in research design and methodology, psychologists are in a unique position to enhance the empirical underpinnings of pharmacotherapy in the treatment of pediatric disorders.

The purpose of this chapter is to provide an overview of pediatric psychopharmacology and pharmacology, particularly as they relate to the practice of psychology in medical and clinical settings. First, general considerations that have an impact on the role of the pediatric psychologist in determining the need for and evaluating the efficacy of medication are delineated. Second, the specific uses of psychotropic medications in pediatric populations are reviewed briefly. Third, medications used for conditions such as asthma, diabetes, and chronic pain are reviewed, to explicate the role of pharmacology in the overall treatment of the child or adolescent. Finally, we offer suggestions for research and clinical practice designed to increase the visibility of pediatric psychologists in promoting more effective pharmacotherapeutic practice and in advocating for the use of medications in the context of multimodal intervention programs.

THE ROLE OF THE PEDIATRIC PSYCHOLOGIST IN PHARMACOTHERAPY

Regardless of the specific medication employed, a number of factors have an impact on the role of the pediatric psychologist, both prior to and in the course of pharmacotherapy with children. Specific issues discussed here include (1) determining when to use medication, (2) considering developmental factors, (3) consulting with physicians in the assessment of medication response, and (4) promoting compliance with medication regimens.

When to Use Medication

Determining when and how to prescribe medication is a complex decision, especially (as in most cases) when multiple interventions are utilized to treat a specific condition. Unfortunately, there are few empirically based guidelines for making such decisions. Nevertheless, Werry (1999, pp. 14–20) outlined several principles for the use of psychotropic medications that can serve as guidelines in determining the necessity of pharmacotherapy in treating both physical and psychopathological disorders. These principles are reviewed briefly in adapted form as follows:

1. *"When in doubt, don't prescribe."* Caution should be employed before medication is prescribed (Werry, 1999). If psychosocial interventions can be effective in the absence of medication, then the former are the interventions of first choice.
2. *"Make the right choice."* Practitioners should be highly knowledgeable about childhood disorders and the medications that could be effective in treating specific conditions (Werry, 1999). Medication choices should be guided by knowledge of empirical data identifying the best agent for a specific disorder. In the absence of a clearly identified choice, the practitioner must balance the knowledge of the properties (i.e., behavioral effects and side

effects) of each medication against the physical and psychological profile of the child to be treated.

3. *"Keep medication in perspective."* Rarely is pharmacotherapy alone the optimal treatment for most childhood disorders. Rather than deciding whether to use medication *or* an alternative intervention, the practitioner should make efforts to utilize pharmacotherapy *and* other treatment modalities, in order to promote possible synergistic effects.

4. *"Keep it simple."* Consistent adherence with medication regimens is often difficult to obtain in the treatment of childhood disorders (Brown & Sawyer, 1998; Litt, 1992). One factor that may enhance treatment adherence is to keep medication administration simple (e.g., using only one drug at a time; Werry, 1999).

5. *"Make an effort to communicate."* Throughout the course of the medication decision-making process, the practitioner should take care to build a communicative relationship with the patient and his or her parents (Werry, 1999). The parent(s) should be fully informed as to the advantages and disadvantages of medications being considered. In the case of psychotropic medications, the child or adolescent should understand that behavioral changes are not solely attributable to pharmacotherapy, that the medication is merely a means to the desired result of clinical improvement that is obtained through a number of interventions.

6. *"Take it slow."* Whenever possible, the decision to prescribe a particular medication should be made within an appropriate time interval that allows for careful consideration of all treatment alternatives.

7. *"Look out for the child's best interests."* Children often have minimal input into treatment decisions that affect their lives. The relative costs and benefits of pharmacological treatment must be weighed carefully before prescribing (Werry, 1999).

Developmental Factors in Pharmacotherapy

Age-related or developmental factors have been virtually ignored in the child pharmacological literature. Prescription practices are often based on empirical data obtained from adult patients, with minimal information about the effects of medication on different age groups. Given that the body's metabolism rate fluctuates with age and that a child's body is changing and developing at a rapid pace, the differences between children and adults in responses to medication must be empirically determined to guide practice. Within the child domain in general, there is also a need to consider whether specific medications are differentially effective at various age levels.

The two developmental stages that require specific attention are the preschool period (i.e., under the age of 5 years) and adolescence. The use of medications with preschool-age children is controversial in some cases because of a lack of empirical data on medication response in this population, particularly when psychotropic agents are used (Greenhill, 1998; Zito et al., 2000). In addition, given the physical immaturity of children at this age level, the possibility of a greater number and severity of side effects must be considered for many medications (Firestone, Musten, Pisterman, Mercer, & Bennett, 1998).

The pharmacological treatment of adolescents involves two unique aspects. First, the adolescent must be willing to participate in symptom evaluation and, eventually, to accept the intervention to ensure compliance with the therapeutic regimen (Gadow, 1986). Thus the importance of establishing a communicative relationship with adolescent patients is underscored. In addition, the rationale for medication use, as well as possible benefits and side effects, must be carefully reviewed with the patients. The second factor to be considered is that adolescents are at high risk for medication overdose (Gadow, 1986). Thus psychoactive medications should be employed cautiously with those teenagers who are at higher risk for substance abuse (e.g., those exhibiting symptoms of conduct disorder) or who exhibit signs of suicidal ideation.

Assessment of Medication Response

Medication response can be assessed across physiological, behavioral, and affective domains (Brown & Sawyer, 1998; Phelps, Brown, & Power, 2002; Werry & Aman, 1999). Unfortunately, all too often in clinical practice, titration of medication dosage and assessment of treatment efficacy are based solely on the subjective reports of parents and not on behavioral assessment data, which are critical methods in evaluating response to psychotropic medications such as stimulants (DuPaul & Barkley, 1993; Northup & Gulley, 2001). Behavioral assessment techniques (e.g., direct observations of behavior) have been used quite successfully in evaluating the stimulant medication response of individual children across numerous areas of functioning (e.g., Evans et al., 2001; Northup & Gulley, 2001). Behavioral assessment measures have the advantage of assessing behaviors with greater ecological validity and clinical importance than those behaviors tapped by traditional laboratory measures (DuPaul & Barkley, 1993).

A number of factors related to the efficacy of medication regimens lend further credence to the incorporation of behavioral assessment methodologies in evaluating treatment response. First, medication-related changes in a specific behavioral realm typically vary across dose in a systematic fashion. For example, the behavioral effects of stimulant medications are found to increase linearly in association with dosage increments, at least at the group level of analysis (e.g., Denney & Rapport, 2001). Therefore, measures that are reliable and valid for repeated administrations across dose are needed to assess individual response. Second, at an individual level of analysis, separate classes of behavior may be affected differently by a medication, even at the same dose (e.g., Northup, Gulley, Edwards, & Fountain, 2001). For instance, a child may show the greatest improvement in academic performance at a different dose of methylphenidate from that which is optimal for impulse control or sustained attention. This difference implies the need for multiple assessment measures collected across areas of functioning and settings. Finally, although dose–response effects may be consistent at the group level of analysis, individual children may vary considerably with respect to behavior change across doses (Evans et al., 2001). Therefore, behavioral change must be evaluated across doses on an individual basis, ideally by employing single-subject design methodologies.

Given the prevalence of stimulant treatment for ADHD, several "models" for the assessment of psychostimulant effects have been proposed over the years (e.g., Barkley, Connor, & Kwasnik, 2000; Gadow, Nolan, Paoliccelli, & Sprafkin, 1991). These assessment models share a number of core features that could be adapted for use in evaluating a variety of medications, such as:

1. The use of placebo controls and double-blind methodology to reduce possible biases in the reports of parents and teachers.
2. Randomization of dose order across participants to control for possible order effects, at least at the group level of analysis.

3. Inclusion of multiple assessment measures, using a variety of methodologies (e.g., parent and teacher ratings of symptoms, observations of classroom behavior or performance on clinic analogue tasks, productivity and accuracy on academic tasks).
4. Collection of assessment data at a time when medication effects are most prominent.
5. Evaluation of possible side effects during both medication and nonmedication conditions.

Furthermore, the most comprehensive models involve the assessment of children's functioning across behavioral, social, and academic domains.

In many instances, practitioners do not have the resources and time to conduct comprehensive, placebo-controlled medication evaluations as described previously. Nevertheless, the pediatric psychologist and physician can, as a team, collect objective data in a cost-effective fashion that will greatly aid them in making medication-related decisions. This process is accomplished by collecting several measures of treatment response (e.g., parent and teacher ratings) and assessing possible side effects across dosage conditions. If possible, those adults who are evaluating changes in the child's performance (e.g., teachers) should be kept "blind" to the medication condition. For instance, even during a nonmedication phase, the child may continue to go to the nurse's office at the same time to receive "medication" and take a vitamin instead. Finally, although behavioral assessment techniques are quite useful in the clinical evaluation of medication effects, this methodology is limited by the fact that dosage selection rules are rarely operationalized in an objective manner (Gadow et al., 1991). Ultimately, the decision as to whether a specific psychotropic medication works for an individual and what dose is "optimal" is reached through a subjective process (i.e., clinical judgment). Thus medication assessment models, particularly for psychoactive agents, must be refined through systematic research comparing the advantages and disadvantages of various decision-making models that employ explicit criteria for determining a child's optimal dose in an effort to enhance the reliability of treatment decisions based on clinical judgment (DuPaul & Barkley, 1993).

Adherence with Medication Regimens

Inconsistent adherence to medication administration schedules is apparently a widespread problem in child pharmacotherapy, as the mean nonadherence rate for patients in pediatric clinics has been estimated to be 50% (Lemanek, Kamps, & Chung, 2001). Some authors have asserted that nonadherence to treatment is the major reason why some individuals are not found to respond to medication regimens (Zametkin & Yamada, 1999). Several types of nonadherence with medication regimens have been identified, including complete failure to follow a medication regimen, ingesting medication at improper time intervals, and/or ingesting too large or too small amounts of medication relative to the prescribed dosage (Litt, 1992). Pediatric psychologists are often asked to design interventions that will enhance a patient's adherence with prescribed treatment procedures, including medication (see La Greca & Bearman, Chapter 8, this volume). Specific strategies may include providing education about medication to the patient and his or her family, simplifying the treatment regimen, using packaging that provides cues for medication administration (e.g., calendar packs), and peer support (Litt, 1992). In particular, behavior modification techniques, such as contingency management, have been among the most effective methods to encourage adherence to specific aspects of the treatment regimen, such as pill taking and/or pill swallowing (Lemanek et al., 2001).

PSYCHOPHARMACOLOGY

Attention-Deficit/Hyperactivity Disorder and Conduct Disorder

ADHD is the most common disorder treated with psychotropic medications. The most popular medications prescribed for ADHD are central nervous system (CNS) stimulants, including methylphenidate (MPH; Ritalin, Concerta, Metadate CD), amphetamine compounds (Adderall), dextroamphetamine (Dexedrine), and pemoline (Cylert), with MPH being the most commonly prescribed (DuPaul, Barkley, & Connor, 1998; Pelham et al., 2001; Wilens & Spencer, 2000; see Table 14.1). A number of other medications have been used in the treatment of ADHD, including tricyclic antidepressants (e.g., desipramine), bupropion, clonidine, and guanfacine (Connor, 1998). None of these agents, however, have been found to be superior to stimulants; thus the stimulants are typically tried first, and alternative substances are utilized only when necessary.

The behavioral effects of stimulants in the treatment of children with ADHD are the most widely researched and documented in the field of pharmacotherapy for childhood mental health disorders (Wilens & Spencer, 2000). The short-term behavioral effects of stimulants on children with ADHD include improvements in social, behavioral, and academic functioning. Reductions in classroom disruptiveness and increases in on-task behavior are among the most thoroughly documented results of stimulant treatment (DuPaul et al., 1998). Interactions with teachers, parents, and peers are improved by reductions in impulsivity, interruptions, and, in some cases, aggression (Pelham et al., 2001; Wilens & Spencer, 2000). Although the short-term behavioral effects are numerous, the long-term effects of stimulant use need to be explored further. The scant research in existence provides no evidence that stimulants, when used in isolation, improve the long-term outcome of children with ADHD (DuPaul et al., 1998).

Approximately 70–80% of children and 60% of adolescents with ADHD will respond positively to stimulant medication (Barkley et al., 2000). Stimulant response among preschoolers is not as well documented, but it is presumed to be less positive than that exhibited by older children (Wilens & Spencer, 2000). The behavioral effects of stimulants are idiosyncratic and have been found to vary as a function of dose and target behavior. Each of these issues suggests the need for careful monitoring of medication effects and the use of adjunctive interventions (e.g., behavior modification) contemporaneous with pharmacotherapy.

Adverse effects from the use of stimulant medications in the treatment of ADHD are numerous but benign. At the onset of treatment, children may exhibit insomnia, loss of appetite, headaches, stomachaches, nausea, moodiness, irritability, and increased talkativeness (DuPaul et al., 1998; Wilens & Spencer, 2000). In addition, pemoline may cause damage to the liver and is not considered a first-line medication for this disorder. Approximately 33% of children treated with MPH may experience a behavioral rebound (i.e., worsening of symptoms beyond those observed without medication) in late afternoon (DuPaul et al., 1998). Fortunately, most of these adverse side effects can be controlled by monitoring the children closely and making corrections in the dosage as necessary. To date, the only long-term side effect that has been identified is possible inhibition of growth in both height and weight. The growth suppression effect is dose related, more prevalent with dextroamphetamine than with MPH, more likely to occur during the first year of treatment, and may be reversed when medication is discontinued (DuPaul et al., 1998).

Several different medications have been suggested for the treatment of conduct disorder; no single medication has been clearly proven to be effective. Lithium carbonate has

TABLE 14.1. Medications Used to Treat Child and Adolescent Disorders

Disorder	Class of medication	Specific medication
Attention-deficit/hyperactivity disorder	CNS stimulants	Methylphenidate Amphetamine compounds Dextroamphetamine Pemoline
	Tricyclic antidepressants	Imipramine Desipramine
	Antihypertensives	Clonidine Guanfacine
Conduct disorder	Antimanics	Lithium carbonate
	CNS stimulants	Methylphenidate
Depression	Tricyclic antidepressants	Imipramine Desipramine
	Selective serotonin reuptake inhibitors	Fluoxetine Paroxetine
Bipolar disorder	Antimanics	Lithium carbonate
Anxiety disorders	Anxiolytics	Clonazepam Chlordiazepoxide
	Tricyclic antidepressants	Imipramine Desipramine
Obsessive–compulsive disorder	Serotonin reuptake inhibitors	Clomipramine Fluoxetine Fluvoxamine Sertraline
Schizophrenia	Antipsychotics (neuroleptics)	Haloperidol Clozapine
Pervasive developmental disorders	Antipsychotics (neuroleptics)	Haloperidol Pimozide Trifluoperazine
Tic disorders	Antipsychotics (neuroleptics)	Haloperidol Pimozide
	Antihypertensives	Clonidine
Nocturnal enuresis	Tricyclic antidepressants	Imipramine
	Prostaglandin synthesis inhibitors	Indomethacin Diclofenac sodium
	Antidiuretic hormone	Desmopressin acetate (DDAVP)
Seizure disorders	Anticonvulsants	Phenytoin Carbamazepine Valproate Ethosuximide Lamotrigine
Asthma	Bronchodilator antiasthma drugs	Albuterol Salbutamol Terbutaline Salmeterol Theophylline Atropine sulfate Ipratropium bromide

(*continued*)

TABLE 14.1. (*continued*)

Disorder	Class of medication	Specific medication
Asthma (*continued*)	Nonbronchodilator antiasthma drugs	Cromolyn sodium Prednisone Beclomethasone dipropionate Fluticasone propionate
	Leukotriene modifiers	Zileuton Montelukast Zafirlukast
Diabetes	Anabolic hormones	Insulin
Pediatric pain	Local anesthetics	Prilocaine Lignocaine Amethocaine
	Systemic analgesics	Morphine Codeine Acetaminophen Ibuprofen
	Anxiolytics	Clonazepam
	Tricyclic antidepressants	Imipramine Desipramine
Cancer	Antineoplastics	Cyclophosphamide Actinomycin-D Vincristine Doxorubicin
	Biological agents	Interferons Interleukins

been suggested as an effective treatment but has several disadvantages, such as concerns about toxicity and the related need for careful monitoring. MPH has been found to reduce aggression, stealing, and property destruction in children with ADHD and comorbid conduct disorder (Stoewe, Kruesi, & Lelio, 1995), but this finding has yet to be replicated in a sample of children exhibiting conduct disorder in the absence of ADHD. Clonidine and the neuroleptics (e.g., haloperidol) may also result in improvements in aggression and arousal, although further study is necessary (Stoewe, Kruesi, & Lelio, 1995).

Mood and Anxiety Disorders

Unipolar depression in children is less responsive to medical treatment than in adults, although the same medications are often used to treat both groups (Wilens, Spencer, Frazier, & Biederman, 1998; see Table 14.1). Tricyclic antidepressants (TCAs; e.g., imipramine and desipramine) have shown positive results in open-label studies of children with depression; however, results have been less positive in placebo-controlled studies (for review, see Wagner & Ambrosini, 2001). Side effects of TCAs include dry mouth, blurred vision, constipation, and negative effects on cardiovascular functioning (e.g., cardiac arrhythmia). Due to these side effects and the fact that TCAs may not be very effective in pediatric populations, the selective serotonin reuptake inhibitors (SSRIs; e.g., fluoxetine [Prozac], paroxetine [Paxil]) have become the medications of choice for the treatment of unipolar depression in children. Results of double-blind studies of fluoxetine and paroxetine for treatment of children with depression are promising (Wagner & Ambrosini, 2001). In addition, the SSRIs may result in fewer and less serious side effects than the TCAs (Wilens et al., 1998).

The primary medication in the treatment of children with bipolar disorder is lithium carbonate, although there are few controlled studies of its use in the pediatric population. In addition, sodium valproate may be as effective as lithium carbonate, particularly in cases of rapid cycling, but further study is necessary to confirm these results (James & Javaloyes, 2001). A high rate of relapse occurs when medical treatment is discontinued, so lithium is often used as a prophylaxis. Given the potential toxicity of this substance, however, it is important to keep lithium blood levels to a minimum while achieving clinical effects (James & Javaloyes, 2001).

The treatment of anxiety disorders in children is complicated due to the lack of reliable assessment tools and diagnostic criteria and the high rates of comorbid disorders. However, it is assumed that children's responses to treatment will be similar to that of adults with anxiety disorders. The few double-blind placebo-controlled studies involving children and adolescents suggest that anxiolytic (e.g., clonazepam and chlordiazepoxide) and tricyclic antidepressant medications (e.g., imipramine and desipramine) may be effective in treating childhood anxiety disorders (for review, see Hawkridge & Stein, 1998). In addition, based on preliminary research, it seems that SSRIs (e.g., fluoxetine and sertraline) may reduce some of the symptoms of childhood anxiety disorders, although further study is necessary before widespread use of these agents can be recommended (Hawkridge & Stein, 1998).

Various psychoactive medications, particularly serotonin reuptake inhibitors (SRIs), have been found to be effective in the treatment of obsessive–compulsive disorder (OCD) in adults (Park, Jefferson, & Greist, 1997), and SRIs (e.g., clomipramine) are currently considered the treatment of choice for OCD in children and adolescents (Rapoport & Inoff-Germain, 2000). The SSRIs (e.g., fluoxetine [Prozac], fluvoxamine, and sertraline) have also received some attention for the treatment of OCD in children and adolescents, and preliminary results are positive (Rapoport & Inoff-Germain, 2000). Although side effects are typically minimal, treatment with SSRIs should begin with a low dose that is slowly increased until maximum symptom reduction is achieved (Park et al., 1997).

Pervasive Developmental Disorders and Childhood Schizophrenia

Antipsychotics (or neuroleptics) are the most commonly prescribed medications for the treatment of pervasive developmental disorders (PDDs) and childhood-onset schizophrenia (Jacobsen & Rapoport, 1998; Posey & McDougle, 2000; see Table 14.1). The most widely studied medication in the treatment of childhood schizophrenia is haloperidol (Haldol), although clozapine is becoming the subject of increased scrutiny. Clozapine may result in greater improvements on measures of psychosis than haloperidol, and it is associated with fewer extrapyramidal side effects (Jacobsen & Rapoport, 1998; Posey & McDougle, 2000). At this time, other neuroleptics (e.g., risperidone and olanzapine) have been subjected only to open-label trials, but researchers are hopeful that these medications will be as effective as clozapine (Jacobsen & Rapoport, 1998).

In the treatment of PDD, many medications have been tried, but none have been found to lead to complete diminution of symptoms. Instead, medication is used to reduce the occurrence of particular symptoms and to potentially enhance the effectiveness of other components of a multimodal treatment plan (Posey & McDougle, 2000). SRIs are receiving some attention for the treatment of PDDs, and preliminary results are promising (Posey & McDougle, 2000). In addition, high-potency antipsychotic medications, such as haloperidol, pimozide, and trifluoperazine, have been shown to enhance interpersonal communication and reduce many of the maladaptive behaviors (e.g., aggressiveness, sterotypies, and social withdrawal) associated with PDDs (Posey & McDougle, 2000).

The extrapyramidal side effects of antipsychotic medications include acute dystonia (e.g., neck twisted to the side, eyes rolled back under lids), parkinsonism (e.g., drooling and pill rolling), and tardive dyskinesia. In addition, these medications may result in excessive sedation, irritability, and weight gain, as well as adverse effects on cognitive functioning (Posey & McDougle, 2000). Although some of these side effects can be reduced with treatment (e.g., antiparkinsonian medications), children should be treated with the minimum effective dose to reduce the severity of adverse reactions.

Tic Disorders and Tourette's Disorder

Psychoactive medications can be effective in the reduction of motor and vocal tics, with the neuroleptics haloperidol and pimozide being the treatments of choice (Chappell, Leckman, & Riddle, 1995; Wilens et al., 1998; see Table 14.1). Haloperidol and pimozide are effective at low doses and can eliminate symptoms of tic disorders (including Tourette's disorder; Wilens et al., 1998). The side effects of these medications have been enumerated in the preceding section. Given the potential adverse effects of haloperidol, clonidine (Catapres) has become the medication of choice in some treatment centers, particularly for children evidencing tics of mild to moderate severity (Chappell et al., 1995; Wilens et al., 1998). Clonidine may prove beneficial in avoiding some of the side effects of haloperidol, but patient responses to this medication are inconsistent (Chappell et al., 1995). In addition, tricyclic antidepressants (e.g., desipramine, nortriptyline), atypical neuroleptics (e.g., sulpiride, tiapride), and guanfacine (Tenex) are receiving increased attention in the treatment of tic disorders; however, these have been evaluated primarily in the context of open, uncontrolled trials (Chappell et al., 1995; Wilens et al., 1998).

Nocturnal Enuresis

The medications that have been found to be most effective in the treatment of nocturnal enuresis have been the tricyclic antidepressants (e.g., imipramine) and desmopressin acetate (DDAVP; see Table 14.1). In addition, preliminary studies show that prostaglandin synthesis inhibitors (e.g., indomethacin and diclofenac sodium) may be effective in increasing bladder control and enhancing vasopressin, particularly in combination with imipramine (Moffatt, 1997). Until recently, imipramine (Tofranil) was the most widely prescribed medical treatment for nocturnal enuresis. However, due to potential side effects (e.g., mood and sleep disturbance, decreased appetite, anxiety, and fatigue) and the risk of overdose, imipramine is no longer prescribed as frequently (Moffatt, 1997). Therefore, DDAVP may be the medical treatment of choice for the control of nocturnal enuresis in children. DDAVP is an antidiuretic hormone analogue, available as a nasal spray and in oral form, which acts on the kidneys to suppress urine output while sleeping (Moffatt, 1997). This effect is reversed when the medication is discontinued. In general, pharmacological treatment of enuresis is usually less effective than nonmedical, behavioral treatments (e.g., the urine alarm); thus medication is rarely used in isolation as a treatment for this disorder (Moffatt, 1997).

Seizure Disorders

Pharmacotherapy for the effective treatment of seizure disorders often includes a variety of medications, depending on the type of seizure, although traditional anticonvulsant medications (e.g., valproate and carbamazepine) are typically the first line of treatment. Newer anticonvulsant medications (e.g., lamotrigine and felbamate) may be prescribed when adequate seizure control is not achieved with traditional medications or when side effects are intolerable (Williams & Sharp, 2000). Anticonvulsant medications that have been found effective in the control of tonic–clonic (grand mal) seizures include phenobarbital, phenytoin (Dilantin), carbamazepine (Tegretol), and valproate (Depakote, Depakene; see Table 14.1). The treatments of choice for absence (petit mal) seizures are ethosuximide (Zarontin) or valproate. Finally, first-line treatments for partial seizures include carbamazepine, phenytoin, and valproate. Gabapentin (Neurontin), or felbamate (Felbatol) are prescribed as second-line treatments when necessary (Williams & Sharp, 2000). Anticonvulsant medications should be prescribed in the smallest dose that allows for maximum seizure control, and medication for the treatment of seizures should begin as monotherapy. If seizures cannot be adequately controlled with only one medication, polypharmacy may be considered. In addition, all of the anticonvulsants may impair cognitive functioning, and thus effects on learning and school performance should be monitored closely.

PEDIATRIC PHARMACOLOGY

The pharmacotherapy of several medical disorders that pediatric psychologists are most likely to encounter is discussed in the following sections. These disorders include asthma, diabetes, pediatric pain, and cancer. In addition, the psychoactive effects of various medication regimens are delineated.

Asthma

Although advances have been made in regard to establishing the etiology of asthma, the lack of a clearly defined causal mechanism continues to hamper treatment efforts (see McQuaid & Walders, Chapter 16, this volume). The medications that have been found effective include various bronchodilator antiasthma agents (e.g., ß-adrenergic agonists and theophylline), nonbronchodilator antiasthma medications (e.g., cromolyn, corticosteroids), and leukotriene modifiers (e.g., leukotriene synthesis inhibitors and leukotriene receptor antagonists; see Table 14.1).

The strongest bronchodilators are the ß-adrenergic agonists, including albuterol (Proventil, Ventolin), metaproterenol (Alupent), salbutamol, terbutaline, salmeterol, and formoterol (Szefler 2000). ß-Adrenergic agonists can be successfully used to treat a variety of asthmatic conditions, including mild asthma, exercise-induced breathing difficulties, and chronic or acute asthmatic conditions (Szefler, 2000). The long-acting ß-adrenergic agonists (e.g., salmeterol and formoterol) may be used as prophylactic medications or to control nocturnal asthma, and the most effective long-term treatment of asthma may be a combination of inhaled ß-adrenergic agonists and inhaled corticosteroids.

Theophylline has been proven to be effective in the control of asthma, and the availability of sustained-release forms (e.g., Theo-Dur) resulted in enhanced control of nighttime asthma symptoms (Szefler, 2000). Historically, theophylline was the treatment of choice for acute, severe asthma; however, other agents (e.g., early use of corticosteroids and leukotriene modifiers) may be preferred at the present time (Bender, 1999; Szefler, 2000).

When administered alone, anticholinergics (e.g., atropine sulfate) have a slower onset of action and are not as effective as the ß-adrenergic agonists. However, when combined with ß-adrenergic agonists, bronchodilation may be improved, and hospitalization of patients with asthma may be reduced. Cromolyn sodium or disodium cromoglycate inhibits constriction of airways in reaction to exercise, cold air, or allergens, although the specific mechanism of action is unknown (Szefler, 2000). Because the effects of this substance may take up to 4 weeks to appear, cromolyn therapy may be used as a prophylaxis once asthma symptoms are controlled with another medication, such as an inhaled ß-adrenergic agonist and/or a corticosteroid (Bender, 1999).

The corticosteroids used for the treatment of childhood asthma include methylprednisolone, beclomethasone, and prednisone (Bender, 1999). These agents prevent and/or inhibit inflammation of the airways and mucus secretion (Bender, 1999), and early intervention with corticosteroids may prevent the progression of asthma (Szefler, 2000). Inhaled corticosteroids, such as beclomethasone dipropionate and fluticasone propionate, may be more effective than orally administered steroids and are also associated with less severe systemic effects (Price, 2000).

The leukotriene modifiers, including leukotriene synthesis inhibitors (e.g., zileuton) and leukotriene receptor antagonists (e.g., montelukast [Singulair], zafirlukast), may counteract the release of leukotrienes, thereby preventing airway inflammation. The leukotriene receptor antagonists have received the most attention for the treatment of children with asthma. In fact, montelukast has been found to be effective in children as young as 2 years old (Szefler, 2000).

Diabetes

A deficiency of insulin, a major anabolic hormone that regulates the use and storage of nutrient fuels in the body, leads to diabetes mellitus (see Wyscocki, Greco, & Buckloh, Chapter 18, this volume). Fortunately, several varieties of insulin are available and effective in the treatment of diabetes (Owens, Zinman, & Bolli, 2001). Purified insulin was initially the treatment of choice for individuals with diabetes, but insulin analogues with improved pharmacokinetics have recently been developed (Owens et al., 2001). Insulin analogues offer several advantages over purified and human insulin. Due to the rapid action, insulin analogues may be injected up to 15 minutes after the start of a meal and will still be as effective as soluble insulin that is injected 30 minutes before eating. In addition, there is less variation in the absorption of insulin analogues, which may result in fewer episodes of hypoglycemia, particularly nocturnal hypoglycemia (Owens et al., 2001). Potential complications arising from insulin therapy include diabetic ketoacidosis and hypoglycemia, the latter of which is usually attributable to administration of an inappropriate dosage or to extraneous factors (e.g., missing a meal). Given the seriousness of diabetes, insulin therapy is usually embedded in the context of a multimodal treatment regimen that also includes family education (e.g., methods of blood glucose self-testing, steps to insulin administration, and facts about diabetes) and dietary modifications (Owens et al., 2001).

Pediatric Pain

A number of pharmacological agents have been used in the management of pediatric pain associated with surgery or illness (see Dahlquist & Switkin, Chapter 12, and Blount, Piira,

& Cohen, Chapter 13, this volume). Drugs used to reduce pain have included local anesthetics, opioid analgesics, non-narcotic analgesics, nonsteroidal anti-inflammatory agents, and psychotropic medications (see Table 14.1).

Local anesthetics are typically the first line of treatment for procedural pain (i.e., pain associated with venous or lumbar puncture), and they are thought to be one of the safest methods of pain control for children in these situations (Morton, 1998). Intravenous or intramuscular morphine is one of the most commonly used opioid analgesics, although codeine is often preferred due to the fact that it can be administered orally (Brown, Tanaka, & Donegan, 1998). Opioid analgesics are used only for the treatment of severe pain, given possible adverse effects that include constipation, urinary retention, nausea and vomiting, dizziness, and respiratory depression. If children are monitored carefully while receiving opioid analgesics for severe pain, addiction is rare (Brown et al., 1998); however, abrupt discontinuance of these medications can lead to significant withdrawal symptoms. Acetaminophen is the non-narcotic analgesic most frequently used with children, because it has been found effective in reducing moderate pain associated with headache, otitis media, or minor injuries (Brown et al., 1998; Tarnowski, Brown, Dingle, & Dreelin, 1998). However, it has poor anti-inflammatory properties. The typical doses (10 mg/kg every 6 hours) of acetaminophen are rarely associated with side effects, and these are usually benign (e.g., rash). The nonsteroidal anti-inflammatory medications are particularly effective pain relievers when inflammation (e.g., juvenile rheumatoid arthritis) is the primary cause of discomfort (Tarnowski et al., 1998), and they are also commonly used for postoperative pain relief (Morton, 1998). Adverse treatment emergent effects can include gastritis, bleeding in the gastrointestinal tract, anemia, and iron deficiency (Brown et al., 1998).

Psychopharmacological medications, such as antidepressants and anxiolytics, are sometimes combined with analgesics in the treatment of pain. In addition, psychotropic medications, such as neuroleptics and anxiolytics, may be helpful in treating anxiety related to pain (e.g., before invasive procedures), and tricyclic antidepressants may be combined with cognitive behavioral techniques to decrease mild pain (e.g., headaches). The combination of medication and cognitive-behavioral interventions (e.g., distraction strategies) represents the most typical treatment package.

Cancer

Cancer is a heterogeneous group of illnesses, as there are approximately 100 different types of cancer, including leukemia, brain tumors, and lymphoma (see Vannatta & Gerhardt, Chapter 20, this volume). Leukemia is the most common childhood cancer, and acute lymphocytic leukemia is the most common subtype (Handler & DuPaul, 1999). Various antineoplastic medications are used to treat cancer in children (see Table 14.1). In addition, intrathecal and systemic drugs or steroids may be used in combination to minimize the use of radiation (Waber & Mullenix, 2000). Frequently, the combination of medications is preferred over the use of a single agent, in order to increase cellular sites of action and perhaps to reduce the probability of the development of a drug-resistant clone of cells (Chan & Erlichman, 1993).

The pharmacotherapy of cancer in children differs from medication treatment for other disorders in two ways (Chan & Erlichman, 1993). First, toxic side effects commonly occur in conjunction with treatment, because of a narrow therapeutic index. Second, the purpose of treatment is to administer maximal doses of medication to provoke some toxicity. Thus adverse effects, such as a failure to gain weight or grow in linear height, are not uncommon during treatment, although a growth rebound typically occurs on cessation of chemotherapy. Therefore, patients must be monitored frequently and closely to prevent significant side effects.

As in the treatment of other disorders reviewed in this chapter, single-treatment modalities are rarely used in isolation. Other treatment options besides medication include surgery and radiation therapy, especially when the tumor load is greatest (Chan & Erlichman, 1993). Because the long-term neuropsychological outcomes for children who undergo chemotherapy and radiation treatments are still relatively unknown, children who have been cured need to be monitored to detect and treat any long-term adverse effects of intervention.

Behavioral Effects of Pediatric Medicines

Many of the medications used to treat various childhood disorders can adversely affect behavioral, emotional, or cognitive functioning. Although this phenomenon has not been extensively studied in the research literature, available data indicate that deleterious effects on CNS functioning accounted for approximately 18% of the adverse responses reported to be experienced by children and adolescents between 1985 and 1989 (Arnold, Janke, Waters & Milch, 1999). Adverse CNS effects were more likely to be caused by antibiotics than other medications, more likely to affect boys than girls, and more likely to be exhibited by children under the age of 5 years. Commonly used pediatric medicines can lead to intoxication, delirium, delusions, hallucinations, mood disturbance, anxiety, or interference with learning (Arnold et al., 1999). For instance, antihistamines, opioid analgesics, and corticosteroids have been associated with impairment in perception, cognition, and/or mood in some children.

When changes in behavioral, emotional, or cognitive functioning are evidenced, the first step is to determine whether the reactions can be attributed to the medication or to extraneous variables (e.g., stress, disturbance in family relationships). Several factors increase the probability that observed behavioral reactions are medication related: (1) The child has ingested a very high dosage; (2) the specific medication acts directly on CNS functioning or easily crosses the blood–brain barrier; (3) the child has a developmental disability or psychopathological disorder; (4) multiple agents are being used to treat the child; and (5) dose changes are being made in a rapid fashion, without allowing for habituation to occur (Arnold et al., 1999). Although adverse effects on CNS functioning are not common, they occur frequently enough that medical practitioners must familiarize themselves with potential psychoactive effects of a wide range of medications (Arnold et al., 1999).

CONCLUSIONS AND RECOMMENDATIONS FOR FUTURE RESEARCH

This chapter has provided a brief overview of the pharmacological treatment of a variety of childhood disorders. Medication is a major component of intervention for both physical and psychopathological conditions, despite a lack of strong empirical underpinnings for this practice in some cases. Pediatric psychologists can serve as important members of the medication treatment team by assisting physicians both in determining the need for pharmacotherapy and in evaluating the behavioral and affective outcomes associated with medication treatment (see also Brown & Sammons, 2002). It is important for psychologists to provide a developmental perspective on the treatment regimen, particularly as it affects the cognitive, emotional, and social functioning of ill children. Given that adherence with medication regimens can be inconsistent, behavioral consultation designed to increase treatment adherence is a crucial component of an intervention program, especially when chronic pharmacotherapy is necessary.

Despite the widespread use of medication in treating a variety of childhood disorders, surprisingly few empirical data are available to guide practice (Brown & Sammons, 2002). In particular, investigations into new psychoactive substances should be driven by symptomatology exhibited by children rather than by extrapolations from adult psychopharmacology (Werry, 1999). In addition, the impact of all pediatric medicines on social, psychological, and biological development, as well as on peer and family relationships, needs to be studied in detail (Werry, 1999). Of greatest concern is the fact that many of the medications reviewed in this chapter have the potential to disrupt learning and cognitive functioning. Yet the field knows little about the specific cognitive effects of most of the medications that are typically used in clinical practice. In similar fashion, pharmacotherapy is generally used in the context of multimodal interventions; however, there is a dearth of information about the interaction of medications and other therapies in the treatment of childhood disorders. The specific relationship among type of medication, dosage, and type of psychosocial intervention should be explicated whenever possible. Finally, longitudinal studies of pharmacotherapeutic effects must be conducted, particularly for children exhibiting those disorders (e.g., ADHD and asthma) that frequently require chronic treatment with medication (Werry, 1999). With an expanding assessment technology and knowledge of the importance of behavioral and developmental factors, it is likely that significant advances in child pharmacotherapy will be forthcoming.

REFERENCES

Arnold, L. E., Janke, I., Waters, B., & Milch, A. (1999). Psychoactive effects of medical drugs. In J. S. Werry & M. G. Aman (Eds.), *Practitioner's guide to psychoactive drugs for children and adolescents* (2nd ed., pp. 387–412). New York: Plenum Press.

Barkley, R. A., Connor, D. F., & Kwasnik, D. (2000). Challenges to determining adolescent medication response in an outpatient clinical setting: Comparing Adderall and methylphenidate for ADHD. *Journal of Attention Disorders, 4*, 102–113.

Bender, B. G. (1999). Learning disorders associated with asthma and allergies. *School Psychology Review, 28*, 204–214.

Brown, R. T., & Sammons, M. T. (2002). Pediatric psychopharmacology: A review of new developments and recent research. *Professional Psychology: Research and Practice, 33*, 135–147.

Brown, R. T., & Sawyer, M. G. (1998). *Medications for school-age children: Effects on learning and behavior.* New York: Guilford Press.

Brown, R. T., Tanaka, O. F., & Donegan, J. E. (1998). Pain management. In L. Phelps (Ed.), *Health-related disorders in children and adolescents: A guidebook for understanding and educating* (pp. 501–513). Washington, DC: American Psychological Association.

Chan, H. S. L., & Erlichman, C. (1993). Cancer chemotherapy in pediatric malignancies. In I. C. Raddle & S. M. MacLeod (Eds.), *Pediatric pharmacology and therapeutics* (pp. 515–528). St. Louis, MO: Mosby.

Chappell, P. B., Leckman, J. F., & Riddle, M. A. (1995). The pharmacologic treatment of tic disorders. *Child and Adolescent Psychiatric Clinics of North America, 4*, 197–216.

Connor, D. F. (1998). Other medications in the treatment of child and adolescent ADHD. In R. A. Barkley (Ed.), *Attention-deficit hyperactivity disorder: A handbook for diagnosis and treatment* (2nd ed., pp. 564–581). New York: Guilford Press.

Denney, C. B., & Rapport, M. D. (2001). Cognitive pharmacology of stimulants in children with ADHD. In M. V. Solanto, A. F. T. Arnsten, & F. X. Castellanos (Eds.), *Stimulant drugs and ADHD: Basic and clinical neuroscience* (pp. 283–302). New York: Oxford University Press.

DuPaul, G. J., & Barkley, R. A. (1993). Behavioral contributions to pharmacotherapy: The utility of behavioral methodology in medication treatment of children with attention deficit hyperactivity disorder. *Behavior Therapy, 24*, 47–65.

DuPaul, G. J., Barkley, R. A., & Connor, D. F. (1998). Stimulants. In R. A. Barkley (Ed.), *Attention-deficit hyperactivity disorder: A handbook for diagnosis and treatment* (2nd ed., pp. 510–551). New York: Guilford Press.

Evans, S. W., Pelham, W. E., Smith, B. H., Bukstein, O., Gnagy, E. M., Greiner, A. R., et al. (2001). Dose–response effects of methylphenidate on ecologically valid measures of academic performance and classroom behavior in adolescents with ADHD. *Experimental and Clinical Psychopharmacology, 9*, 163–175.

Firestone, P., Musten, L. M., Pisterman, S., Mercer, J., & Bennett, S. (1998). Short-term side effects of stimulant medication are increased in preschool children with attention-deficit/hyperactivity disorder: A double blind placebo-controlled study. *Journal of Child and Adolescent Psychopharmacology, 8*, 13–25.

Gadow, K. D. (1986). *Children on medication: Vol. 1. Hyperactivity, learning disabilities, and mental retardation.* San Diego: College Hill Press.

Gadow, K. D. (1999). Prevalence of drug therapy. In J. S. Werry & M. G. Aman (Eds.), *Practitioner's guide to psychoactive drugs for children and adolescents* (2nd ed., pp. 51–67). New York: Plenum Press.

Gadow, K. D., Nolan, E. E., Paoliccelli, L. M., & Sprafkin, J. (1991). A procedure for assessing the effects of methylphenidate on hyperactive children in public school settings. *Journal of Clinical Child Psychology, 20*, 268–276.

Greenhill, L. L. (1998). The use of psychotropic medication in preschoolers: Indications, safety, and efficacy. *Canadian Journal of Psychiatry, 43*, 576–581.

Gutierrez, P. M., & Silk, K. R. (1998). Prescription privileges for psychologists: A review of the psychological literature. *Professional Psychology: Research and Practice, 29*, 213–222.

Handler, M. W., & DuPaul, G. J. (1999). Pharmacological issues and iatrogenic effects on learning. In R. T. Brown (Ed.), *Cognitive aspects of chronic illness in children* (pp. 355–385). New York: Guilford Press.

Hawkridge, S. M., & Stein, D. J. (1998). A risk–benefit assessment of pharmacotherapy for anxiety disorders in children and adolescents. *Drug Safety, 19*, 283–297.

Jacobsen, L. K., & Rapoport, J. L. (1998). Childhood-onset schizophrenia: Implications of clinical and neurobiological research. *Journal of Child Psychology and Psychiatry, 39*, 101–113.

James, A. C., & Javaloyes, A. M. (2001). Practitioner review: The treatment of bipolar disorder in children and adolescents. *Journal of Child Psychology and Psychiatry, 42*, 439–449.

Lemanek, K. L., Kamps, J., & Chung, N. B. (2001). Empirically supported treatments in pediatric psychology: Regimen adherence. *Journal of Pediatric Psychology, 26*, 253–275.

Litt, I. F. (1992). Compliance with pediatric medication regimens. In S. J. Yaffe & J. V. Aranda (Eds.), *Pediatric pharmacology: Therapeutic principles in practice* (pp. 45–54). Philadelphia: Saunders.

Moffatt, M. E. (1997). Nocturnal enuresis: A review of the efficacy of treatments and practical advice for clinicians. *Developmental and Behavioral Pediatrics, 18*, 49–56.

Morton, N. S. (1998). Prevention and control of pain in children. *Pain Reviews, 5*, 1–15.

Northup, J., & Gulley, V. (2001). Some contributions of functional analysis to the assessment of behaviors associated with attention deficit hyperactivity disorder and the effects of stimulant medication. *School Psychology Review, 30*, 227–238.

Northup, J., Gulley, V., Edwards, S., & Fountain, L. (2001). The effects of methylphenidate in the classroom: What dosage, for which children, for what problems? *School Psychology Quarterly, 16*, 303–323.

Owens, D. R., Zinman, B., & Bolli, G. B. (2001). Insulins today and beyond. *The Lancet, 358*, 739–746.

Park, L. T., Jefferson, J. W., & Greist, J. H. (1997). Obsessive–compulsive disorder: Treatment options. *CNS Drugs, 7*, 187–202.

Pelham, W. E., Gnagy, E. M., Burrows-Maclean, L., Williams, A., Fabiano, G. A., Morrisey, S. M., et al. (2001). Once-a-day Concerta methylphenidate versus three-times-daily methylphenidate in laboratory and natural settings. *Pediatrics, 107*(6), e105. Retrieved September 19, 2001, from *http://www.pediatrics.org/cgi/content/full/107/6/e105*

Phelps, L., Brown, R. T., & Power, T. J. (2002). *Pediatric psychopharmacology: Combining medical and psychosocial interventions.* Washington, DC: American Psychological Association.

Posey, D. J., & McDougle, C. J. (2000). The pharmacotherapy of target symptoms associated with autistic disorder and other pervasive developmental disorders. *Harvard Review of Psychiatry, 8*, 45–63.

Price, J. (2000). The role of inhaled corticosteroids in children with asthma. *Archives of Disease in Childhood, 82*, 10–14.

Rapoport, J. L., & Inoff-Germain, G. (2000). Practitioner review: Treatment of obsessive–compulsive disorder in children and adolescents. *Journal of Child Psychology and Psychiatry, 41*, 419–431.

Safer, D. J., & Zito, J. M. (2000). Pharmacoepidemiology of methylphenidate and other stimulants for the treatment of attention deficit hyperactivity disorder. In L. L. Greenhill & B. B. Osman (Eds.), *Ritalin: Theory and practice* (2nd ed., pp. 7–26). Larchmont, NY: Liebert.

Stoewe, J. K., Kruesi, M. J. P., & Lelio, D. F. (1995). Psychopharmacology of aggressive states and features of conduct disorder. *Child and Adolescent Psychiatric Clinics of North America, 4*, 359–379.

Szefler, S. J. (2000). Asthma: The new advances. *Advances in Pediatrics, 47*, 273–308.

Tarnowski, K. J., Brown, R. T., Dingle, A. D., & Dreelin, E. (1998). Pain management. In R. T. Ammerman & J. V. Campo (Eds.), *Handbook of pediatric psychology and psychiatry: Vol. II. Disease, injury, and illness* (pp. 1–15). Boston: Allyn & Bacon.

Waber, D. P., & Mullenix, P. J. (2000). Acute lymphoblastic leukemia. In K. O. Yeates, M. D. Ris, & H. G. Taylor (Eds.), *Pediatric neuropsychology: Research, theory, and practice* (pp. 300–319). New York: Guilford Press.

Wagner, K. D., & Ambrosini, P. J. (2001). Childhood depression: Pharmacological therapy/treatment (Pharmacotherapy of childhood depression). *Journal of Clinical Child Psychology, 30*, 88–97.

Werry, J. S. (1999). Introduction: A guide for practitioners, professionals, and public. In J. S. Werry & M. G. Aman (Eds.), *Practitioner's guide to psychoactive drugs for children and adolescents* (2nd ed., pp. 3–22). New York: Plenum Press.

Werry, J. S., & Aman, M. G. (1999). Anxiolytics, sedatives, and miscellaneous drugs. In J. S. Werry & M. G. Aman (Eds.), *Practitioner's guide to psychoactive drugs for children and adolescents* (2nd ed., pp. 433–469). New York: Plenum Press.

Wilens, T. E., & Spencer, T. J. (2000). The stimulants revisited. *Child & Adolescent Psychiatric Clinics of North America, 9*, 573–603.

Wilens, T. E., Spencer, T. J., Frazier, J., & Biederman, J. (1998). Child and adolescent psychopharmacology. In T. H. Ollendick & M. Hersen (Eds.), *Handbook of child psychopathology* (3rd ed., pp. 603–636). New York: Plenum Press.

Williams, J., & Sharp, G. B. (2000). Epilepsy. In K. O. Yeates, M. D. Ris, & H. G. Taylor (Eds.), *Pediatric neuropsychology: Research, theory, and practice* (pp. 47–73). New York: Guilford Press.

Zametkin, A. J., & Yamada, E. M. (1999). Monitoring and measuring drug effects: I. Physical effects. In J. S. Werry & M. G. Aman (Eds.), *Practitioner's guide to psychoactive drugs for children and adolescents* (2nd ed., pp. 3–22). New York: Plenum Press.

Zito, J. M., Safer, D. J., dosReis, S., Gardner, J. F., Boles, M., & Lynch, F. (2000). Trends in the prescribing of psychotropic medications to preschoolers. *Journal of the American Medical Association, 283*, 1025–1030.

Part III

CHRONIC MEDICAL CONDITIONS: RESEARCH AND CLINICAL APPLICATIONS

15

Neonatology, Prematurity, NICU, and Developmental Issues

GLEN P. AYLWARD

Pediatric psychologists are frequently involved in the care and assessment of children who are born at biological risk. Such risk includes prematurity (< 37 weeks gestational age) and low birthweight, as well as exposure to potential central nervous system (CNS) insults such as asphyxia, prenatal drug use, or maternal infections during pregnancy. The range of involvement includes developmental assessment, infant stimulation, family consultation, early intervention services, longitudinal follow-up, addressing subsequent health-related issues, or identification of later cognitive, neuropsychological, academic, or behavioral problems (Aylward, 1997). Services are provided in neonatal nurseries, follow-up clinics, developmental diagnostic programs, outpatient ambulatory settings, or schools.

Improved survival rates of low birthweight (LBW; < 2,500 grams), very low birthweight (VLBW; < 1,500 grams), and extremely low birthweight (ELBW; < 1,000 grams) babies have increased the need for services in this population. LBW accounts for approximately 7.4% of births. With regard to survival, 49% of babies born in the 501- to 750-grams weight range, 85% of those 751 to 1,000 grams, 93% born at 1,001 to 1,250 grams, and 95% in the 1,251- to 1,500-gram range survive (Stevenson et al., 1998). Survival rates in smaller ELBW babies (i.e., those < 800 grams), and those born at 23–24 weeks gestation have more than doubled (Hack, Friedman, & Fanaroff, 1996). Much of the improvement in survival of these smaller babies is attributable to increased use of antenatal steroids, more aggressive approaches to delivery room resuscitation, and surfactant replacement (Hack & Fanaroff, 1999). However, infants born between 501 and 1,500 grams contribute disproportionately to perinatal mortality and morbidity rates, despite accounting for approximately 1% of deliveries (Stevenson et al., 1998). Improvements in medical technology also have enhanced survival rates of larger babies who have sustained CNS insults, raising concern that the increase in the absolute number of infants exposed to potential CNS damage who now survive will produce a higher rate of neurodevelopmental morbidity (Bregman, 1998).

Children with LBW make up a heterogeneous group that includes preterm infants, as well as babies born at term but who are below normal in weight due to abnormal maternal or fetal conditions. Prior to the 1990s, infants were primarily grouped by birthweight versus gestational age, due to inaccuracy in obstetrical estimation of gestational age or postnatal assessment. With refinement of fetal ultrasound techniques, estimation of gestational age has become more precise, and gestational age is a stronger determinant of organ/system maturation and viability than is birthweight. Sole use of a birthweight cutoff as the prime descriptor is confounded because it could include (1) extremely preterm infants who are average for gestational age (AGA); (2) less-preterm infants who are small for gestational age (SGA; < 3rd or < 10th percentile, depending on cutoff employed); or (3) older preterm or full-term infants who are extremely SGA (Touwen, 1986). SGA babies often have better survival rates than their AGA counterparts because of a higher gestational age and corresponding degree of maturity; conversely, they often have higher developmental morbidity (particularly SGA preterm babies) than their AGA counterparts with the same gestational age (Bos, Einspieler, & Prechtl, 2001). Therefore, birthweight and gestational age are critical considerations.

A gradient of developmental sequelae exists in children that is inversely related to decreasing birthweight. The smaller the baby, the greater the likelihood of problems. However, when considering this gradient, birthweight must be viewed in conjunction with other biomedical and environmental risks. The incidence of major disabilities, which include moderate to severe mental retardation, sensorineural hearing loss or blindness, cerebral palsy, and epilepsy, is 6–8% in babies with LBW, 14–17% in infants with VLBW, and 20–25% in children born with ELBW. In comparison, major handicaps occur in 5% of full-term infants (Bennett & Scott, 1997; Halsey, Collin, & Anderson, 1993; Hack, Taylor, & Klein, 1995). These rates of handicap have remained relatively constant over the past decade. However, the nature of impairment may be changing, with significant problems frequently being found in infants previously considered to be "nondisabled." These high-prevalence–low-severity dysfunctions appear to be increasing, and they include learning disabilities, borderline mental retardation, attention-deficit/hyperactivity disorders, specific neuropsychological deficits (e.g., visual motor integration), and behavioral problems. These high-prevalence–low-severity dysfunctions occur in 50–70% of infants with VLBW, again with an inverse birthweight gradient being found (Goyen, Lui, & Woods, 1998; O'Callaghan et al., 1996; Msall et al., 1991; Taylor, Klein, & Hack, 2000). More than one-half of children born at VLBW will require special education services, 20% or more will need a self-contained learning disabilities placement, and 16–20% will repeat at least one grade. However, the situation is compounded by the fact that the social, ethnic, and educational backgrounds of mothers of these infants may also influence the prevalence of these disabilities.

Whereas major disabilities are often identified during infancy, high-prevalence–low-severity dysfunctions become more obvious at school entry and later. There are no good predictors of these more subtle problems that can be identified during infancy or preschool age. It is extremely difficult to determine early on whether identified problems are indicative of continuing recovery or catch-up from the negative effects of extremely low gestational age and birthweight or of the emergence of the true impact of a more permanent handicap. This difficulty is due to continued cortical development, as well as to increased demands for performance in areas previously not emphasized.

Multiple factors are associated with a condition such as ELBW or intrauterine exposure to cocaine. These include severity of neonatal course (days in hospital, other medical conditions), sociodemographic factors (socioeconomic status, social support, race), subsequent illness (hospitalizations), maternal physical and mental health, and environmental exposures to positive and negative experiences (early intervention, lead, smoking in household). Neurodevelopmental, cognitive, behavioral, health-related quality of life (HRQL), functional, and social outcomes (social development, self-concept) are also of concern.

Various risk scores and neonatal admission severity scores for physiological status and intensity of therapeutic intervention have been developed (e.g., Brazy, Eckerman, Oehler, Goldstein, & O'Rand, 1991; Korner et al., 1993; Richardson, Gray, McCormick, Workman-Daniels, & Goldmann, 1993). These often prove helpful in clarifying an infant's medical course and the likelihood of sequelae. The major sources of morbidity in the neonatal period are intracranial events, pulmonary immaturity, and infections (McCormick, 1989). Therefore, severe ultrasound abnormality (Grades III or IV intraventricular hemorrhage [IVH], periventricular leukomalacia [PVL], periventricular hemorrhagic infarction [PVI]—discussed subsequently), septicemia, necrotizing enterocolitis, chronic lung disease (oxygen dependence ≥ 36 weeks conceptional age [age, corrected for prematurity]) and bronchopulmonary dysplasia (BPD), apnea of prematurity, and signs of asphyxia such as seizures, are indicators of increased risk for problems. Number of days the infant remains hospitalized after birth is often considered a marker for biological risk. However, this marker is disproportionately affected by infants with extremely low gestational ages. Medical status postdischarge is important, as subsequent hospitalizations are associated with lower verbal, visual–perceptual, and visual–motor scores and less positive teacher ratings (Zelkowitz, Papageorgiou & Allard, 1994). Nutritional adequacy is also a critical postnatal influence because of the developing brain's need for folic acid, iron, vitamins, fatty acids, and other nutrients.

Age correction for prematurity (subtracting the weeks of prematurity from the child's chronological age) is applied when preterm infants are followed longitudinally; however, correction is controversial. The general consensus, though not unanimous, is that correction should occur arguably up to 2 years of age (Blasco, 1989; Hunt & Rhodes, 1977; Lems, Hopkins, & Sampson, 1993). Age correction reflects a biological/maturational perspective, whereas use of chronological age represents an environmentally based orientation. Adjustment for prematurity is assumed to differentiate transient effects of preterm birth from more persistent deficits, although some argue that it simply masks deficits. Imprecise gestational age estimation, concomitant medical issues, and a lack of consensus regarding whether to correct to 37 or 40 weeks are additional confounds. Although correction is considered less of an issue at ages 6 to 8 years, the mean increment in the Verbal IQ with adjustment was 5.2 points (range 2–8), the increment in Performance IQ was 7 points (range 4–11), and the average increase in the Full Scale IQ was 5.8 points (range 2–10; Aylward, Pfeiffer, Wright, & Verhulst, 1989). Conclusions about later functioning of infants with VLBW and ELBW will differ, depending on whether corrected or uncorrected scores are employed.

Finally, it is difficult to accurately determine probabilities of later outcomes for premature infants and those at biological risk because the literature is not consistent. Variations in medical management techniques in different neonatal intensive care units (NICUs), varying foci of study, diversity in study populations, mediating and moderating effects of the environment, type of follow-up assessments, and duration of follow-up preclude easy interpretation (Aylward, 2002a).

With regard to developmental issues in infants born preterm, subsequent outcome is the result of an interchange between normal developmental processes, recovery of neurodevelopmental function in response to varying CNS insults, improvement in physical status, and environmental influences (Aylward, 1997). Moreover, reciprocal, bidirectional influences exist between the infant and environment: The infant can influence the caretaker, just as the caretaker can influence the infant. There is a transaction over time between infant and environment, with the infant bringing behavioral predispositions such as temperament or consequences of CNS or physical insults (e.g., irritability) to such transactions. A supportive environment can facilitate self-righting in the child (Sameroff & Chandler, 1975). Therefore, characteristics of either the child or the environment can potentially be either protective or risk producing in nature. An accumulation of risk factors—child-related, environmental, or both—increases the draw toward less optimal outcomes (Wolraich, Felice, & Drotar, 1996).

THE CONCEPT OF RISK IN INFANCY

Risk refers to variables whose presence have a potentially negative influence on development. There are three categories of risk: established, biological, and environmental (Tjossem, 1976). Established risks are medical conditions of a known etiology whose compromised developmental outcome is well documented (e.g., genetic disorders, HIV in infancy). As indicated previously, biological risks include exposure to potentially noxious prenatal, perinatal, or postnatal events such as IVH, hypoxic–ischemic encephalopathy (HIE), or LBW. Environmental risks include the quality of the caregiver–infant interaction, opportunities for developmental and cognitive stimulation, and health care. Adverse environmental risks such as low socioeconomic status (SES) and poor social support can increase the likelihood of compromised outcome. Relationships between social class, perinatal complications, and cognitive development are complex and intertwined. As a result, many children are exposed to both biological and environmental risk, this combination sometimes being referred to as "double jeopardy" or "double hazard" (Escalona, 1982; Parker, Greer, & Zuckerman, 1988). In these cases, nonoptimal biological and environmental risks work synergistically to negatively affect later function (Aylward, 1990, 1992). There is a ceiling effect, in which a severe degree of biological risk will minimize the impact of environmental influences. This effect has been shown in the follow-up of smaller infants with ELBW (e.g., < 750 grams) or babies with LBW involved in the Infant Health and Development Program intervention study (Aylward, 1996; McCormick, McCarton, Brooks-Gunn, Belt, & Gross, 1998; Taylor, Klein, Minich, & Hack, 2000).

Established and Biological Risks

There are many causes for developmental problems in neonates and infants. These include infections and genetic, nutritional, metabolic, traumatic, intoxicant, maternal prenatal disease-related, anoxic–hypoxic, or idiopathic factors (Risser & Edgell, 1988). The timing of exposure to these etiological agents is important (Aylward, 1997). A *critical period* is the time during which the action of a specific internal or external influence is necessary (critical) for normal development. A *sensitive period* is the time during which the CNS is highly susceptible to the effects of harmful or deleterious internal or external conditions. A critical period occurs when certain conditions are necessary for the CNS to develop normally; a sensitive period is the time in which damage to the CNS can lead to alterations, reorganization, and potential disruptions in the system. Critical periods generally are very circumscribed, whereas sensitive periods are more variable (e.g., Capone, 1996).

Approximately 3% of births show evidence of major malformations (Paneth, 1995), and these often develop during critical periods. In the prenatal period, problems in the *dor-*

sal induction phase of CNS development (3–4 weeks gestation; closure of the neural tube) result in so-called neural tube problems such as anencephaly (open skull with missing parts of the brain), encephalocele (protruding brain tissue), myelomeningocele (spina bifida; incomplete closure of the spinal cord), or congenital hydrocephalus (increased pressure and enlarged ventricles due to fluid backup). Problems in the *ventral induction phase* (5–6 weeks; major portions of the brain are formed) result in abnormalities of the face or brain and include holoprosencephaly (single-lobed brain) or Dandy Walker malformation (agenesis of cerebellar hemispheres). Disruptions in the *proliferation phase* (2–4 months; production of nerve cells) result in too many or too few neurons being produced, causing conditions such as microcephaly or megalencephaly (macrocephaly). Disruptions in the *migration phase* (3–5 months; movement of nerve cells from site of origin [germinal matrix] to final position) produce anomalous formation of the cortical plate, resulting in disorders such as schizencephaly (thickened cortical mantle with seams or clefts), lissencephaly (absence of gyri, resulting in a smooth brain), polymicrogyria (small gyri with shallow convolutions), heterotopias (neuronal migration to wrong locations), or agenesis of the corpus callosum. Problems in *organization/differentiation* of the brain (peak age 6 months gestation through third postnatal year; dendritic, axonal, and synaptic development) result in disorders in neural differentiation or in the development of synapses, causing aberrant cortical circuitry. Finally, disruptions in *myelination* (occurring over a prolonged period from sixth month of gestation into adulthood) result in nerve conduction problems and include cerebral white matter hypoplasia (underdevelopment). In addition, amino acid deficits (e.g., phenylketonuria), inborn errors of metabolism, degenerative diseases (e.g., adrenoleukodystrophy), and early malnutrition can affect myelin development. Dorsal and ventral induction and proliferation occur prenatally, whereas migration may occur postnatally in preterm infants. Organization/differentiation and myelination occur prenatally and postnatally in all babies (Giedd, 1997). Established or environmental risks can affect any of the stages discussed, and the areas having the highest metabolic activity at the time of exposure will be most affected.

Low Birthweight

It becomes difficult to separate out biological risk that arises solely as a consequence of preterm birth from the specific effects attributable to perinatal insults such as IVH or HIE. These latter insults most likely are moderators of prematurity per se. Even in the absence of identifiable nonoptimal CNS events, preterm birth is characterized by a failure of brain structures to proceed in a predictable temporal and spatial sequence. More specifically, there is a disruption of organizational events. Being born LBW or smaller most likely also has an effect on biosynthesis of neurotransmitters such as dopamine. Some data suggest that neonatal ultrasounds are not sensitive enough to detect subtle injury to gray or white matter that becomes more apparent on magnetic resonance imaging (MRI) performed in adolescence (Stewart et al., 1999). These abnormalities are more prevalent in individuals born very preterm than in full-term controls. Even preterm infants without IVH have smaller volumes than controls in brain structures such as the basal ganglia, corpus callosum, amygdala, and hippocampus (Peterson et al., 2000). It appears that subplate neurons, the basal ganglia, the thalamus, and the hippocampus are particular areas of vulnerability (Perlman, 2001). Disruptions in white matter involve myelination and dendritic connections and would have an impact on cortical and subcortical circuits. Therefore, the brain of the baby born prematurely is not organized in the same manner as that of a full-term infant. Reduced size of the posterior body of the corpus callosum may be related to later IQ deficits due to poor interhemispheric interaction; disruption of circuits connecting frontal, striatal, and thalamic regions may be associated with dysregulation of attention and arousal (attention deficits and executive dysfunction), whereas reduced hippocampal volume is associated with memory deficits and weaknesses in numeracy (Isaacs et al., 2000). Moreover, prematurity itself may be a reflection of preexisting risk conditions that have affected the fetus prior to preterm birth—conditions that negatively affect brain development of the fetus and cause the mother to deliver prematurely. Undoubtedly, there exists a gradient in which disruption in corticogenesis and connectivity is inversely related to birthweight and/or to gestational age (particularly less than 33 weeks), even in the absence of other concomitant biomedical risks such as IVH.

Asphyxia

The spectrum of CNS disorders following perinatal insults is determined by the brain's maturational stage at the time of the insult, as well as the nature and severity of the insult (Aylward, 1997; Hill & Volpe, 1989). As a result, the effects of a particular type of CNS event will differ in preterm and full-term infants. Pediatric psychologists will encounter several terms that are related to biological risk during the perinatal period. *Hypoxemia* is a reduction of oxygen in the blood (brain hypoxia is a reduction of oxygen to brain tissue). *Ischemia* is defined as reduced blood flow to the brain, while *asphyxia* is a disturbed exchange of oxygen and carbon dioxide due to an interruption in respiration that results in hypoxemia, hypercarbia (increased carbon dioxide), and acidemia (decreased blood pH). Asphyxia is accompanied by multisystem organ dysfunction (cardiovascular, gastrointestinal, pulmonary, and renal). Hypoxic–ischemic encephalopathy (HIE) refers to a deprivation of oxygen to the brain due to the combined effects of hypoxemia and ischemia. *Anoxia* refers to complete lack of oxygen.

Asphyxia has traditionally been indexed as a low Apgar score (range 0–10, based on heart rate, respiratory effort, reflex irritability, muscle tone, and color). However, Apgar scores have been misused and are not predictive of subsequent outcome. A low 1-minute Apgar score does not correlate with later outcome (American Academy of Pediatrics, 1996; Aylward, 1993), and even a low 5-minute score has limited utility. This score may be more useful if change between 1 and 5 minutes is considered. Apgar scores should simply be considered indicative of the infant's condition during and immediately after birth—the original purpose of the score. In fact, normal Apgar scores are found in 75% of children who later are diagnosed with cerebral palsy. Therefore, caution should be exercised when considering low Apgar scores as the cause of later intellectual or academic problems in children; in fact, much of the injury could have occurred prior to birth. However, asphyxia is the precipitating event for HIE, and perinatal HIE is the major cause of neurodevelopmental morbidity in the neonatal period (Volpe, 1998).

In full-term infants, HIE causes cell death in the cerebral cortex, diencephalon, brainstem, and cerebellum. Injury to the basal ganglia and thalamus also occurs. Moderate and severe HIE in term infants is associated with a high incidence of cognitive and motor dysfunction, including microcephaly, mental retardation, epilepsy, and cerebral palsy. Mild HIE (Stage I) lasts less than 24 hours, and the infant displays hyperalertness, uninhibited reflexes, irritability, and jitteriness. Later cognitive and academic problems are minimal. Moderate HIE (Stage II) is characterized by lethargy, stupor, hypotonia, depressed primitive reflexes, seizures, and decreased movements. This persists for approximately 1 week, and 20–

40% of these babies will have sequelae. Severe HIE (Stage III) involves coma, flaccid tone, seizures, increased intracranial pressure, and suppressed brainstem function. Virtually all survivors have significant cognitive and psychoeducational sequelae.

In the preterm infant, HIE causes cell death deeper within the brain, namely, in the white matter behind and to the side of the lateral ventricles (periventricular leukomalacia; PVL). There is less effect on gray matter in preterm than in full-term infants, and this insult is more often associated with spasticity, neurosensory, and motor problems than with cognitive deficits per se. *Periventricular/intraventricular hemorrhage* (PVH/IVH) involves bleeding into the subependymal germinal matrix (site of cell proliferation), and this occurs in 35–45% of infants under 32 weeks' gestational age, with even higher percentages found in babies with lower gestational ages. HIE, respiratory distress, or circulatory problems can produce PVH/IVH, and obstructive hydrocephalus is a frequent result. IVH is graded (I–IV) based on the amount of blood in the ventricles and degree of distention, with grades III and IV being considered severe. Grade I involves subependymal/germinal matrix hemorrhage with no or minimal IVH (< 10% of ventricular area); Grade II involves 10–50% of the ventricular area without ventricular dilatation; and Grade III involves more than 50% of the ventricular area, with distension of the lateral ventricles. Grade IV includes intracerebral involvement or other parenchymal lesion (with 60% mortality rate), and it is thought not to be on a continuum, reflecting *periventricular hemorrhagic infarction* (PVI). PVI involves death of periventricular white matter, is large and asymmetric, and involves frontal–parieto–occipital regions with alterations in hemispheric connectivity (see Aylward, 1997). The risk of disability at preschool and school age increases directly in relation to the grade of IVH: 5–10% of children with Grade I, 15–20% with Grade II, 35–50% with Grade III, and greater than 90% with Grade IV will have school problems.

The consequences of HIE are due to a so-called neurotoxic cascade in which the excitatory amino acid, glutamate, is released, binds to receptors, hyperexcites the cell, and depletes it of energy. There is an influx of calcium into the cell, and this, coupled with continued excitation, causes "death by calcium" (Dammann & Leviton, 1999). Essentially, there is necrosis (cell swells, ruptures, or bursts, and its contents cause inflammation to adjacent cells) and apoptosis (shrinkage of the cell, similar to programmed cell death). The second wave of damage occurs with reperfusion, in which free radicals (unpaired outer orbital electron) and nitric oxide cause more injury, and granulocytes plug microvessels. The scenario is further compounded by several developmental components in preterm babies: (1) immature blood-brain barriers, (2) incomplete myelination, and (3) suboptimal levels of endogenous cell neuroprotectors (called neurotrophins or oligotrophins). This course of events produces white matter damage. Maternal infections during pregnancy will release proinflammatory cytokines that prompt premature labor and produce white matter damage in the premature infant, as discussed previously (Perlman, 1998). In fact, the combination of maternal infection and HIE increases the rate of cerebral palsy seventyfold in full-term infants. Therefore, the same insult may have a different pattern of damage as one moves away from the focal site of injury, depending on the gradient of necrosis and apoptosis.

CNS Infections

Cytomegalovirus (CMV) is the most common viral disease transmitted in utero. It results in intrauterine growth retardation (IUGR), microcephaly, seizures, mental retardation, retinal problems, and hearing loss, particularly if symptoms are evident at birth (90% are asymptomatic at birth). The virus is particularly devastating to rapidly growing germinal cells, leading to periventricular lesions. *Toxoplasmosis* is caused by a protozoan parasite (often introduced by cats) to asymptomatic mothers who then transmit the parasite to the fetus after the second month of gestation. Resultant problems include prematurity, microcephaly, hydrocephalus, seizures, CNS calcifications, and chorioretinitis (eye damage). Later emergence of intellectual deficits may occur. *Congenital rubella* is characterized by IUGR, cataracts and other eye problems, microcephaly, hearing deficits, and other organ involvement. Approximately 25% of exposed infants have neurological symptoms at birth, and 33–40% display psychomotor retardation by the end of the first year. Timing of infection is critical, as severe CNS malformation occurs if the virus is introduced before the 12th week of gestation, deafness if introduced at 13–16 weeks, and mental retardation with introduction in the second trimester. *Herpes simplex virus* (HSV) Type 2 affects the fetus in the first 20 weeks of pregnancy and, more frequently, at birth; severe brain abnormalities, mental retardation, and seizures may occur. Maternal transmission of *human immunodeficiency virus* (HIV) to the developing fetus occurs in 30% of cases, and vertical transmission (prenatal, perinatal, or postnatal mother–child transmission) accounts for the largest number of cases. Although virtually all infants born to HIV-positive mothers test positive for the virus at birth, they may not actually be infected—infants passively acquire maternal antibodies in utero. Many infected infants die by 12–18 months; survival time after diagnosis depends on a number of variables: timing of infection, premature birth, route of transmission (vertical or horizontal), and other acquired infections. The terms "HIV encephalopathy" or "neuroaids" are used to refer to children with delayed motor and/or mental milestones, abnormal motor signs, weakness, disordered brainstem function, ataxia, blindness, secondary microcephaly, and seizures. Three patterns of developmental decline emerge: (1) infants who demonstrate symptoms very early, with a progressive decline and plummeting loss of developmental milestones; (2) those who develop deterioration in early childhood or school age (median age, 6 years), with attentional and academic difficulties being markers of a deteriorating course; and (3) children who display a more subacute course, interrupted by plateaus, with milestone acquisition being initially slow, followed by a protracted plateau without newly acquired skills, accompanied by mild spasticity. The developmental course of HIV is affected by drug treatment.

Drugs

A variety of drugs can have teratogenic effects on the development and function of the CNS; however, outcome is affected by a complex matrix of environmental, physiological, and timing and chronicity issues. For example, *cocaine hydrochloride* crosses the placenta easily and affects nerve endings and chemical messenger transmission (dopamine). Indirect injury occurs as a result of drug effects on maternal physiology (rise in maternal and fetal systolic blood pressure, reduction in uterine blood flow, decreased fetal oxygenation). Direct injury is the result of the influence of the drug on fetal and peripheral nervous system development (e.g., dopamine depletion). The drug affects the regions of the brain crucial for learning, memory, behavioral, and cognitive functions. As a result, infants have problems of state modulation, increased irritability, poor habituation, and behavior (Bendersky & Lewis, 1998; Phillips, Sharma, Premachandra, Vaughn, & Reyes-Lee, 1996). *Ethanol* exposure can lead to full-blown fetal alcohol syndrome (FAS), more subtle fetal alcohol effects (FAE), or alcohol-related neurodevelopmental disorder (ARND; Sampson et al., 1997). The effects of prenatal alcohol exposure should be considered to occur on a continuum, with FAE occurring more than twice as frequently as FAS. Ethanol exposure may affect all organ systems and induce fetal hypoxia. The diagnosis of FAS is made when a recognizable pattern of malformation is noted; FAE is less specific. Many infants are SGA, and during infancy, 75% show irritability, tremulousness, difficulties with sucking, and hypotonia. Microcephaly, learning disabilities, perceptual problems, mild mental retardation, delayed adaptive behavior, ADHD, and behavior problems may occur. Amount, timing, duration, and polydrug usage in conjunction with alcohol will determine the type and severity of sequelae. In addition, some *antiepileptic medications* may cause CNS malformations, IUGR, and later behavioral and cognitive changes. *Narcotics* (heroin, methadone, codeine) may produce IUGR, premature birth, withdrawal symptoms, and microcephaly.

In summary, biological and established risks entail genetic disturbances, trauma, hemorrhage, stroke, infection, hypoxia and ischemia, and toxins. Each directly and indirectly affects some portion of the brain or prevents normal development and maturation (Aylward, 1997).

Environmental Risk

Environmental risk is a powerful moderator of development in infancy, and IQ scores in children from disadvantaged families are typically 0.5 to 1 standard deviation below average. Socioeconomic status (SES) is typically represented by maternal education and occupational status. However, SES is highly variable within middle- and lower-class categories. Social support includes tangible components (e.g., housing) and intangible components (e.g., attitudes, encouragement to achieve). The environment involves both process and status features. Process features are more proximal aspects of the environment that are experienced most directly (mother–infant interaction). Status features are distal and broader, involving more indirectly experienced environmental aspects (e.g., social class, location of residence). Environmental effects become increasingly apparent between 18 and 36 months, with 24 months being an age that is cited frequently (Murphy, Nichter, & Liden, 1982). Process or proximal environmental variables are more predictive of subsequent outcome early on; status or distal factors are more predictive at school age or later (Aylward, 1990, 1992, 1996). Measurement of occupational status or other distal variables in isolation may not accurately reflect the type of parenting to which a child is exposed, nor does it provide appreciation of everyday stresses or day-to-day positive aspects of the environment that may serve to buffer the infant from negative factors associated with global environmental risk.

Therefore, the components of environmental risk are complex and include family risk (social support, parent–child interaction, stressful life events, organization) and social-class risk (SES, parental education; Bendersky & Lewis, 1994). Certain aspects of the environment mediate the effects of other environmental variables on outcome, varying by the age of the child. For example, in a recent investigation, environmental risks (unemployment, high family density, depression in parent, stressful life events) influenced outcome at 1 to 3 years, poverty (family income) exerted influence at 2 and 3 years, and neighborhood affluence influenced development at age 3 (Kato-Klebanov, Brooks-Gunn, McCarton, & McCormick, 1998). Isolated or single environmental factors have a small, incremental effect on later cognitive function. The accumulation of risk factors is the major contributor to developmental morbidity (Sameroff, Seifer, Barocas, Zax, & Greenspan, 1987). Hence, negative components of the environment have a synergistic or additive effect on infants who are biologically vulnerable vis-à-vis the transactional (Sameroff & Chandler, 1975) or "risk-route" models (Aylward & Kenny, 1979). Both models assume that a degree of plasticity exists in both the child and the environment. The child is constantly reorganizing and self-righting, and the environment can facilitate or impede resiliency, leading to a "continuum of caretaking casualty" (Sameroff & Chandler, 1975). Therefore, environment and resilience processes (Masten, 2001) must be considered as part of the mix when working with children with biomedical and environmental risk factors.

Medical and biological factors were found to determine whether a developmental problem occurred, but environmental factors had a tempering or exacerbating effect on the degree of the problem (Hunt, Cooper, & Tooley, 1988). However, there is a gradient between more severe biological risk such as ELBW and outcome in which environmental effects are minimized, probably because of the overwhelming impact of biomedical issues (Hack, Taylor, Klein, & Minich,, 2000). Similar limiting effects of biological risk were found in the Infant Health and Development Program (IHDP; Infant Health and Development Program, 1990). This multisite study, evaluating the effects of early intervention over 8 years, found that, although there was a main effect for intervention, when the LBW group was divided into heavier (2,001–2,500 grams) and lighter (< 2,001 grams) subgroups, differences between intervention and control groups varied and were generally evident only in the heavier babies (McCormick et al., 1998). The biomedical and environmental risk interaction becomes highly complex when one considers school and functional outcomes. In general, biomedical variables are related to neurological, neuromotor, neuropsychological, and perceptual-performance functions. Environmental variables are more strongly associated with verbal, academic, and IQ measures. However, with regard to psychoeducational issues, recent data suggest that perinatal variables are related to physical impairment, sensory impairment, and profound and trainable mental handicap; sociodemographic influences are associated with emotional handicap and speech and language impairment. Both biomedical and environmental risks are related to educable mental handicap and specific learning impairment (Resnick et al., 1998).

OUTCOMES

Later outcome is perhaps the primary issue facing pediatric psychologists who work with children born prematurely. There exists an array of possible outcomes of interest: medical/physical, neurological, cognitive, academic, motor, neuropsychological, social competency, and behavioral (Aylward, 2002b). Recently, there has been increased emphasis on a broader, multidimensional conceptualization of outcome, namely, functional and health-related quality of life (HRQL; McCormick, 1997; Vohr & Msall, 1997). Unfortunately, the follow-up literature contains methodological problems that make it difficult to distill findings and identify meaningful trends (Aylward, 2002a; Aylward et al., 1989). Moreover, there is no true "gold standard" in developmental assessment. Therefore, sensitivity and specificity are not appropriate; instead, "copositivity" and "conegativity" are more accurate in situations in which scores on one test are compared with those obtained on another reference standard. The Bayley Scales of Infant Development (BSID) and the more recent BSID-II are typically considered the best criterion measures during infancy, although controversy surrounds the BSID-II regarding which beginning item set should be used (based on corrected or uncorrected scores; Gauthier, Bauer, Messinger, & Closius, 1999; Washington, Scott, Johnson, Wendel, & Hay, 1998). It is also estimated that mean IQ/DQ (developmental quotient) on a given test increases one-half point per year, or 3–5 points per decade (Flynn, 1999). Therefore, the mean score of a test developed in the 1970s conceivably could increase by as much as 15 points. School entry or beyond is the best endpoint for determination of outcome because HRQL, academic achievement, and other high prevalence–low-severity dysfunctions are better identified at that time. These issues must be considered when summarizing outcomes of children born prematurely.

Intelligence Quotients

Comparison of infants born LBW with smaller infants and controls has consistently produced a 0.3 to 0.6 standard deviation decrease in IQ in children born prematurely. The decrement (excluding children with major handicaps) generally ranges from 3.8 to 9.3 IQ points, with some outliers having 12- to 17-point differences (Aylward et al., 1989; Breslau, DelDotto, & Brown, 1994; Whitfield, Eckstein, & Grunau, 1997). Higher percentages of borderline IQ have been reported in the ELBW population, with estimates ranging from 13–15% (Whitfield et al., 1997) and with some estimates being as high as 37% at age 2 years (Vohr et al., 2000). A gradient or linear trend exists in which heavier birthweights are associated with higher IQ scores; more than double the number of LBW and smaller infants have IQ scores that are 1 *SD* below the mean. In one study, the likelihood of a later-measured IQ being less than 70 was 9.54 times greater in infants under 750 grams and 2.15 times greater in infants 750–1,499 grams than in normal birthweight babies (Hack et al., 2000; Taylor et al., 2000). Therefore, children born ELBW and VLBW who do not have major handicaps have mean group IQ scores that fall in the borderline to average range of intelligence, with the majority of studies suggesting that low average scores are the mode (Aylward, 2002b).

Visual–Motor Skills

The majority of ELBW and VLBW babies appear to manifest some type of visual-motor problem (Dewey, Crawford, Creighton, & Sauve, 1999; Goyen et al., 1998; Whitfield et al., 1997). Deficits are apparent on neuropsychological tasks such as copying, perceptual matching, spatial processing, finger tapping, pegboard performance, visual memory, and visual–sequential memory. Once again, the lower the birthweight, the greater the likelihood of problems. Estimates of visual–perceptual and visual–motor integrative problems are in the 11–20% range, and fine motor problems are as high as 71% in children with ELBW (Goyen et al., 1998). Fine motor problems are thought to be the basis for these visual–motor deficits. Even in children with VLBW who showed no developmental problems at age 3, motor and visual–motor deficits were found at school age, suggesting a strong link with prematurity per se (Dewey et al., 1999).

Language

Many language functions (particularly vocabulary and receptive language) are reasonably intact in children with LBW. However, more complex verbal processes, such as understanding of syntax, abstract verbal skills, verb production, and mean length of utterance (MLU), have been found deficient in comparison with normal birthweight peers (Le Normand & Cohen, 1999). These deficits are subtle but critical in social and academic endeavors.

School/Learning Difficulties

More than one-half of children with VLBW and 60–70% of children with ELBW require special assistance in school. By middle-school age, children with ELBW are 3 to 5 times more likely to have learning problems in reading, mathematics, spelling, or writing (O'Callaghan et al., 1996). By adolescence there is an eight- to tenfold increase in the necessity for remedial education resources or special educational needs in comparison with full-term controls (Saigal, Stoskopf, Streiner, & Burrows, 2001; Taylor et al., 2000). An inverse gradient is found with respect to learning difficulties: 50–63% in those born under 750 grams, 30–38% in those 750–1,499 grams, and a 7–18% rate in full-term infants (Breslau, 1995; Halsey, Collin, & Anderson, 1996; Taylor et al., 2000). Many of these children display nonverbal learning disabilities (NVLD). More specifically, verbal cognitive skills are better than nonverbal abilities; visual–motor integrative abilities, visual perception, mathematics, spatial skills, and fine motor speed are affected. Verbal abstracting, reading comprehension, written output, and social skills are additional areas of deficit. A higher prevalence of problems in executive function, such as organization, planning, problem solving, and abstracting, has been reported.

Behavioral Issues

Symptoms suggestive of attention-deficit/hyperactivity disorder (ADHD) are reported to occur 2.6 times more frequently in children born with VLBW or ELBW, with some estimates indicating a sixfold increase; 9–10% of adolescents born with ELBW are reported to have ADHD (Breslau, 1995; Saigal et al., 2001; Taylor, Hack, & Klein, 1998). It is hypothesized that prematurity and its effects act through association with health, cognitive, and neuromotor function to explain behavioral and emotional problems at school age (e.g., Nadeau, Boivin, Tessier, LeFebvre, & Robacy, 2001). The link between extremely preterm birth and later internalizing and externalizing behavioral problems is indirect. Behavioral, ADHD, and other social-interactive and emotional concerns surface as the result of the mediating effect of both neuromotor and cognitive deficits (e.g., language, executive function) that are sequelae of prematurity. Similarly, an infant with LBW who has lung disease has a high likelihood of bronchopulmonary dysplasia, which, in turn, increases the risk of later reactive airway disease or asthma. Related restrictions in ability to engage in usual childhood activities and slower physical growth would then interfere with socioemotional development, self-concept, and later school performance. There are multiple reports of increased stress in the families of children born prematurely. This stress would affect the child's emotional status because of bidirectional influences. Stress is higher if the child has a functional handicap, increased medical concerns, or low developmental functioning. Parents frequently articulate concerns about the child's self-esteem, acceptance by peers, and his or her future, as well as the child's impact on other family members (e.g., increased need for supervision, altered family routines; Taylor et al., 2000).

Outcome Status over Time

Of concern is the trend that outcome for children born with ELBW or VLBW worsens over time, this being a so-called sleeper effect. In one study of children with ELBW, 52% were functioning in the normal range at 4 years of age. However, by age 8, only 31% did not have problems. The prevalence of so-called minor disabilities increased from 31% at age 4 years to 53% by age 8 (Monset-Couchard, de Belhmann, & Kastler, 1996). Other studies suggest that rates of normality at age 6 are more than halved by age 8 in very premature infants (e.g., Saigal, Szatmari, Rosenbaum, Campbell, & King, 1990). Mild to moderate disabilities may be identified later than more severe problems because these less severe sequelae become apparent when demands for higher level skills cannot be met because of the underlying, subtle cognitive deficiencies. Children with ELBW or VLBW may be less likely to take advantage of learning opportunities because of these deficits in basic skills, and these children subsequently become increasingly frustrated and less responsive to interventions, and they lose motivation (Aylward, 2002b; Dewey et al., 1999; O'Callaghan et al., 1996; Taylor et al., 2000). It appears that areas of development such as motor and neurological function show lags (early delays but with subsequent catch-up), whereas others, such as cognitive and expressive language, may represent deficits (early delays that reflect persistent problems). There are linear and nonlinear patterns of development, and development may follow divergent paths as a result of medical complications such as BPD or IVH. Velocity and continuity of change (process), as well as endpoint function in a given area (products), should be evaluated (Aylward, 2002b; Miller et al., 1995).

SUMMARY

Although major brain pathways in the infant are specified in the genome, the connections between brain and behavior are fashioned by a complex interplay of the effects of disruption of CNS organization due to prematurity, actual CNS damage, recovery, and social experience. Social experience can affect the structure of the brain in that subsequent experience (activity) selects out synapses that will persist, whereas lack of experience (inactivity) will produce regression and cell death (Eisenberg, 1999). Besides clinical factors such as chronic lung disease, transient hypothyroxemia of prematurity (low thyroid hormone), or glucocorticoid exposure, stressful environmental conditions (ranging from bright lights and noise in the NICU to the mother–child interaction to "social niche") will affect the developing brain (Eisenberg, 1999; Perlman, 2001).

The spectrum of sequelae found in children born at biological risk or combined biological and environmental risk does not differ dramatically from problems found in those born at normal birthweight. What is different is the disproportionately greater incidence and complexity of these problems and the specific profiles of deficits. Although both biomedical and environmental factors affect outcome, the impact of biomedical factors intensifies as birthweight or gestational age decreases. This suggests the need for pediatric psychologists to be well versed in outcomes that are particularly associated with biomedical risk, as well as those linked to environmental factors. Because summary scores may grossly underestimate the complex nature and long-range impact of these deficits on the individual child, pediatric psychologists must develop improved assessment techniques to evaluate more specific functions and to better understand the complex dynamics of altered brain development, actual damage, and brain plasticity.

REFERENCES

American Academy of Pediatrics, Committee on Fetus and Newborn. (1996). Use and abuse of the Apgar score. *Pediatrics, 98*, 141–142.

Aylward, G. P. (1990). Environmental influences on the developmental outcome of children at risk. *Infants and Young Children, 2*, 1–9.

Aylward, G. P. (1992). The relationship between environmental risk and developmental outcome. *Journal of Developmental and Behavioral Pediatrics, 13*, 222–229.

Aylward, G. P. (1993). Perinatal asphyxia: Effects of biologic and environmental risks. *Clinics in Perinatology, 20*, 433–449.

Aylward, G. P. (1996). Environmental risk, intervention and developmental outcome. *Ambulatory Child Health, 2,* 161–170.

Aylward, G. P. (1997). *Infant and early childhood neuropsychology.* New York: Plenum Press.

Aylward, G. P. (2002a). Methodological issues in outcome studies of at-risk infants. *Journal of Pediatric Psychology, 27,* 37–45.

Aylward, G. P. (2002b). Cognitive and neuropsychological outcome: More than IQ scores. *Mental Retardation and Developmental Disabilities Research and Reviews, 8,* 234–240.

Aylward, G. P., & Kenny, T. J. (1979). Developmental follow-up: Inherent problems and a conceptual model. *Journal of Pediatric Psychology, 4,* 331–343.

Aylward, G. P., Pfeiffer, S. I., Wright, A., & Verhulst, S. J. (1989). Outcome studies of low birth weight infants published in the last decade: A meta-analysis. *Journal of Pediatrics, 115,* 515–521.

Bendersky, M., & Lewis, M. (1994). Environmental risk, biological risk, and developmental outcome. *Developmental Psychology, 30,* 484–494.

Bendersky, M., & Lewis, M. (1998). Arousal modulation in cocaine-exposed infants. *Developmental Psychology, 34,* 555–564.

Bennett, F. C., & Scott, D. T. (1997). Long-term perspective on premature infant outcome and contemporary intervention issues. *Seminars in Perinatology, 21,* 190–201.

Blasco, P. A. (1989). Preterm birth: To correct or not to correct. *Developmental Medicine and Child Neurology, 31,* 816–826.

Bos, A. F., Einspieler, C., & Prechtl, H. F. R. (2001). Intrauterine growth retardation, general movements, and neurodevelopmental outcome: A review. *Developmental Medicine and Child Neurology, 43,* 61–68.

Brazy, J. E., Eckerman, C. O., Oehler, J. M., Goldstein, R. F., & O'Rand, M. A. (1991). Nursery Neurobiologic Risk Score: Important factors in predicting outcome in very low birth weight infants. *Journal of Pediatrics, 118,* 783–792.

Bregman, J. (1998). Developmental outcome in very low birth weight infants: Current status and future trends. *Pediatric Clinics of North America, 45,* 673–690.

Breslau, N. (1995). Psychiatric sequelae of low birthweight. *Epidemiologic Reviews, 17,* 96–106.

Breslau, N., DelDotto, J. E., & Brown, G. (1994). A gradient relationship between low birth weight and IQ at age 6 years. *Archives of Pediatric and Adolescent Medicine, 148,* 377–383.

Capone, G. T. (1996). Human brain development. In A. J. Capute & P. J. Accardo (Eds.), *Developmental disabilities in infancy and childhood*: Vol. 1. Neurodevelopmental diagnosis and treatment (2nd ed., pp. 25–75). Baltimore: Brookes.

Dammann, O., & Leviton, A. (1999). Brain damage in preterm newborns: Might enhancement of developmentally regulated endogenous protection open a door for prevention? *Pediatrics, 104,* 541–550.

Dewey, D., Crawford, S. G., Creighton, D. E., & Sauve, R. S. (1999). Long-term neuropsychological outcomes in very low birth weight children free of sensorineural impairments. *Journal of Clinical and Experimental Neuropsychology, 21,* 851–865.

Eisenberg, L. (1999). Experience, brain and behavior: The importance of a head start. *Pediatrics, 103,* 1031–1035.

Escalona, S. K. (1982). Babies at double hazard: Early development of infants at biologic and social risk *Pediatrics, 70,* 670–676.

Flynn, J. R. (1999). Searching for justice: The discovery of IQ gains over time. *American Psychologist, 54,* 5–20.

Gauthier, S. M., Bauer, C. R., Messinger, D. S., & Closius, J. M. (1999). The Bayley Scales of Infant Development—II: Where to start? *Journal of Developmental and Behavioral Pediatrics, 20,* 75–79.

Geidd, J. N. (1997). Normal development. *Child and Adolescent Psychiatric Clinics of North America, 6,* 265–282.

Goyen, T., Lui, K., & Woods, R. (1998). Visual-motor, visual-perceptual, and fine-motor outcomes in very-low-birthweight children at 5 years. *Developmental Medicine and Child Neurology, 40,* 76–81.

Hack, M., & Fanaroff, A. A. (1999). Outcomes of children of extremely low birthweight and gestational age in the 1990s. *Early Human Development, 53,* 193–218.

Hack, M., Friedman, H., & Fanaroff, A. A. (1996). Outcomes of extremely low birth weight infants. *Pediatrics, 98,* 931–937.

Hack, M., Taylor, H. G., & Klein, N. (1995). Long term developmental outcome of low birthweight infants. In P. Shiono & R. Behrman (Eds.), *The future of children: Low birthweight* (Vol. 5, pp. 176–196). Los Altos, CA: Packard Foundation.

Hack, M., Taylor, H. G., Klein, N., & Minich, N. M. (2000). Functional limitations and special health care needs of 10– to 14–year-old children weighing less than 750 grams at birth. *Pediatrics, 106,* 554–559.

Halsey, C. L., Collin, M. F., & Anderson, C. L. (1993). Extremely low birth weight children and their peers: A comparison of preschool performance. *Pediatrics, 91,* 807–811.

Halsey, C. L., Collin, M. F., & Anderson, C. L. (1996). Extremely low birth weight children and their peers. *Archives of Pediatric and Adolescent Medicine, 150,* 790–794.

Hill, A., & Volpe, J. J. (1989). Perinatal asphyxia: Clinical aspects. *Clinics in Perinatology, 16*, 435–457.

Hunt, J. V., Cooper, B. A. B., & Tooley, W. H. (1988). Very low birth weight infants at 8 and 11 years of age: Role of neonatal illness and family status. *Pediatrics, 82*, 596–603.

Hunt, J. V., & Rhodes, L. (1977). Mental development of preterm infants during the first year. *Child Development, 48*, 204–210.

Infant Health and Development Program. (1990). Enhancing the outcomes of low birth weight, premature infants: A multisite, randomized trial. *Journal of the American Medical Association, 263*, 3035–3042.

Isaacs, E. B., Lucas, A., Chong, W. K., Wood, S. J., Johnson, C. L., Marshall, C., et al. (2000). Hippocampal volume and everyday memory in children of very low birth weight. *Pediatric Research, 47*, 713–720.

Kato-Klebanov, P., Brooks-Gunn, J., McCarton, C., & McCormick, M. (1998). The contribution of neighborhood and family income to developmental test scores over the first three years of life. *Child Development, 69*, 1420–1436.

Korner, A. F., Stevenson, D. K., Kraemer, H. C., Spiker, D., Scott, D. T., Constantinou, J., et al. (1993). Prediction of the development of low birth weight preterm infants by a new Neonatal Medical Index. *Journal of Developmental and Behavioral Pediatrics, 14*, 106–111.

Le Normand, M. T., & Cohen, H. (1999). The delayed emergence of lexical morphology in preterm children: The case of verbs. *Journal of Neurolinguistics, 12*, 235–246.

Lems, W., Hopkins, B., & Sampson, J. F. (1993). Mental and motor development in preterm infants: The issue of corrected age. *Early Human Development, 34*, 113–123.

Masten, A. S. (2001). Ordinary magic: Resilience processes in development. *American Psychologist, 56*, 227–238.

McCormick, M. C. (1989). Long-term follow-up of infants discharged from neonatal intensive care units. *Journal of the American Medical Association, 261*, 1767–1772.

McCormick, M. C. (1997). Quality of care: An overdue agenda. *Pediatrics, 99*, 249–250.

McCormick, M. C., McCarton, C., Brooks-Gunn, J., Belt, P., & Gross, R. T. (1998). The Infant Health and Development Program: Interim summary. *Journal of Developmental and Behavioral Pediatrics, 19*, 359–370.

Miller, C. L., Landry, S. H., Smith, K. E., Wildin, S. R., Anderson, A. E., & Swank, P. R. (1995). Developmental change in the neuropsychological functioning of very low birth weight infants. *Child Neuropsychology, 1*, 224–236.

Monset-Couchard, M., de Belhmann, O., & Kastler, B. (1996). Mid- and long-term outcome of 89 premature infants weighing less than 1000 g. at birth, all appropriate for gestational age. *Biology of the Neonate, 70*, 328–338.

Msall, M. E., Buck, G. M., Rogers, B. T., Merke, D., Catanzaro, N. L., & Zorn, W. A. (1991). Risk factors for major neurodevelopmental impairments and need for special education resources in extremely premature infants. *Journal of Pediatrics, 119*, 606–614.

Murphy, T. F., Nichter, C. A., & Liden, C. B. (1982). Developmental outcome of the high-risk infant: A review of methodological issues. *Seminars in Perinatology, 6*, 353–364.

Nadeau, L., Boivin, M., Tessier, R., LeFebvre, F., & Robacy, P. (2001). Mediators of behavioral problems in 7–year-old children born after 24 to 28 weeks of gestation. *Journal of Developmental and Behavioral Pediatrics, 22*, 1–10.

O'Callaghan, M. J., Burns, Y. R., Gray, P. H., Harvey, J. M., Mohay, H., Rogers, Y. M., et al. (1996). School performance of ELBW children: A controlled study. *Developmental Medicine and Child Neurology, 38*, 917–926.

Paneth, N. S. (1995). The problem of low birth weight. In P. Shiono & R. Behrman (Eds.), *The future of children: Low birth weight* (Vol. 5, pp. 11–34). Los Altos, CA: Packard Foundation.

Parker, S., Greer, S., & Zuckerman, B. (1988). Double jeopardy: The impact of poverty on early child development. *Pediatric Clinics of North America, 35*, 1227–1240.

Perlman, J. M. (1998). White matter injury in the preterm infant: An important determination of abnormal neurodevelopmental outcome. *Early Human Development, 53*, 99–120.

Perlman, J. M. (2001). Neurobehavioral deficits in premature graduates of intensive care: Potential medical and neonatal environmental risk factors. *Pediatrics, 108*, 1339–1348.

Peterson, B. S., Vohr, B., Staib, L. H., Cannistraci, C. J., Dolberg, B. A., Schneider, K. C., et al. (2000). Regional brain volume abnormalities and long-term cognitive outcome in preterm infants. *Journal of the American Medical Association, 284*, 1939–1947.

Phillips, R. B., Sharma, R., Premachandra, B. R., Vaughn, A. J., & Reyes-Lee, M. (1996). Intrauterine exposure to cocaine: Effect on neurobehavior of neonates. *Infant Behavior and Development, 19*, 71–81.

Resnick, M. B., Gomatam, S. V., Carter, R. L., Ariet, M., Roth, J., Kilgore, K. L., et al. (1998). Educational disabilities of neonatal intensive care graduates. *Pediatrics, 102*, 308–316.

Richardson, D. K., Gray, J. E., McCormick, M. C., Workman-Daniels, K., & Goldmann, D. A. (1993). Score for acute neonatal physiology (SNAP): A physiologic severity index for neonatal intensive care. *Pediatrics, 91*, 617–623.

Risser, A. H., & Edgell, D. (1988). Neuropsychology of the developing brain: Implications for neuropsychological assessment. In M. Tramontana & S. Hooper (Eds.), *Assessment issues in child neuropsychology* (pp. 41–65), New York: Plenum Press.

Saigal, S., Stoskopf, B. L., Streiner, D. L., & Burrows, E. (2001). Physical growth and current health status of infants who were of extremely low birth weight and controls at adolescence. *Pediatrics, 108*, 407–415.

Saigal, S., Szatmari, P., Rosenbaum, P., Campbell, D., & King, S. (1990). Intellectual and functional status at school entry of children who weighed 1000 grams or less at birth: A regional perspective of births in the 1980's. *Journal of Pediatrics, 116,* 409–416.

Sameroff, A. J., & Chandler, M. J. (1975). Reproductive risk and the continuum of caretaking casualty. In F. D. Horowitz (Ed.), *Review of child development research* (Vol. 4, pp. 187–244). Chicago: University of Chicago Press.

Sameroff, A. J., Seifer, R., Barocas, R., Zax, M., & Greenspan, S. (1987). Intelligence quotient scores of 4–year-old children: Social environmental risk factors. *Pediatrics, 79*, 343–349.

Sampson, P. D., Streissguth, A. P., Bookstein, F. L., Little, R. E., Clarren, S. K., Dehaene, P., et al. (1997). Incidence of fetal alcohol syndrome and prevalence of alcohol-related neurodevelopmental disorder. *Teratology, 56,* 317–326.

Stevenson, D. K., Wright, L. L., Lemons, J. A., Oh, W., Korones, S. B., Papile, L., et al. (1998). Very low birth weight outcomes of the National Institute of Child Health and Human Development Neonatal Research Network, January 1993 through December 1994. *American Journal of Obstetrics and Gynecology, 179,* 1632–1640.

Stewart, A. L., Rifkin, L., Amess, P. N., Kirkbride, V., Townsend, J. P., Miller, D. H., et al. (1999). Brain structure and neurocognitive and behavioral function in adolescents who were born very preterm. *The Lancet, 353,* 1635–1657.

Taylor, H. G., Hack, M., & Klein, N. K. (1998). Attention deficits in children with < 750 g. birth weight. *Developmental Neuropsychology, 4*, 21–34.

Taylor, H. G., Klein, N., & Hack, M. (2000). School-age consequences of birth weight less than 750 grams: A review and update. *Developmental Neuropsychology, 17*, 289–321.

Taylor, H. G., Klein, N., Minich, N. M., & Hack, M. (2000). Middle-school-age outcomes in children with very low birthweight. *Child Development, 71*, 1495–1511.

Tjossem, T. (1976). *Intervention strategies for high risk infants and young children.* Baltimore: University Park Press.

Touwen, B. C. L. (1986). Very low birth weight infants. *European Journal of Pediatrics, 145*, 460.

Vohr, B., & Msall, M. E. (1997). Neuropsychological and functional outcomes of very low birth weight infants. *Seminars in Perinatology, 21*, 202–220.

Vohr, B., Wright, L. L., Dusick, A. M., Mele, L., Verter, J., Steichen, J. J., et al. (2000). Neurodevelopmental and functional outcomes of extremely low birth weight infants in the National Institute of Child Health and Human Development Neonatal Research Network, 1993–1994. *Pediatrics, 105*, 1216–1226.

Volpe, J. J. (1998). Neurologic outcome of prematurity. *Archives of Neurology, 55,* 297–300.

Washington, K., Scott, D. T., Johnson, K. A., Wendel, S., & Hay, A. E. (1998). The Bayley Scales of Infant Development—II and children with developmental delays: A clinical perspective. *Journal of Developmental and Behavioral Pediatrics, 19,* 346–349.

Whitfield, M. F., Eckstein, R. V., & Grunau, L. H. (1997). Extremely premature (≤ 800 g.) school children: Multiple areas of hidden disability. *Archives of Disease in Childhood, 77*, F85–F90.

Wolraich, M. L., Felice, M. E., & Drotar, D. (1996). *The classification of child and adolescent mental diagnoses in primary care: Diagnostic and statistical manual for primary care (DSM-PC) child and adolescent version.* Elk Grove Village, IL: American Academy of Pediatrics.

Zelkowitz, P., Papageorgiou, A., & Allard, M. (1994). Relationship of rehospitalization to cognitive and behavioral outcomes in very low birth weight and normal birthweight children. *Journal of Developmental and Behavioral Pediatrics, 15,* 179–185.

16

Pediatric Asthma

ELIZABETH L. MCQUAID
NATALIE WALDERS

For reasons that are not completely understood, the prevalence of asthma has increased dramatically over the course of the past several decades (Centers for Disease Control and Prevention [CDC], 1995). Concomitant rises in asthma morbidity and mortality have also been documented and appear to be disproportionately greater in the pediatric population (CDC, 1995; Sly, 1994). These increases in morbidity and mortality have persisted despite considerable advances in the pharmacological management of asthma, a contradiction that has earned asthma the label of a "modern health paradox" (Clark et al., 1998). In response to the dramatic increases in asthma, national and international efforts have been mobilized to generate a consensus regarding diagnostic criteria and treatment for the disease (American Academy of Allergy, Asthma, and Immunology [AAAAI], 1999; National Institutes of Health [NIH], 1997). Asthma is now recognized as a complex disease, with both episodic and chronic features. It has long been accepted that the central characteristics of asthma include airway hyperresponsiveness and reversible airway obstruction (Larsen, 1992). More recent definitions also emphasize chronic inflammation of the airways, even in milder forms of the disease (NIH, 1997). Accordingly, treatment approaches now underscore the need for ongoing management, even in the absence of active symptoms.

The shift in emphasis from episodic management to ongoing, preventive management places greater responsibility on the family of a child with asthma. Families of children with asthma, particularly when symptoms are persistent, face an array of management tasks, including daily medication use, identification and avoidance of triggers, and management of exacerbations (Klinnert, McQuaid, & Gavin, 1997). Adherence to treatment recommendations presumably leads to greater symptom control, decreased health care utilization, and enhanced quality of life. Families tend to experience more substantial treatment adherence challenges in relationship to the complexity of management plans. Not surprisingly, nonadherence to asthma treatment regimens is a pervasive problem (Bender et al., 2000; Rand & Wise, 1995).

The changes in pediatric asthma treatment have yielded an expanded role for pediatric psychologists. Multiple points for effective intervention exist, including assisting practitioners in identifying children at higher risk for asthma complications, providing psychosocial interventions to children and families, and consulting with professionals regarding the most effective family-based approaches for treatment. Although the research base regarding emotional and behavioral variables in pediatric asthma is growing, much empirical work remains to be done. Further investigation of family influences that facilitate asthma management, research regarding the effects of asthma on individual and family adaptation, and controlled trials investigating psychosocial treatments are all required to advance our understanding of how to best help children and families cope with asthma.

PEDIATRIC ASTHMA: DEFINITION AND SCOPE OF THE PROBLEM

Defining Characteristics of Asthma

Asthma is characterized as a chronic inflammatory disorder of the airways that involves intermittent and variable periods of airway obstruction (NIH, 1997). The pathophysiology of asthma involves many cell pathways and contributes to multiple processes, including chronic inflammation, airway hyperresponsiveness, bronchoconstriction, swelling of the airways, and mucus plugging. Although the exact cause of asthma onset in any individual is not known, several variables are thought to contribute to its inception. These include genetic variables such as a predisposition to allergy (Cookson, 1999), environmental influences such as exposure to infectious agents, allergens, or irritants (Busse & Lemanske, 2001), and psychological influences such as stress (Mrazek & Klinnert, 1991). The etiology of asthma is likely due to a complex interaction among a range of these variables.

The course of asthma is intermittent and variable. It involves chronic underlying inflammation, which may not produce noticeable symptoms, and exacerbations, which are characterized by active symptoms. Typically, symptoms occur as a result of airway hyperresponsiveness to a variety of triggers. Asthma triggers include airborne irritants (e.g., cigarette smoke), as well as allergens that elicit symptoms among individuals with specific immunological hypersensitivity (e.g., animal dander). Common types of asthma triggers include environmental (e.g., dust), seasonal (e.g., weather changes), and infectious factors (e.g., respiratory infections). Triggers vary by individual, and sensitivity can change over the course of illness. This complexity underscores the need for individualized treatment plans that highlight the specific profile of triggers, symptoms, and medication needs for a particular patient.

During an asthma exacerbation, patients experience a range of processes that contribute to breathing difficulty, including constriction of the bronchial smooth muscles, swelling of bronchial tissues, and increased mucus secretion (Taitel, Allen, & Creer, 1998). Asthma exacerbations can vary in severity and duration but are commonly marked by symptoms of coughing, shortness of breath, wheezing, and chest tightness. Although the airway obstruction associated with asthma is typically reversible without lung damage, more permanent "remodeling" of the airways has been recognized as a potential consequence of the disease (AAAAI, 1999). Recent research suggests that early recognition and treatment of the disease during the first 5 years of life may play a role in preventing the progressive loss of lung function later in childhood (Martinez, 1999).

Asthma Prevalence and Morbidity

Asthma is the most common chronic illness in childhood and adolescence, affecting nearly 5 million individuals under age 18 in the United States (CDC, 1996). The overall prevalence of the disease has increased, with national statistics of asthma prevalence increasing approximately 58.6% between 1982 and 1996 (CDC, 1995). More recent epidemiological data suggest that rising asthma prevalence rates reached a plateau in the late 1990s (American Lung Association [ALA], 2000), but the general trend over the past several decades has been toward a marked increase. Although no clear explanation for this increase exists, some have theorized it may be due to greater exposure to indoor allergens due to overall lifestyle changes (Platts-Mills, Blumenthal, Perzanowski, & Woodfolk, 2000). Others have proposed that frequent use of antibiotics and decreased exposure to infections early in life might alter the immune response that, paradoxically, could lead to an increased likelihood of developing asthma, the so-called hygiene hypothesis (Mattes & Karmaus, 1999; Strachan, 1989).

The extensive prevalence of asthma, although demonstrated across the lifespan, is most critically a pediatric concern. Asthma is over 40% more prevalent in children and adolescents than in the general population (CDC, 1995). This prevalence is associated with extensive functional morbidity and is a leading cause of hospitalizations, emergency department visits, and activity restriction for children and adolescents (Taylor & Newacheck, 1992; Weiss, Gergen, & Hodgson, 1992). Asthma accounts for more than 3 million doctor visits and more than 500,000 emergency room visits on an annual basis for children under age 15 (AAAAI, 1999). In addition, an estimated 164,000 hospitalizations for asthma occur each year (AAAAI, 1999). Asthma is also the leading cause of school absences, with approximately 10 million school days missed per year due to asthma symptoms (Taylor & Newacheck, 1992).

Asthma poses a substantial economic burden on the health care system in the United States, with annual expenditures for asthma estimated to exceed $12 billion (ALA, 2000). A large proportion of asthma health care costs are allocated for serious consequences of the disease, such as hospitalizations and emergency room visits, which could potentially be avoided through the implementation of optimal pharmacological intervention and self-management techniques (Smith et al., 1997). Indirect costs are also substantial; economic losses from lost work days and diminished productivity associated with missed school days from asthma are estimated to total $1.5 billion annually (ALA, 2000).

Asthma Mortality

Although asthma-related fatalities are relatively rare compared with other pediatric chronic illnesses, death rates from pediatric asthma have actually risen considerably in recent years (Weiss & Wagener, 1990). According to national data, the asthma death rate for individuals under age 19 years increased by nearly 80% between 1980 and 1993 (CDC, 1996). Deaths from asthma have been linked to a number of risk factors, including medication nonadherence and inadequate skills in perceiving the severity of symptoms (NIH, 1995). One investigation of a cluster of asthma-related deaths in an urban area identified African American minority status, low socioeconomic status (SES) background, adolescence, and lack of family involvement with medication as risk factors for asthma mortality (Birkhead, Olfaway, Strunk, Townsend, & Teutsch, 1989).

Disproportionate Impact of Asthma

Although asthma is a widespread public health concern, the morbidity and mortality associated with pediatric asthma disproportionately affect ethnic minority youth, urban communities, and low-income populations (Crain, Kercsmar, Weiss, Mitchell, & Lynn, 1998; Evans, 1992). Asthma risk factors characteristic of urban communities and often found among low-income populations include environmental exposure to indoor and outdoor allergens and inadequate access to health care services (Crain et al., 1998; Rosenstreich et al., 1997). Ethnic minorities demonstrate higher rates of asthma, more frequent health care utilization, and more fatalities from asthma than Caucasians (Lozano, Connell, & Koepsell, 1995; Weiss et al., 1992). African Americans with asthma are at a particularly increased risk of activity restriction and hospitalization and are 6 times more likely than Caucasians to suffer fatal asthma episodes (Weitzman, Gortmaker, Sobel, & Perrin, 1992). Substantially higher prevalence of asthma and consequences of asthma have also been identified among Puerto Ricans (Carter-Pokras & Gergen, 1993). Although some researchers caution that the disproportionate impact of asthma on ethnic minorities may reflect health disparities associated with poverty and urban communities, higher asthma rates and risks have been identified among ethnic minority groups after controlling for these factors (Joseph, Ownby, Peterson, & Johnson, 2000; Miller, 2000; Nelson et al., 1997).

PSYCHOLOGICAL ASPECTS OF PEDIATRIC ASTHMA

Asthma Onset

Psychological factors have long been recognized in the development and course of pediatric asthma. Before the advent of modern immunology and the recognition of allergic phenomena, asthma was considered primarily a "nervous disease" and was actually referred to in early medical textbooks as "asthma nervosa" (Alexander, 1950). In the middle of the twentieth century, psychosomatic models of illness attempted an integration of biological and psychological influences on the expression of asthma (Alexander, 1950). These conceptualizations were heavily dependent on psychodynamic models of functioning and viewed the central conflict in asthma as "excessive unresolved dependence on the mother," in which "everything which threatens to separate the patient from the protective mother or her substitute is apt to precipitate an asthma attack" (Alexander, 1950, p. 134). Over the past several decades, transformations in the field have emphasized a complex integration of genetic, immunological, and psychosocial factors in both the onset and expression of asthma.

A child's risk for developing asthma is clearly influenced by heredity (Larsen, 1992; Mrazek & Klinnert, 1991). Research has indicated that psychosocial and behavioral factors also play a role in asthma onset (Klinnert et al., 2001; Wright, Rodriguez, & Cohen, 1998). Some distinct parental behaviors have been demonstrated to have an effect on a child's risk for developing asthma. These behaviors include maternal smoking during pregnancy and child exposure to environmental tobacco smoke (Environmental Protection Agency [EPA], 1992). There is also evidence that psychological stress may influence the development and pathophysiology of asthma through increased risk of respiratory infections (Wright et al., 1998).

Some recent research has suggested that maternal factors such as difficulties in parenting may increase asthma risk (Klinnert & Mrazek, 1994; Klinnert et al., 2001). Klinnert and colleagues (2001) conducted a prospective longitudinal study of asthma onset in children at genetic risk for developing the illness due to maternal asthma, investigating physiological and psychological influences. Two early indicators, an index of allergy and an index of global parenting difficulty at infant age 3 weeks, were independent predictors of asthma status between ages 6 and 8 years. The authors suggested that developmentally relevant stressful events and/or the quality of the caregiving may, in fact, alter the emotional and physiological regulation of the infant in the direction of increased allergic response. In this way, the development and course of asthma may be affected by genetic risk, environmental exposure, and psychological factors such as parent–child interactions.

Emotions and Asthma Course

Emotions have long been recognized as having a role in initiating asthma episodes for some individuals, a phenomenon that may have lent credence to early conceptualizations of asthma attacks as largely psychogenic in origin. Reviews of the literature indicate that for a portion of individuals with asthma (approximately 15–30%), stress and emotions are identified as triggers for asthma episodes (Isenberg, Lehrer, & Hochron, 1992; Wright et al., 1998). Experimental manipulations of the impact of stress on airway function in asthma have yielded similar findings. Specifically, a portion of individuals with asthma react with bronchoconstriction when subjected to stressful experiences such as performing mental arithmetic (Miklich, Rewey, Weiss, & Kolton, 1973), watching emotionally charged films (Miller & Wood, 1994), and speaking about an embarrassing event (McQuaid et al., 2000).

The psychophysiological mechanism that links emotional processes to asthma exacerbations is not clear, although some preliminary models to explain this association have been posed. The research that documents some association between emotional stimulation and pulmonary function is largely based on the assumption that the autonomic nervous system mediates the effects of emotions on asthma. Specifically, for some individuals, increased activity of the vagus nerve and stimulation of the parasympathetic nervous system may result in bronchoconstriction in the large airways (see Isenberg et al., 1992, for a review). Miller and Wood (1994) have proposed a pattern of emotional responsivity and physiological reactivity, linked through cholinergic pathways, which may affect airway function for some children with asthma. The risk for emotionally induced asthma is increased when a child's asthma is psychophysiologically reactive and when the child is exposed to significant life stress or emotional challenge. Theories such as these that investigate physiological processes, psychological vulnerability, and life circumstances in explaining the relationships between emotions and asthma are useful models in guiding future research.

Behavioral Adjustment in Pediatric Asthma

The question of whether or not children with asthma have more behavior problems than their healthy peers has also been a topic of some debate. Early clinical impressions characterized children with asthma as having difficulties in separation from parents and anxiety (Alexander, 1950). Subsequent research has been somewhat contradictory. Some studies have documented minimal behavioral differences between children with asthma and healthy controls (Graham, Rutter, Yule, & Pless, 1967), whereas others have found that children with asthma demonstrate more internalizing behavior problems relative to norms (Klinnert, McQuaid, McCormick, Adinoff, & Bryant, 2000; Wamboldt, Fritz, Mansell, McQuaid, & Klein, 1998) and controls (Austin, Smith, Risinger, & McNelis, 1994). Additionally, there is some evidence that children with more severe asthma have more behavior problems relative to those with milder forms of the disease (Klinnert et al., 2000; MacLean, Perrin, Gortmaker, & Pierre, 1992; Wamboldt et al., 1998). A recent meta-analysis of behavioral adjustment in children with asthma concluded that, in general, children with asthma do have more behavioral difficulties than their peers and that these difficulties are more pronounced in the internalizing domain (McQuaid, Kopel, & Nassau, 2001). Disease severity moderated this relationship such that children with mild forms of the illness were not significantly different from healthy peers, but with increasing disease severity behavioral difficulties were more evident (McQuaid, Kopel, & Nassau, 2001).

There is clear evidence that having psychological difficulties puts children with asthma at risk for increased morbidity. Psychological distress in pediatric asthma has been associated with asthma that is challenging to manage, with more problematic adherence (Creer, 1993), and requiring higher doses of steroids (Fritz & Overholser, 1989). Children with asthma who have comorbid behavior problems and/or reported depressive symptoms tend to have more frequent and prolonged hospital admissions (Kaptien, 1982) and more functional impairment due to asthma (Gustadt, Gillette, & Mrazek, 1989). Although the overall mortality rate for asthma is low, psychological distress has been found to be a risk factor for asthma mortality (Sears, Rea, & Fenwich, 1986; Strunk, Mrazek, Wolfson Fuhrmann, & LaBrecque, 1985). Given these issues, identification of comorbid behavior problems in children with asthma and appropriate referral for treatment, if indicated, should be clear priorities for health care providers.

Developmental and Family Implications

A number of works have summarized the developmental implications of childhood chronic illness, documenting effects in various domains of functioning (Midence, 1994). A chronic illness such as asthma has the potential to affect the achievement of age-appropriate developmental tasks, such as individuation from parents, socialization outside the family, the establishment of peer relationships, and the formation of a positive self-image (Garrison & McQuiston, 1989). The extent to which asthma exerts influence in these domains is likely moderated by disease severity, with children who have more severe and persistent forms of asthma most affected (Fritz & McQuaid, 2000). Additionally, the course of asthma may vary across childhood. Although the misconception that many children "outgrow" asthma persists, asthma typically presents with a chronic and fluctuating course, with periods of exacerbation and remission (Larsen, 1992).

Some research suggests that school-age children with asthma have many misperceptions about the illness and the preventive use of medications (Kieckhefer & Spitzer, 1995; McQuaid, Howard, Kopel, Rosenblum, & Bibace, 2002). Asthma is characterized by a complex presentation, with a varying course of symptoms that wax and wane in response to allergic, environmental, and psychological factors. Treatment recommendations can also be varied and complex, including multiple medications and a range of strategies for disease prevention. This situation results in a clinical picture that may be difficult for even adults to understand. As a result, educational efforts need to be developmentally appropriate and reinforced regularly by physicians and other health care providers to ensure adequate understanding of disease and management strategies (McQuaid et al., 2002).

The implementation of skills for effective pediatric asthma management results from a complex set of interactions between parent and child. Children's active participation may vary widely by age, developmental maturity, and attitude toward illness (McQuaid, Kopel, & Nassau, 2001). Optimally, parents involve children in the disease management process by providing direct guidance, then supervising task performance, and eventually allowing the child to perform the skill independently (Brown, Avery, Mobley, Boccuti, & Golbach, 1996). Research in other chronic illnesses, specifically diabetes and cystic fibrosis, has demonstrated that as children progress through middle childhood, they do gradually assume more responsibility for illness management (Anderson, Auslander, Jung, Miller, & Santiago, 1990; Drotar & Ievers, 1994). In the pediatric asthma population, preadolescent children tend to assume responsibility for tasks of identifying and managing symptoms when they occur. They are less likely to assume responsibility for tasks of preventive management, such as avoiding triggers or taking regular medications (McQuaid, Penza-Clyve, et al., 2001). Families often face challenges in optimally distributing responsibilities for asthma management tasks between parents and children, particularly during periods of developmental transitions. Some research has demonstrated that adherence may be compromised when parents overestimate the asthma self-management behaviors of adolescents (Walders, Drotar, & Kercsmar, 2000).

Adolescence brings significant challenges with regard to the management of chronic illness, as teenagers may exert their growing independence in ways that can be life threatening, such as through nonadherence to medication regimens and minimization of acute symptoms. Consistent with research regarding other chronic illnesses, adolescence is a time in which difficulties in adherence to asthma medications can become more pronounced (Bender, Milgrom, Rand, & Ackerson, 1998). Adolescents with severe asthma are also at higher risk for mortality from the disease relative to their younger counterparts (Birkhead et al., 1989; Rich & Schneider, 1996). Specification of developmental expectations for children's self-management of illness and identification of children at particular risk because of psychological or developmental factors are key roles for psychologists.

INTERDISCIPLINARY MANAGEMENT OF ASTHMA

The value of merging medical, behavioral, and educational approaches in asthma management has been recognized through research and clinical practice experiences (Clark et al., 1998). Numerous intervention studies have found empirical support for interdisciplinary approaches to asthma management that integrate the expertise of a variety of providers such as physicians, psychologists, nurses, and health educators (Bratton et al., 2001; Evans et al., 1999; Weinstein, Faust, McKee, & Padman, 1992). In addition to establishing criteria for the medical management of asthma, the NIH guidelines (1997) recognize the benefits of an interdisciplinary approach to asthma management in a variety of situations, such as comorbid psychiatric distress, family problems, or nonadherence that may jeopardize appropriate management of the condition.

Basic Medical Approach

The primary step in successful asthma management is the involvement of a physician skilled in asthma diagnosis, treatment, and symptom monitoring. The NIH (1997) guidelines for the treatment of asthma provides level-of-care recommendations according to illness severity and related functional morbidity. Depending on the severity and course of the condition, childhood asthma may be medically managed by a primary care pediatrician or may necessitate the involvement of a specialty provider, such as a pulmonologist or an allergist. Pediatric asthma specialists are uniquely qualified to manage challenging asthma cases that require complicated medication management and involve a high risk for morbidity (Legorreta et al., 1998). In general, practice guidelines for asthma recommend an appropriate, timely response to acute exacerbations at all stages, including preventing disease progression by avoiding asthma triggers and using long-term-control medications to reduce underlying airway inflammation. A central feature of practice guidelines involves a written asthma "action plan" that incorporates medications to prevent symptoms and to reduce acute symptoms, as well as instruction regarding appropriate health care utilization according to symptom severity. Significant developments in options for the pharmacological management of asthma have been developed and disseminated in recent years. The NIH (1997) divides the pharmacological management of asthma into two categories: quick-relief medications and long-term-control medications. Table 16.1 includes an overview of available medications and a description of their indications. Quick-relief medications are used to provide rapid relief of symptoms associated with bronchoconstriction found in all forms of asthma. Quick-relief medications are not intended for use on a regular basis to control symptoms, but rather on a periodic, or as-needed basis. For patients with intermittent asthma that involves infrequent exacerbations, a quick-relief medication, such as a short-acting $ß_2$-agonist, may be the only form of indicated treatment. Systemic corticosteroids are also considered quick-relief medications but are generally used to reverse serious exacerbations when other medications have been ineffective. Excessive reliance on quick-relief medications is a key indicator that asthma is insufficiently managed and that more aggressive treatment, such as the addition of a long-term-control medication, is warranted.

In contrast to quick-relief medications, long-term-control medications are taken on a daily basis to control persistent asthma symptoms. Patients with persistent forms of asthma, marked by underlying inflammation of the airways, generally require both quick-relief medication and long-term-control medication. Several forms of long-term-control medications are available. Inhaled corticosteroids, which are regarded as an effective anti-inflammatory technique for daily control of symptoms, are commonly prescribed (NIH, 1997). Other preventive medications include cromolyn sodium (prescribed in inhaler form) and leukotriene modifiers (prescribed in pill form). In addition, long-acting $ß_2$-agonists may be administered in conjunction with anti-inflammatory medications to provide sustained symptom control. A new form of medication (e.g., Advair) offers a dual delivery of inhaled corticosteriod along with a long-acting $ß_2$-agonist in a single therapeutic dose for patients who require both forms of medication.

Role of Pediatric Psychology

The unique contribution of clinical psychology and behavioral techniques in working with children with asthma has been emphasized in the research literature (Creer, 2000). Psychologists can provide valuable consultation to physicians on an outpatient basis, on inpatient units, and through informal consultation. Due to the prevalence of pediatric asthma, along with the identified comorbidity between asthma and behavioral conditions, many clinical child psychologists will encounter patients with asthma within their general practices. This situation underscores the importance of facilitating asthma awareness and competencies among psychologists, whether they specialize in pediatric or clinical child psychology practice. A number of roles for pediatric psychologists in facilitating asthma management are emphasized: (1) providing patient and family asthma education, (2) identification and treatment of psychosocial barriers to effective asthma management, and (3) implementation of psychosocial intervention techniques to promote effective family-based asthma management behaviors.

TABLE 16.1. Asthma Medications

Name	Indications	Notes
	Quick-relief medications	
Albuterol (e.g., Ventolin, Proventil, Airet)	• Relief of acute symptoms through smooth muscle relaxation. • Prevention of bronchoconstriction prior to exercise.	• May be administered in inhaled or nebulized form. • Overreliance on albuterol (e.g., more than one canister per month) indicates inadequate asthma control and need for additional preventive measures.
Levalbuterol (Xopenex)	Same as above	Same as above
Pirbuterol (e.g., Maxair)	Same as above	• Only available in nebulizer form.
Anticholinergics, ipratropium bromide (e.g., Atrovent)	• Relief of acute bronchospasm.	• May be administered in inhaled or nebulized form. • Not intended for use with exercise-induced symptoms. • Alternative medication for patients unable to take ß$_2$-agonists.
Oral corticosteriods (e.g., prednisone, Prelone, Medrol)	• Treatment of moderate to severe exacerbations to provide quicker and more sustained relief from airflow obstruction and prevention of relapse. • Typically prescribed in short courses or "bursts."	• Administered in tablet or liquid form. • Significant side effects associated with long-term use require monitoring.
	Long-term-control medications	
Inhaled corticosteriods (e.g., Flovent, Beclovent, Pulmicort, Azmacort)	• Long-term prevention of symptom exacerbations. • Reduce the need for quick-relief medications. • Reduce airway inflammation.	• Administered through metered dose inhalers (MDIs), nebulizers, or dry power inhalers (DPIs). • Use of a spacer is recommended for MDIs. • Mouth rinsing after inhalations is recommended.
Oral/systemic corticosteriods (e.g., Prednisone, Prelone, Orapred)	• Typically provided in short-term "burst" dosages to gain control over acute symptoms. • May be used to control chronic symptoms through daily or every-other-day administration.	• Administration of the lowest effective dose is recommended. • Monitoring of side effects recommended, particularly when administered for sustained periods of time.
Cromolyn sodium/nedoromil sodium (e.g., Intal, Tilade)	• Long-term prevention of symptoms and initiated prior to exposure to known triggers or allergens.	• Administered in inhaled or nebulized form. • Less effective anti-inflammatory properties than corticosteroids.
Leukotriene modifiers (e.g., Singulair, Accolate, Zyflo)	• Long-term prevention of symptom exacerbations.	• Administered in tablet form with once-daily dosing. • Particularly beneficial for control of nocturnal symptoms.

(*continued*)

TABLE 16.1. (*continued*)

Name	Indications	Notes
Long-acting ß$_2$-Agonists (e.g., Serevent, Volmax, Foradil)	• Used in conjunction with anti-inflammatory medications. • Provides long-standing control of nocturnal symptoms and exercise-induced bronchospasm.	• Administered through MDIs or DPIs. • Not indicated for the treatment of acute exacerbations. • Not intended for long-term-control use in isolation from anti-inflammatory agents.
Combined long-acting ß$_2$-agonist and long-acting corticosteroid (e.g., Advair)	• Delivers combination of anti-inflammatory medication and long-term-control relief of bronchospasm.	• Administered in DPI format only. • Condenses the delivery of two forms of medication into a single dose administered twice daily.
Methylxanthines (e.g., theophylline, Slo-Bid, Theodur)	• Long-term control of persistent symptoms, particularly nocturnal symptoms. • Minimal evidence of improved symptom control compared with other long-term-control medications.	• Administered in tablet form. • Numerous adverse effects are reported. • Monitoring of serum concentration levels is required to ensure optimal dosing.

Note. Adapted from National Institutes of Health (1997) and American Academy of Allergy, Asthma, and Immunology (1999).

Patient and Family Education

Research has demonstrated insufficient asthma knowledge among pediatric patients and families, inaccuracies regarding the type and use of medications, lack of understanding concerning the etiology and course of asthma, and incorrect beliefs concerning asthma management techniques (Celano, Geller, Phillips, & Ziman, 1998; Clark, 1998; Zimmerman, Bonner, Evans, & Mellins, 1999). Numerous educational programs for asthma have been developed in response to documented deficiencies in asthma knowledge, with somewhat mixed results. Some educational efforts have resulted in reductions in asthma morbidity and improved adherence (e.g., Fitzpatrick, Coughlin, & Chamberlin, 1992). However, a meta-analysis addressing the impact of educational programs on pediatric asthma morbidity demonstrated minimal effects (Bernard-Bonnin, Stachenko, Bonin, Charette, & Rousseau, 1995). One interpretation of the equivocal results of educational programs is that providing asthma education without incorporating strategies for translating knowledge into healthy behavioral patterns is largely insufficient (Clark & Gong, 2000).

Pediatric psychologists can take several roles in promoting asthma awareness and addressing the challenges involved in changing asthma management behaviors through increasing asthma knowledge. First, pediatric psychologists are in a position to identify knowledge deficits that may not be recognized by medical staff or family members. On identification of insufficient asthma knowledge, psychologists can refer patients to existing educational programs, to advocacy organizations (e.g., American Lung Association), or to the medical team for education. Pediatric psychologists are also uniquely qualified to deliver asthma education in a developmentally appropriate manner and are skilled in working closely with families to optimize behaviors.

An additional role for psychologists involves the development of new educational resources or the refinement of existing educational programs to reflect empirically supported behavioral principles (Chambless & Hollon, 1988). Clinical psychologists possess the specialized training in behavioral techniques necessary to combine factual knowledge with strategies for implementing and adjusting asthma management behaviors. This task may be accomplished on an individual basis by supplementing educational materials with behavioral intervention to help families modify asthma management patterns more effectively while expanding their knowledge base. The goal of expanding education to incorporate behavioral modification may also be achieved on a more widespread basis by consulting with educational programs to infuse behavioral features into asthma education curricula.

Identification and Treatment of Psychosocial Barriers to Effective Asthma Management

A range of psychosocial stressors have been identified as risk factors for exacerbating the morbidity and mortality associated with asthma (Lara, Allen, & Lange, 1999). For instance, family mental health problems (Weil et al., 1999), limited problem-solving skills (Wade, Holden, Lynn, Mitchell, & Ewart, 2000), and family dysfunction have been identified as risk factors for morbidity (Strunk, 1987). Medical professionals involved in asthma care typically do not have expertise in recognizing psychosocial risk factors. Moreover, medical professionals do not have the training or the resources to modify psychosocial stressors once identified. As a result, collaborative relationships between psychologists and medical staff represent a valuable model for improving asthma outcomes (Sobel, 1995; Walders, Nobile, & Drotar, 2000).

Psychosocial Intervention Techniques

In contrast to asthma education efforts that seek to address gaps in asthma knowledge, psychosocial interventions attempt to foster new skills in managing the symptoms and treatments of asthma. The term "asthma self-management" is often used to describe the skills necessary to cope with the treatment demands of asthma and the obligations of patient-directed, rather than physician-facilitated care (Creer, 2000). In contrast to adult asthma, in which the individual patient is the central figure, self-management in pediatric asthma recognizes the family context of management behaviors. The cooperation between patient, family, and provider in asthma self-management is pivotal in accomplishing optimal outcomes (Bauman, 2000). Psychosocial interventions can identify and address treatment barriers to promote mastery over complex asthma management tasks and maximize adherence (Rapoff, 1999).

Numerous psychosocial interventions for asthma have been published in the literature and implemented in clinical practice, including self-management training, problem-solving techniques, family-based interventions, and psychophysiological modalities (i.e., relaxation training and biofeedback). Psychosocial interventions may be offered to patients singularly or in combination, depending on the particular patient and family needs. Psychosocial interventions may be delivered in an inpatient pediatric setting through consultation and liaison work or on an outpatient basis to patients referred specifically for asthma-related concerns. Alternatively, these techniques may be delivered to patients in therapy for other issues who are simultaneously coping with asthma. Psychosocial interventions appear to be particularly effective in maximizing treatment adherence, facilitating cooperation between families and physicians, and delivering asthma education in an optimal manner (Lemanek, Kamps, & Chung, 2001).

Deficits in problem-solving skills have been identified among families coping with asthma (Wade et al., 2000), resulting in the recommendation to identify and modify ineffective problem-solving strategies among children and families. A substantive body of research has developed and empirically evaluated problem-solving techniques (e.g., Nezu, Nezu, Friedman, Faddis, & Houts, 1998). Family-based asthma interventions have gained increasing recognition in the literature as a tool to promote effective asthma management among families (e.g., Gebert et al., 1998; Gustafsson, Kjellman, & Cederblad, 1986). Family-based intervention principles involve encouraging developmentally appropriate distribution of management tasks between family members, promoting a balance between child self-management and parental involvement or supervision and enhancing asthma awareness among family members (Tal, Gil-Spielberg, Antonovsky, Tal, & Moaz, 1990; Weinstein et al., 1992).

Psychophysiological tools, including relaxation training and biofeedback, have also been evaluated as adjunctive treatments for asthma symptoms. Relaxation training involves the use of relaxation through breathing techniques, progressive/passive muscle relaxation, or another modality in an attempt to reduce autonomic arousal and emotional distress during an asthma exacerbation (McQuaid & Nassau, 1999). Biofeedback is based on the technique of teaching patients to modify physical symptoms by receiving consistent feedback concerning the exacerbation or reduction of physiological symptoms. McQuaid and Nassau (1999) examined several different forms of biofeedback applications for pediatric asthma and concluded that some forms of biofeedback to modify asthma symptoms are empirically supported but that more research is needed to determine if these strategies effect changes that are clinically significant.

CONCLUSION

Research and practice in the management of pediatric asthma is at a crossroads. In recent years, spiraling estimates of prevalence and morbidity have engendered coordinated efforts on national and local levels to diagnose and manage the illness more effectively. Guidelines from national organizations provide recommendations for accurate diagnosis and effective management of the disease (NIH, 1997). The pace of development and dissemination of new asthma medications has been steadily increasing. Despite these advances, asthma remains a critical public health problem with significant morbidity and health care costs. Implementation of the recommendations for asthma management is a difficult task for health care professionals and families—and a significant gap remains between these recommendations and actual practice. Many families still conceive of asthma as episodic and believe that they are treating asthma effectively by managing the symptoms of the illness rather than recognizing the chronicity of asthma and attempting to prevent future episodes (Glaxo-Wellcome, 1998). Misconceptions about the nature and function of asthma medications persist among children and adults (Kieckhefer & Spitzer, 1995; McQuaid et al., 2002). Even though the majority of physicians report that they regularly prepare action plans for their asthma patients, very few patients recall ever receiving a written action plan from their doctors. Adherence to medications, which are regularly prescribed for children with persistent asthma, remains poor (Bender et al., 2000). In order to accomplish reductions in asthma morbidity and improvements in asthma management, research and clinical advances are necessary, and health care policy considerations are relevant. The field of pediatric psychology is uniquely suited to contribute to each of these areas.

Although behavioral research in pediatric asthma has made great strides in the past decades, further empirical work is needed in many areas. Investigations of risk for asthma onset utilizing a biopsychosocial framework can lead to integrated approaches to asthma prevention. Research addressing the complex interactions between stress and emotions, immune function, and asthma exacerbations may lead to new nonpharmacological approaches to asthma control. Further research is needed to explain the gap between physician recommendations for asthma management and families' actual implementation of asthma management practices. Research frameworks that identify individual and systems factors that support adaptive asthma management are necessary and will serve to inform the development of future interventions. Rigorous evaluation of existing psychosocial interventions through randomized, controlled trials will help refine existing programs and promote best-practice guidelines.

Psychologists and other mental health professionals can serve many key roles in working directly with families of children with asthma. Increased collaboration with pediatricians and specialists can facilitate effective asthma care. Specifically, psychologists can help physicians identify family barriers to adherence and help construct asthma management plans that take family barriers and strengths into account. Individual and family psychological intervention can be critical in preventing mental health problems from complicating treatment adherence or exacerbating physical symptoms, in cases of comorbid psychiatric and medical concerns. Moreover, psychologists can participate in the programming and implementation of educational interventions, emphasizing developmental and family approaches. The interventions provided by psychologists and other mental health professionals can help to "bridge the gap" between provider and patient—to assist families in understanding asthma, to help them solve problems related to adherence, and to support them in following their management plan.

Because of the high prevalence and risks of asthma, along with the disproportionate impact of asthma on ethnic minorities, low-income families, and inner-city communities, asthma treatment represents an important public health priority. Through mobilizing communities and health care systems to recognize the complexities of asthma management, psychologists can serve as influential advocates for patients and families. Examples include the many asthma coalitions that have been formed on local levels with mental health representation to promote access to optimal and interdisciplinary asthma care for patients and families.

Pediatric asthma remains a significant health care problem on local, national, and international levels. Research that integrates medical and behavioral aspects of the disease is necessary to increase professional understanding of the illness. Multidisciplinary approaches to clinical care are particularly useful for children with severe asthma and in cases in which psychosocial barriers impede asthma care. As a result, there is a growing role for psychologists and mental health professionals who work with children who have asthma and their families. As clinical issues can serve to inform research agendas, empirical findings should help health care professionals continue to develop guidelines for effective psychosocial interventions to assist the population of children with pediatric asthma. Psychologists are encouraged to evaluate the effectiveness of collaborative care approaches to asthma in order to document improvements in clinical outcome and cost offset associated with interdisciplinary asthma management. These data are instrumental in securing payment for pediatric psychology services and in promoting the value-added benefit of collaborative care models.

REFERENCES

Alexander, F. G. (1950). *Psychosomatic medicine: Its principles and applications.* New York: Norton.

American Academy of Allergy, Asthma, and Immunology. (1999). *Asthma promoting best practice: Guide for managing asthma in children.* Milwaukee, WI: Author.

American Lung Association. (2000). *Trends in asthma morbidity and mortality: Epidemiology and statistics unit.* New York: Author.

Anderson, B. J., Auslander, W. F., Jung, K. C., Miller, P., & Santiago, J. V. (1990). Assessing family sharing of diabetes responsibilities. *Journal of Pediatric Psychology, 15*, 477–492.

Austin, J. K., Smith, M. S., Risinger, M. W., & McNelis, A. M. (1994). Childhood epilepsy and asthma: Comparison of quality of life. *Epilepsia, 35*, 608–615.

Bauman, L. J. (2000). A patient-centered approach to adherence: Risks for nonadherence. In D. Drotar (Ed.), *Promoting adherence to medical treatment in childhood chronic illness: Concepts, methods, and interventions* (pp. 71–94). Mahwah, NJ: Erlbaum.

Bender, B., Milgrom, H., Rand, C., & Ackerson, L. (1998). Psychological factors associated with medication nonadherence in asthmatic children. *Journal of Asthma, 35*, 347–353.

Bender, B., Wamboldt, F. S., O'Connor, S. L., Rand, C., Szefler, S., Milgrom, H., & Wamboldt, M. Z. (2000). Measurement of children's asthma medication adherence by self-report, mother report, canister weight, and Doser CT. *Annals of Allergy, Asthma, and Immunology, 85*, 416–421.

Bernard-Bonnin, A., Stachenko, S., Bonin, D., Charette, C., & Rousseau, E. (1995). Self-management teaching programs and morbidity of pediatric asthma: A meta-analysis. *Journal of Allergy and Clinical Immunology, 90*, 135–138.

Birkhead, B., Olfaway, N. J., Strunk, R. C., Townsend, M. C., & Teutsch, S. (1989). Investigation of a cluster of deaths of adolescents with asthma: Evidence implicating inadequate treatment and poor patient adherence with medications. *Journal of Allergy and Clinical Immunology, 84*, 484–491.

Bratton, D. L., Price, M., Gavin, L., Glenn, K., Brenner, M., Gelfand, E. W., & Klinnert, M. D. (2001). Impact of a multidisciplinary day program on disease and healthcare costs in children and adolescents with severe asthma: A two-year follow-up study. *Pediatric Pulmonology, 31*, 177–189.

Brown, J. V., Avery, E., Mobley, C., Boccuti, L., & Golbach, T. (1996). Asthma management by preschool children and their families: A developmental framework. *Journal of Asthma, 33*, 299–311.

Busse, W. W., & Lemanske, R. F. J. (2001). Advances in immunology: Asthma. *New England Journal of Medicine, 344*, 350–362.

Carter-Pokras, O. D., & Gergen, P. J. (1993). Reported asthma among Puerto Rican, Mexican-American, and Cuban children, 1982 through 1984. *American Journal of Public Health, 83*, 580–582.

Celano, M., Geller, R. J., Phillips, K. M., & Ziman, R. (1998). Treatment adherence among low-income children with asthma. *Journal of Pediatric Psychology, 23*, 345–349.

Centers for Disease Control and Prevention. (1995). *Vital and Health Statistics, Current Estimates From the National Health Interview Survey, 1994* (DHHS Publication No. PHS 96–1521). Washington, DC: U. S. Government Printing Office.

Centers for Disease Control and Prevention. (1996). Asthma morbidity and hospitalization among children and young adults: US 1980–1993. *Morbidity and Mortality Weekly, 45*, 350–353.

Chambless, D. L., & Hollon, S. D. (1998). Defining empirically supported therapies. *Journal of Consulting and Clinical Psychology, 66*, 7–18.

Clark, N. M. (1998). Management of asthma by parents and children. In A. H. Kotses (Ed.), *Self-management of asthma* (Vol. 113, pp. 271–292). New York: Marcel Dekker.

Clark, N. M., & Gong, M. (2000). Management of chronic disease by practitioners and patients: Are we teaching the wrong things? *British Medical Journal, 320*, 572–575.

Clark, N. M., Gong, M., Schork, M. A., Evans, D., Roloff, D., Hurwitz, M., et al. (1998). Impact of education on patient outcomes. *Pediatrics, 101*, 831–836.

Cookson, W. (1999). The alliance of genes and environment in asthma and allergy. *Nature, 402*, B5–B11.

Crain, E. F., Kercsmar, C., Weiss, K. B., Mitchell, H., & Lynn, H. (1998). Reported difficulties in access to quality care for children with asthma in the inner city. *Archives of Pediatric and Adolescent Medicine, 151*, 333–339.

Creer, T. L. (1993). Medication compliance and childhood asthma. In N. A. Krasneger (Ed.), *Developmental aspects of health compliance behavior* (pp. 303–333). Hillsdale, NJ: Erlbaum.

Creer, T. L. (2000). Self-management and the control of chronic pediatric illness. In D. Drotar (Ed.), *Promoting adherence to medical treatment in chronic illness: Concepts, methods, and interventions* (pp. 95–130). Mahwah, NJ: Erlbaum.

Drotar, D., & Ievers, C. (1994). Age differences in parent and child responsibilities for management of cystic fibrosis and insulin-dependent diabetes mellitus. *Developmental and Behavioral Pediatrics, 15*, 265–272.

Environmental Protection Agency. (1992). *Respiratory health effects of passive smoking: Lung cancer and other disorders* (EPA Publication No. EPA/600/6–90–006F). Washington, DC: Author.

Evans, I. (1992). Asthma among minority children: A growing problem. *Chest, 101*, 368S–371S.

Evans, R., Gergen, P. J., Mitchell, H., Kattan, M., Kercsmar, C., Crain, E., et al. (1999). A randomized clinical trial to reduce asthma morbidity among inner-city children: Results of the National Cooperative Inner-City Asthma Study. *Journal of Pediatrics, 135*, 332–338.

Fitzpatrick, S. B., Coughlin, S. S., & Chamberlin, J. (1992). A novel asthma camp intervention for childhood asthma among urban blacks. *Journal of the National Medical Association, 84*, 233–237.

Fritz, G. K., & McQuaid, E. L. (2000). Chronic medical conditions: Impact on development. In A. J. Sameroff, M. Lewis, & S. M. Miller (Ed.), *Handbook of developmental psychopathology* (2nd ed., pp. 277–289). New York: Kluwer Academic/Plenum Press.

Fritz, G. K., & Overholser, J. C. (1989). Patterns of response to childhood asthma. *Psychosomatic Medicine, 51*, 347–355.

Garrison, W. T., & McQuiston, S. (1989). *Chronic illness during childhood and adolescence: Psychological aspects*. Beverly Hills, CA: Sage.

Gebert, N., Hummelink, R., Konning, J., Staab, D., Schmidt, S., Szczepanski, R., et al. (1998). Efficacy of a self-management program for childhood asthma: A prospective controlled study. *Patient Education and Counseling, 35*, 213–220.

Glaxo-Wellcome. (1998). *Asthma in America: A landmark survey, executive summary*. Research Triangle Park, NC: Author.

Graham, P. J., Rutter, M. L., Yule, W., & Pless, I. B. (1967). Childhood asthma: A psychosomatic disorder? Some epidemiological considerations. *British Journal of Preventive and Social Medicine, 21*, 78–85.

Gustadt, L. B., Gillette, J. W., & Mrazek, D. A. (1989). Determinants of school performance in children with chronic asthma. *American Journal of Disease of Childhood, 143*, 471–475.

Gustafsson, P. A., Kjellman, N. I., & Cederblad, M. (1986). Family therapy in the treatment of severe childhood asthma. *Journal of Psychosomatic Research, 30*, 369–374.

Isenberg, S. A., Lehrer, P. M., & Hochron, S. (1992). The effects of suggestion and emotional arousal on pulmonary function in asthma: A review and a hypothesis regarding vagal mediation. *Psychosomatic Medicine, 54*, 192–216.

Joseph, C. L., Ownby, D. R., Peterson, E. L., & Johnson, C. C. (2000). Racial differences in physiologic parameters related to asthma among middle-class children. *Chest, 117*, 1336–1344.

Kaptien, A. A. (1982). Psychological correlates of length of hospitalization and rehospitalization in patients with acute, severe asthma. *Social Science Medicine, 16*, 725–729.

Kieckhefer, G. M., & Spitzer, A. (1995). School-age children's understanding of the relations between their behavior and their asthma management. *Clinical Nursing Research, 4*, 149–167.

Klinnert, M., & Mrazek, D. A. (1994). Early asthma onset: The interaction between family stressors and adaptive parenting. *Psychiatry, 57*, 51–61.

Klinnert, M. D., McQuaid, E. L., McCormick, D., Adinoff, A. D., & Bryant, N. E. (2000). A multimethod assessment of behavioral and emotional adjustment in children with asthma. *Journal of Pediatric Psychology, 25*, 35–46.

Klinnert, M. D., Nelson, H. S., Price, M. R., Adinoff, A. D., Leung, D. Y. M., & Marzek, D. A. (2001). Onset and persistence of childhood asthma: Predictors from infancy. *Pediatrics, 108*, e69–77.

Klinnert, M. K., McQuaid, E. L., & Gavin, L. (1997). Assessing the family asthma management system. *Journal of Asthma, 34*, 77–88.

Lara, M., Allen, F., & Lange, L. (1999). Physician perceptions of barriers to care for inner-city Latino children with asthma. *Journal of Health Care for the Poor and Underserved, 10*, 27–44.

Larsen, G. L. (1992). Asthma in children. *New England Journal of Medicine, 326*, 1540–1545.

Legorreta, A. P., Christian-Herman, J., O'Connor, R. D., Hasan, M. M., Evans, R., & Leung, K. M. (1998). Compliance with national asthma management guidelines and specialty care. *Archives of Internal Medicine, 158*, 457–464.

Lemanek, K. L., Kamps, J., & Chung, N. B. (2001). Empirically supported treatments in pediatric psychology: Regimen adherence. *Journal of Pediatric Psychology, 26*, 279–282.

Lozano, P., Connell, F. A., & Koepsell, T. D. (1995). Use of health services by African-American children with asthma on Medicaid. *Journal of the American Medical Association, 274*, 469–473.

MacLean, W. E. J., Perrin, J. M., Gortmaker, S., & Pierre, C. B. (1992). Psychological adjustment of children with asthma: Effects of illness severity and recent stressful life events. *Journal of Pediatric Psychology, 17*, 159–171.

Martinez, F. D. (1999). Maturation of immune responses at the beginning of asthma. *Journal of Allergy and Clinical Immunology, 103*, 355–361.

Mattes, J., & Karmaus, W. (1999). The use of antibiotics in the first year of life and the development of asthma: Which comes first? *Clinical and Experimental Allergy, 29*, 729–732.

McQuaid, E. L., Fritz, G. K., Nassau, J. H., Mansell, A., Lilly, M. K., & Klein, R. (2000). Stress and airway resistance in children with asthma. *Journal of Psychosomatic Research, 49*, 239–245.

McQuaid, E. L., Howard, K., Kopel, S. J., Rosenblum, K., & Bibace, R. (2002). Developmental concepts of asthma: Reasoning about illness and strategies for prevention. *Applied Developmental Psychology, 23*, 179–194.

McQuaid, E. L., Kopel, S. J., & Nassau, J. H. (2001). Behavioral adjustment in children with asthma: A meta-analysis. *Journal of Developmental and Behavioral Pediatrics, 22*, 430–439.

McQuaid, E. L., & Nassau, J. H. (1999). Empirically supported treatments of disease-related symptoms in pediatric psychology: Asthma, diabetes, and cancer. *Journal of Pediatric Psychology, 24*, 306–328.

McQuaid, E. L., Penza-Clyve, S., Nassau, J. H., Fritz, G. K., Klein, R., O'Connor, S., et al. (2001). Sharing family responsibility for asthma management tasks. *Children's Health Care, 30*, 183–199.

Midence, K. (1994). The effects of chronic illness on children and their families: An overview. *Genetic, Social, and General Psychology Monographs, 120*, 311–326.

Miklich, D. R., Rewey, H. H., Weiss, J. H., & Kolton, S. (1973). A preliminary investigation of psychophysiological responses to stress among different subgroups of asthmatic children. *Journal of Psychosomatic Research, 17*, 1–8.

Miller, B. D., & Wood, B. L. (1994). Psychophysiologic reactivity in asthmatic children: A cholinergically mediated confluence of pathways. *Journal of the American Academy of Child and Adolescent Psychiatry, 33*, 1236–1245.

Miller, J. E. (2000). The effects of race/ethnicity and income on early childhood asthma prevalence and health care issues. *American Journal of Public Health, 90*, 428–430.

Mrazek, D. A., & Klinnert, M. (1991). *Asthma: Psychoneuroimmunologic considerations* (2nd ed.). San Diego: Academic Press.

National Institutes of Health. (1995). *Asthma management in minority children: Practical insights for clinicians, researchers and public health planners* (DHHS Publication No. 95–3675). Washington, DC: U.S. Government Printing Office.

National Institutes of Health. (1997). *National Asthma Education and Prevention Program (National Heart, Lung, and Blood Institute) Second Expert Panel on the Management of Asthma. Expert Panel Report 2: Guidelines for the diagnosis and management of asthma* (DHHS Publication No. 97–4051). Bethesda, MA: Author.

Nelson, D. A., Johnson, C. C., Divine, G. W., Strauchman, C., Joseph, C. L., & Ownby, D. R. (1997). Ethnic differences in the prevalence of asthma in middle class children. *Annals of Allergy, Asthma, and Immunology, 78*, 21–26.

Nezu, A. M., Nezu, C. M., Friedman, S. H., Faddis, S., & Houts, P. S. (1998). *A problem-solving approach: Helping cancer patients cope*. Washington, DC: American Psychological Association.

Platts-Mills, T. A., Blumenthal, K., Perzanowski, M., & Woodfolk, T. A. (2000). Determinants of clinical allergic disease: The relevance of indoor allergens to the increase in asthma. *American Journal of Respiratory and Critical Care Medicine, 162*, S128–S133.

Rapoff, M. A. (1999). *Adherence to pediatric medical regimens*. New York: Kluwer Academic/Plenum Publishers.

Rand, C. S., & Wise, R. A. (1995). *Adherence with asthma therapy in the management of asthma*. New York: Marcel Dekker.

Rich, M., & Schneider, L. (1996). Managing asthma with the adolescent. *Current Opinions in Pediatrics, 8*, 301–309.

Rosenstreich, D. L., Eggleston, P., Kattan, M., Baker, D., Slavin, R. G., Gergen. P., et al. (1997). The role of cockroach allergy and exposure to cockroach allergen in causing morbidity among inner-city children with asthma. *New England Journal of Medicine, 336*, 1356–1363.

Sears, M. R., Rea, H. H., & Fenwich, J. (1986). Deaths from asthma in New Zealand. *Archives of Disease in Childhood, 61*, 6–10.

Sly, R. (1994). Changing asthma mortality. *Annals of Allergy, 73*, 259–268.

Smith, D. H., Malone, D. C., Lawson, K. A., Okamoto, L. J., Battista, C., & Saunders, W. B. (1997). A national estimate of the economic cost of asthma. *American Journal of Respiratory and Critical Care Medicine, 156*, 787–793.

Sobel, D. S. (1995). Rethinking medicine: Improving health outcomes with cost-effective psychosocial interventions. *Psychosomatic Medicine, 57*, 234–244.

Strachan, D. P. (1989). Hayfever, hygiene, and household size. *British Medical Journal, 299*, 1259–1260.

Strunk, R. C. (1987). Asthma deaths in childhood: Identification of patients at risk and intervention. *Journal of Allergy and Clinical Immunology, 80*, 472–477.

Strunk, R. C., Mrazek, D. A., Wolfson Fuhrmann, G. S., & LaBrecque, J. F. (1985). Physiologic and psychological characteristics associated with deaths due to asthma in childhood: A case-controlled study. *Journal of the American Medical Association, 254*, 1193–1198.

Taitel, M. S., Allen, L., & Creer, T. L. (1998). *The impact of asthma on the patient, family, and society*. New York: Marcel Dekker.

Tal, D., Gil-Spielberg, R., Antonovsky, H., Tal, A., & Moaz, B. (1990). Teaching families to cope with childhood asthma. *Family Systems Medicine, 8*, 135–144.

Taylor, W. R., & Newacheck, P. W. (1992). The impact of childhood asthma on health. *Pediatrics, 90*, 657–662.

Wade, S. L., Holden, G., Lynn, H., Mitchell, H., & Ewart, C. (2000). Cognitive-behavioral predictors of asthma morbidity in inner-city children. *Developmental and Behavioral Pediatrics, 21*, 340–346.

Walders, N., Drotar, D., & Kercsmar, C. (2000). The allocation of family responsibility for asthma management tasks in African-American adolescents. *Journal of Asthma, 37*, 89–99.

Walders, N., Nobile, C., & Drotar, D. (2000). *Promoting adherence to medical treatment in childhood chronic illness: Challenges in a managed care environment.* Mahwah, NJ: Erlbaum.

Wamboldt, M. Z., Fritz, G. K., Mansell, A., McQuaid, E. L., & Klein, R. B. (1998). Relationship of asthma severity and psychological problems in children. *Journal of the American Academy of Child and Adolescent Psychiatry, 37*, 943–950.

Weil, C. M., Wade, S. L., Bauman, L. J., Lynn, H., Mitchell, H., & Lavigne, J. (1999). The relationship between psychosocial factors and asthma morbidity in inner-city children with asthma. *Pediatrics, 104*, 1274–1280.

Weinstein, A. G., Faust, D. S., McKee, L., & Padman, R. (1992). Outcome of short-term hospitalization for children with severe asthma. *Journal of Allergy and Clinical Immunology, 90*, 66–75.

Weiss, K. B., Gergen, P. J., & Hodgson, T. A. (1992). An economic evaluation of asthma in the United States. *New England Journal of Medicine, 326*, 862–866.

Weiss, K. B., & Wagener, D. K. (1990). Changing patterns of asthma mortality: Identifying target populations at high risk. *Journal of the American Medical Association, 264*, 1683–1687.

Weitzman, M., Gortmaker, S. L., Sobel, A. M., & Perrin, J. M. (1992). Recent trends in the prevalence and severity of childhood asthma. *Journal of the American Medical Association, 268*, 2673–2677.

Wright, R., Rodriguez, M., & Cohen, S. (1998). Review of psychosocial stress and asthma: An integrated biopsychosocial approach. *Thorax, 53*, 1066–1074.

Zimmerman, B. J., Bonner, S., Evans, D., & Mellins, R. B. (1999). Self-regulating childhood asthma: A developmental model of family change. *Health Education and Behavior, 26*, 55–71.

17

Cystic Fibrosis

LORI J. STARK
LAURA M. MACKNER
SUSANA R. PATTON
JAMES D. ACTON

Cystic fibrosis (CF) is a genetically inherited disease that affects approximately 25,000 to 30,000 individuals in the United States, primarily Caucasians (Cystic Fibrosis Foundation, 2001). It is transmitted in an autosomal recessive pattern, and an estimated 4-5% of Caucasian Americans are carriers of at least one CF gene. CF affects the exocrine or secretory glands of several major organs in the respiratory, gastrointestinal, and reproductive systems, as well as in the skin. In addition to an elevated sweat chloride concentration, it is most commonly characterized by pancreatic insufficiency and chronic progressive pulmonary disease, which results in early death due to cardiorespiratory failure or complications. With recent advances in therapies, the mean life expectancy is 32.2 years, and the percentage of adult patients with CF has risen from 32% in 1990 to 39% in 2000 (Cystic Fibrosis Foundation, 2001). This increase in longevity is an exciting outcome of improved therapies, but it has posed new challenges in the management of disease and lifestyle choices. New therapies, while contributing to improved survival, have complicated an already arduous self-management regimen. Additionally, in order to maximize the benefit from therapies such as lung transplantation and, potentially, gene replacement therapy, it is important to optimize adherence to currently available therapies in order to minimize progression of the disease. Thus this chapter provides a general overview of CF and its treatment, information on adherence to disease management, and the impact of this chronic disease on affected individuals.

ETIOLOGY

The basic defect occurs in a single gene located on the short arm of chromosome 7. This gene produces a protein called the cystic fibrosis transmembrane conductance regulator

(CFTR) that plays a major role in transporting chloride and water across the cell membrane. The most common defect is named Delta F508. In 2000, CF genotype had been determined for 75% of patients seen at CF centers. Initially, there was hope that by characterizing an individual's specific genetic mutations, the corresponding phenotypic expression of their disease severity (e.g. "mild" or "severe") could be predicted. Although some associations have been demonstrated between certain mutations and the likelihood of pancreatic insufficiency, this has not been the case with respect to the severity of lung disease.

DIAGNOSIS

To meet diagnostic criteria for CF, an individual must have both suggestive clinical findings and laboratory evidence of CFTR dysfunction. Clinical findings may be respiratory (e.g., chronic cough, recurrent pneumonia, chronic sinusitis), digestive (e.g., failure to thrive, malabsorption, intestinal obstruction), or associated with dysfunction of other systems (e.g., infertility, hypochloremic dehydration). The sweat test is the standard test for confirming the diagnosis of CF. Although more than 50% of children are diagnosed by age 6 months and more than 70% by 1 year of age, the dependence on clinical suspicion can delay the diagnosis, creating emotional difficulties for families and delaying treatment for the child. Neonatal screening for CF is available in only a few states due to the cost and expertise needed and the high rate of false positives of the screening test. The Wisconsin CF Neonatal Screening Project (Farrell et al., 1997) has found that infants diagnosed through neonatal screening were younger at age of diagnosis and had significantly higher weight and height for age percentiles, both at the time of their diagnosis and at ages 5–6 years (Farrell et al., 1997), and greater height for age *z*-scores at age 12 years (Farrell et al., 2001). These data demonstrate the potential of neonatal screening programs to improve growth; however, no evidence exists that neonatal testing can affect survival.

MECHANISM OF DISEASE AND TREATMENT

Decreased production of or decrease in function of CFTR in epithelial cells that line the airways, intestines, pancreatic ducts, hepatic ducts and vas deferens cause decreased transportation of chloride ions and insufficient fluid secretion. This results in the production of abnormally thick and sticky mucus that obstructs airways and ducts, and ultimately leads to chronic injury and dysfunction of the involved organs. Because there is no cure for CF, treatment typically targets symptoms of the disease, primarily in the lungs and pancreas. Although the lungs of patients with CF are normal at birth, the production of thick, viscid mucus impedes the normal cleaning mechanism and leaves the lungs vulnerable to infection by microorganisms. Microorganisms such as *P. aeruginosa* and *B. cepacia* can never be permanently eliminated once established in the CF lung. Thus, individuals with CF have chronic bacterial infection with bouts of pulmonary exacerbations that result in progressive damage to the airways and eventually to respiratory failure.

Given the progression of CF in the lungs, treatment has traditionally focused on assisting the patient in clearing the mucus from the lungs and treating infections. To clear mucus from the lungs, chest physiotherapy (CPT) techniques are employed that involve a caregiver clapping on up to 11 sections of the patient's chest and the patient coughing up and expectorating the mucus dislodged from the airways. CPT is recommended two to four times daily and can last up to 30 minutes. To assist in clearing the mucus the patient may use inhaled or nebulized bronchodilators to open the airways and/or mucolytic agents to thin the mucus prior to CPT. The addition of these agents can add another 15 to 20 minutes to CPT. Over the past 5 years several advances have been made that allow the patient with CF a little more independence in performing airway clearance. Specifically, two devices, the Flutter and the high-frequency chest compression vest (HFCC; ThAIRapy vest), have been developed that allow patients to do airway clearance without someone doing the clapping. The Flutter is an inexpensive, small plastic handheld device that loosens mucus and accelerates airflow in the mid- and large airways by vibrating airway walls when the patient exhales into it. The HFCC vest loosens mucus by delivering sharp compression pulses to the entire chest via an inflatable vest worn by the patient. The vest is clinically effective compared with standard CPT but expensive, as it must be rented and is not always covered by health insurance. Another advance in airway clearance is the development of rhDNase to decrease the viscosity of lung secretions. RhDNase, administered by aerosol one to two times daily, has been shown to significantly improve pulmonary function in patients with pulmonary exacerbation (Willmott et al., 1996).

Antibiotic treatment is also a mainstay of CF treatment for bronchial infection. There are two theories on the use of antibiotics: (1) prophylactically to reduce the frequency of infections; or (2) only for pulmonary exacerbations. The prophylactic use of antibiotics is coming into question as more long-term studies are being completed that show no benefit (Beardsmore et al., 1994) and potential negative effects (Ramsey, 1996). However, a recently completed study of the use of aerolized tobramycin (TOBI) demonstrated improved pulmonary function, reduced sputum bacterial density, reduced need for intravenous antibiotics, and reduced hospitalization when used daily on an every-other-month schedule (Ramsey et al., 1999). As with the use of antibiotics in general, it remains controversial in CF when to initiate treatment: when clinically indicated or only after documented colonization of *P. aeruginosa*. In addition to routine use of antibiotics, a better understanding of the role of inflammation in lung destruction has led to investigation of anti-inflammatory therapy, including steroids such as predisone and nonsteroidal anti-inflammatory agents such as ibuprofen. Although the long-term side effects of steroids, such as growth failure and insulin-dependent diabetes (Eigan, Rosenstein, FitzSimmons, & Schidlow, 1995), preclude the use of these agents on a routine or long-term basis, high-dose ibuprofen with appropriate drug level assessment appears promising (Konstan, Byard, Hoppel, & Davis, 1995).

Treatment for pulmonary symptoms takes a substantial amount of time and effort to coordinate and complete. During episodes of pulmonary exacerbation, the antibiotic regimen is intensified, as are airway clearance treatments. Pulmonary exacerbation is indicated by symptoms of fatigue, reduced pulmonary function, change in chest X-ray or physical exam, worsening of appetite and weight loss, increased cough and sputum production, and sometimes fever. If symptoms do not respond to increased oral or inhaled antibiotics, intravenous antibiotics are initiated, typically in the hospital. Approximately 37 to 40% of patients with CF have one or more acute exacerbations a year, resulting in a mean hospital stay of 10 to 12 days (Cystic Fibrosis Foundation, 2001).

Unlike in the lungs, the damage in the pancreas begins before birth (Mueller, Aubrei, Gasser, Duchatel, & Boue, 1985) as the accumulation of mucus secretions obstruct the pancreatic ducts, resulting in tissue damage that leads to inadequate secretion of digestive enzymes. Eighty-five to ninety percent of individuals with CF are pancreatic insufficient at diagnosis. Even patients who are pancreatic sufficient may later convert to being pancreatic insufficient. Pancreatic insufficiency prevents digestion of fat, protein, and fat-soluble vitamins. Pancreatic replacement enzymes are prescribed to aid in digestion but do not totally correct for malabsorption. Thus, to offset the energy loss from malabsorption and the energy demands due to lung disease, individuals with CF are recommended to consume 120–150% of the recommended daily allowance (RDA) of energy for healthy individuals and a regimen of fat-soluble vitamins (Ramsey, Farrell, & Pencharz, 1992).

MEDICAL COMPLICATIONS OF CF AS THE PATIENT AGES

The progressive nature of CF causes many patients to experience a number of complications as they grow older. CF-related diabetes (CFRD) has become an increasing problem for patients with CF, with the average age of onset between 18 and 21 years (Rosenecker, Eichler, Kuhn, Harms, & von der Hardt, 1995). CFRD is typically associated with more severe disease symptoms and earlier death in affected patients, and findings suggest that the deterioration in patients' health may precede the diagnosis of CFRD by 2 to 4 years (Lanng, Thorsteinsson, Nerup, & Koch, 1994). CFRD shares features of both Type 1 and Type 2 diabetes but is a distinct entity. In addition to the increased intake of calories and fats typically recommended for patients with CF, the treatment regimen involves regular glucose monitoring, insulin administration, tracking of carbohydrate intake, and consistent meals and snacks. Defects in CFTR can also cause liver disease in patients with CF. The prevalence rate for liver disease is 5.3% among Americans with CF (Cystic Fibrosis Foundation, 2001). Treatment for CF-related liver disease includes oral bile acid medication, sclerotherapy and vasopressin to treat hypertension and/or bleeding in the liver, and, occasionally, transplantation. Osteoporosis is another problem that has received increased attention as survival rates for CF have improved. Bone mineral density (BMD) is the marker for osteoporosis. Adults with CF have average BMD values around 2.5 *SD*s below the mean and have a significantly higher rate of fractures compared with healthy adults (Aris et al., 1998). Lowered BMD begins in childhood in CF (Henderson & Madsen, 1996). Treatment guidelines have not been established for osteoporosis in CF, but exceeding recommendations for calcium intake has been suggested (Ott & Aitken, 1998).

Although not a complication of aging per se, many patients with CF experience fertility problems as a result of the disease. Although male potency is typically normal, 98% of men with CF are missing or have a dysfunctional vas deferens, making it difficult or impossible to conceive a baby with a woman without intervention. The pathophysiology behind this abnormality is not well understood, but it may be due to either a congenital abnormality or to the consequence of collecting mucus and other secretions (Bolyard, 2001). This abnormality cannot be surgically corrected, but conception can be assisted through in vitro fertilization (McCallum et al., 2000). Science has also made strides in assisting women with CF who wish to become mothers. Unlike their male counterparts, women with CF usually have anatomically normal reproductive organs. However, when compared with healthy peers, their fertility rate is typically lower (Bolyard, 2001). The reason for this difference is not well understood, but it may be related to disruptions in ovulation or possibly abnormally thick cervical mucus, which may prevent sperm from penetrating into the cervix and achieving conception. Historically, women with CF were advised not to become pregnant because of the potential health risks they might face due to the strain of pregnancy. More recent studies have demonstrated improved outcomes for mothers with CF and their infants (Gilljam et al., 2000).

ADHERENCE TO TREATMENT

Assessment

Clearly, the patient with CF must follow a complex, arduous daily regimen, the complexity of which typically increases as the patient ages and develops new complications. Adherence to CF treatment is critically important to optimal health and longevity (Patterson, Budd, Goetz, & Warwick, 1993). In addition, although new therapies being developed hold promise for halting the progression of lung disease in patients with CF, lung damage cannot be reversed once it has occurred. Despite the importance of adherence, very few studies examine adherence or the reasons for poor adherence within this disease. In addition, most of the studies are limited in the information that they provide because of their reliance on self-reported adherence and the use of broad definitions of compliance (Eddy et al., 1998; Passero, Remor, & Solomon, 1981). The overreliance on self-report is problematic because of the discrepancy found between self-report and electronic monitoring of adherence in other populations with pediatric chronic illnesses. In the literature on adherence in CF, self-report of adherence to medication and vitamins has been quite high (82–90%) whereas self-report of adherence to CPT and diet has been found to be much lower (40% and 20%, respectively, Passero et al., 1981; 51% and 12%, respectively, Eddy et al., 1998). However, in the one study that assessed adherence to pancreatic enzyme replacement therapy independent of other medications, 19% of patients were found to be taking pancreatic enzymes at the most ineffective time, after meals (Rusakow, Miller, McCarthy, Gershan, & Splaingard, 1998). Findings such as these have led to conclusions that overall adherence to treatment in CF is generally good, but that adherence to CPT and diet are difficult (Gudas, Koocher, & Wypij, 1991).

Recently, investigators have attempted to improve on self-report methodologies by obtaining more detailed information on adherence. For example, the Treatment Adherence Questionnaire—Cystic Fibrosis (TAQ-CF) is a self-report measure that assesses frequency and *duration* of airway clearance, aerosol treatment, and pancreatic enzymes (Quittner et al., 1996). Employing this measure, Ievers et al. (1999) found a high correlation between mother's report and physician prescription for the frequency of airway clearance but only a moderate correlation for the duration of treatment. In addition, they found only moderate correlations between mothers' self-reports of their children's adherence to the frequency of taking aerosol mediations and pancreatic enzymes and physician recommendations. The correlations between child self-report and physician recommendations were even lower across all treatment components.

Use of 24-hour recall of daily activities, including the performance of treatment, is a relatively sophisticated and powerful self-report methodology for assessing adherence to treatment in children with diabetes that has been relatively underutilized in assessing adherence in other chronic conditions, including CF. Employing this methodology, Ricker, Delameter, and Hsu (1998) found that adherence to CPT was lower than for the other components and that the range of adherence within each component of the regimen was large: 65–100% for CPT (mean 76.54%), 75–100% for antibiotics (mean 88.56%), and 88–100% for multivitamins (mean 91.18%).

Because of the complexity of the treatment regimen for CF, it is important to examine not only whether the treatment was performed but also whether it was performed correctly, for the right amount of time, and at the recommended interval. Electronic monitoring provides a way of assessing adherence more precisely but has rarely been used in CF, probably because of the absence of electronic monitoring capabilities for many aspects of the CF regimen. Nonetheless, the limited data available indicate that in order to truly understand the challenges to adherence, advances in assessment are needed. For example, using electronic monitoring to assess adherence to nebulized rhDNase in children with CF, Wilkinson and Paton (1999) found that an average of only 51.8% of doses were taken at the correct time for a minimum of 5 minutes. Failure to administer nebulized medications for a sufficient amount of time results in inadequate dosing for a therapeutic effect.

Whereas self-report of good adherence is suspect, self-report of poor adherence is generally assumed more accurate, because there is less motivation for patients to "fake bad." In self-report adherence studies, adherence to diet and CPT are typically rated low by patients and their families (Eddy et al., 1998; Passero et al., 1981). Studies assessing adherence to dietary recommendations in children with CF using 3- to 5-day diet diaries generally agree with the self-report data. On average only 15–23% of children have been found to be meeting their dietary treatment needs of at least 120% of the RDA for energy (Anthony, Paxton, Bines, & Phelan, 1999; Stark, Jelalian, Mulvihill et al., 1995; Tomezsko, Stallings, & Scanlin, 1992). For CPT, new forms of airway clearance such as the Flutter or ThAIRapy vest may result in better adherence because they are less imposing and therefore more acceptable to patients. However, little empirical investigation exists regarding adherence to these airway clearance methods, and no relationship has been found between adherence and satisfaction with CPT technique (Oermann, Swank, & Sockrider, 2000).

Variables Associated with Adherence

Despite the difficulties involved in assessing adherence to the CF treatment regimen, the literature does provide some insight into the variables associated with adherence and nonadherence. In general, global knowledge of CF does not appear to influence adherence (Parcel et al., 1994), but specific understanding of the treatment regimen has been found to be associated with better adherence (Henley & Hill, 1990; Ievers et al., 1999). Age is also strongly related to adherence, as older children and adolescents with CF have been found to be less adherent than younger children (DiGirolamo, Quittner, Ackerman, & Stevens, 1997; Quittner et al., 1996; Ricker et al., 1998). Adolescence appears to be a particularly difficult period during which to ensure adherence, and the trajectory of nonadherence into adulthood is not well understood. In adults with CF, individuals who report more "worry" about their disease report greater adherence to airway clearance and pancreatic enzyme usage (Abbott, Dodd, & Webb, 1996), and individuals who score higher on optimism and hopefulness showed better adherence than those who endorsed more avoidant coping strategies (Abbott, Dodd, Gee, & Webb, 2001).

Variables associated with dietary adherence have received the most attention, as researchers have attempted to identify barriers that may be targeted in subsequent intervention studies to improve adherence to diet. In a series of studies across toddlers, preschoolers, and school-age children with CF, parent and child mealtime behaviors were examined (Powers et al., 2002; Stark, Jelalian, Mulvihill et al., 1995; Stark et al., 1997). In these studies children with CF were found to consume similar amounts of calories per day as children without CF, but not enough to meet the CF dietary recommendations. Children with CF were also found to take significantly longer to eat than control children, and parents of children with CF reported more mealtime problems of dawdling and refusing food than parents of control children. Direct observation of behaviors of parents and preschool-age children (Stark et al., 2000) found that children with CF showed a greater frequency of behaviors incompatible with eating than children without CF and that parents of children with CF demonstrated a greater frequency of behaviors to encourage eating. Subsequent evaluation of these differences on family functioning during mealtime indicated that this increased frequency of parent and child behaviors may have negative effects. Spieth et al. (2001) found that the families of preschool children with CF scored significantly lower on six out of seven domains of family functioning than families of children without CF and that they scored in the "unhealthy" range on all seven domains, whereas families of the controls scored in the "healthy" range. These findings indicate that families of children with CF may face additional challenges when feeding their children and that commonly used strategies may have negative effects on family functioning at meals.

Intervention

Although little research has been done on assessing compliance in CF, even less has been done to directly intervene to improve adherence. Only two published studies target improved adherence to CPT (Hagopian & Thompson, 1999; Stark, Miller, Plienes, & Drabman, 1987), three published studies target improved adherence to diet (Stark, Bowen, Tyc, Evans, & Passero, 1990; Stark et al., 1993; Stark et al., 1996), three studies examine home-based exercise (de Jong, Grevink, Roorda, Kaptein, & van der Schans, 1994; Holzer, Schnall, & Landau, 1984; Schneiderman-Walker et al., 2000), and two studies consider adherence across the CF treatment regimen (Bartholomew et al., 1997; Goldbeck & Babka, 2001). Each of the interventions for adherence to CPT were single case studies, and one study was conducted with a child with CF who had comorbid disorders of mental retardation and autism (Hagopian & Thompson, 1999), thus limiting the generalizability of the findings to the CF population. Only one of the three studies on home-based exercise intervention provides a measure of adherence to treatment (Schneiderman-Walker et al., 2000), and none of the studies adequately describes interventions to improve adherence.

The nutrition intervention studies (Stark et al., 1990; Stark et al., 1993; Stark et al., 1996) have all implemented a group behavioral treatment that targeted adherence difficulties described by parents and children ages 3 to 12 years. Children participating in these studies have consistently increased their daily caloric intake by an average of 900 cal/day and demonstrated an average weight gain of 1.47 kg. A meta-analysis comparing the effects of behavioral intervention with medical interventions of parenteral and enteral nutrition found the gains reported for the behavioral treatment to be comparable to medical intervention for weight gain and caloric intake (Jelalian, Stark, Reynolds, & Seifer, 1998).

A psychoeducational program recently developed and evaluated under a demonstration grant targeted adherence to self-management across the entire treatment regimen in CF (Bartholomew et al., 1997). The Cystic Fibrosis Family Education Program is a self-paced, print curriculum that provides instructional information on all aspects of self-management in CF and instructs families on the use of goal setting, reinforcement, and self-monitoring. A variety of outcome measures focusing on knowledge, self-efficacy, and self-management were obtained from patients from birth to 18 years of age. Although the study reports significant effects for self-management scores, it is not clear whether actual behavior change occurred because self-management was measured via questionnaire rather than objective measures of adherence. Goldbeck and Babka (2001) evaluated the impact of a multifamily educational program for children with CF age 12 and under. Treatment sessions focused on a specific management or educational area for CF, and all members of the treatment team participated, but no changes were found on any of the measures of adherence or coping.

In general, the literature on treatment adherence in CF is limited in the number and scope of studies, both in assessment and treatment outcome. Studies typically rely on single self-report measures to assess the impact of intervention on improved adherence. Further, most studies are limited in sample size or do not employ a control group. In the exercise literature, interventions were implemented with no measure of adherence. If the field is to advance its understanding of effective treatments to increase adherence in CF, clinical researchers need to employ randomized clinical designs with sufficient participants to evaluate interventions and rigorous outcome measures that provide objective, as well as self-report data on adherence. Currently Quittner and Drotar are comparing Behavioral–Family Systems Therapy to education only to improve CPT and medication adherence in adolescents with CF (Quittner & Drotar, 1997). This study is unique in that it specifically targets and measures adherence to three separate components of treatment (enzyme use, inhaled medications, and airway clearance) and employs multiple measures of adherence on each outcome variable, including self-report and electronic monitoring (Quittner, Drotar et al., 2000). With a projected enrollment of 120 adolescents with CF, data from this clinical trial will be useful not only in determining the efficacy of the intervention but also in providing data on baseline adherence to CF treatment regimens.

PSYCHOLOGICAL ADJUSTMENT

A child with CF must cope with multiple demands and potential stressors. The nature of these demands and the child's ability to cope with them likely differs at different developmental levels. The following section describes developmental issues a child with CF might face and the research on the psychological adjustment of these children. Due to recent advances in medical care, this section focuses on recent work on the psychosocial functioning of children with CF.

Infancy and Preschool Age

Infants and preschoolers with CF typically experience few health problems related to their illness. However, adherence during this period is important to maintain good health. Developmentally, the infancy and preschool years are characterized by conflict between dependence on the caregiver and independence. Feeding and eating issues may be foremost during this time, and medication administration may also be difficult as a toddler asserts autonomy. Goldberg and colleagues have conducted a line of research investigating the psychological adjustment and health status of children with CF from infancy to age 4 and found that children with CF are at higher risk for insecure attachment when compared with norms but not when compared with a healthy comparison group (Simmons, Goldberg, Washington, Fischer-Fay, & Maclusky, 1995) or to children with congenital heart disease (CHD; Goldberg, Gotowiec, & Simmons, 1995). In addition, children with CF who had insecure attachments showed lower nutritional status through age 3 years than children with CF who had secure attachments. The authors suggested that this relationship may be due to stress related specifically to the feeding interaction or to underlying attachment patterns (Goldberg et al., 1995). Behavior problems among the children with CF, however, were comparable to those of healthy children and children with CHD through age 4. Thus Simmons and Goldberg (2001) concluded that infants and preschoolers with CF generally do well in the area of psychological adjustment. However, they suggested that three subgroups fare less well: children with insecure attachments who are at risk for feeding problems and nutritional deficiencies, children who do not respond to treatment and have continual poor physical health, and children who develop significant behavior problems, with no evidence that their behavior problems are related to their medical problems. Clinically, these findings highlight the need for prevention or intervention emphasizing the development of secure attachment, appropriate feeding strategies, and support for parents, especially those who have children with severe disease.

School Age

School-age children face the developmental challenges of continuing autonomy and developing psychosocial competence. As children with CF enter school, they may become more aware of the impact of CF on their lives and of their differences when compared with other children. In a qualitative study of children with CF, themes that emerged include developing an understanding of the disease, concerns about being teased by peers, telling others about the disease, and competing physically with peers (D'Auria, Christian, & Richardson, 1997). Although the majority of school-age children with CF continue to enjoy good health during this period, many may be hospitalized for the first time. Also, with increasing demands related to school, sports, and social activities, fitting daily CF treatments into their schedules can become a challenge for many families.

A prior review of the psychological adjustment of school-age children and adolescents reported that, overall, children with CF do not demonstrate difficulty in adjustment but may be at risk for anxiety-related concerns and somatic complaints (Stark, Jelalian, & Miller, 1995). More recent studies have also found a risk for anxiety in children and adolescents with CF, as well as a risk for behavioral disturbances (Thompson, Gustafson, Gil, Godfrey, & Bennett-Murphy, 1998; Thompson, Gustafson, Hamlett, & Spock, 1992). Low self-worth, high maternal anxiety, high levels of perceived stress, low levels of perceived efficacy, and low levels of internal health locus of control were significant predictors of children's symptoms (Thompson et al., 1998; Thompson et al., 1992). However, two studies found a reduction in symptoms over time for children with CF (Thompson, Gustafson, Gil, Kinney, & Spock, 1999; Wilson, Fosson, Kanga, & D'Angelo, 1996). These studies suggest that symptoms of poor psychological adjustment may be transitory for many children with CF and may resolve naturally as children grow older.

Among studies with combined samples of children and adolescents, two studies found CBCL scores to be in the normal range, suggesting few externalizing or internalizing behavior problems in children and adolescents with CF (Czyzewski & Bartholomew, 1998; Pumariega, Pearson, & Seilheimer, 1993). However, Pumariega et al. (1993) also found 11% of children with CF to have clinically significant depression scores and 9% to have clinically significant trait anxiety scores, as measured by the Child Depression Inventory and the State–Trait Anxiety Inventory for Children. These seemingly contradictory findings suggest that children's level of functioning may vary widely depending on how it is assessed; thus multimethod assessments are needed to ensure greater accuracy. Although CBCL scores were in the normal range, Czyzewski and Bartholomew (1998) found that children's adaptive behavior composite subscales and daily living and socialization skills subscales were significantly below the standardization mean. However, by parent report, 73% of children had no functional limitations.

Although prior research on the psychological adjustment of school-age children has found children with CF to report greater anxiety and somatic complaints, research conducted in the past 10 years has proven mixed. Although one study reported high rates of poor psychological adjustment for school-age children with CF (Thompson et al., 1992), others report functioning in the normal range (Czyzewski & Bartholomew, 1998; Pumariega et al., 1993). Additionally, there is some evidence for improved functioning over time, suggesting that symptoms may be transient and easily resolved for many children (Thompson et al., 1999; Wilson et al., 1996). Children with a greater number of stressors, fewer coping strategies, and anxious mothers appeared to be at higher risk for psychological difficulty (Thompson et al., 1998; Thompson et al., 1992). Also, children themselves reported increasing concerns about peers and the impact that their disease may have on their physical abilities (D'Auria et al., 1997). Because many of these studies lacked comparison groups, their overall conclusions are limited. Many of these studies also used mixed samples of children and adolescents, which is unfortunate because developmental and health-related issues are different for these two groups. Future prospective studies investigating risk factors associated with children's psychological adjustment are important, as prevention and intervention strategies will likely be most successful if they focus on helping children develop strategies for coping with stress and peer relations.

Adolescence

Adolescence is a period of identity formation during which social functioning and peer acceptance are of primary importance. Adolescents with CF may be physically smaller than their peers and may have delayed puberty, which can have effects on self-esteem and peer relations. Adherence to medical regimens is also typically lowest during adolescence, which can contribute to declines in health. During this time, children and families begin to look toward the future and to make plans for education or for a vocation. Adolescents with CF face these important decisions, as well as the challenges of becoming an adult with a chronic, fatal disease. Overall, the research with adolescents with CF has focused on two main areas: adolescents' psychological adjustment and their personal experience of living with CF. Looking at psychological adjustment, past research with adolescents with CF has found them to be comparable to their peers with regard to their psychological adjustment (Stark, Jelalian, & Miller, 1995). However, more recent studies have been mixed. Blair, Cull, and Freeman (1994) found that adolescents with CF were not significantly more distressed than healthy or anorexic adolescents, whereas Thompson, Gustafson, and Gil (1995) found that 51% of adolescents met criteria for DSM diagnoses of anxiety disorder or oppositional behavior. DiGirolamo et al. (1997) found that 9% of adolescents in their sample had clinically significant symptoms of depression; however, patients' overall self-esteem was in the normal range. In contrast, Sawyer, Rosier, Phelan, and Bowes (1995) found that adolescent girls with CF reported self-images that were significantly below norms, particularly in the area of body image, whereas adolescent boys with CF reported self-images that were within the normal range.

Related to psychological adjustment, two studies have examined specific psychosocial concerns for adolescents with CF. In a qualitative study, D'Auria, Christian, Henderson, and Haynes (2000) reported concerns about worsening of symptoms, feeling "out of the loop" at school due to absences, finding new friends among other adolescents with CF, and dealing with the implications of a lifelong disease. DiGirolamo et al. (1997) reported that the most commonly mentioned problem areas were school (making up missed schoolwork, experiencing symptoms at school), medications and treatment, and parent–teen relationships and that the problem area rated as most difficult was clinic and hospital visits. Although social ties play an important part in the lives of adolescents, only one study specifically examined social support among adolescents with CF, it found that adolescents reported more support from family members than from friends (Graetz, Shute, & Sawyer, 2000). Clearly, more research is needed to investigate how adolescents with CF may perceive the support that they receive from family and friends, as well as the role that support may play in their overall functioning. In addition, more efforts are needed to develop psychosocial treatments, as only one such study was found in the literature (Hains, Davies, Behrens, & Biller, 1997) and the results of that study were mixed concerning improved coping and decreased anxiety for five adolescents with CF.

In general, studies are limited by a lack of healthy comparison groups, and the results are mixed. Illness severity and worsening health are a concern to adolescents (D'Auria et al., 2000) and may contribute to poor psychological adjustment (Thompson et al., 1995). Other areas of concern to adolescents with CF include peer and family relationships, school, and treatment. These concerns are not surprising given the developmental importance of peers and the worsening health these adolescents often experience. Adolescents who experience health difficulties and school absences should be given ample opportunity to interact with peers when possible, and they may benefit from interventions that target coping with CF-related stressors.

FAMILY ADAPTATION AND FUNCTIONING

Having a family member with CF involves a significant burden of care. Parents of children with CF are responsible for administering a complex treatment regimen, for managing the emotional distress associated with a fatal, chronic medical condition, and for managing the feelings of siblings who may perceive differential treatment. CF can affect every member of the family. Research in this area has primarily focused on parental and family functioning, with some work in sibling adaptation.

Family Functioning

Ievers and Drotar (1996) recently reviewed studies on parental and family functioning published from 1981 to 1994. This section reviews their findings and adds findings from more recent studies. Ievers and Drotar concluded that parents of children with CF experience significantly more overall stress and more illness-related stress than parents of healthy children, and two of three studies reviewed indicated that mothers of children with CF had significantly greater psychological distress. However, most studies did not find significant differences between families with a child with CF and families with healthy children in child-rearing practices or in general family functioning. Ievers and Drotar reported that concerns most commonly cited by parents of children with CF included the chronic burden of care, the terminal nature of the illness, and disruptions in family relationships, such as marital relationships. Recent work by Quittner et al. (1998) lends additional support for the findings that parents of a child with CF experience more stress than parents of healthy children. Parents of children with CF displayed significantly more marital conflict over child rearing, a greater burden of child care and medical care, fewer positive daily interactions between spouses, more frustration over the spousal division of labor, and less recreational time than parents of healthy children. Two additional studies investigated variables related to stressors in families with a child with CF. One study found that younger age of the child was significantly related to more stress associated with typical routines and that better health was significantly related to stress associated with illness routines (Eiser, Zoritch, Hiller, Havermans, & Billig, 1995). The other study found poor maternal perception of physical well-being to be significantly associated with treatment adherence problems, poor peer relations, and poor sibling relations in the family (Foster, Bryon, & Eiser, 1998).

Although studies have found greater stress in families of a child with CF, four studies indicate that general family functioning and maternal well-being is similar to that of families with healthy children (Blair et al., 1994; Blair, Freeman, & Cull, 1995; Darke & Goldberg, 1994; Foster et al., 1998). However, differences in specific aspects of family functioning have been identified. Parents of children with CF were found to be more overinvolved, controlling, and serious and less encouraging in their interactions with their children than parents of healthy children (Blair et al., 1995; Solomon & Breton, 1999). Children with CF were found to be more demanding and whiny than healthy children, and their cues were more difficult to read. The literature on family functioning is fairly consistent: Families with a child with CF experience more stress, but parental and family functioning is generally not significantly different from that in families with healthy children. However, differences in specific aspects of family functioning may exist. For example, families with a child with CF may be more involved or controlling than families with healthy children, which is not surprising given the treatment demands.

Sibling Adjustment

Most studies on siblings of children with CF have focused on differential treatment or attention among the child with CF and healthy siblings. One qualitative study reported that 60% of children felt that their sibling with CF received special attention (Derouin & Jessee, 1996). Foster et al. (2001) found that parents reported treating their child with CF differently, especially when that child was ill. Children with CF reported that they felt that their parents were more lenient when disciplining them compared with their siblings, and both parents and children with CF felt that siblings were resentful or jealous of the extra attention the child with CF received. However, neither of these studies employed a control group. Davies (1993) used a questionnaire to compare the amount of maternal care given to healthy siblings in families with a child with CF to the amount of care given in families with only healthy children and found no significant differences. Quittner and Opipari (1994) used daily phone interviews to assess the amount of time mothers spent with children in families with a child with CF compared with families with only healthy children. Mothers in the CF group spent significantly more time with their children with CF than with their healthy children, and they rated the quality of the time with the healthy child as more negative than mothers in the comparison group. Mothers in the comparison group did not spend a significantly greater amount of time with any one healthy child, and there was little difference in their ratings of the quality of the time with each child. Overall, the body of literature on siblings of children with CF is small and inconsistent, and conclusions cannot be made about sibling adjustment without further research.

NEW CHALLENGES AND NEW FRONTIERS IN CF

In order for pediatric psychologists to provide innovative care and conduct meaningful research in CF, they must have a comprehensive understanding of what the advances in the treatment of the disease mean for individuals growing up with CF. This understanding includes knowledge of adult outcome in terms of psychosocial functioning, transitioning to adult care, and the impact of new therapies on quality of life at all developmental levels, including adulthood.

Adults with CF: Psychosocial Outcome

As improved medical treatments have increased the life expectancy of patients with CF, personal and professional development becomes increasingly important to understand. In the United States, only a small percentage of adults with CF describe themselves as unemployed (9%) or disabled (13%). Approximately 28% of adults report having a college degree, an additional 24% describe themselves as full-time students, and 50% report that they are employed either full or part time. In addition to achieving educational and professional goals, 36% of adults with CF report that they are married or living with someone, although the majority (59%) are single (Cystic Fibrosis Foundation, 2001).

Studies specifically examining the psychosocial functioning and adaptation of adult patients with CF have yielded variable results. The most recent research reported relatively normal functioning in adult patients (Anderson, Flume, & Hardy, 2001; Blair et al., 1994), whereas an earlier review of studies suggests that adults with CF may experience clinically elevated symptoms of depression and anxiety and noteworthy eating disturbances (Stark, Jelalian, & Miller, 1995). Because the symptoms of CF tend to worsen with age, the pervasiveness of psychopathology and emotional distress in older patients with CF may be a function of their disease status rather than their age. Anderson et al. (2001) examined the psychological functioning of adults with CF and related this functioning to patients' age, gender, and disease severity. Overall, the researchers found the adult sample to be within the normal range on symptoms of depression and anxiety. However, when placed in predictor models to determine variables that may predict poorer psychological functioning, significant main effects were found for patient health status variables. Separate univariate analysis of variance revealed that patients lower in lung functioning reported increased anxiety scores. Interestingly, patients with lower percentage of ideal body weight (e.g., an indication of more severe nutritional disease) reported lower levels of anxiety than patients with more normal body weight, a finding that was contrary to expectations.

Overall, the recent research investigating psychosocial well-being has found adults with CF to be functioning independently and within the normal range for symptoms of depression and anxiety. Risk factors for psychosocial problems in adults with CF are unclear; some evidence suggests that patients' age and disease status may contribute to greater vulnerability to distress (Anderson et al., 2001). Today, adults with CF balance a number of competing demands, including school or work demands, family or parenting demands, social demands, and treatment demands. Understanding and preparing patients with CF to manage these demands is a new area requiring both clinical and research attention.

Transition from Pediatric to Adult Care

One way to enhance adaptation and disease management as the life expectancy of the patient with CF lengthens may be to facilitate transition from pediatric care teams to adult care teams. Currently, there are 44 adult CF programs in the United States that have specific accreditation from the CF Foundation. These programs are staffed by medical professionals with experience in caring for adult patients, as well as specialized training in the management of CF. Adult CF centers can offer patients comprehensive medical care that is sensitive to their changing needs, such as issues regarding birth control and family planning. To assist patients in managing social and vocational challenges due to acute disease exacerbation or a chronic decline in health status, many centers employ social workers who can advise patients on issues of disability, health insurance, and other financial matters. The typical age of transition for patients is about 18 years (Flume, Anderson, Hardy, & Gray, 2001). No specific guidelines direct the transition of patients from pediatric to adult CF centers. However, a number of factors have been identified that may predict better transitions, including a lengthy transition period and early involvement of both the pediatric and adult CF teams in the patient's care (Flume et al., 2001). Given their background in child development, pediatric psychologists may play an active role in the transition process for adolescents and young adults with CF by providing information regarding emotional and cognitive development and an assessment of the adolescent's readiness to assume a more active role in self-management of his or her disease. One study on self-management found adolescents (ages 11 to 14 years) with CF to be comparable to adolescents with insulin-dependent diabetes mellitus on their level of independence for treatment responsibilities. Although child age was positively associated with increased responsibility, parents of adolescents with CF continued to have sole responsibility for 37% of treatment-related tasks, and shared responsibility was relatively stable across the age groups of 8–10 years and 11–14 years (Drotar & Ievers, 1994). Studies such as this one could be expanded to evaluate older adolescents in order to assist with transition planning to adult care.

Health-Related Quality of Life in CF

Most studies of children with CF have used general measures of health-related quality of life (HRQL) and found it to be related to general health status (Czyzewski, Mariotto, Bartholomew, LeCompte, & Sockrider, 1994) and pulmonary function (Quittner, Sweeny, et al., 2000). Epker and Maddrey (1998) found that HRQL scores for children with CF were significantly worse than those found in previously published data from children with juvenile rheumatoid arthritis and asthma but similar to those of children with epilepsy. Children with CF and their parents reported the most impairment in the areas of general health perceptions and family cohesion. Assessing HRQL will become increasingly important as the life expectancy of patients with CF increases. Understanding the impact of new treatments on HRQL will be important for individuals in weighing the burden of adherence to tasks against potential benefits. For example, in a comparison of home-based versus hospital-based intravenous antibiotics, Wolter, Bowler, Nolan, and McCormack (1997) found that hospitalized patients reported significantly better HRQL in the areas of fatigue, mastery, and overall HRQL. However, home-based patients reported significantly better HRQL in the areas of disruption to family, self, sleep, eating, and total disruption. Thus various treatments and the delivery of treatment affect HRQL differently. Better ways to measure HRQL will be critical to developing the best methods of care for patients with CF.

CONCLUSIONS

Medical treatments for CF continue to advance. However, based on the current review, psychological assessment and intervention for CF appears to lag behind the research on other chronic conditions, such as diabetes, in the sheer number of studies conducted and the methodological sophistication employed. In general, except for small areas of CF treatment, such as diet, the field has little understanding of adherence and how to improve it. On the positive side, there are currently two multisite studies of behavioral interventions to improve adherence (Quittner, Drotar et al., 2000; Stark et al., 1996). Research on psychological adjustment and family functioning continues to support the notion that increased risk for adjustment difficulties, but not overt psychopathology, is associated with CF. There is even evidence to support increased adaptation over time. Unfortunately, very little research has been devoted to interventions aimed at improving adaptation and coping in children or adolescents identified as having difficulty in these areas. Recently, the Cochrane Library approved a protocol for a review of studies on the effects of psychological interventions for CF. Resources such as this one can be critical in keeping abreast of new and/or effective treatments in the area. In addition, emerging areas of research are transition to adult care and HRQL. Increased life expectancy and the rapidly expanding new treatments for patients with CF make these areas of critical importance to both researchers and clinicians and have direct implications for adherence, as well as for the general health and adjustment of patients with CF.

REFERENCES

Abbott, J., Dodd, M., Gee, L., & Webb, K. (2001). Ways of coping with cystic fibrosis: Implications for treatment adherence. *Disability and Rehabilitation, 23*, 315–324.

Abbott, J., Dodd, M., & Webb, A. K. (1996). Health perceptions and treatment adherence in adults with cystic fibrosis. *Thorax, 51*, 1233–1238.

Anderson, D. L., Flume, P. A., & Hardy, K. K. (2001). Psychological functioning of adults with cystic fibrosis. *Chest, 119*, 1079–1084.

Anthony, H., Paxton, S., Bines, J., & Phelan, P. (1999). Psychosocial predictors of adherence to nutritional recommendations and growth outcomes in children with cystic fibrosis. *Journal of Psychosomatic Research, 47*, 623–634.

Aris, R. M., Renner, J. B., Winders, A. D., Buell, H. E., Riggs, D. B., Lester, G. E., & Ontjes, D. A. (1998). Increased rate of fractures and severe kyphosis: Sequelae of living into adulthood with cystic fibrosis. *Annals of Internal Medicine, 128*, 186–193.

Bartholomew, L. K., Czyzewski, D. I., Parcel, G. S., Swank, P. R., Sockrider, M. M., Mariotto, M. J., et al. (1997). Self-management of cystic fibrosis: Short-term outcomes of the Cystic Fibrosis Family Education Program. *Health Education and Behavior, 24*, 652–666.

Beardsmore, C. S., Thompson, J. R., Williams, A., McArdle, E. K., Gregory, G. A., Weaver, L. T., & Simpson, H. (1994). Pulmonary functioning in infants with cystic fibrosis: The effect of antibiotic treatment. *Archives of Disease in Childhood, 71*, 133–137.

Blair, C., Cull, A., & Freeman, C. P. (1994). Psychosocial functioning of young adults with cystic fibrosis and their families. *Thorax, 49*, 798–802.

Blair, C., Freeman, C., & Cull, A. (1995). The families of anorexia nervosa and cystic fibrosis patients. *Psychological Medicine, 25*, 985–993.

Bolyard, D. R. (2001). Sexuality and cystic fibrosis. *MCN, American Journal of Maternal Child Nursing, 26*, 39–41.

Cystic Fibrosis Foundation. (2001, September). *Patient registry 2000 annual data report*. Bethesda, MD: Author.

Czyzewski, D. I., & Bartholomew, L. K. (1998). Quality of life outcomes in children and adolescents with cystic fibrosis. In D. Drotar (Ed.), *Measuring health-related quality of life in children and adolescents* (pp. 203–218). Mahwah, NJ: Erlbaum.

Czyzewski, D. I., Mariotto, M. J., Bartholomew, L. K., LeCompte, S. H., & Sockrider, M. M. (1994). Measurement of quality of well-being in a child and adolescent cystic fibrosis population. *Medical Care, 32*, 965–972.

Darke, P. R., & Goldberg, S. (1994). Father–infant interaction and parent stress with healthy and medically compromised infants. *Infant Behavior and Development, 17*, 3–14.

D'Auria, J. P., Christian, B. J., Henderson, Z. G., & Haynes, B. (2000). The company they keep: The influence of peer relationships on adjustment to cystic fibrosis during adolescence. *Journal of Pediatric Nursing, 15*, 175–182.

D'Auria, J. P., Christian, B. J., & Richardson, L. F. (1997). Through the looking glass: Children's perceptions of growing up with cystic fibrosis. *Canadian Journal of Nursing Research, 29*, 99–112.

Davies, L. K. (1993). Comparison of dependent-care activities for well siblings of children with cystic fibrosis and well siblings in families without children with chronic illness. *Issues in Comprehensive Pediatric Nursing, 16*, 91–98.

de Jong, P. T., Grevink, R. G., Roorda, R. J., Kaptein, A. A., & van der Schans, G. P. (1994). Effect of a home exercise training program in patients with cystic fibrosis. *Chest, 5*, 463–468.

Derouin, D., & Jessee, P. O. (1996). Impact of a chronic illness in childhood: Siblings' perceptions. *Issues in Comprehensive Pediatric Nursing, 19*, 135–147.

DiGirolamo, A. M., Quittner, A. L., Ackerman, V., & Stevens, J. (1997). Identification and assessment of ongoing stressors in adolescents with a chronic illness: An application of the Behavior-Analytic Model. *Journal of Clinical Child Psychology, 26*, 53–66.

Drotar, D., & Ievers, C. E. (1994). Age differences in parent and child responsibilities for management of cystic fibrosis and insulin-dependent diabetes mellitus. *Developmental and Behavioral Pediatrics, 15*, 265–272.

Eddy, M. E., Carter, B. D., Kronenberger, W. G., Conradsen, S., Eid, N. S., Bourland, S. L., & Adams, G. (1998). Parent relationships and compliance in cystic fibrosis. *Journal of Pediatric Health Care, 12*, 196–202.

Eigan, H., Rosenstein, B. J., FitzSimmons, S., & Schidlow, D. V. (1995). A multicenter study of alternated prednisone in patients with cystic fibrosis. *Journal of Pediatrics, 126*, 515–523.

Eiser, C., Zoritch, B., Hiller, J., Havermans, T., & Billig, S. (1995). Routine stresses in caring for a child with cystic fibrosis. *Journal of Psychosomatic Research, 39*, 641–646.

Epker, J., & Maddrey, A. M. (1998). Quality of life in pediatric patients with cystic fibrosis. *International Journal of Rehabilitation and Health, 4*, 215–222.

Farrell, P. M., Kosorok, M. R., Laxova, A., Shen, G., Koscik, R. E., Bruns, W. T., et al. (1997). Nutritional benefits of neonatal screening for cystic fibrosis. *The New England Journal of Medicine, 337*, 963–969.

Farrell, P. M., Kosorok, M. R., Rock, M. J., Laxova, A., Zeng, L., Lai, H. C., et al. (2001). Early diagnosis of cystic fibrosis through neonatal screening prevents severe malnutrition and improves long-term growth. *Pediatrics, 107*, 1–13.

Flume, P. A., Anderson, D. L., Hardy, K. K., & Gray, S. (2001). Transition programs in cystic fibrosis centers: Perceptions of pediatric and adult program directors. *Pediatric Pulmonology, 31*, 443–450.

Foster, C., Bryon, M., & Eiser, C. (1998). Correlates of well-being in mothers of children and adolescents with cystic fibrosis. *Child: Care, Health, and Development, 24*, 41–56.

Foster, C., Eiser, C., Oades, P., Sheldon, C., Tripp, J., Goldman, P., et al. (2001). Treatment demands and differential treatment of patients with cystic fibrosis and their siblings: Patient, parent and sibling accounts. *Child: Care, Health and Development, 27*, 349–364.

Gilljam, M., Antoniou, M., Shin, J., Dupuis, A., Corey, M., & Tullis, D. E. (2000). Pregnancy in cystic fibrosis. *Chest, 118*, 85–92.

Goldbeck, L., & Babka, C. (2001). Development and evaluation of a multi-family psychoeducational program for cystic fibrosis. *Patient Education and Counseling, 44*, 187–192.

Goldberg, S., Gotowiec, A., & Simmons, R. J. (1995). Infant–mother attachment and behavior problems in healthy and chronically ill preschoolers. *Development and Psychopathology, 7*, 267–282.

Graetz, B. W., Shute, R. H., & Sawyer, M. G. (2000). An Australian study of adolescents with cystic fibrosis: Perceived supportive and nonsupportive behaviors from families and friends and psychological adjustment. *Journal of Adolescent Health, 26*, 64–69.

Gudas, L. J., Koocher, G. P., & Wypij, D. (1991). Perceptions of medical compliance in children and adolescents with cystic fibrosis. *Journal of Developmental and Behavioral Pediatrics, 12*, 236–242.

Hagopian, L. P., & Thompson, R. H. (1999). Reinforcement of compliance with respiratory treatment in a child with cystic fibrosis. *Journal of Applied Behavior Analysis, 32*, 233–236.

Hains, A. A., Davies, W. H., Behrens, D., & Biller, J. A. (1997). Cognitive behavioral interventions for adolescents with cystic fibrosis. *Journal of Pediatric Psychology, 22*, 669–687.

Henderson, R. C., & Madsen, C. D. (1996). Bone density in children and adolescents with cystic fibrosis. *Journal of Pediatrics, 128*, 28–34.

Henley, L. D., & Hill, I. D. (1990). Errors, gaps, and misconceptions in the disease-related knowledge of cystic fibrosis patients and their families. *Pediatrics, 85*, 1008–1014.

Holzer, F. J., Schnall, R., & Landau, L. I. (1984). The effect of a home exercise programme in children with cystic fibrosis and asthma. *Australian Paediatric Journal, 20*, 297–302.

Ievers, C. E., Brown, R. T., Drotar, D., Caplan, D., Pishevar, B. S., & Lambert, R. G. (1999). Knowledge of physician prescriptions and adherence to treatment among children with cystic fibrosis and their mothers. *Developmental and Behavioral Pediatrics, 20*, 335–343.

Ievers, C. E., & Drotar, D. (1996). Family and parental functioning in cystic fibrosis. *Developmental and Behavioral Pediatrics, 17*, 48–55.

Jelalian, E., Stark, L. J., Reynolds, L., & Seifer, R. (1998). Nutrition intervention for weight gain in cystic fibrosis: A meta-analysis. *Journal of Pediatrics, 132*, 486–492.

Konstan, M. W., Byard, P. J., Hoppel, C. L., & Davis, P. B. (1995). Effect of high-dose ibuprofen in patients with cystic fibrosis. *New England Journal of Medicine, 332*, 848–854.

Lanng, S., Thorsteinsson, B., Nerup, J., & Koch, C. (1994). Diabetes mellitus in cystic fibrosis: Effect of insulin therapy on lung function and infections. *Acta Paediatrica, 83*, 849–853.

McCallum, T. J., Milunsky, J. M., Cunningham, D. L., Harris, D. H., Maher, T. A., & Oates, R. D. (2000). Fertility in men with cystic fibrosis: An update on current surgical practices and outcomes. *Chest, 118*, 1059–1062.

Mueller, F., Aubrei, M. C., Gasser, B., Duchatel, F., & Boue, A. (1985). Prenatal diagnosis of cystic fibrosis 11: Meconium ileus in affected fetuses. *Prenatal Diagnosis, 5*, 104–117.

Oermann, C. M., Swank, P. R., & Sockrider, M. M. (2000). Validation of an instrument measuring patient satisfaction with chest physiotherapy techniques in cystic fibrosis. *Chest, 118*, 92–97.

Ott, S. M., & Aitken, M. L. (1998). Osteoporosis in patients with cystic fibrosis. *Clinics in Chest Medicine, 19*, 555–567.

Parcel, G. S., Swank, P. R., Mariotto, M. J., Bartholomew, L. K., Czyzewski, D. I., Sockrider, M. M., & Seilheimer, D. K. (1994). Self-management of cystic fibrosis: A structural model for educational and behavioral variables. *Social Science and Medicine, 38*, 1307–1315.

Passero, M. A., Remor, B., & Solomon, J. (1981). Patient-reported compliance with cystic fibrosis therapy. *Clinical Pediatrics, 20*, 264–268.

Patterson, J. M., Budd, J., Goetz, D., & Warwick, W. J. (1993). Family correlates of a 10–year pulmonary health trend in cystic fibrosis. *Pediatrics, 91*, 383–389.

Powers, S. W., Patton, S. R., Byars, K. C., Mitchell, M. M., Jelalian, E., Mulvihill, M. M., et al. (2002). Caloric intake and eating behavior in infants and toddlers with cystic fibrosis. *Pediatrics, 109*, 1–10.

Pumariega, A. J., Pearson, D. A., & Seilheimer, D. K. (1993). Family and childhood adjustment in cystic fibrosis. *Journal of Child and Family Studies, 2*, 109–118.

Quittner, A. L., & Drotar, D. (1997). *Controlled trial of family interventions for cystic fibrosis*. National Institutes of Health Grant No. R01 HL47064.

Quittner, A. L., Drotar, D., Ievers-Landis, C., Slocum, N., Seidner, D., & Jacobsen, J. (2000). Adherence to medical treatments in adolescents with cystic fibrosis: The development and evaluation of family-based interventions. In D. Drotar (Ed.), *Promoting adherence to medical treatment in chronic childhood illness: Concepts, methods, and interventions* (pp. 383–408). Mahwah, NJ: Erlbaum.

Quittner, A. L., & Opipari, L. C. (1994). Differential treatment of siblings: Interview and diary analyses comparing two family contexts. *Child Development, 65*, 800–814.

Quittner, A. L., Opipari, L. C., Espelage, D. L., Carter, B., Eid, N., & Eigen, H. (1998). Role strain in couples with and without a child with a chronic illness: Associations with marital satisfaction, intimacy, and daily mood. *Health Psychology, 17*, 112–124.

Quittner, A. L., Sweeny, S., Watrous, M., Munzenberger, P., Bearss, K., Gibson Nitza, A., Fisher, L. A., et al. (2000). Translation and linguistic validation of a disease-specific quality of life measure for cystic fibrosis. *Journal of Pediatric Psychology, 25*, 403–414.

Quittner, A. L., Tolbert, V. E., Regoli, M. J., Orenstein, D. M., Hollingsworth, J. L., & Eigen, H. (1996). Development of the Role-Play Inventory of Situations and Coping Strategies for Parents of Children with Cystic Fibrosis. *Journal of Pediatric Psychology, 21*, 209–235.

Ramsey, B. (1996). Management of pulmonary disease in patients with cystic fibrosis. *New England Journal of Medicine, 335*, 179–188.

Ramsey, B., Farrell, P., & Pencharz, P. (1992). Nutritional assessment and management in cystic fibrosis: Consensus conference. *American Journal of Clinical Nutrition, 55*, 108–116.

Ramsey, B., Pepe, M. S., Quan, J. M., Otto, K. L., Montgomery, A. B., Williams-Warren, J., et al. (1999). Intermittent administration of inhaled tobramycin in patients with cystic fibrosis. *New England Journal of Medicine, 340*, 23–30.

Ricker, J. H., Delameter, A. M., & Hsu, J. (1998). Correlates of regimen adherence in cystic fibrosis. *Journal of Clinical Psychology in Medical Settings, 5*, 159–172.

Rosenecker, J., Eichler, I., Kuhn, L., Harms, H. K., & von der Hardt, H. (1995). Genetic determination of diabetes mellitus in patients with cystic fibrosis: Multicenter Cystic Fibrosis Study Group. *Journal of Pediatrics, 127*, 441–443.

Rusakow, L. S., Miller, T., McCarthy, C. A., Gershan, W. M., & Splaingard, M. L. (1998). Unsuspected nonadherence with recommended pancreatic enzyme administration in patients with cystic fibrosis. *Children's Health Care, 27*, 259–264.

Sawyer, S. M., Rosier, M. J., Phelan, P. D., & Bowes, G. (1995). The self-image of adolescents with cystic fibrosis. *Journal of Adolescent Health, 16*, 204–208.

Schneiderman-Walker, J., Pollock, S. L., Corey, M., Wilkes, D. D., Canny, G. J., Pedder, L., & Reisman, J. J. (2000). A randomized controlled trial of a 3–year home exercise program in cystic fibrosis. *Journal of Pediatrics, 136*, 304–310.

Simmons, R. J., & Goldberg, S. (2001). Infants and pre-school children. In M. Bluebond-Langner, B. Lask, & D. B. Angst (Eds.), *Psychosocial aspects of cystic fibrosis* (pp. 110–124). New York: Oxford University Press.

Simmons, R. J., Goldberg, S., Washington, J., Fischer-Fay, A., & Maclusky, I. (1995). Infant–mother attachment and nutrition in children with cystic fibrosis. *Journal of Developmental and Behavioral Pediatrics, 16*, 183–186.

Solomon, C. R., & Breton, J. J. (1999). Early warning signals in relationships between parents and young children with cystic fibrosis. *Children's Health Care, 28*, 221–240.

Spieth, L., Stark, L. J., Mitchell, M. J., Schiller, M., Cohen, L. L., Mulvihill, M. M., & Hovell, M. (2001). Observational assessment of family functioning at mealtime in preschool children with cystic fibrosis. *Journal of Pediatric Psychology, 26*, 215–224.

Stark, L. J., Bowen, A. M., Tyc, V. L., Evans, S., & Passero, M. A. (1990). A behavioral approach to increasing calorie consumption in children with cystic fibrosis. *Journal of Pediatric Psychology, 15*, 309–326.

Stark, L. J., Jelalian, E., & Miller, D. L. (1995). Cystic fibrosis. In M. C. Roberts (Ed.), *Handbook of pediatric psychology* (2nd ed., pp. 241–262). New York: Guilford Press.

Stark, L. J., Jelalian, E., Mulvihill, M. M., Powers, S. W., Bowen, A. M., Spieth, L. E., et al. (1995). Eating in preschool children with cystic fibrosis and healthy peers: Behavioral analysis. *Pediatrics, 95*, 210–215.

Stark, L. J., Jelalian, E., Powers, S. W., Mulvihill, M. M., Opipari, L. C., Bowen, A., et al. (2000). Parent and child mealtime behavior in families of children with cystic fibrosis. *Journal of Pediatrics, 136*, 195–200.

Stark, L. J., Knapp, L. G., Bowen, A. M., Powers, S. W., Jelalian, E., Evans, S., et al. (1993). Increasing calorie consumption in children with cystic fibrosis: Replication with 2-year follow-up. *Journal of Applied Behavior Analysis, 26*, 435–450.

Stark, L. J., Miller, S. T., Plienes, A. J., & Drabman, R. S. (1987). Behavioral contracting to increase chest physiotherapy. *Behavior Modification, 11*, 75–86.

Stark, L. J., Mulvihill, M. M., Jelalian, E., Bowen, A. M., Powers, S. W., Tao, S., et al. (1997). Descriptive analysis of eating behavior in school-age children with cystic fibrosis and healthy control children. *Pediatrics, 99*, 665–671.

Stark, L. J., Mulvihill, M. M., Powers, S. W., Jelalian, E., Keating, K., Creveling, S., et al. (1996). Behavioral intervention to improve calorie intake of children with cystic fibrosis: Treatment versus wait list control. *Journal of Pediatric Gastroenterology and Nutrition, 22*, 240–253.

Thompson, R. J., Jr., Gustafson, K. E., & Gil, K. M. (1995). Psychological adjustment of adolescents with cystic fibrosis or sickle cell disease and their mothers. In J. L. Wallander & L. J. Siegel (Eds.), *Adolescent health problems: Behavioral perspectives* (pp. 232–247). New York: Guilford Press.

Thompson, R. J., Jr., Gustafson, K. E., Gil, K. M., Godfrey, J., & Bennett-Murphy, L. M. (1998). Illness specific patterns of psychological adjustment and cognitive adaptational processes in children with cystic fibrosis and sickle cell disease. *Journal of Clinical Psychology, 54*, 121–128.

Thompson, R. J., Jr., Gustafson, K. E., Gil, K. M., Kinney, T. R., & Spock, A. (1999). Change in the psychological adjustment of children with cystic fibrosis or sickle cell disease and their mothers. *Journal of Clinical Psychology in Medical Settings, 6*, 373–391.

Thompson, R. J., Jr., Gustafson, K. E., Hamlett, K. W., & Spock, A. (1992). Psychological adjustment of children with cystic fibrosis: The role of child cognitive processes and maternal adjustment. *Journal of Pediatric Psychology, 17*, 741–755.

Tomezsko, J. L., Stallings, V. A., & Scanlin, T. F. (1992). Dietary intake of healthy children with cystic fibrosis compared with normal control children. *Pediatrics, 90*, 547–553.

Wilkinson, J. D., & Paton, J. Y. (1999). Compliance with nebulised RhDNase in children with cystic fibrosis [Abstract]. *Netherlands Journal of Medicine, 54*, S82.

Willmott, R. W., Amin, R. S., Colin, A. A., DeVault, A., Dozor, A. J., Eigen, H., et al. (1996). Aerosolized recombinant human DNase in hospitalized cystic fibrosis patients with acute pulmonary exacerbations. *American Journal of Respiratory and Critical Care Medicine, 153*, 1914–1917.

Wilson, J., Fosson, A., Kanga, J. F., & D'Angelo, S. L. (1996). Homostatic interactions: A longitudinal study of biological, psychosocial, and family variables in children with cystic fibrosis. *Journal of Family Therapy, 18*, 123–139.

Wolter, J. M., Bowler, S. D., Nolan, P. J., & McCormack, J. G. (1997). Home intravenous therapy in cystic fibrosis: A prospective randomized trial examining clinical, quality of life and cost aspects. *European Respiratory Journal, 10*, 896–900.

18

Childhood Diabetes in Psychological Context

TIM WYSOCKI
PEGGY GRECO
LISA M. BUCKLOH

This chapter surveys three broad domains of research on the adaptation of youth and families to childhood diabetes: (1) research on diabetes knowledge, skills, and treatment adherence; (2) studies of stress, coping, and psychological sequelae of diabetes; and (3) investigations of the social context of diabetes. The chapter reviews selected research, especially intervention studies, in the context of modern therapy for this chronic disease.

DIABETES MELLITUS IN CHILDREN AND ADOLESCENTS

Diabetes mellitus is a common pediatric chronic disease (University of Michigan Diabetes Research and Training Center, 1998). Type 1 diabetes mellitus (DM1), previously known as insulin-dependent diabetes mellitus, juvenile diabetes, or childhood diabetes, occurs in about 1 in 500–600 children. Onset peaks in middle childhood, but it can be diagnosed through middle adulthood. DM1 results from autoimmune destruction of pancreatic islet cells that produce insulin, resulting in permanent insulin deficiency. Insulin regulates glucose metabolism, which is essential for growth, activity, wound healing, and brain function. Thus people with DM1 cannot survive without insulin replacement. DM1 is treated with either multiple daily insulin injections or the use of an insulin pump, which infuses a constant rate of insulin through a catheter, with "bolus" doses before meals.

Previously uncommon in children, Type 2 diabetes mellitus (DM2), formerly known as non-insulin-dependent diabetes mellitus, now accounts for 10–20% of new cases of diabetes in youth. The incidence of DM2 is disproportionately higher among African American, Native American, and Hispanic populations. Rather than insulin deficiency, as in DM1, insulin resistance occurs in DM2, impairing cellular uptake of insulin. DM2 often progresses to islet cell failure and insulin deficiency, with symptoms similar to those of DM1. For some youths, DM2 may be managed with diet and exercise alone or with oral medications. However, many youths with DM2 require insulin injections, and so their treatment is virtually identical to that for DM1.

These therapies restore glucose metabolism, but blood glucose often deviates from the normal range (70–120 mg/dl). So patients perform daily self-monitoring of blood glucose (SMBG) by pricking a finger with a lancet, putting blood on a test strip, and inserting it into a glucose meter that displays, then stores, the results in memory. Most patients are asked to perform SMBG before meals, at bedtime, and at other times to evaluate glucose fluctuations and to adjust their regimens accordingly. The glycosylated hemoglobin test (HbA_{1C}) reflects average blood glucose levels over the prior 2–3 months and is commonly obtained at diabetes clinic visits. Nutrition and exercise also affect blood glucose levels. The most common current dietary regimen is based on "carbohydrate counting," in which patients are to eat a specified number of grams of carbohydrates at each meal and scheduled snack. In modern dietary management of diabetes, children may eat limited quantities of refined sweets if these are included in the daily carbohydrate allowance and if glycemic targets are reached. Regular exercise is also crucial to modern diabetes management because it may reduce insulin requirements, promote cardiovascular health, facilitate weight control, and yield psychological benefits.

Modern therapy allows patients to live quite normally, yet it only crudely approximates normal metabolism. Abnormally high (hyperglycemia) or low (hypoglycemia) blood glucose levels must be detected and corrected. Hyperglycemia results from underdosing or omitting insulin injections or oral medications, overeating, stress, and infections. Prolonged hyperglycemia can lead to hospitalization for diabetic ketoacidosis (Glasgow et al., 1991; Gray, Marrero, Godfrey, Orr, & Golden, 1988). Hypoglycemia results from injecting too much insulin, undereating, or extraordinary physical exertion. Symptoms may include trembling, nausea, sweating, dizziness, and confusion. Mild to moderate hypoglycemia is treated by ingesting carbohydrates. Severe hypoglycemia is often treated by injection of glucagon, a hormone that blocks insulin and raises blood glucose. Severe hypoglycemia is often predictable and preventable (Cox et al., 1994) through careful attention to SMBG results.

Many youths with diabetes become overweight due in part to chronically high levels of insulin. Youths with DM1 may gain weight as a result of striving for tight diabetic control. In DM2, weight control may obviate the need for insulin injections, permitting some patients to be managed on oral medications, diet, and/or exercise. Both DM1 and DM2 raise the long-term risks of damage to the heart, kidneys, eyes, and nerves. Major studies of DM1 (Diabetes Control and Complications Trial Research Group, 1994) and DM2 (United Kingdom Prospective Diabetes Study, 1998) proved that complication risks increase linearly with HbA_{1C} levels. Maintaining near-normal HbA_{1C} can reduce the risks of complications to levels that equal those of the general population. Since these major studies were done, care for youths with diabetes now emphasizes more aggressively the maintenance of near-normal HbA_{1C} (Tamborlane, Gatcomb, Held, & Ahern, 1994). This is done by increased use of insulin pumps and of three or more daily insulin injections; by training patients and families to adjust their regimens to prevent or correct blood glucose fluctuations; by more frequent blood glucose testing; and by placing a greater emphasis on the family as the center of a multidisciplinary team. Both DM1 and DM2 require the patient and family to cope with, implement, monitor, and regulate a very complex medical regimen. These demands affect and are affected by many psychological processes. This chapter reviews the scientific evidence of these interactions.

DIABETES MANAGEMENT: KNOWLEDGE, SKILLS, AND TREATMENT ADHERENCE

Accurate knowledge about diabetes and its treatment may be a prerequisite to both treatment adherence (Hanson, Henggeler, & Burghen, 1987) and metabolic control (Gray et al., 1988). Diabetes knowledge increases with the age of the child (Johnson, 1995; Wysocki, Meinhold, et al., 1996). But diabetes knowledge and technical skills tend to deteriorate over time and often drift from ideal standards. Youths with diabetes and their parents are prone to performance errors in dietary management (Schmidt, Klover, Arfken, Delamater, & Hobson, 1992), SMBG testing (Delamater, Davis et al., 1988), insulin administration (Weissberg-Benchell et al., 1995) and managing hypoglycemia and hyperglycemia (Johnson, Perwein, & Silverstein, 2000). Thus it is important that diabetes knowledge and skills be reevaluated and refined regularly (Johnson, 1995). The importance of knowledge in preventing diabetes mismanagement was shown in studies of the relationship between diabetes knowledge and regimen adherence. Christensen (1983) noted a strong relationship between diabetes knowledge and diabetes self-care in children. Knowledge was associated with HbA_{1C} in some studies (e.g., Harkavy et al.,1983) but not others (e.g., Anderson, Miller, Auslander, & Santiago, 1981; Johnson, 1995). Health care professionals are often perplexed when a knowledgeable patient is in poor metabolic control. However, the weak association between diabetes knowledge and diabetic control should not be surprising, because the latter is influenced by many other variables, including treatment adherence, adequacy of the diabetes regimen, the family's relationship with health care professionals, parent–child communication about diabetes and the sophistication of the family's diabetes problem-solving skills. Youths and their families often receive diabetes education at the time of diagnosis and at diabetes summer camps. Although patient knowledge may increase at summer camps, Harkavy and colleagues (1983) reported that 12- to 14-year-olds benefited more from instruction during diabetes summer camp than did 10- to 11-year-olds. Diabetes summer camps may also improve psychosocial functioning; in one study, youths with several chronic diseases had improved attitudes toward their illnesses and less anxiety after a summer camp program (Briery & Rabian, 1999). A multicomponent, behaviorally oriented summer camp improved the self-efficacy, problem-solving skills, and coping strategies of adolescents with diabetes despite producing no change in diabetes knowledge or skills (Schlundt, Flannery, Davis, Kinzer, & Pichert, 1999).

Many behavioral, psychological, and medical variables can contribute to the metabolic status of youth with DM1, but perhaps the most critical is regimen adherence. Adherence with a proper regimen may prevent or delay the long-term complications of diabetes (Diabetes Control and Complications Trial Research Group, 1994), but the complexity of this regimen makes strict adherence very difficult. Glasgow, McCaul, and Schafer (1986) assessed the frequency of barriers (environmental and cognitive events that are obstacles to regimen adherence) in adolescents and adults with DM1. They noted that there are many barriers to adherence and that more barriers surround tasks that require greater lifestyle changes, such as diet and exercise. They found that adherence to an aspect of the diabetes regimen relates inversely to the degree of lifestyle change required by the task (Glasgow, McCaul, & Schafer, 1987) and to the number and severity of barriers to completing that task (Glasgow et al., 1986).

Various methods of assessing adherence are available. Patients may rate their adherence to specific regimen components (e.g., Hanson et al., 1987; La Greca & Skyler, 1991), record adherence behaviors in a diary, or be interviewed about diabetes-related activities (Harris et al., 2000; Johnson, Silverstein, Rosenbloom, Carter, & Cunningham, 1986). Most of these tools conceptualize adherence as an inter-related network of regimen behaviors rather than a single trait (Glasgow et al., 1987; Glasgow, Wilson, & McCaul, 1985; Johnson et al., 1986). For example, youth may adhere to one regimen task, such as insulin administration, but not to others, such as blood glucose testing or exercise. Similarly, adherence with specific regimen tasks may vary over time. Employing multiple methods and sources of information may improve the measurement of adherence (Quittner, Espelage, Ievers-Landis, & Drotar, 2000).

Research has not revealed a consistent, robust relationship between treatment adherence and HbA_{1C} (e.g., Johnson, Freund, Silverstein, Hansen, & Malone, 1990; Glasgow et al., 1987). Following are some possible reasons for these findings:

1. Adherence and diabetic control may be measured over differing time frames. Adherence tends to be measured over short periods (e.g., 3 days over 2 weeks; Johnson et al., 1986) relative to the HbA_{1C}, which reflects average blood glucose over 2–3 months
2. Regimen instructions and measures used to assess adherence may not correspond; for example, a child is told to "eat more vegetables," whereas adherence is measured as the percent of calories from fat (Glasgow, Wilson, & McCaul, 1985).
3. Youths may adhere to a regimen that is inappropriate or inaccurately recalled.
4. Measures may assess behaviors that have little direct effect on diabetic control (e.g., wearing diabetic identification).
5. Measures of adherence may be biased by social desirability or other factors that impede accurate recall. Drotar and Riekert (1999) found that nonparticipants in research on adherence had significantly worse adherence than did those who participated in such studies. This finding may dilute the statistical relationship between adherence and metabolic control, but it does not reduce the importance of assessing and working to improve adherence in youths with diabetes.

Adherence has also been associated with many family characteristics, such as diabetes knowledge and family relations (Hanson et al., 1987; Seiffge-Krenke, 1998), environmental support (McCaul, Glasgow, & Schafer, 1987), and family communication and conflict (Bobrow, AvRuskin, & Siller, 1985; Hauser et al., 1990). Hence, family-focused intervention may improve diabetes management (see Delamater et al., 2001; Grey, 2000; Hampson et al., 2001, for recent reviews). For example, we have reported on the adaptation of Robin and Foster's (1989) behavioral family systems therapy to target communication and problem-solving skills in families of adolescents with DM1. This intervention improved family communication and conflict resolution (Wysocki et al., 2000), enhanced directly observed family communication skills (Wysocki et al., 1999), and had durable benefits (Wysocki, Greco, Harris, Bubb, & White, 2001). We are now evaluating an adapted version of this therapy designed to enhance its impact on treatment adherence and diabetic control.

Other interventions that can improve adherence or diabetic control include behavioral contracting (Wysocki, Green, & Huxtable, 1989), facilitation of parental involvement in adolescents' diabetes management (Anderson, Ho, Brackett, Finkelstein, & Laffel, 1997), progressively intrusive family intervention (Gray et al., 1988), group coping-skills training (Grey, Boland, Davidson, Li, & Tamborlane, 2000), behavioral family therapy (Ryden et al., 1994), and a diabetes/psychiatry inpatient program (Geffken et al., 1997).

Despite its central role in DM1 therapy, family use of SMBG data has inspired little research. The test results should enhance evaluation and adjustment of the treatment regimen by health professionals, anticipation and prevention of hypoglycemia and hyperglycemia by patients and families, appreciation of the glycemic effects of daily activities, and flexibility in daily living (University of Michigan Diabetes Research & Training Center, 1998). Delamater, Davis, and colleagues (1988) found that families of adolescents with DM1 rarely used SMBG data for adjusting insulin doses or injection–meal intervals. The benefit of doing so is clear: Peyrot and Rubin (1988) found that adults who reported more frequent use of SMBG data for insulin self-regulation were in better diabetic control. Wysocki, Hough, Ward, Allen, and Murgai (1992) studied use of SMBG data by 47 families of youths with DM1 over 4 weeks. Parents recorded daily their specific uses of such SMBG data as adjustments in insulin, diet, or exercise; evaluation of hypoglycemia; and decisions to complete urine ketone tests. Families who used SMBG data more often had less conflict about diabetes, better diabetes knowledge, and better adherence. Training in active use of SMBG data may enhance diabetes self-management.

Two interventions targeting diabetes problem solving based on SMBG data have been evaluated. Delamater and colleagues (1990) randomized 36 youths newly diagnosed with DM1 to either conventional therapy (CT), supportive counseling (SC), or self-management training (SMT). SMT yielded significantly lower HbA_{1C} than CT over a 2-year follow-up. Similarly, Anderson, Wolf, Burkhart, Cornell, and Bacon (1989) described a peer group intervention targeting family use of SMBG data and showed that this treatment improved HbA_{1C} compared with standard care. Others have studied patients' accuracy in estimating their blood glucose levels based on subjective physical symptoms. Like adults, youths are quite inaccurate at estimating their current blood glucose levels (Freund, Johnson, Rosenbloom, Alexander, & Hansen, 1986; Gonder-Frederick, Snyder, & Clarke, 1991). But they can become more accurate by evaluating which physical symptoms are truly predictive of blood glucose (Nurick & Johnson, 1991). Many adolescents may base self-care decisions on subjective estimates of blood glucose levels, and many such decisions may be unsafe. Diabetes knowledge, skills, and treatment adherence are critical to growing up healthy despite having diabetes. But youths with diabetes and their families also face challenges of coping with stress and being at higher risks of certain types of psychopathology.

STRESS, COPING, AND PSYCHOLOGICAL ADJUSTMENT

Stress may affect glycemic control and adherence; neuroendocrine responses to stress can directly alter metabolic functioning. Support for this process was provided by Chase and Jackson (1981), who noted that the frequency of stressful events reported by children with DM1 was associated with triglyceride, cholesterol, and serum glucose levels. Hanson, Henggeler, and Burghen (1987) also showed a direct effect of stress on metabolic control in adolescents with DM1. It has been postulated that stress can have either direct effects through physiological mechanisms or mediated effects through processes such as regimen adherence (e.g., Aikens, Wallander, Bell, & Cole, 1992), but there has been inconsistent support for adherence as a mediating variable. Hanson and colleagues (1987) noted that, rather than the relationship between stress and metabolic control being mediated by adherence, chronic stress and adherence were both *directly* linked to metabolic control. Aikens and colleagues (1992) also found that adherence was not a mediator of the relationship between stress and metabolic control.

Severe stress may also impede family management of diabetes. In a retrospective study of psychosocial stress factors in children with DM1, White, Kolman, Wexler, Polin, and Winter (1984) noted that stress in families with limited problem-solving skills was a major variable in poorly controlled diabetes. As the authors pointed out, the presence of stress itself does not always result in poor diabetic control; how families respond to stressors also influences their impact. This idea has received empirical support; patients who are in poor metabolic control have been found to use maladaptive ways of coping with stress to a greater extent than youths in good metabolic control (Delamater, Kurtz, Bubb, White, & Santiago, 1987; Hanson et al., 1989). Thus, not only do adolescents and their families need to recognize the presence and effects of stress, but they also may benefit both psychologically and physiologically from learning to cope adaptively with stress.

Some studies suggest that stress management and coping skills can have positive effects for adolescents with diabetes. Boardway, Delamater, Tomakowsky, and Gutai (1993) found that after stress management training adolescents reported decreased diabetes-specific stress but did not exhibit changes in metabolic control, regimen adherence, coping styles, or self-efficacy about diabetes. Grey and colleagues (2000) taught adolescents coping skills consisting of problem solving, conflict resolution, and cognitive behavior modification and found that the adolescents had better metabolic control and self-efficacy after 6 months than did controls.

Children and adolescents with diabetes are at increased risk for psychiatric problems such as depression, anxiety, and eating disorders. Kovacs, Goldston, Obrosky, and Bonar (1997) showed prospectively that 27% of youths had an episode of major depression and 13% had anxiety disorders during the 10 years after onset of diabetes. Depression may impede treatment adherence; treating it may lower HbA_{1c} levels (Lustman, Griffith, & Clouse, 1996).

Adolescents with DM1 also may be at higher risk of eating disorders. This elevated risk may be due in part to the weight gain associated with the initiation of insulin treatment, particularly in females with high body dissatisfaction (Colton, Rodin, Olmsted, & Daneman, 1999). Higher risk may also be related to the focus on dietary management of this chronic disease (Antisdel & Chrisler, 2000). Children and adolescents who engage in binge eating may compensate by insulin omission, often resulting in high HbA_{1c} levels (Takii et al., 1999). The percentage of female adolescents and adults who purposefully omit insulin has been reported to be as high as 31%, although less than 9% report frequent omission (Polonsky et al., 1994). In adolescents with comorbid diabetes and eating disorders, multidisciplinary assessment and treatment of the complex combination of psychological and medical aspects of both of these disorders is required.

Diabetes may threaten the psychological adjustment of patients themselves, but it also appears that the treatment burden may have adverse psychological effects on other family members, particularly mothers. Given the importance of family cooperation and support for effective diabetes management, families must also recognize and contend with these risks. There is ample evidence that mothers assume the brunt of the behavioral and emotional burden of diabetes management. Studies by Hodges and Parker (1987), Banion, Miles, and Carter (1983), Wysocki, Huxtable, Linscheid, and Wayne (1989), and Hauenstein, Marvin, Snyder, and Clarke (1989) confirmed that mothers of children with DM1 report more parenting stress than do mothers of healthy children, that the uncertainties associated with DM1 are important contributors to that stress, and that parenting these children is more complex and challenging than parenting healthy children. Thus it is not surprising that mothers show an elevated incidence of depression during the first year of DM1 (Kovacs et al., 1985) and that maternal depressive symptoms may manifest long after diagnosis as diabetes-specific "burnout" syndrome (Kovacs et al., 1990). The extent to which maternal stress, anxiety, and depression adversely affect DM1 management is unknown, but it is likely that these symptoms could impede adherence and self-regulation in some families.

The impact of diabetes on fathers and their roles in diabetes management have been researched infrequently. Kovacs and colleagues (1985) found that fathers did not demonstrate increased depressive symptomatology during the first year after diagnosis of childhood DM1. Wysocki (1993) reported that father–adolescent communication and problem-solving skills were equally robust predictors of adolescents' diabetic control and treatment adherence as were mother–adolescent interactions, but fathers' reports about other aspects of parent–adolescent relationships correlated more weakly with diabetes outcomes than did mothers' reports. Hanson, Henggeler, Rodrigue, Burghen, and Murphy (1988) found that youths from father-absent families were at risk of poorer glycemic control. No studies have explored the impact of fathers' involvement in DM1 management on diabetes outcomes or determined whether it serves as a protective factor for the emergence of maternal depression. Given the important role of social support as a determinant of health outcomes in other medical conditions, it is likely that fathers' involvement in daily disease management would facilitate better diabetic control and family adaptation to DM1.

In addition to the potential emotional and behavioral effects of diabetes, individuals with diabetes may experience adverse cognitive effects of the disease on an acute and chronic basis. Children with early DM1 onset (before 5 to 7 years in age) are at risk for developing learning disabilities, although no consistent pattern of neuropsychological findings has emerged (Rovet & Fernandes, 1998; Ryan, 1997). Because diabetes duration, frequency of hypoglycemia, frequency of ketoacidosis, and chronicity of hyperglycemia are intercorrelated, a causative relationship between any of these etiological variables and cognitive sequelae has been difficult to confirm. Even mild hypoglycemia can lead to acute deterioration of mental acuity, and deterioration in cognitive function may persist for several days following severe hypoglycemia (Ryan et al., 1990). Given these findings, many youth with diabetes merit an evaluation of cognitive functioning. It also is particularly important in younger children who are at risk of diabetes-associated cognitive impairment to minimize the frequency of hypoglycemia and prolonged hyperglycemia. It is important to consider cognitive impairment as a possible variable contributing to ineffective diabetes self-management in youth.

Children and adolescents with diabetes and their families face multiple threats to their psychological adjustment and functioning. Although it is important to address these individual issues, it is also important to understand individuals within their social contexts, including their involvement with peers, school, and the health care team.

SOCIAL CONTEXT OF CHILDHOOD DIABETES

The treatment and monitoring demands imposed by DM1 pervade daily life; management of diabetes requires adherence to multiple daily tasks in the home, school, and community. Thus the involvement of family, friends, teachers, and health care professionals is integral to successful diabetes management. Several recent studies have indicated that parental involvement in diabetes care is predictive of achievement of treatment goals (Grey, Davidson, Boland, & Tamborlane, 2001), as well as decreased family conflict and improved glycemic control (Anderson, Brackett, & Laffel, 1999). Maintaining parental involvement need not be complicated; a recent study found that low-intensity intervention integrated into diabetes clinic visits strengthened parent involvement in diabetes management (Anderson et al., 1999).

However, parental involvement in diabetes care should be appropriate for the child's maturity level. A healthy balance of self-care autonomy and psychological maturity may result in DM1-specific self-sufficiency and maximize treatment safety and efficacy (e.g., La Greca, Follansbee, & Skyler, 1990). Deviation from this balance may have adverse effects; La Greca and colleagues (1990) found that children with greater responsibility, particularly for insulin administration, were in poorer diabetic control. Adolescents with excessive self-care autonomy relative to their psychological maturity demonstrate worse treatment adherence and more diabetes-related hospitalizations than those whose responsibilities are more appropriate developmentally (Wysocki, Taylor et al., 1996). These findings sound a note of caution regarding the encouragement of maximal self-care autonomy among adolescents with DM1 and imply that families who maintain more parental involvement in diabetes care during adolescence may enjoy better outcomes.

Beyond parental involvement in diabetes care, consideration of the family environment is essential. Dimensions of family functioning are important predictors of family adaptation to diabetes regimen demands (Blechman & Delamater, 1993). For example, Wysocki (1993) found that family communication, problem solving, and conflict resolution skills were important correlates of treatment adherence, diabetic control, and adolescents' emotional adjustment to DM1. Authoritative parenting, characterized by support and affection, may be advantageous for regimen adherence and glycemic control of children with diabetes (Davis et al., 2001), whereas conflict, specifically mother–daughter conflict, is associated with poorly controlled DM1 (Bobrow et al., 1985).

These cross-sectional studies yielded consistent results, but their findings have been bolstered further by the work of Hauser, Jacobson, and their colleagues in a longitudinal study of children enrolled at diagnosis of DM1. Reports from this series indicate that premorbid family function was a significant predictor of initial coping with the diagnosis (Wertlieb, Hauser, & Jacobson, 1986), with adherence over intervals as long as 4 years (Hauser et al., 1990; Jacobson et al., 1987, 1990), and with diabetic control over the same intervals (Jacobson et al., 1994). The prospective nature of these studies bolsters the conclusion that family function is associated causally with diabetes outcomes, rather than simply being a correlate of those outcomes.

Positive dimensions of family functioning, such as the provision of social support, may also have a profound impact on adaptation to diabetes. Parental support and adolescent social competence buffer the adverse effects of stress on glycemic control (Hanson et al., 1987). Further, social support from family and friends may be predictive of better self-care (Skinner, John, & Hampson, 2000). Diabetes-specific social support provided by family members may vary by regimen task; family members tend to offer the most support for maintaining a meal plan and for insulin administration (Greco et al., 1991; La Greca et al., 1995). Family members are also more likely to offer tangible support such as reminding, assisting, or doing diabetes-related tasks for the child. The value of this tangible support offered by family members is evidenced by better treatment adherence for those adolescents reporting higher levels of family support (La Greca et al., 1995).

Siblings are also an important part of the family environment. Siblings of children with DM1 may be in a unique position to influence diabetes management, either positively or negatively; however, this issue has received little empirical attention. Resentment over inequitable parental attention given to the child with DM1, the imposition of dietary constraints on the entire family, and the impact of DM1 on family finances could aggravate conflicts among healthy siblings and children with diabetes. Alternatively, disease-specific social support from siblings may have positive effects on children with DM1 in terms of treatment adherence, managing hypoglycemia, and facilitating adaptation to diabetes within the peer group.

Social relationships outside of the family become increasingly important throughout childhood and adolescence and also may affect adaptation to diabetes. Greater interest in peer relations and increased desire for independence from parents may negatively influence diabetes care (e.g., Jacobson et al., 1990). Children and adolescents display poor dietary adherence when with friends (at school, in restaurants), with a significant negative impact on metabolic control (Delamater, Smith, Kurtz, & White, 1988). In adolescence, accommodating peers may be more important than complying with regimen demands. Peer pressure appears to peak in midadolescence (Berndt, 1992) and, correspondingly, adolescents with diabetes in this age range evidence decreases in adherence in exchange for peer acceptance (Thomas, Peterson, & Goldstein, 1997).

Conversely, peers can be an asset to diabetes care; peers may serve as a vital source of constructive support. Social support from peers is rated as important by adolescents with Type 1 diabetes (Greco et al., 1991). In addition, peer support may play a unique and positive role; peers are more likely than family members to provide adolescents with companionship and emotional support in relation to diabetes care (La Greca et al., 1995). Further, improved social skills and relationships may be reflected in adherence (Citrin, La Greca, & Skyler, 1985; Gross, 1987), as well as in better glycemic control (Kaplan, Chadwick, & Schimmel, 1985). However, adolescents with diabetes may construct a barrier to receiving and benefiting from positive support offered by peers. Jacobson and colleagues (1986) noted that among newly diagnosed children and adolescents with diabetes, more than one-half did not talk about diabetes with their peers, and more than one-third believed that their peers would like them less if they knew about their diagnosis.

The difficulties that adolescents have with regimen demands may not reflect deficient knowledge or problem-solving ability. Adolescents have greater cognitive maturity and problem-solving ability than younger children, yet they display lower levels of adherence than younger children (Band, 1990; Thomas et al., 1997), in part due to peer pressure. Traditional knowledge-based and problem-solving approaches to intervention, although effective (e.g., Anderson et al., 1989), may not address adolescents' vulnerability to peer pressure. Thomas and colleagues (1997) instead suggest a focus on managing peer impressions as a more developmentally appropriate strategy for adolescents with diabetes. A recent evaluation of a structured short-term group program for integrating peers into the diabetes care of their adolescent friends indicates promise for this approach (Greco, Shroff Pendley, McDonell, & Reeves, 2001). Adolescents with diabetes and their best friends participated in a group intervention aimed at increasing diabetes knowledge and social support of diabetes care. Following the intervention, adolescents and their friends demonstrated higher levels of knowledge about diabetes and support and a higher ratio of peer to family support, and the friends demonstrated improved self-perception. Parents also reported improved family functioning and decreased diabetes-related conflict following the intervention.

Children and adolescents with DM1 and their families must also learn to advocate for the child's special needs and to deal adaptively with DM1 in schools, in day care settings, and in athletic or recreational programs. Adults in these settings may benefit from (1) general information about DM1, (2) a description of the child's regimen and the impact that it will have in that setting, (3) discussion of barriers within that particular setting that may interfere with regimen adherence, and (4) a means for addressing problems that may arise within the system.

The degree to which the parent or youth takes responsibility for this process depends on variables related to maturity, as well as to age. Anderson and colleagues (Anderson, Auslander, Jung, Miller, & Santiago, 1990) devised a measure of family sharing of diabetes responsibilities, part of which examines the sharing of information about diabetes in social systems other than the family. Older children, especially girls, assumed greater responsibility for informing others about their diabetes in multiple contexts. The authors postulated that this pattern reflected a general shift of responsibility for DM1-related tasks as children mature. Gender differences in maturation rate and parental expectations for responsibility may account for the reported differences in boys' and girls' responsibilities in these areas. Overall, there is a paucity of empirical studies of the presumed benefit to children from the sharing of information and advocating for the diabetes regimen in various social contexts. Families should advocate for their child's diabetes-related needs while remaining sensitive to individual differences (e.g., age, maturation, shyness or embarrassment over disclosure) that might influence this process.

The health care system is another social system within which the child and his or her family must learn to function adaptively. Despite the potential importance of these processes, little research has been done on the variables that influence children's socialization as health care consumers, their internalization of attitudes toward health care delivery and health professionals, and their achievement of autonomous relationships with health care providers. Nonetheless, every child with DM1 must be prepared to face a lifetime of interactions with health professionals and to cultivate a partnership founded on trust and communication. For example, Marrero and colleagues (1989) reported that patient and physician collaboration in the computerized review of recent SMBG results was an effective and valued educational experience. However, clinical encounters with children with DM1 carry the potential for generating counterproductive and deceptive interactions between youths and health professionals. Social demand characteristics of typical clinical encounters may influence many children with DM1 to report erroneous blood glucose test results, presumably to avoid disapproval or criticism (Delamater, Kurtz, White, & Santiago, 1988). Wilson and Endres (1986) reported a higher frequency of distorted SMBG results recorded in children's log books compared with automated recording of true test results by reflectance meters with memory .

The few studies that have focused on health care utilization during early adulthood suggest that young adults visit health care providers infrequently for routine or proactive services and are far more prone to utilize health care services episodically or in response to specific crises (Bartsch, Barnes, Jarrett, & Lindsay, 1989; Wysocki, Hough, Ward, & Green, 1992). Older adolescents may become isolated as they establish independence from family life, withdrawing from regular health care (Olsen & Sutton, 1998). When asked how health professionals can best care for them, adolescents stressed eight themes: (1) treat me like a person, (2) try to understand, (3) don't treat me differently, (4) give me some encouragement, (5) don't force me, (6) give me options, (7) have a sense of humor, and (8) know what you are doing (Woodgate, 1998).

A DIABETES RESEARCH AGENDA FOR PEDIATRIC PSYCHOLOGY

Much has been learned about psychological factors in diabetes, but much remains to be clarified. Five broad areas represent particularly exciting avenues for future exploration.

Psychological Variables in the Etiology and Management of Type 2 Diabetes

DM2 has become an epidemic in the pediatric age group in the past decade. The presumed etiological factors include genetic propensity, obesity, and sedentary lifestyle. Pediatric psychologists could contribute to the prevention of DM2 in at-risk youths by testing behavioral interventions that encourage weight control and regular physical exercise (Epstein, Valoski, Wing, & McCurley, 1994). Similarly, youths who have already been diagnosed with DM2 may benefit from these same interventions through better long-term health status and possible avoidance of daily insulin injections.

Maintenance of Parental Involvement in Diabetes Management

Several studies show that many adolescents are unable to manage diabetes completely independently and that excessive self-care responsibility relative to psychological maturity is associated with poor diabetes outcomes (Anderson et al., 1990; Ingersoll, Orr, Herrold, & Golden, 1986; Wysocki, Taylor, et al., 1996). Thus maintaining parental involvement in diabetes care may counter the deterioration in treatment adherence and diabetic control that typify adolescence. However, the precise nature of that parental involvement and of the factors that affect it remain to be specified.

Variables Affecting Higher Level Diabetes Self-Regulation Skills

Research on the relationship between treatment adherence and diabetic control has not emphasized families' day-to-day self-regulation of the regimen. Earlier studies suggest underuse of SMBG data for treatment adjustments, particularly in a proactive sense (Delamater, Davis et al., 1988; Wysocki et al., 1992). Research on variables that affect the frequency and proficiency of family self-regulation of the regimen is desperately needed. Little is known about how interactions between families and health professionals affect the therapeutic use of SMBG data. This process might be critical for families who lack the prerequisite cognitive or motivational attributes needed for high-level diabetes self-management.

Adaptation to New Technologies

Many scientific and technical advances have appeared or are on the horizon. These include insulin pump therapy, minimally invasive devices that measure blood glucose continuously, new methods of insulin delivery, computerized insulin-dosing algorithms, closed-loop systems that adjust insulin doses to glucose levels automatically, and autoantibody testing to quantify levels of risk for DM1. Pediatric psychologists can help to clarify the psychological effects of these advances to optimize their clinical benefits (e.g., Johnson, 2001).

Efficiency and Cost-Effectiveness of Intensive Therapy

The high cost of intensive therapy versus standard medical care for diabetes, the long-term nature of this investment, and the short-term focus of health care cost containment efforts make it unlikely that funding sources will support the widespread use of intensified therapy. These same observations imply that studies to enhance the efficiency of intensive therapy would be valued. Component analyses of intensive therapy could identify the critical elements of a less expensive, but possibly equally effective, treatment. Empirically validated identification of patients who are likely to benefit from intensive therapy could permit targeted allocation of scarce resources. Researchers could also identify critical self-management behaviors that mediate successful intensive therapy, facilitating optimal treatment outcomes among those who initiate intensified therapy.

CLINICAL IMPLICATIONS

This chapter has summarized many consistent research findings that should influence the clinical practice of pediatric psychology with this population. Childhood diabetes places an enormous cognitive, affective, and behavioral burden on children and adolescents and their families. They must learn and maintain a variety of skills in the face of significant developmental changes. Diabetes knowledge is necessary but not sufficient for adequate treatment adherence and metabolic control. Adherence is a multifactorial construct rather than a stable trait that reflects a complex interaction among many demographic, psychological, and social factors. There are several validated behavioral interventions that have been shown to improve treatment adherence in children and adolescents with diabetes. Unfortunately, improved treatment adherence does not guarantee improved metabolic control.

Aside from the burden of diabetes self-management, children and adolescents must cope with an array of stresses and are at increased risk for psychopathology. It is important to be aware of this increased risk and to screen patients for problems such as anxiety, depression, and eating disorders. Many patients need psychological intervention for treatment of these problems. Cognitive-behavioral treatment consisting of stress management techniques, problem solving, and conflict resolution can improve psychological adjustment and metabolic control. Family members, especially mothers, are also at risk for psychological problems. Their needs should be addressed as well. In addition, children and adolescents may be at risk for adverse cognitive sequelae of diabetes. Some children may warrant cognitive evaluation, especially children diagnosed at very young ages. Cognitive impairment may be contributing to ineffective diabetes self-management in some children and adolescents.

Family variables are integral to the treatment of a child or adolescent with diabetes. Parental involvement is very important and predictive of the achievement of treatment goals, decreased family conflict, and improved glycemic control. Children and adolescents' self-care independence must be balanced with their psychological maturity, as a mismatch can have negative effects on adjustment and treatment adherence. Family environmental factors such as parental support, social competence, family communication, problem solving, and conflict resolution skills are correlates of physical and psychological adjustment and are areas for intervention with families. In adolescence, accommodating peers becomes increasingly important. Peers can be an asset in the treatment process and can provide an important and different type of social support from that given by family members. Finally, patients and families must advocate for their special needs in a variety of social contexts, including school and the health care environment. Health care professionals can help adolescents with diabetes by being competent, encouraging, empathetic, good humored, flexible, and inclusive of the patient in the treatment process.

REFERENCES

Aikens, J. E., Wallander, J. L., Bell, D. S. H., & Cole, J. A. (1992). Daily stress variability, learned resourcefulness, regimen adherence, and metabolic control in Type I diabetes mellitus: Evaluation of a path model. *Journal of Consulting and Clinical Psychology, 60*, 113–118.

Anderson, B. J., Auslander, W. F., Jung, K. C., Miller, J. P., & Santiago, J. V. (1990). Assessing family sharing of diabetes responsibilities. *Journal of Pediatric Psychology, 15*, 477–492.

Anderson, B. J., Brackett, J., & Laffel, L. M. (1999). An office-based intervention to maintain parent-adolescent teamwork in diabetes management: Impact on parent involvement, family conflict, and subsequent glycemic control. *Diabetes Care, 22*, 713–721.

Anderson, B. J., Ho, J., Brackett, J., Finkelstein, D., & Laffel, L. (1997). Parental involvement in diabetes management tasks: Relationships to blood glucose monitoring adherence and metabolic control in young adolescents with insulin-dependent diabetes mellitus. *Journal of Pediatrics, 130*, 257–265.

Anderson, B. J., Miller, B., Auslander, W. F., & Santiago, J. V. (1981). Family characteristics of diabetic adolescents: Relationships to metabolic control. *Diabetes Care, 4*, 586–594.

Anderson, B. J., Wolf, F. M., Burkhart, M. T., Cornell, R. G., & Bacon, G. E. (1989). Effects of peer group intervention on metabolic control of adolescents with DM1: Randomized outpatient study. *Diabetes Care,12*, 179–184.

Antisdel, J. E., & Chrisler, J. C. (2000). Comparison of eating attitudes and behaviors among adolescent and young women with Type 1 diabetes mellitus and phenylketonuria. *Journal of Developmental and Behavioral Pediatrics, 21*, 81–86.

Band, E. B. (1990). Children's coping with diabetes: Understanding the role of cognitive development. *Journal of Pediatric Psychology, 15*, 27–41.

Banion, C., Miles, M., & Carter, M. (1983). Problems of mothers in the management of children with diabetes. *Diabetes Care, 6*, 548–551.

Bartsch, C., Barnes, B., Jarrett, L., & Lindsay, R. (1989). Where did they go? Life after teen diabetes clinic [Abstract]. *Diabetes, 38*(Suppl. 2), 40A.

Berndt, T. J. (1992). Friendship and friend's influence in adolescents. *Current Directions in Psychological Science, 1*, 156–159.

Blechman, E. A., & Delamater, A. M. (1993). Family communication and Type I diabetes: A window on the social environment of chronically ill children. In R. E. Cole & D. Reiss (Eds.), *How do families cope with chronic illness?* (pp. 1–24). Hillsdale, NJ: Erlbaum.

Boardway, R. H., Delamater, A. M., Tomakowsky, J., & Gutai, J. P. (1993). Stress management training for adolescents with diabetes. *Journal of Pediatric Psychology, 18*, 29–45.

Bobrow, E. S., AvRuskin, T. W., & Siller, J. (1985). Mother–daughter interaction and adherence to diabetes regimens. *Diabetes Care, 8*, 146–151.

Briery, B. G., & Rabian, B. (1999). Psychosocial changes associated with participation in a pediatric summer camp. *Journal of Pediatric Psychology, 24*, 183–190.

Chase, H. P., & Jackson, G. G. (1981) Stress and sugar control in children with insulin-dependent diabetes mellitus. *Journal of Pediatrics, 98*, 1011–1013.

Christensen, K. (1983). Self-management in diabetic children. *Diabetes Care, 6*, 552–555.

Citrin, W., La Greca, A. M., & Skyler, J. S. (1985). Group intervention in Type I diabetes mellitus. In P. I. Ahmed & N. Ahmed (Eds.), *Coping with juvenile diabetes* (pp. 181–204). Springfield, IL: Thomas.

Colton, P. A., Rodin, G. M., Olmsted, M. P., & Daneman, D. (1999). Eating disturbances in young women with Type 1 diabetes mellitus: Mechanisms and consequences. *Psychiatric Annals, 29*, 213–218.

Cox, D. J., Kovatchev, B. P., Julian, D. M., Gonder-Frederick, L. A., Polonsky, W. H., Schlundt, D. G., & Clarke, W. L. (1994). Frequency of severe hypoglycemia in insulin-dependent diabetes mellitus can be predicted from self-monitoring blood glucose data. *Journal of Clinical Endocrinology and Metabolism, 79*, 1659–1662.

Davis, C. L., Delamater, A. M., Shaw, K. H., La Greca, A. M., Widson, M., Perez-Rodriguez, J. E., & Nemery, R. (2001). Parenting styles, regimen adherence, and glycemic control in 4- to 10-year-old children with diabetes. *Journal of Pediatric Psychology*, 26, 123–129.

Delamater, A. M., Bubb, J., Davis, S., Smith, J. A., Schmidt, L., White, N. H., & Santiago, J. V. (1990). Randomized prospective study of self-management training with newly diagnosed diabetic children. *Diabetes Care, 13*, 492–498.

Delamater, A. M., Davis, S., Bubb, J., Smith, J., White, N. H., & Santiago, J. V. (1988). Self-monitoring of blood glucose by adolescents with diabetes: Technical skills and utilization of data. *Diabetes Educator, 15*, 56–61.

Delamater, A. M., Jacobson, A. M., Anderson, B. J., Cox, D. J., Fisher, L., Lustman, P., et al. (2001). Psychosocial therapies in diabetes: Report of the psychosocial therapies working group. *Diabetes Care, 24*, 1286–1292.

Delamater, A. M., Kurtz, S., Bubb, J., White, N. H., & Santiago, J. V. (1987). Stress and coping in relation to metabolic control of adolescents with Type I diabetes mellitus. *Journal of Developmental and Behavioral Pediatrics, 8*, 136–140.

Delamater, A. M., Kurtz, S. M., White, N. H., & Santiago, J. V. (1988). Effects of social demand on reports of self-monitored blood glucose in adolescents with Type I diabetes mellitus. *Journal of Applied Social Psychology, 18*, 491–502.

Delamater, A. M., Smith, J. A., Kurtz, S. M., & White, N. H. (1988). Dietary skills and adherence in children with Type 1 diabetes mellitus. *Diabetes Educator, 14*, 33–36.

Diabetes Control and Complications Trial Research Group. (1994). Effect of intensive treatment on the development and progression of long-term complications in adolescents with insulin-dependent diabetes mellitus. *Journal of Pediatrics, 125*, 177–188.

Drotar, D., & Riekert, K. (1999). Who participates in research on adherence to treatment in insulin-dependent diabetes mellitus: Implications and recommendations for research. *Journal of Pediatric Psychology, 24*, 253–258.

Epstein, L., Valoski, A., Wing, R., & McCurley, J. (1994). Ten-year outcomes of behavioral family-based treatment for childhood obesity. *Health Psychology, 13*, 373–383.

Freund, A., Johnson, S. B., Rosenbloom, A., Alexander, B., & Hansen, C. A. (1986). Subjective symptoms, blood glucose estimation, and blood glucose concentrations in adolescents with diabetes. *Diabetes Care, 9*, 236–243.

Geffken, G., Lewis, C., Johnson, S., Silverstein, J., Rosenbloom, A., & Monaco, L. (1997). Residential treatment for youngsters with difficult to manage insulin-dependent diabetes mellitus. *Journal of Clinical Endocrinology and Metabolism, 10*, 517–527.

Glasgow, A. M., Weissberg-Benchell, D. R., Tynan, W. D., Epstein, S. F., Driscoll, C., Terek, J., & Beliveau, E. (1991). Re-admissions of children with diabetes mellitus to a children's hospital. *Pediatrics, 88*, 98–104.

Glasgow, R. E., McCaul, K. D., & Schafer, L. C. (1986). Barriers to regimen adherence among persons with insulin-dependent diabetes. *Journal of Behavioral Medicine, 9*, 65–77.

Glasgow, R. E., McCaul, K. D., & Schafer, L. C. (1987). Self-care behaviors and glycemic control in Type I diabetes. *Journal of Chronic Disease, 40*, 399–417.

Glasgow, R. E., Wilson, W., & McCaul, K. D. (1985). Regimen adherence: A problematic construct in diabetes research [Editorial]. *Diabetes Care, 8*, 300–301.

Gonder-Frederick, L. A., Snyder, A. L., & Clarke, W. L. (1991). Accuracy of blood glucose estimation by children with IDDM and their parents. *Diabetes Care, 14*, 565–570.

Gray, D. L., Marrero, D. G., Godfrey, C., Orr, D. P., & Golden, M. P. (1988). Chronic poor metabolic control in the pediatric population: A stepwise intervention program. *Diabetes Educator, 14*, 516–520.

Greco, P., La Greca, A. M., Auslander, W. F., Spetter, D., Skyler, J. S., Fisher, E., & Santiago, J. V. (1991). Family and peer support of diabetes care among adolescents [Abstract]. *Diabetes, 40*(Suppl. 1), 537A.

Greco, P., Shroff Pendley, J., McDonell, K., & Reeves, G. (2001). A peer group intervention for adolescents with Type 1 diabetes and their best friends. *Journal of Pediatric Psychology, 26*, 485–490.

Grey, M. (2000). Interventions for children with diabetes and their families. *Annual Review of Nursing Research, 18*, 149–170.

Grey, M., Boland, E. A., Davidson, M., Li, J., & Tamborlane, W. V. (2000). Coping skills training for youth with poorly controlled diabetes mellitus has long-lasting effects on metabolic control and quality of life. *Journal of Pediatrics, 137*, 107–113.

Grey, M., Davidson, M., Boland, E. A., & Tamborlane, W. V. (2001). Clinical and psychosocial factors associated with achievement of treatment goals in adolescents with diabetes mellitus. *Journal of Adolescent Health, 28*, 377–385.

Gross, A. M. (1987). A behavioral approach to the compliance problems of young diabetics. *Journal of Compliance in Health Care, 2*, 7–21.

Hampson, S., Skinner, T. C., Hart, J., Storey, L., Gage, H., Foxcroft, D., et al. (2001). Effect of psychoeducational and psychosocial interventions for adolescents with diabetes: A systematic review. *Health Technology Assessment, 5*, 1–79.

Hanson, C. L., Cigrang, J. A., Harris, M. A., Carle, D. L., Relyea, G., & Burghen, G. (1989). Coping styles in youths with insulin-dependent diabetes mellitus. *Journal of Consulting and Clinical Psychology, 57*, 644–651.

Hanson, C. L., Henggeler, S. W., & Burghen, G. (1987). Social competence and parental support as mediators of the link between stress and metabolic control in adolescents with insulin-dependent diabetes mellitus. *Journal of Consulting and Clinical Psychology, 55*, 529–533.

Hanson, C. L., Henggeler, S. W., Rodrigue, J. R., Burghen, G. A., & Murphy, W. D. (1988). Father-absent adolescents with insulin-dependent diabetes mellitus: A population at special risk? *Journal of Applied Developmental Psychology, 9*, 243–252.

Harkavy, J., Johnson, S. B., Silverstein, J. H., Spillar, R., McCallum, M., & Rosenbloom, A. (1983). Who learns what at diabetes summer camp? *Journal of Pediatric Psychology, 8*, 143–153.

Harris, M. A., Wysocki, T., Sadler, M., Wilkinson, K., Harvey, L. M., Buckloh, L. M., et al. (2000). Validation of a structured interview for the assessment of diabetes self management. *Diabetes Care, 23*, 1301–1304.

Hauenstein, E., Marvin, R., Snyder, A., & Clarke, W. L. (1989). Stress in parents of children with diabetes mellitus. *Diabetes Care, 12*, 18–23.

Hauser, S., Jacobson, A. M., Lavori, P., Wolfsdorf, J., Herskowitz, R., Milley, J., et al. (1990). Adherence among children and adolescents with insulin-dependent diabetes mellitus over a four-year longitudinal follow-up: Immediate and long-term linkages with the family milieu. *Journal of Pediatric Psychology, 15*, 527–542.

Hodges, L., & Parker, J. (1987). Concerns of parents with diabetic children. *Pediatric Nursing, 13*, 22–24.

Ingersoll, G., Orr, D. P., Herrold, A., & Golden, M. P. (1986). Cognitive maturity and self-management among adolescents with insulin-dependent diabetes mellitus. *Journal of Pediatrics, 108*, 620–623.

Jacobson, A. M., Hauser, S. T., Lavori, P., Willett, J., Cole, C., Wolfsdorf, J. I., et al. (1994). Family environment and glycemic control: A four-year prospective study of children and adolescents with DM1. *Psychosomatic Medicine, 17*, 267–274.

Jacobson, A. M., Hauser, S. T., Lavori, P., Wolfsdorf, J. I., Herskowitz, R. D., Milley, J., et al. (1990). Adherence among children and adolescents with DM1 over a four-year longitudinal follow-up: The influence of patient coping and adjustment. *Journal of Pediatric Psychology, 15*, 511–526.

Jacobson, A. M., Hauser, S. T., Wertlieb, D., Wolfsdorf, J., Orelans, J., & Vieyra, M. (1986). Psychological adjustment of children with recently diagnosed diabetes mellitus. *Diabetes Care, 9*, 323–329.

Jacobson, A. M., Hauser, S. T., Wolfsdorf, J., Houlihan, J., Milley, J. E., Herskowitz, R. D., et al. (1987). Psychologic predictors of compliance in children with recent onset of diabetes. *Journal of Pediatrics, 110*, 805–811.

Johnson, S. B. (1995). Insulin-dependent diabetes mellitus in childhood. In M. C. Roberts (Ed.), *Handbook of pediatric psychology* (2nd ed., pp. 263–285). New York: Guilford Press.

Johnson, S. B. (2001). Screening programs to identify children at risk for diabetes mellitus: Psychological impact on children and parents. *Journal of Clinical Endocrinology and Metabolism, 14*(Suppl. 1), 653–659.

Johnson, S. B., Freund, A., Silverstein, J. H., Hansen, C. A., & Malone, J. I. (1990). Adherence-health status relationships in childhood diabetes. *Health Psychology, 9*, 606–631.

Johnson, S. B., Perwein, A. R., & Silverstein, J. H. (2000). Response to hypo- and hyperglycemia in adolescents with Type 1 diabetes. *Journal of Pediatric Psychology, 25*, 171–178.

Johnson, S. B., Silverstein, J., Rosenbloom, A., Carter, R., & Cunningham, W. (1986). Assessing daily management in childhood diabetes. *Health Psychology, 5*, 545–564.

Kaplan, R. M., Chadwick, M. W., & Schimmel, L. E. (1985). Social learning intervention to improve metabolic control in Type 1 diabetes mellitus. *Diabetes Care, 8*, 152–155.

Kovacs, M., Finkelstein, R., Feinberg, T. L., Crouse-Novak, M., Paulauskas, S., & Pollock, M. (1985). Initial psychologic responses of parents to the diagnosis of insulin-dependent diabetes mellitus in their children. *Diabetes Care, 8*, 568–575.

Kovacs, M., Goldston, D., Obrosky, D. S., & Bonar, L. K. (1997). Psychiatric disorders in youths with IDDM: Rates and risk factors. *Diabetes Care, 20*, 36–44.

Kovacs, M., Iyengar, S., Goldston, D., Obrosky, D. S., Stewart, J., & Marsh, J. (1990). Psychological functioning among mothers of children with insulin-dependent diabetes mellitus: A longitudinal study. *Journal of Consulting and Clinical Psychology, 58*, 159–165.

La Greca, A. M., Auslander, W. F., Greco, P., Spetter, D., Fisher, E. B., & Santiago, J. V. (1995). I get by with a little help from my family and friends: Adolescents' support for diabetes care. *Journal of Pediatric Psychology, 21*, 449–476.

La Greca, A. M., Follansbee, D. M., & Skyler, J. S. (1990). Developmental and behavioral aspects of diabetes management in youngsters. *Children's Health Care, 19*, 132–139.

La Greca, A. M., & Skyler, J. S. (1991). Psychosocial aspects of DM1: A multivariate framework. In P. McCabe, T. Field, & N. Schneiderman (Eds.), *Stress, coping, and disease* (pp. 169–190). Hillsdale, NJ: Erlbaum.

Lustman, P. J., Griffith, L. S., & Clouse, R. E. (1996). Recognizing and managing depression in patients with diabetes. In B. J. Anderson & R. R. Rubin (Eds.), *Practical psychology for diabetes clinicians* (pp. 143–152). Alexandria, VA: American Diabetes Association.

Marrero, D. G., Kronz, K. K., Golden, M. P., Wright, J. C., Wright, J. C., Orr, D. P., & Fineberg, N. S. (1989). Clinical evaluation of computer-assisted self-monitoring of blood glucose system. *Diabetes Care, 12*, 351–356.

McCaul, K. D., Glasgow, R. E., & Schafer, L. C. (1987). Diabetes regimen behaviors predicting adherence. *Medical Care, 25*, 868–881.

Nurick, M., & Johnson, S. B. (1991). Enhancing blood glucose awareness in adolescents and young adults with IDDM. *Diabetes Care, 14*, 1–7.

Olsen, R., & Sutton, J. (1998). More hassle, more alone: Adolescents with diabetes and the role of formal and informal support. *Child: Care, Health, and Development, 24*, 31–39.

Peyrot, M., & Rubin, R. R. (1988). Insulin self-regulation predicts better glycemic control [Abstract]. *Diabetes, 37*(Suppl. 1), 53A.

Polonsky, W. H., Anderson, B. J., Lohrer, P. A., Aponte, J. E., Jacobson, A. M., & Cole, C. F. (1994). Insulin omission in women with IDDM. *Diabetes Care, 17,* 1178–1185.

Quittner, A. L., Espelage, D. L., Ievers-Landis, C., & Drotar, D. (2000). Measuring adherence to medical treatments in chronic childhood illness: Considering multiple methods and sources of information. *Journal of Clinical Psychology in Medical Settings, 7,* 41–54.

Robin, A. L., & Foster, S. L. (1989). *Negotiating parent–adolescent conflict: A behavioral–family systems approach.* New York: Guilford Press.

Rovet, J., & Fernandes, C. (1998). Insulin-dependent diabetes mellitus. In R. T. Brown (Ed.), *Cognitive aspects of chronic illness in children* (pp. 142–171). New York: Guilford Press.

Ryan, C. M. (1997). Effects of diabetes mellitus on neuropsychological function: A lifespan perspective. *Seminars in Clinical Neuropsychiatry, 2,* 4–14.

Ryan, C. M., Atchison, J., Puczynski, S., Puczynski, M., Arslanian, S., & Becker, D. M. (1990). Mild hypoglycemia associated with deterioration of mental efficiency in children with insulin-dependent diabetes mellitus. *Journal of Pediatrics, 117,* 32–38.

Ryden, O., Nevander, L., Johnsson, P., Hansson, K., Kronvall, P., Sjoblad, S., & Westbom, L. (1994). Family therapy in poorly controlled juvenile DM1: Effects on diabetic control, self-evaluation and behavioral symptoms. *Acta Paediatrica, 83,* 285–291.

Schlundt, D. G, Flannery, M. E., Davis, D. L., Kinzer, C. K., & Pichert, J. W. (1999). Evaluation of a multicomponent, behaviorally oriented, problem-based, "summer school" program for adolescents with diabetes. *Behavior Modification, 23,* 79–105.

Schmidt, L. E., Klover, R. V., Arfken, C. L., Delamater, A. M., & Hobson, D. (1992). Compliance with dietary prescriptions in children and adolescents with insulin-dependent diabetes mellitus. *Journal of the American Dietetic Association, 92,* 567–570.

Seiffge-Krenke, I. (1998). The highly structured family in families of adolescents with diabetes: Functional or dysfunctional for metabolic control? *Journal of Pediatric Psychology, 23,* 313–322.

Skinner, T. C., John, M., & Hampson, S. E. (2000). Social support and personal models of diabetes as predictors of self-care and well-being: A longitudinal study of adolescents with diabetes. *Journal of Pediatric Psychology, 25,* 257–267.

Takii, M., Komaki, G., Uchigata, Y., Maeda, M., Omori, Y., & Kubo, C. (1999). Differences between bulimia nervosa and binge-eating disorder in females with Type 1 diabetes: The important role of insulin omission. *Journal of Psychosomatic Research, 47,* 221–231.

Tamborlane, W. V., Gatcomb, P., Held, N., & Ahern, J. (1994, September/October). Implications of the DCCT results in treating children and adolescents with diabetes. *Clinical Diabetes,* 115–116.

Thomas, A. M., Peterson, L., & Goldstein, D. (1997). Problem solving and diabetes regimen adherence by children and adolescents with IDDM in social pressure situations: A reflection of normal development. *Journal of Pediatric Psychology, 22,* 541–561.

United Kingdom Prospective Diabetes Study Group. (1998). Intensive blood glucose control with sulphonylureas or insulin compared with conventional treatment and risk of complications in patients with Type 2 diabetes (UKPDS 33). *Lancet, 352,* 837–853.

University of Michigan Diabetes Research and Training Center. (1998). *Teenagers with Type 1 diabetes: A curriculum for adolescents and their families.* Alexandria, VA: American Diabetes Association.

Weissberg-Benchell, J., Glasgow, A., Tynan, W., Wirtz, P., Turek, J., & Ward, J. (1995). Adolescent diabetes management and mismanagement. *Diabetes Care, 18,* 77–82.

Wertlieb, D., Hauser, S. T., & Jacobson, A. M. (1986). Adaptation to diabetes: Behavior symptoms and family context. *Journal of Pediatric Psychology, 11,* 463–479.

White, K., Kolman, M. L., Wexler, P., Polin, G., & Winter, R. J. (1984). Unstable diabetes and unstable families: A psychosocial evaluation of children with recurrent diabetic ketoacidosis. *Pediatrics, 73,* 749–755.

Wilson, D. P., & Endres, R. K. (1986). Compliance with blood glucose monitoring in children with Type I diabetes mellitus. *Journal of Pediatrics, 108,* 1022–1024.

Woodgate, R. L. (1998). Health professionals caring for chronically ill adolescents: Adolescents' perspectives. *Journal of the Society of Pediatric Nurses, 3,* 57–68.

Wysocki, T. (1993). Associations among parent–adolescent relationships, metabolic control and adjustment to diabetes in adolescents. *Journal of Pediatric Psychology, 18,* 443–454.

Wysocki, T., Greco, P., Harris, M. A., Bubb, J., & White, N. H. (2001). Behavior therapy for families of adolescents with diabetes: Maintenance of treatment effects. *Diabetes Care, 24*(3), 441–446.

Wysocki, T., Green, L. B., & Huxtable, K. (1989). Blood glucose monitoring by diabetic adolescents: Compliance and metabolic control. *Health Psychology, 8,* 267–284.

Wysocki, T., Harris, M. A., Greco, P., Bubb, J., Elder, C. L., Harvey, L. M., et al. (2000). Randomized, controlled trial of behavior therapy for families of adolescents with insulin-dependent diabetes mellitus. *Journal of Pediatric Psychology, 25,* 23–33.

Wysocki, T., Hough, B. S., Ward, K. M., Allen, A. A., & Murgai, N. (1992). Use of blood glucose data by families of children and adolescents with DM1. *Diabetes Care, 15*, 1041–1044.

Wysocki, T., Hough, B. S., Ward, K. M., & Green, L. B. (1992). Diabetes mellitus in the transition to adulthood: Adjustment, self-care and health status. *Journal of Developmental and Behavioral Pediatrics, 13*, 194–201.

Wysocki, T., Huxtable, K., Linscheid, T. R., & Wayne, W. (1989). Adjustment to diabetes mellitus in preschoolers and their mothers. *Diabetes Care, 12*, 524–529.

Wysocki, T., Meinhold, P., Taylor, A., Hough, B. S., Barnard, M. U., Clarke, W. L., et al. (1996). Psychometric properties and normative data for the parent version of the Diabetes Independence Survey. *Diabetes Educator, 22*, 587–591.

Wysocki, T., Miller, K. M., Greco, P., Harris, M. A., Harvey, L. M., Elder-Danda, C. L., et al. (1999). Behavior therapy for families of adolescents with diabetes: Effects on directly observed family interactions. *Behavior Therapy, 30*, 496–515.

Wysocki, T., Taylor, A., Hough, B. S., Linscheid, T. R., Yeates, K. O., & Naglieri, J. A. (1996). Deviation from developmentally appropriate self-care autonomy: Association with diabetes outcomes. *Diabetes Care, 19*, 119–125.

19

Diseases of the Blood

Sickle Cell Disease and Hemophilia

KATHLEEN L. LEMANEK
MARK A. RANALLI
KELLY GREEN
CHARMAINE BIEGA
CLAUDIA LUPIA

Research on the adaptation of children and adolescents with sickle cell disease (SCD) and hemophilia has grown steadily. However, this growth has not been consistent across areas of adaptation. The majority of studies have focused on improving the understanding of the pathophysiology of these disorders and advancements in their treatment. With respect to SCD, a surge also has been evident in studies on the neurocognitive functioning of children from preschool age through adolescence. This chapter reviews the literature on the psychosocial and medical adaptation of children and adolescents with SCD or hemophilia. The review of medical adaptation includes discussion of the prevalence, pathophysiology, clinical manifestations, and approaches to treatment. Studies on the psychological, the social, and the academic adaptation of children and adolescents with SCD and hemophilia are then reviewed. The chapter concludes with recommendations for future research and practice as part of a comprehensive and family-centered system of care.

SICKLE CELL DISEASE

SCD represents a spectrum of inherited disorders of the oxygen-carrying red blood cell protein, hemoglobin. Although the gene for SCD is found principally in individuals of African ancestry, this disorder is encountered with increasing frequency in descendants of individuals from Turkey, Greece, southern Mediterranean regions, Saudi Arabia, India, the Caribbean, and Latin America. In the United States, approximately 72,000 people are affected by

SCD. The disease occurs in approximately 1 in every 500 African American births and in 1 in every 1,000 to 1,400 Hispanic American births (National Heart, Lung, and Blood Institute, 1996).

Medical Aspects

Genetics and Molecular Biology

Normal hemoglobin in humans, called hemoglobin A (HbA), is found almost exclusively in the red blood cells and is composed of two alpha globin and two beta globin chains. The genetic change responsible for the sickle cell syndromes involves a single amino acid substitution within the beta globin gene of hemoglobin (Ingram, 1956). The SCD gene has persisted presumably because of the survival advantage that young heterozygous patients experience when infected by malaria (Allison, 1954). The most common and the most severe SCD genotype occurs when individuals inherit two sickle beta globin genes (HbSS). Disease of reduced severity results when other mutant forms of the beta gene are inherited in combination with a sickle gene, including HbC and HbE. Another variant, sickle cell thalassemia, involves a functionally normal HbA beta chain that is made in lower amounts than usual. Patients with "sickle cell trait" inherit one normal and one sickle beta gene. Approximately 2 million Americans (1 in 12 African Americans) have sickle cell trait (National Heart, Lung, and Blood Institute, 1996). In general, these individuals are completely asymptomatic, except under rare and extreme conditions, and enjoy a lifespan that is similar to that of the non-SCD population.

Pathophysiology

The sickling process is a multicellular and polygenic phenomenon. Under conditions of hypoxia and acidosis, sickle hemoglobin molecules coalesce with each other into large polymers that damage the erythrocyte membrane, causing the characteristic sickled red blood cell shape (Eaton & Hofrichter, 1990). These rigid and deformed red blood cells are unable to pass through the narrowest blood vessels. A red blood cell "logjam" results, with reduced blood flow through this obstruction. The resulting oxygen and nutrient starvation, combined with the accumulation of toxic waste products, produce the acute and chronic symptoms seen clinically.

Clinical Manifestations

The variable severity of SCD complications depends on the sickle cell genotype; alterations in nonhemoglobin genes; the existence of comorbid illnesses such as asthma, infections, or renal disease; knowledge and adherence to prescribed therapy; and psychosocial factors. After 6 months of age, fetal hemoglobin levels fall and sickle hemoglobin levels climb, with the resulting appearance of clinically evident disease (Goldberg, Husson, & Bunn, 1977). Individuals who experience acute symptoms earlier tend to have more clinically virulent disease (Miller et al., 2001).

Pain. Children and adolescents with SCD typically experience an average of 5 to 7 pain episodes or vaso-occulsive crises (VOC) per year (Shapiro, 1993). Pain episodes may last 1 day, 3 or more days, or be chronic. Pain is often described as aching, tiring, and uncomfortable; severe pain is represented by red and green in descriptions and drawings on a body diagram (Walco & Dampeir, 1990). Pain occurs most commonly in an extremity, in the back, the chest, or the abdomen and interferes with academic demands (i.e., completing school assignments, school attendance), sleep, and social activities (Gil, Porter, Ready, Workman, Sedway, & Anthony, 2000; Shapiro et al., 1995). These disruptions of daily activities seem dependent on the level of pain experienced (Gil et al., 2000). Narcotic medications and health care services are used more often as pain ratings increase to 6 or 7 on a 10-point scale, and school, household, and social activities decrease or stop at these ratings. Dehydration, illness, extremes in temperature, or emotional stress may trigger pain episodes. Approximately 90% of pain episodes are managed at home, with one to two hospitalizations occurring per year (Shapiro et al., 1995; Walco & Dampier, 1990). Currently, there is no standard management for sickle cell pain.

Pulmonary and Cardiac Complications. Acute pulmonary events are a major cause of mortality and are a common reason for hospitalization (Kirkpatrick & Bass, 1989). Over 50% of individuals possess the combination of SCD and asthma and may benefit from asthma management (Leong, Dampier, Varlotta, & Allen, 1997). The "acute chest syndrome" (ACS) is described as a new infiltrate and chest pain in the presence of symptoms of respiratory compromise. Cardiac complications may account for 10–30% of deaths (Gerry, Bulkley, & Hutchins, 1978). Myocardial infarctions also have been described in adults with SCD in the absence of atherosclerotic disease.

Cerebral Vascular Accidents. Ten percent of individuals with SCD will experience a stroke before the age of 20 years (Frempong, 1991). Strokes result from sickling within the large arteries of the brain. Silent infarcts also are commonly seen in neurologically intact individuals with SCD. These individuals are at a heightened risk for developing further silent and clinically evident strokes (Miller et al., 2001). Without proper management, upward of 50% of individuals with SCD and stroke experience progression of cerebrovascular injury. Transcranial Doppler ultrasonography (TCD) may assist in the early identification of individuals who are at risk of stroke before they occur (Adams et al., 1998).

Infectious Complications. Poor or absent splenic function seen in SCD prevents the clearance of bacterial organisms, resulting in infections that are rapidly fatal, even if diagnosed properly (Fernbach & Burdine, 1970). The use of daily penicillin prophylaxis and the adoption of aggressive treatment algorithms for patients with fever over the past two decades have substantially reduced early death in children with SCD and improved life expectancy overall (Gaston et al., 1986).

Skeletal Complications, Growth, and Puberty. Skeletal complications are common in individuals with SCD and include weakened bones that easily fracture and degenerative joint disease that involves chronic pain and disability. SCD is associated with delayed growth and sexual maturation due to the demands of profound anemia and psychosocial, nutritional, and hormonal factors (Phebus, Gloninger, & Maciak, 1984). Most children with SCD achieve adult heights within expected norms for adults without SCD. The majority of adolescents also experience full pubertal development, although this process may not be complete until age 20.

Hepatobiliary and Genitourinary Complications. Bilirubin stones, resulting from the increased blood cell turnover in SCD, form in the gallbladder and cause pain, jaundice, and, if untreated, infection. Individuals with SCD who are chronically transfused are at risk for hepatitis virus infection, with chronic liver injury, and possible death from liver failure. Renal dysfunction in individuals with SCD is common and related to high blood flow through the kidneys and to chronic sickling within the renal medulla (Kontessis, Mayopoulou-Symvoulidis, Symvoulidis, & Kontopoulou-Griva, 1992). Males may experience prolonged painful erections due to sickling within the penile tissues that ultimately produce scarring and impotence. In women with SCD, amenorrhea and infertility are not uncommon, and pregnancy is accompanied by a substantially increased risk of maternal and fetal complications.

Treatment Approaches

Advances in the understanding of sickle cell pathophysiology and improvements in supportive care have translated into improvements in quality of life and life expectancy. Early identification through newborn screening for SCD also has had favorable impact on such outcomes (Leikin et al., 1989). Whereas past management has focused largely on symptom control and not on symptom prevention, new treatment approaches show promise as preventative strategies.

Supportive Care. Hydration and analgesia are employed in the management of acute SCD complications. Nonsteroidal anti-inflammatory medications and patient-controlled analgesia units are used with increasingly frequency. Supervised incentive spirometry and early ambulation show promise in preventing progression of acute pulmonary exacerbations. Transfusions are indicated for the management of strokes, pulmonary complications, and chronic pain. However, their use in the treatment of acute pain episodes is controversial. The use of phenotypically similar blood and automated exchange transfusions reduces the risk of iron overload, a potentially fatal complication.

Novel Agents. Hydroxyurea (HU) and butyrate are medications that increase (protective) fetal hemoglobin levels (Platt et al., 1984). The chronic use of HU has produced a reduction in the duration of hospital stays, the frequency of VOC events, and the number of required transfusions (Charache et al., 1995). Infants tolerate HU well, but its safety and efficacy are still to be proven in this age group (Wang et al., 2001). Butyrate's use as a chronic medication remains to be elucidated.

Bone Marrow Transplantation and Gene Replacement Therapy. Bone marrow transplantation (BMT) offers the prospect of a cure for patients with SCD. Unfortunately, current BMT-associated mortality rates approach 5–20%. BMT has thus far been reserved for patients with clinically aggressive SCD who have failed maximal medical therapy. Gene therapy is still in its preclinical phases of investigation.

Psychological Aspects

Previous research on the psychological status of children with SCD revealed similarities in self-concepts with their healthy peers. However, adolescents with SCD were at risk of developing negative self-concepts and poor peer relationships due to the physical manifestations of the disorder (e.g., delayed sexual maturation) and its activity limitations (e.g., participation in sports). In addition, children and adolescents with SCD were at risk of developing internalizing behavior problems, especially depression and anxiety (Thompson, Gil, Burbach, Keith, & Kinney, 1993a; Williams, Earles, & Pack, 1983). Recommendations for future research included observation of peer and family interactions and use of cross-informants, especially peer ratings, to assess specific domains of functioning and stability of adaptation. Recent studies have incorporated some of these recommendations into their designs, with a particular focus on family adaptation and child-rearing patterns.

Interpersonal Functioning

Predictors of adjustment have highlighted interpersonal, stress-processing, and social-ecological factors, but not disease-related factors (Burlew, Telfair, Colangelo, & Wright, 2000).

Individual Differences. Findings from recent studies have continued to show that children and adolescents with SCD are at risk of developing internalizing problems (Gartstein, Short, Vannatta, & Noll, 1999; Thompson, Gustafson, Gil, Godfrey, & Murphy, 1998). Parents of males with SCD also have continued to report more parenting concerns (e.g., medical and daily care), increased internalizing behavior problems, and greater restriction of activities than parents of females with SCD (Brown & Lambert, 1999; Hill & Zimmerman, 1995; Ievers-Landis et al., 2001). The heightened risk for both males and females has been identified primarily through parent reports of behavior problems and shown less consistently through child reports of symptomatology. For example, two studies (Gartstein et al., 1999; Noll et al., 1996) have not found elevations on measures of anxiety and depression completed by youths with SCD compared with their classmates. Gender differences also have been shown in peer ratings. In the one recent study on peer relationships (Noll et al., 1996), females with SCD were seen by their peers as less sociable and less well accepted, whereas males were viewed as less aggressive.

Stability of Adjustment. Recent studies have attempted to delineate illness-specific patterns of short-term and long-term adjustment based on stress and coping models (Thompson et al., 1994; Thompson et al., 1998; Thompson, Gustafson, Gil, Kinney, & Spock, 1999). In the 1998 study, self-reported cognitive processes, including stress appraisal and self-worth, accounted for 21% and 12%, respectively, of short-term adjustment in children with SCD. Over a 2-year period, coping strategies characterized by negative thinking and few efforts at coping accounted for a significant proportion of variance in child-reported adjustment problems and lower self-worth (Thompson, Gustafson, et al., 1999). Instability in child-reported problems also was found, as evidenced by a consistency of only 32% in adjustment classification for child-reported problems and 66% for mother-reported problems.

Few intervention studies have been conducted to foster interpersonal functioning or to reduce problems in adjustment. Improved psychosocial adjustment has, though, been obtained for adolescents through interventions that address strengthening social support networks while they are hospitalized (Hazzard, Celano, Collins, & Markov, 2002) or as outpatients (Telfair & Gardner, 1999).

Parent and Family Functioning

Researchers have examined parent and family functioning within stress and coping models to identify risk and protective factors, as well as processing factors.

Parent Adjustment. Research has revealed increased psychological distress in parents of children and adolescents with SCD compared with parents of healthy children (Thompson, Gil, Burbach, Keith, & Kinney, 1993b; Thompson, Gustafson, et al., 1999; Thompson, Gustafson, Bonner, & Ware, 2002). For example, Thompson and colleagues (Thompson, Gustafson, et al., 1999; Thompson et al., 2002) found that poorer parent adjustment, especially maternal anxiety, was related to higher levels of daily stress, lower expectations of illness efficacy, and decreased knowledge of child development. Noll et al. (1994), however, did not find significant differences between caregivers of children with SCD and comparison caregivers on self-reported measures of psychological distress or family conflict. Distress in caregivers was related to perceived family conflict, but not to a diagnosis of SCD or social support.

Family Functioning. Research has shown relationships among parent coping, family functioning, self-reported distress, and parent-reported internalizing and externalizing behavior problems in youths with SCD (Brown, Lambert, et al., 2000; Kliewer & Lewis, 1995; Thompson, Armstrong, et al., 1999). For example, Brown, Lambert, et al. (2000) found a relationship between caregiver adjustment and their coping strategies, with less use of disengagement coping (e.g., wishful thinking, social withdrawal) predicting better adjustment. Kliewer and Lewis (1995) revealed that parent coping accounted for 40% of the variance in child coping. The influence of family functioning on adaptation may be dependent on the reliability between caretaker and youth ratings. Brown and Lambert (1999) found higher endorsement of depression symptoms (e.g., hopelessness, negative self-appraisal) in youth with SCD when both caretakers and youth rated their families as low on cohesiveness.

Child-rearing practices and parenting concerns have received increased attention in the literature. In general, few differences have been found in child-rearing practices and parenting concerns in families of children with SCD compared with families of healthy children. In one study (Noll, McKellop, Vannatta, & Kalinyak, 1998) the only difference between parents of children with SCD and parents of their classmates was that the former reported greater concerns about their children's health and about being seen as different from peers. Other studies also have identified health, increased supervision and adherence to medical management, and emotional reactions to SCD as ongoing concerns of parents with children and adolescents with SCD (Ievers-Landis et al., 2001; Rao & Kramer, 1993). In addition, parents report problems related to typical child-rearing tasks and parenting, such as sleep problems, child care, academic difficulties, and economic stress.

There is a paucity of intervention studies in this area overall. In one published study (Kaslow et al., 2000), improvements in disease knowledge were found following a six-session psychoeducational family intervention and at a 6-month follow-up for the intervention group compared with a standard-care group. But no differences were obtained on measures of family functioning and support or child internalizing or externalizing behavior problems as reported by parents and the youth.

Pain

Vaso-occlusive pain episodes are the most common complaint of SCD. Research in this area has focused on describing the natural history of these pain episodes and their effects on daily activities and events and on the accurate assessment of pain. Various studies support the perception that children and adolescents can be accurate reporters of their pain experiences when using age-appropriate pain assessment devices (e.g., pain diary; Gil et al., 2000; Walco & Dampier, 1990). Unfortunately, few studies have been published on establishing effective treatment approaches for pain prevention and management

Individual Differences. Individual differences of age and gender have been inconsistently reported in recent studies of pain. Some studies, involving children ranging from 3 or 4 years old to 18 years old, find that older children and adolescents report higher levels of pain than younger children (Conner-Warren, 1996; Jackson, Sporrer, Agner, Laver, & Abbound, 1994). The coping strategies used by children also have not been stable across an 18-month period, compared with those of adolescents and adults (Gil, Wilson, & Edens, 1997). Reports of gender differences in pain reports have been mixed, with girls reporting more pain than boys in some studies (Shapiro et al., 1995) but not others (Conner-Warren, 1996).

Coping Strategies. Previous research has consistently identified a relationship among coping strategies, psychosocial adjustment, and health care use. In general, children whose coping is characterized by negative thinking and passive strategies are less active in school and social situations, use more health care services, and evidence more psychological problems than those whose coping is active (Gil, Williams, Thompson, & Kinney, 1991; Thompson et al., 1994). These relationships appear to be stable over short and longer periods of time (e.g., 10 months). Coping strategies used by parents also have been associated with children's coping and the presence of behavior problems. For example, Gil and colleagues (1991) found a relationship between parents' negative thinking and passive coping and children's activity reduction and behavior problems. More recently, Sharpe and associates (Sharpe, Brown, Thompson, & Eckman, 1994) showed that family adaptability was associated with mothers' endorsement of engagement coping strategies to manage pain, whereas internalizing behavior problems and negative thinking in the children were associated with mothers' use of disengagement coping.

Pain Management. Previous studies have emphasized designing home-based treatments, due to frequency of home management and the disruptive nature of pain on daily activities (Shapiro et al., 1995). In addition, the inclusion of parents to provide pain intensity ratings and to coach children and adolescents in their attempts to control pain have been encouraged (Gil et al., 2000). Finally, interventions should focus on teaching active coping strategies and/or modifying maladaptive coping strategies early rather than waiting for maladaptive strategies to become stable. The typical pain management protocol includes hydration, use of nonsteroidal anti-inflammatory drugs (e.g., Advil [ibuprofen]), and changes to opiods if the pain is not relieved (e.g., Tylenol with codeine, Dilaudid). Increasingly, alternative pain management strategies, such as massage, distraction, and relaxation techniques, have been incorporated into pain protocols. Previous research has provided preliminary support for cognitive-behavioral techniques (i.e., biofeedback, relaxation training, hypnosis, pain behavior contracts) in reducing pain and decreasing the number and duration of hospitalizations, especially when included as part of a multidisciplinary intervention program (e.g., Cozzi, Tryon, & Sedlacek, 1987; Dinges et al., 1997).

Recent intervention studies have followed a skills training approach, with a focus on teaching cognitive-behavioral pain management strategies to children (e.g., deep breathing, imagery; Gil, Wilson, Edens, Workman, et al., 1997; Gil et al., 2001; Powers, Mitchell, Graumlich, Byars, & Kalinyak, 2002). Results have been generally positive in terms of decreases in negative thinking, increases in active coping, and decreased disruption in daily activities (e.g., school attendance, hours slept). However, results have not been consistent across children or time periods (i.e., immediate posttreatment, 1- to 3-month follow-up).

A pilot study is currently being completed by Lemanek, Ranalli, and Wentz (2002) that examines the effects of massage therapy on pain management in children with SCD. Parents of young children are being taught traditional massage techniques, with various psychological (e.g., anxiety) and disease-related variables (e.g., utilization rates, medication usage) being monitored. Although adequate pain assessment and management continues to be a serious problem for youths with SCD, few studies have been implemented to examine the most effective treatment strategies.

Neurocognitive Functioning

Earlier research on the cognitive functioning of children and adolescents with SCD showed mixed results in terms of global intellectual deficits (Swift et al., 1989) or domain-specific deficits (Brown et al., 1993). Recent studies have attempted to correct earlier methodological flaws, including variance in disease variables (i.e., Hb type) and instrument selection. Children and adolescents with SCD are considered at risk of developing academic difficulties because of several factors. A primary factor has been the frequent school absences reported for many youths due to minor infections, clinic visits or hospitalizations, or medical complications (e.g., pain; Shapiro et al., 1995). In addition, sleep may be negatively affected by pain at night, with subsequent effects of the poor sleep on the child's day-to-day functioning, including fatigue and inattentiveness (Gil, Wilson, & Edens, 1997a; Noll et al., 2001). Finally, parents may perceive their children and adolescents as vulnerable and unable to attend school on a regular basis (Shapiro et al., 1995).

This section summarizes information on the cognitive functioning of children and adolescents with SCD. Detailed descriptions of neurological and neuropsychological studies, disease-specific models of deficits, and clinical and research implications can be found in reviews by Bonner, Gustafson, Schumacher, and Thompson (1999) and Kral, Brown, and Hynd (2001). The neurocognitive functioning of children and adolescents with overt and silent strokes have received the most attention in recent studies due to the potentially pervasive and lifelong impact of impairment.

Recent studies on the neurocognitive functioning of youths with SCD have included as participants a combination of youths with SCD with documented strokes, those with silent strokes, and classmates or siblings. Documentation of these overt or silent strokes has been verified through magnetic resonance imaging (MRI). When comparing youths with SCD but no evidence of stroke with classmates or siblings, global deficits and specific deficits in attention have been found, but no differences in such areas as academic achievement (Brown et al., 1993; Noll et al., 2001). Evidence also suggests that deficits in cognitive functioning may be present during the first 3 years of life (Thompson et al., 2002). In this cooperative study of infants and toddlers with SCD, decreases in cognitive functioning were found, especially between the 12- and 24-month assessments, with poorer cognitive functioning associated with parenting risk (i.e., learned helplessness) and biomedical risk (i.e., HbSS).

Differential performance has been found in children with SCD and overt strokes and those with silent strokes compared with classmates or siblings. In general, deficits on measures of general intelligence, language abilities, visual-motor skills, academic achievement, and sequential memory have been found for children with SCD and overt strokes in a cooperative study of SCD (Armstrong et al., 1996). Other studies (e.g., Brown, Davis, et al., 2000; DeBaun et al., 1998) have revealed deficits in more specific areas of executive functioning, including attention, with the frontal lobe proposed as the site of injury. Deficits in social-emotional functioning (e.g., errors in decoding emotions and subtle social cues) have been identified in children with HbSS and strokes compared with children without central nervous system involvement or children with HbSC (Boni, Brown, Davis, Hsu, & Hopkins, 2001). These studies indicate that specific domains of functioning should be examined in youth with overt and silent strokes. Poor school performance has been identified in children with silent infarcts, with 80% showing clinically significant cognitive deficits and 35% demonstrating deficits in academic skills (Schatz, Brown, Pascual, Hsu, & DeBaun, 2001). Decreased performance also has been found on measures of visual-motor speed, mathematics, and vocabulary (Armstrong et al., 1996).

The work of Schatz and colleagues (Schatz et al., 1999) has indicated that the location of the lesion and the volume of the infarct (i.e., size of lesion) have direct relevance to the impairments identified in children with overt or silent strokes. Children with SCD who sustained anterior cerebral infarcts had deficits on neurocognitive measures of attention and executive functioning, whereas children with more widespread infarcts showed additional problems in visual-spatial skills. In addition, the volume of the cerebral infarction was associated with spatial and language performance deficits but not with performance deficits in other cognitive domains. The authors suggest that global measures of cognitive functioning cannot isolate injuries to the frontal lobe, necessitating comprehensive neuropsychological testing.

HEMOPHILIA

Hemophilia is an X-linked genetic coagulation disorder resulting in a deficiency of clotting factors. There are a total of nine known clotting factors that aid in the process of clot formation. The most common deficiencies are Hemophilia A, or classic hemophilia (Factor VIII deficiency), and Hemophilia B, or Christmas disease (Factor IX deficiency). Hemophilia A occurs in 1 of 5,000 male births, and Hemophilia B occurs in 1 of 30,000 male births (Mannucci & Tuddenham, 2001). Hemophilia affects all racial and ethnic groups and is worldwide in distribution. Rarely do females have hemophilia, but carriers may be considered symptomatic.

Medical Aspects

Diagnosis

The diagnosis of hemophilia is made through a laboratory test that measures the circulating factor VIII and IX level within the blood. A suspicion of hemophilia is considered when children have prolonged bleeding from circumcision, hematomas, or mouth bleeding. Individuals with mild hemophilia may remain undiagnosed for a number of years until they undergo a surgical procedure or dental work or sustain a trauma-related injury. Hemophilia is often confused with nonaccidental injury, but prompt diagnosis can avoid unnecessary suspicion and investigation (Harley, 1997).

Pathophysiology

Patients with hemophilia have decreased levels of clotting factor in their blood, resulting in prolonged bleeding after injury. Bleeding episodes involve skin, mouth, joints, muscles (e.g., arms, legs), and viscera (Aledort, 1996). Hemarthrosis, or joint bleeding, originates from the synovial membrane and causes decreased range of motion, warmth, pain, and swelling. Repeated bleeding into the same joint may produce a target joint, which is a joint that bleeds frequently and may do so spontaneously. Target joints can lead to the development of synovitis, progression of chronic arthritis, and disability. Life-threatening bleeds include intracranial, neck, spinal cord, and abdomen.

Clinical Manifestations

Severity of Bleeding. Bleeding in hemophilia can be predicted from the level of factor coagulant (Cohen, 2000; Venkateswaran, Williams, Jones, & Nuss, 1998). Severe hemophilia is diagnosed when less than 1% of deficient factor is present. Bleeding episodes can occur frequently after minor trauma, spontaneously, or both. Individuals with moderate hemophilia have factor levels between 1 and 5%, with bleeding usually occurring in response to minor trauma. Those individuals with factor levels greater than 5% have mild hemophilia, with fewer bleeding episodes that are usually associated with severe trauma or surgery.

Developmental Age. In children and adolescents, bleeding is closely related to stages of development and physical activity. Newborns with hemophilia present with intracranial and extracranial hemorrhage and bleeding after circumcision. However, intracranial hemorrhages are often preventable through appropriate diagnosis and treatment. Infants and toddlers may evidence mouth bleeding, bleeding from erupting teeth, and hematomas from related injuries (Lemanek, Buckloh, Woods, & Butler, 1995). In adults, bleeding is related to activity, trauma, and lifestyles.

Inhibitor Development. Inhibitor development continues to be a serious complication in individuals with hemophilia. Inhibitors are antibodies that function to destroy either factor VIII or IX. When the factor is infused into individuals, their bodies react to the infused factor as if it were a foreign substance, thus preventing the blood from clotting. Incidence of inhibitor development occurs most often in individuals with severe disease, with the most common appearing in individuals with Hemophilia A (Damiano, Hutter, & Tri-Regional Nursing Group, 2000). Immune tolerance is the usual treatment of choice by most hemophilia treatment centers and involves the use of repeated massive doses of factor.

Treatment Approaches

Factor Replacement Therapy. Treatment of bleeding episodes in hemophilia is done by replacement of the deficient clotting factor and involves an injection of factor given intravenously. Treatment is used to prevent bleeds or to minimize the effects of bleeding episodes (World Federation of Hemophilia, 1998). Factor replacement has undergone numerous changes over the years, with transfusion of whole blood being the treatment of choice until the early 1960s. Factor concentrates were then developed that allowed individuals to be treated sooner, thereby decreasing hospital stays and visits to emergency rooms. Prompt treatment decreased damage to joints and complications of bleeding and increased life expectancy and quality of life. Many individuals with hemophilia who received products between 1979 and 1985 developed HIV and hepatitis through contaminated factor products.

Since 1985, efforts have been made to free factor concentrates of viral contamination.

The use of recombinant products is the recommended treatment of choice, especially in young children and newly diagnosed individuals who have not been previously treated with blood- or plasma-derived products (National Hemophilia Foundation Medical and Scientific Advisory Council [MASAC], 2000). Since the advent of recombinant factor, prophylaxis is considered the optimal therapy for individuals with severe hemophilia to reduce joint disease and to enhance quality of life.

Gene Therapy. The newest treatment on the horizon is gene therapy. Gene therapy is the correction of a gene defect by placing a nondefective gene into cells. Individuals with hemophilia are good candidates for gene therapy, with progress being made through a small group of clinical trials.

Comprehensive Care. Comprehensive care is a model that uses a team approach to provide optimal care for individuals with hemophilia and their families. Care is given by a multidisciplinary team, which provides diagnosis, assessment, treatment, education, data collection, research, and advocacy. Treatment at home has increased since the inception of treatment centers across the country, resulting in decreased hospital stays and fewer missed days from school. Families and individuals are taught to recognize early signs of bleeding and to administer appropriate treatment at the onset of an episode, thereby reducing the overall cost of hemophilia care (Green, 1999). As such, involvement of individuals and families as functioning members of the team reduces complications and promotes the quality of life. The efficacy of hemophilia treatment centers is seen by the lower mortality rates in individuals with more severe disease. (Soucie et al., 2000).

Psychological Aspects

A range of psychological and social problems have been reported in the literature on children and adolescents with bleeding disorders, including functional disability, depression and anxiety, skewed peer relationships, and altered family dynamics (Dudley, Kocik, & Atwood, 1998). Extremes of timidity and risk taking, preoccupations with health, and difficulties with intimacy and social isolation also have been identified in individuals with hemophilia (Agle, Gluck, & Pierce, 1987; Nimorwicz & Klein, 1982).

Disease-Related Variables

A few studies have found a relationship between psychological adaptation and level of disability (Bussing & Johnson, 1992; Triemstra et al., 1998). Triemstra and colleagues (1998) showed that feelings of competence at managing their own physical health and attention to psychological health moderate the negative impact of disability on the life satisfaction of patients. Bussing and Johnson (1992) also found that increased severity of hemophilia has a heightened impact on psychological adaptation, particularly depression and anxiety.

Anecdotal evidence suggests a relationship between psychological stress and the severity and frequency of bleeds (Markova, 1997). Investigators have reported cases in which bleeds apparently occurred in advance of an anticipated traumatic event or were not associated with any predisposing trauma (Baird & Wassen, 1985). These bleeds have thus been associated with anxiety and stress. However, there is little evidence of dysfunctional adaptation in children and adolescents with hemophilia when using empirically based assessment (Logan, Gibson, Hann, & Parry Jones, 1993). Studies using structured interviews or standardized questionnaires have identified few, if any, differences in individuals with hemophilia in personality and social functioning (Bussing & Johnson, 1992).

Self-Concept

The diagnosis of hemophilia complicates the developmental process of becoming a distinct independent self. Adolescents with hemophilia must integrate into their sense of self the developmental and physical changes that are inherent within a bleeding disorder. For example, individuals with hemophilia have substantial swelling and bruising or impaired mobility from joint or muscle bleeds. Limited participation in school and peer activities also may affect one's sense of self. Haas, Schultz, and Rigdon (1997) have asserted that children and adolescents with hemophilia are at risk of developing an identity as "crippled or fragile" due to such changes and limitations. Although being different is inherent in a diagnosis of chronic illness, caregivers of youths with bleeding disorders must guard against their defining themselves by their illness (Green, 1999).

Peer Relationships

DeMaio and Nimorwicz Siewers (1996) have stated that peer relationships have a major impact on youths' social adjustment and sense of self. A significant variable for children and adolescents with hemophilia in developing peer relationships is their individual awareness of the visibility of hemophilia. Shelley (1985) found children's and adolescents' perceptions that peers are focusing on their "condition" is correlated with anxiety about interactions and difficulty making close friends. Carroll, Robinson, Schatz, and McRedmond (2002) revealed that up to 46% of adolescents with hemophilia have difficulty developing healthy peer relationships. Children and adolescents with hemophilia also report concerns about peers' ignorance about hemophilia, especially the fear that they will bleed to death with a superficial injury. The emergence as an "untouchable" among peers can fill a child or adolescent with a sense of "powerlessness and stinging humiliation" (Massie, 1985). The ability to self-infuse significantly enhances opportunities to avoid peer scrutiny and stigmatization, thereby helping to foster healthy and lasting peer relationships (Jones, 1995; Markova, 1997). Self-treating also provides opportunities to determine how and what to tell peers, which increases control over specific outcomes. Finally, self-treating relieves and prevents pain, thus freeing youths to concentrate on schoolwork and friends.

Family Relationships

Findings from research on the impact of chronic illness on marital relations and the family is unclear. However, the social and personal impingement of hemophilia on family members has been characterized as dramatic (Haas et al., 1997). Nimorwicz and Klein (1982) claim that it is virtually impossible for families to anticipate how the complex issues associated with this disease will affect their lives. The burden caused by hemophilia appears to be greater with regard to psychological stress than to the medical management of the disease (Markova, 1997). Hemophilia can have an impact on unaffected family members in both substantial and subtle ways (Sargent, 1983). One way is through financial burdens. For example, a self-insured company that employs a parent of a child with hemophilia can incur as much as $1 million worth of factor and medical care during the first 4 years of life. Adding to the weight of this burden is the possible pressure that parents feel to perform at work and children's and adolescents' feelings of being responsible for the financial costs.

Studies suggest that mothers of children and adolescents with hemophilia suffer more psychological distress and depression than mothers of healthy children (Handford, Mayes, Bixler, & Mattison, 1986). Mothers reportedly express feelings of guilt stemming from their status as genetic carriers of hemophilia. Both parents mention adjusting their expectations for their children's and adolescents' futures (DeMaio & Nimorwicz Siewers, 1996). Generalized stress on marital relations has been reported, as well as specific parent distress, including an ever-present fear of bleeds, concern about children's and adolescents' future, and restrictions on family activities (Daria, 2001).

Academic Skills

Medical advances in treatment have increased the life expectancy of children and adolescents with hemophilia (Ell & Reardon, 1990). With these advances have come concerns about attaining academic and life skill competencies to avoid negative outcomes in adulthood. The introduction of home factor therapy has effectively reduced school absenteeism in children and adolescents with hemophilia. But school absences remain a salient issue, as children and adolescents with hemophilia miss an average of 18 days per year compared with the national average of 4 days (Woolf et al., 1989). Hemophilia treatment centers and families of children and adolescents with hemophilia enlist schools as full members of the comprehensive care team. The goal of this collaboration is to reduce health risk by teaching school personnel about hemophilia, to minimize any stigmatization from the disease (e.g., swelling and bruising, use of crutches), and to foster participation in school-related activities.

Limited data have shown a correlation between hemophilia and school performance. Woolf and colleagues (1989) found deficiencies in math and reading for boys with hemophilia, who were studied between the ages of 8 and 19 years. Most studies, however, have identified few, if any, correlations (Kvist, Kvist, & Rajantie, 1990; Markova, 1997). A clear exception is the impact of an undiagnosed and/or untreated head bleed that most often occurs during birth or infancy. Although these conditions occur infrequently, such trauma can be neurologically devastating.

Medical and Psychosocial Care

Obtaining and maintaining psychosocial adaptation while living with hemophilia can be very difficult. Medical and psychosocial care for children and adolescents with hemophilia is often a fragmented, confusing conglomerate of funding, programming, expertise, and treatment strategy (Ell & Reardon, 1990). However, a number of current treatment strategies have provided unique opportunities to accomplish developmental tasks. A comprehensive treatment team, home infusion, and prophylaxis treatment have given caregivers the tools to enhance their youth's psychosocial adaptation.

Comprehensive Treatment Team. Similarities in quality of life between children with hemophilia and matched controls have been attributed to the impact of comprehensive treatment centers and advances in medical care (Boelsen, 1997). Centers have successfully shifted the approach to care from episodic to long-term health maintenance. Studies by

Smith and colleagues (Smith & Levine, 1984; Smith, Keyes, & Forman, 1982) have illuminated the success of the treatment center model. These authors have found the number of days missed from school, the average number of hospital admissions, the number of inpatient days, and the overall cost of care for children and adolescents with hemophilia to be significantly reduced.

Treatment centers are often confronted with parents who assume an intense caregiver identity, which may then hinder children's and adolescents' development of independence. Anxiety, overprotection, and guilt reported by parents makes it difficult to balance necessary protection and unnecessary restrictions (Haas et al., 1997). Treatment centers may generate opportunities for children and adolescents to practice independent skills in a sympathetic environment (DeMaio & Nimorwicz Siewers, 1996). In general, hemophilia treatment centers may assist parents in determining when and how much independence their youth can assume regarding their medical management.

Home Infusion. Self-treating helps children and adolescents assume a new independent identity as the family expert on hemophilia (Evans, 1997). Children and adolescents may schedule their own appointments and choose whether parents attend these appointments. They also may manage their own factor inventory. Finally, they may be able to learn medical and first aid skills that could be beneficial to them and their families, thereby fostering a sense of mastery.

Prophylaxis Treatment. A prophylaxis treatment strategy has altered the impact of hemophilia on children and adolescents and their families. Including factor as part of a regimen frees youths to be more physically active because they can treat themselves prior to an activity (Gilbert, 1996). Treatment before the start of an activity substantially reduces the risk of bleeds. Physical therapists in treatment centers have thus been promoting fitness programs that focus on flexibility and maximizing joint movement. These types of programs in turn minimize the impact of social isolation due to the inability to participate.

HIV and HCV. Approximately 70% of individuals who used blood products prior to 1985 were infected with HIV (Augustiniak, 1990). Although many of these individuals have died from complications of HIV/AIDS, many other individuals have survived due in part to advanced treatment strategies. Unfortunately, a large percentage of these individuals have not developed the life skills required to be functioning, productive adults. The HIV crisis also has affected treatment center staff. For example, caregiver burnout has been correlated with level of mistrust by individuals with hemophilia and their caregivers following the hemophilia HIV crisis (Brown et al., 2002). Hepatitis C (HCV) is endemic in the hemophilia community, yet there appears to be a dearth of literature on its psychosocial impact compared with that of HIV (Haas et al., 1997). Liver-compromising medications and diffuse symptoms contribute to the psychosocial implications of living with hepatitis.

Other Intervention Strategies. Empirically supported noninvasive interventions with children and adolescents with hemophilia have included hypnosis and relaxation training used to decrease the frequency of bleeds (Bussing & Johnson, 1992). Hypnosis also has been used effectively to reduce blood flow and to manage pain (Chaves, 1989). Progressive muscular relaxation, meditative breathing, and imagery have been identified as successful in managing pain in hemophilia (Varni, 1981).

CONCLUSIONS

SCD

SCD is an inherited hemoglobinopathy, with recurrent pain being the most common complication. The occurrence of infections and strokes also are of significant concern to health care providers and to families of young children with SCD. The mortality rate for SCD has declined sharply over the past 25 years due to the institution of newborn screening, penicillin prophylaxis, and pneumococcal vaccines (Davis, Schoendorf, Gergen, & Moore, 1997). Although new approaches (e.g., HU, TCD) are being developed to reduce or manage medical complications, a cure appears possible only in the distant future. The majority of studies on the psychological aspects of SCD have examined correlates or predictors of adaptation in children and adolescents with SCD and their parents. In general, youths with SCD, especially adolescent males, and their parents are at risk of developing primarily internalizing behavior problems and symptoms. This heightened risk appears related to disease-specific stress in managing SCD, especially pain, daily hassles, and limited family cohesion and support. The influence of parents' coping on children's coping is evident, with disengagement or passive coping strategies negatively affecting management of pain and adaptation in general. Academic difficulties may be due to a variety of factors, such as frequent absences and the negative effect of pain on sleep. In addition, the significant effects of overt strokes and silent strokes on children and adolescents are now being documented by cooperative group studies.

Future research in SCD should continue to focus on isolating individual difference variables that may affect changes in adaptation in general and coping in particular of youths and their parents. These individual difference variables should move beyond gender and disease severity to include developmental factors, such as chronological age, cognitive level, and social functioning (Gil, Wilson, & Edens, 1997; Sharpe et al., 1994). In particular, the role played by these developmental factors in parents' caretaking of sons versus daughters and on the management of disease-related tasks should be emphasized in future research. Changes in treatment status or increases in other stresses also should be monitored as potential precursors associated with transition into and out of "good" adjustment rather than as markers of risk and resiliency (Gil et al., 1997; Thompson, Gustafson, et al., 1999). Neuroimaging and neuropsychological testing, specifically tests that measure sustained attention and problem-solving skills, should be a part of standard care for children at risk of developing strokes. In addition, decision-making algorithms should be designed to identify all children likely to experience a stroke or who show specific CNS pathology on neuroimaging (Brown, Davis, et al., 2000; Schatz et al., 1999).

Several factors pertaining to African American families have not been considered when examining family influence on youth's adjustment, according to Barbarin (1994). For instance, such factors as African American families' social location, racial discrimination, and restricted access to education and employment, along with the role of religion and integration of single-adult and extended-family structures, should be included in future research and clinical practice. These factors should then be incorporated into delineating risk and protective factors to identify those families in need of social and psychological services. Issues regarding the lack of culturally sensitive measures of adaptation and family functioning will need to be addressed when identifying at risk families. A more thorough description of family caregiving styles and cultural experiences, especially in families immigrating to the United States, also will be necessary to understand how youths and families respond to a diagnosis of SCD and its management (Sterling, Peterson, & Weekes, 1997).

Future research should emphasize, in particular, the design and implementation of interventions that prevent or modify the development of maladaptive behaviors and coping styles. Early screening should be mandatory for young children with SCD to obtain a baseline index of their cognitive abilities, social-emotional development, and family functioning. Early intervention efforts can then be instituted for those children in need of educational or social services. Intervention efforts also should be directed at developing more adaptive coping responses, such as problem solving and seeking social support, as well as pain management strategies that incorporate pharmacological and nonpharmacological approaches (e.g., distraction, visual imagery, massage). However, all intervention efforts will need to be validated to confirm their empirical support. Research on interventions can be extended by supplementing quantitative analyses with qualitative analyses (see Barbarin, 1994; Hill & Zimmerman, 1995) to provide more accurate services to youth with SCD and their families.

Hemophilia

Nearly 18,000 individuals in the United States live with hemophilia. Children and adolescents with hemophilia can live with significant recurrent bleeds that most often occur in the joints. These recurrent bleeds may result in a life of pain, reduced joint mobility, and chronic arthritis. Although the exact psychosocial impact of living with hemophilia is debated, most would agree that it is significant and may affect social functioning, self-concept, and peer and family relationships. Home factor replacement, increased product safety, and a comprehensive care team help mitigate the impact of living with hemophilia. Medical and psychosocial outcomes have improved in correlation with the development of these intervention strategies. Individuals with hemophilia are, in fact, living longer than ever before and are more effectively negotiating daily life tasks related and unrelated to their disease.

Clearly many questions remain to be studied. There is a need for more current studies measuring academic achievement for children and adolescents with hemophilia. There is also a need for longitudinal studies in which both physical and psychosocial interventions can be repeatedly assessed. This approach will facilitate more effective evaluation of the impact of hemophilia and treatment strategies on overall and disease-specific adaptation. Other research is needed on the development of HCV drugs that are more effective and less damaging to the liver. Finally, Phase II trials will begin on the efficacy of gene therapy as a cure for hemophilia. Although the community remains excited, global impact is not imminent.

General

SCD or hemophilia affects children's or adolescents' medical, personal, social, and educational functioning, as well as that of their families. The chronic nature of these disorders requires a shift in the philosophy of the health care system from tertiary care to prevention. Programs that provide medical training and care to children and adolescents with SCD or hemophilia and their families should be designed to prevent challenges and problems across all areas of functioning rather than to treat complications after they have developed. Secondary care in terms of moderating the effect of risk factors also should receive attention in future training and service programs. This shift in philosophy is consistent with the comprehensive care approach being proposed and refined for children with all chronic illnesses. For this shift in philosophy to change health care patterns and practices of those caring for individuals with SCD or hemophilia, funding allocations and priorities in budget distributions will need to be made in federal, state, and local institutions and agencies across the country.

REFERENCES

Adams, R. J., McKie, V. C., Hsu, L., Files, B., Vichinsky, E., Pegelow, C., et al. (1998). Prevention of a first stroke by transfusions in children with sickle cell anemia and abnormal results on transcranial Doppler ultrasonography. *New England Journal of Medicine, 339,* 5–11.

Agle, D. P., Gluck, H., & Pierce, G. F. (1987). The risk of AIDS: Psychologic impact on the hemophilia population. *General Hospital Psychiatry, 9,* 11–17.

Aledort, L. M. (1996). Hemophilia: Yesterday, today and tomorrow. *Mount Sinai Journal of Medicine, 63,* 225–235.

Allison, A. C. (1954). Incidence of malarial parasitaemia in African children with and without sickle cell trait. *British Medical Journal, 1,* 290–294.

Armstrong, F. D., Thompson, R. J., Wang, W., Zimmerman, R., Pegelow, C. H., Miller, S., et al. (1996). Cognitive functioning and brain magnetic resonance imaging in children with sickle cell disease. *Pediatrics, 97,* 864–870.

Augustiniak, L. (1990, June). *U. S. Seroconversion Survelliance Project: Regional seropositivity rates for HIV infection in patients with hemophilia.* Paper presented at the Sixth International Conference on AIDS, San Francisco, CA.

Baird, P., & Wassen, T. A. (1985). Effects of life stressors on blood usage in hemophiliac patients: A pilot study. *International Journal of Psychosomatics, 32,* 3–5.

Barbarin, O. A. (1994). Risk and resilience in adjustment to sickle cell disease: Integrating focus groups, case reviews, and quantitative methods. *Journal of Health and Social Policy, 5,* 97–121.

Boelsen, R. (1997, January). Quality of life issues in children and adolescents with hemophilia. *Hemaware,* 25–27.

Boni, L. A., Brown, R. T., Davis, P. C., Hsu, L., & Hopkins, K. (2001). Social information processing and magnetic resonance imaging in children with sickle cell disease. *Journal of Pediatric Psychology, 26,* 309–319.

Bonner, M. J., Gustafson, K. E., Schumacher, E., & Thompson, R. J. (1999). The impact of sickle cell disease on cognitive functioning and learning. *School Psychology Review, 28,* 182–193.

Brown, R. T., Buchanan, I., Doepke, K., Eckman, J. R., Baldwin, K., Goonan, B., & Schoenherr, S. (1993). Cognitive and academic functioning in children with sickle cell disease. *Journal of Clinical Child Psychology, 22,* 207–218.

Brown, R. T., Davis, P. C., Lambert, R., Hsu, L., Hopkins, K., & Eckman, J. (2000). Neurocognitive functioning and magnetic resonance imaging in children with sickle cell disease. *Journal of Pediatric Psychology, 25,* 503–513.

Brown, R. T., & Lambert, R. (1999). Family functioning and children's adjustment in the presence of a chronic illness: Concordance between children with sickle cell disease and caretakers. *Families, Systems, and Health, 17,* 165–179.

Brown, R. T., Lambert, R., Devine, D., Baldwin, K., Casey, R., Doepke, K., et al. (2000). Risk-resistance adaptation model for caregivers and their children with sickle cell syndromes. *Annals of Behavioral Medicine, 22,* 158–169.

Brown, L. K., Schultz, J. R., Forsberg, A. D., King, G., Kocik, S. M., & Butler, R. B. (2002). Predictors of retention among HIV/hemophilia health care professionals. *General Hospital Psychiatry, 24,* 48–54.

Burlew, K., Telfair, J., Colangelo, I., & Wright, E. C. (2000). Factors that influence adolescent adaptation to sickle cell disease. *Journal of Pediatric Psychology, 25,* 287–299.

Bussing, R., & Johnson, S. B. (1992). Psychosocial issues in hemophilia before and after the HIV crisis: A review of current research. *General Hospital Psychiatry, 14,* 387–403.

Carroll, B. A., Robinson, J. S., Schatz, J., & McRedmond, K. (2002, January–February). Moving from a model to a program: Applying developmental counseling for vocational success. *Hemaware,* 20–24.

Charache, S., Terrin, M. L., Moore, R. D., Dover, G. J., Barton, F. B., Eckert, S. V., et al. (1995). Effect of hydroxyurea on the frequency of painful crises in sickle cell anemia. *New England Journal of Medicine, 332,* 1317–1322.

Chaves, J. F. (1989). Hypnotic control of clinical pain. In N. P. Spanos & J. F. Chaves (Eds.), *Hypnosis: The cognitive behavioral perspective* (pp. 188–193). Buffalo, NY: Proetheus Books.

Cohen, A. (2000). Hematologic emergencies. In G. Fleischer & S. Ludwig (Eds.), *Textbook of pediatric emergency medicine* (pp. 877–879). New York: Lippincott.

Conner-Warren, R. L. (1996). Pain intensity and home pain management of children with sickle cell disease. *Issues in Comprehensive Pediatric Nursing, 19,* 183–195.

Cozzi, L., Tryon, W. W., & Sedlacek, K. (1987). The effectiveness of biofeedback-assisted relaxation in modifying sickle cell crises. *Biofeedback and Self-Regulation, 12,* 51–61.

Damiano, M. L., Hutter, J. J., & the Tri-Regional Nursing Group. (2000). Immune tolerance for haemaophilia patients with inhibitors: Analysis of the western United States experience. *Haemophilia, 6,* 526–532.

Daria, I. (2001, July). A family triumphs. *Hemalog*, 19–22.

Davis, H., Schoendorf, K. C., Gergen, P. J., & Moore, R. M. (1997). National trends in the mortality of children with sickle cell disease, 1968 through 1992. *American Journal of Public Health, 87,* 1317–1322.

DeBaun, M. R., Schatz, J., Siegel, M. J., Koby, M., Craft, S., Resar, L., et al. (1998). Cognitive screening examinations for silent cerebral infarcts in sickle cell disease. *American Academy of Neurology, 50,* 1678–1682.

DeMaio, D., & Nimorwicz Siewers, P. (1996). Clinical and psychosocial issues in hemophilia. In National Hemophilia Foundation (Eds.), *Orientation manual for hemophilia healthcare professionals* (pp. 9–14). New York: National Hemophilia Foundation.

Dinges, D., Whitehouse, W., Orne, E. C., Bloom, P., Carlin, M., Bauer, N., et al. (1997). Self-hypnosis training as an adjunct treatment in the management of pain associated with sickle-cell disease. *International Journal of Clinical and Experimental Hypnosis, 45,* 417–432.

Dudley, B., Kocik, S., & Atwood, R. (1998, October). Social work and hemophilia care: A look back. *Hemaware, 59–75.*

Eaton, W. A., & Hofrichter, J. (1990). Sickle cell hemoglobin polymerization. *Advances in Protein Chemistry, 40,* 63–79.

Ell, K. O., & Reardon, K. K. (1990). Psychosocial care for the chronically ill adolescent: Challenges and opportunities. *Health Social Work, 15,* 272–282.

Evans, S. (1997, January). Teens and parents: A success strategy. *Hemalog,* 24–27.

Fernbach, D. J., & Burdine, J. A., Jr. (1970). Sepsis and functional asplenia. *New England Journal of Medicine, 282,* 691.

Frempong, K. O. (1991). Stroke in sickle cell disease: Demographic, clinical and therapeutic considerations. *Seminars in Hematology, 28,* 213–219.

Gartstein, M. A., Short, A. D., Vannatta, K., & Noll, R. B. (1999). Psychosocial adjustment of children with chronic illness: An evaluation of three models. *Journal of Developmental and Behavioral Pediatrics, 20,* 157–163.

Gaston, M. H., Verter, J. I., Woods, G., Pegelow, C., Kelleher, J., Presbury, G., et al. (1986). Prophylaxis with oral penicillin in children with sickle cell anemia: A randomized trial. *New England Journal of Medicine, 314,* 1593–1599.

Gerry, J. L., Bulkley, B. H., & Hutchins, G. M. (1978). Clinical analysis of cardiac dysfunction in 52 patients with sickle cell anemia. *American Journal of Cardiology, 42,* 211–216.

Gil, K. M., Anthony, K. K., Carson, J. W., Redding-Lallinger, R., Daeschner, C. W., & Ware, R. E. (2001). Daily coping practice predicts treatment effects in children with sickle cell disease. *Journal of Pediatric Psychology, 26,* 163–173.

Gil, K. M., Porter, L., Ready, J., Workman, E., Sedway, J., & Anthony, K. K. (2000). Pain in children and adolescents with sickle cell disease: An analysis of daily pain diaries. *Children's Health Care, 29,* 225–241.

Gil, K. M., Williams, D. A., Thompson, R. J., & Kinney, T. R. (1991). Sickle cell disease in children and adolescents: The relation of child and parent pain coping strategies to adjustment. *Journal of Pediatric Psychology, 16,* 643–663.

Gil, K. M., Wilson, J. J., & Edens, J. L. (1997). The stability of pain coping strategies in young children, adolescents, and adults with sickle cell disease over an 18-month period. *Clinical Journal of Pain, 13,* 110–115.

Gil, K. M., Wilson, J. J., Edens, J. L., Workman, E., Ready, Y., Sedway, J., et al. (1997). Cognitive coping skills training in children with sickle cell disease. *International Journal of Behavioral Medicine, 4,* 365–378.

Gilbert, M. S. (1996). *Hemophilia, sports, and exercise.* Pasadena, CA: National Hemophilia Foundation.

Goldberg, M. A., Husson, M. A., & Bunn, H. F. (1977). Participation of hemoglobins A and F in polymerization f sickle hemoglobin. *Journal of Biological Chemistry, 252,* 3414–3421.

Green, K. (1999). Treatment strategies for adolescents with hemophilia: Opportunities to enhance development. *Adolescent Medicine: State of the Art Reviews, 10,* 369–376.

Haas, L. J., Schultz, J. R., & Rigdon, M. A. (1997). Psychosocial services of hemophilia. *Hemophilia, 30,* 355–366.

Handford, H. A., Mayes, S. D., Bixler, E. O., & Mattison, R. E. (1986). Personality traits of hemophilic boys. *Journal of Developmental and Behavioral Pediatrics, 7,* 224–229.

Harley, J. R. (1997). Disorders of coagulation misdiagnosed as nonaccidental bruising. *Pediatric Emergency Care, 13,* 347–349.

Hazzard, A., Celano, M., Collins, M., & Markov, Y. (2002). Effects of STARBRIGHT World on knowledge, social support, and coping in hospitalized children with sickle cell disease and asthma. *Children's Health Care, 31,* 69–86.

Hill, S. A., & Zimmerman, M. K. (1995). Valiant girls and vulnerable boys: The impact of gender and race on mothers' caregiving for chronically ill children. *Journal of Marriage and the Family, 57,* 43–53.

Ievers-Landis, C. E., Brown, R. T., Drotar, D., Bunke, V., Lambert, R. G., & Walker, A. A. (2001). Situational analysis of parenting problems for caregivers of children with sickle cell syndromes. *Journal of Developmental and Behavioral Pediatrics, 22,* 169–178.

Ingram, V. M. (1956). A specific chemical difference between globins of normal and sickle-cell anemia hemoglobins. *Nature, 178,* 792–794.

Jackson, S. M., Sporrer, K. A., Agner, S. A., Laver, J. H., & Abboud, M. R. (1994, March). *Pain in children and adolescents with sickle cell anemia: A prospective study utilizing self-reporting.* Paper presented at the annual meeting of the National Sickle Cell Disease Program, New York.

Jones, P. (1995). *Growing up with hemophilia: Four articles on childhood.* Los Angeles, CA: World Federation of Hemophilia.

Kaslow, N. J., Collins, M. H., Rashid, F., Baskin, M. L., Griffith, J. R., Hollins, L., & Eckman, J. E. (2000). The efficacy of a pilot family psychoeducational intervention for pediatric sickle cell disease (SCD). *Families, Systems, and Health, 18,* 381–404.

Kirkpatrick, M. B., & Bass, J. B. (1989). Pulmonary complications in adults with sickle cell disease. *Pulmonary Perspectives, 6,* 6–10.

Kliewer, W., & Lewis, H. (1995). Family influences on coping processes in children and adolescents with sickle cell disease. *Journal of Pediatric Psychology, 20,* 511–525.

Kontessis, P., Mayopoulou-Symvoulidis, D., Symvoulidis, A., & Kontopoulou-Griva, I. (1992). Renal involvement in sickle cell-beta thalassemia. *Nephronology, 61,* 10–15.

Kral, M. C., Brown, R. T., & Hynd, G. W. (2001). Neuropsychological aspects of pediatric sickle cell disease. *Neuropsychological Review, 11,* 179–196.

Kvist, B., Kvist, M., & Rajantie, J. (1990). School absences, school achievement and personality traits of the haemophilia child. *Scandanavian Journal of Social Medicine, 18,* 125–132.

Leikin, S. L., Gallagher, D., Kinney, T. R., Sloane, D., Klug, P., & Rida, W. (1989). Mortality in children and adolescents with sickle cell disease: Cooperative study of sickle cell disease. *Pediatrics, 84,* 500–508.

Lemanek, K. L., Buckloh, L. M., Woods, G., & Butler, R. (1995). Diseases of the circulatory system: Sickle cell disease and hemophilia. In M. C. Roberts (Ed.), *Handbook of pediatric psychology* (2nd ed., pp. 286–309). New York: Guilford Press.

Lemanek, K. L., Ranalli, M., & Wentz, P. (2002, September). *The benefits of massage therapy in enhancing coping in children with sickle cell disease.* Paper presented at the annual meeting of the National Sickle Cell Disease Program, Washington, DC.

Leong, M. A., Dampier, C., Varlotta, L., & Allen, J. L. (1997). Airway hyperreactivity in children with sickle cell disease. *Journal of Pediatrics, 131,* 278–283.

Logan, F. A., Gibson, B., Hann, I. M., & Parry Jones, W. L. (1993). Children with hemophilia: Same or different? *Child: Care, Health and Development, 19,* 261–273.

Mannucci, P. M., & Tuddenham, E. G. D. (2001). The hemophilias: From royal genes to gene therapy. *New England Journal of Medicine, 344,* 1773–1779.

Markova, I. (1997). The family and hemophilia. *Hemophilia, 28,* 335–346. Massie, R. K. (1985). The constant shadow: Reflections on the life of a chronically ill child. In N. Hobbs & J. M. Perrin (Eds.), *Issues in the care of children with chronic illness* (pp. 13–23). San Francisco, CA: Jossey-Bass.

Miller, S. T., Macklin, E. A., Pegelow, C. H., Kinney, T. R., Sleeper, L. A., Bello, J. A., et al. (2001). Silent infarction as a risk factor for overt stroke in children with sickle cell anemia: A report from the Cooperative Study of Sickle Cell Disease. *Journal of Pediatrics, 139,* 385–390.

National Heart, Lung, and Blood Institute. (1996). *Sickle cell anemia* (NIH Publication No. 96-4057). Washington, DC: U.S. Government Printing Office.

National Hemophilia Foundation Medical and Scientific Advisory Council. (2001). *Prophylaxis (Prophylactic administration of clotting factor concentrate to prevent bleeding)* (Medical Bulletin No. 117). New York: Author.

Nimorwicz, P., & Klein, P. H. (1982). Psychosocial aspects of hemophilia in families. 2: Intervention strategies and procedure. *Clinical Psychology Review, 2,* 171–181.

Noll, R. B., McKellop, J. M., Vannatta, K., & Kalinyak, K. (1998). Child rearing practices of primary caregivers of children with sickle cell disease: The perspectives of professionals and caregivers. *Journal of Pediatric Psychology, 23,* 131–140.

Noll, R. B., Stith, L., Gartstein, M. A., Ris, M. D., Grueneich, R., Vannatta, K., & Kalinyak, K. (2001). Neuropsychological functioning of youths with sickle cell disease: Comparisons with non-chronically ill peers. *Journal of Pediatric Psychology, 26,* 69–78.

Noll, R. B., Swiecki, E., Garstein, M., Vannatta, K., Kalinyak, K., Davies, W. H., & Bukowski, W. M. (1994). Parental distress, family conflict, and role of social support for caregivers with or without a child with sickle cell disease. *Family Systems Medicine, 12,* 281–294.

Noll, R. B., Vannatta, K., Koontz, K., Kalinyak, K., Bukowski, W. M., & Davies, W. H. (1996). Peer relationships and emotional well-being of youngsters with sickle cell disease. *Child Development, 67,* 423–436. Phebus, C. K., Gloninger, M. F., & Maciak, B. J. (1984). Growth patterns by age and sex in children with sickle cell disease. *Journal of Pediatrics, 105,* 28–33.

Platt, O. S., Orkin, S. H., Dover, G., Beardsley, G. P., Miller, B., & Nathan, D. G. (1984). Hydroxyurea enhances fetal hemoglobin production in sickle cell anemia. *Journal of Clinical Investigation, 74,* 652–656.

Powers, S. W., Mitchell, M. J., Graumlich, S. E., Byars, K. C., & Kalinyak, K. (2002). Longitudinal assessment of pain, coping, and daily functioning in children with sickle cell disease receiving pain management skills training. *Journal of Clinical Psychology in Medical Settings, 9,* 109–119.

Rao, R. P., & Kramer, L. (1993). Stress and coping among mothers of infants with a sickle cell condition. *Children's Health Care, 22,* 169–188.

Sargent, J. (1983). The sick child: Family complications. *Journal of Developmental and Behavioral Pediatrics, 4,* 50–52.

Schatz, J., Brown, R. T., Pascual, J. M., Hsu, L., & DeBaun, M. R. (2001). Poor school and cognitive functioning with silent cerebral infarcts and sickle cell disease. *Neurology, 56,* 1109–1111.

Schatz, J., Craft, S., Koby, M., Siegel, M. J., Resar, L., Lee, R. R., et al. (1999). Neuropsychologic deficits in children with sickle cell disease and cerebral infarction: Role of lesion site and volume. *Child Neuropsychology, 5,* 92–103.

Shapiro, B. (1993). Management of painful episodes in sickle cell disease. In N. L. Schechter, C. B. Berde, & M. Yaster (Eds.), *Pain in infants, children, and adolescents* (pp. 385–410). Baltimore, MD: Williams & Wilkins.

Shapiro, B. S., Dinges, D. F., Orne, E. C., Bauer, N., Reilly, L. B., Whitehouse, W. G., et al. (1995). Home management of sickle cell-related pain in children and adolescents: Natural history and impact on school attendance. *Pain, 61,* 139–144.

Sharpe, J. N., Brown, R. T., Thompson, N. J., & Eckman, J. (1994). Predictors of pain in mothers and their children with sickle cell syndrome. *Journal of the American Academy of Child and Adolescent Psychiatry, 33,* 1246–1255.

Shelley, L. F. (1985). *Touch me who dares.* London: Gromer Press.

Smith, P. S., Keyes, N. C., & Forman, E. W. (1982). Socioeconomic evaluation of a state funded comprehensive hemophilia care program. *New England Journal of Medicine, 306,* 575–579.

Smith, P. S., & Levine, P. H. (1984). The benefits of comprehensive care of hemophilia: A 5–year study of outcomes. *American Journal of Public Health, 74,* 616–617.

Soucie, J. M, Nuss, R., Evatt, B., Abdelhak, A., Cowan, L., Hill, H., et al. (2000). Mortality among males with hemophilia: Relations with source of medical care. *Blood, 96,* 437–442.

Sterling, Y. M., Peterson, J., & Weekes, D. P. (1997). African-American families with chronically ill children: Oversights and insights. *Journal of Pediatric Nursing, 12,* 292–300.

Swift, A. V., Cohen, M. J., Hynd, G. W., Wisenbaker, J. M., McKie, K. M., Makari, G., & McKie, V. C. (1989). Neuropsychologic impairment in children with sickle cell anemia. *Pediatrics, 84,* 1077–1085.

Telfair, J., & Gardner, M. M. (1999). African American adolescents with sickle cell disease: Support groups and psychological well-being. *Journal of Black Psychology, 25,* 378–390.

Thompson, R. J., Armstrong, F. D., Kronenberger, W. G., Scott, D., McCabe, M. A., Smith, B., et al. (1999). Family functioning, neurocognitive functioning, and behavior problems in children with sickle cell disease. *Journal of Pediatric Psychology, 24,* 491–498.

Thompson, R. J., Gil, K. M., Burbach, D. J., Keith, B. R., & Kinney, T. R. (1993a). Role of child and maternal processes in the psychological adjustment of children with sickle cell disease. *Journal of Consulting and Clinical Psychology, 61,* 468–474.

Thompson, R. J., Gil, K. M., Burbach, D. J., Keith, B. R., & Kinney, T. R. (1993b). Psychological adjustment of mothers of children and adolescents with sickle cell disease: The role of stress, coping methods, and family functioning. *Journal of Pediatric Psychology, 18,* 549–559.

Thompson, R. J., Gil, K. M., Keith, B. R., Gustafson, K. E., George, L. K., & Kinney, T. R. (1994). Psychological adjustment of children with sickle cell disease: Stability and change over a 10–month period. *Journal of Counseling and Clinical Psychology, 62,* 856–860.

Thompson, R. J., Gustafson, K. E., Bonner, M. J., & Ware, R. E. (2002). Neurocognitive development of young children with sickle cell disease through three years of age. *Journal of Pediatric Psychology, 27,* 235–244.

Thompson, R. J., Gustafson, K. E., Gil, K. M., Godfrey, J., & Murphy, L. M. B. (1998). Illness specific patterns of psychological adjustment and cognitive adaptational processes in children with cystic fibrosis and sickle cell disease. *Journal of Clinical Psychology, 54,* 121–128.

Thompson, R. J., Gustafson, K. E., Gil, K. M., Kinney, T. R., & Spock, A. (1999). Change in the psychological adjustment of children with cystic fibrosis or sickle cell disease and their mothers. *Journal of Clinical Psychology in Medical Settings, 6,* 373–392.

Triemstra, A. H. M., Van Der Ploeg, H. M., Smit, C., Breit, E., Ader, H. J., & Rosendaal, F. R. (1998). Well-being of hemophilia patients: A model for direct and indirect effects of medical parameters on the physical and psychosocial functioning. *Social Science Medicine, 47,* 581–593.

Varni, J. W. (1981). Self regulation techniques in the management of chronic arthritic pain in hemophilia. *Behavior Therapy, 12,* 185–194.

Venkateswaran, L., Williams, J. A., Jones, D. J., & Nuss, R. (1998). Mild hemophilia in children: Prevalence, complications and treatment. *Journal of Pediatric Hematology/Oncology, 20*, 32–35.

Walco, G., & Dampier, C. (1990). Pain in children and adolescents with sickle cell disease: A descriptive study. *Journal of Pediatric Psychology, 15*, 643–658.

Wang, W. C., Wynn, L. W., Rogers, Z. R., Scott, J. P., Lane, P. A., & Ware, R. E. (2001). A two-year pilot trial of hydroxyurea in very young children with sickle-cell anemia. *Journal of Pediatrics, 139*, 790–796.

Williams, I., Earles, A. N., & Pack, B. (1983). Psychological considerations in sickle cell disease. *Nursing Clinics of North America, 18*, 215–229.

Woolf, A., Rappaport, L., Reardon, P., Ciborowski, J., D'Angelo, E., & Bessette, J. (1989). School functioning and disease severity in boys with hemophilia. *Journal of Developmental and Behavioral Pediatrics, 10*, 81–85.

World Federation of Hemophilia. (1998). *Key issues in hemophilia treatment: Part 1. Products* (Vol. 1). Montreal, Quebec, Canada: Author.

20

Pediatric Oncology

Psychosocial Outcomes for Children and Families

KATHRYN VANNATTA
CYNTHIA A. GERHARDT

Pediatric psychologists make valuable contributions to the understanding and care of families faced with pediatric malignancies. As members of multidisciplinary teams, they help to determine how children and parents cope with a cancer diagnosis, manage ongoing treatment demands, and adjust in the face of uncertain treatment outcomes. In addition, pediatric psychologists have expertise in research design and assessment that can improve professionals' understanding of the impact of cancer on children and families and inform the development of empirically based interventions to ameliorate difficulties.

Pediatric malignancies are the leading cause of death by disease for children in the United States under age 15. One in every 330 children develops cancer before age 19 (Ross, Severson, Pollock, & Robinson, 1996), and the incidence of childhood cancer is rising (Miller, Young, & Nivakovic, 1995). Although children typically have more advanced disease at diagnosis than adults, childhood cancers are more responsive to therapy (Percy, 1995). Advances in treatment over the past 30 years have improved the overall 5-year survival rate to almost 75% (National Cancer Institute [NCI], 2002). Unfortunately, improvements in survival rates have not come without costs. Current treatment regimens are quite intense, often combining surgery, radiation, and chemotherapy. Multiagent chemotherapy is administered in higher doses for longer periods (Crist & Kun, 1991), and concern is often noted that improved survival may occur at the expense of social, emotional, or behavioral quality of life for these children.

PSYCHOSOCIAL ADJUSTMENT OF CHILDREN UNDERGOING TREATMENT FOR CANCER

Previous work has suggested that children undergoing cancer treatment may be at risk for psychosocial difficulties in two principal domains: (1) social adjustment with peers (Katz, Rubinstein, Hubert, & Blew, 1988; Larcombe et al., 1991) and (2) emotional well-being (Bennett, 1994; Canning, Hanser, Shade, & Boyce, 1992; Dolgin, Katz, Zeltzer, & Landsverk, 1989; Lavigne & Faier-Routman, 1992; Varni, Katz, Colegrove, & Dolgin, 1995). Unfortunately, confidence in these conclusions is undermined by limitations in the design of many of these studies. In general, studies that have used rigorous, controlled designs, multiple information sources, and standardized measures of social functioning, emotional well-being, and behavioral functioning have not found the same evidence of difficulties that had been reported previously (Noll et al., 1999; Eiser, Hill, & Vance, 2000).

This is not to say that there are no reports of difficulties among children with cancer. Longitudinal work suggests that children who have been recently diagnosed and are in the early stage of treatment experience increased levels of distress compared with healthy comparison children (Sawyer, et al., 1995; Sawyer, Antoniou, Toogood, & Rice, 1997). These elevations in distress may reflect adjustment to the immediate disruption caused by hospitalization and initiation of treatment, invasive procedures, and somatic and mood disturbances associated with intensive chemotherapy. Emotional difficulties do not appear to be pervasive or long lasting, and most children function similarly to comparison children without cancer after returning to school (Noll et al., 1999) or by 1 year postdiagnosis (Sawyer et al., 1995, 1997). In addition, data from peers and teachers, as well as child self-reports, regarding peer relationships suggest that children undergoing cancer treatment have levels of social functioning that are comparable to classmates and may even reflect enhancement of social reputation and acceptance (Noll et al., 1999).

An alternative explanation has been posited for the low level of affective distress reported by children undergoing cancer treatment. Building on findings that these children may report lower levels of depression than healthy children, Phipps and Srivastava (1997) have reported an increased incidence of a repressive adaptive style among pediatric cancer patients and that this adaptive style is associated with lower self-report of depressive symptoms. Recent work suggests that repressive style may characterize children prior to cancer onset rather than represent a response to traumatic stress (Phipps, Steele, Hall, & Leigh, 2001).

PSYCHOSOCIAL LATE EFFECTS FOR PEDIATRIC CANCER SURVIVORS

Adverse effects of cancer and its treatment can develop as a child matures and may emerge as long-standing difficulties after treatment is completed and a "cure" has been achieved (VonEssen, Enskar, Kreuger, Larsson, & Sjoden, 2000). Survivors of pediatric malignancies remain at risk for a recurrence, and 3–12% develop a secondary cancer within 20 years of their initial diagnosis. Children who have completed treatment are at increased risk for physical limitations, including endocrine and thyroid complications (e.g., growth problems, obesity, and reproductive difficulties), cardiac, pulmonary, renal/urological, gastrointestinal, ocular, and dental problems (DeLaat & Lampkin, 1992; Lackner et al., 2000; Oeffinger, Eshelman, Tomlinson, Buchanan, & Foster, 2000). Cosmetic impairments have been documented in as many as two-thirds of long-term survivors, and functional limitations (e.g., diminished stamina) have been noted in one-third (Mulhern, Wasserman, Friedman, & Fairclough, 1989). The full impact of cosmetic, medical, and functional limitations may not be apparent immediately after completion of cancer treatment, but they may occur as "late effects" among survivors. In addition, the significance of these deficits and their impact on development may evolve over time.

As with investigations of the short-term psychosocial consequences of cancer treatment, methodological limitations have characterized the extant work on survivorship. Studies have yielded mixed results, with evidence of considerable hardiness for survivors in more rigorously designed investigations (Eiser et al., 2000). Given the traumatic nature of cancer treatment, several researchers have investigated the occurrence of posttraumatic stress symptoms (PTSS) among survivors. Stuber and colleagues (1997) have reported that PTSS among survivors of pediatric cancer are predicted by retrospective appraisals of treatment as "hard" or "scary" and life threatening, by general level of anxiety, by history of other stressful experiences, and by social support. In addition, increased PTSS were experienced by children who had more recently completed treatment. Levels of PTSS for survivors have also been reported to be elevated relative to instrument norms (Stuber, Christakis, Houskamp, & Kazak, 1996). However, other reports indicate that similar levels of PTSS are reported by demographically matched samples of survivors and controls (Barakat et al., 1997; Butler, Rizzi, & Handwerger, 1996; Kazak et al., 1997).

A reliance on deficits-based measures has generally led to a neglect of more subtle aspects of cancer survivorship, such as attaining normal developmental goals and life achievements. To fully understand survivorship, a shift from the sole use of measures of psychopathology to the use of more subtle measures of developmental outcomes will be important. Although some studies have shown no differences between pediatric cancer survivors and either sibling controls or the general population, most studies have suggested that survivors struggle in multiple developmental domains (Chang, 1991; Eisner & Havermans, 1994). Numerous studies have indicated that pediatric cancer survivors experience job discrimination, rejection from the military, and less job success, especially among females (Chang, Nesbit, Youngren, & Robison, 1987; Makipernaa, 1989; Zeltzer et al., 1997). Cancer survivors have also reported changes in educational and career goals, repeating grades, missing school days, and experiencing other learning and school problems (Chang et al., 1987; Gray et al., 1992; Lansky, List, & Ritter-Sterr, 1986).

Other researchers have focused on the long-term impact of cancer treatment on identity development and self-concept. Madan-Swain and colleagues (2000) reported that adolescent cancer survivors were more likely than healthy adolescents to display a foreclosed identity status, characterized by internalization of the values and beliefs of significant adults without extensive exploration of alternative points of view. Furthermore, foreclosure was positively associated with disease severity, length of treatment, and length of time off therapy. Although significant associations were not found between identity formation and level of PTSS, the authors speculate that premature foreclosure may reflect an adaptive process in response to the cancer experience to minimize distress and reduce ambiguity. Other researchers have voiced concern about the impact of cancer on adult attachment, romantic relationships, psychosexual functioning, and reproductive decisions, especially among females (Green, Zevon, & Hall, 1991; Joubert et al., 2001; Makipernaa, 1989; Meadows, McKee, & Kazak, 1989; Shover, 1999; Anderson, 1999). However, more research using strong designs (e.g., control groups) is clearly needed in this area.

Finally, an area of behavioral functioning that deserves attention is the involvement of survivors in high-risk or health-compromising behaviors. Adolescence and early adulthood are developmental periods in which some experimentation with high-risk behaviors, such as sexual activity and substance use, is normative (Irwin, 1993). Unfortunately, involvement in these behaviors, even at an experimental level, can have significant long-term consequences for physical and psychosocial health (e.g., sexually transmitted diseases, drunken driving accidents; Schwarzer, Jerusalem, & Kleine, 1990). These consequences may be especially problematic for youths with a history of health problems, such as cancer. For example, cancer survivors may have pulmonary or liver toxicities that, when coupled with tobacco or alcohol use, could increase their vulnerability to further health problems or secondary malignancies.

Data from at least one study suggest that pediatric cancer survivors may engage in less aggressive and risk-taking behavior (e.g., illegal drug use) than controls (Verrill, Schafer, Vannatta, & Noll, 2000). Further, Tyc, Hadley, and Crockett (2001) reported that survivors generally understand the health risks of tobacco use and perceive themselves as vulnerable to these risks, with older and less informed survivors reporting the greatest intention to use tobacco products. Unfortunately, young adult survivors of pediatric cancer may be just as likely as peers to smoke (Verrill et al., 2000). Furthermore, Chen et al. (1998) provides evidence that the impact of cancer treatment on health-compromising behaviors may be a complicated process of direct and indirect effects. Among leukemia survivors, they found that more intensive treatment (e.g., cranial radiation and intrathecal chemotherapy) was associated with decreased educational attainment that, in turn, predicted heightened risk of behavior such as cigarette and drug use. Additional research is needed to examine the impact of parental monitoring, increased exposure to health education, and peer involvement (Dishion, Capaldi, & Yoerger, 1999) on the health-related behavior of pediatric cancer survivors. In addition, work is needed to improve the health promotion practices of cancer survivors (e.g., compliance with medical follow-up regarding late effects and detection of secondary malignancies, diet, and exercise).

SUBGROUPS AT INCREASED RISK FOR PSYCHOSOCIAL DIFFICULTIES

Many aspects of pediatric cancer can be conceptualized as experiences shared to some extent by most children diagnosed with a malignancy (e.g., the unexpected diagnosis of a serious or life-threatening condition, invasive medical treatment, and disruption in normative activities and routines). Considerable variation in the severity and duration of these experiences would, of course, have the potential to affect psychosocial outcomes. In general, there is little evidence that variability in general treatment intensity is associated with the degree of psychosocial difficulty displayed by children (Noll et al., 1999). This finding, along with a lack of significant differences between groups of children with cancer and healthy comparison children, suggests that these general factors do not affect psychosocial adjustment beyond the initial postdiagnosis stage. Rather, subgroups of children may be at increased risk for psychosocial morbidity as a function of specific individual, diagnostic, or treatment factors.

Considerable evidence exists that children with brain tumors (BT) are at increased risk for neurocognitive difficulties, as are children who receive cranial radiation and intrathecal chemotherapy to prevent CNS occurrence of acute lymphoblastic leukemia (see Powers, Vannatta, Noll, Cool, & Stehbens, 1995, for a review). Although declines in functioning are not reported by all studies, considerable evidence exists for deleterious effects on full-scale IQ, memory, attention, and academic functioning (e.g., Lockwood, Bell, & Coegrove, 1999; Raymond-Speden, Tripp, Lawrence, & Holdaway, 2000; Schatz, Kramer, Ablin, & Matthay, 2000). Problems emerge as late effects of CNS treatment and appear to be more severe for children who are younger at the time they receive treatment. Recent work has used longitudinal designs to document emergence and continuation of neuropsychological impairments for long-term survivors (e.g., Brown, Sawyer, Antoniou, Toogood, & Rice, 1999). Evaluation of the cognitive effects of cancer and its treatment constitutes one of the largest domains of behavioral research in pediatric oncology, and excellent review articles (Moleski, 2000; Powers et al., 1995), methodological critiques (Butler & Copeland, 1993), and discussion of practical implications for educators and clinicians (Armstrong, Blumberg, & Toledano, 1999) are available.

Difficulties for children with CNS malignancies appear to expand beyond neurocognitive functioning to include broader domains of adjustment such as social functioning and peer relationships, including diminished involvement in social activities, social withdrawal, and diminished friendships (Carpentieri, Mulhern, Douglas, Hanna, & Fairclough, 1993; Radcliffe, Bennett, Kazak, Foley, & Phillips, 1996; Vannatta, Gartstein, Short, & Noll, 1998). Poorer outcomes for children surviving BT as opposed to other forms of cancer is consistent with evidence of greater disruptions in the psychosocial functioning of children who have sustained traumatic brain versus orthopedic injuries (Andrews, Rose, & Johnson, 1998; Bloom et al., 2001). In addition, theoretical perspectives on resilience suggest that social and behavioral development are affected in enduring ways only by environmental threats that either alter CNS functioning or alter the child's primary caregiving system (Masten, Best, & Garmezy, 1990).

Unfortunately, information regarding the emotional and behavioral functioning of children treated for BT is somewhat limited. Elevations in parent reports of behavior problems and internalizing difficulties have been found by some but not all researchers (Carlson-Green, Morris, & Krawiecki, 1995; Carpentieri et al., 1993; LeBaron, Zeltzer, Zeltzer, Scott, & Marlin, 1988). Early work (Hirsh, Renier, Czernichow, Benveniste, & Pierre-Kahn, 1979) described survivors of BT as emotionally regressed and inhibited, and more recent efforts have found increased rates of loneliness (Fossen, Abranhamsen, & Storm-Mathisen, 1999). However, conflicting results have been reported using parent and self-report measures of emotional functioning for a sample of pediatric BT survivors (Radcliffe et al., 1996). Child-reported depression scores were actually lower than instrument norms, and self-concept scores were similar to normative values (Radcliffe et al., 1996). It is unclear whether the inconsistent evidence of emotional distress among BT survivors reflects: (1) methodological issues related to the comparison of clinical samples to instrument norms, (2) parental report of distress that BT survivors do not in fact experience, or (3) a repressive adaptive style similar to that of other children with cancer (Phipps et al. 2001).

Additional research has examined the psychosocial correlates of CNS prophylactic treatment for children with acute lymphoblastic leukemia (ALL). In general, broad indices of behavioral and emotional adjustment have not demonstrated consistent associations with either the dose or type of neurotoxic treatment children have received (Butler, Rizzi, & Bandilla, 1999; Noll et al., 1997). There is evidence, however, that social functioning (e.g., sociability, isolation, numbers of friends) may be affected by the intensity of neurotoxic treatment, especially for children who are younger at the time of treatment (Chen et al., 1998; Hill et al., 1998; Vannatta, Zeller, Noll, & Koontz, 1998; Vannatta, Gerhardt, & Noll, 1999).

PARENT, SIBLING, AND FAMILY ADJUSTMENT

A child's diagnosis and treatment for cancer occurs within the context of the family system and has great potential for affecting parent, sibling, and family functioning (Grootenhuis & Last, 1997; Wallander & Varni, 1998). The common values, rules, and beliefs within the family provide a framework for how individuals interpret and respond to the many challenges presented when a child has cancer. Although efforts have historically focused on children with cancer and their mothers, more recent efforts have expanded to include fathers and, to a lesser degree, sibling and family factors. This shift in focus has occurred in response to calls for a broader conceptualization of family-centered care and research in pediatric psychology (e.g., Seagull, 2000).

Caring for a child with cancer can require a significant change in the family system, with much of the family's attention and resources focused on the affected child. In addition to fears of loss and the threat to the child's physical well-being, cancer treatment can introduce multiple daily hassles and stressful life events (e.g., Dockerty, Williams, McGee, & Skegg, 2000). Traditionally, mothers assume the greatest responsibility for the day-to-day aspects of their child's care (e.g., medications, appointments, and hospital stays), whereas fathers often assume primary financial responsibilities (Chesler & Parry, 2001; Quittner, Opipari, Regoli, Jacobsen, & Eigen, 1992; Quittner et al., 1998). Siblings also may need to adjust to the decreased availability of their parents and assume greater responsibilities at home.

Evidence of the emotional toll on parents is mixed. In general, prospective studies indicate that parental distress, particularly anxiety and depression, may be higher near diagnosis for both mothers and fathers relative to controls or norms; however, symptoms typically decline to normal levels after the first year (Hoekstra-Weebers, Jaspers, Kamps, & Klip, 1998; Kupst et al., 1995; Sawyer et al., 1997; Sawyer, Antoniou, Toogood, Rice, & Baghurst, 2000). Other studies indicate that this pattern is true only for mothers, whereas fathers have reported consistently low scores at both intervals (Dahlquist, Czyzewski, & Jones, 1996; Noll et al., 1995). Although scores for parental distress may be significantly higher than norms or those of controls in the initial year of treatment, they typically fall in the mild to moderate range and well below clinical cutoffs (e.g., Noll et al., 1995). Parents may still benefit from intervention to alleviate distress, however, as subclinical symptoms of anxiety and depression can be associated with other concurrent and future difficulties (Gerhardt, Compas, Connor, & Achenbach, 1999; Gotlieb, Lewinsohn, & Seeley, 1995).

Researchers have suggested that the long-term adjustment of parents can be best conceptualized within the context of posttraumatic stress symptoms (PTSS; Stuber, Kazak, Meeske, & Barakat, 1998). Approximately 6–10% of parents of pediatric cancer survivors have endorsed severe or high levels of PTSS, with an additional 20–40% exhibiting subclinical but moderate levels (Kazak et al., 1997; Manne, Du Hamel, Gallelli, Sorgen, & Redd, 1998; Stuber et al., 1998). In two studies, parents of pediatric cancer survivors have reported significantly higher levels of PTSS than comparisons (Barakat et al., 1997; Kazak et al., 1997). For example, Kazak et al. (1997) found that both mothers and fathers of survivors reported more intrusive thoughts and higher reaction index scores, with fathers of survivors also reporting more avoidance than comparisons.

A recent review has highlighted increased concern regarding the adjustment of siblings of children with cancer and the shortage of well-designed studies in this area (Houtzager, Grootenhuis, & Last, 1999). Qualitative and descriptive studies indicate that siblings may be at risk for emotional and behavioral problems but that they can also exhibit positive traits, such as being more sensitive and thoughtful of others (e.g., Heffernan & Zanelli, 1997). A novel body of work from seven collaborative sites has evaluated the adjustment of 254 siblings of children diagnosed with cancer nearly 2 years earlier (Sahler et al., 1994). In these studies, siblings were noted to have more emotional and behavioral problems than matched controls obtained from national survey data (Sahler et al., 1994). In addition, siblings reported more somatic complaints, especially problems with appetite and sleep, and their parents were less likely than controls to seek health care for them (Zeltzer et al., 1996). Other work has suggested that 6 months or more after diagnosis, siblings in the United States and China may have higher rates of scores in a clinical range on standardized measures of adjustment (Sloper & White, 1996; Wang & Martinson, 1996) and lower scores on indicators of social competence (Wang & Martinson, 1996). However, data from a Dutch sample suggests that over the long run, sibling adjustment is comparable to controls (Van Dongen-Melman, De Groot, Hahlen, & Verhulst, 1995).

Despite the potential for significant disruption, previous research has indicated that family adjustment is generally satisfactory and consistent among families of children with cancer (Grootenhuis & Last, 1997). Multiple indicators of family adjustment have been reported as being similar to controls or norms near diagnosis (Manne et al., 1995; Sawyer et al., 1997), after therapy (Noll et al., 1995; Sawyer et al., 1997), and long term (Kazak et al., 1997; Sawyer et al., 2000). One exception was that fathers of children who were off therapy scored significantly lower on controlling factors than controls indicating fewer family rules and greater emphasis on independence (Noll et al., 1995). Few studies have included information about dyadic relationships within the family (e.g., parent–child, marital relationships), but one study noted that marital satisfaction and overall adjustment were stable and within the normal range for parents of children with cancer at diagnosis and 20 months later (Dahlquist et al., 1996).

Multiple studies have investigated the individual and environmental variables that may be associated with adjustment for parents and families. Such variables may include disease indicators (e.g., time since diagnosis, type of diagnosis), demographic characteristics (e.g., age, gender), and individual and family process variables (e.g., parental distress, coping, social support). Parent and family factors can influence child outcomes, with current data suggesting that more adaptive parent and family adjustment may predict better child adjustment (Drotar, 1997; Sawyer, Streiner, Antoniou, Toogood, & Rice, 1998). Although we were unable to find any recent longitudinal work to document specific predictors of sibling adjustment, several predictors of parent and family adjustment were identified. For example, distress among mothers of children with cancer may be predicted by earlier trait anxiety and pleasant events (Hoekstra-Weebers, Jaspers, Kamps, & Klip, 1999), as well as appraisal of illness strain and family cohesion (Sloper, 2000). For fathers, distress may be predicted by earlier trait anxiety and social support (Hoekstra-Weebers et al., 1999; Hoekstra-Weebers, Jaspers, Kamps, & Klip, 2001). Another study indicated that marital satisfaction at 20 months postdiagnosis was predicted by depression and spouse's satisfaction near diagnosis for both mothers and fathers (Dahlquist et al., 1996). Thus the literature tends to support a transactional model in which predictive factors tend to influence one another across time.

END OF LIFE CARE AND BEREAVEMENT

Despite improved survival rates, over one-fourth of children with cancer, or approximately 1,700 children annually, will die from their disease or from side effects of treatment (National Cancer Institute, 2002). Although much attention and resources have been dedicated to the study of quality of life and survivorship, research on end-of-life (EOL) care and bereavement has lagged behind in terms of quantity and quality (Dijkstra & Stroebe, 1998; Oliver, 1999).

Several novel papers have begun to address the importance of providing education to health care providers on EOL care (Sahler, Frager, Levetown, Cohn, & Lipson, 2000), assessing the impact of health care provider attitudes and practices on EOL care (Hilden et al., 2001), communicating with families about the prognosis in a timely manner (Wolfe, Klar, et al., 2000), and providing effective palliative treatment (Cooley et al., 2000; Wolfe, Griere, et al., 2000). Guidelines for discussing EOL care with families include: (1) sharing information in a cognitively and developmentally appropriate manner; (2) incorporating the ethical principles of self-determination and best interests of the patient; (3) early recognition and minimization of physical and emotional pain; (4) partnering with families to support their caregiving efforts; and (5) addressing the personal and professional challenges faced by providers (Sahler et al., 2000).

Current research indicates that the death of a child may be one of the most difficult and profound experiences for parents and siblings. Bereaved parents have reported internalizing difficulties and family disruption that may endure for years. For example, bereaved parents may be at risk for depression, anxiety, guilt, posttraumatic stress, and anger (Hazzard, Weston, Gutterres, 1992; Miles & Demi, 1992; Murphy et al., 1999). They routinely score worse on most scales of adjustment, especially internalizing problems, compared with norms and controls (Lehman, Wortman, & Williams, 1987; Roskin, 1985).

Families also undergo significant changes following the death of a child (Martinson, McClowry, Davies, & Kuhlenkamp, 1994). Although bereaved families have reported higher levels of cohesion than controls (Davies, 1988), other studies suggest less family cohesion and increased parental and marital strain (Lehman, Lang, Wortman, & Sorenson, 1989; Martinson et al., 1994; West, Sandler, Pillow, Baca, & Gersten, 1991). Bereaved parents have reported less marital satisfaction, less sexual intimacy, more frequent thoughts of separation, and higher rates of divorce than nonbereaved parents (Lang & Gottlieb, 1991, 1993; Gottlieb, Lang, & Amsel, 1996; Najman et al., 1993).

With regard to parent–child relationships, bereaved parents may be so preoccupied with their own grief that they may unintentionally "overlook" surviving children (Rosen, 1985), or they may become closer to and overprotective of surviving children (Lehman et al., 1989). Bereaved parents also tend to report higher levels of parenting stress than controls (Lehman et al., 1987) and generally report feeling overwhelmed by their day-to-day parental responsibilities (Lehman et al., 1989). Bereaved siblings also report a general lack of communication, decreased availability, and less support from parents after the death (Rosen, 1985).

Surviving siblings may have a variety of psychosocial difficulties after the death. They have reported feelings of isolation and social withdrawal at home and with peers (Davies, 1991; Martinson & Campos, 1991; Rosen, 1985), in addition to feeling guilty, anxious, and depressed (Fanos & Nickerson, 1991; Rosen, 1985). Parents have noted similar problems in their children, including anxiety, sleep problems, nightmares, and posttraumatic stress symptoms (Applebaum & Burns, 1991; Powell, 1991). Compared with instrument norms and controls, bereaved siblings have been reported by parents and teachers to have significantly lower social competence and higher internalizing and externalizing scores within 2 years of the death (Birenbaum, Robinson, Phillips, Stewart, & McCown, 1989; Hutton & Bradley, 1994; McCown & Davies, 1995).

Clearly, more research is needed that addresses the prospective course of grief, risk and resistance factors. Future improvements in the methodological rigor of bereavement research will best inform the design and evaluation of empirically based interventions and aftercare programs. Because not all families may need or want services, the identification of subgroups or targets for intervention would optimize the delivery and cost of services.

PSYCHOSOCIAL INTERVENTION WITH CHILDREN AND FAMILIES AFFECTED BY PEDIATRIC CANCER

The Children's Oncology Group (COG) guidelines for standard psychosocial care (Noll & Kazak, 1997) includes recommendations for services across all phases of treatment, including: ongoing attention to clear communication with families about the disease, elements of treatment, and medical decision making; management of affective (e.g., anxiety), behavioral (e.g., adherence), and physical (e.g., pain, nausea) difficulties associated with invasive procedures and chemotherapy; school reentry and other academic needs; and coping with relapse, death, and bereavement. The needs of both families and patients must be given consideration; assistance should focus not just on financial needs and challenges but on behavioral and mental health needs as well. Considerable challenges exist, however, to providing routine, comprehensive psychosocial care in the current climate of health care economics. Whitsett, Pelletier, and Scott-Lane (1999) made suggestions for stretching resources by combining traditional means of psychosocial service delivery with group-oriented services and printed materials for patients and families.

Published data are not available regarding the efficacy of such comprehensive models of psychosocial care; however, several components of these models have been subjected to empirical evaluation. Kazak (1999) has emphasized that documentation of treatment efficacy is a necessary step in promoting psychosocial care in pediatric oncology. Considerable literature supports the use of behavioral interventions such as relaxation and distraction for reducing chemotherapy side effects and anticipatory nausea (see McQuaid & Nassau, 1999, for a review). Similarly, behavioral pain management and relaxation have been empirically validated for reduction of anxiety and pain during invasive medical procedures, such as starting peripheral intravenous lines, lumbar punctures, and bone marrow aspirations (Powers, 1999).

Other research has attempted to inform intervention efforts by delineating how common difficulties among pediatric oncology patients develop and are maintained (e.g., Stockhorst et al., 2000). Chen, Zeltzer, Craske, and Katz (2000) have reported interesting findings regarding the role of memory for event details in children's emotional distress during repeated lumbar punctures. Accuracy of recall was associated with child's age but unrelated to the use of medication commonly believed to have amnesic effects. Exaggerations of negative memories were predictive of higher affective distress during subsequent procedures, leading Chen et al. (2000) to suggest intervention strategies to reduce procedural distress by targeting the children's recall of prior procedures. This research group has provided initial evidence that this may be a productive direction for intervention research (Chen, Zeltzer, Craske, & Katz, 1999).

During recent years, several research groups have developed novel intervention programs to test by randomized clinical trials. Butler (1998) and colleagues have developed a multisite program to remediate neuropsychological and academic deficits in children who have had a CNS cancer or received cancer treatment with CNS effects. The intervention adapts techniques developed for training attentional skills for individuals who have sustained traumatic brain injuries while also training academic skills for approaching tasks and understanding concepts for arithmetic. An alternative approach that uses pharmacological treatment with methylphenidate to treat cognitive sequelae of CNS treatment has also been undergoing evaluation (Thomson et al., 2001). Sahler and colleagues (2002) have conducted a multisite, randomized clinical trial of a problem-solving intervention to reduce distress for mothers of children diagnosed with cancer. Mothers reported reduced negative affect, and this effect was associated with targeted changes in problem-solving skills. Finally, Kazak and colleagues (1999) have begun to publish results from a family-oriented program, Surviving Cancer Competently: An Intervention Program (SCCIP). Adolescent cancer survivors, parents, and siblings participate in group sessions that focus on reducing subsequent posttraumatic stress symptoms. Preliminary data (Kazak et al., 1999) support the feasibility of the program, family satisfaction with the intervention, and a reduction in PTSS 6 months after the intervention.

These innovative intervention programs were created to address areas of difficulty identified by prior research in pediatric oncology. In each case, intervention techniques were extrapolated from existing clinical literature regarding similar problems in different populations. In addition to identifying targets for new intervention efforts, well-designed descriptive research has the potential to identify the mechanisms or pathways that mediate the development of psychosocial difficulties for pediatric oncology patients and their families. In instances in which multiple mechanisms (e.g., social problem-solving deficits, functional limitations, parental involvement) could lead to the emergence of an identified problem (e.g, social isolation and withdrawal among BT survivors), it would be highly beneficial to empirically delineate pathways through tests of mediating processes. Results could then be used to select intervention strategies.

Unfortunately, little research has adequately tested mediation of psychosocial outcomes in pediatric oncology. Confusion about how to define mediation and test its operation is common in pediatric psychology literature (Holmbeck, 1997). Simple correlations between potential explanatory processes and outcomes within samples of patients do not demonstrate mediation of the impact of illness on adjustment. Clear demonstration of mediation requires data on specific outcomes and potential mediators both for children receiving treatment and for case controls (e.g., Vannatta, Zeller, Noll, & Koontz, 1998). This further emphasizes the need for methodologically rigorous study design in pediatric psychology.

SUMMARY

The diagnosis and treatment of pediatric cancer has the potential to be traumatic or disruptive to children, parents, and siblings. It appears, however, that disruptions in psychosocial functioning are not normative and primarily occur immediately following diagnosis and initiation of treatment. Subgroups of children, particularly those whose disease or treatment affects the CNS, may be at risk for poorer outcomes. Additional research is needed regarding subgroups at risk, as well as more subtle aspects of survivorship that may emerge as late effects. The impact of pediatric cancer on families, both when medical treatment does and does not result in a cure, should be an additional domain addressed by future research. Carefully designed studies should identify pathways that explain the emergence and maintenance of different outcomes. Such work has enormous potential to inform the development of intervention trials that can be integrated into ongoing clinical care.

ACKNOWLEDGMENTS

We wish to acknowledge Robert B. Noll for his support and mentorship of their work in pediatric oncology.

REFERENCES

Anderson, B. (1999). Surviving cancer: The importance of sexual self-concept. *Medical and Pediatric Oncology, 33,* 15–23.

Andrews, T. K., Rose, F. D., & Johnson, D. A. (1998). Social and behavioral effects of traumatic brain injury in children. *Brain Injury, 12,* 133–138.

Applebaum, D. R., & Burns, B. G. (1991). Unexpected childhood death: Post-traumatic stress disorder in surviving siblings and parents. *Journal of Clinical Child Psychology, 20,* 114–120.

Armstrong, F. D., Blumberg, M. J., & Toledano, S. R. (1999). Neurobehavioral issues in childhood cancer. *School Psychology Review, 28,* 194–203.

Barakat, L. P., Kazak, A. E., Meadows, A. T., Casey, R., Meeske, K., & Stuber, M. L. (1997). Families surviving childhood cancer: A comparison of posttraumatic stress symptoms with families of healthy children. *Journal of Pediatric Psychology, 22,* 843–859.

Bennett, D. S. (1994). Depression among children with chronic medical problems: A meta-analysis. *Journal of Pediatric Psychology, 19,* 149–170

Birenbaum, L. K., Robinson, M. A., Phillips, D. S., Stewart, B. J., & McCown, D. E. (1989). The response of children to the dying and death of a sibling. *Omega, 20,* 213–228.

Bloom, D. R., Levin, H. S., Ewing-Cobbs, L., Saunders, A. E., Song, J., & Kowatch, R. A. (2001). Lifetime and novel psychiatric disorders after pediatric traumatic brain injury. *American Academy of Child and Adolescent Psychiatry, 40,* 572–579.

Brown, R. T., Sawyer, M. G., Antoniou, G., Toogood, I., & Rice, M. (1999). Longitudinal follow-up of the intellectual and academic functioning of children receiving central nervous system prophylactic chemotherapy for leukemia: A four-year final report. *Developmental and Behavioral Pediatrics, 20,* 373–377.

Butler, R. W. (1998). Attentional processes and their remediation in childhood cancer. *Medical and Pediatric Oncology Supplement, 1,* 75–78.

Butler, R. W., & Copeland, D. R. (1993). Neuropsychological effects of central nervous system prophylactic treatment in childhood leukemia: Methodological considerations. *Journal of Pediatric Psychology, 18,* 319–338.

Butler, R. W., Rizzi, L. P., & Bandilla, E. B. (1999). The effects of childhood cancer and its treatment on two objective measures for psychological functioning. *Children's Health Care, 28,* 311–327.

Butler, R. W., Rizzi, L. P., & Handwerger, B. A. (1996). Brief report: The assessment of posttraumatic stress disorder in pediatric cancer patients and survivors. *Journal of Pediatric Psychology, 21,* 499–504.

Canning, E. H., Hanser, S. B., Shade, K. A., & Boyce, W. T. (1992). Mental disorders in chronically ill children: Parent–child discrepancy and physician identification. *Pediatrics, 90,* 692–696.

Carlson-Green, B., Morris, R. D., & Krawiecki, N. (1995). Family and illness predictors of outcomes in pediatric brain tumors. *Journal of Pediatric Psychology, 20,* 769–784.

Carpentieri, S. C., Mulhern, R. K., Douglas, S., Hanna, S., & Fairclough, D. L. (1993). Behavioral resiliency among children surviving brain tumors: A longitudinal study. *Journal of Clinical Child Psychology, 22,* 236–246.

Chang, P. (1991). Psychosocial needs of long-term childhood cancer survivors: A review of literature. *Pediatrician, 18,* 20–24.

Chang, P., Nesbit, M. E., Youngren N., & Robison, L. L. (1987). Personality characteristics and psychosocial adjustment of long-term survivors of childhood cancer. *Journal of Psychosocial Oncology, 5,* 43–58.

Chen, E., Zeltzer, L. K., Bentler, P. M., Byrne, J., Nicholson, H. S., Meadows, A. T., et al. (1998). Pathways linking treatment intensity and psychosocial outcomes among adult survivors of childhood leukemia. *Journal of Health Psychology, 3,* 23–38.

Chen, E., Zeltzer, L. K., Craske, M. G., & Katz, E. R. (1999). Alteration of memory in the reduction of children's distress during repeated aversive medical procedures. *Journal of Consulting and Clinical Psychology, 67,* 481–490.

Chen, E., Zeltzer, L. K., Craske, M. G., & Katz, E. R. (2000). Children's memories for painful cancer treatment procedures: Implications for distress. *Child Development, 71,* 933–947.

Chesler, M. A., & Parry, C. (2001). Gender roles and/or styles in crisis: An integrative analysis of the experiences of fathers of children with cancer. *Qualitative Health Research, 11,* 363–384.

Cooley, C., Adeodu, S., Aldred, H., Beesley, S., Leung, A., & Thacker, L. (2000). Paediatric palliative care: A lack of research-based evidence. *International Journal of Palliative Nursing, 6,* 346–351.

Crist, W. M., & Kun, L. E. (1991). Common solid tumors of childhood. *New England Journal of Medicine, 324,* 461–469.

Dahlquist, L. M., Czyzewski, D. I., & Jones, C. L. (1996). Parents of children with cancer: A longitudinal study of emotional distress, coping style, and marital adjustment two and twenty months after diagnosis. *Journal of Pediatric Psychology, 21,* 541–554.

Davies, B. (1988). The family environment in bereaved families and its relationship to surviving sibling behavior. *Children's Health Care, 17,* 22–31.

Davies, B. (1991). Long-term outcomes of adolescent sibling bereavement. *Journal of Adolescent Research, 6,* 83–96.

DeLaat, C. A., & Lampkin, B. C. (1992). Long-term survivors of childhood cancer: Evaluation and identification of sequelae of treatment. *Cancer: A Cancer Journal for Clinicians, 40,* 263–282.

Dijkstra, I. C., & Stroebe, M. S. (1998). The impact of a child's death on parents: A myth (not yet) disproved? *Journal of Family Studies, 4,* 159–185.

Dishion, T. J., Capaldi, D. M., & Yoerger, K. (1999). Middle childhood antecedents to progressions in male adolescent substance use: An ecological analysis of risk and protection. *Journal of Adolescent Research, 14,* 175–205.

Dockerty, J. D., Williams, S. M., McGee, R., & Skegg, D. C. G. (2000). Impact of childhood cancer on the mental health of parents. *Medical and Pediatric Oncology, 35,* 475–483.

Dolgin, M. J., Katz, E. R., Zeltzer, L. K., & Landsverk, J. (1989). Behavioral distress in pediatric patients with cancer receiving chemotherapy. *Pediatrics, 84,* 103–110.

Drotar, D. (1997). Relating parent and family functioning to the psychological adjustment of children with chronic health conditions: What have we learned? What do we need to know? *Journal of Pediatric Psychology, 22,* 149–165.

Eiser, C., & Havermans, T. (1994). Long term social adjustment after treatment for childhood cancer. *Archives of Disability in Children, 70,* 66–70.

Eiser, C., Hill, J. J., & Vance, Y. H. (2000). Examining the psychological consequences of surviving childhood cancer: Systematic review as a research method in pediatric psychology. *Journal of Pediatric Psychology, 25,* 449–460.

Fanos, J. H., & Nickerson, B. G. (1991). Long-term effects of sibling death during adolescence. *Journal of Adolescent Research, 6,* 70–82.

Fossen, A., Abranhamsen, T. G., & Storm-Mathisen, I. (1999). Psychological outcome in children treated for brain tumor. *Pediatric Hematology and Oncology, 15,* 479–488.

Gerhardt, C. A., Compas, B. E., Connor, J. K., & Achenbach, T. M. (1999). Association of mixed anxiety–depression syndrome and symptoms of major depressive disorder during adolescence. *Journal of Youth and Adolescence, 28,* 305–323.

Gotlieb, I. H., Lewinsohn, P. M., & Seeley, J. R. (1995). Symptoms versus a diagnosis of depression: Differences in psychosocial functioning. *Journal of Consulting and Clinical Psychology, 65,* 90–100.

Gottlieb, L., Lang, A., & Amsel, R. (1996). The long-term effects of grief on marital intimacy following infant death. *Omega, 33,* 1–19.

Gray, R. E., Doan, B. D., Shermer, P., Fitzgerald, A. V., Berry, M. P., Jenkin, D., & Doherty, M. A. (1992). Psychological adaptation of survivors of childhood cancer. *Cancer, 70,* 2713–2721.

Green, D. M., Zevon, M. A., & Hall, B. (1991). Achievement of life-goals by adult survivors of modern treatment for childhood cancer. *Cancer, 67,* 206–213.

Grootenhuis, M. A., & Last, B. F. (1997). Adjustment and coping by parents of children with cancer: A review of the literature. *Supportive Care in Cancer, 5,* 466–484.

Hazzard, A., Weston, J., & Gutterres, C. (1992). After a child's death: Factors related to parental bereavement. *Developmental and Behavioral Pediatrics, 13,* 24–30.

Heffernan, S. M., & Zanelli, A. S. (1997). Behavior changes exhibited by siblings of pediatric oncology patients: A comparison between maternal and sibling descriptions. *Journal of Pediatric Oncology Nursing, 14,* 3–14.

Hilden, J. M., Emanuel, E. J., Fairclough, D. L., Link, M. P., Foley, K. M., Clarridge, B. C., et al. (2001). Attitudes and practices among pediatric oncologists regarding end-of-life care: Results of the 1998 American Society of Clinical Oncology survey. *Journal of Clinical Oncology, 19,* 205–212.

Hill, J. M., Kornblith, A. B., Jones, D., Freeman, A., Holland, J. F., Glicksman, A. S., et al. (1998). A comparative study of the long term psychosocial functioning of childhood acute lymphoblastic leukemia survivors treated by intrathecal methotrexate with or without cranial radiation. *Cancer, 82,* 208–218.

Hirsh, J. F., Renier, D., Czernichow, R., Benveniste, L., & Pierre-Kahn, A. (1979). Medulloblastoma in childhood: Survival and functional results. *Acta Neurochirurgica, 48,* 1–15.

Hoekstra-Weebers, J. E. H. M., Jaspers, J. P. C., Kamps, W. A., & Klip, E. C. (1998). Gender differences in psychological adaptation and coping in parents of pediatric cancer patients. *Psycho-oncology, 7,* 26–36.

Hoekstra-Weebers, J. E. H. M., Jaspers, J. P. C., Kamps, W. A., & Klip, E. C. (1999). Risk factors for psychological maladjustment of parents of children with cancer. *Journal of the American Academy of Child and Adolescent Psychiatry, 38,* 1526–1535.

Hoekstra-Weebers, J. E. H. M., Jaspers, J. P. C., Kamps, W. A., & Klip, E. C. (2001). Psychological adaptation and social support of parents of pediatric cancer patients: A prospective longitudinal study. *Journal of Pediatric Psychology, 26,* 225–235.

Holmbeck, G. N. (1997). Toward terminological, conceptual, and statistical clarity in the study of mediators and moderators: Examples from the child-clinical and pediatric psychology literatures. *Journal of Consulting and Clinical Psychology, 65,* 599–610.

Houtzager, B. A., Grootenhuis, M. A., & Last, B. F. (1999). Adjustment of siblings to childhood cancer: A literature review. *Supportive Care in Cancer, 7,* 302–320.

Hutton, C. J., & Bradley, B. S. (1994). Effects of sudden infant death on bereaved siblings: A comparative study. *Journal of Child Psychology and Psychiatry, 35,* 723–732.

Irwin, C. E. (1993). Adolescence and risk taking: How are they related? In N. J. Bell & R. W. Bell (Eds.), *Adolescent risk taking* (pp. 7–28). Newbury Park, CA: Sage.

Joubert, D., Sadeghi, M. R., Elliott, M., Devins, G. M., Laperriere, N., & Rodin, G. (2001). Physical sequelae and self-perceived attachment in adult survivors of childhood cancer. *Psycho-oncology, 10,* 284–292.

Katz, E. R., Rubinstein, C. L., Hubert, N. C., & Blew, A. (1988). School and social reintegration of children with cancer. *Journal of Psychosocial Oncology, 6,* 123–140

Kazak, A. E. (1999). Effective psychosocial intervention for children with cancer and their families. *Medical and Pediatric Oncology, 32,* 292–293.

Kazak, A. E., Meeske, K., Penati, B., Barakat, L. P., Christakis, D., Meadows, A. T., Casey, R., & Stuber, M. L. (1997). Posttraumatic stress, family functioning, and social support in survivors of childhood leukemia and their mothers and fathers. *Journal of Consulting and Clinical Psychology, 65,* 120–129.

Kazak, A. E., Simms, S., Barakat, L., Hobbie, W., Foley, B., Golomb, V., & Best, M. (1999). Surviving Cancer Competently Intervention Program (SCCIP): A cognitive-behavioral and family therapy intervention for adolescent survivors of childhood cancer and their families. *Family Process, 38,* 175–191.

Kupst, M. J., Natta, M. B., Richardson, C. C., Schulman, J. L., Lavigne, J. V., & Das, L. (1995). Family coping with pediatric leukemia: Ten years after treatment. *Journal of Pediatric Psychology, 20,* 601–617.

Lackner, H., Benesch, M., Schagerl, S., Kerbl, R., Schwinger, W., & Urban, C. (2000). Prospective evaluation of late effects after childhood cancer therapy with a follow-up over 9 years. *European Journal of Pediatrics, 159,* 750–758.

Lang, A., & Gottlieb, L. (1991). Marital intimacy in bereaved and nonbereaved couples: A comparative study. In D. Papadatou & C. Papadatos (Eds.), *Children and death* (pp. 267–275). New York: Hemisphere.

Lang, A., & Gottlieb, L. (1993). Parental grief reactions and marital intimacy following infant death. *Death Studies, 17,* 233–255.

Lansky, S. B., List, M. A., & Ritter-Sterr, C. (1986). Psychosocial consequences of cure. *Cancer, 58,* 529–533.

Larcombe, I. J., Walker, J., Charlton, A., Meller, S., Jones, P. M., & Mott, M. G. (1991). Impact of childhood cancer on return to normal schooling. *British Medical Journal, 301,* 169–171.

Lavigne, J. V., & Faier-Routman, J. (1992). Psychological adjustment to pediatric physical disorders: A meta-analytic review. *Journal of Pediatric Psychology, 17,* 133–157.

LeBaron, S., Zeltzer, P. L., Zeltzer, L. K., Scott, S. E., & Marlin, A. E. (1988). Assessment of quality of survival in children with medulloblastoma and cerebellar astrocytoma. *Cancer, 62,* 1215–1222.

Lehman, D. R., Lang, E. R., Wortman, C. B., & Sorenson, S. B. (1989). Long-term effects of sudden bereavement: Marital and parent–child relationships and children's reactions. *Journal of Family Psychology, 2,* 344–367.

Lehman, D. R., Wortman, C. B., & Williams, A. F. (1987). Long-term effects of losing a spouse or child in a motor vehicle crash. *Journal of Personality and Social Psychology, 52,* 218–231.

Lockwood, K. A., Bell, T. S., & Coegrove, R. W. (1999). Long-term effects of cranial radiation therapy on attention functioning in survivors of childhood leukemia. *Journal of Pediatric Psychology, 24,* 55–66.

Madan-Swain, A., Brown, R. T., Foster, M. A., Vega, R., Byars, K., Rodenberger, W., et al. (2000). Identity in adolescent survivors of childhood cancer. *Journal of Pediatric Psychology, 25,* 105–115.

Makipernaa, A. (1989). Long term quality of life and psychosocial coping after treatment of solid tumors in childhood. *Acta Paediatric Scandanavia,78,* 728–735.

Manne, S. L., Du Hamel, K., Gallelli, K., Sorgen, K., & Redd, W. H. (1998). Posttraumatic stress disorder among mothers of pediatric cancer survivors: Diagnosis, comorbidity, and utility of the PTSD checklist as a screening instrument. *Journal of Pediatric Psychology, 23,* 357–366.

Manne, S. L., Lesanies, D., Meyers, P., Wollner, N., Steinherz, P., & Redd, W. (1995). Predictors of depressive symptomatology among parents of newly diagnosed children with cancer. *Journal of Pediatric Psychology, 20,* 491–510.

Martinson, I. M., & Campos, R. G. (1991). Adolescent bereavement: Long-term responses to a sibling's death from cancer. *Journal of Adolescent Research, 6,* 54–69.

Martinson, I. M., McClowry, S. G., Davies, B., & Kuhlenkamp, E. J. (1994). Changes over time: A study of family bereavement following childhood cancer. *Journal of Palliative Care, 10,* 19–25.

Masten, A. S., Best, K. M., & Garmezy, N. (1990). Resilience and development: Contributions from the study of children who overcome adversity. *Development and Psychopathology, 2,* 425–444.

McCown, D. E., & Davies, B. (1995). Patterns of grief in young children following the death of a sibling. *Death Studies, 19,* 41–53.

McQuaid, E. L., & Nassau, J. H. (1999). Empirically supported treatments of disease-related symptoms in pediatric psychology: Asthma, diabetes, and cancer. *Journal of Pediatric Psychology, 24,* 305–328.

Meadows, A. T., McKee, L., & Kazak, A. E. (1989). Psychological status of young adult survivors of childhood cancer: A survey. *Medical and Pediatric Oncology, 17,* 466–470.

Miles, M. S., & Demi, A. S. (1992). A comparison of guilt in bereaved parents whose children died by suicide, accident, or chronic disease. *Omega, 24,* 203–215.

Miller, R. W., Young, J. L., & Nivakovic, B. (1995). Childhood cancer. *Cancer, 75,* 395–405.

Moleski, M. (2000). Neuropsychological, neuroanatomical, and neurophysiological consequences of CNS chemotherapy for acute lymphoblastic leukemia. *Archives of Clinical Neuropsychology, 15,* 603–630.

Mulhern, R. K., Wasserman, A. L., Friedman, A. G., & Fairclough, D. (1989). Social competence and behavioral adjustment of children who are long-term survivors of cancer. *Pediatrics, 83,* 18–25.

Murphy, S. A., Braun, T., Tillery, L., Cain, K. C., Johnson, L. C., & Beaton, R. D. (1999). PTSD among bereaved parents following the violent deaths of their 12– to 28–year-old children: A longitudinal prospective analysis. *Journal of Traumatic Stress, 12,* 273–291.

Najman, J., Vance, J., Boyle, F., Embleton, G., Foster, B., & Thearle, J. (1993). The impact of a child death on marital adjustment. *Social Science and Medicine, 37,* 1005–1010.

National Cancer Institute (2002, January). Cancer facts. Retrieved November 20002, from *http://nci. nih. gov*

Noll, R. B., Gartstein, M. A., Hawkins, A., Vannatta, K., Davies, W. H., & Bukowski, W. M. (1995). Comparing parental distress for families with children who have cancer and matched comparison families without children with cancer. *Family Systems Medicine, 13,* 11–27.

Noll, R. B., Gartstein, M. A., Vannatta, K., Correll, J., Bukowski, W. M., & Davies, W. H. (1999). Social, emotional, and behavioral functioning of children with cancer. *Pediatrics, 103,*71–78.

Noll, R. B., & Kazak, A. (1997). Standards for psychosocial care. In A. R. Ablin (Ed.) *Supportive care of children with cancer* (pp. 263–273). Baltimore: Johns Hopkins Press.

Noll, R. B., Stehbens, J. A., MacLean, W. E., Waskerwitz, M. J., Whitt, J. K., Ruymann, F. B., et al. (1997). Behavioral adjustment and social functioning of long-term survivors of childhood leukemia: Parent and teacher reports. *Journal of Pediatric Psychology, 22,* 827–841.

Oeffinger, K. C., Eshelman, D. A., Tomlinson, G. E., Buchanan, G. R., & Foster, B. M. (2000). Grading late effects in young adult survivors of childhood cancer followed in an ambulatory adult setting. *Cancer, 88,* 1687–1695.

Oliver, L. E. (1999). Effects of a child's death on the marital relationship: A review. *Omega, 39,* 197–227.

Percy, C. (1995). Introduction. *Cancer, 75,* 140–146.

Phipps, S., & Srivastava, D. K. (1997). Repressive adaptation in children with cancer. *Health Psychology, 16,* 521–528.

Phipps, S., Steele, R. G., Hall, K., & Leigh, L. (2001). Repressive adaptation in children with cancer: A replication and extension. *Health Psychology, 20,* 445–451.

Powell, M. (1991). The psychosocial impact of sudden infant death syndrome on siblings. *Irish Journal of Psychology, 12,* 235–247.

Powers, S. W. (1999). Empirically supported treatments in pediatric psychology: Procedure related pain. *Journal of Pediatric Psychology, 24,* 131–145.

Powers, S. W., Vannatta, K., Noll, R. B., Cool, V. A., & Stehbens, J. A. (1995). Leukemia and other childhood cancers. In M. C. Roberts (Ed.), *Handbook of pediatric psychology* (2nd ed., pp. 310–326). New York: Guilford Press.

Quittner, A. L., Espelage, D. L., Opipari, L. C., Carter, B., Eid, N., & Eigen, H. (1998). Role strain in couples with and without a child with a chronic illness: Associations with marital satisfaction, intimacy, and daily mood. *Health Psychology, 17,* 112–124.

Quittner, A. L., Opipari, L. C., Regoli, M. J., Jacobsen, J., & Eigen, H. (1992). The impact of caregiving and role strain on family life: Comparisons between mothers of children with cystic fibrosis and matched controls. *Rehabilitation Psychology, 37,* 275–290.

Radcliffe, J., Bennett, D., Kazak, A. E., Foley, B., & Phillips, P. C. (1996). Adjustment in childhood brain tumor survival: Child, mother, and teacher report. *Journal of Pediatric Psychology, 21,* 529–539.

Raymond-Speden, E., Tripp, G., Lawrence, B., & Holdaway, D. (2000). Intellectual, neuropsychological, and academic functioning in long-term survivors of leukemia. *Journal of Pediatric Psychology, 25,* 59–68.

Rosen, H. (1985). Prohibitions against mourning in childhood sibling loss. *Omega, 15,* 307–316.

Roskin, M. (1985). Emotional reactions among bereaving Israeli parents. *Israel Journal of Psychiatry and Related Sciences, 21,* 73–84.

Ross, J. A., Severson, R. K., Pollock, B. H., & Robinson, L. L. (1996). Childhood cancer in the United States. *Cancer, 77,* 201–207.

Sahler, O. J., Frager, G., Levetown, M., Cohn, F. G., & Lipson, M. A. (2000). Medical education about end-of-life care in the pediatric setting: Principles, challenges, and opportunities. *Pediatrics, 105,* 575–584.

Sahler, O. J., Roghmann, K. J., Carpenter, P. J., Mulhern, R. K., Dolgin, M. J., Sargent, J. R., et al. (1994). Sibling adaptation to childhood cancer collaborative study: Prevalence of sibling distress and definition of adaptation levels. *Journal of Developmental and Behavioral Pediatrics, 15,* 353–366.

Sahler, O. J. Z., Varni, J. W., Fairclough, D. L., Butler, R. W., Noll, R. B., Dolgin, M. J., et al. (2002). Problem solving skills training for mothers of children with newly diagnosed cancer: A randomized trial. *Journal of Developmental and Behavioral Pediatrics, 23,* 77–86.

Sawyer, M. G., Antoniou, G., Nguyen, A. M., Toogood, I., Rice, M., & Baghurst, P. (1995). A prospective study of the psychological adjustment of children with cancer. *American Journal of Pediatric Hematology Oncology, 17,* 39–45.

Sawyer, M., Antoniou, G., Toogood, I., & Rice, M. (1997). Childhood cancer: A two-year prospective study of the psychological adjustment of children and parents. *Journal of the American Academy of Child and Adolescent Psychiatry, 36,* 1736–1743.

Sawyer, M., Antoniou, G., Toogood, I., Rice, M., & Baghurst, P. (2000). Childhood cancer: A 4-year prospective study of the psychological adjustment of children and parents. *Journal of Pediatric Hematology/Oncology, 22,* 214–220.

Sawyer, M. G., Streiner, D. L., Antoniou, G., Toogood, I., & Rice, M. (1998). Influence of parental and family adjustment on the later psychological adjustment of children treated for cancer. *Journal of the American Academy of Child and Adolescent Psychiatry, 37,* 815–822.

Schatz, J., Kramer, J. H., Ablin, A., & Matthay, K. K. (2000). Processing speed, working memory, and IQ: A developmental model of cognitive deficits following radiation therapy. *Neuropsychology, 14,* 189–200.

Schwarzer, R., Jerusalem, M., & Kleine, D. (1990). Predicting adolescent health complaints by personality and behaviors. *Psychology and Health, 4,* 233–244.

Seagull, E. A. (2000). Beyond mothers and children: Finding the family in pediatric psychology. *Journal of Pediatric Psychology, 25,* 161–169.

Shover, L. R. (1999). Psychosocial aspects of infertility and decisions about reproduction in young cancer survivors: A review. *Medical and Pediatric Oncology, 33,* 53–59.

Sloper, P. (2000). Predictors of distress in parents of children with cancer: A prospective study. *Journal of Pediatric Psychology, 25,* 79–91.

Sloper, P., & White, D. (1996). Risk factors in the adjustment of siblings of children with cancer. *Journal of Child Psychology and Psychiatry, 37,* 597–607.

Stockhorst, U., Spennes-Saleh, S., Korholz, D., Gobel, U., Schneider, M. E., Steingruber, H. J., & Klosterhalfen, S. (2000). Anticipatory symptoms and anticipatory immune responses in pediatric cancer patients receiving chemotherapy: Features of a classically conditioned response? *Brain, Behavior, and Immunity, 14,* 198–218.

Stuber, M. L., Christakis, D., Houskamp, B., & Kazak, A. E. (1996). Posttraumatic symptoms in childhood leukemia survivors and their parents. *Psychosomatics, 37,* 254–261.

Stuber, M. L., Kazak, A. E., Meeske, K., & Barakat, L. (1998). Is posttraumatic stress a viable model for understanding responses to childhood cancer? *Child and Adolescent Psychiatric Clinics of North America, 7,* 169–182.

Stuber, M. L. Kazak, A. E., Meeske, K., Barakat, L., Guthrie, D., Garnier, H., et al. (1997). Predictors of posttraumatic stress symptoms in childhood cancer survivors. *Pediatrics, 100,* 958–964.

Thomson, S. J., Leigh, L., Christensen, R., Xiang, X., Kun, L. E., Heiderman, R. L., et al. (2001). Immediate neurocognitive effects of methylphenidate on learning impaired survivors of childhood cancer. *Journal of Clinical Oncology, 19,* 1802–1808.

Tyc, V. L., Hadley, W., & Crockett, G. (2001). Predictors of intentions to use tobacco among adolescent survivors of cancer. *Journal of Pediatric Psychology, 26,* 117–121.

Van Dongen-Melman, J. E. W. M., De Groot, A., Hahlen, K., & Verhulst, F. C. (1995). Siblings of childhood cancer survivors: How does this "forgotten" group of children adjust after cessation of successful cancer treatment? *European Journal of Cancer, 31A,* 2277–2283.

Vannatta, K., Gartstein, M. A., Short, A., & Noll, R. B. (1998). A controlled study of peer relationships of children surviving brain tumors: Teacher, peer, and self ratings. *Journal of Pediatric Psychology, 23,* 279–288.

Vannatta, K., Gerhardt, C. A., & Noll, R. B. (1999) Neurotoxicity of treatment for pediatric cancer: Implications for social behavior and peer acceptance. *Journal of Developmental and Behavioral Pediatrics, 20*, 401–402.

Vannatta, K., Zeller, M., Noll, R. B., & Koontz, K. (1998). Social functioning of children surviving bone marrow transplantation. *Journal of Pediatric Psychology, 23*, 169–178.

Varni, J. W., Katz, E. R., Colegrove, R., & Dolgin, M. (1995). Perceived physical appearance and adjustment of children with newly diagnosed cancer: A path analytic model. *Journal of Behavioral Medicine, 18,* 261–278.

Verrill, J. R., Schafer, J., Vannatta, K., & Noll, R. B. (2000). Aggression, antisocial behavior, and substance abuse in survivors of pediatric cancer: Possible protective effects of cancer and its treatment. *Journal of Pediatric Psychology, 25*, 493–502.

VonEssen, L., Enskar, K., Kreuger, A., Larsson, B., & Sjoden, P. O. (2000). Self-esteem, depression, and anxiety among Swedish children and adolescents on and off cancer treatment. *Acta Paediatrica, 89*, 229–236.

Wallander, J. L., & Varni, J. W. (1998). Effects of pediatric chronic physical disorders on child and family adjustment. *Journal of Child Psychology and Psychiatry, 39*, 29–46.

Wang, R. H., & Martinson, I. M. (1996). Behavioral responses of healthy Chinese siblings to the stress of childhood cancer in the family: A longitudinal study. *Journal of Pediatric Nursing, 11,* 383–391.

West, S. G., Sandler, I., Pillow, D. R., Baca, L., & Gersten, J. (1991). The use of structural equation modeling in generative research: Toward the design of preventive intervention for bereaved children. *American Journal of Community Psychology, 19*, 459–480.

Whitsett, S. F., Pelletier, W., & Scott-Lane, L. (1999). Meeting impossible psychosocial demands in pediatric oncology: Creative solutions to universal challenges. *Medical and Pediatric Oncology, 32*, 289–291.

Wolfe, J., Grier, H. E., Klar, N., Levin, S. B., Ellenbogen, J. M., Salem-Schatz, S., et al. (2000). Symptoms and suffering at the end of life in children with cancer. *New England Journal of Medicine, 342,* 326–333.

Wolfe, J., Klar, N., Grier, H. E., Duncan, J., Salem-Schatz, S., Emanuel, E. J., & Weeks, J. C. (2000). Understanding of prognosis among parents of children who died of cancer: Impact on treatment goals and integration of palliative care. *Journal of the American Medical Association, 284,* 2469–2475.

Zeltzer, L. K., Chen, E., Weiss, R., Guo, M. D., Robison, L. L., Meadows A. T., et al. (1997). Comparison of psychologic outcome in adult survivors of childhood acute lymphoblastic leukemia versus sibling controls: A cooperative children's cancer group and NIH study. *Journal of Clinical Oncology, 15,* 547–556.

Zeltzer, L. K., Dolgin, M. J., Sahler, O. J., Roghmann, K., Barbarin, O. A., Carpenter, P. J., et al. (1996). Sibling adaptation to childhood cancer collaborative study: Health outcomes of siblings of children with cancer. *Medical and Pediatric Oncology, 27,* 98–107.

21

HIV and AIDS in Children and Adolescents

F. DANIEL ARMSTRONG
ELIZABETH J. WILLEN
KAREN SORGEN

In 1982, the Centers for Disease Control and Prevention (CDC) reported the first cases of pediatric AIDS in the United States (Chadwick & Yogev, 1995). Since that time, women of childbearing age and children have experienced dramatic increases in rates of HIV infection and AIDS. In the United States, approximately 8,900 children under age 13 have HIV or AIDS, and 91% acquired the infection by vertical transmission from their mothers. Transmission by drug use or sexual contact remains a significant concern for older children and adolescents. HIV infection in young women and children in United States overwhelmingly (78%) affects those living in poverty and representing ethnic minority groups. Fortunately, deaths of children due to HIV are declining, down from 554 deaths in 1993 to 74 in 2000 (Centers for Disease Control and Prevention, 2001). However, the epidemic among mothers and children in the United States is dwarfed by the international experience. The World Health Organization has estimated that more than 3–4 million children may be HIV-infected in sub-Saharan Africa alone (Morison, 2001; Stoneburner, Sato, & Burton, 1994).

Much has been learned about the effects of HIV on children's development, psychological functioning, and adaptation. Advances in the treatment of HIV and AIDS have led to significant reductions in the rate of vertical transmission (Connor et al., 1994), better management of symptoms (Mintz, 1999), and significant improvements in the ability to reduce the presence of the virus using highly active anti-retroviral therapy (HAART; Brown, Lourie, & Pao, 2000; Mintz, 1999). With these improvements in treatment, HIV in children has changed from a uniformly deadly disease early in childhood to one involving chronic management well into adolescence (Chiriboga, 2002; Gray, Newell, Thorne, Peckham, & Levy, 2001). We provide a basic understanding of the pathophysiology of HIV/AIDS, give an overview of the theoretical and empirical underpinnings of current therapy, and then review the major psychological outcomes that have been identified over the past 20 years. Observations about psychological functioning have changed over time, as the natural history of the disease has been affected by significant changes in the way it is treated and managed. Corresponding to these changes in medical care have been significant changes in the perception and approach to individuals with HIV in our society. Because this is an emerging area of scientific and social importance, we conclude with a discussion of emerging concerns for psychologists working with children with HIV and their families.

THE BIOLOGY OF HIV

Virology and Immunology

The human immunodeficiency virus (HIV) is a single-stranded RNA retrovirus that is attracted to the CD4 surface molecule of T-cells, which are part of the human immune system. There are two types of T-cells: (1) helper T-cells (CD4+) and (2) suppressor T-cells (CD8+) that guard against immune overactivation. The HIV becomes incorporated into the DNA of the T-cell, replicates HIV-specific RNA proteins, kills the T-cell, and releases new HIV to continue the infection process. As the immune system attempts to protect itself from the loss of helper T-cells, it produces new T-cells. As this process continues, increasing numbers of T-cells are destroyed, the viral load of HIV increases, and immune function is seriously impaired (Hanson & Shearer, 1998).

Clinical Manifestations

The clinical manifestations of this process include many opportunistic infections (those that occur because of the absence of an effective immune system), direct effects on central nervous system development, wasting syndromes, lung disease, and malignant disease, most commonly lymphoma. During the early phases of the epidemic, and currently in the developing world, one of the most significant symptoms of HIV in young children has been CNS encephalopathy, characterized by developmental plateau or rapid progressive decline, changes in the frontal cortex and basal ganglia, motor hypo- or hypertonicity, and sometimes early death (Hanson & Shearer, 1998; Mitchell, 2001). Fortunately, the development of HAART therapies has reduced the occurrence of the symptoms in many children treated in United States today.

Treatment Considerations

Current treatment approaches to HIV in children fall into three areas: (1) prevention, (2) symptom management, and (3) HAART therapy. Primary prevention involves treatment of the mother during pregnancy, labor, and delivery, followed by brief treatment of the newborn. This approach resulted in a dramatic reduction, from nearly 30% of children acquiring HIV through vertical transmission to approximately 7% when this treatment is provided (Connor et al., 1994). Symptom management involves both preventive (use of prophylactic antibiotics) and aggressive use of antibiotics and antiviral medications to treat opportunistic infections (Mintz, 1999). Treatment of HIV has evolved rapidly. Early treatment relied on single agents (e.g., zidovidine) or combinations of agents, but this strategy was generally ineffective in either reducing or eliminating the presence of HIV (viral load) or sustaining treatment effects over time. Between 1997 and 1999, new approaches to treatment using combination antiretroviral medications and protease inhibitors (HAART) became widespread and resulted not only in prevention of symptoms but also in reduction or elimination of detectable levels of the virus (Gray et al., 2001). This approach has dramatically improved children's quality of life.

PSYCHOLOGICAL AND BEHAVIORAL ASPECTS OF PEDIATRIC HIV/AIDS

Early research on pediatric HIV focused on early neurological and neurodevelopmental consequences of the illness (e.g., Armstrong, Seidel, & Swales, 1993) or on the implications of stigma associated with having a diagnosis of HIV (e.g., Hardy, Armstrong, Routh, Albrecht, & Davis, 1994). Today, the neurocognitive effect of HIV remains the area of greatest focus, but other issues associated with the transition from acute, terminal illness to chronic illness have gradually moved to the forefront of the field. Concerns with stigma have gradually been replaced by concerns about appropriate disclosure of HIV information to children (American Academy of Pediatrics Committee on Pediatric AIDS, 1999; Wiener, Battles, Heilman, Sigelman, & Pizzo, 1996). The focus on care of the child with HIV and his or her family has shifted from terminal care to management of symptoms that affect treatment outcome and quality of life (Mialky, Vagnoni, & Rutstein, 2001; Pontali et al., 2001; Van Dyke et al., 2002).

HIV/AIDS AND CENTRAL NERVOUS SYSTEM DEVELOPMENT

HIV infection can have a profound effect on the development of the central nervous system, with associated cognitive, social, and emotional consequences that become evident over the course of the child's life. If inadequately treated, neurocognitive and developmental difficulties may be noted early in infancy, may present as subtle difficulties during the preschool and school-age years, or may only become evident during the preteen and teenage years. Deficits may be global in nature, affecting multiple areas of neurocognitive functioning, or very specific, affecting isolated functions and sparing others. Some types of cognitive impairment may be acute, some may resolve with active therapy, and some may be delayed effects of earlier CNS infection. Further, the specific pattern of neurocognitive deficits seen in any individual child appear dependent on (1) medical factors, such as viral load and CD4 count (Mintz, 1999; Mitchell, 2001), (2) the age at which a child experienced CNS infection (Coscia, Christensen, & Henry, 1997), (3) whether CNS damage was related to an isolated event or was the consequence of prolonged CNS disease (Mitchell, 2001), (4) whether and when HAART therapy was initiated (Mintz, 1999), (5) the time interval between CNS damage and assessment of function (Armstrong & Mulhern, 1999), (6) the age of the child at the time of assessment (Armstrong & Mulhern, 1999), and (7) the neurocognitive abilities that a child should have developmentally acquired at the time an assessment is conducted (Armstrong & Mulhern, 1999). Therefore, neurocognitive difficulties in children with HIV/AIDS may be seen at any age, and the neurocognitive performance of a child with HIV may vary substantially over repeated assessments. For some children, a distinctive pattern of neurodevelopment may be noted; for others, improvements and declines may occur in a less predictable fashion depending on the natural history of the disease and the effectiveness of available therapy. In many cases, rapid or significant declines in neurocognitive function may represent the earliest indication of advancing disease and/or failure of current medical treatment (Pearson et al., 2000).

Neurological Manifestations

The primary mechanism for neurological compromise and pediatric HIV is believed to be related to the ability of the virus to infect macrophages and microglia, causing a release of toxic substances into the brain. The result is damage to the white matter of the brain, demyelination of nerve tracks, and alterations in the blood–brain barrier (Mintz, 1999; Mitchell, 2001). This process ultimately produces (1) cerebral atrophy, (2) ventricular enlargements, (3) calcifications in the basal ganglia, cerebellum, and subcortical frontal white matter, (4) cerebral atrophy associated with a reduction in white matter, and (5) demyelination (Mintz, 1999). Other significant events may occur, including vascular injury, metabolic abnormalities, hypoxia, and sensory impairment related to repeated infections (Armstrong et al., 1993). Although secondary infections of the CNS due to HIV-immuno-compromise and subsequent opportunistic infection have been well documented, these types of infections occur rarely in infants and young children (Mintz, 1999). Older children and adolescents are at greater risk, as repeated, severe infections that affect the brain, such as toxoplasmosis, herpes simplex, and cytomegalovirus, may have substantial impact on brain structure and function over time (Mintz, 1999; Mitchell, 2001).

Clinical manifestations of CNS encephalopathy in untreated infants and children have commonly involved slowed brain development, a plateau (failure to develop) in brain development, or, in extreme cases, a progressive deterioration of developed brain structures (Mintz, 1999; Mitchell, 2001). These patterns were common during the early part of the HIV epidemic, but this pattern is seldom seen now in the United States. However, the plateau or progressive deterioration in brain development remains a significant concern with children in developing nations who do not have access to HAART therapies (Bailey, Kamenga, Nsuami, Nieburg, & St. Louis, 1999), and thus remains a focus of significant, current concern.

Static encephalopathy is more common in the United States and does not involve an insidious deterioration of attained brain development; rather, it is characterized by significantly delayed brain development. The cognitive abilities of children with static encephalopathy often range from low average to markedly impaired, depending on their individual rates of neurodevelopment (Armstrong et al., 1993; Brouwers, Belman, & Epstein, 1994; Brown et al., 2000). Fortunately, there is a subset of children with HIV infection who appear to experience minimal CNS effects of the illness (Gay et al., 1995; Mitchell, 2001).

Neurodevelopmental Manifestations

The effects of HIV on the developing CNS are seen in the behavior of and acquisition of skills by infants and children who are infected. However, there are other critical factors associated with HIV that may also contribute to delays in cognitive, social, and emotional functioning. Children with HIV are overwhelmingly poor, culturally and ethnically of minority backgrounds, may have been prenatally exposed to drugs and alcohol, may be raised by parents who are dealing with the consequences of their own HIV/AIDS, may have lost parents due to death and live with relatives or in foster care, may lack opportunities for stimulation during critical periods of development, and may have learning or developmental disabilities unrelated to HIV (Armstrong et al., 1993; Brown et al., 2000; Coscia et al., 2001). Recognizing the potential contribution of these factors to a child's neurodevelopment, it nonetheless appears that HIV independently results in significant risk for cognitive, social, and emotional difficulties, particularly for children who acquired the disease through vertical transmission.

Because many children died during the first few years of life during the first years of the HIV epidemic, most of the research on neurodevelopment in children with HIV has focused on infants. Neurodevelopmental outcomes were included in the earliest clinical trials conducted by the Pediatric AIDS Clinical Trials Group (PACTG), and in a number of studies neurocognitive functioning was considered a primary outcome of the clinical trial. As children have survived into the school-age and adolescent years, studies are being completed that address the functioning of these older children, although the number of completed trials is limited.

Infancy

Most studies of neurodevelopment in children vertically infected with HIV have compared children with documented HIV infection with those who, at birth, had detectable levels of maternal antibodies that then disappeared as the children acquired their own antibodies (seroreverters) or with children who were never exposed to HIV (seronegative, or nonexposed). Some studies included children who both were drug-exposed and had HIV (Chase et al., 2000; Englund et al., 1996), whereas others have excluded children with a previous history of drug exposure (Gay et al., 1995; Knight, Mellins, Levenson, Arpadi, & Kairam, 2000; Pollack et al., 1996). Early studies of HIV in infancy found significant delays in global cognitive and motor functioning, with substantial numbers of children meeting criteria for developmental disability and mental retardation (Armstrong et al., 1993; Englund et al., 1996). Most of the studies reflected patterns of neurodevelopment in untreated or minimally treated children. As children began to be treated with AZT and other simple combination therapies, differences between HIV-infected seroreverters and nonexposed children continued to be noted on measures of cognitive, motor, and emotional expressiveness (Chase et al., 2000; Gay et al., 1995; Macmillan et al., 2001; Moss, Wolters, Brouwers, Hendricks, & Pizzo, 1996; Pearson et al., 2000; Smith et al., 2000). These patterns have been associated with abnormalities detected on biological markers (Brouwers, Civitello, DeCarli, Wolters, & Sei, 2000), neuroimaging (Brouwers et al., 1995), and growth (Macmillan et al., 2001). Early encephalopathy with developmental delay has also been associated with early mortality (Rigardetto et al., 1999). Fortunately, the magnitude of these deficits appears less severe for children who have received more aggressive treatment than for those who experienced CNS disease early in the epidemic (Mintz, 1999), and not all children with HIV experience significant developmental delay during infancy (Gay et al., 1995). Early-treatment studies with single or combination drug therapies suggested improvement in cognitive function and development (Butler et al., 1991; DeCarli et al., 1991), and HAART also appears to result in neurocognitive improvement (Gray et al., 2001) and prevention of further declines.

Although factors such as prenatal drug exposure, differential exposure to HIV treatment, and cultural or ethnic factors may influence development, the effects of HIV appear to independently affect development (Blanchette, Smith, Fernandes-Penney, King, & Read, 2001; Chase et al., 2000; Mellins, Levenson, Zawadzki, Kairam, & Weston, 1994). Developmental cognitive and motor delays have also been identified as significant predictors of disease progression (Pearson et al., 2000). Fortunately, not all infected children experience early CNS disease and delay (Gay et al., 1995).

Preschool- and School-Age Children

With prolonged survival, investigations of neurocognitive functioning began to focus on children in the preschool- and school-age range. In contrast to the finding for infants, substantial developmental delays in the area of general neurocognitive functioning have typically not been reported (Bisiacchi, Suppiej, & Laverda, 2000; Moss et al., 1996; Wolters, Brouwers, Civitello, & Moss, 1997). Two factors may be associated with this finding. First, many of the children with the earliest signs of HIV and AIDS-related symptoms did not survive into the school years. Second, most of the survivors have benefited from progress in the use of antiretroviral medications, and many of the CNS-related features of the illness improved after the initiation of antiretroviral therapy (Havens, Whitaker, Feldman, Alvarado, & Ehrhardt, 1993). As with the studies on infancy, impaired neurocognitive functioning has been associated with a greater degree of encephalopathy and symptomatology, and this group remains at risk for significant neurocognitive impairment when treatment is ineffective. However, for children who are clinically asymptomatic, specific and subtle neurocognitive impairment may be noted. Although global cognitive deficits are not usually seen in these children, specific functional deficits have been identified, and these are associated with difficulties in school performance that result in more than 50% of these children requiring special education services (Mialky et al., 2001).

Although some studies have identified significantly poorer functioning in the areas of memory (Bisiacchi et al., 2000; Fundaro et al., 1998), processing speed (Cohen et al., 1991), motor abilities (Boivin et al., 1995; Moss et al., 1996), and executive functioning (Bisiacchi et al., 2000), the most common areas of deficit had been reported in the areas of visual-spatial and perceptual organization (Bisiacchi et al., 2000; Fundaro et al., 1998; Tardieu et al., 1995), social emotional regulation (Moss et al., 1996; Tardieu et al., 1995), and language development (Brouwers et al., 2001; Coplan et al., 1998; Moss et al., 1996; Tardieu et al., 1995; Wolters et al., 1997). Attention problems are common in preschool children, but several investigators have found particularly high rates of attention problems in children with HIV infection (Brouwers et al., 1994), leading to the speculation that HIV may affect specific attention mechanisms in the development of the brain. Other investigators have reported delays in expressive and receptive language (Wolters et al., 1997), but others found this to improve after the initiation of antiretroviral therapy (Coplan et al., 1998).

As more children survive into late childhood and early adolescence, new research should further illuminate the neurocognitive effects of HIV on the developing brain. Although it is clear that early CNS disease and related neurodevelopmental impairment is associated with an overall poorer prognosis (Pearson et al., 2000), the empirical literature so far suggests that subtle neurocognitive impairment may exist even for those children who are asymptomatic.

Late Adolescence and Adulthood

Given the progressive and debilitating course of HIV/AIDS and potential long-term limitations of antiretroviral therapy, it is anticipated that vertically infected adolescents will eventually experience greater neurocognitive decline and symptoms consistent with the AIDS-related dementia complex reported in the adult HIV literature (Melton, Kirkwood, &

Ghaemi, 1997). Adult AIDS-related dementia is characterized by cognitive, motor, and behavioral slowing, progressive memory impairments, apathy and withdrawal, and deficits in frontal lobe functions, including impaired judgment and reasoning skills (Simpson & Berger, 1996).

Children Infected by Transfusion, Sexual Transmission, or Drug Use

Because of new screening procedures for blood products, the majority of young children with HIV since 1985 were infected by vertical or perinatal transmission (Llorente, LoPresti, & Satz, 1997). Horizontal transmission refers to infection through other modalities, including transfusions and sexual activity. Although an increasing and alarming number of young people are becoming infected through unprotected sex, it is expected that their neurocognitive profiles will be similar to those of adults infected through sexual activity or needle sharing, because the virus is introduced into the brain after most of neurodevelopment has occurred. Therefore, the developmental impact of this disease may not be experienced in the same way as in children with vertically acquired HIV. However, early in the history of the epidemic, a number of infants and children were infected through blood transfusions, most notably children with hemophilia.

Although infection may have occurred as early as in the first few weeks of life in some children infected through transfusion, subsequent neurodevelopmental profiles have varied from the typical course noted in vertical infection. Some investigators (e.g., Brouwers, Belman & Epstein, 1994) suggest a differential course for the disease and initial onset of symptoms, depending on mode of transmission. Others (Cohen et al., 1991; Loveland et al., 1994; Loveland et al., 2000) identified a shorter and more similar course to what is observed in adults infected with HIV. Cohen and colleagues (1991) found neurocognitive deficits in children horizontally infected with HIV when compared with healthy peers but also found no differences in overall cognitive functioning between the two groups for as long as 8 ½ years postinfection. Compared with vertically infected children with no evidence of encephalopathy early in development, the horizontally infected children may have been spared the early developmental impact of HIV on brain function that has been associated with later neurocognitive problems. Similar findings were noted in a large multicenter study of children with hemophilia (Stehbens et al., 1997). Baseline evaluations yielded no differences between HIV-infected and uninfected controls on overall neurocognitive functioning. Because these boys had been infected for an average of 6 years, it was suggested that the neurodevelopmental course of HIV in children with hemophilia is more similar to the adult course of the disease. At least one other major study found better overall neurocognitive functioning in horizontally versus vertically infected children with HIV (Englund et al., 1996), although similar CNS abnormalities were identified in both groups. However, in a large multicenter study of HIV-positive or negative boys with hemophilia, boys infected with HIV differed from those who were noninfected over time in overall intellectual functioning, visual-spatial and perceptual skills, nonverbal memory, academic achievement, and language skills (Loveland et al., 2000). Declines in performance appeared substantially related to increasingly compromised immune functioning.

The neurocognitive impact of HIV infection in children infected by blood transfusion appears less severe, and these children may maintain relatively normal functioning for an extended time period. Unfortunately, few data are available about the functioning of adolescents who acquire HIV through sexual contact or drug use, even though these behaviors may place these adolescents at greater risk for poorer immune functioning and therefore at elevated risk for more severe and earlier neurocognitive impairment than those infected by blood transfusion.

HIV/AIDS AND PSYCHOSOCIAL ISSUES

The psychological implications for children living with HIV have changed dramatically over the past decade as treatment has improved. With decreased mortality, psychosocial and behavioral consequences of the disease and its treatment have gained importance. Children with HIV often deal with multigenerational loss, stigmatization, and the stressors of living in impoverished neighborhoods (Lewis, 2001), increasing their risk for acute and long-term coping and adjustment difficulties.

The Social Context of Pediatric HIV: Caregivers

Most children who are vertically infected with HIV are confronted with multiple challenges unrelated to the disease. These children are largely from minority cultural and ethnic backgrounds, predominantly African American and Hispanic, and from families living in poverty (Centers for Disease Control and Prevention, 2001). Children may live with their birth parents, with grandparents and other family members, or in foster or adoptive care. Mothers are frequently single parents, and in the case of those with children who acquired HIV through vertical transmission, are themselves HIV infected (Mellins & Ehrhardt, 1994). Those parents who are HIV infected report being socially isolated, having few financial or social resources, and experiencing significant burden caring for themselves and their infected and uninfected children (Antle, Wells, Goldie, DeMatteo, & King, 2001; Mellins et al., 1994). The caregiving burden is complicated by the fact that more than half may meet diagnostic criteria for a psychiatric disorder (Murphy, Koranyi, Crim, & Whited, 1999). However, at least one study found that, although nearly one-third of parents of children with HIV experienced clinical levels of psychological distress, this frequency was similar to that of parents who were uninfected and whose children were uninfected (Bachanas, Kullgren, Schwartz, McDaniel, et al., 2001). Thus all considerations of psychological distress in children infected with HIV must occur in the context of poverty, stigma, burden, and other environmental stressors and limitations.

Psychological Adjustment and Coping: Children and Adolescents

Despite significant concerns about the risk of psychological maladjustment in children infected with HIV, most studies to date have found no differences in the self-reported psychological adjustment of children with HIV compared with those who serorevert or were never exposed (Bachanas, Kullgren, Schwartz, Lanier, et al., 2001; Moss, Bose, Wolters, & Brouwers, 1998; Thorne et al., 2002). However, caregivers report higher levels of subjective distress in children infected with HIV (Bachanas, Kullgren, Schwartz, Lanier, et al., 2001; Havens, Whitaker, Feldman, & Ehrhardt, 1994). Rates of clinically significant behavioral and emotional problems in children and adolescents infected with HIV exceed those expected in the general population (Bachanas, Kullgren, Schwartz, Lanier, et al., 2001; Havens et al., 1994) but are still lower than the rates of comparison groups of noninfected children. This suggests that the risk factors associated with poverty, socioeconomic status, and living environment are far more important to psychological adjustment than HIV (Bachanas, Kullgren, Schwartz, Lanier, et al., 2001).

Changes in behavior and emotional functioning noted in children with HIV may be due to the direct effects of the illness and medications or to difficulties coping with the illness or both. Behavior changes can be seen in children with encephalopathy or other HIV-related central nervous system diseases. Side effects of some antiretroviral medications include depression and anxiety (New York State Department of Health, 2001). Other side effects (e.g., impaired concentration, changes in appetite, sleep disturbances) may also be erroneously attributed to depression. Living with a life-threatening disease can cause feelings of sadness and hopelessness. Moreover, some children experience body changes such as wasting, atopic dermatitis, ringworm, and/or insertion of a tube to allow for medication access. Small stature and descended stomachs are other bodily characteristics seen in some children with HIV that can have psychological implications, including poor self-image and feelings of being different (Lewis, Haiken, & Hoyt, 1994). In addition to symptoms of depression, fear of death, isolation, fear of rejection, repeated hospitalizations and medical procedures can contribute to symptoms of anxiety.

Older children and adolescents with HIV, whether the infection is vertically or behaviorally acquired, have greater risk for adjustment problems (Bachanas, Kullgren, Schwartz, Lanier, et al., 2001) and psychiatric diagnoses, greater history of sexual abuse, and higher current substance abuse (Pao et al., 2000). Nearly half of adolescents with behaviorally acquired HIV may experience depression (Pao et al., 2000), and adolescents whose parents die of HIV have a significant increase in the risk for depression (Battles & Wiener, 2002). Other factors associated with elevated levels of psychological adjustment problems include (1) disease progression (Bose, Moss, Brouwers, Pizzo, & Lorion, 1994; Moss et al., 1998), (2) being reminded about the disease and its implications for normal behavior (Brown, Schultz, & Gragg, 1995), (3) an increased number of negative life events (Moss et al., 1998), and (4) high levels of caregiver distress (Bachanas, Kullgren, Schwartz, McDaniel, et al., 2001; Forehand et al., 1998). Changes in the pattern of psychological adjustment may be affected by the effectiveness of treatment, with at least one investigation finding that the adaptive behavior of children improved significantly after the initiation of zidovudine (Wolters, Brouwers, Moss, & Pizzo, 1994).

The approach used to cope with the illness has also been associated with psychological adjustment outcome. Coping that focuses primarily on emotional management has been associated with elevated levels of adjustment problems (Bachanas, Kullgren, Schwartz, Lanier, et al., 2001), as has coping that utilizes all types of strategies at high levels (Brown et al., 1995). On the other hand, adolescents with hemophilia and HIV reported that active cognitive and behavioral coping strategies were considered most effective and resulted in better perceptions of psychological adjustment (Brown et al., 1995).

Disclosure of HIV Status

Disclosure of HIV status is an issue for children receiving information about their own diagnosis and for children receiving information about the diagnoses of a parent. Early in the epidemic, Hardy and colleagues (Hardy et al., 1994) found significant differences in the frequency of disclosure about diagnoses between preschool children with HIV and children with cancer, with almost no children with HIV having received their diagnosis and almost all children with cancer having received their diagnosis. More recent studies suggest that between 17 and 66% of children with HIV have received full or partial disclosure about their diagnosis (Instone, 2000; Mialky et al., 2001) but that disclosure took place 2–8 years after diagnosis (Instone, 2000). Between 30 and 57% of children whose mothers are infected with HIV have been informed about their mothers' diagnosis (Murphy, Steers, & Dello Stritto, 2001; Simoni, Davis, Drossman, & Weinberg, 2000) . Disclosure of the child's diagnosis to the child has been associated with lower subsequent levels of behavior problems (Battles & Wiener, 2002), and nondisclosure has been associated with elevated levels of behavior problems (Bachanas, Kullgren, Schwartz, Lanier, et al., 2001). Lower levels of aggression and higher levels of self-esteem have been observed in children who are informed about their parent's diagnosis, whereas those who are told to keep the information a secret have subsequently been identified as having significantly more behavior problems (Murphy et al., 2001).

Unlike with other childhood medical illnesses, disclosure of disease to the child with HIV may also involve disclosure of other sensitive issues, such as maternal HIV status, maternal IV drug use, infidelity, and/or adoption (Lipson, 1994). Parents have reported a need for secrecy (Funck-Brentano et al., 1997), fear about the stigma of AIDS (Wiener et al., 1996), and a need to be ready to disclose (Ledlie, 1999) as factors associated with the decision to disclose either maternal or child diagnosis. Other factors associated with the decision to disclose include a perceived severity of symptoms (Armistead, Tannenbaum, Forehand, Morse, & Morse, 2001), high perceived stress (Murphy et al., 1999), low parenting efficacy (Murphy et al., 1999), and high levels of social support (Murphy et al., 2001), although these relationships have not occurred in every study (Simoni et al., 2000).

One of the reasons that disclosure is such a challenging and controversial issue is that there is no agreement about the age at which disclosure should take place. The American Academy of Pediatrics Committee on Pediatric AIDS recommends that disclosure of HIV infection should take a child's age and psychosocial maturity into consideration (American Academy of Pediatrics Committee on Pediatric AIDS, 1999). If it is suspected that the child is sexually active, disclosure becomes critical so that discussions of sexual responsibility can be incorporated into the child's treatment plan. This is particularly important because at least one study found that 58% of boys with hemophilia and HIV who were sexually active had not disclosed their HIV status to their sexual partners (Geary, King, Forsberg, Delaronde, & Parsons, 1996). It is also important to disclose if there is suspicion or evidence that the child knows about his or her status.

Caregiver Factors Related to Disclosure

It is not uncommon for health care professionals and caregivers to have different ideas about when to inform children about their illness. The child's age (Wiener et al., 1996), maternal depression (Wiener et al., 1996), perceived social support (Murphy et al., 2001), and disease severity (Armistead et al., 2001) have been documented as factors related to caregivers' decision to disclose. Parents also express concern about adverse impact of disease knowledge on their child's emotional functioning and physical well-being (Lewis et al., 1994).

Behavioral Medicine Issues: Adherence

The primary challenge for children treated with HAART is adhering to a very complicated and demanding treatment regimen. Most children with HIV have adherence rates of 50–70% (Pontali et al., 2001; Rapoff & Barnard, 1991; Van Dyke et al., 2002; Watson &

Farley, 1999), but even partial nonadherence may have significant consequences associated with increased viral load and development of resistance to the primary medications (Brown et al., 2000; Watson & Farley, 1999). There is a clear relationship between adherence and health, with full adherence associated with significantly lower or nonexistent viral load (Van Dyke et al., 2002; Watson & Farley, 1999).

HAART regimens typically involve two, three, or four medications, each administered up to eight times per day. Some of the regimens also require significant food restrictions and alterations (Pontali et al., 2001). In the majority of cases, parents are responsible for maintaining these regimens, although older children sometimes take personal responsibility. Parents and children have reported a number of barriers to adherence, including too many medications, scheduling problems, child behavior problems and refusal, poor taste and food interactions, and difficulty with pill swallowing or invasive medical procedures (Pontali et al., 2001; Van Dyke et al., 2002).

Strategies to improve adherence have included maintaining written medication schedules, improving the formulations of the antiretroviral medications, and using counseling to tailor the medication regimen to the specific needs and practices of individual families (Pontali et al., 2001). Children with HIV infection are more likely to adhere if they participate in the development of their treatment plans. Changes in routines, such as sleeping late on weekends, must be addressed and planned for to prevent declines in adherence. As children reach school age, they begin spending more time away from home and with their friends or extended family members who may not be aware of their status. Giving children a choice between liquid or pill form of the medication may increase adherence. Pill charts displaying stickers of each medication, the prescribed dose, and food requirements may also be helpful. Visual aids and rewards are valuable tools, particularly for younger children or for non-English-speaking or illiterate families.

For adolescents who are behaviorally infected with HIV and newly diagnosed, initiating HAART regimens can be even more demanding. Living arrangements, storage of medication, and support must be addressed. Some newly diagnosed teens do not disclose to family members right away, which can interfere with adherence as these teens may not have the needed support and monitoring for good adherence. Because poor adherence carries an increased risk for drug resistance, physicians may begin with placebo medications while the teen adjusts to the regimen.

Pain intervention strategies, such as use of cognitive-behavioral pain management strategies and topical analgesics, have proven effective in reducing distress and improving adherence with the blood drawing that is necessary with HAART (Schiff, Holtz, Peterson, & Rakusan, 2001). Although not reported in the literature, a number of immunology clinics have also implemented specific training in pill swallowing to facilitate adherence. Concrete, behavioral approaches appear most effective in addressing these issues.

Isolation/Stigmatization

The psychological ramifications of HIV infection are similar to those of other childhood chronic illnesses. Children with HIV experience repeated and painful medical procedures, recurring hospitalizations and medical visits, frequent school absences, and disruptions in daily routines. However, for the HIV-infected child, these stressors may be further complicated by feelings of shame about the disease, social stigma, and possible isolation. After disease disclosure to the child takes place, children are often instructed to keep their HIV status a secret from others. Families fear that they will be treated differently by the community and school. Fear of rejection by extended family members and friends is also a great concern. The burden of secrecy and feelings of being different from their peers put children at increased risk for significant feelings of shame and subsequent social withdrawal. Despite evidence about HIV modes of transmission, some families continue to be ostracized by other family members, landlords, employees, or friends who fear contagion (Steiner & Boyd-Franklin, 1995).

COMPREHENSIVE APPROACH TO SERVICES

As the system of care for pediatric HIV has evolved, the need for integrated, multidisciplinary approaches has been clearly recognized. Many programs now include specialists and primary care physicians, nurses, case managers, social workers, nutritionists, and psychologists. Besides just having these professionals available, a number of programs have developed new models for integrating services based on a recognition of the complex interactions between disease, treatment, environment, and development (Armstrong et al., 1999; Draimin, Gamble, Shire, & Hudis, 1998; Gerson et al., 2001; Ledlie, 2001). Although these models have not been subjected to rigid program evaluation and outcome comparisons, they represent innovative approaches to HIV care that may have relevance for dealing with other illnesses.

CURRENT ISSUES AND FUTURE CONSIDERATIONS

The face of pediatric HIV/AIDS has changed dramatically over the past 10 years. Although a cure for the illness is not yet available, HAART has transformed the disease from one inevitably causing significant illness and neurological consequences to one that can be managed with a reasonably good quality of life. Much of the research in the area of pediatric HIV/AIDS has involved very small samples, perhaps limiting the generalizability of findings. Research focusing on the effects of HIV in the HAART era will be even more challenging than in the past. With the success of early treatment and prevention of HIV transmission during labor and delivery, significantly fewer children will require treatment for vertically acquired HIV. Clearly, understanding the effects of HIV on the development of children will require complex models that examine the influence of the disease, development of the central nervous system, immunological parameters, and the influence of very significant environmental factors. It is unlikely that this kind of research can be conducted without multidisciplinary collaboration and collaboration among investigators working at different sites and centers across the country (Armstrong & Drotar, 2000; Stehbens et al., 1997).

In the United States much of the stigma associated with HIV is diminishing. However, the focus on "superconfidentiality" related to HIV and AIDS remains in place to protect the civil rights of infected individuals. The rights of children and adolescents to know about their diagnosis and anticipated consequences of their disease are being recognized, but these rights often conflict with the rights of parents. Sometimes the conflict is an emotional one, based on the parents' fear that the information will have a negative effect on the child. In other cases, the conflict is a legal one involving unconsented disclosure of the parent's diagnosis when the child with vertically acquired HIV is told his or her diagnosis. It is likely that this issue will involve court challenges, lawsuits, and ethics deliberations over the coming years. For psychologists, the lack of disclosure raises another important ethical concern. As we have noted, HIV is associated with significant neurocognitive impairment, and specific patterns of difficulty may emerge over time. The failure to disclose diagnostic information may, in many cases, serve as a barrier to access for needed special education services at a time when the services may be most helpful.

Finally, the primary focus on pediatric AIDS is likely to shift from the boundaries of the United States to focus on the world. At the current time, nearly one-third of the individuals living in sub-Saharan Africa are HIV infected, and the numbers of children who are infected is largely unknown. Most of these children and their parents have limited access to even basic antiretroviral therapy, much less HAART (Gow, 2002; Morison, 2001). Some investigators (Boivin et al., 1995; Drotar et al., 1997) have already expanded research efforts in these populations. Opportunities to better investigate and influence the psychological factors associated with prevention of HIV transmission, neurocognitive development in infected children, and access to effective care once it is available are likely to be rapidly expanding. The establishment of collaborations and development of expertise with international colleagues from multiple disciplines will be essential to the advancement of our understanding of HIV, treatment and intervention, and prevention on a worldwide basis over the coming decade.

ACKNOWLEDGMENTS

Preparation of this chapter was supported in part by the following grants: 2-U01-A12-756006, MCJ-129147-05-09, 90DD0408, and HA660862 Sub 03.

REFERENCES

American Academy of Pediatrics Committee on Pediatric AIDS. (1999). Disclosure of illness status to children and adolescents with HIV infection. *Pediatrics, 103,* 164–166.

Antle, B. J., Wells, L. M., Goldie, R. S., DeMatteo, D., & King, S. M. (2001). Challenges of parenting for families living with HIV/AIDS. *Social Work, 46,* 159–169.

Armistead, L., Tannenbaum, L., Forehand, R., Morse, E., & Morse, P. (2001). Disclosing HIV status: Are mothers telling their children? *Journal of Pediatric Psychology, 26,* 11–20.

Armstrong, F. D., & Drotar, D. (2000). Multi-institutional and multi-disciplinary research collaboration: Strategies and lessons from cooperative trials. In D. Drotar (Ed.), *Handbook of research in pediatric and clinical child psychology* (pp. 281–303). New York: Kluwer Academic/Plenum.

Armstrong, F. D., Harris, L. L., Thompson, W., Semrad, J. L., Jensen, M. M., Lee, D. Y., et al. (1999). The Outpatient Developmental Services Project: Integration of pediatric psychology with primary medical care for children infected with HIV. *Journal of Pediatric Psychology, 24,* 381–391.

Armstrong, F. D., & Mulhern, R. K. (1999). Acute lymphoblastic leukemia and brain tumors. In R.T. Brown (Ed.), *Cognitive aspects of chronic illness in children* (pp. 47–77). New York: Guilford Press.

Armstrong, F. D., Seidel, J. F., & Swales, T. P. (1993). Pediatric HIV infection: A neuropsychological and educational challenge. *Journal of Learning Disabilities, 26,* 92–103.

Bachanas, P. J., Kullgren, K. A., Schwartz, K. S., Lanier, B., McDaniel, J. S., Smith, J., & Nesheim, S. (2001). Predictors of psychological adjustment in school-age children infected with HIV. *Journal of Pediatric Psychology, 26,* 343–352.

Bachanas, P. J., Kullgren, K. A., Schwartz, K. S., McDaniel, J. S., Smith, J., & Nesheim, S. (2001). Psychological adjustment in caregivers of school-age children infected with HIV: Stress, coping, and family factors. *Journal of Pediatric Psychology, 26,* 331–342.

Bailey, R. C., Kamenga, M. C., Nsuami, M. J., Nieburg, P., & St. Louis, M. E. (1999). Growth of children according to maternal and child HIV, immunological and disease characteristics: A prospective cohort study in Kinshasa, Democratic Republic of Congo. *International Journal of Epidemiology, 28,* 532–540.

Battles, H. B., & Wiener, L. S. (2002). From adolescence through young adulthood: Psychosocial adjustment associated with long-term survival of HIV. *Journal of Adolescent Health, 30,* 161–168.

Bisiacchi, P. S., Suppiej, A., & Laverda, A. (2000). Neuropsychological evaluation of neurologically asymptomatic HIV-infected children. *Brain and Cognition, 43,* 49–52.

Blanchette, N., Smith, M. L., Fernandes-Penney, A., King, S., & Read, S. (2001). Cognitive and motor development in children with vertically transmitted HIV infection. *Brain and Cognition, 46,* 50–53.

Boivin, M. J., Green, S. D., Davies, A. G., Giordani, B., Mokili, J. K., & Cutting, W. A. (1995). A preliminary evaluation of the cognitive and motor effects of pediatric HIV infection in Zairian children. *Health Psychology, 14,* 13–21.

Bose, S., Moss, H. A., Brouwers, P., Pizzo, P., & Lorion, R. (1994). Psychologic adjustment of human immunodeficiency virus-infected school-age children. *Journal of Developmental and Behavioral Pediatrics, 15,* S26–S33.

Brouwers, P., Belman, A. L., & Epstein, L. G. (1994). Central nervous system involvement: Manifestations, evaluation, and pathogenesis. In P. A. Pizzo & C. M. Wilfert (Eds.), *Pediatric AIDS: The challenge of HIV infection in infants, children, and adolescents* (2nd ed., pp. 433–455). Baltimore: Williams & Wilkins.

Brouwers, P., Civitello, L., DeCarli, C., Wolters, P., & Sei, S. (2000). Cerebrospinal fluid viral load is related to cortical atrophy and not to intracerebral calcifications in children with symptomatic HIV disease. *Journal of Neurovirology, 6,* 390–397.

Brouwers, P., DeCarli, C., Civitello, L., Moss, H., Wolters, P., & Pizzo, P. (1995). Correlation between computed tomographic brain scan abnormalities and neuropsychological function in children with symptomatic human immunodeficiency virus disease. *Archives of Neurology, 52,* 39–44.

Brouwers, P., van Engelen, M., Lalonde, F., Perez, L., de Haan, E., Wolters, P., & Martin, A. (2001). Abnormally increased semantic priming in children with symptomatic HIV-1 disease: Evidence for impaired development of semantics? *Journal of the International Neuropsychology Society, 7,* 491–501.

Brown, L. K., Lourie, K. J., & Pao, M. (2000). Children and adolescents living with HIV and AIDS: A review. *Journal of Child Psychology and Psychiatry, 41,* 81–96.

Brown, L. K., Schultz, J. R., & Gragg, R. A. (1995). HIV-infected adolescents with hemophilia: Adaptation and coping: The Hemophilia Behavioral Intervention Evaluation Project. *Pediatrics, 96,* 459–463.

Butler, K. M., Husson, R. N., Balis, F. M., Brouwers, P., Eddy, J., el Amin, D., et al. (1991). Dideoxyinosine in children with symptomatic human immunodeficiency virus infection. *New England Journal of Medicine, 324,* 137–144.

Centers for Disease Control and Prevention. (2001). *HIV/AIDS Surveillance Report* (13th ed.). Atlanta, GA: Department of Health and Human Services, Public Health Service.

Chadwick, E.G., & Yogev, R. (1995). Pediatric AIDS. *Pediatric Clinics of North America, 42,* 969–992.

Chase, C., Ware, J., Hittelman, J., Blasini, I., Smith, R., Llorente, A., et al. (2000). Early cognitive and motor development among infants born to women infected with human immunodeficiency virus: Women and Infants Transmission Study Group. *Pediatrics, 106,* E25.

Chiriboga, C. A. (2002). Human immunodeficiency virus (HIV) in children. *Current Treatment Options in Neurology, 4,* 213–224.

Cohen, S. E., Mundy, T., Karassik, B., Lieb, L., Ludwig, D. D., & Ward, J. (1991). Neuropsychological functioning in human immunodeficiency virus Type 1 seropositive children infected through neonatal blood transfusion. *Pediatrics, 88,* 58–68.

Connor, E. M., Sperling, R. S., Gelber, R., Kiselev, P., Scott, G., O'Sullivan, M. J., et al. (1994). Reduction of maternal–infant transmission of human immunodeficiency virus Type 1 with zidovudine treatment: Pediatric AIDS Clinical Trials Group Protocol 076 Study Group. *New England Journal of Medicine, 331,* 1173–1180.

Coplan, J., Contello, K. A., Cunningham, C. K., Weiner, L. B., Dye, T. D., Roberge, L., et al. (1998). Early language development in children exposed to or infected with human immunodeficiency virus. *Pediatrics, 102,* e8.

Coscia, J. M., Christensen, B. K., & Henry, R. R. (1997). Risk and resilience in the cognitive functioning of children born to HIV-1–infected mothers: A preliminary report. *Pediatric AIDS and HIV Infection, 8,* 108–113.

Coscia, J. M., Christensen, B. K., Henry, R. R., Wallston, K., Radcliffe, J., & Rutstein, R. (2001). Effects of home environment, socioeconomic status, and health status on cognitive functioning in children with HIV-1 infection. *Journal of Pediatric Psychology, 26,* 321–329.

DeCarli, C., Fugate, L., Falloon, J., Eddy, J., Katz, D. A., Friedland, R. P., et al. (1991). Brain growth and cognitive improvement in children with human immunodeficiency virus–induced encephalopathy after 6 months of continuous infusion zidovudine therapy. *Journal of Acquired Immune Deficiency Syndrome, 4,* 585–592.

Draimin, B. H., Gamble, I., Shire, A., & Hudis, J. (1998). Improving permanency planning in families with HIV disease. *Child Welfare, 77,* 180–194.

Drotar, D., Olness, K., Wiznitzer, M., Guay, L., Marum, L., Svilar, G., et al. (1997). Neurodevelopmental outcomes of Ugandan infants with human immunodeficiency virus Type 1 infection. *Pediatrics, 100,* e5.

Englund, J. A., Baker, C. J., Raskino, C., McKinney, R. E., Lifschitz, M. H., Petrie, B., et al. (1996). Clinical and laboratory characteristics of a large cohort of symptomatic, human immunodeficiency virus-infected infants and children: AIDS Clinical Trials Group Protocol 152 Study Team. *Pediatric Infectious Disease Journal, 15,* 1025–1036.

Forehand, R., Steele, R., Armistead, L., Morse, E., Simon, P., & Clark, L. (1998). The Family Health Project: Psychosocial adjustment of children whose mothers are HIV infected. *Journal of Consulting and Clinical Psychology, 66,* 513–520.

Funck-Brentano, I., Costagliola, D., Seibel, N., Straub, E., Tardieu, M., & Blanche, S. (1997). Patterns of disclosure and perceptions of the human immunodeficiency virus in infected elementary school-age children. *Archives of Pediatric and Adolescent Medicine, 151,* 978–985.

Fundaro, C., Miccinesi, N., Baldieri, N. F., Genovese, O., Rendeli, C., & Segni, G. (1998). Cognitive impairment in school-age children with asymptomatic HIV infection. *AIDS Patient Care and STDs, 12,* 135–140.

Gay, C. L., Armstrong, F. D., Cohen, D., Lai, S., Hardy, M. D., Swales, T. P., et al. (1995). The effects of HIV on cognitive and motor development in children born to HIV-seropositive women with no reported drug use: Birth to 24 months. *Pediatrics, 96,* 1078–1082.

Geary, M. K., King, G., Forsberg, A. D., Delaronde, S. R., & Parsons, J. (1996). Issues of disclosure and condom use in adolescents with hemophilia and HIV: Hemophilia Behavioral Evaluative Intervention Project Staff. *Pediatric AIDS and HIV Infection, 7,* 418–423.

Gerson, A. C., Joyner, M., Fosarelli, P., Butz, A., Wissow, L., Lee, S., et al. (2001). Disclosure of HIV diagnosis to children: When, where, why, and how. *Journal of Pediatric Health Care, 15,* 161–167.

Gow, J. (2002). The HIV/AIDS epidemic in Africa: Implications for U.S. policy. *Health Affiliations, 21,* 57–69.

Gray, L., Newell, M. L., Thorne, C., Peckham, C., & Levy, J. (2001). Fluctuations in symptoms in human immunodeficiency virus–infected children: The first 10 years of life. *Pediatrics, 108,* 116–122.

Hanson, I. C., & Shearer, W. T. (1998). AIDS and other acquired immunodeficiency diseases. In R. D. Feigin & J. D. Cherry (Eds.), *Textbook of pediatric infectious diseases* (4th ed., pp. 954–979). Philadelphia: Saunders.

Hardy, M. S., Armstrong, F. D., Routh, D. K., Albrecht, J., & Davis, J. (1994). Coping and communication among parents and children with human immunodeficiency virus and cancer. *Journal of Developmental and Behavioral Pediatrics, 15,* S49–S53.

Havens, J., Whitaker, A., Feldman, J., Alvarado, L., & Ehrhardt, A. (1993). A controlled study of cognitive and language function in school-aged HIV-infected children. *Annals of the .New York Academy of Sciences, 693,* 249–251.

Havens, J. F., Whitaker, A. H., Feldman, J. F., & Ehrhardt, A. A. (1994). Psychiatric morbidity in school-age children with congenital human immunodeficiency virus infection: A pilot study. *Journal of Developmental and Behavioral Pediatrics, 15,* S18–S25.

Instone, S. L. (2000). Perceptions of children with HIV infection when not told for so long: Implications for diagnosis disclosure. *Journal of Pediatric Health Care, 14,* 235–243.

Knight, W. G., Mellins, C. A., Levenson, R. L., Jr., Arpadi, S. M., & Kairam, R. (2000). Brief report: Effects of pediatric HIV infection on mental and psychomotor development. *Journal of Pediatric Psychology, 25,* 583–587.

Ledlie, S. W. (1999). Diagnosis disclosure by family caregivers to children who have perinatally acquired HIV disease: When the time comes. *Nursing Research, 48,* 141–149.

Ledlie, S. W. (2001). The psychosocial issues of children with perinatally acquired HIV disease becoming adolescents: A growing challenge for providers. *AIDS Patient Care and STDs, 15,* 231–236.

Lewis, S. Y. (2001). Coping over the long haul: Understanding and supporting children and families affected by HIV disease [Commentary]. *Journal of Pediatric Psychology, 26,* 359–361.

Lewis, S. Y., Haiken, H. J., & Hoyt, L. G. (1994). Living beyond the odds: A psychosocial perspective on long-term survivors of pediatric human immunodeficiency virus infection. *Journal of Developmental and Behavioral Pediatrics, 15,* S12–S17.

Lipson, M. (1994). Disclosure of diagnosis to children with human immunodeficiency virus or acquired immunodeficiency syndrome. *Journal of Developmental Pediatrics, 15,* S61–S65.

Llorente, A. M., LoPresti, C. M., & Satz, P. (1997). Neuropsychological and neurobehavioral sequeale associated with pediatric HIV infection. In C. R. Reynolds & E. Fletcher-Janzen (Eds.), *Handbook of clinical child neuropsychology* (2nd ed., pp. 634–650). New York: Plenum Press.

Loveland, K. A., Stehbens, J., Contant, C., Bordeaux, J. D., Sirois, P., Bell, T. S., et al. (1994). Hemophilia growth and development study: Baseline neurodevelopmental findings. *Journal of Pediatric Psychology, 19,* 223–239.

Loveland, K. A., Stehbens, J. A., Mahoney, E. M., Sirois, P. A., Nichols, S., Bordeaux, J. D., et al. (2000). Declining immune function in children and adolescents with hemophilia and HIV infection: Effects on neuropsychological performance: Hemophilia Growth and Development Study. *Journal of Pediatric Psychology, 25,* 309–322.

Macmillan, C., Magder, L. S., Brouwers, P., Chase, C., Hittelman, J., Lasky, T., et al. (2001). Head growth and neurodevelopment of infants born to HIV-1–infected drug-using women. *Neurology, 57,* 1402–1411.

Mellins, C. A., & Ehrhardt, A. A. (1994). Families affected by pediatric acquired immunodeficiency syndrome: Sources of stress and coping. *Journal of Developmental and Behavioral Pediatrics, 15,* S54–S60.

Mellins, C. A., Levenson, R. L., Jr., Zawadzki, R., Kairam, R., & Weston, M. (1994). Effects of pediatric HIV infection and prenatal drug exposure on mental and psychomotor development. *Journal of Pediatric Psychology, 19,* 617–627.

Melton, S. T., Kirkwood, C. K., & Ghaemi, S. N. (1997). Pharmacotherapy of HIV dementia. *Annals of Pharmacotherapy, 31,* 457–473.

Mialky, E., Vagnoni, J., & Rutstein, R. (2001). School-age children with perinatally acquired HIV infection: Medical and psychosocial issues in a Philadelphia cohort. *AIDS Patient Care and STDs, 15,* 575–579.

Mintz, M. (1999). Clinical features and treatment interventions for human immunodeficiency virus–associated neurologic disease in children. *Seminars in Neurology, 19,* 165–176.

Mitchell, W. (2001). Neurological and developmental effects of HIV and AIDS in children and adolescents. *Mental Retardation and Developmental Disabilities Research Reviews, 7,* 211–216.

Morison, L. (2001). The global epidemiology of HIV/AIDS. *British Medical Bulletin, 58,* 7–18.

Moss, H., Bose, S., Wolters, P., & Brouwers, P. (1998). A preliminary study of factors associated with psychological adjustment and disease course in school-age children infected with the human immunodeficiency virus. *Journal of Developmental and Behavioral Pediatrics, 19,* 18–25.

Moss, H. A., Wolters, P. L., Brouwers, P., Hendricks, M. L., & Pizzo, P. A. (1996). Impairment of expressive behavior in pediatric HIV-infected patients with evidence of CNS disease. *Journal of Pediatric Psychology, 21,* 379–400.

Murphy, D. A., Steers, W. N., & Dello Stritto, M. E. (2001). Maternal disclosure of mothers' HIV serostatus to their young children. *Journal of Family Psychology, 15,* 441–450.

Murphy, L. M., Koranyi, K., Crim, L., & Whited, S. (1999). Disclosure, stress, and psychological adjustment among mothers affected by HIV. *AIDS Patient Care and STDs, 13,* 111–118.

New York State Department of Health. (2001). *Mental health care for people with HIV infection: HIV clinical guidelines for the primary care practitioner.* New York: New York State Department of Health AIDS Institute.

Pao, M., Lyon, M., D'Angelo, L. J., Schuman, W. B., Tipnis, T., & Mrazek, D. A. (2000). Psychiatric diagnoses in adolescents seropositive for the human immunodeficiency virus. *Archives of Pediatric and Adolescent Medicine, 154,* 240–244.

Pearson, D. A., McGrath, N. M., Nozyce, M., Nichols, S. L., Raskino, C., Brouwers, P., et al. (2000). Predicting HIV disease progression in children using measures of neuropsychological and neurological functioning: Pediatric AIDS Clinical Trials 152 Study Team. *Pediatrics, 106,* e76.

Pollack, H., Kuchuk, A., Cowan, L., Hacimamutoglu, S., Glasberg, H., David, R., et al. (1996). Neurodevelopment, growth, and viral load in HIV-infected infants. *Brain and Behavioral Immunology, 10,* 298–312.

Pontali, E., Feasi, M., Toscanini, F., Bassetti, M., De Gol, P., Nuzzolese, A., & Bassetti, D. (2001). Adherence to combination antiretroviral treatment in children. *HIV Clinical Trials, 2,* 466–473.

Rapoff, M. A., & Barnard, M. U. (1991). Compliance with pediatric medical regimens. In J. A. Cramer & B. Spilker (Eds.), *Patient compliance in medical practice and clinical trials* (pp. 73–98). New York: Raven Press.

Rigardetto, R., Vigliano, P., Boffi, P., Marotta, C., Raino, E., Arfelli, P., et al. (1999). Evolution of HIV-1 encephalopathy in children. *Panminerva Medicina, 41,* 221–226.

Schiff, W. B., Holtz, K. D., Peterson, N., & Rakusan, T. (2001). Effect of an intervention to reduce procedural pain and distress for children with HIV infection. *Journal of Pediatric Psychology, 26,* 417–427.

Simoni, J. M., Davis, M. L., Drossman, J. A., & Weinberg, B. A. (2000). Mothers with HIV/AIDS and their children: Disclosure and guardianship issues. *Women's Health, 31,* 39–54.

Simpson, D. M., & Berger, J. R. (1996). Neurologic manifestations of HIV infection. *Medical Clinics of North America, 80,* 1363–1394.

Smith, R., Malee, K., Charurat, M., Magder, L., Mellins, C., Macmillan, C., et al. (2000). Timing of perinatal human immunodeficiency virus Type 1 infection and rate of neurodevelopment: The Women and Infant Transmission Study Group. *Pediatric Infectious Disease Journal, 19,* 862–871.

Stehbens, J., Loveland, K. A., Bordeaux, J. D., Contant, C., Schiller, M., Scott, A., et al. (1997). A collaborative model for research: Neurodevelomental effects of HIV-1 in children and adolescents with hemophilia and an example. *Children's Health Care, 26,* 115–135.

Steiner, G. L., Boyd-Franklin, N., & Boland, M. (1995). Rationale and overview of the book. In N. Boyd-Franklin, G. Steiner, & M. G. Boland (Eds.), *Children, families, and HIV/AIDS: Psychosocial and therapeutic issues* (pp. 4–7). New York: Guilford Press.

Stoneburner, R., Sato, R., & Burton, A. (1994). The global HIV pandemic. *Acta Paediatrica, 400*(Suppl.), 1–4.

Tardieu, M., Mayaux, M. J., Seibel, N., Funck-Brentano, I., Straub, E., Teglas, J. P., & Blanche, S. (1995). Cognitive assessment of school-age children infected with maternally transmitted human immunodeficiency virus Type 1. *Journal of Pediatrics, 126,* 375–379.

Thorne, C., Newell, M. L., Botet, F. A., Bohlin, A. B., Ferrazin, A., Giaquinto, C., et al. (2002). Older children and adolescents surviving with vertically acquired HIV infection. *Journal of Acquired Immune Deficiency Syndrome, 29,* 396–401.

Van Dyke, R. B., Lee, S., Johnson, G. M., Wiznia, A., Mohan, K., Stanley, K., et al. (2002). Reported adherence as a determinant of response to highly active antiretroviral therapy in children who have human immunodeficiency virus infection. *Pediatrics, 109,* e61.

Watson, D. C., & Farley, J. J. (1999). Efficacy of and adherence to highly active antiretroviral therapy in children infected with human immunodeficiency virus Type 1. *Pediatric Infectious Disease Journal, 18,* 682–689.

Wiener, L. S., Battles, H. B., Heilman, N., Sigelman, C. K., & Pizzo, P. A. (1996). Factors associated with disclosure of diagnosis to children with HIV/AIDS. *Pediatric AIDS and HIV Infection, 7,* 310–324.

Wolters, P. L., Brouwers, P., Civitello, L., & Moss, H. A. (1997). Receptive and expressive language function of children with symptomatic HIV infection and relationship with disease parameters: A longitudinal 24-month follow-up study. *AIDS, 11,* 1135–1144.

Wolters, P. L., Brouwers, P., Moss, H. A., & Pizzo, P. A. (1994). Adaptive behavior of children with symptomatic HIV infection before and after zidovudine therapy. *Journal of Pediatric Psychology, 19,* 47–61.

22

Pediatric Neurological Conditions

Brain and Spinal Cord Injury and Muscular Dystrophy

SETH WARSCHAUSKY
DONALD G. KEWMAN
ANNE BRADLEY
PAMELA DIXON

This chapter includes overviews of a diverse set of pediatric neurological conditions with differing onsets, types of cognitive and/or motoric impairments, and prognoses. Traumatic brain injury (TBI) and spinal cord injury (SCI) have an acute onset and prolonged course of recovery, frequently resulting in chronic residual problems. Muscular dystrophies (MD) have variable courses, including fatal outcomes. These conditions present both overlapping and specific psychological challenges to children and their families. In developing effective psychological interventions for children with these conditions and their families, the pediatric rehabilitation psychologist must draw on a broad set of clinical skills and condition-specific knowledge.

TRAUMATIC BRAIN INJURY

Children with traumatic brain injury (TBI) are at increased risk for cognitive, behavioral, and emotional morbidities. Although severity of injury has been shown to be the most consistent determinant of the cognitive effects of injury, nonmedical factors account for a significant portion of the variance in behavioral outcomes. The neurobehavioral recovery of children from TBI is multiply determined by interrelated factors such as family functioning and child characteristics, both before and after injury.

Epidemiology and Etiology

Wide variability in pediatric TBI incidence and prevalence rates has been reported in studies within the United States, as well as between countries. The average incidence rate reported in studies reviewed by Kraus (1995) is approximately 180 per 100,000 children under 15 years of age. Among hospital-treated cases, approximately 75% are mild in severity, whereas 13% are severe (Lescohier & DiScala, 1993). There are significant changes in the risk associated with gender at different ages, with similar risk among children under age 5 and rising risk for boys through childhood and adolescence (Kraus, 1995). Causes of injury vary with age. Younger children are more likely to be injured in falls and violence associated with abuse, and older children and adolescents more likely to be injured in collisions, sports activities, and other types of violence (Kraus, 1995).

Pathophysiology

Distinctions are made between primary effects of injury that include contusions and hemorrhage and secondary effects, such as swelling and edema that arise subsequent to the trauma. Recent years have brought greater understanding of biochemical reactions following brain injury that lead to a significant portion of diffuse axonal injury noted macro- and microscopically in brain tissue. Severe TBI frequently leads to elevated intracranial pressure, and when pressure exceeds a critical value, cerebral blood flow diminishes and ischemic/hypoxic injury can occur. TBI includes increased risk of posttraumatic seizures, but development of an epileptic condition occurs in only about 2% of the population (McLean et al., 1995).

Assessment of Severity

Severity of TBI is determined by a number of key indicators, including depth of coma, neuropathology such as focal and diffuse injury, severity of elevated intracranial pressure, length of posttraumatic amnesia, presence or absence of hypoxic insult, and pupillary reactivity. Depth of coma is assessed with the Glasgow Coma Scale (GCS; Teasdale & Jennett, 1974), a rating typically first performed in the emergency room. The GCS includes specific ratings of eye opening and movement and verbal and motoric responses. In the research literature, length of coma often is described in terms of amount of time before the patient began to follow commands. With moderate to severe injury, in particular, neuroimaging typically involves a CT scan, with some centers also using MRI. Posttraumatic amnesia (PTA) is the period during which the patient's ability to lay down new memories is impaired. A number of instruments are used to assess PTA, including the Children's Orientation and Amnesia Test (COAT; Ewing-Cobbs, Levin, Fletcher, Minerm, & Eisenberg, 1990), a brief set of questions that can be administered to the patient on a daily basis.

Numerous studies have shown that severity of injury as assessed with depth of coma and presence of lesions predicts gross outcome, with severe injury producing much greater risk than mild or moderate. At this point, there is not conclusive evidence that mild injury entails increased risk of chronic neurobehavioral impairments, though early postconcussive symptoms are not unusual (Yeates et al., 1999).

Neurobehavioral Sequelae

In recent years, superb overviews of the neuropsychology of pediatric TBI have been published (e.g., Broman & Michel, 1995; Yeates, 2000). As the literature is quite complex, the reader is encouraged to refer to these resources. The early stages of recovery often are characterized using the Rancho Los Amigos Scale (Hagen, Malkmus, & Durham, 1972), an ordinal description of levels of cognitive and behavioral recovery from coma to purposeful/appropriate functioning. It is particularly helpful for families to have some understanding of these stages in early recovery, as behavioral symptoms, such as agitation, that may be quite disturbing may also reflect improvement in status.

One of the most robust findings with pediatric TBI is slowed processing speed. The processing speed index of the WISC-III is the most sensitive of the four index scores, showing strong associations with severity of injury as indicated by depth and length of coma (Donders, 1997). Tests of span of apprehension, such as digit span, are not particularly sensitive to TBI (Warschausky, Kewman, & Selim, 1996). There has been recent interest in pediatric TBI as entailing risk for an "acquired ADHD," but the very limited research to date suggests important group differences in the nature of inhibitory response deficits (Konrad, Gauggel, Manz, & Scholl, 2000).

Executive dysfunction also is common after moderate to severe TBI. Recent work has begun to shed light on both the primary nature of these dysfunctions and the functional correlates of specific deficits. Levin et al. (1997) have shown that severity of injury is associated with executive dysfunction and that brain lesion volume size and location are differentially associated with performance on different executive function tasks.

Although evidence exists that pediatric TBI is associated with risk of memory impairments, little is known about the specific nature of those impairments or the subtypes of impairments associated with specific types of injury (Hoffman, Donders, & Thompson, 2000). Severity of injury is associated with the magnitude of memory impairment as indicated by general performance on the California Verbal Learning Test—Children's Version (Delis, Kramer, Kaplan, & Ober, 1994). Some evidence exists for specific effects of pediatric TBI on the storage, retention, and retrieval processes.

Surprisingly little work documents the types of academic achievement difficulties associated with TBI. Although no evidence exists of a specific learning disability pattern associated with TBI, deficits in the areas of attention and executive functions, as well as memory, can have profound effects on academic functioning. Verbal IQ, however, appears to be one of the strongest predictors of academic placement and the need for special education services (Donders, 1994). Moderate to severe injury is associated with a decline in general adaptive functioning; assessment of adaptive behavior is a critical component in comprehensive neuropsychological evaluations (Max, Koele, Lindgren, et al., 1998).

Some evidence shows that, early in recovery, nonverbal functions, including visuoperceptual and visuoconstructive skill and ability, are impaired to a greater extent than are basic verbal functions. Early work by Chadwick, Rutter, Brown, Shaffer, and Traub (1981) indicated significant verbal–nonverbal discrepancies early in recovery, with closing of the gap over the first year following injury. Donders (1997) has shown the strong association between the WISC-III perceptual organization index and severity of injury.

Despite the apparent relative sparing of aspects of verbal intellect and vocabulary early in recovery, language functions such as discourse cohesion and inferencing have been shown to be impaired following injury (Chapman et al., 1992; Barnes & Dennis, 2001). In turn, these impairments may have specific adverse effects on aspects of social competence and social integration.

Psychological and Social Effects of TBI

Child Psychopathology

Traumatic brain injury can lead to marked psychological, behavioral, and social changes. Symptoms such as affective instability, aggression and rage, inattention, impaired social judgment, and apathy are significantly higher among children with severe TBI compared with orthopedic controls or groups with mild to moderate TBI (Brown, Chadwick, Shaffer, Rutter, & Traub, 1981; Taylor et al., 1999). Postinjury depressive symptomatology and diagnoses have been reported as occurring in up to 25% of children with severe injuries (Kirkwood et al., 2000; Max, Koele, Smith, et al., 1998). Max and colleagues found that almost 40% of their samples with severe injuries developed persistent personality change due to a TBI (Max et al., 2000). Early in recovery, however, it is important to differentiate between acute brain injury effects on affective expression and initiation and those of a depressive affective disorder.

Family Functioning

Caregivers of children with severe TBI, typically mothers, experience considerable psychological distress, family burden, and injury-related stress (Wade, Taylor, Drotar, Stancin, & Yeates, 1998). Wade and colleagues (1998) reported that 41% of the caregivers in their sample experienced significant distress, four times the level reported in normative samples. Changes in child behavior as a result of severe injury, such as increased dependence, fatigue, argumentativeness, and decreased concentration, are associated with increases in family strain (Rivara et al., 1996). Postinjury family functioning is most strongly predicted by preinjury family functioning, as well as by the development of postinjury psychological disorders in the child (Max, Castillo, et al., 1998).

Recent findings provide strong support for a bidirectional relationship between child and family functioning. Family variables such as structure, warmth, and marital conflict have effects on children's psychological and behavioral status (Wade, Drotar, Taylor, & Stancin, 1995). Taylor and colleagues found that postinjury parental distress and burden predict more behavior problems and lower levels of adaptive behavior; in turn, more child behavior problems are associated with subsequent increases in parental distress and burden (Taylor et al., 2001).

The preinjury functioning of families is an important predictor of the psychological resources available to families to help with coping and adaptation through the initial trauma and phases of recovery. High preinjury general family functioning predicts positive postinjury child adaptive functioning, social competence, and overall psychological/behavioral functioning at 1 year post-TBI (Rivara et al., 1993). Yeates et al. (1997) found that high preinjury family functioning buffered the behavioral effects of the injury and that low family functioning exacerbated effects.

Rehabilitation and Reintegration after TBI

Psychological and Behavioral Interventions

There are a small number of outcome studies of psychological intervention for children with TBI, largely consisting of case studies of behavioral intervention for externalizing behaviors or strategies for cognitive skill acquisition (Kehle, Clark, & Jenson, 1996). Misconceptions about interventions with children with TBI include assumed intractability of behaviors associated with organicity and the biased focus on addressing maladaptive rather than adaptive behavior (Deaton, 1987).

Aggression and Disinhibition

Aggressive behavior can be exhibited while a child is agitated, both in the acute stages of recovery and as a long-term consequence of TBI. Operant conditioning has been used successfully to address aggression, screaming, and noncompliance prior to full resolution of posttraumatic amnesia (PTA; Slifer et al., 1996) These studies suggest that memory impairments associated with PTA do not preclude the application of behavioral treatments. Feeney and Ylvisaker (1995) have described a school-based behavioral intervention that was successful in reducing or eliminating aggressive behavior. However, in their study, aggressive behavior resumed on withdrawal of treatment, indicating the necessity for ongoing intervention.

Anxiety and Depression

Both pharmacological and psychotherapeutic treatment of internalizing symptoms occur in most settings, yet little information is available regarding the applicability or need for modification of these treatments in cases of TBI. Intervention frequently focuses on depression and bereavement associated with loss of function or the loss of a loved one in the accident. Anxiety, though not well studied, is sometimes exhibited acutely following TBI or can emerge later in recovery. Although anxiety can be transient, sustained reactions require systematic intervention, commonly cognitive and behavioral interventions, sometimes in combination with pharmacological treatment.

Social Interventions

Children with TBI are at risk for impaired social skills and isolation (Bohnert, Parker, & Warschausky, 1997; Warschausky, Cohen, Parker, Levendosky, & Okun, 1997). Social skills programs in school settings include general skills training and targeted interventions that largely focus on aggression. These school-based programs often are derived from cognitive-behavioral models that assume either intact cognitive abilities or global mental impairment. Children who sustain TBI tend to lack assertiveness skills and have a complex set of cognitive difficulties. Thus programs frequently do not target needed content and are not tailored to the unique cognitive deficits of persons with acquired brain dysfunction.

The "Building Friendships" program is an example of a collaborative social integration program that includes the child, parent, school staff, and peers (Cooley, Glang, & Voss, 1997). Limited outcome study data indicate that the program increased participant social contact (Glang, Todis, Cooley, Wells, & Voss, 1997). Importantly, follow-up data indicated that the social improvements were not maintained after facilitation was withdrawn. School-based social integration interventions appear quite promising, but it is essential to include generalization and maintenance strategies in these programmatic interventions (Lloyd & Cuvo, 1994).

Parent Training and Intervention

Treatment of parental distress following a child's TBI can address both the well-being of parents and the potential adverse effects of parent distress on the recovery of the child. Indirect effects of distress can include compromised functioning in new roles, such as case manager and rehabilitation team member. In a small exploratory study comparing types of parent interventions, a stress management–support group exhibited greater reduction in depression and anxiety than an information–support group (Singer et al., 1994).

School Reentry

The potential motor, language, cognitive, and behavioral sequelae of TBI necessitate planning for the child's reentry into school. The Individuals with Disabilities Education Act (IDEA) mandates that TBI be considered a distinct disability category. As a result, children who exhibit TBI-associated cognitive impairments are eligible and entitled to services that will facilitate their education in an effort to maximize their participation in school, though states differ in how TBI fits into state special education eligibility categories.

Research suggests that classmates are more supportive of the reentering child when they have been educated about the particular illness or injury and that they demonstrate more positive behavioral intentions toward children with disabilities when they are exposed to programs that promote acceptance (Morgan, Bieberich, Walker, & Schwerdtfeger, 1998). School personnel can benefit from general information about TBI, as well as specific recommendations for the child, based on neuropsychological test findings and physical needs.

SPINAL CORD INJURY

The overall prevalence of SCI has been conservatively estimated at approximately 721 per 1 million persons (Harvey, Rothchild, Asmann, & Stripling, 1990), or approximately 206,000, based on a current U.S. population estimate of 286 million. Children 0–15 years make up only about 4% of those newly injured (Nobunaga, Go, & Karunas, 1999); however, older adolescents and young adults ages 16–30 comprise the largest group of newly injured (54.1%). Males slightly outnumber females, 1.5:1, before age 9, but by the ages of 16–20 the ratio is approximately 5:1 (Vogel & DeVivo, 1996).

Motor vehicle accidents are the most common cause of SCI, accounting for about 41% of injuries in both children and adults and about one-half in those below age 21. In those under 21 years of age, trauma from sports accidents is the second leading cause of SCI (22.9%), followed by violence (18.6%). However, etiology varies between demographic groups. For example, violence is the cause of injury in more than one-half of African Americans ages 0–20 (Vogel & DeVivo, 1996). Etiology also varies by age. For instance, child abuse and birth trauma are causes of SCI unique to the neonate and infant populations.

In adolescents and adults, spinal cord injuries most frequently result from a vertebral fracture or dislocation that impinges on the spinal cord, causing bruising, tearing, or bleeding. In contrast, 50% of children under age 10 receive traction, contusion, or ischemic injury to the spinal cord, with no radiological evidence of fracture or dislocation (Boyd & Perrin, 1992). Approximately 70% of those injured before age 9 have thoracic lumbar or sacral injuries that result in paraplegia, whereas those ages 9–20 have a much higher proportion of cervical injuries (53–54%) that result in tetraplegia (Vogel & DeVivo, 1996.) A high percentage of SCIs in young children are complete injuries, including both sensory and motoric loss (Dickman & Rekate, 1993), with a 0–10% prognosis for functional recovery. Approximately 40% of children with SCIs who were injured in motor vehicle accidents have associated head injuries (Eleraky, Theodore, Adams, Rekate, & Sonntag, 2000).

Changes in the acute medical treatment of SCI and rehabilitative treatment have improved the functional capabilities of children and adolescents with SCI. Such innovations can also have a positive impact on quality of life (e.g., Pontari et al., 2000). Improvements in the ability of children to demonstrate gains in functional skill involving residual motor abilities has been found to occur more rapidly during inpatient rehabilitation after SCI in adolescents ages 16–18 than in younger children ages 7–15 (Dixon, Warschausky, Tate, & Karunas, 2001).

Complications

Children with complete injuries will usually lose normal sensation, as well as use of muscles controlled by nerves below the level of injury. Those with lesions at or above C3 (the third cervical vertebra) will usually be unable to breathe without mechanical ventilation. Most children will have neurogenic bowels and bladders, with a resulting inability to control defecation and urination in the usual fashion. Boys often lose their ability to have psychogenic erections and their ability to ejaculate; however, they may be able to obtain reflex erections. Girls maintain their fertility but often lose normal genital sensation. Children with sensory loss due to SCI are prone to decubitus ulcers (i.e., pressure sores) on their legs, buttocks, or bony prominences, which can lead to serious infections. The most serious and immediately life-threatening complication of SCI above the T6 (the sixth thoracic vertebra) is autonomic dysreflexia, a sudden and extreme elevation in blood pressure (Boyd & Perrin, 1992). The experience of acute anxiety has been known to be associated with autonomic dysreflexia; therefore, careful evaluation of anxiety complaints to rule out associated dysreflexia is important.

Psychosocial Adjustment of Children

The literature about the psychosocial effects of SCI on children is sparse and largely theoretical (Warschausky, Engel, Kewman, & Nelson, 1996). The early effects of SCI may give rise to bizarre experiences that are difficult for a child to comprehend or integrate. The child loses bodily sensations and may initially experience the sense that his or her head is free-floating or legs are twisted in an unnatural fashion (Boyd & Perrin, 1992). Children may exhibit a range of reactions to their SCI, including becoming noncommunicative, irritable, withdrawn, aggressive, and noncompliant, refusing to eat, engaging in passive self-destructive behavior, having difficulty sleeping, or exhibiting regressive behavior.

Psychosocial Adjustment of Adolescents

Psychological adjustment to SCI may be most difficult for adolescents. Adolescents' initial reactions may include a period of withdrawal, slowed thought processes, and depersonalization. This period often is followed by the adolescent's conviction that he or she will walk again. Upon acknowledging his or her paralysis and its sequelae, the adolescent may experience rage, intense grief, and humiliation. The adolescent may believe that the injury is punishment for real or imagined faults. As rehabilitation hospitalizations have become shorter in recent years, much of the emotional adjustment to SCI occurs after discharge.

Children and adolescents with SCI run a higher risk of developing a posttraumatic stress disorder (PTSD). In one study of persons with SCI ages 11–24, 25% met diagnostic criteria for PTSD (Boyer, Knolls, Kafkalas, & Tollen, 2000). Traumatic experiences in life prior to an SCI have been shown to increase the risk of developing PTSD after an SCI in adults (Radnitz, Schlein, & Hsu, 2000). It is quite possible that these findings also extend to the younger population with SCI. In addition, a child whose SCI was caused by violence, such as a gunshot, were frequently involved in alcohol and drug use at the time of their injury (Graham & Weingarden, 1989). Many of these youngsters were reluctant to discuss the circumstances of their injuries. Families of these children report feelings of isolation and ongoing fears of further violence (Havel & Lawrence, 1993).

In general, adolescents with SCIs struggle to cope with their physical changes. They compare their bodies with those of their nondisabled peers and can develop a negative view of themselves (Mulcahey, 1992). Participants in Dewis's (1989) study were focused on obtaining a superficial sense of physical normality, making great efforts to cover up evidence of their disabilities with clothing and to hide any sign of discomfort, pain, or fatigue related to their injuries. Several studies indicate that loss of bowel and bladder control was an important concern for most of the participants, and many expressed shame and embarrassment about bowel programs and urinary catheterization to empty their bladders (Dewis, 1989; Mulcahey, 1992).

SCI and resulting impaired mobility diminish the adolescent's freedom and ability to interact with his or her peers (Rutledge & Dick, 1983). Social withdrawal may lead to diminished social experience and subsequent failure to develop mature social skills.

Long-Term Psychological Consequences

Studies have found that, in the long term, young people with either an SCI or spina bifida had a positive sense of self and global self-worth that was similar to that of nondisabled peers. Furthermore, the level of self-worth was not associated with severity of disability. It was, however, strongly related to perceived social support from parents (Antle, 2000). The long-term outcomes for adults who incurred a pediatric SCI show that life satisfaction is associated with greater education, income, satisfaction with employment and social and recreational opportunities, and fewer medical complications. Life satisfaction was not associated with severity of injury or age of injury (Vogel, Klaas, Lubicky, & Anderson, 1998). Measures of psychopathology and health often do not differ significantly between participants with pediatric versus adult-onset SCI or physically healthy controls (Sammallahti, Kannisto, & Aalberg, 1996).

Effects on the Family

The SCI of a family member disrupts family task organization, sometimes causing role strain. In her study of changes in family roles after a family member's SCI, Killen (1990) found that the injury predisposed family members toward more traditional, familiar roles. Respondents to Killen's study reported that a child's SCI was initially viewed as a severe crisis that would lessen gradually over time; yet the sense of crisis never dissipated for a majority of family members. At the same time, many respondents to the study reported that the child's SCI increased their family's strength and solidarity.

Mothers and fathers tended to view the traumatic experience of SCI as more frightening and causing greater feelings of helplessness than did their injured children (Boyer et al., 2000). Boyer et al. (2000) found that 41% of mothers and 35.6% of fathers of children with SCI met diagnostic criteria for PTSD. Mothers' posttraumatic stress scores were most highly correlated with their injured child's score and the father's score, whereas fathers' scores were not strongly correlated with their child's score.

Conflict centering on different views of the injured child's abilities may arise between parents and the child; for example, an adolescent is likely to rebel against a parent who infantilizes him or her because of his or her SCI. Iannacconi (1994) reported that 24% of adolescents with SCI feel infantilized and overprotected by their parents. Parental overprotection is a common barrier to emotional and physical rehabilitation.

Treatment Issues in Child and Family Adaptation to SCI

Research on perceptions and attributions of children and adults with SCI reveals that greater passivity and dependence are associated with poorer outcomes in adulthood. Among adults who sustained injuries in childhood, a greater sense of internal locus of control and less perception of powerful others as sources of control were associated with better outcomes, including greater subjective sense of well-being and physical health, respectively (Krause, Stanwyck, & Maides, 1998). Studies of adults who sustained injuries as children suggest that measures of psychological well-being, including depression, self-esteem, self-perception, and "life satisfaction," were not significantly related to level of injury (Vogel et al., 1998). The same is true among adolescents and children for self-esteem (Antle, 2000). However, the level of injury may influence the processes that are used to achieve this adaptation. Sammallahti et al. (1996) found that less severely injured adults with pediatric SCI onset were more likely to use task orientation as an adaptive coping mechanism than more severely injured participants. Quality of peer and family social relations is also related to psychological outcome in SCI and may facilitate adaptation. Antle (2000) found that feelings of self-worth were significantly associated with perceived social support of friends and parents.

Compliance with Medical Treatment and Psychological Well-Being

Medical complications often have a negative impact on global perceptions of well-being and functional independence. Vogel et al. (1998) found that measures of life satisfaction in adults with pediatric SCI onset were negatively related to medical complications. Muscle spasticity in children tends to be more severe than in adults and is more likely to be associated with pain or discomfort. Interventions that assist in identifying and avoiding noxious stimuli, vigilance with range of motion exercises, and proper body positioning are helpful in managing spasticity. Pain and distress management interventions would likely be helpful, as well.

Skin integrity is another common medical complication that interferes with functionality. Pressure sores are more likely in children with paraplegia than tetraplegia and in children who are 8 to 12 years of age. Hickey, Anderson, and Vogel (1999) hypothesize that adults' expectations that children at 8 to 9 years of age can take on higher levels of responsibility for self-care may exceed their capacity to follow through with the high degree of consistency needed for SCI self-care.

Treatment of PTSD in Children with SCI and Their Families

As noted, children with SCI and their parents run a higher risk of acute and chronic traumatic stress symptoms. Empirical evidence for effective treatment of PTSD tends to support cognitive behavioral approaches over other therapeutic approaches or medication management alone (Cohen, Berliner, & March, 2000). Cohen, Mannarino, Berliner, and Esther (2000) identify four major aspects of cognitive-behavioral treatment that, used in combination, were associated with a decrease in PTSD symptoms in children. These include exposure techniques (details of the traumatic event are reviewed or imagined), addressing cognitive distortions (i.e., self-blame, survivor guilt, and change in worldview), replacing automatic negative thoughts, and teaching stress management strategies (i.e., relaxation techniques and thought stopping or replacement). Treatment of parental PTSD symptoms is considered the fourth important component in treatment of children with PTSD.

Issues in Sexuality Counseling and Education

Important issues in sexuality counseling and education specific to SCI include providing education regarding the impact of SCI on sexual and reproductive functioning, identifying and challenging perceptions and attributions that impede successful adaptation to changes in psychosexual functions, identifying risk factors for delayed sexual development and solving problems, and developing skills and tools to reduce the risk of sexual and physical abuse.

The impact of SCI on sexual arousal is as variable as the injuries sustained (Sipski, 1997). The exact nature of changes in genital and other erogenous zone sensation and response varies with level and completeness of SCI. Areas of the body both above and below the level of injury can be responsive to sexual arousal. Male infertility is common due to ejaculation difficulties, low sperm counts, and poor sperm motility. Improvements in assisted reproductive technology can often overcome these barriers. A short-term cessation of menstruation is common in postpubertal females just post-SCI onset, but it resumes, and females often return to premorbid reproductive capacities. However, rates for pregnancies vary depending on level of injury sustained, with fewer pregnancies at higher levels and with more complete injuries (Charlifue, Gerhart, Menter, Whiteneck, & Manley, 1992).

Children and adolescents with SCI run a risk of delayed psychosexual development due to such factors as lack of access to peers related to social isolation and the impact of medical and therapeutic regimens on time available for social activities, lack of knowledge about sexuality in general and their own sexual and reproductive capabilities in particular, parenting issues such as constraints on the development of independence, and parental doubts about the adolescent's capabilities and potential (Kewman, Warschausky, Engel, & Warzak, 1997). Lack of role models has been identified as an inhibiting factor in sexual identity development for people with disabilities. Kewman et al. (1997) and Hwang (1997) highlight the increased risk for sexual and physical abuse in people with physical disabilities. Providing education and counseling in matters of assertive behavior, identifying warning signs of abusive relationships, and avoiding or eliciting assistance in problematic situations is thus indicated.

Reentry and Reintegration into the Larger Community

Research highlights the importance of educational, vocational, social, and recreational opportunities for children, adolescents, and adults to their psychological well-being and their relative lack of access to these opportunities. However, little research is available that identifies important factors or interventions to promote integration. Dudgeon, Massagli, and Ross (1997) surveyed children with SCI and their teachers and found that accommodations in schools, such as human assistance, assistive technology, and curriculum modifications, were often geared toward participation rather than quality of performance and degree of productivity. They expressed concern that the emphasis on participation may fail to prepare children for the quality and productivity requirements in the workplace. Employment or student status in adults with SCI also is associated with quality-of-life indices (Krause & Anson, 1997). The employment rate for persons with SCI who were injured before age 25 was approximately 32% in one multicenter study (Krause et al., 1999).

MUSCULAR DYSTROPHY

The common types of muscular dystrophy (MD) that present in childhood include Duchenne/Becker muscular dystrophy, myotonic dystrophy, congenital muscular dystrophy, limb girdle muscular dystrophy, facioscapulohumeral dystrophy, and Emery-Dreifuss muscular dystrophy (Roland, 2000). The mode of inheritance varies, with Duchenne/Becker and Emery-Dreifuss being X-linked recessive, congenital muscular dystrophies being autosomal recessive, and the others being autosomal dominant. X-linked muscular dystrophies affect only males, with very rare exceptions, whereas other types affect both sexes. There has been rapid progress in identifying the locations of gene defects associated with the different types of MD. Duchenne MD mRNA has been found in brain tissue (Nudel, Robzyk, & Yaffe, 1988; Chamberlain, 1988), with evidence of differences in the mRNA in brain versus muscle (Nudel et al., 1989). The associated dystrophin deficiency in the brain is thought to have complex effects on brain development and integrity of synaptic membranes (Mehler, 2000).

Duchenne muscular dystrophy (DMD), an X-linked form, accounts for approximately 45–55% of the incidence of MD worldwide, with incidence rates typically in the range of 20–30 per 100,000 male births and a prevalence of 3 per 100,000 in the general population (Walton & Gardner-Medwin, 1988). Although the incidence rate of each type of muscular dystrophy reportedly has declined since the 1950s, the prevalence rates have been increasing, probably due to improvements in medical care and increased life expectancy. Diagnosis of muscular dystrophy typically stems from developmental history, levels of serum creatine kinase, electromyography, and muscle biopsy. Duchenne and Becker types are distinguished by the presence of dystrophin that, although abnormal, is much higher in the latter disorder.

Onset and progression of illness varies with subtype. DMD symptoms usually are not noted prior to age 2. At ages 2–3, clumsiness, toe-walk, and falls may be noted, and hypertrophy begins to appear. At ages 3–6, gross motor signs, such as frequent falling and increased difficulty climbing stairs, become more prominent. Around age 7, decline becomes precipitous; most children use wheelchairs for ambulation by middle childhood. Physical therapy, orthotics, and surgery can prolong ambulation, but it is very rare to see ambulation beyond age 12. Cardiomyopathy is prevalent. Respiratory difficulty increases, and contractures develop. Following loss of ambulation, 95% of children develop scoliosis. Death usually is due to respiratory failure. There have been advances in pharmacological treatments for DMD, including use of corticosteroids to slow progression of the disease, and current treatment research directions include work to develop gene therapies (Bertolini, 2001).

A number of authors have developed functional classifications of stages of DMD deterioration, the extent to which ambulation is independent is a key variable (Vignos, 1977; Zellweger & Hanson, 1967). The Becker type illness has a later onset than DMD, usually around age 11. Course of illness is more benign, and the cognitive deficits often noted in DMD are not prominent. Course of illness in the autosomal recessive and facioscapulohumeral types is quite variable, with significant differences in symptoms and rapidity of decline among lower subtypes.

DMD and Cognition

Duchenne's (Duchenne de Boulogne, 1868) initial descriptions of DMD included observations of diminished intellect. Cotton, Voudouris, and Greenwood (2001) demonstrated that IQs are normally distributed around a mean of 80.2. Intelligence does not appear to correlate with degree of physical disability or cortical atrophy. Although children with DMD tend to exhibit increased head circumference, there is no correlation between circumference and either intellect or degree of physical disability. Associations between intelligence and DNA deletions have been inconclusive, though recent evidence is promising (Al-Qudah, Kobayashi, Chuang, Dennis, & Ray, 1990; Felisari et al., 2000). Findings regarding the stability of level of intellect in DMD have been inconsistent, and some researchers have speculated that a number of intellectual profiles may be associated with DMD subtypes (Cotton et al., 2001).

Neuropsychological studies remain sparse, but initial findings suggest areas of deficit apart from level of intellect, as well as changes in the neuropsychological profile with development. Children with DMD have been found to exhibit specific deficits in attention, verbal fluency, and aspects of memory, but findings are too sparse and preliminary to be summarized as an identifiable profile (Cotton, Crowe, & Voudouris, 1998). Recent evidence of specific verbal working memory deficits is particularly promising (Hinton, De Vivo, Nereo, Goldstein, & Stern, 2001). Decreases in visual-motor functions with age appear to be specifically related to decreased motor speed (Cotton et al., 2001; Sollee, Latham, Kindlon, & Bresnan, 1985).

Psychological and Social Functioning

There are indications that the psychological adjustment of children with muscular dystrophies may be related to type of illness, age, and physical decline. Consistent with general findings regarding children with disabilities (Lavigne & Faier-Routman, 1992), children with DMD exhibit greater prevalence of clinically significant distress, with predominant internalizing features, when compared with peers without physical or cognitive impairments. Thompson, Zeman, Fanurik, & Sirotkin-Roses (1992) found a very high percentage (89%) of parent-reported behavior problems in this population; however, findings regarding the psychological adjustment of older versus younger boys with DMD are inconsistent. Harper (1983) found that although MMPI profiles of adolescents with DMD were similar to those of a comparison group with mixed orthopedic conditions, emotional distress and social withdrawal were noted with physical deterioration. MMPI profiles of individuals with noncongenital myotonic muscular dystrophy fall within normal limits (Franzese et al., 1991); however, subclinical concerns included dysthymic features.

DMD, as a debilitating, progressive, and ultimately fatal condition in which caregiving demands increase over time, is associated with a high percentage of parents reporting significant psychological distress. Stressors identified by parents include difficulties obtaining adequate resources, practical difficulties in providing care (e.g., lifting and toileting), and emotional reactions (Firth, Gardner-Medwin, Hosking, & Wilkinson, 1983). Thompson et al. (1992) found that 57% of parents with a child with DMD reported poor adjustment. Mediating variables include palliative versus adaptive coping and family conflict. Parental stress appraisals, palliative coping, and distress are associated with children's behavioral problems. Importantly, parents report significant concerns about how to discuss DMD with their affected sons (Buchanan, LaBarbera, Roelofs, & Olson, 1979; Firth et al., 1983).

Respiratory failure due to muscle fatigue, atelectasis, pneumonia, or retained secretions is the major cause of death in DMD. Deterioration in respiratory status correlates with functional class and peripheral muscle strength. In later-stage illness, patient and family may face decisions regarding mechanical ventilation. Patients and family members generally preferred to receive information regarding mechanical ventilation prior to the onset of respiratory failure (Miller, Colbert, & Osberg, 1990). Knowledge regarding the disease process, resources, and the difficulties inherent in discontinuing ventilator support, once initiated, are cited by families as important in decisions regarding ventilator dependency. Physicians' beliefs and practices regarding disclosure of long-term mechanical ventilation options with families sometimes are influenced by the physician's determination of the patient's quality of life rather than the principle of assuring informed consent and decision making.

Ventilator dependency appears to have a more negative impact on family members than on patients, as social lives and recreation are restricted. Mothers typically discontinue employment to become full-time caregivers with onset of ventilator dependency. A significant body of literature addresses family stress in home care of ventilator-dependent children, with repeated emphasis on the importance of resources, including adequate home care staffing and respite options to buffer stress.

CONCLUSIONS

This diverse set of conditions entails differing degrees and types of psychological risk. Children with brain injury appear to be at greater risk for long-term emotional, behavioral, and social difficulties than children with SCI or muscular dystrophy. With TBI, unlike many other medical conditions, severity of condition is associated with increased risk of psychopathology; neuropsychologically informed intervention planning is essential. That said, family functioning is a critical predictor of psychological and behavioral outcome after TBI and remains a central focus for pediatric psychological assessment and intervention. SCI and muscular dystrophy involve physical disabilities, and psychological risks tend to be associated with specific medical and developmental phases. Sustaining an SCI in adolescence appears to be associated with greater initial psychological risk, though long-term adjustment typically is quite positive. As discussed, the relatively high risk for PTSD warrants specific focus for assessment. There can be periods during recovery, development, or deterioration of condition during which the psychological needs of parents may be as significant as or more significant than those of the child.

The three neurological conditions described are associated with chronic childhood disability. The pediatric psychologist has an important role as an advocate in facilitating community integration and highlighting the importance of access to social activities for healthy child adjustment and development. Often, specific advocacy is needed to help with school planning. Apart from addressing acute stress and affective and behavioral dysfunction, a key goal is to empower the child and family by helping to develop their knowledge of disability rights and accessible community activities.

REFERENCES

Al-Qudah, A. A., Kobayashi, J., Chuang, S., Dennis, M., & Ray, P. (1990). Etiology of intellectual impairment in Duchenne muscular dystrophy. *Pediatric Neurology, 6*, 57–59.

Antle, B. J. (2000). Seeking strengths in young people with physical disabilities: Learning from the self-perceptions of children and young adults. *Dissertation Abstracts International, 60*(10-A), 3795.

Barnes, M. A., & Dennis M. (2001). Knowledge-based inferencing after childhood head injury. *Brain and Language, 76,* 253–265.

Bertolini, T. E. (2001). Muscular dystrophies. In R. Pourmand (Ed.), *Neuromuscular diseases* (pp. 227–293). Woburn, MA: Butterworth-Heinemann.

Bohnert, A., Parker, J., & Warschausky, S. (1997) Friendship adjustment in children following traumatic brain injury. *Developmental Neuropsychology, 13,* 477–486.

Boyd, J., & Perrin, J. C. S. (1992). Spinal cord injury. In E. Molnar (Ed.), *Pediatric rehabilitation* (2nd ed., pp. 336–362). Baltimore: Williams & Wilkins.

Boyer, B. A., Knolls, M. L., Kafkalas, C. M., & Tollen, L. G. (2000). What is the trauma?: Patients', mothers' and fathers' fear and helplessness related to post-traumatic aspects of pediatric SCI. *Topics in Spinal Cord Injury Rehabilitation, 6*(Suppl.), 134–147.

Broman, S. H., & Michel, M. E. (1995). *Traumatic head injury in children.* New York: Oxford University Press.

Brown, G., Chadwick, O., Shaffer, D., Rutter, M., & Traub, M. (1981). A prospective study of children with head injuries: III. Psychiatric sequelae. *Psychological Medicine, 11,* 63–78.

Buchanan, D. C., LaBarbera, C. J., Roelofs, R., & Olson, W. (1979). Reactions of families to children with Duchenne muscular dystrophy. *General Hospital Psychiatry, 1,* 262–269.

Chadwick, O., Rutter, M., Brown, G., Shaffer, D., & Traub, M. (1981). A prospective study of children with head injuries: II. Cognitive sequelae. *Psychological Medicine, 11,* 49–61.

Chamberlain, J. S. (1988). Expression of the murine Duchenne muscular dystrophy gene in muscle and brain. *Science, 239,* 1416–1418.

Chapman, S. B., Culhane, K. A., Levin, H. S., Harard, H., Mendelsohn, D., Weing-Cobbs, L., et al. (1992). Narrative discourse after closed head injury in children and adolescents. *Brain and Language, 43,* 42–65.

Charlifue, W. W., Gerhart, K. A., Menter, R. R., Whiteneck, G. G., & Manley, M. S. (1992). Sexual issues of women with spinal cord injuries. *Paraplegia, 30,* 192–199.

Cohen, J., Mannarino, A., Berliner, L., & Deblinger, E. (2000). Trauma-focused cognitive behavioral therapy for children and adolescents: An empirical update. *Journal of Interpersonal Violence, 15,* 1202–1223.

Cohen, J. A., Berliner, L. M., & March, J. S. (2000). Treatment of children and adolescents. In E. B. Foa, T. M. Keane, & M. J. Friedman (Eds.), *Effective treatments for PTSD: Practice guidelines from the International Society for Traumatic Stress Studies* (pp. 330–332). New York: Guilford Press.

Cooley, E. A., Glang, A., & Voss, J. (1997) Making connections: Helping children with ABI build friendships. In A. Glang, G. H. S. Singer & B. Todis (Eds.), *Students with acquired brain injury: The school's response* (pp. 255–275). Baltimore: Brookes.

Cotton, S., Crowe, S. F., & Voudouris, N. (1998). Neuropsychological profile of Duchenne muscular dystrophy. *Child Neuropsychology, 4*(2), 110–117.

Cotton, S., Voudouris, N. J., & Greenwood, K. M. (2001). Intelligence and Duchenne muscular dystrophy: Full Scale, Verbal and Performance intelligence quotients. *Developmental Medicine and Child Neurology, 43,* 497–501.

Deaton, A. V. (1987). Behavioral change strategies for children and adolescents with severe brain injury. *Journal of Learning Disabilities, 20*(10), 581–589.

Delis, D. C., Kramer, J. H., Kaplan, E., & Ober, B. A. (1994). *California Verbal Learning Test—Children's Version.* San Antonio, TX: Psychological Corporation.

Dewis, M. E. (1989). Spinal cord injured adolescents and young adults: The meaning of body changes. *Journal of Advanced Nursing, 14,* 389–396.

Dickman, C. A., & Rekate, H. L. (1993). Spinal trauma. In M. R. Eichelberger (Ed.), *Pediatric trauma: Prevention, acute care, rehabilitation* (pp. 362–377). St Louis, MO: Mosby-Year Book.

Dixon, P. J., Warschausky, S. A., Tate, D., & Karunas, R. (2001). Recovery of functional independence in children with spinal cord injury. *SCI Psychosocial Process, 14*(2), 68–73.

Donders, J. (1994). Academic placement after traumatic brain injury. *Journal of School Psychology, 32*(1), 53–65.

Donders, J. (1997). Sensitivity of the WISC-III to injury severity in children with traumatic head injury. *Assessment, 4,* 107–109.

Duchenne de Boulogne, G. V. A. (1868). *De l'electrisation localisee et de son application à la pathologie et à la therapeutique* (3rd ed). Paris: Bailliere et Fils.

Dudgeon, B., Massagli, T., & Ross, B. (1997). Educational participation of children with spinal cord injury. *American Journal of Occupational Therapy, 51,* 553–561.

Eleraky, M. A., Theodore, N., Adams, M., Rekate, H. L., & Sonntag, V. K. H. (2000). Pediatric cervical spine injuries: Reprint of 102 cases and review of the literature. *Journal of Neurosurgery, 92*(1), 12–17.

Ewing-Cobbs, L., Levin, H. S., Fletcher, J. M., Minerm, M. E., & Eisenberg, H. M. (1990). The Children's Orientation and Amnesia Test: Relationship to severity of acute head injury and to recovery of memory. *Neurosurgery, 27,* 683–691.

Feeney, T. J., & Ylvisaker, M. (1995). Choice and routine: Antecedent behavioral interventions for adolescents with severe traumatic brain injury. *Journal of Head Trauma Rehabilitation, 10*(3), 67–86.

Felisari, B., Boneschi, F. M., Bardoni, A., Sironi, M., Comi, G. P., Robotti, M., et al. (2000). Loss of Dp140 dystrophin isoform and intellectual impairment in Duchenne dystrophy. *Neurology, 55*(4), 559–564.

Firth, M., Gardner-Medwin, D., Hosking, G., & Wilkinson, E. (1983). Interviews with parents of boys suffering from Duchenne muscular dystrophy. *Developmental Medicine and Child Neurology, 25,* 466–471.

Franzese, A., Antonini, G., Iannelli, M., Leardi, M. G., Spada, S., Vichi, R., et al. (1991). Intellectual functions and personality in subjects with noncongenital myotonic muscular dystrophy. *Psychological Reports, 68,* 723–732.

Glang, A., Todis, B., Cooley, E., Wells, J., & Voss, J. (1997) Building social networks for children and adolescents with traumatic brain injury: A school-based intervention. *Journal of Head Trauma Rehabilitation, 12*(2), 32–47.

Graham, P. M., & Weingarden, S. I. (1989) Victims of gun shootings: A retrospective study of 36 spinal cord injured adolescents. *Journal of Adolescent Health Care, 10,* 534–536.

Hagen, C., Malkmus, D., & Durham, P. (1972). *Levels of cognitive functioning.* Downey, CA: Rancho Los Amigos Hospital.

Harper, D. (1983). Personality correlates and degree of impairment in male adolescents with progressive and nonprogressive physical disorders. *Journal of Clinical Psychology, 39,* 858–867.

Harvey, C., Rothchild, B. B., Asmann, A. J., & Stripling, T. (1990). New estimates of traumatic SCI prevalence: A survey-based approach. *Paraplegia, 28,* 537–544.

Havel, M. O., & Lawrence, D. W. (1993) Implications for discharge of adolescents with spinal cord injuries due to violence. *SCI Psychosocial Process, 6,* 9–11.

Hickey, K. J, Anderson, C. J., & Vogel, L. C. (1999). Pressure ulcers in pediatric spinal cord injury. *Topics in Spinal Cord Injury Rehabilitation, 6,* 85–90.

Hinton, V. J,. De Vivo, D. C., Nereo, N. E., Goldstein, E., & Stern, Y. (2001). Selective deficits in verbal working memory associated with a known neuropsychological profile of Duchenne muscular dystrophy. *Journal of the International Neuropsychological Society, 7*(1), 45–54.

Hoffman, N., Donders, J., & Thompson, E. H. (2000) Novel learning abilities after traumatic head injury in children. *Archives of Clinical Neuropsychology, 15*(1), 47–58.

Hwang, K. (1997). Living with a disability: A woman's perspective. In M. L. Sipski & C. J. Alexander (Eds.), *Sexual function in people with disability and chronic illness: A health professional's guide* (pp. 119–132). Gaithersburg, MD: Aspen.

Iannaccone, S. (1994). Pediatric aspects of spinal rehabilitation. *Journal of Neurologic Rehabilitation, 8*(1), 41–46.

Kehle, T. J., Clark, E., & Jenson, W. R. (1996). Interventions for students with traumatic brain injury: Managing behavioral disturbances. *Journal of Learning Disabilities, 29*(6), 633–642.

Kewman, D., Warschausky, S., Engel, L., & Warzak, W. (1997). Sexual development of children and adolescents. In M. Sipski & C. J. Alexander (Eds.), *Sexual function in people with disability and chronic illness: A health professional's guide* (pp. 355–378). Gaithersburg, MD: Aspen.

Killen, J. M. (1990). Role stabilization in families after spinal cord injury. *Rehabilitation Nursing, 15*(1), 19–21.

Kirkwood, M., Janusz, J., Yeates, K. O., Taylor, H. G., Wade, S. L., Stancin, T., & Drotar, D. (2000). Prevalence and correlates of depressive symptoms following traumatic brain injuries in children. *Child Neuropsychology, 6*(3), 195–208.

Konrad, K., Gauggel, S., Manz, A., & Scholl, M. (2000). Lack of inhibition: A motivational deficit in children with attention deficit/hyperactivity disorder and children with traumatic brain injury. *Child Neuropsychology, 6*(4), 286–296.

Kraus, J. F. (1995). Epidemiological features of brain injury in children: Occurrence, children at risk, causes and manner of injury, severity and outcomes. In S. H. Broman & M. E. Michel (Eds.), *Traumatic head injury in children* (pp. 22–39). New York: Oxford University Press.

Krause, J., & Anson, C. (1997). Adjustment after spinal cord injury: Relationship to participation in employment or educational activities. *Rehabilitation Counseling Bulletin, 40,* 202–214.

Krause, J., Stanwyck, C., & Maides, J. (1998). Locus of control and life adjustment: Relationship among people with spinal cord injury. *Rehabilitation Counseling Bulletin, 41,* 162–172.

Krause, J. S., Kewman, D. G., DeVivo, M. J., Maynard, F., Coker, J., Roach, M. J., & Ducharme, S. (1999). Employment after spinal cord injury: An analysis of cases from the model spinal injury systems. *Archives of Physical Medicine and Rehabilitation, 80*(11), 1492–1500.

Lavigne, J. V., & Faier-Routman, J. (1992). Psychological adjustment to pediatric physical disorders: A meta-analytic review. *Journal of Pediatric Psychology, 17,* 133–157.

Lescohier, I., & DiScala, C. (1993). Blunt trauma in children: Causes and outcomes of head versus intracranial injury. *Pediatrics, 91,* 721–725.

Levin, H. S., Song, J., Scheibel, R. S, Fletcher, J. M., Harward, H., Lilly, M., & Goldstein, F. (1997). Concept formation and problem-solving following closed head injury in children. *Journal of the International Neuropsychology Society, 3*, 598–607.

Lloyd, L. F., & Cuvo, A. J. (1994). Maintenance and generalization of behaviours after treatment of persons with traumatic brain injury. *Brain Injury, 8*(6), 529–540.

Max, J. E., Castillo, C. S., Robin, D. A., Lindgren, S. D., Smith, W. L., Sato, Y., et al. (1998). Predictors of family functioning after TBI in children and adolescents. *American Academy of Child and Adolescent Psychiatry, 37*(1), 83–90.

Max, J. E., Koele, S., Castillo, C. C., Lindgren, S. D., Arndt, S., Bokura, H., et al. (2000). Personality change disorder in children and adolescents following TBI. *Journal of the International Neuropsychological Society, 6*(3), 279–289.

Max, J. E., Koele, S., Lindgren, S. D., Robin, D. A., Smith, W. L., Sato, Y., & Arndt, S. (1998). Adaptive functioning following TBI and orthopedic injury: A controlled study. *Archives of Physical Medicine and Rehabilitation, 79*, 893–899.

Max, J. E., Koele, S. L., Smith, W. L., Sato, Y., Lindgren, S. D., Robin, D. A., & Arndt, S. (1998). Psychiatric disorders in children and adolescents after severe TBI: A controlled study. *Journal of the American Academy of Child and Adolescent Psychiatry, 37*(8), 832–840.

McLean, D. E., Kaitz, E. S., Kennan, C. J., Dabney, K., Cawley, M. F., & Alexander, M. A. (1995). Medical and surgical complications of pediatric brain injury. *Journal of Head Trauma Rehabilitation, 10*, 1–12.

Mehler, M. F. (2000). Brain dystrophin, neurogenetics and mental retardation. *Brain Research Reviews, 32*, 277–307.

Miller, J. R., Colbert, A. P., & Osberg, J. S. (1990). Ventilator dependency: Decision making, daily functioning and quality of life for patients with Duchenne muscular dystrophy. *Developmental Medicine and Child Neurology, 32*, 1078–1086.

Morgan, S. B., Bieberich, A. A., Walker, M., & Schwerdtfeger, H. (1998). Children's willingness to share activities with a physically handicapped peer: Am I more willing than my classmate? *Journal of Pediatric Psychology, 23*(6), 367–375.

Mulcahey, M. J. (1992). Returning to school after a spinal cord injury: Perspectives from four adolescents. *American Journal of Occupational Therapy, 46*(4), 305–312.

Nobunaga, A. I., Go, B. K., & Karunas, R. B. (1999). Recent demographic and injury trends in people served by the model spinal cord injury care systems. *Archives of Physical Medicine and Rehabilitation, 80*, 1372–1382.

Nudel, U., Robzyk, K., & Yaffe, D. (1988). Expression of the putative Duchenne muscular dystrophy gene in differentiated myogenic cell cultures and in the brain. *Nature, 331*, 635–638.

Nudel, U., Zuk, D., Einat, P., Zeelon, E., Levy, Z., Neuman, S., & Yaffe, D. (1989). Duchenne muscular dystrophy gene product is not identical in muscle and brain. *Nature, 337*(6202), 76–78.

Pontari, M. A., Weibel, B., Morales, V., Dean, G., Gaughan, J., & Betz, R. R. (2000). Improved quality of life after continent urinary diversion in pediatric patients with tetraplegia after spinal cord injury. *Topics in Spinal Cord Injury Rehabilitation*, 6(Suppl.), 25–29.

Radnitz, C. L., Schlein, I. S., & Hsu, L., (2000) The effects of prior trauma exposure on the development of PTSD following spinal cord injury. *Journal of Anxiety Disorders 14*(3), 313–324.

Rivara, J. M. B., Jaffe, K. M., Fay, G. C., Polissar, N. L., Martin, K. M., Shurtleff, H. A., & Liao, S. (1993). Family functioning and injury severity as predictors of child functioning one year following TBI. *Archives of Physical Medicine and Rehabilitation, 74*, 1047–1055.

Rivara, J. M. B., Jaffe, K. M., Polissar, N. L., Fay, G. C., Liao, S., & Martin, K. M. (1996). Predictors of family functioning and change 3 years after TBI in children. *Archives of Physical Medicine and Rehabilitation, 77*, 754–764.

Roland, E. H. (2000). Muscular dystrophy. *Pediatrics in Review, 21*(7), 1–8.

Rutledge, D. N., & Dick, G. (1983). Spinal cord injury in adolescence. *Rehabilitation Nursing, 8*(6), 18–21.

Sammallahti, P., Kannisto, M., & Aalberg, V. (1996). Psychological defenses and psychiatric symptoms in adults with pediatric spinal cord injuries. *Spinal Cord, 34*, 669–672.

Singer, G. H. S., Glang, A., Nixon, C., Cooley, E., Kerns, K. A., Williams, D., & Powers, L. E. (1994). A comparison of two psychosocial interventions for parents of children with acquired injury: An exploratory study. *Journal of Head Trauma Rehabilitation, 9*(4), 38–94.

Sipski, M. L. (1997). Spinal cord injury and sexual function: An educational model. In M. L. Sipski & C. J. Alexander (Eds.), *Sexual function in people with disability and chronic illness: A health professional's guide* (pp. 149–176). Gaithersburg, MD: Aspen.

Slifer, K. J., Tucker, C. L., Gerson, A. C., Cataldo, M. D., Sevier, R. C., Suter, A. H., & Kane, A. C. (1996). Operant conditioning for behavior management during post-traumatic amnesia in children and adolescents with brain injury. *Journal of Head Trauma Rehabilitation, 11*(1), 39–50.

Sollee, N. D., Latham, E. E., Kindlon, D. J., & Bresnan, M. J. (1985). Neuropsychological impairment in Duchenne muscular dystrophy. *Journal of Clinical and Experimental Neuropsychology, 7*, 486–496.

Taylor, H. G., Yeates, K. O., Wade, S. L., Drotar, D., Stancin, T., & Burant, C. (2001). Bidirectional child–family influences on outcomes of traumatic brain injury in children. *Journal of the International Neuropsychological Society, 7*(6), 755–767.

Taylor, H. G., Yeates, K. O., Wade, S. L., Drotar, D., Klein, S. K., & Stancin, T. (1999). Influences on first-year recovery from TBI in children. *Neuropsychology, 13*(1), 76–89.

Teasdale, G., & Jennett, G. (1974). Assessment of coma and impaired consciousness. *Lancet, 2,* 81.

Thompson, R. J., Zeman, J. L., Fanurik, D., & Sirotkin-Roses, M. (1992). The role of parent stress and coping and family functioning in parent and child adjustment to Duchenne muscular dystrophy. *Journal of Clinical Psychology, 48,* 11–19.

Vignos, P. (1977). Respiratory function and pulmonary infection in Duchenne muscular dystrophy. *Israeli Journal of Medical Science, 13,* 207–214.

Vogel, L., Klaas, S., Lubicky, J., & Anderson, C. (1998). Long-term outcomes and life satisfaction of adults who had pediatric spinal cord injuries. *Archives of Physical Medicine and Rehabilitation, 79,* 1496–1503.

Vogel, L. C., & DeVivo, M. J. (1996) Etiology and demographics. In R. R. Betz & M. J. Mulcahey (Eds.), *The child with a spinal cord injury* (pp. 3–12). Rosemont, IL: American Academy of Orthopaedic Surgeons.

Wade, S., Drotar, D., Taylor, H. G., & Stancin, T. (1995). Assessing the effects of TBI on family functioning: Conceptual and methodological issues. *Journal of Pediatric Psychology, 20*(6), 737–752.

Wade, S. L., Taylor, H. G., Drotar, D., Stancin, T., & Yeates, K. O. (1998). Family burden and adaptation during the intial year after BI in children. *Pediatrics, 102*(1), 110–116.

Walton, J., & Gardner-Medwin, D. (1988). Progressive muscular dystrophy and the myotomic disorders. In J. N. Walton (Ed.), *Disorders of voluntary muscle* (5th ed.). Edinburgh, UK: Churchill Livingstone.

Warschausky, S., Cohen, E., Parker, J., Levendosky, A. A., & Okun, A. (1997). Social problem-solving skills of children with traumatic brain injury. *Pediatric Rehabilitation, 1*(2), 77–81.

Warschausky, S., Engel, L., Kewman, D. G., & Nelson, V. (1996). Psychosocial factors in rehabilitation of a child with a spinal cord injury. In R. R. Betz & M. J. Mulcahey (Eds.), *The child with a spinal cord injury* (pp. 471–482). Rosemont, IL: American Academy of Orthopaedic Surgeons.

Warschausky, S., Kewman, D., & Selim, A. (1996). Attentional performance of children with traumatic brain injury: A quantitative and qualitative analysis of digit span. *Archives of Clinical Neuropsychology, 11*(2), 147–153.

Yeates, K. O. (2000). Closed head injury. In K. O. Yeates, M. D. Ris, & H. G. Taylor (Eds.), *Pediatric neuropsychology: Research, theory, and practice* (pp. 92–116). New York: Guilford Press.

Yeates, K. O., Luria, J., Bartkowski, H., Rusin, J., Martin, L., & Bigler, E. D. (1999). Postconcussive symptoms in children with mild closed head injuries. *Journal of Head Trauma Rehabilitation, 14*(4), 337–350.

Yeates, K. O., Taylor, H. G., Drotar, D., Wade, S. L., Klein, S., Stancin, T., & Schatschneider, C. (1997). Preinjury family environment as a determinant of recovery from traumatic brain injuries in school-age children. *Journal of the International Neuropsychological Society, 3,* 617–630.

Zellweger, H., & Hanson, J. W. (1967). Psychometric studies in muscular dystrophy type IIIa (Duchenne). *Developmental Medicine and Child Neurology, 9,* 576–581.

23

Medical and Psychosocial Aspects of Juvenile Rheumatoid Arthritis

MICHAEL A. RAPOFF
ANN M. McGRATH
CAROL B. LINDSLEY

Pediatric rheumatic diseases are chronic multisystem disorders that involve acute and chronic tissue inflammation of the musculoskeletal system, blood vessels, and skin. Juvenile rheumatoid arthritis (JRA) is the most common pediatric rheumatic disease and a major cause of short- and long-term disability among chronic pediatric diseases (Cassidy & Petty, 2001). Children with JRA and their families have to adhere to complex daily medical regimens and cope with pain and the psychosocial impact of living with a chronic disease. This chapter reviews the medical and psychosocial aspects of JRA, including adherence to medical regimens, chronic pain, and psychosocial adjustment and coping. Clinical and research implications are reviewed at the end of each section.

MEDICAL ASPECTS

The etiology of JRA is not known, although variables thought to be important in the pathophysiology of the disease include genetic predisposition, unknown environmental triggers, and immune reactivity. The hallmark of the disease is synovitis (inflammation of the synovial membrane of a joint). There are three subtypes of JRA; the categorization is made according to the symptomatology that occurs over the first 6 months of disease (Cassidy & Petty, 2001).

Systemic-Onset JRA

This subtype affects approximately 10% of children with JRA and is defined by the presence of a characteristic rash or high cyclic fevers, along with joint symptoms, either arthritis or arthralgias. These children also frequently show other manifestations, such as lymphadenopathy (inflammation of lymph nodes), hepatosplenomegaly (enlargement of the liver and spleen), pericarditis (inflammation of the pericardium or sac enclosing the heart), serositis (inflammation of a serous membrane), and marked laboratory abnormalities. The systemic symptoms will generally reverse over the first few months of disease as the joint symptoms persist and often progress. These children often are admitted to the hospital to establish a firm diagnosis and begin therapy. The pericarditis is a potentially life-threatening manifestation. Most children will respond to appropriate therapy, however, this subtype remains the most difficult group to treat, and up to 25% of children have a poor prognosis with continually active and poorly responsive disease. The severest involvement is generally in the hands, hips, and neck, so both mobility and dexterity are at risk.

Polyarticular JRA

This subtype occurs in about 40% of children with JRA and is defined as involvement of more than four joints. Usually these include hands, wrists, knees, ankles, and neck. If the disease begins at an early age, there may be involvement of the mandibular growth centers that leads to facial asymmetry. About 25% of these children have a positive rheumatoid factor test, which is a marker for more severe disease.

Pauciarticular (Oligoarticular) JRA

This subtype occurs in 40–50% of children with JRA and is defined as involvement of four or fewer joints, with the joints most frequently involved being the knees or ankles. There are two subgroups of patients: (1) young girls who test positive for ANA (antinuclear antibody) and have a high risk for eye involvement (uveitis), and (2) older boys who have a long-term risk for developing involvement of the axial skeleton, hips, and back. The diagnosis is made with the demonstration of persistent arthritis in one or more joints for a minimum of 6 weeks and with the exclusion of other diagnoses. Early, accurate diagnosis is critical to achieving optimal outcome in these children.

Treatment

Once the diagnosis is established, most children require regular therapy. The specific therapy used depends on the age of the child and the severity of the arthritis. Nonsteroidal anti-inflammatory agents (NSAIDS) are the standard first-line therapy. Well-established drugs such as naproxen or ibuprofen are used in young children and longer acting, once-a-day drugs such as nambutome or the newer COX-2 inhibitors such as celicoxib or rofecoxib are often used in older children and adolescents. The less frequently dosed drugs make adherence easier.

Most children with pauciarticular disease respond to NSAIDs, but intra-articular corticosteroids may be needed for unresponsive joints, and occasionally second-line agents such as sulfasalzaine are added. In polyarticular disease, NSAIDs are initial therapy, with second-line agents or disease-modifying antirheumatic drugs (DMARDs), such as hydroxychloroquine, sulfasalazaine, or methotrexate, added for poorly responsive or unresponsive disease after weeks to months. Low-dose short-term corticosteroid therapy may be used as "bridge therapy" to control symptoms during a transitional period, as DMARDs take weeks to months to be effective. In systemic disease, DMARDs such as hydroxychloroquine or methotrexate may be added early in the disease course, and daily corticosteroids may be required for pericarditis or unresponsive disease. Children with eye involvement are generally treated with corticosteroid eye drops and dilating agents. The activity of the eye disease does not usually fluctuate with that of the joint disease. Every effort is made to avoid long-term corticosteroid therapy in children because of their serious effects of toxicity, including growth retardation, iatrogenic Cushing's disease, osteoporosis, fractures, obesity, and hypertension. Patients with persistent, severe polyarticular or systemic disease who do not respond to methotrexate therapy are candidates for antitumor necrosis factor drugs, enteracept or infliximab.

In addition to drug therapy, children with JRA must be carefully monitored for growth abnormalities, nutrition, vision, and school and social functioning as well as psychological and emotional health. Therapeutic exercise programs with professional supervision may be needed to maximize joint motion and minimize muscle atrophy. Overall, the disease outcomes have markedly improved over the past two decades, and most children with JRA who have early diagnosis and receive appropriate treatment will have minimal joint deformity and can lead active, normal lives.

ADHERENCE TO MEDICAL REGIMENS

Children with JRA and their parents are usually asked to adhere consistently and over a long period of time to a variety of therapeutic regimens, most notably, medications, therapeutic exercises, and splinting of joints. Many of these regimens may have delayed beneficial effects and in the short term may cause unwanted side effects, such as gastrointestinal irritation and pain. Factors associated with JRA and its treatment (i.e., the need for consistent adherence over a long period of time, delayed beneficial effects, and negative side effects) have been predictive of greater adherence problems to medical regimens for pediatric chronic diseases (Rapoff, 1999).

Adherence Rates to Regimens for JRA

Few studies have specifically addressed adherence to regimens for JRA. Two retrospective studies by Litt and colleagues found that only 55% of children and adolescents with JRA were adherent to salicylate medications, as determined by serum assays (Litt & Cuskey, 1981; Litt, Cuskey, & Rosenberg, 1982). In three separate within-subject design studies involving five patients with JRA (ages 3 to 14 years), baseline adherence with medications as assessed by parental observations or pill counts ranged from 38 to 59% (Rapoff, Lindsley, & Christophersen, 1984; Rapoff, Purviance, & Lindsley, 1988a, 1988b). Two survey studies found that adherence problems were more common with prescribed exercises than medications or splint wearing (Hayford & Ross, 1988; Rapoff, Lindsley, & Christophersen, 1985). In the aggregate, these data suggest that the extent of adherence to medications for JRA can vary widely across different patient samples and methods of assessing adherence but appears to be less than optimal, as is the case with other chronic pediatric diseases (Rapoff, 1999). The two survey studies would suggest that adherence to therapeutic exercises for JRA is more problematic than adherence to medications. Interventions to improve adherence with regimens for JRA could lead to better disease control and enhanced quality of life. A few studies have targeted improvements in adherence to regimens (primarily medications) for JRA.

Adherence Intervention Studies

Two studies have examined the efficacy of parent-managed token reinforcement programs in altering adherence to regimens for JRA. The first study (Rapoff et al., 1984) focused on improving adherence to medications, splint wearing, and prone lying (to prevent hip contractures) for a 7-year-old female with severe systemic-onset JRA. Adherence was assessed by parental observations, with acceptable interobserver reliability (94%) obtained with an investigator conducting independent observations in the home. Mean baseline adherence was low for medications (59%) and nil (0%) for both splint wearing and prone lying. Introduction of the token system increased adherence to 95% for medications, 77% for splint wearing, and 71% for prone lying. At the 10-week follow-up (with the token system withdrawn), adherence to medications, splint wearing, and prone lying averaged 90%, 91%, and 80%, respectively. Although they were not formally assessed, the pediatric rheumatologist anecdotally noted concomitant improvements in function for this patient, such as greater hip extension.

The second study (Rapoff et al., 1988a) also tested the efficacy of a token system program in improving adherence to medications for a 14-year-old male with polyarticular JRA. Adherence was assessed by weekly pill counts obtained from the patient's mother over the phone, with independent counts by an investigator in the clinic (agreement with the mother's count was 100%). A withdrawal (reversal) single-subject design was employed to evaluate the effects of the intervention on adherence and several clinical outcome parameters (e.g., active joint counts). Medication adherence averaged 44% during baseline, increased to an average of 59% during a simplified regimen condition (in which the dosage was reduced from four to three times a day), and further increased and remained at 100% during the first token system phase. Adherence decreased during a token system withdrawal phase (mean = 77%), increased during the second token system phase (mean = 99%), and averaged 92% during the maintenance phase (in which the token system was not in effect but could be reinstated if adherence dropped below 80% for 2 consecutive weeks). At the 9-month follow-up (no token system in effect and no contingency for reinstatement), adherence averaged 97%. Though not as straightforward as the adherence results, improvements were shown in clinical outcomes during the token system and follow-up phases (e.g., five active joints) relative to baseline and the token system withdrawal phase (e.g., ten active joints).

Although the previously mentioned studies showed that token systems could be effective in improving adherence, they are labor intensive for families and require well-trained personnel to implement and monitor. One study (Rapoff et al., 1988b) evaluated less complex behavioral strategies (such as self-monitoring and positive verbal feedback) combined with educational strategies (verbal and written information about medications and the importance of adherence and strategies for improving adherence). This study involved three female patients with JRA, ages 3, 10, and 13, years and adherence was again assessed by weekly pill counts obtained from parents over the phone, with independent counts by one of the investigators in the clinic (agreement was 100%). A multiple baseline across-subjects design was used to evaluate the efficacy of the intervention. Baseline medication adherence averaged 38% and 54% for two of the patients and increased during the intervention phase to an average of 97% and 92%, respectively. Adherence increased only slightly for the third patient, from an average of 44% during baseline to an average of 49% during the intervention phase. Adherence decreased for all three patients at 4-month follow-up (means ranged from 24 to 89%). Interestingly, the patient for whom the intervention was least effective was a 13-year-old who had less parental supervision of her regimen and whose mother admitted she was nonadherent to medications prescribed to treat her arthritis. Unfortunately, clinical outcomes were not reported for these patients.

A recently completed randomized controlled trial experimentally validated a nurse-implemented, clinic-based intervention to prevent medication adherence problems among children and adolescents who were newly diagnosed with JRA (Rapoff, 2000). A total of 54 patients were entered in the study and produced some useable data ($N = 29$ in the experimental group and $N = 25$ in the control group). Mean age of the total sample was 7.8 years (range of 2 to 16 years), and 74% were female. About half the sample (52%) had polyarticular JRA, 31% had pauciarticular JRA, and 17% had systemic-onset JRA.

Patients were matched by age and type of JRA and then randomly assigned to the experimental or (attention-placebo) control groups. Patients and parents in the experimental group were given verbal, written, and audiovisual information from a nurse about adherence improvement strategies, including prompting, monitoring, positive reinforcement, and discipline techniques (see Rapoff, 1998). Control group patients and parents were given verbal, written, and audiovisual information about JRA and treatments by the same nurse but no specific information about adherence improvement strategies. Patients and parents in both groups received their respective interventions during a 1½-hour clinic visit and were telephoned by the nurse, biweekly for 2 months and then monthly for 10 months. The content of the phone calls centered on the information presented during the initial clinic visit.

Analysis of covariance (ANCOVA) for repeated measures (with baseline adherence as the covariate) showed a significant group ($p = .016$) and group × time interaction ($p = .047$) on adherence (assessed by electronic monitoring) in favor of the experimental group patients, but no significant differences between the experimental and control groups on disease activity/limitations or on direct or indirect health care costs.

The adherence results supported the prediction that a nurse-administered adherence intervention can significantly enhance adherence to medications for newly diagnosed patients with JRA relative to an attention-placebo control condition. This finding was encouraging because most pediatric rheumatology treatment centers have a nurse clinician as a central member of the medical team and because nurses are in a unique position to offer patients and their families guidance about maintaining adherence to prescribed treatments. The lack of significant differences in disease-related outcomes may have been due to "floor effects" (or low disease activity levels at baseline) that may have prevented improvements that could be differentially attributed to the adherence intervention. The lack of significant differences in health care costs may be due to the faulty assumption that increased adherence would lower costs, when, in fact, adherent patients and families may be more consistent in pursuing medical follow-up and purchasing medications, at least in the short run. Distinguishing unnecessary health care costs (the costs of diagnostic and treatment services because of poor adherence) from necessary costs may be useful to determine whether improved adherence reduces unnecessary costs.

Clinical and Research Implications

Few adherence intervention studies target medical regimens for children with JRA, especially for therapeutic exercises. The studies that have been done suggest a three-tiered approach to minimizing nonadherence: primary, secondary, and tertiary prevention (Rapoff, 2000). *Primary prevention* efforts would be most relevant for those patients who have not yet exhibited clinically significant nonadherence (inconsistencies in following a particular regimen that may result in compromised health and well-being); possibly those recently diagnosed or those who are able to sustain adequate adherence over time. Interventions at this level would involve educational (e.g., stressing the importance of adherence), organizational (e.g., simplifying regimens), and relatively simple behavioral strategies (e.g., monitoring of regimen adherence by providers or parents). *Secondary prevention* might be most applicable to those patients for whom clinically significant nonadherence has been identified early on in the disease course or has yet to compromise their health and well-being. Interventions at this level might include more frequent monitoring of regimen adherence by parents and patients, specific and consistent positive social reinforcement for adherence, and general discipline strategies (e.g., time-out for younger children). Pediatric psychologists could train primary health care providers, particularly nurses, to implement primary and secondary level interventions. *Tertiary prevention* efforts would apply to patients with an ongoing pattern of clinically significant nonadherence. Strategies at this level might include token system programs, contingency contracting, self-management training (e.g., problem solving to anticipate and manage obstacles to adherence), and possibly psychotherapy. Because of the demanding and technical nature of these strategies, pediatric psychologists would be responsible for implementing strategies at this level.

Implementing and evaluating primary, secondary, and tertiary prevention approaches to medical nonadherence depends on a number of factors. First, prevention efforts require a valid, reliable, and clinically feasible way to detect or assess nonadherence. Although no such "ideal" measure exists, 24-hour recall interviews (in clinics or by phone) may be the best option in that they have been shown to be reliable, valid, and feasible for routine and serial assessments of adherence to regimens for diabetes and cystic fibrosis and could be easily be adapted for JRA regimens (Rapoff, 1999). Second, information obtained from routine and serial assessments of adherence should also allow for the detection of clinically significant nonadherence. Previous attempts at determining the levels of adherence necessary to prevent deleterious health outcomes have been arbitrary and not biologically based (e.g., adequate adherence defined as consuming 80% of prescribed medication doses). Third, because the desired outcome of adherence interventions is that patients get better, feel better, and do better, there is a need for both traditional (e.g., clinical signs and symptoms) and quality-of-life measures of disease and health status that are valid, reliable, and clinically feasible (Rapoff, 1999). Finally, because JRA affects relatively small numbers of children and adolescents, empirical validation of primary, secondary, and tertiary prevention interventions will require multicenter collaborative research studies.

PAIN IN JRA

Chronic pain is a primary clinical manifestation of JRA (Cassidy & Petty, 2001). Children with JRA often report mild to moderate levels of pain intensity (Gragg et al., 1996; Hagglund, Schopp, Alberts, Cassidy, & Frank, 1995; Ilowite, Walco, & Pochaczevsky, 1992; Thompson, Varni, & Hanson, 1987; Varni, Rapoff, Waldron, Gragg, Bernstein, & Lindsley, 1996a) and some (14% in one study) even report no pain (Sherry, Bohnsack, Salmonson, Wallace, & Mellins, 1990). However, about 25 to 30% report pain intensities in the moderate to severe range (Ross, Lavigne, Hayford, Dyer, & Pachman, 1989; Schanberg, Lefebvre, Keefe, Kredich, & Gil, 1997) and, in one study (Benestad, Vinje,

Veierød, & Vandvik, 1996), 82% of children with JRA reported pain lasting from 30 minutes to 24 hours a day, with a mean of 4.3 hours per day. Also, a recent long-term follow-up study from the Mayo Clinic found that the adults who were diagnosed with JRA reported significantly greater pain, fatigue, and disability relative to gender-matched healthy cases (Peterson, Mason, Nelson, O'Fallon, & Gabriel, 1997). Thus pain is a significant problem for some children with JRA that persists into adulthood and is associated with greater disability.

Biobehavioral Model of Pain

The most widely accepted definition of pain ("an unpleasant sensory and emotional experience associated with actual or potential tissue damage") acknowledges that pain is simultaneously a physiological and psychological experience (International Association for the Study of Pain, 1979, p. 250). Beginning with the introduction of the gate control theory of pain (Melzack & Wall, 1965), researchers have gravitated to a biobehavioral model of pain that focuses on the unique and interactive components of nociceptive activity, emotions, cognitions, and behavior in the experience of pain (Rapoff & Lindsley, 2000).

Nociception

There are physiological, anatomical, and chemical properties of the nervous system that contribute to the perception of pain. Nociceptive afferents (nerve fibers) in the joint are located in the joint capsule and ligaments, bone, periosteum, articular fat pads, and perivascular sites and respond to noxious mechanical, thermal, and chemical stimulation (Randich, 1993). The enhanced pain associated with arthritis is probably due to the response of joint afferents to mechanical and heat stimulation present during inflammation and chemical mediators of joint inflammation, such as prostaglandins, that sensitize joint afferent fibers (Meyer, Campbell, & Raja, 1994).

This inflammation-induced sensitization of articular afferents likely contributes to hyperalgesia, an increased response to stimuli that are typically painful, and allodynia, pain due to stimuli that do not typically provoke pain (Levine & Taiwo, 1994). Also, studies of experimentally induced pain found reduced pain threshold in inflamed and noninflamed joints of children with active arthritis and, to a lesser degree, in the joints of children in remission (Hogeweg et al., 1995; Hogeweg, Kuis, Oostendorp, & Helders, 1995; Thastum, Zachariae, Schøler, Bjerring, & Herlin, 1997). The persistence of lowered pain threshold, even after nociceptive input to the joint might be expected to cease, suggests a role for long-lasting structural and functional changes, or "neuroplastic alterations" due to "central sensitization" (Coderre & Katz, 1997; Kuis, Heijnen, Hogeweg, Sinnema, & Helders, 1997). Thus peripheral and central sensitization mechanisms may be operative in arthritis-related pain.

Emotions

It is widely accepted that pain is an emotional, as well as a sensory, experience (Banks & Kerns, 1996). Some researchers have even suggested that people in pain do not suffer unless they experience emotional distress (Craig, 1994). There is strong correlational support for the link between negative emotions, particularly anxiety and depression, and increased pain intensity and interference in the lives of children with JRA (Gragg et al., 1996; Hagglund et al., 1995; Ross et al., 1993; Thompson et al., 1987; Varni et al., 1996a; Varni, Rapoff, Waldron, Gragg, Bernstein, & Lindsley, 1996b).

Although an inextricable link exists between pain and emotional distress, studies supporting this link are usually correlational and cross-sectional, thus precluding any clear explication of causal mechanisms. However, several major links between emotional distress and pain have been proposed (Banks & Kerns, 1996; Gamsa, 1990): (1) emotional distress can cause pain (e.g., depression can lead to increased preoccupation with bodily sensations such as pain, thus lowering the pain threshold); (2) emotional distress as a consequence of pain (e.g., increased pain results in reductions in social and recreational activities, which in turn fosters a state of depression); and (3) emotional distress and pain occur concurrently and may share common etiological factors (e.g., biogenic amines, such as serotonin and norepinephrine, are thought to play a role in depression and pain). The "compromise" position among these three proposed links (and the one most consistent with a biobehavioral model of pain) is that emotional distress and pain are reciprocally linked (e.g., increased anxiety can induce muscle tension, thereby directly inducing or exacerbating musculoskeletal pain, or increased pain can induce anxiety about future prognosis or interference with life activities).

Cognitions

This variable is concerned with how people attend to and think about the experience of pain. The focus in the pain literature has been on maladaptive rather than adaptive thinking. Cognitive processing of pain can be maladaptive in at least two ways: (1) people can fail to attend to information or generate self-talk that might be helpful in coping with pain (less "forethought"), or (2) people can engage in dysfunctional thinking that leads to maladaptive coping and greater pain (such as wishful or catastrophic thinking).

Catastrophizing (defined as "an exaggerated negative orientation toward noxious stimuli") may be the most "toxic" type of dysfunctional thinking related to pain and seems to include three components: (1) rumination (preoccupation with pain-related thoughts); (2) magnification (exaggeration of the threat value of pain); and (3) helplessness (adopting a helpless orientation to coping with pain, such as thinking one cannot do anything about pain that is unrelenting; Sullivan, Bishop, & Pivik, 1995).

Consistent evidence from the literature on pain and adjustment of adults with rheumatoid arthritis demonstrates that catastrophizing and wishful thinking are associated with poorer outcomes, such as greater pain, depression, anxiety, and functional limitations (Zautra & Manne, 1992). In contrast, relatively few studies have investigated cognitive coping strategies in children with JRA, most likely because few pain coping instruments have been developed. Varni, Waldron, et al. (1996) found that "cognitive self-instruction" (primarily wishful thinking) was related to greater emotional distress and that "cognitive refocusing" (engaging in activities as a distraction from pain) was related to less pain intensity and emotional distress. Another study (Schanberg et al., 1997) found that "pain control and rational thinking" (controlling and decreasing pain while avoiding catastrophizing) predicted lower pain intensity. Reid, Gilbert, and McGrath (1998) found that "emotion-focused avoidance" coping (catastrophizing and expressing negative emotions) was associated with greater pain intensity, pain duration, and anxiety. A study in Denmark (Thastum, Zachariae, Schøler, & Herlin, 1998) found that internalizing/catastrophizing coping was associated with higher experimental pain intensity (using a cold pressor paradigm) and that distraction and positive self-statements were related to lower experimental pain intensity.

Behavior

When children are in pain, they exhibit a wide variety of pain behaviors, such as limping, grimacing, crying, resting, or asking for medication. How others respond to these pain displays or behaviors can be adaptive or maladaptive for the child experiencing pain. Pain behaviors such as guarding and malpositioning of affected joints may be maladaptive for children with JRA (Cassidy & Petty, 2001). Caregivers' responses to children's pain-related behaviors may also be maladaptive, such as when parents allow children to avoid attending school, resulting in low academic performance and missed opportunities for social interactions. Conversely, if children engage in "well" behaviors (e.g., positive coping strategies) and parents reinforce adaptive behaviors, then children would be expected to experience less pain and disability from pain. There is ample support for this operant behavioral perspective in the adult pain literature, mostly with people who have chronic back pain (Keefe & Lefebvre, 1994), but fewer studies have been done with children (McGrath, 1990). One study did find that children with JRA who reported resting more and withdrawing from activities showed higher levels of pain and emotional distress (Varni, Waldron, et al., 1996). Another study found that children with JRA who engaged in "approach" coping (including talking to a friend or family member about how they felt) showed less functional disability (Reid et al., 1998).

Clinical and Research Implications

A biobehavioral model of pain would suggest a number of treatment options (Rapoff & Lindsley, 2000). Early and aggressive pharmacological treatment of JRA could lead to enhanced pain relief and function, both short term and long term, via a reduction in peripheral and central sensitization mechanisms. Neurochemical mechanisms also suggest the value of nonpharmacological therapies in the treatment of arthritis-related pain, such as cooling and resting inflamed joints (to control nociceptive inputs and avoid peripheral sensitization) and relaxation or other psychological treatments.

Psychological interventions that reduce negative emotional states would be expected to directly or indirectly reduce pain intensity and pain interference. Helping children to manage disease-related stressors (e.g., relaxation and problem-solving techniques) should result in concomitant reductions in negative emotions and pain. Enlisting the social support and reinforcement of family and friends should foster greater participation in social and recreational activities by patients, thereby reducing emotional distress and preoccupation with pain and suffering.

Cognitive restructuring may be helpful in countering maladaptive thinking about pain by having children identify negative thoughts (e.g., "I can't do anything to make my pain better"), challenge or question these thoughts, and substitute more helpful thoughts (e.g., "I can distract myself or do relaxation exercises to reduce my pain"). Imagery techniques (e.g., vividly imagining a relaxing place or experience) combined with relaxation exercises are often helpful in diverting attention from pain, thereby reducing pain.

Parents are important role models for their children, and they need to be made aware of how they cope with their own pain (such as headaches) and thereby influence how their children cope with pain (Rapoff & Lindsley, 2000). Parents can be taught more adaptive strategies for coping with pain so that they can model these strategies for their children (e.g., not avoiding responsibilities because of pain and using effective medical or psychological therapies to control pain). Family members and friends can be taught to respond adaptively to pain behaviors, including not being overly solicitous and attentive to pain behaviors and reinforcing alternative and adaptive coping strategies. Children with JRA can be helped to find ways (in spite of their pain) to do what they want and need to do.

There is a need for well-controlled, multisite pain intervention trials for children with JRA. Studies to date have been promising but have involved small samples and no control or alternative-treatment comparison groups (Lavigne, Ross, Berry, Hayford, & Pachman, 1992; Walco, Varni, & Ilowite, 1992).

PSYCHOSOCIAL ADJUSTMENT AND COPING

A substantial body of research exists on the psychosocial adjustment and coping of children and adolescents with JRA (for other reviews, see Bradley, 1985; Hoyeraal, 1987; Lavigne & Faier-Routman, 1992; Quirk & Young, 1990). Early studies of children with JRA suggested increased psychosocial problems, but these studies involved small sample sizes, hospitalized children, and the use of nonstandardized measures (Cleveland, Reitman, & Brewer, 1965; Rimon, Belmaker, & Ebstein, 1977). More recent studies tend to include larger samples, standardized measures, and more sophisticated statistical approaches, and they often examine predictors of adjustment from a specific theoretical perspective. In addition, studies have also expanded their focus to include the parents and siblings of children and adolescents with JRA.

Social and Emotional Adjustment

Some studies have found significant differences between the psychosocial functioning of children with JRA and control children (McAnarney, Pless, Satterwhite, & Friedman, 1974). However, the majority of studies have found no significant psychosocial deficits in children with JRA compared with normative or healthy control samples.

Kellerman, Zeltzer, Ellenberg, Dash, and Rigler (1980) assessed 168 chronically ill adolescents (30 with rheumatic disease) and 349 healthy controls and found no significant differences between healthy and ill adolescents or between illness subgroups on measures of anxiety or self-esteem. Brace, Smith, McCauley, and Sherry (2000) compared adolescents with JRA to healthy adolescents and adolescents with chronic fatigue syndrome (CFS). The adolescents with CFS scored significantly higher on measures of internalizing problems (e.g., depression), school absences, and parental reinforcement of illness behavior than did the healthy adolescents. Adolescents with JRA scored in the intermediate range, between adolescents with CFS and healthy adolescents, on most measures, with the exception that adolescents with JRA had the lowest parental reinforcement of illness behavior.

Noll and colleagues (2000) compared 74 children with JRA with 74 case-control classmates and found no significant differences between groups on any of the 10 measures used to assess social and emotional functioning, with both groups scoring in the normative range on all measures. Huygen, Kuis, and Sinnema (2000) conducted a study of 47 Dutch patients with JRA, 52 healthy peers, and their parents. Results indicated that self-esteem, perceived competence, body image, social competence, social support, and psychopathology were equivalent across groups despite children with JRA having less ability to participate in sports, less frequent opportunities to play with friends, and lower perceived athletic competence. Thus the majority of research indicates that children with JRA have no significant social or emotional difficulties when compared with healthy children.

School Adjustment

An early epidemiological study indicated that chronically ill children were significantly delayed in school achievement when compared with their peers, possibly due to increased school absences (Pless & Roughmann, 1971). Studies addressing school absence have found that children with JRA tend to be absent significantly more often than their healthy peers (Fowler, Johnson, & Atkinson, 1985). However, this scenario is not necessarily the case, and it seems that disease severity is related to school absence. In a study of 113 children and adolescents with JRA, Sturge, Garralda, Boissin, Dore, and Woo (1997) found the mean school attendance rate to be 92%. Children with more severe forms of JRA were significantly more likely to miss school.

Long-Term Psychosocial Adjustment

Miller, Spitz, Simpson, and Williams (1982) conducted a follow-up study of 121 individuals with JRA who had reached at least the age of 18 years and found that most of them were working, attending school full time, or a combination of the two. The authors also compared 50 patients with their siblings and found no significant differences on any demographic or psychosocial variables. However, Peterson et al. (1997) conducted a 25-year follow-up study of 44 individuals diagnosed with JRA (M = 33.5 years) and 102 age- and sex-matched controls. Results indicated that people with JRA had significantly lower functional status, more physical disability, higher unemployment, and less ability to exercise than controls. The major differences between these two studies are the age at assessment and the type of control group used. Miller et al. (1982) studied children with JRA around 18 years of age, whereas Peterson et al. (1997) studied patients around 33 years of age. Therefore, it is possible that children with JRA function fairly typically through the age of dependence (when they typically live with their families) but tend to have more difficulty as they progress through life. Also, the Miller et al. (1982) study compared children with JRA with their siblings, where Peterson et al. (1997) used an age- and sex-matched control group. It is possible, therefore, that using the nonsibling control group allowed other demographic features (i.e., socioeconomic status) to increase the differences between groups that were found in the Peterson et al. (1997) study.

Theoretical Models and Prediction of Adjustment

Several studies have tested theoretical models developed to predict the psychosocial adjustment of children with JRA and other chronic health conditions. Gartstein, Short, Vannatta, and Noll (1999) evaluated three models: (1) the *discrete disease model* (children with different diseases experience different stressors); (2) the *noncategorical model* (children with different diseases experience similar stressors); and (3) the *mixed model* (a mixture of the discrete and noncategorical models). A sample of 169 children with chronic illnesses (35 with JRA) was compared with 168 classroom comparison peers on demographic, parental, and self-report variables. Findings supported the noncategorical model, in that regardless of specific chronic illness category, children with chronic illness experienced similar social functioning and internalizing and externalizing difficulties as children with other types of chronic illness.

A representative noncategorical model, which has received the greatest attention in the literature on psychosocial adjustment of children with chronic illness, is the disability–

stress–coping model proposed by Wallander and Varni (1992). This model specifies categories of risk (e.g., daily hassles) and resistance (e.g., social support) factors that predict adjustment to chronic illness, over and above demographic and disease-related variables. Several studies have tested this model on samples of children and adolescents with JRA. Varni, Wilcox, and Hanson (1988) assessed the effects of family social support on adjustment in 23 children with JRA, after controlling for disease activity and peer social support. Higher family social support significantly predicted lower internalizing and externalizing behavior problems. Wallander, Varni, Babani, Banis, and Wilcox (1989) studied 153 children with a chronic health condition (23 children with JRA) and found that both family psychological resources (e.g., family cohesion) and family utilitarian resources (e.g., family income) were related to more positive child adjustment. Also, family psychological resources contributed unique variance to child adjustment beyond that accounted for by utilitarian family resources. Using the same sample of 153 children with a chronic health condition, Wallander and Varni (1989) found that children who received high levels of social support from both parents and peers tended to show better adjustment than those children who received high social support from only one source, either parents or peers. Thus research on the disability–stress–coping model indicates that children with JRA who have more family social support, more family psychological resources, and higher parent social support tend to fare better than children with JRA who do not.

von Weiss et al. (2002) specifically focused on one risk factor (daily hassles) and one resistance factor (social support) with a sample of 160 children and adolescents with rheumatic disease (67.5% diagnosed with JRA). Results failed to support the hypothesis that social support moderated the relationship between daily hassles and adjustment problems, but rather indicated that higher social support (particularly from parents and peers) predicted fewer adjustment problems regardless of the level of stress experienced by children and adolescents with JRA.

Several studies have specifically examined age (as a proxy for developmental factors) and disease severity as predictors of adjustment in children with JRA. Ungerer, Horgan, Chaitow, and Champion (1988) conducted a study of 363 children, adolescents, and young adults with JRA. There were no differences in self-esteem among the three groups of patients with JRA compared with normative samples. However, the authors did find developmental differences in that social isolation, psychological problems (e.g., feeling lonely), and greater disease severity were associated with lower self-esteem for the child and adolescent groups but not for young adults. In an early study of 42 children with rheumatic disease and 42 healthy controls, McAnarney et al. (1974) found that children with mild disease had lower levels of psychosocial functioning than children with more severe disease. In contrast, Billings, Moos, Miller, and Gottlieb (1987) compared 52 children with mild or inactive rheumatic disease, 43 children with severe disease, and 93 control children (patients with JRA composed 82% of the rheumatic disease sample). Parents reported children with severe disease to have significantly more psychological symptoms than children with mild or inactive rheumatic disease and controls. Other studies have also found a positive relationship between disease severity and adjustment problems (Daltroy et al., 1992).

Schanberg et al. (2000) investigated daily variation in mood, stressful events, and physical symptoms in children with rheumatic diseases. Twelve children (10 girls, ages 7 to 15 years) completed a daily diary booklet for a 7-day period rating their overall mood, negative daily events (e.g., "got in trouble"), symptoms (pain, fatigue, and stiffness), and interference of disease with daily activities. Compliance with the daily diaries was high (97.6%). Children also completed the Children's Depression Inventory (CDI). Children showed variability in daily mood (generally moderately positive), frequency of daily stressful events (average of two events per day), and daily symptoms (generally low to middle level on pain and stiffness). More negative daily mood and more daily stressful events significantly predicted increased reports of fatigue, stiffness, and reduction in daily activities. Negative daily mood also predicted increased reports of pain. Unexpectedly, daily stressful events were unrelated to daily mood. None of the 12 children scored in the clinically significant range on the CDI. The results regarding the relationship between disease severity and psychosocial functioning are difficult to interpret, as some studies indicate a positive association between the two variables and some indicate the lack of a relationship at all. Future research needs to be completed to determine if these ambivalent findings are due to measurement issues, definitions of functioning and disease severity, or some other source.

Parents and Siblings of Children with JRA

Henoch, Batson, and Baum (1978) compared a sample of 88 children with JRA to 2,952 control children and found that families of children with JRA were significantly more likely to have unmarried parents due to divorce, separation, or death; and they experienced adoption in their families three times more frequently than the control population. In a study of maternal functioning, Manuel (2001) assessed 92 mothers of children with JRA. Compared with normative groups, mothers of children with JRA reported significantly higher levels of emotional distress. Regression analyses showed that daily hassles and illness-related stressors were both significant predictors of emotional distress among mothers of children with JRA. Maternal education and appraisal of the impact of the child's illness on the family served to buffer against psychological distress. That is, more positive appraisal was associated with decreased distress, even when illness stress was high; and higher levels of education were associated with decreased distress, even when daily hassles stress was high.

Daniels, Miller, Billings, and Moos (1986) compared 72 children with a rheumatic disease (58 with JRA) and their siblings with 60 demographically matched siblings of healthy children on parent measures of psychological functioning and family functioning. Results indicated no differences between groups on any measures, with siblings of JRA children and siblings of healthy children functioning equally well. In a later study, the authors (Daniels, Moos, Billings, & Miller, 1987) compared 93 children with rheumatic disease and 72 of their siblings with 93 demographically matched siblings of healthy controls. The authors found that across all three groups maternal depressed mood and JRA physical symptoms predicted greater adjustment problems and that high family cohesion and expressiveness were related to better functioning. Thus research indicates that JRA has little effect on siblings but likely causes stress to mothers, especially when JRA symptoms are high, daily hassles are high, illness appraisal is elevated, and maternal education levels are low.

Clinical and Research Implications

The bulk of the empirical evidence suggests that children and adolescents with JRA do not appear to be at any greater risk of developing clinically significant adjustment problems. However, it is possible that this risk has been underestimated due to underreporting of psychosocial difficulties or fluctuations in psychosocial functioning concomitant with fluctuations in disease severity that may not be captured in cross-sectional studies. Also, there are clearly some children who are at greater risk for adjustment problems (e.g., those with more severe disease). This situation calls for longitudinal studies to assess psychosocial adjustment and coping among children and adolescents with JRA coupled with well-timed psychosocial interventions for those determined to be at risk or experiencing significant distress or disruption in their daily lives. Studies on adjustment and coping should include measures of adaptive or protective constructs; instruments to assess these types of constructs will need to be developed and validated. For example, Barlow and associates have recently reported on the development and preliminary validation of parent and child arthritis self-efficacy scales (Barlow, Shaw, & Wright, 2000, 2001). Instead of duplicating efforts to develop new instruments to measure these constructs, investigators should collaborate and pool reliability and validity data across sites. Innovative and potentially more useful approaches to assess variability in adjustment and coping might involve within-person research to examine daily fluctuations and associations between daily measures of stress, mood, and disease symptoms (as was done by Schanberg et al., 2000). Such daily measures would also provide more detailed outcome data for psychosocial intervention trials.

REFERENCES

Banks, S. M., & Kerns, R. D. (1996). Explaining high rates of depression in chronic pain: A diathesis–stress framework. *Psychological Bulletin, 119,* 95–110.

Barlow, J. H., Shaw, K. L., & Wright, C. C. (2000). Development and preliminary validation of a self-efficacy measure for use among parents of children with juvenile idiopathic arthritis. *Arthritis Care and Research, 13,* 227–236.

Barlow, J. H., Shaw, K. L., & Wright, C. C. (2001). Development and preliminary validation of a children's arthritis self-efficacy scale. *Arthritis Care and Research, 45,* 159–166.

Benestad, B., Vinje, O., Veierød, M. B., & Vandvik, I. H. (1996). Quantitative and qualitative assessments of pain in children with juvenile chronic arthritis based on the Norwegian version of the Pediatric Pain Questionnaire. *Scandinavian Journal of Rheumatology, 25,* 293–299.

Billings, A. G., Moos, R. H., Miller, J. J., & Gottlieb, J. E. (1987). Psychosocial adaptation in juvenile rheumatic disease: A controlled evaluation. *Health Psychology, 6,* 343–359.

Brace, M. J., Smith, M. S., McCauley, E., & Sherry, D. D. (2000). Family reinforcement of illness behavior: A comparison of adolescents with chronic fatigue syndrome, juvenile arthritis, and healthy controls. *Journal of Developmental and Behavioral Pediatrics, 21,* 332–339.

Bradley, L. A. (1985). Psychological aspects of arthritis. *Bulletin on the Rheumatic Diseases, 35,* 1–12.

Cassidy, J. T., & Petty, R. E. (2001). *Textbook of pediatric rheumatology* (4th ed.). Philadelphia: Saunders.

Cleveland, S. E., Reitman, E. E., & Brewer, E. J. (1965). Psychological factors in juvenile rheumatoid arthritis. *Arthritis and Rheumatism, 8,* 1152–1158.

Coderre, T. J., & Katz, J. (1997). Peripheral and central hyperexcitability: Differential signs and symptoms in persistent pain. *Behavioral and Brain Sciences, 20,* 404–419.

Craig, K. D. (1994). Emotional aspects of pain. In P. D. Wall & R. Melzack (Eds), *Textbook of pain* (3rd ed., pp. 261–274). Edinburgh, UK: Churchill Livingstone.

Daltroy, L. H., Larson, M. G., Eaton, H. M., Partridge, A. J., Pless, I. B., Rogers, M. P., et al., (1992). Psychosocial adjustment in juvenile arthritis. *Journal of Pediatric Psychology, 17,* 277–289.

Daniels, D., Miller, J. J., Billings, A. G., & Moos, R. H. (1986). Psychosocial functioning of siblings of children with rheumatic disease. *Journal of Pediatrics, 109,* 379–383.

Daniels, D., Moos, R. H., Billings, A. G., & Miller, J. J. (1987). Psychosocial risk and resistance factors among children with chronic illness, healthy siblings, and healthy controls. *Journal of Abnormal Child Psychology, 15,* 295–308.

Fowler, M. G., Johnson, M. P., & Atkinson, S. S. (1985). School achievement and absence in children with chronic health conditions. *Journal of Pediatrics, 106,* 683–687.

Gamsa, A. (1990). Is emotional disturbance a precipitator or a consequence of chronic pain? *Pain, 42,* 183–195.

Gartstein, M. A., Short, A. D., Vannatta, K., & Noll, R. B. (1999). Psychosocial adjustment of children with chronic illness: An evaluation of three models. *Journal of Developmental and Behavioral Pediatrics, 20,* 157–163.

Gragg, R. A., Rapoff, M. A., Danovsky, M. B., Lindsley, C. B., Varni, J. W., Waldron, S. A., et al. (1996). Assessing chronic musculoskeletal pain associated with rheumatic disease: Further validation of the Pediatric Pain Questionnaire. *Journal of Pediatric Psychology, 21,* 237–250.

Hagglund, K. J., Schopp, L. M., Alberts, K. R., Cassidy, J. T., & Frank, R. G. (1995). Predicting pain among children with juvenile rheumatoid arthritis. *Arthritis Care and Research, 8*, 36–42.

Hayford, J. R., & Ross, C. K. (1988). Medical compliance in juvenile rheumatoid arthritis: Problems and perspectives. *Arthritis Care and Research, 1*, 190–197.

Henoch, M. J., Batson, J. W., & Baum, J. (1978). Psychosocial factors in juvenile rheumatoid arthritis. *Arthritis and Rheumatism, 21*, 229–233.

Hogeweg, J. A., Huygen, A. C. J., De Jong-De Vos Van Steenwijk, C., Bernards, A. T. M., Oostendorp, R. A. B., & Helders, P. J. M. (1995). The pain threshold in juvenile chronic arthritis. *British Journal of Rheumatology, 34*, 61–67.

Hogeweg, J. A., Kuis, W., Oostendorp, R. A. B., & Helders, P. J .M. (1995). General and segmental reduced pain thresholds in juvenile chronic arthritis. *Pain, 62*, 11–17.

Hoyeraal, H. M. (1987). Methodological problems: Juvenile chronic arthritis. *Scandanavian Journal of Rheumatology, 66*, 69–74.

Huygen, A. C. J., Kuis, W., & Sinnema, G. (2000). Psychological, behavioral, and social adjustment in children and adolescents with juvenile chronic arthritis. *Annals of Rheumatic Disease, 59*, 276–282.

Ilowite, N. T., Walco, G. A., & Pochaczevsky, R. (1992). Assessment of pain in patients with juvenile rheumatoid arthritis: Relation between pain intensity and degree of joint inflammation. *Annals of the Rheumatic Diseases, 51*, 343–346.

International Association for the Study of Pain. (1979). Pain terms: A list with definitions and notes on usage: Recommended by the IASP subcommittee on taxonomy. *Pain, 6*, 249–252.

Keefe, F. J., & Lefebvre, J. C. (1994). Behaviour therapy. In P. D. Wall & R. Melzack (Eds.), *Textbook of pain* (3rd edition, pp. 1367–1380). Edinburgh, UK: Churchill Livingstone.

Kellerman, J., Zeltzer, L., Ellenberg, L., Dash, J., & Rigler, D. (1980). Psychological effects of illness in adolescence: I. Anxiety, self-esteem, and perception of control. *Journal of Pediatrics, 97*, 126–131.

Kuis, W., Heijnen, C. J., Hogeweg, J. A., Sinnema, G., & Helders, P. J. M. (1997). How painful is juvenile chronic arthritis? *Archives of Disease in Childhood, 77*, 451–453.

Lavigne, J. V., & Faier-Routman, J. (1992). Psychological adjustment to pediatric physical disorders: A meta-analytic review. *Journal of Pediatric Psychology, 17*, 133–157.

Lavigne, J. V., Ross, C. K., Berry, S. L., Hayford, J. R., & Pachman, L. M (1992). Evaluation of a psychological treatment package for treating pain in juvenile rheumatoid arthritis. *Arthritis Care and Research, 5*, 101–110.

Levine, J., & Taiwo, Y. (1994). Inflammatory pain. In P. D. Wall & R. Melzack (Eds), *Textbook of pain* (3rd ed., pp. 45–56). Edinburgh, UK: Churchill Livingstone.

Litt, I. F., & Cuskey, W. R. (1981). Compliance with salicylate therapy in adolescents with juvenile rheumatoid arthritis. *American Journal of Diseases of Children, 135*, 434–436.

Litt, I. F., Cuskey, W. R., & Rosenberg, A. (1982). Role of self-esteem and autonomy in determining medication compliance among adolescents with juvenile rheumatoid arthritis. *Pediatrics, 69*, 15–17.

Manuel, J. C. (2001). Risk and resistance factors in the adaptation in mothers of children with juvenile rheumatoid arthritis. *Journal of Pediatric Psychology, 26*, 237–246.

McAnarney, E. R., Pless, I. B., Satterwhite, B., & Friedman, S. B. (1974). Psychological problems of children with chronic juvenile arthritis. *Pediatrics, 53*, 523–528.

McGrath, P. A. (1990). *Pain in children: Nature, assessment and treatment*. New York: Guilford Press.

Melzack, R., & Wall, P. D. (1965). Pain and mechanisms: A new theory. *Science, 150*, 971–979.

Meyer, R. A., Campbell, J. N., & Raja, S. N. (1994). Peripheral neural mechanisms of nociception. In P. D. Wall & R. Melzack (Eds.), *Textbook of pain* (3rd ed., pp. 13–44). Edinburgh, UK: Churchill Livingstone.

Miller, J. J., Spitz, P. W., Simpson, U., & Williams, G. F. (1982). The social functioning of young adults who had arthritis in childhood. *Journal of Pediatrics, 100*, 378–382.

Noll, R. B., Kozlowski, K., Gerhardt, C., Vannatta, K., Taylor, J., & Passo, M. (2000). Social, emotional, and behavioral functioning of children with juvenile rheumatoid arthritis. *Arthritis and Rheumatism, 43*, 1387–1396.

Peterson, L. S., Mason, T., Nelson, A. M., O'Fallon, W. M., & Gabriel, S. E. (1997). Psychosocial outcomes and health status of adults who have had juvenile rheumatoid arthritis. *Arthritis and Rheumatism, 40*, 2235–2240.

Pless, K. B., & Roughmann, K. J. (1971). Chronic illness and its consequences: Observations based on three epidemiologic surveys. *Journal of Pediatrics, 79*, 351–359.

Quirk, M. E., & Young, M. H. (1990). The impact of JRA on children, adolescents, and their families; Current research and implications for future studies. *Arthritis Care and Research, 3*, 36–43.

Randich, A. (1993). Neural substrates of pain and analgesia. *Arthritis Care and Research, 6*, 171–177.

Rapoff, M. A. (1998). *Helping children follow their medical treatment program: Guidelines for parents of children with rheumatic diseases*. (Available from the author, University of Kansas Medical Center, Department of Pediatrics, 3901 Rainbow Boulevard, Kansas City, KS 66160–7330).

Rapoff, M. A. (1999). *Adherence to pediatric medical regimens.* New York: Kluwer/Plenum.

Rapoff, M. A. (2000). Facilitating adherence to medical regimens for pediatric rheumatic diseases: Primary, secondary, and tertiary prevention. In D. Drotar (Ed.), *Promoting adherence to medical treatment in chronic childhood illness: Concepts, methods, and interventions* (pp. 329–345). Mahwah, NJ: Erlbaum.

Rapoff, M. A., & Lindsley, C. B. (2000). The pain puzzle: A visual and conceptual metaphor for understanding and treating pain in pediatric rheumatic disease. *Journal of Rheumatology, 58*(Suppl.), 29–33.

Rapoff, M. A., Lindsley, C. B., & Christophersen, E. R. (1984). Improving compliance with medical regimens: Case study with juvenile rheumatoid arthritis. *Archives of Physical Medicine and Rehabilitation, 65,* 267–269.

Rapoff, M. A., Lindsley, C. B., & Christophersen, E. R. (1985). Parent perceptions of problems experienced by their children in complying with treatments for juvenile rheumatoid arthritis. *Archives of Physical Medicine and Rehabilitation, 66,* 427–430.

Rapoff, M. A., Purviance, M. R., & Lindsley, C. B. (1988a). Improving medication compliance for juvenile rheumatoid arthritis and its effect on clinical outcome: A single-subject analysis. *Arthritis Care and Research, 1,* 12–16.

Rapoff, M. A., Purviance, M. R., & Lindsley, C. B. (1988b). Educational and behavioral strategies for improving medication compliance in juvenile rheumatoid arthritis. *Archives of Physical Medicine and Rehabilitation, 69,* 439–441.

Reid, G. J., Gilbert, C. A., & McGrath, P. J. (1998). The Pain Coping Questionnaire: Preliminary validation. *Pain, 76,* 83–96.

Rimon, R., Belmaker, R. H., & Ebstein, R. (1977). Psychosomatic aspects of juvenile rheumatoid arthritis. *Scandinavian Journal of Rheumatology, 6,* 1–10.

Ross, C. K., Lavigne, J. V., Hayford, J. R., Berry, S. L., Sinacore, J. M., & Pachman, L. M. (1993). Psychological factors affecting reported pain in juvenile rheumatoid arthritis. *Journal of Pediatric Psychology, 18,* 561–573.

Ross, C. K., Lavigne, J. V., Hayford, J. R., Dyer, A. R., & Pachman, L. M. (1989). Validity of reported pain as a measure of clinical state in juvenile rheumatoid arthritis. *Annals of the Rheumatic Diseases, 48,* 817–819.

Schanberg, L. E., Lefebvre, J. C., Keefe, F. J., Kredich, D. W., & Gil, K. M. (1997). Pain coping and the pain experience in children with juvenile chronic arthritis. *Pain, 73,* 181–189.

Schanberg, L. E., Sandstrom, M. J., Starr, K., Gil, K. M., Lefebvre, J. C., Keefe, F. J., et al. (2000). The relationship of daily mood and stressful events to symptoms in juvenile rheumatic disease. *Arthritis Care and Research, 13,* 33–41.

Sherry, D. D., Bohnsack, J., Salmonson, K., Wallace, C. A., & Mellins, E. (1990). Painless juvenile rheumatoid arthritis. *Journal of Pediatrics, 116,* 921–923.

Sturge, C., Garralda, M. E., Boissin, M., Dore, C. J., & Woo, P. (1997). School attendance and juvenile chronic arthritis. *British Journal of Rheumatology, 36,* 1218–1223.

Sullivan, M. J. L., Bishop, S. R,, & Pivik, J. (1995). The Pain Catastrophizing Scale: Development and validation. *Psychological Assessment, 7,* 524–532.

Thastum, M., Zachariae, R., Schøler, M., Bjerring, P., & Herlin, T. (1997). Cold pressor pain: Comparing responses of juvenile arthritis patients and their parents. *Scandinavian Journal of Rheumatology, 26,* 272–279.

Thastum, M., Zachariae, R., Schøler, M., & Herlin, T. (1998). A Danish adaptation of the Pain Coping Questionnaire for children: Preliminary data concerning reliability and validity. *Acta Paediatrica, 88,* 132–138.

Thompson, K. L., Varni, J. W., & Hanson, V. (1987). Comprehensive assessment of pain in juvenile rheumatoid arthritis: An empirical model. *Journal of Pediatric Psychology, 12,* 241–255.

Ungerer, J. A., Horgan, B., Chaitow, J., & Champion, G. D. (1988). Psychosocial functioning in children and young adults with juvenile arthritis. *Pediatrics, 81,* 195–202.

Varni, J. W., Rapoff, M. A., Waldron, S. A., Gragg, R. A., Bernstein, B. H., & Lindsley, C. B. (1996a). Chronic pain and emotional distress in children and adolescents. *Journal of Developmental and Behavioral Pediatrics, 17,* 154–161.

Varni, J. W., Rapoff, M. A., Waldron, S. A., Gragg, R. A., Bernstein, B. H., & Lindsley, C. B. (1996b). Effects of perceived stress on pediatric chronic pain. *Journal of Behavioral Medicine, 19,* 515–528.

Varni, J. W., Waldron, S. A., Gragg, R. A., Rapoff, M. A., Bernstein, B. H., Lindsley, C. B., et al. (1996). Development of the Waldron/Varni Pediatric Pain Coping Inventory. *Pain, 67,* 141–150.

Varni, J. W., Wilcox, K. T., & Hanson, V. (1988). Mediating effects of family social support on child psychological adjustment in juvenile rheumatoid arthritis. *Health Psychology, 7,* 421–431.

von Weiss, R. T., Rapoff, M. A., Varni, J. W., Lindsley, C. B., Olson, N. Y., Madson, K. L., et al. (2002). Daily hassles and social support as predictors of adjustment in children with pediatric rheumatic disease. *Journal of Pediatric Psychology, 27,* 155–165.

Walco, G. A., Varni, J. W., & Ilowite, N. T. (1992). Cognitive behavioral pain management in children with juvenile rheumatoid arthritis. *Pediatrics, 89,* 1075–1079.

Wallander, J. L., & Varni, J. W. (1989). Social support and adjustment in chronically ill and handicapped children. *American Journal of Community Psychology, 17,* 185–201.

Wallander, J. L., & Varni, J. W. (1992). Adjustment in children with chronic physical disorders: Programmatic research on a disability–stress–coping model. In A. M. La Greca, L. J. Siegel, J. L. Wallander, & C. E. Walker (Eds.), *Stress and coping in child health* (pp. 279–298). New York: Guilford Press.

Wallander, J. L., Varni, J. W., Babani, L., Banis, H. T., & Wilcox, K. T. (1989). Family resources as resistance factors for psychological maladjustment in chronically ill and handicapped children. *Journal of Pediatric Psychology, 14,* 157–173.

Zautra, A., & Manne, S. L. (1992). Coping with rheumatoid arthritis: A review of a decade of research. *Annals of Behavioral Medicine, 14,* 31–39.

24

Cardiovascular Disease

ALAN M. DELAMATER

Cardiovascular disease in children includes congenital heart disease (CHD), acquired heart disease, and arrhythmias, as well as systemic hypertension. In recent years, surgical and medical advances have allowed many children with cardiovascular disease who previously would have died to survive. The increased longevity of pediatric cardiac patients, along with the stress associated with diagnosis, treatment, and ongoing management, has inspired many studies to determine the psychological and cognitive effects of cardiovascular disease in children. This chapter considers pediatric cardiac disorders and pediatric risk factors for adult-onset cardiovascular disease. The various types of pediatric cardiac disease and their medical management are described, followed by sections reviewing the effects of cardiac disease on cognitive development and behavioral and emotional functioning. Most of these studies have been conducted with children with CHD. The last part of the chapter reviews pediatric risk factors for adult-onset acquired cardiovascular disease, as well as interventions to reduce later risk of cardiovascular disease.

PEDIATRIC CARDIAC DISORDERS

Medical Aspects

Congenital Heart Disease

CHD refers to a variety of disorders involving structural defects to the heart or the coronary blood vessels that occur during fetal development. The etiology in most cases is not known, but it is presumed to be due to a combination of genetic and environmental factors. The incidence of CHD is approximately 8 in 1,000 live births (Gersony, 1987), and most cases are diagnosed during infancy. CHD is grouped into acyanotic and cyanotic subtypes. Oxygenation of blood is significantly reduced in cyanotic CHD. As reviewed later in the chapter, cyanosis can be an important factor in children's cognitive and psychological development.

Acynaotic CHD. The most common type of CHD involves holes in the walls of the heart chambers, the effect of which is to shunt blood away from the body and to the lungs. These disorders include ventricular septal defects (about 28% of CHD cases), atrial septal–atrial ventricular canal defects and patent ductus arteriosis (each about 10% of CHD cases), and coarctation (i.e., constriction) of the aorta (about 5% of CHD cases). Valvular lesions (which obstruct blood flow at the valves) may result in either pulmonic stenosis (about 10% of cases) or aortic stenosis (about 7% of cases). Cardiomyopathy (i.e., disease of the heart muscle) is another type of acyanotic CHD (Gersony, 1987).

Cyanotic CHD. Cyanotic CHD involves communication between the systemic and pulmonary circulations, with a shunting of blood away from the lungs; this process results in reduced oxygenation of the blood, or cyanosis. Examples of these defects include pulmonary atresia and tetralogy of Fallot, each of which account for about 10% of CHD cases. An additional 5% of CHD cases involve transposition of the great arteries, in which there is a reversal of the aorta and pulmonary arteries, leading to mixing of oxygenated and deoxygenated blood.

Medical management. Children and adolescents with CHD may show a number of symptoms, including fatigue, dyspnea (shortness of breath), growth failure, cough, cyanosis, or chest pain, depending on the type of lesion. The majority of patients with CHD have mild disease requiring no treatment. Although many patients with moderate to severe disease could be expected to function normally, those with severe disease will have decreased exercise tolerance and restricted physical activity. Patients with cyanotic CHD may be especially susceptible to fatigue, headaches, and dizziness and should avoid high altitudes, abrupt changes in temperature, and situations in which dehydration could occur. Females with mild or moderate disease who have had corrective surgery can have normal pregnancies; however, those with severe cyanotic CHD are at high risk for problems related to pregnancy.

Surgical advances over the past decades allow most severe defects to be corrected with low mortality rates. However, neurological complications of cardiac surgery are not uncommon and may significantly affect functioning, including mental retardation, language and learning disorders, and movement and seizure disorders (Ferry, 1987). In recent years there have been several important developments for surgical and medical interventions of CHD. One trend is primary repair of CHD during the neonatal period. Another trend has been the utilization of low-flow cardiopulmonary bypass rather than hypothermic circulatory arrest as a support technique during cardiac surgery, as the latter has been associated with greater central nervous system complications postoperatively. When children decompensate after open-heart surgery, extracorporeal membrane oxygenation (ECMO) has been successfully used in life-threatening situations. Interventional catheterization (i.e., angioplasty and valvuloplasty) has been increasingly used as an alternative to open-heart surgery for repair of certain types of CHD, including recurrent coarctation of the aorta, atrial septal defects, patent ductus arteriosus, and pulmonic and aortic stenosis. Heart transplantation has become an accepted treatment approach in cases of severe end-stage heart disease without other treatment options. More than 3,500 pediatric heart transplantations have been conducted by various centers throughout the world since 1982, with 1-year survival rates of 75 to 85% and 4-year survival rates of 65%.

Most patients with CHD require medical follow-up at regular intervals. Depending on the status of the lesion, patients may be seen from once a week to once a month or once a year. Many cases followed by pediatric cardiologists include older children and adolescents with complex, severe defects that were corrected in early childhood. Routine tests for evaluation and monitoring include chest radiographs, electrocardiograms, echocardiography, exercise testing, radionuclide studies, and cardiac catheterization. Because invasive procedures may be stressful to young patients, routine clinical practice for most patients involves heavy sedation. After surgical repair, some patients and parents may fear recurrence of heart-related problems or have unrealistic perceptions concerning physical activity restrictions. Residual problems may exist, requiring further interventions, including surgery. Additional information on the medical aspects of CHD can be found in Fyler (1992).

Acquired Heart Disease

Acquired heart disease in childhood includes a variety of disorders, generally resulting from bacterial and/or viral infections that damage the heart. These disorders include infective endocarditis, rheumatic heart disease, and diseases of the myocardium and pericardium (Gersony, 1987). Normal children may acquire these diseases, but children with CHD may be particularly susceptible. Another type of acquired heart disease is coronary artery disease secondary to Kawasaki syndrome. Medical treatment for acquired heart disease includes prophylactic drug regimens, and sometimes cardiac surgery is required to repair the structural damage to the heart. When other treatment options are exhausted in severe cases, heart transplantation may be undertaken as a last resort. Acquired heart disease is a significant cause of morbidity and mortality among children. With early diagnosis and effective treatment, however, mortality is low. Preventive interventions are therefore very important in the medical management of acquired heart disease. One of the major problems seen in clinical practice with this patient population is nonadherence with prophylactic drug regimens. Unfortunately, empirical studies with this population are lacking. Because these diseases pose a considerable health risk for children, more research addressing regimen adherence of children with acquired heart diseases is needed.

Arrhythmias

Childhood cardiac rhythm disturbances or arrhythmias can result from CHD (both acyanotic and cyanotic subtypes), acquired heart diseases, or acquired systemic disorders. The main risk associated with an arrhythmia is severe tachycardia (fast heart rate) or bradycardia (slow heart rate), resulting in decreased cardiac output; severe untreated arrhythmia may lead to sudden death. Some rhythm disturbances, such as premature atrial and ventricular beats, are common in children but are not associated with significant health risks in the majority of cases. The most common significant arrhythmias are bypass tracts such as Wolff–Parkinson–White (pre-excitation) syndrome (i.e., a type of supraventricular tachyarrhythmia) and congenital heartblock (i.e., a type of bradyarrhythmia; Gersony, 1987). Arrhythmias are identified more often now in children because of improved diagnostic methods with electrocardiogram. There are also more survivors of cardiac surgery for CHD who are at increased risk for arrhythmias. Treatments include pharmacological agents, surgery to remove bypass tracts, implanted pacemakers and defibrillators, and heart transplantation for extreme cases unresponsive to other interventions. Problems with dosage of medications, variable responses, side effects, and medication adherence are significant issues in the treatment of pediatric arrhythmias. Relatively few studies of psychological and behavioral factors have been conducted with these patients.

Effects on Cognitive Development

A number of studies have examined cognitive development of children with CHD. The results of these studies generally suggest that lesions resulting in cyanosis may have an adverse effect on cognitive development, presumably due to inadequate oxygenation of the brain during early development. In addition, findings support the idea that surgery conducted at earlier ages is associated with improved cognitive functioning.

In a study of cyanotic children who had corrective surgery for transposition of the great arteries (TGA) prior to testing, Newburger, Silbert, Buckley, and Fyler (1984) found IQ to be in the normal range. There was no difference compared with a group of children with acyanotic CHD (all with ventricular septal defect) who had also received corrective surgery. Although a significant inverse correlation was observed between age at repair (reflecting duration of hypoxia) and IQ for the cyanotic children, there was no relationship between age at repair and IQ for the acyanotic group.

O'Dougherty, Wright, Garmezy, Loewenson, and Torres (1983) evaluated a group of school-age children with TGA on standardized measures of intelligence, perceptual–motor functioning, and academic achievement. The children had open-heart surgical repair during early childhood. Although the mean IQ of the group was in the normal range, the distribution was bimodal, with more children than expected having borderline or lower intelligence (13%) or superior or very superior intelligence (16%). An inverse correlation was obtained between age at surgery and IQ, perceptual–motor function, and academic achievement, suggesting that chronic hypoxia has adverse effects on cognitive development. Forty-two percent of the sample required special education programs. In another report on these same children, O'Dougherty, Wright, Loewenson, and Torres (1985) compared them to a sample of control children matched for age, race, and socioeconomic status but with no history of sensory, neurological, or learning problems. The cyanotic CHD group scored significantly lower on the WISC-R Freedom from Distractibility factor than would be expected based on the standardization sample, and they performed more poorly on a continuous performance test of attention. In addition, 23% of the CHD sample versus only 4% of the WISC-R standardization sample had a 30-point discrepancy between Verbal and Performance IQ.

Aram, Ekelman, Ben-Schachar, and Levinsohn (1985) found that children with cyanotic CHD had significantly lower IQ scores than children with acyanotic CHD. DeMaso, Beardslee, Silbert, and Fyler (1990) evaluated the intellectual functioning of children with TGA, children with tetralogy of Fallot (TOF), and a group of children originally diagnosed with acyanotic CHD who experienced spontaneous recovery without medical intervention. Significantly lower IQ scores were found in both cyanotic groups than in the controls. Fourteen percent of children with TGA and 22% of children with TOF had IQ scores less than 79, as compared with only 3% of the acyanotic children. In addition, 40% of children with TGA and 45% of children with TOF had clinically significant CNS impairment.

The effects of surviving a cardiac arrest on the cognitive functioning of children with CHD has also been examined. Morris, Krawiecki, Wright, and Walter (1993) found that more children than expected scored less than one standard deviation below the normative means for the various neuropsychological tests used in the study. In addition, a longer duration of cardiac arrest was associated with worse performance. A control group was not studied, and it could not be determined whether the observed deficits were due to cyanotic CHD or to cardiac arrest. Bloom, Wright, Morris, Campbell, and Krawiecki (1997) compared children with CHD who had sustained a cardiac arrest in the hospital with a medically similar group of children with CHD to examine the additive impact of cardiac arrest on the functioning of children with CHD. The children in the cardiac-arrest group had significantly lower scores on measures of general cognitive, motor, and adaptive behavior functioning, as well as greater disease severity. Forty-four percent of the cardiac-arrest group performed at least one standard deviation below the mean on the general cognitive index .as compared with only 6% of the children who had not sustained a cardiac arrest. These findings suggest that children who survive cardiac arrest may be at increased risk for cognitive difficulties.

A study was conducted by Chinese researchers to determine the impact of acyanotic CHD on intellectual development of children (Yang, Liu, & Townes, 1994). The findings revealed significantly lower cognitive abilities—particularly complex integrative brain function—in the children with acyanotic CHD than in a control group of children matched for age, educational level, and social class.

Relatively few studies have examined the school performance of children with CHD. Wright and Nolan (1994) compared the school performance of a group of children with surgically corrected cyanotic lesions with that of a group of children who had innocent murmurs. The findings showed poorer performance in all academic areas in the children with cyanotic CHD. Previous studies with small samples have shown moderate cognitive impairment in young children with hypoplastic left heart syndrome (e.g., Kern, Hinton, Nereo, Hayes, & Gersony, 1998). A recent study of developmental outcomes in a larger sample of children with this disease was conducted by Mahle and colleagues (2000). Parent questionnaires indicated that one-third of the children had been diagnosed with a learning disability and were receiving special education, with 19% having been held back in school. Standardized intellectual testing was performed with a subsample of these patients, revealing a median IQ of 86, with 18% of patients in the mentally retarded range and 36% in the borderline range. Multivariate analyses indicated that lower full-scale IQ and verbal IQ was predicted by history of preoperative seizure activity and that lower performance IQ was predicted by preoperative seizures and longer duration of cardiopulmonary bypass during surgery.

Behavioral and Emotional Functioning

A number of studies have examined the behavioral and emotional functioning of children with CHD. Early studies suggested a negative impact on behavior, emotions, and family functioning. Generally, more recent studies indicate several specific problems observed during early childhood but fairly adaptive functioning later in childhood.

Children with CHD may have impaired growth and have been described as having difficulty with feeding. Lobo (1992) examined parent–infant interaction during feeding of infants with various types of CHD compared with healthy controls matched for age and birthweight. The findings suggested that the behavior of infants with CHD may make feeding difficult, increasing the risk of growth problems. One factor that may contribute to behavioral difficulties is temperament. Marino and Lipshitz (1991) examined parent-rated temperament in a group of infants and toddlers with CHD and compared their scores with norms from standardized scales. Results indicated that infants with CHD were more withdrawn and intense in emotional reactions and had lower thresholds for stimulation. Toddlers with CDH were rated as less active, rhythmic, and intense and more negative in mood. However, there was no relationship between severity of CHD (as determined by oxygen saturation levels and physician ratings) and temperament. In another study related to temperament and parent–child interaction, Bradford (1990) examined factors related to young children's distress during diagnostic procedures. Children were observed with their mothers present while they underwent radiological examination for possible CHD. Stranger sociability and parental discipline were also measured using accepted methods. Nearly half of the sample did not exhibit significant distress during the procedure. Child distress was associated with low stranger sociability and negative parenting style (i.e., use of force and reinforcement of dependency).

DeMaso et al. (1990) examined psychological functioning as part of their study of children with cyanotic CHD, described earlier. Both groups of children with cyanotic CHD (i.e., TGA and TOF) were rated as having poorer psychological functioning than the control group of healthy children who had spontaneous recovery of their heart problems. There was no difference between the cyanotic subgroups. Multiple regression analysis revealed that psychological functioning was predicted by degree of CNS impairment and IQ. DeMaso et al. (1991) examined the effect of maternal perceptions and CHD severity on the behavioral–emotional adjustment of children. The total Behavior Problems score from the Child Behavior Checklist was used as the criterion measure. Predictor variables included the Parenting Stress Index, Parental Locus of Control Scale, and a measure of disease severity. Results showed good overall behavioral functioning for the children. Similarly, scores for parenting stress and locus of control were very close to the means from the norms for these measures. The majority of variance in child adjustment was accounted for by maternal perceptions, with medical severity explaining very little variance. The Morris et al. (1993) study of children who survived cardiac arrest, described earlier, included two measures of behavioral and emotional functioning. Although behavioral problems were not observed, a significant proportion of the sample scored less than a standard deviation below the mean for norms on a measure of adaptive behavior.

Spurkland, Bjornstad, Lindberg, and Seem (1993) examined psychosocial functioning in adolescents with "complex" (i.e., cyanotic) CHD compared with adolescents who had repaired atrial septal defects and were in good health. Measures included behavioral ratings by parents, standardized clinical interviews for diagnosis of psychiatric disorders, and interviews with parents to assess family functioning. Physical capacity was quantified by a standardized bicycle ergometer stress test. Significant differences in physical capacity and psychiatric status were observed between the groups. Forty-two percent of the youths with complex CHD were given DSM-III diagnoses versus 27% of the acyanotic patients. The most common diagnoses were overanxious disorder and dysthymic disorder. Among youths with complex CHD, only one-third were functioning normally, with one-third having minor to moderate problems and another third having serious dysfunction. In the acyanotic group, only 4% had a major psychiatric disorder, with 54% functioning normally and 42% having minor to moderate problems. Greater psychopathology was associated with more severe physical impairment. Parent behavior ratings revealed clinically significant problems in 19% of the complex group versus only 4% in the acyanotic group. Family difficulties were associated with psychosocial functioning of adolescents, but similar levels of chronic family difficulties were evident in both groups.

Yang et al. (1994) studied the behavioral adjustment of children with acyanotic CHD. Behavioral ratings made by parents indicated more behavioral problems in patients with CHD than in controls. Casey, Sykes, Craig, Power, and Mulholland (1996) examined the behavioral adjustment of children with surgically corrected complex CHD compared with healthy children with innocent heart murmurs. Behavior ratings by teachers indicated that children with CHD were more withdrawn and more likely to have academic achievement problems. Degree of family strain and exercise tolerance were significant predictors of teacher-rated school performance. Ratings by parents revealed that children with CHD were more withdrawn, had more social problems, and engaged in fewer activities.

Few studies have considered longer term psychological adjustment of children with CHD. Baer, Freedman, and Garson (1984) reported a study of psychological functioning in young adults who had surgical correction for TOF during childhood. Patients were divided into two groups, based on early or later age at surgery. Results suggested that children receiving later surgery described their current personalities as more timid and reserved, less venturesome, and more apprehensive than those who had surgery earlier in childhood. Long-term psychosocial functioning was also evaluated by Utens and colleagues (1994). This study is noteworthy because of the large sample, including 288 young adult patients who were evaluated at a mean follow-up interval of 16 years after surgical correction for CHD in childhood. Compared with reference groups, CHD patients reported favorable psychosocial adjustment, with fewer emotional symptoms and better self-esteem, and no negative effects in terms of school or employment. There were no differences among patients with various types of CHD. Another study of long-term psychological outcomes was reported by Alden, Gilljam, and Gillberg (1998). These investigators studied adolescents with TGA who had had surgical correction on average 11.5 years earlier. Children completed measures of self-esteem and body image, and parents completed a measure of family functioning and were interviewed regarding their child's psychiatric status. Although the findings generally indicated good psychosocial functioning for these patients and their families, 19% of the patients had significant symptoms, most with internalizing disorders. Poorer cardiac function was associated with more emotional symptoms.

The studies reviewed here have all considered the behavioral and emotional adjustment of children with CHD. However, few studies are available concerning the psychosocial functioning of children with other types of cardiovascular disorders. Schneider, Davis, Boxer, Fisher, and Friedman (1990) evaluated psychosocial functioning in adolescent patients with Marfan syndrome. Patients and their parents were interviewed, and patients completed a measure of self-image. Although good psychosocial adaptation was reported, patients did indicate negative effects of their disease on physical activities and self-image. There was also evidence of problems with adherence to the medical regimen.

Another cardiovascular disease that has received little research attention is arrhythmias. DeMaso and colleagues (2000) examined psychological functioning in children and adolescents both before and 3 months after they underwent radiofrequency catheter ablation to correct their arrhythmias. Normal psychological functioning was observed before ablation. After ablation, patients reported reductions in cardiac-related anxiety and increased enjoyment, with better functioning reported by patients who had curative ablation, suggesting improved quality of life following ablation.

A recent study by Schneider, Delamater, Geith, Young, and Wolff (2001) specifically examined disease-related quality of life in children with arrhythmias. Patients completed a new measure of quality of life designed to assess issues related to having an arrhythmia. The majority of children reported their health to be excellent or good. Children who had had previous surgery for their cardiac condition reported increased worries regarding their arrhythmias. Greater frequency of daily medications was associated with more worries about their arrhythmias and greater impact of the arrhythmias on their lives. These findings suggest that past surgical history and current regimen complexity are associated with disease-specific quality of life in young patients with cardiac arrhythmias.

Impact of Newer Medical Interventions

Several new developments have occurred in recent years regarding medical and surgical interventions for cardiac disease in children. Surgical repair for CHD is now commonly undertaken during the neonatal period, as studies have demonstrated the advantages of early repair. Regarding newer support techniques during surgery, low-flow cardiopulmonary bypass has advantages over hypothermic circulatory arrest in terms of perioperative neurological effects, although longer term effects have not yet been determined. In this section the few studies evaluating the psychological effects of low-flow cardiopulmonary bypass, ECMO, heart transplantation, and pacemakers are discussed.

Hypothermic Circulatory and Low-Flow Cardiopulmonary Bypass

Several studies have shown the use of low-flow cardiopulmonary bypass to be associated with reduced neurological sequelae. Bellinger et al. (1995) conducted a randomized clinical trial of children with TGA that had been repaired by an arterial switch operation that used either predominantly total circulatory arrest or continuous low-flow cardiopulmonary bypass. Developmental and neurological evaluations were performed at 1 year of age. Infants who received circulatory arrest had lower mean scores on the Psychomotor Development index of the Bayley Scales of Infant Development and a higher proportion had scores less than 80 (27 vs. 12%). The score on the Psychomotor Development index was inversely related to the duration of circulatory arrest. Neurological abnormalities were more common among the children assigned to circulatory arrest, and the risk of neurological abnormalities increased with the duration of circulatory arrest. In a follow-up study, Bellinger, Rappaport, Wypij, Wernovsky, and Newburger (1997) examined these children's developmental status based on parent-completed questionnaires when the children were 2½ years of age. Results indicated that the children in the circulatory arrest group showed poorer expressive language. Oates, Simpson, Turnbull, and Cartmill (1995) compared children who had had their defects repaired with the use of deep hypothermia and circulatory arrest to those who had had repair with the use of cardiopulmonary bypass. Children's cognitive abilities were examined at an average of 9 to 10 years after the operations. Shorter reaction times were observed for children in the bypass group than for those in the hypothermic circulatory arrest group. Although there were no significant differences in intelligence scores between the groups, a relationship was observed between IQ scores and arrest time, indicating a significant decrease in IQ with increasing arrest time.

Extracorporeal Membrane Oxygenation

Extracorporeal membrane oxygenation (ECMO) is a surgical procedure involving cardiopulmonary bypass of blood via cannulation of the right common carotid artery and right internal jugular vein. This is a life-saving technique used for children whose risk of survival is less than 20% without ECMO. ECMO is considered a standard therapy for neonatal respiratory failure that is unresponsive to other interventions. Several studies have examined the developmental course of these young children. Generally, results have shown that children treated with ECMO develop at or just below age-expected levels, in terms of growth and intellectual functioning, up to 3 years of age. Longer term follow-up studies into middle childhood similarly indicate that most children demonstrated normal growth and development but that neurological complications occurred in nearly 20% of cases.

ECMO has also been applied to children whose cardiopulmonary status deteriorates rapidly following surgery for repair of CHD. This latter group of patients is usually older, ranging from infants to preschoolers. Little is known, however, about children who have received ECMO after cardiac surgery. Tindall, Rothermel, Delamater, Pinsky, and Klein (1999) examined neuropsychological functioning in young children who had ECMO after cardiac surgery 4 years previous to the study, compared with cardiac controls (without ECMO) and normal control children. Patients who had ECMO had significantly more impairment than the other groups, including abstract reasoning and lateralized motor impairment (left hand), as well as lower visual memory and visual-spatial constructive skills, compared with both cardiac and normal controls.

Heart Transplantation

Very ill children with severe CHD, acquired cardiac disease, or intractable arrhythmias may require heart transplantation. This procedure was first performed successfully in children over 25 years ago. In recent years more pediatric heart transplants have been performed, and techniques have been refined. Survival rates and quality of life have improved so dramatically that this treatment is now considered an accepted modality for patients whose disease is at end stage and for whom there are no alternative treatments. However, approximately 20% of children may have neurological complications following heart transplantation. Descriptive clinical reports suggest that children do not have major abnormalities and that rehabilitation is good as children return to school and engage in age-appropriate activities (e.g., Backer et al., 1992). Several studies have examined the cognitive development and psychological adjustment of children following heart transplantation and have indicated that some patients may be at risk for cognitive and psychosocial problems following transplantation (Todaro, Fennell, Sears, Rodrigue, & Roche, 2000).

Cognitive Development. Trimm (1991) used the Bayley Scales of Infant Development to evaluate the development of infants who received heart transplantation before 4 months of age. The majority of children had Mental Development index scores in the normal range over the follow-up period. However, 41% had scores less than 84 on the Psychomotor Development index. In another study of neurodevelopmental outcomes of children receiving transplants during infancy, Baum et al. (1993) found a mean Bayley Mental Developmental index of 87 and Psychomotor Developmental index of 90, with 67% of the sample having scores in the normal range. Wray and Yacoub (1991) compared children who received heart transplantation with children who had corrective open-heart surgery and healthy control children. Developmental evaluations indicated that the transplant group scored lower than the healthy controls but that mean scores were within normal limits. For children older than 5 years of age, however, the transplant group was significantly lower than both groups on developmental and academic achievement scores. Those with a history of cyanotic CHD, regardless of transplant or open-heart surgery, did worse. In another report, Wray, Pot-Mees, Zeitlin, Radley-Smith, and Yacoub (1994) found that, about 1 year after transplantation, children with heart transplants had lower developmental functioning than healthy controls and lower intellectual abilities and spelling achievement than both healthy controls and children with CHD who had received open-heart surgery. A recent report evaluated neurodevelopmental outcomes in 18 children who had heart transplantation during infancy (Fleisher et al., 2002). Compared with an age-matched group of children who had received cardiac surgery for CHD, children who had transplants had more difficulties with growth and development, neurological abnormalities, hearing problems, and speech and language delays.

Psychosocial Adjustment. Uzark and colleagues (1992) examined psychosocial adjustment nearly 2 years after heart transplant in a group of children. Parent behavior ratings indicated that these children had significantly lower levels of social competence and more behavior problems than the normative population, with depression noted as the most common psychological problem among these patients. Psychosocial problems of children were associated with greater family stress and fewer family coping resources. Wray et al. (1994) also found more behavior problems among children who had heart transplants, compared with children with CHD who had corrective surgery or healthy controls. Significant behavior problems were noted in 24% of the sample of children who had transplants. DeMaso, Twente, Spratt, and O'Brien (1995) evaluated psychosocial functioning of children both before and 1 year after heart transplantation. Psychosocial adjustment was noted to improve markedly at follow-up, although 20% of patients still had some symptoms of psychological distress. Patients with more psychosocial difficulties prior to transplantation had more hospitalizations after transplantation. Serrano-Ikkos, Lask, Whitehead, Rees, and Graham (1999) also examined the psychosocial adjustment of children both before and 1 year after heart transplants and compared them with children receiving conventional surgery for CHD. Before surgery, psychiatric disorder was observed in 26% of children in both groups; after surgery, psychiatric disorder decreased to 6% in the conventional surgery group but remained elevated in the transplant group.

Little is known about the school performance of children after they have received heart transplants, although one recent study addressing this issue was reported by Wray, Long, Radley-Smith, and Yacoub (2001). Children returned to school on average about 6 months after transplantation. Although complete data were not available on all children throughout the 5-year follow-up phase, findings indicated that children who had had heart transplants were more likely to be underachieving in reading and arithmetic; this finding was attributable to school absences. In addition, although behavior problems were noted by teachers in only 6% of the heart-transplant group at 6 months posttransplant, significant behavior problems were noted in 29% at 3 years and in 27% at 5 years after transplant.

The posttransplantation regimen is stressful, including daily doses of immunosuppressive medications that may have considerable side effects, as well as extensive medical follow-up, including endomyocardial biopsy. Adherence problems may become an issue, yet few studies have addressed this issue. Studies indicate that 20% (Douglas, Hsu, & Addonizio, 1993) to 30% (Serrano-Ikkos, Lask, Whitehead, & Eisler, 1998) of pediatric patients have significant adherence problems, increasing the chances of graft rejection. Similarly, in a study of adult patients, those who were nonadherent had higher incidences of hospital readmission and higher total medical costs (Paris, Muchmore, Pribil, Zuhdi, & Cooper, 1994).

Pacemakers

More children are receiving pacemakers for heart rhythm disturbances, but little is known about psychosocial functioning in this patient population. Alpern, Uzark, and Dick (1989) conducted a study of children with CHD who required pacemakers, 33% of whom had cyanotic CHD. Comparison groups included CHD patients without pacemakers (50% with cyanotic CHD) and healthy children. Standardized measures of trait anxiety, self-competence, and locus of control were obtained. No differences were observed for anxiety and self-competence, but children with pacemakers reported a more external locus of control. Content analysis of interviews with the children revealed those with pacemakers had heightened fears of pacemaker failure and social rejection. However, although the nonpacemaker group and healthy controls viewed children with pacemakers as having significant emotional and social differences, children with pacemakers perceived themselves as no different from their peers. These findings suggest relatively healthy psychological adaptation in children with CHD who have pacemakers, but these children may be at risk for difficulties with autonomy and social isolation and rejection.

Summary and Implications for Future Research

Research findings indicate that children with cyanotic CHD are at risk for having lower intellectual abilities than children with acyanotic CHD, particularly if their disease is severe and if their corrective surgery is not completed within the first few years of life. It is important to note, however, that mean IQ scores of children with cyanotic CHD have consistently been in the normal range and that lower IQ scores have been associated with significant CNS involvement. It appears that corrective surgery, particularly when conducted at younger ages, has significant benefits on intellectual functioning, presumably due to better oxygenation of the brain during early development. Even after surgery, however, these children may still be at risk for learning problems, as some evidence indicates greater distractibility and attention deficits and lower levels of academic achievement. Children treated with ECMO after cardiac surgery appear to experience both general cognitive impairment and lateralized deficits of functions performed by the right hemisphere. After heart transplantation, children's cognitive development appears to proceed normally, but children receiving transplantation at older ages do less well than those treated earlier.

The research literature on behavioral and emotional functioning suggests that infants with CHD have temperamental characteristics that may make feeding difficult. This finding could partly explain the tendency for children with CHD to show abnormal growth. Some evidence shows parent–infant interaction problems during feeding. With regard to psychosocial adjustment later in childhood, the findings are mixed, with some reports of adjustment difficulties in the children with more severe cyanotic CHD. Older children may have concerns with social anxiety, autonomy, and feelings of vulnerability. When standardized behavioral ratings are reported, mean scores for the group have typically been within the normal range. In general, the data suggest that the risk of adjustment problems increases when corrective surgery occurs later in childhood or when physical capacity remains limited and cyanosis persists.

The research literature on CHD is limited by several methodological problems. Study samples are usually small, raising concerns about sampling bias. When sociodemographic characteristics of the sample are reported, in most cases the sample is predominantly white and in the middle range of socioeconomic status. Additionally, samples are often heterogeneous with regard to type of cardiac defect. Several studies did not use control groups, relying instead on comparisons with test norms. This approach is not appropriate because any differences observed cannot necessarily be attributed to CHD; rather, differences can be due to having a chronic disease that involves frequent contact with health care professionals.

Few controlled studies have been reported with respect to the developmental outcomes of children receiving cardiac transplantation or ECMO. Further studies with larger samples are needed to more precisely determine the longer term neurodevelopmental outcomes of children. More studies of medication adherence are needed following cardiac transplantation. Although the development and psychosocial adjustment of children after heart transplantation appears normal, a significant number of children may have learning difficulties, and there is some evidence of increased depression and lower social competence among school-age children. This issue remains important for future studies.

Very little intervention research has been reported. A clinical report by Bullock and Shaddy (1993) suggests that relaxation and imagery techniques without sedation are helpful for pediatric heart transplant patients during endomyocardial biopsy. In a controlled study, Campbell, Kirkpatrick, Berry, and Lamberti (1995) found that a family-based cognitive-behavioral treatment including relaxation and problem solving resulted in better adjustment in the hospital, as well as at home and school after discharge.

The research findings suggest a number of issues to consider in clinical practice. Parents should be counseled, while their child is still an infant, regarding the risk of temperamental difficulties and associated feeding problems during infancy and early childhood. Specific training in feeding skills could be initiated early and may help prevent growth problems commonly observed among CHD children. In addition, counseling regarding potential academic difficulties may be useful, particularly for school-age children with more severe disease; these children should have comprehensive psychoeducational evaluations and individual educational plans made as needed to facilitate optimal academic performance.

Many parents and patients may have unrealistic perceptions concerning the risk of sudden death, leading to unnecessary restrictions for the child and greater distress for all. Studies with mothers of children with CHD reveal a number of concerns and issues for their own adjustment (Davis, Brown, Bakeman, & Campbell, 1998; Van Horn, DeMaso, Gonzalez-Heydrich, & Erickson, 2001). Given the potentially disabling effects of cyanotic CHD, counseling is needed about reasonable expectations for age-appropriate activities, including participation in sports. For older girls anticipating parenthood, counseling is also indicated regarding the significant risks associated with pregnancy.

In terms of acquired heart disease of childhood, little systematic research has been reported. This area needs more attention from pediatric psychologists. Research studies should particularly target adherence to prophylactic drug regimens, as this is a significant clinical issue related to morbidity of children and clinical decisions regarding transplantation.

PEDIATRIC RISK FACTORS FOR ADULT-ONSET HEART DISEASE

Despite the decline in mortality due to cardiovascular disease in adults over the past few decades, coronary heart disease remains the major cause of death in the United States (Sytkowski, Kannel, & D'Agostino, 1990). Epidemiological research conducted with adults has established elevated levels of blood pressure, serum cholesterol, cigarette smoking, diabetes mellitus, advancing age, and family history of heart disease as primary risk factors for coronary heart disease (Kannel, McGee, & Gordon, 1976). Although the Type A behavior pattern had been proposed as another independent risk factor for adult heart disease, hostility has been identified as the cardiotoxic component of the Type A behavior pattern (e.g., Barefoot, Dahlstrom, & Williams, 1983).

A substantial literature exists that addresses the development in childhood of risk factors for later cardiovascular disease in adulthood. Coronary heart disease generally makes its first clinical appearance in middle age, but evidence indicates that the atherosclerotic process begins during childhood (Berenson et al., 1980). Recent studies have shown the presence of atherosclerosis in the aorta and coronary arteries in adolescents who died and underwent autopsy (e.g., Berenson et al., 1998). A number of risk factors for coronary heart disease have been identified in healthy children, including elevated blood pressure, high cholesterol, and obesity (Lauer, Connor, Leaverton, Reiter, & Clarke, 1975), as well as cigarette smoking and hostility. Therefore, much research has addressed the question of how to prevent coronary heart disease by implementing health promotion programs during childhood. The following sections provide an overview of risk factors in childhood for cardiovascular disease of adulthood and health promotion interventions to prevent adult cardiovascular disease.

High Blood Pressure

The prevalence of clinical hypertension in children is relatively infrequent and is generally secondary to disorders in the renal, vascular, or endocrine systems. Secondary hypertension is generally more common among younger children, with about 75% due to a renal abnormality. Primary, or essential, hypertension refers to elevated blood pressure without a known etiology that can explain it, and it is more common in adolescents than in younger children. It is important to note that in unselected pediatric samples, causes of hypertension are identifiable only in a very small percentage of cases. Many factors are thought to be involved in the development of essential hypertension, including heredity, obesity, salt sensitivity, and stress.

A number of studies have established that high blood pressure in childhood can predict essential hypertension in adulthood (e.g., Lauer & Clarke, 1989). Blood pressure levels have been observed in longitudinal studies to track fairly well throughout childhood, particularly at the higher levels (e.g., Lauer, Clarke, & Beaglehole, 1984). Resting blood pressure, blood pressure reactivity to laboratory stressors, and obesity have been shown to predict ambulatory blood pressure 2½ years later in young adolescents (Del Rosario, Treiber, Harshfield, Davis, & Strong, 1998). Obesity and blood pressure reactivity were also predictive of left ventricular hypertrophy at follow-up in these adolescents (Murdison et al., 1998). High blood pressure in children has clearly been shown to be related to being overweight. For example, in the Bogalusa study the odds ratios for overweight children having high diastolic and systolic blood pressure were 2.4 and 4.5, respectively (Freedman, Dietz, Srinivasan, & Berenson, 1999).

According to the National High Blood Pressure Education Program Working Group on Hypertension Control in Children and Adolescents (1996), estimates of the prevalence of pediatric hypertension have varied due to inconsistencies in definitions and measurement across studies. Normal blood pressure is considered to be less than the 90th percentile for age and sex for both systolic and diastolic blood pressure; high normal is defined as either systolic or diastolic blood pressure or both being between the 90th and 95th percentiles for age and sex; high blood pressure (significant hypertension) is defined as average systolic and/or diastolic blood pressure greater than or equal to the 95th percentile for age and sex measured on at least three occasions; severe hypertension exceeds the 99th percentile. The prevalence of significant hypertension is overestimated when using only a few screenings. Most large screening studies have found a prevalence of about 1–2% after multiple evaluations (e.g., Sinaiko, Gomez-Marin, & Prineas, 1989).

High Cholesterol

Epidemiological studies have demonstrated that elevated blood cholesterol levels, particularly low-density lipoprotein (LDL) cholesterol, increase risk for coronary heart disease (e.g., Castelli et al., 1986). Clinical trials with adults have shown significantly reduced risk of coronary heart disease via lowering of blood cholesterol. High cholesterol early in life plays an important role in the development of adult coronary heart disease. In a study of 35 individuals from the Bogalusa heart study who died at a mean age of 18 years, autopsy results showed a significant association of serum total and LDL cholesterol with degree of aortic fatty streaks (Newman et al., 1986). The distributions of blood lipid levels in childhood and adolescence have been described in epidemiological studies (Berenson et al., 1980; Lauer et al., 1975). Studies have also shown relatively good tracking of blood cholesterol levels, so that children who have high levels are likely to also have high levels as adults (Lauer & Clarke, 1990).

The report of the Expert Panel on Blood Cholesterol Levels in Children and Adolescents (1992) made the following conclusions: (1) children and adolescents in the United States have higher levels of blood cholesterol than children in other countries; (2) autopsy studies have shown that early coronary atherosclerosis begins in childhood and adolescence; (3) high blood total cholesterol, low-density lipoprotein cholesterol and very low-density lipoprotein cholesterol, and low high-density lipoprotein cholesterol are associated with early atherosclerotic lesions; (4) children and adolescents with high cholesterol levels often have positive family histories for coronary heart disease; (5) familial aggregation for high blood cholesterol may result from both genetic and environmental factors; and (6) children and adolescents with high cholesterol have an increased probability of high cholesterol levels as adults. According to the report, total cholesterol levels less than 170 mg/dL and LDL cholesterol less than 110 mg/dL are in the acceptable range; 170–199 for total cholesterol and 110–129 for LDL cholesterol are borderline; 200 for total cholesterol and 130 LDL cholesterol are classified as high (95th percentile), warranting further evaluation. In light of the considerable data relating high cholesterol to increased risk of coronary heart disease and the association between dietary intake and blood cholesterol levels in children (Morrison et al., 1980), the report of the Expert Panel (1992) made the following nutrition recommendations for healthy children and adolescents: saturated fats should be less than 10% of total calories; total fat should average no more than 30% of total calories; and dietary cholesterol should be less than 300 mg/day.

Cigarette Smoking

Despite the well-known health hazards associated with smoking, significant numbers of adolescents smoke tobacco. In a study reported in 1981, about one-fourth of high school seniors reporting daily cigarette smoking (Johnston, Bachman, & O'Malley, 1981). Ten years later, a study of students in the sixth through ninth grades showed a prevalence of 25% for cigarette smoking and 12% for smokeless tobacco (Gottlieb, Pope, Rickert, & Hardin, 1993). Smoking has increased among girls, so that their smoking rate is about equal to that of boys, and cigarette smoking has remained high among adolescents in recent years. Use of smokeless tobacco is increasing among children and adolescents (Brownson, DiLorenzo, Van Tuinen, & Finger, 1990). Peer and parental influences appear to be most significant in youths' smoking acquisition (Biglan, McConnell, Severson, Bavry, & Ary, 1984; Noland et al., 1990). Given the difficulties that adolescents have in quitting cigarette smoking (Burt & Peterson, 1998; Zhu, Sun, Billings, Choi, & Malarcher, 1999) and the role of smoking in atherosclerosis (Berenson et al., 1998), as well as in lung cancer, efforts to prevent tobacco use among youths remains a significant concern.

Obesity and Diabetes

Relatively few children develop Type 1 diabetes mellitus, but many more are likely to develop Type 2 later in adolescence or early adulthood (American Diabetes Association, 2000; Fagot-Campagna, et al., 2000). Recent studies have shown the incidence of Type 2 diabetes to have increased dramatically in the past decade (Neufeld, Raffel, Landon, Chen, & Vadheim, 1998; Pinhas-Hamiel et al., 1996). Because diabetes is a major risk factor for cardiovascular disease, prevention efforts have focused on behaviors that increase risk of Type 2 diabetes. One variable known to increase risk for Type 2 diabetes is obesity. Besides Type 2 diabetes, obesity in childhood has been associated with a variety of other health problems, including hypertension and hyperlipidemia (Freedman et al., 1999; Freedman, Khan, Dietz, Srinivasan, & Berenson, 2001). It is thought that the association of these disorders may be due to the same disease process and that obesity and related insulin resistance may be critical etiological factors (Reaven, 1988). Previously this underlying disease process was termed "syndrome X," but it is now referred to as the "metabolic syndrome" or "insulin resistance" syndrome, a precursor to both Type 2 diabetes and cardiovascular disease. Research has recently shown these risk factors to be present in many children, particularly in minority Hispanic and African American children (Batey et al., 1997; Lindquist, Gower, & Goran, 2000; Treviño et al., 1999; Young-Hyman, Schlundt, Herman, De Luca, & Counts, 2001).

Recent studies indicate that the prevalence of obesity in children is very high, about 25%, and the incidence appears to be increasing (Troiano & Flegal, 1998). Obesity in childhood is associated with increased risk of continued obesity into adolescence and adulthood (Freedman et al., 2001) and long-term adverse health effects (Must, Jacques, Dallai, Bajema, & Dietz, 1992). Studies of blood pressure in children have shown a consistent relationship between weight and blood pressure, as well as serum lipids (Freedman et al., 1999). Thus childhood obesity is a significant health problem that creates increased risk for the metabolic syndrome and eventual Type 2 diabetes and cardiovascular disease. Prevention of and early intervention with childhood obesity is therefore an important goal for the prevention of cardiovascular disease.

Studies of the determinants of obesity in children have shown a relationship between child and parental obesity that can be explained by both genetic and environmental-behavioral factors. Specific behavioral factors include consumption of high fat diets and physical inactivity (Gortmaker, Dietz, & Cheung, 1990). In addition, childhood obesity has been associated with excessive TV viewing (Dietz & Gortmaker, 1985), presumably through its influence on diet and physical activity (Taras, Sallis, Patterson, Nader, & Nelson, 1989) and lowering of metabolic rate (Klesges, Shelton, & Klesges, 1993).

Type A Behavior, Anger, and Hostility

Early studies suggested that the Type A behavior pattern was associated with increased risk of cardiovascular disease, but more recent studies have identified hostility as the most significant component of the pattern in terms of cardiovascular risk (Barefoot et al., 1983). Because cardiovascular risk factors are evident during childhood, a number of studies have investigated Type A behavior in children and its cardiovascular consequences, but less pediatric research has focused specifically on anger and hostility and its association with cardiovascular risk. Several reports have shown that Type A children, like their adult counterparts, exhibit elevated cardiovascular reactivity to stressful laboratory tasks (Matthews & Jennings, 1984). This finding is important because one of the mechanisms linking these behaviors and later cardiovascular consequences is increased cardiovascular reactivity mediated by the sympathetic nervous system (Frederickson & Matthews, 1990). Stability of systolic blood pressure reactivity has been observed in early childhood (Jemerin & Boyce, 1990; Sallis et al., 1989). The Type A behavior pattern also appears to be relatively stable during childhood (Visintainer & Matthews, 1987) and from childhood to adulthood (Bergman & Magnusson, 1986).

Siegel (1984) examined the relationship between anger and cardiovascular risk in a cross-sectional study of 213 adolescents. Results showed that frequent anger directed outward was associated with higher systolic and diastolic blood pressure, as well as with greater likelihood of cigarette smoking and less leisure physical activity. These associations were stronger for boys than for girls. Anger was not related to serum cholesterol or obesity. A recent study by Schneider, Nicolotti, and Delamater (2002) found that after controlling for traditional risk factors such as body mass index and family history, aggressiveness in children was associated with increased blood pressure responses.

Interventions to Reduce Cardiovascular Risk

Interventions to reduce the risk of cardiovascular disease have focused on modification of diet to reduce fat content and physical activity levels to promote improved cardiovascular fitness. Achieving these goals also serves to decrease obesity, thus reducing a number of later health risks. Research efforts have also been directed toward smoking prevention programs for children. A selected review of pediatric intervention programs to reduce cardiovascular risk factors follows. Health promotion interventions are reviewed more extensively by Wilson and Evans (Chapter 5, this volume).

Studies have shown familial aggregation with regard to physical activity (Sallis, Patterson, Buono, Atkins, & Nader, 1988) and dietary habits (Patterson, Rupp, Sallis, Atkins, & Nader, 1988), blood pressure (Zinner, Levy, & Kass, 1971), serum lipoproteins (Morrison, Namboodiri, Green, Martin, & Glueck, 1983), cigarette smoking (Noland et al., 1990), obesity (Stunkard, Foch, & Hrubek, 1986), and hostility (Matthews, Rosenman, Dembroski, Harris, & MacDougall, 1984). Other studies have shown an association of family stress with increased anger and cardiovascular risk factors in youths (Weidner, Hutt, Connor, & Mendell, 1992; Woodall & Matthews, 1989). These findings indicate that health promotion programs targeting cardiovascular risk should be family based for optimal effects. Empirical support for this approach has been provided in controlled treatment–outcome studies (e.g., Epstein, Wing, Koeske, & Valoski, 1987; Jelalian & Saelens, 1999).

A variety of health promotion strategies have been examined. For example, interventions have been conducted with individual high-risk families or groups of families in clinical settings or at school sites, administered by teachers as part of educational curricula at schools, or with entire communities using combinations of clinic-based, school-based, and media-based interventions. Notable among the individual or group treatment approaches for high-risk children is the work of Epstein and colleagues, who have demonstrated the long-term success of a family-based behavioral program for weight loss in obese children

(Epstein et al., 1987; Epstein, Valoski, Wing, & McCurley, 1990). Reductions in serum triglycerides have also been reported secondary to weight loss in obese children (Epstein, Kuller, Wing, Valoski, & McCurley, 1989).

Several controlled intervention studies have been conducted on reducing cholesterol in children. A home-based, parent–child autotutorial dietary education program was conducted with 4- to 10-year-old children with elevated LDL cholesterol (Shannon et al., 1994). At 3-month follow-up, children in the treatment group reduced their consumption of dietary fat and had lower LDL cholesterol than children in the control group. A recent trial was conducted to evaluate the efficacy of a cholesterol-lowering diet in 8- to 10-year-old children with elevated LDL cholesterol (Obarzanek et al., 2001). In this randomized clinical trial with 663 children, a dietary behavioral intervention resulted in reduced dietary fat consumption and lower blood cholesterol levels in the treated group over a mean 7.4 years of follow-up. These findings indicate that a reduced fat diet can be safely sustained in growing children. Other reports of children treated for hypercholesterolemia have focused on psychosocial concerns of these children and their parents. Although psychosocial functioning of children was in the normal range, 11% of parents reported that they believed their child's quality of life would have been better had they not known their diagnosis; worry about cardiovascular disease was reported by 22% of children (Tonstad, 1996; Tonstad, Novik, & Vandvik, 1996).

School-based group health promotion treatment of families was used in the San Diego Family Health Project (Nader et al., 1992), which is noteworthy for its inclusion of Hispanic families. This program, like other successful programs, is based on social learning theory and principles of self-management. Family diet, exercise, and social support were targeted. Over a 4-year period, better results were observed for dietary behaviors than for physical activity (Nader et al., 1992). Another school-based intervention trial used a teacher-administered health curriculum focusing on diet, physical activity, and cigarette smoking (Walter, Hofman, Vaughan, & Wynder, 1988). In this large-scale primary prevention trial, several thousand children in the fourth through eighth grades in 37 schools around New York City were studied over a 5-year period. Significant reductions in cholesterol were observed after 5 years, and improvements in dietary behavior and health knowledge were also noted. Another major study of this type was the Child and Adolescent Trial for Cardiovascular Health (CATCH), a large multisite study designed to reduce cardiovascular risk in elementary school children through school-based dietary, physical activity, and educational interventions. The results of this trial showed that school-level interventions improved school lunch and physical education programs, increased students' physical activity, and reduced their dietary fat consumption (Nader et al., 1999).

A number of studies have examined the effects of broad-based school health education interventions that target a variety of cardiovascular risk behaviors; the weakest effects of these school-based interventions have been on obesity (Resnicow & Robinson, 1997). However, the school site, because of its accessibility to the community, may be an optimal place for delivery of family-based weight control programs (Story, 1999). Family-based approaches at the school site hold particular promise for interventions with low-income children, whose families may otherwise not have access to a health care team. Community-based cardiovascular risk reduction programs target entire communities for prevention of heart disease. Exemplary among such programs is the Bogalusa heart study (Berenson et al., 1983), which is noteworthy for reducing cardiovascular risk factors in a large biracial sample of children in Louisiana.

Summary and Implications

A substantial amount of research has addressed the development of risk factors in childhood for acquired heart disease later in life. Studies have demonstrated a high prevalence of various cardiovascular risk factors in children, including high blood pressure, high cholesterol, tobacco use, and obesity. In addition, studies have shown the Type A behavior pattern to be relatively common and stable in children and that such children exhibit heightened cardiovascular reactivity to stress. Because studies indicate that hostility is the Type A component most important to cardiovascular outcomes, more pediatric psychology research is needed regarding the developmental antecedents of hostility and its relationship to cardiovascular risk, as well as interventions to reduce hostility. Another priority area for future study is the role of stress in the development of hypertension, as well as preventive stress management programs for youths with high blood pressure.

Interventions to reduce cardiovascular risk in children have taken several approaches, including individual family-based clinical work, family-based group work conducted at the school site, school-based interventions targeting children via the curriculum and modification of the school lunch program, and community-wide interventions targeting entire communities with multiple methods, including the media. Results are encouraging, particularly with effects on diet, but physical activity levels seem more difficult to improve. Because the incidence of obesity in childhood is increasing, because it predicts continued obesity, as well as heightened risk for the metabolic syndrome, Type 2 diabetes, and eventual heart disease, and because established obesity is so difficult to treat, primary prevention of obesity remains a high priority. In terms of public health, this remains one of the most important issues that pediatric psychologists can address.

CONCLUSIONS

Pediatric psychology research in cardiovascular disease of childhood has focused mostly on CHD. Research findings have shown that children with severe forms of CHD are at risk for lower levels of intellectual and academic achievement. For the most part, however, as a group these children can be expected to function in the normal range. To the extent that there is more CNS involvement and cyanosis and that surgical repair is done later in childhood, more serious deficits in cognitive function are more likely. Studies of psychological adjustment of children with CHD have shown similar results, with behavioral rating scores generally in the normal range. Research findings indicate a greater risk for behavioral or emotional difficulties when surgical repair is done later in childhood. More research is needed that focuses on social competence, feelings of vulnerability, and autonomy issues, as these psychological factors may play an important role in the psychological adjustment of children with CHD. Limited intervention research has been conducted in this area. Pediatric psychologists can make significant contributions by designing and evaluating interventions to target feeding difficulties in infants, distress associated with medical procedures, and social adjustment in older children. Very little pediatric psychology research has been conducted focusing on acquired heart disease in children. Studies addressing developmental and psychosocial outcomes and adherence to medical regimens are needed, particularly intervention studies that target regimen adherence.

An extensive literature has documented that the atherosclerotic process begins during childhood. Traditional risk factors for acquired heart disease of adulthood, including hypertension, high cholesterol, use of tobacco, and obesity, have been commonly observed in children and adolescents. These risk factors tend to be fairly stable, so that high levels at young ages can predict similarly high levels at later ages. Studies have also demonstrated familial aggregation of these risk factors, indicating that intervention should target parents, as well as children. Intervention studies have shown greater improvements in health behaviors and outcomes in children when parents are also targeted for treatment. Because obesity is so prevalent in children and adolescents and because Type 2 diabetes is increasing dramatically in youths, effective obesity prevention and treatment programs are a high public health priority.

Clinical interventions with high-risk children will continue to be needed, but the school is an ideal site for family-based group interventions to promote cardiovascular health on a wider scale. In addition, school-based interventions in which the curriculum is modified to include health promotion are a reasonable approach likely to have great public health impact. Studies have already shown this approach to be efficacious, but more work is needed. Relatively little work has been reported thus far with regard to the development of hostility in children and its relationship to cardiovascular risk. Psychoeducational curricula that target hostility as a coping style and attitude should be developed and evaluated in the school setting. More work is also needed to prevent tobacco use in youths, as well as to effectively intervene with cessation programs for those who are already using tobacco products. Community-wide interventions ultimately may have the greatest impact on the primary prevention of cardiovascular disease, but work at the level of schools or individual families will continue to be needed, especially for children with established risk factors.

Cardiovascular disease remains the greatest cause of mortality in this country. Prevention of cardiovascular disease through the implementation of effective health promotion interventions is therefore an issue of high public health significance. Programs with empirically proven efficacy should be disseminated on a wider scale and effectiveness research conducted in community settings. Pediatric psychologists have the opportunity to make tremendous contributions to children's health and well-being by empirical validation of cost-effective programs to reduce cardiovascular risk.

REFERENCES

Alden, B., Gilljam, T., & Gillberg, C. (1998). Long-term psychological outcome of children after surgery for transposition of the great arteries. *Acta Paediatrica*, *87*, 405–410.

Alpern, D., Uzark, K., & Dick, M., II. (1989). Psychosocial responses of children to cardiac pacemakers. *Journal of Pediatrics*, *114*, 494–501.

American Diabetes Association. (2000). Type 2 diabetes in children and adolescents. *Diabetes Care*, *23*, 381–389.

Aram, D. M., Ekelman, B. L., Ben-Shachar, G., & Levinsohn, M. W. (1985). Intelligence and hypoxemia in children with congenital heart disease: Fact or artifact? *Journal of the American College of Cardiology*, *6*, 889–893.

Backer, C. L., Zales, V. R., Idriss, F. S., Lynch, P., Crawford, S., Benson, D. W., Jr., & Mavroudis, C. (1992). Heart transplantation in neonates and children. *Journal of Heart and Lung Transplantation*, *11*, 311–319.

Baer, P. E., Freedman, D. A., & Garson, A., Jr. (1984). Long-term psychological follow-up of patients after corrective surgery for tetralogy of fallot. *Journal of the American Academy of Child Psychiatry*, *23*, 622–625.

Barefoot, J. C., Dahlstrom, W. G., & Williams, W. B. (1983). Hostility, CHD incidence, and total mortality: A 25–year follow-up study of 255 physicians. *Psychosomatic Medicine*, *45*, 59–63.

Batey, L., Goff, D., Tortolero, S., Nichaman, M., Chan, W., et al. (1997). Summary measures of the insulin resistance syndrome are adverse among Mexican-American versus non-Hispanic white children. *Circulation*, *96*, 4319–4325.

Baum, M., Chinnock, R., Ashwal, S., Peverini, R., Trimm, F., & Bailey, L. (1993). Growth and neurodevelopmental outcome of infants undergoing heart transplantation. *Journal of Heart and Lung Tranplantation*, *12*, S211–S217.

Bellinger, D. C., Jonas, R. A., Rappaport, L. A., Wypij, D., Wernovsky, G., Kuban, K., et al. (1995). Developmental and neurologic status of children after heart surgery with hypothermic circulatory arrest or low-flow cardiopulmonary bypass. *New England Journal of Medicine, 332*, 549–555.

Bellinger, D. C., Rappaport, L. A., Wypij, D., Wernovsky, G., & Newburger, J. W. (1997). Patterns of developmental dysfunction after surgery during infancy to correct transposition of the great arteries. *Journal of Developmental and Behavioral Pediatrics, 18*, 75–83.

Berenson, G. S., McMahaan, C., Voors, A., Webber, L., Srinivasan, S., Foster, F. G., & Blonde, C. (1980). *Cardiovascular risk factors in children: The early natural history of atherosclerosis and essential hypertension.* New York: Oxford University Press.

Berenson, G. S., Srinivasan, S. R., Bao, W., Newman, W. P., Tracy, R. E., & Wattigney,W. A. (1998). Association between multiple cardiovascular risk factors and atheroslerosis in children and young adults: The Bogalusa study. *New England Journal of Medicine*, *338*, 1650–1656.

Berenson, G. S., Voors, A. W., Webber, L. S., Frank, G. C., Farris, R. P., Tobian, L., & Aristimuno, G. G. (1983). A model of intervention for prevention of early essential hypertension in the 1980s. *Hypertension*, *5*, 41–53.

Bergman, L. R., & Magnusson, D. (1986). Type A behavior: A longitudinal study from childhood and adulthood. *Psychosomatic Medicine*, *48*, 134–142.

Biglan, A., McConnell, S., Severson, H. H., Bavry, J., & Ary, D. V. (1984). A situational analysis of adolescent smoking. *Journal of Behavioral Medicine*, *7*, 109–114.

Bloom, A. A., Wright, J. A., Morris, R. D., Campbell, R. M., & Krawiecki, N. S. (1997). Additive impact of in-hospital cardiac arrest on the functioning of children with heart disease. *Pediatrics, 99*, 390–398.

Bradford, R. (1990). Short communication: The importance of psychosocial factors in understanding child distress during routine X-ray procedures. *Journal of Child Psychology and Psychiatry, 31*, 973–982.

Brownson, R. C., DiLorenzo, T. M., Van Tuinen, M., & Finger, W. W. (1990). Patterns of cigarette and smokeless tobacco use among children and adolescents. *Preventive Medicine*, *19*, 170–180.

Bullock, E. A., & Shaddy, R. E. (1993). Relaxation and imagery techniques without sedation during right ventricular endomyocardial biopsy in pediatric heart transplant patients. *Journal of Heart and Lung Transplantation, 12*, 59–62.

Burt, R. D., & Peterson, A. V. (1998). Smoking cessation among high school seniors. *Preventive Medicine*, *27*, 319–327.

Campbell, L. A., Kirkpatrick, S. E., Berry, C. C., & Lamberti, J. J. (1995). Preparing children with congenital heart disease for cardiac surgery. *Journal of Pediatric Psychology, 20*, 313–328.

Casey, R. A., Sykes, D. H., Craig, B., Power, R., & Mulholland, H. C. (1996). Behavioral adjustment of children with surgically palliated complex congenital heart disease. *Journal of Pediatric Psychology, 21*, 335–352.

Castelli, W. P., Garrison, R. J., Wilson, P. W. F., Abbott, R. D., Kalousdian, S., & Kannel, W. B. (1986). Incidence of coronary heart disease and lipoprotein cholesterol levels: The Framinghan study. *Journal of the American Medical Association*, *256*, 2835–2838.

Davis, C. C., Brown, R. T., Bakeman, R., & Campbell, R. (1998). Psychological adaptation and adjustment of mothers of children with congenital heart disease: Stress, coping, and family functioning. *Journal of Pediatric Psychology, 23*, 219–228.

Del Rosario, J. D., Treiber, F. A., Harshfield, G. A., Davis, H. S., & Strong, W. B. (1998). Predictors of future ambulatory blood pressure in youth. *Journal of Pediatrics*, *132*, 693–698.

DeMaso, D. R., Beardslee, W. R., Silbert, A. R., & Fyler, D. C. (1990). Psychological functioning in children with cyanotic heart defects. *Journal of Developmental and Behavioral Pediatrics*, *11*, 289–293.

DeMaso, D. R., Campis, L. K., Wypij, D., Bertram, S., Lipshitz, M., & Freed, M. (1991). The impact of maternal perceptions and medical severity on the adjustment of children with congenital heart disease. *Journal of Pediatric Psychology, 16*, 137–149.

DeMaso, D. R., Spratt, E. G., Vaughan, B. L., D'Angelo, E. J., Van der Feen, J. R., & Walsh, E. (2000). Psychological functioning in children and adolescents undergoing radiofrequency catheter ablation. *Psychosomatics*, *41*, 134–139.

DeMaso, D. R., Twente, A. W., Spratt, E. G., & O'Brien, P. (1995). Impact of psychologic functioning, medical severity, and family functioning in pediatric heart transplantation. *Journal of Heart and Lung Transplanation, 14*, 1102–1108.

Dietz, W. H., & Gortmaker, S. L. (1985). Do we fatten our children at the television set? Obesity and television viewing in children and adolescents. *Pediatrics*, *75*, 807–812.

Douglas, J. F., Hsu, D. T., & Addonizio, L. J. (1993). Noncompliance in pediatric heart transplant patients. *Journal of Heart and Lung Transplantation*, *12*, S92.

Epstein, L. H., Kuller, L. H., Wing, R., Valoski, A. V., & McCurley, J. (1989). The effect of weight control on lipid changes in obese children. *American Journal of Diseases of Children*, *143*, 454–457.

Epstein, L. H., Valoski, A., Wing, R., & McCurley, J. (1990). Ten-year follow-up of behavioral family based treatment for obese children. *Journal of American Medicine*, *264*, 2519–2523.

Epstein, L. H., Wing, R. R., Koeske, R., & Valoski, A. (1987). Long term effects of family-based treatment of childhood obesity. *Journal of Clinical and Consulting Psychology, 55*, 91–95.

Expert Panel on Blood Cholesterol Levels in Children and Adolescents. (1992). National Cholesterol Education Program Report. *Pediatrics, 89*(Suppl.), 525–584.

Fagot-Campagna, A., Pettitt, D., Engelgau, M., Rios Burrows, N., Geiss, L., Valdez, R., et al. (2000). Type 2 diabetes among North American children and adolescents: An epidemiologic review and public health perspective. *Journal of Pediatrics, 136*, 664–672.

Ferry, P. C. (1987). Neurological sequelae of cardiac surgery in children. *American Journal of Diseases of Children, 141*, 309–312.

Fleisher, B. E., Baum, D., Brudos, G., Burge, M., Carson, E., Constantinou, J., et al. (2002). Infant heart transplantation at Stanford: Growth and neurodevelopmental outcome. *Pediatrics, 109*, 1–7.

Frederickson, M., & Matthews, K. A. (1990). Cardiovascular responses to behavioral stress and hypertension: A meta-analytic review. *Annals of Behavioral Medicine, 12*, 30–39.

Freedman, D. S., Dietz, W. H., Srinivasan, S. R., & Berenson, G. S. (1999). The relation of overweight to cardiovascular risk factors among children and adolescents: The Bogalusa heart study. *Pediatrics, 103*, 1175–1182.

Freedman, D. S., Khan, L. K., Dietz, W. H., Srinivasan, S. R., & Berenson, G. S. (2001). Relationship of childhood obesity to coronary heart disease risk factors in adulthood: The Bogalusa heart study. *Pediatrics, 108*, 712–718.

Fyler, D. C. (Ed.). (1992). *Nadas' pediatric cardiology.* Philadelphia: Hanley & Belfus.

Gersony, W. M. (1987). The cardiovascular system. In R. E. Behrman & V. C. Vaughan (Eds.), *Nelson textbook of pediatrics* (13th ed., pp. 943–1026). Philadelphia: Saunders.

Gortmaker, S. L., Dietz, W. H., & Cheung, L. W. (1990). Inactivity, diet, and the fattening of America. *Journal of American Dietetic Association.* , *90*, 1247–1255.

Gottlieb, A., Pope, S. K., Rickert, V. I., & Hardin, B. H. (1993). Patterns of smokeless tobacco use by young adolescents. *Pediatrics, 91*, 75–78.

Jelalian, E., & Saelens, B. E. (1999). Empirically supported treatments in pediatric psychology: Pediatric obesity. *Journal of Pediatric Psychology, 24*, 223–248.

Jemerin, J. M., & Boyce, W. T. (1990). Psychobiological differences in childhood stress response: II. Cardiovascular markers of vulnerability. *Journal of Developmental and Behavioral Pediatrics, 11*, 140–150.

Johnston, L. D., Bachman, J. G., & O'Malley, P. M. (1981). *Student drug use in America 1975–1981* (DHHS Publication No. ADM82–1221). Washington, DC: U.S. Government Printing Office.

Kannel, W. B., McGee, D., & Gordon, T. (1976). A general cardiovascular risk profile: The Framingham study. *American Journal of Cardiology, 38*, 46–51.

Kern, J. H., Hinton, V. J., Nereo, N. E., Hayes, C. J., & Gersony, W. M. (1998). Early developmental outcome after the Norwood procedure for hypoplastic left heart syndrome. *Pediatrics, 102*, 1148–1152.

Klesges, R. C., Shelton, M. L., & Klesges, L. M. (1993). Effects of television on metabolic rate: Potential implications for childhood obesity. *Pediatrics, 91*, 281–286.

Lauer, R. M., & Clarke, W. R. (1989). Childhood risk factors for high adult blood pressure: The Muscatine study. *Pediatrics, 84*, 633–641.

Lauer, R. M., & Clarke, W. R. (1990). Use of cholesterol measurements in childhood for the prediction of adult hypercholesterolemia: The Muscatine study. *Journal of the American Medical Association, 264*, 3034–3038.

Lauer, R. M., Clarke, W. R., & Beaglehole, R. (1984). Level, trend and variability of blood pressure during childhood: The Muscatine study. *Circulation, 69*, 242–249.

Lauer, R. M., Connor, W. E., Leaverton, P. E., Reiter, M. A., & Clarke, W. R. (1975). Coronary heart disease risk factors in school children: The Muscatine study. *Journal of Pediatrics, 86*, 697–706.

Lindquist, C. H., Gower, B. A., & Goran, M. I. (2000). Role of dietary factors in ethnic differences in early risk of cardiovascular disease and Type 2 diabetes. *American Journal of Clinical Nutrition, 71*, 725–735.

Lobo, M. L. (1992). Parent–infant interaction during feeding when the infant has congenital heart disease. *Journal of Pediatric Nursing, 7*, 97–105.

Mahle, W. T., Clancy, R. R., Moss, E. M., Gerdes, M., Jobes, D. R., & Wernovsky, G. (2000). Neurodevelopmental outcome and lifestyle assessment in school-aged and adolescent children with hypolastic left heart syndrome. *Pediatrics, 105*, 1082–1089.

Marino, B. L., & Lipshitz, M. (1991). Temperament in infants and toddlers with cardiac disease. *Pediatric Nursing, 17*, 445–448.

Matthews, K. A., & Jennings, J. R. (1984). Cardiovascular responses of boys exhibiting the Type A behavior pattern. *Psychosomatic Medicine, 46*, 484–497.

Matthews, K. A., Rosenman, R. H., Dembroski, T. M., Harris, E. L., & MacDougall, J. M. (1984). Familial resemblance in components of the Type A behavior pattern: A reanalysis of the California Type A twin study. *Psychosomatic Medicine, 46*, 512–522.

Morris, R. D., Krawiecki, N. S., Wright, J. A., & Walter, L. W. (1993). Neuropsychological, academic, and adaptive functioning in children who survive in-hospital cardiac arrest and resuscitation. *Journal of Learning Disabilities*, *26*, 46–51.

Morrison, J. A., Larsen, R., Glatfelter, L., Boggs, D., Burton, K., Smith, C., et al. (1980). Interrelationships between nutrient intake and plasma lipids and lipoproteins in school children aged 6–19: The Princeton School District study. *Pediatrics*, *65*, 727–734.

Morrison, J. A., Namboodiri, K., Green, P., Martin, J., & Glueck, C. J. (1993). Familial aggregation of lipids and lipoproteins and early identification of dyslipoproteinemia. *Journal of the American Medical Association*, *250*, 1860–1868.

Murdison, K. A., Treiber, F. A., Mensah, G., Davis, H., Thompson, W., & Strong, W. B. (1998). Prediction of left ventricular mass in youth with family histories of essential hypertension. *American Journal of the Medical Sciences*, *315*, 118–123.

Must, A., Jacques, P. F., Dallal, G. E., Bajema, C. J., & Dietz, W. H. (1992). Long-term morbidity and mortality of overweight adolescents. *New England Journal of Medicine*, *327*, 1350–1355.

Nader, P. R., Sallis, J. F., Abramson, I. S., Broyles, S. L., Patterson, T. L., Senn, K., et al. (1992). Family-based cardiovascular risk reduction education among Mexican and Anglo-Americans. *Family Community Health*, *15*, 57–74.

Nader, P. R., Stone, E. J., Lytle, L. A., Perry, C. L., Osganian, S. K., Kelder, S., et al. (1999). Three-year maintenance of improved diet and physical activity: The CATCH cohort. *Archives Pediatric and Adolescent Medicine*, *153*, 695–704.

National High Blood Pressure Education Program Working Group on Hypertension Control in Children and Adolescents. (1996). Update on the 1987 task force report on high blood pressure in children and adolescents. *Pediatrics*, *98*, 649–658.

Neufeld, N. D., Raffel, L. J., Landon, C., Chen, Y., & Vadheim, C. M. (1998). Early presentation of Type 2 diabetes in Mexican-American youth. *Diabetes Care*, *21*, 80–86.

Newburger, J. W., Silbert, A. R., Buckley, L. P., & Fyler, D. C. (1984). Cognitive function and age at repair of transportation of the great arteries in children. *New England Journal of Medicine*, *310*, 1495–1499.

Newman, W. P., Freedman, D. S., Voors, A. W., Gard, P. D., Srinivasan, S. R., Cresanta, J. L., et al. (1986). Relation of serum lipoprotein levels and systolic blood pressure to early atherosclerosis. *New England Journal of Medicine*, *314*, 138–144.

Noland, M. P., Kryscio, R. J., Riggs, R. S., Linville, L. H., Perritt, L. J., & Tucker, T. C. (1990). Use of snuff, chewing tobacco, and cigarettes among adolescents in a tobacco producing area. *Addictive Behavior*, *15*, 517–530.

Oates, R. K., Simpson, J. M., Turnbull, J. A., & Cartmill, T. B. (1995). The relationship between intelligence and duration of circulatory arrest with deep hypothermia. *Journal of Thoracic and Cardiovascular Surgery*, *110*, 786–792.

Obzarzanek, E., Kimm, S., Barton, B., Van Horn, L., Kwiterovich, P., Simons-Morton, D., et al. (2001). Long-term safety and efficacy of a cholesterol-lowering diet in children with elevated low-density lipoprotein cholesterol: Seven-year results of the dietary intervention study in children. *Pediatrics*, *107*, 256–264.

O'Dougherty, M., Wright, F. S., Garmezy, N., Loewenson, R. B., & Torres, F. (1983). Later competence and adaptation in infants who survive severe heart defects. *Child Development*, *54*, 1129–1142.

O'Dougherty, M., Wright, F. S., Loewenson, R. B., & Torres, F. (1985). Cerebral dysfunction after chronic hypoxia in children. *Neurology*, *35*, 42–46.

Paris, W., Muchmore, J., Pribil, A., Zuhdi, N., & Cooper, D. (1994). Study of the relative incidences of psychosocial factors before and after heart transplantation and the influence of posttransplantation psychosocial factors on heart transplantation outcome. *Journal of Heart and Lung Transplantation*, *13*, 424–432.

Patterson, T. L., Rupp, J. W., Sallis, J. F., Atkins, C. J., & Nader, P. R. (1988). Aggregation of dietary calories, fats, and sodium in Mexican-American and Anglo families. *American Journal of Preventive Maintenance*, *4*, 75–92.

Pinhas-Hamiel, O., Dolan, L. M., Daniels, S. R., Standiford, D., Khoury, P. R., & Zeitler, P. (1996). Increased incidence of non-insulin-dependent diabetes mellitus among adolescents. *Journal of Pediatrics*, *128*, 608–615.

Reaven, G. M. (1988). Role of insulin resistance in human disease. *Diabetes*, *37*, 1595–1607.

Resnicow, K., & Robinson, T. (1997). School-based cardiovascular disease prevention studies: Review and synthesis. *Annals of Epidemiology*, *S7*, S14–S31.

Sallis, J. F., Patterson, T. L., Buono, M. J., Atkins, C. J., & Nader, P. R. (1988). Aggregation of physical activity habits in Mexican-American and Anglo families. *Journal of Behavioral Medicine*, *11*, 31–41.

Sallis, J. F., Patterson, T. L., McKenzie, T. L., Buono, M. J., Atkins, C. J., & Nader, P. R. (1989). Stability of systolic blood pressure reactivity to exercise in young children. *Journal of Developmental and Behavioral Pediatrics*, *10*, 38–43.

Schneider, M. B., Davis, J. G., Boxer, R. A., Fisher, M., & Friedman, S. B. (1990). Marfan syndrome in adolescents and young adults: Psychosocial functioning and knowledge. *Journal of Developmental and Behavioral Pediatrics*, *11*, 122–127.

Schneider, K., Delamater, A., Geith, T., Young, M., & Wolff, G. (2001) Quality of life in children with cardiac arrhythmia. *Annals of Behavioral Medicine*, *23*(Suppl.), S180.

Schneider, K., Nicolotti, L., & Delamater, A. M. (2002). Aggression and cardiovascular response of children. *Journal of Pediatric Psychology*, *27*, 565–574.

Serrano-Ikkos, E., Lask, B., Whitehead, B., & Eisler, I. (1998). Incomplete adherence after pediatric heart and heart-lung transplantation. *Journal of Heart and Lung Transplantation*, *17*, 1177–1182.

Serrano-Ikkos, E., Lask, B., Whitehead, B., Rees, P., & Graham, P. (1999). Heart or heart-lung transplantation: Psychosocial outcome. *Pediatric Transplantation*, *3*, 301–308.

Shannon, B. M., Tershakovec, A., Martel, J., Achterberg, C., Cortner, J., Smiciklas-Wright, H., et al. (1994). Reduction of elevated LDL-cholesterol levels of 4– to 10–year-old children through home-based dietary education. *Pediatrics*, *94*, 923–927.

Siegel, J. M. (1984). Anger and cardiovascular risk in adolescents. *Health Psychology*, *3*, 293–313.

Sinaiko, A. R., Gomez-Marin, O., & Prineas, R. J. (1989). Prevalence of "significant" hypertension in junior high school-aged children: The children and adolescent blood pressure program. *Journal of Pediatrics*, *114*, 664–669.

Spurkland, I., Bjornstad, P. G., Lindberg, H., & Seem, E. (1993). Mental health and psychosocial functioning in adolescents with congenital heart disease: A comparison between adolescents born with severe heart defect and atrial septal defect. *Acta Paediatrics*, *82*, 71–76.

Story, M. (1999). School-based approaches for preventing and treating obesity. *International Journal of Obesity*, *23*(Suppl. 2), S43–S51.

Stunkard, A. J., Foch, T. T., & Hrubec, Z. (1986). A twin study of human obesity. *Journal of the American Medical Association*, *256*, 51–54.

Sytkowski, P. A., Kannel, W. B., & D'Agostino, R. B. (1990). Changes in risk factors and the decline in mortality from cardiovascular disease. *New England Journal of Medicine*, *322*, 1635–1641.

Taras, H. L., Sallis, J. F., Patterson, T. L., Nader, P. R., & Nelson, J. A. (1989). Television's influence on children's diet and physical activity. *Journal of Developmental and Behavioral Pediatrics*, *10*, 176–180.

Tindall, S., Rothermel, R., Delamater, A. M., Pinsky, W., & Klein, M. (1999). Neuropsychological abilities of children with cardiac disease treated with extracorporeal membrane oxygenation. *Developmental Neuropsychology*, *16*, 101–115.

Todaro, J. F., Fennell, E. B., Sears, S. F., Rodrigue, J. R., & Roche, A. K. (2000). Cognitive and psychological outcomes in pediatric heart transplantation. *Journal of Pediatric Psychology*, *25*, 567–576.

Tonstad, S. (1996). Familial hypercholesterolemia: A pilot study of parents' and children's concerns. *Acta Paediatrica*, *85*, 1307–1313.

Tonstad, S., Novik, T. S., & Vandvik, I. H. (1996). Psychosocial function during treatment for familial hypercholesterolemia. *Pediatrics*, *98*, 249–255.

Treviño, R. P., Marshall, R. M., Hale, D. E., Rodriguez, R., Baker, G., & Gomez, J. (1999). Diabetes risk factors in low-income Mexican-American children. *Diabetes Care*, *22*, 202–207.

Trimm, F. (1991). Physiologic and psychological growth and development in pediatric heart transplant recipients. *Journal of Heart and Lung Transplantation*, *10*, 848–855.

Troiano, R. P., & Flegal, K. M. (1998). Overweight children and adolescents: Description, epidemiology, and demographics. *Pediatrics*, *101*, 497–504.

Utens, E. M., Verhulst, F. C., Erdman, R. A., Meijboom, F. J., Duivenvoorden, H. J., Bos, E., et al. (1994). Psychosocial functioning of young adults after surgical correction for congenital heart disease in childhood: A follow-up study. *Journal of Psychosomatic Research*, *38*, 745–758.

Uzark, K. C., Sauer, S. N., Lawrence, K. S., Miller, J., Addonizio, L., & Crowley, D. C. (1992). The psychosocial impact of pediatric heart transplantation. *Journal of Heart and Lung Tranplantation*, *11*, 1160–1167.

Van Horn, M., DeMaso, D. R., Gonzalez-Heydrich, J., & Erickson, J. D. (2001). Illness-related concerns of mothers of children with congenital heart disease. *Journal of the American Academy of Child and Adolescent Psychiatry*, *40*, 847–854.

Visintainer, P. F., & Matthews, K. A. (1987). Stability of overt Type A behaviors in children: Results from a two- and five-year longitudinal study. *Child Development*, *58*, 1586–1591.

Walter, H. J., Hofman, A., Vaughan, R. D., & Wynder, E. L. (1988). Modification of risk factors for coronary heart disease. *New England Journal of Medicine*, *318*, 1093–1099.

Weidner, G., Hutt, J., Connor, S. L., & Mendell, N. R. (1992). Family stress and coronary risk in children. *Psychosomatic Medicine*, *54*, 471–479.

Woodall, K. L., & Matthews, K. A. (1989). Familial environment associated with Type A behaviors and psychophysiological responses to stress in children. *Health Psychology*, *8*, 403–426.

Wray, J., Long, T., Radley-Smith, R., & Yacoub, M. (2001). Returning to school after heart or heart-lung transplantation: How well do children adjust? *Transplantation*, *72*, 100–106.

Wray, J., Pot-Mees, C., Zeitlin, H., Radley-Smith, R., & Yacoub, M. (1994). Cognitive function and behavioral status in pediatric heart and heart-lung transplant recipients: The Harefield experience. *British Medical Journal, 309*, 837–841.

Wray, J., & Yacoub, M. (1991). Psychosocial evaluation of children after open heart surgery versus cardiac transplantation. In M. Yacoub & J. R. Pepper (Eds.), *Annals of Cardiac Surgery* (Vol. 90–91, pp. 50–55). London: Current Science.

Wright, M., & Nolan, T. (1994). Impact of cyanotic heart disease on school performance. *Archives of Diseases of Children, 71*, 64–69.

Yang, L. L., Liu, M. L., & Townes, B. D. (1994). Neuropsychological and behavioral status of Chinese children with acyanotic congenital heart disease. *International Journal of Neuroscience, 74*, 109–115.

Young-Hyman, D., Schlundt, D., Herman, L., De Luca, F., & Counts, D. (2001). Evaluation of the insulin resistance syndrome in 5- to 10-year-old overweight/obese African American children. *Diabetes Care, 24*, 1359–1364.

Zhu, S. H., Sun, J., Billings, S., Choi, W., & Malarcher, A. (1999). Predictors of smoking cessation in US adolescents. *American Journal of Preventive Medicine, 16*, 202–207.

Zinner, S. H., Levy, P. S., & Kass, E. H. (1971). Familial aggregation of blood pressure in childhood. *New England Journal of Medicine, 284*, 401–404.

25

Pediatric Organ Transplantation in the 21st Century

Emerging Clinical, Ethical, and Research Issues

JAMES R. RODRIGUE
AMANDA B. SOBEL

Major advances in organ transplantation have occurred within the last half century—from innovative surgical techniques to pharmacological improvements that facilitate graft function and optimal preservation of tissue. The notion that transplanting an organ from a brain-dead cadaver to a genetically dissimilar individual with end-stage disease would yield survival and quality of life benefits was revolutionary 50 years ago. Furthermore, what few envisioned then is today's reality—that healthy individuals would volunteer so readily to donate whole organs (e.g., kidney) and parts of organs (e.g., liver, pancreas, lung) to family members, as well as to strangers. Gene transfer is in its infancy, but it offers real possibilities for delivering biologically active molecules to transplanted organs in order to modulate immune activity. Xenotransplantation, the transplantation of tissue from one species to another, is seen by many as the best way to alleviate the severe organ shortage that leads to so many deaths on transplant waiting lists. Of course, as was the case with the pioneers in transplantation, nobody can predict what lies ahead for those who will be affected by end-stage disease a half century from now.

Why is it important for pediatric psychologists to understand the past, present, and future of organ transplantation? First, children have played a central role in the advancement of organ transplantation. They were among the first patients to receive kidney, liver, heart, and intestinal transplants. For instance, an infant received a heart transplant only 3 days after the widely acclaimed first adult heart transplant in 1967 with comparably less fanfare. Second, children are a primary beneficiary of the substantial advances in transplantation. Over 1,700 children in the United States received solid organ transplantation in 2001, and thousands more underwent this lifesaving procedure in other countries. Third, survival brings new clinical challenges into the lives of children and their families, most of which were not the main concern of those trying to save lives through transplantation but are now recognized as being critically important for optimal health outcomes. Pediatric psychologists are best trained to attend clinically and scientifically to these complex developmental, psychological, behavioral health, and family issues. Fourth, living organ donation, most often involving healthy parents donating an organ to their ill child, has enormous clinical, ethical, societal, and health policy implications that pediatric psychologists working in major medical centers will undoubtedly confront in the immediate future. Fifth, pediatric psychologists have the opportunity to be active participants in one of the most exciting and challenging developments in the field of medicine in the last century and to help shape its future.

Several excellent overviews of organ transplantation and its implications for children and families have been written by or for pediatric psychologists in the past several years (Canning & Stuber, 2000; Rodrigue, Gonzalez, & Langham, in press; Schweitzer & Hobbs, 1995; Sexson & Rubenow, 1992; Stewart & Kennard, 1999; Streisand & Tercyak, 2001). These chapters provide very useful information about the range of child and family reactions to transplantation—from cognitive functioning to quality of life—and the roles that psychologists play in clinical assessment and intervention. Extant psychological research in pediatric transplantation is also nicely reviewed in these writings. In this chapter, we seek to highlight and discuss emerging clinical, ethical, and research issues in pediatric transplantation—issues that are pressing in the field of pediatric transplantation now and those that likely will represent prominent themes in the future. Those emerging issues that have received less attention in the writings noted previously present significant clinical and research opportunities for pediatric psychologists. In discussing these issues, we highlight relevant scientific contributions and invoke our own clinical experiences and biases. We also draw heavily on the experiences of our colleagues in other disciplines—pediatrics, surgery, nursing, social work, and bioethics—for this is truly an interdisciplinary effort to enhance the lives of children, adolescents, and families.

OVERVIEW OF PEDIATRIC TRANSPLANTATION

Transplantations of the kidney, heart, liver, lung, and small intestine are now performed at pediatric medical centers worldwide. In the United States alone, there have been more than 18,000 pediatric transplants performed in the past decade, reflecting a 30% increase over the period from 1989 to 2001. The indications for transplantation and patient survival rates, of course, differ by transplant type. Indications for pediatric kidney transplantation include glomerulonephritis, chronic pyelonephritis, and hereditary conditions (e.g., polycystic kidneys). The two primary conditions leading to pediatric heart transplantation are complex congenital heart disease (e.g., including hypoplastic left heart syndrome) and end-stage cardiomyopathy. Biliary atresia (congenital absence or closure of the ducts that drain bile from the liver), metabolic disorders (such as alpha 1-antitrypsin deficiency, cystic fibrosis, and glycogen storage disease), autoimmune hepatitis and other cholestatic diseases (such as Alagille's syndrome) are the most common conditions leading to pediatric liver transplantation. Conditions for which pediatric lung transplantation may be considered most commonly include congenital lung abnormalities in infants and cystic fibrosis in adolescents.

Finally, pediatric intestinal or small bowel transplantation is limited primarily to those children for whom death secondary to complications of protracted parenteral nutrition is likely.

Pediatric transplant outcomes and the management of the young transplant patient have improved over time. Survival rates at all time points are highest for kidney transplant recipients and lowest for lung transplant recipients. In general, survival rates for children are comparable to those for adults. Other outcomes, including physical growth (Studies of Pediatric Liver Transplantation Research Group [SPLIT], 2001; Tejani, Cortes, & Sullivan, 1996), cognitive development (Hobbs & Sexson, 1993; Mendley & Zelko, 1999; Stewart, Kennard, Waller, & Fixler, 1994; Todaro, Fennell, Sears, Rodrigue, & Roche, 2000), neurological functioning (Wijdicks, 1999; Wong, Mallory, Goldstein, Goyal, & Yamada, 1999), academic performance (Kennard et al., 1999), quality of life (Boucek et al., 2001), and the psychological adaptation of children (Demaso, Twente, Spratt, & O'Brien, 1995; Walker, Harris, Baker, Kelly, & Houghton, 1999) and families (Demaso et al., 1995; Rodrigue et al., 1997), are increasingly the focus of investigation within pediatric transplant programs and represent excellent collaborative research opportunities for pediatric psychologists. Unfortunately, the number of children and adolescents awaiting organ transplantation has increased nearly 150% in the past decade. Although waiting times are generally less for children than for adults, the number of deaths of children on the waiting list has jumped about 75% during this same time period and is dramatically higher for infants (United Network for Organ Sharing [UNOS], 2001).

EMERGING CLINICAL ISSUES

Organ transplantation is a process that, for most children and their families, begins with the diagnosis of a serious illness that leads to intensive, prolonged medical and pharmacological interventions and multiple hospitalizations. After months or years of dealing with the rigors and demands of chronic illness and its treatment, referral for transplant evaluation inevitably leads to both excitement and anxiety—excitement about the prospect of living disease free and anxiety about the uncertainty of waiting for a suitable organ. For many children, an organ is eventually procured, and renewed hope for survival follows transplant surgery. Unfortunately, the dynamic process does not end there, as transplant recipients must consume a cocktail of medications on a daily basis (usually for life) and navigate successfully through an assortment of complications that are part of the posttransplant experience. Such complications may include graft rejection, infections, hospital readmissions, various toxicities, and other systemic problems.

Although the point of entry may vary across centers, pediatric psychologists working in large medical centers are often consulted to provide clinical services to children and families at various points along the transplant spectrum. In most programs, the pediatric psychologist conducts a comprehensive psychological evaluation of all transplant candidates. The general purpose of such evaluations is to identify psychological, developmental, and behavioral health strengths and liabilities as they relate to the transplant process. What is the child's understanding of his or her illness and transplantation? Are there any significant behavioral problems or family stressors that could potentially interfere with treatment demands or transplant outcomes if left untreated? Are there any adherence problems that warrant immediate attention to optimize health outcomes? What is the child's current level of cognitive, affective, and academic functioning? Does the child have an available and stable network of family support? What are the other life stressors affecting the family that could potentially interfere with the caregiving demands associated with transplantation? Clinical interviews and some formal testing may serve as the basis for evaluating these questions, as well as the following domains: development, cognitive functioning, academic achievement, psychological adaptation, coping resources, quality of life, adherence, and family functioning (Rodrigue et al., in press; Streisand & Tercyak, 2001). For some children and their families, psychological interventions are necessary to optimize the child's transplant candidacy and to increase the likelihood of positive health outcomes, both before and after transplantation. Pediatric psychologists are in the best position to develop, implement, and evaluate the effectiveness of these interventions.

Although providing evaluation and treatment services to children and families before transplantation is perhaps the most common form of clinical activity for the pediatric psychology consultant, pediatric psychologists can also benefit both the children and the transplant programs they service in several other clinical areas. In this section, we highlight a few key areas in which opportunities are emerging for pediatric psychologists to make substantial and meaningful clinical contributions to the transplant community.

Organ Donation

Without question, the single most pressing issue confronting the field of transplantation as we begin this new century is the severe organ shortage. The lives of many more children could be extended and enhanced if more suitable organs were available for transplantation. The widening gap between the number of people awaiting transplantation and the number of donated organs and how best to reverse this trend has been the focus of considerable dialogue and debate among health professionals, bioethicists, and health policy experts (Howard, 2001; Veatch, 2000). Indeed, on assuming office in 2001, Tommy Thompson, Secretary of the U.S. Department of Health and Human Services, called the organ shortage a national health crisis and launched a nationwide partnership with professional organizations to increase organ donation (U.S. DHHS, 2001). Surprisingly, pediatric psychologists have not routinely been participants in the organ donation dialogue, and psychological associations are noticeably absent in the secretary's initiative to save and enhance the lives of children by increasing organ donation. This omission is unfortunate because two fundamental themes in the secretary's initiative concern the translation of attitudes (about donation) into behavior (consent to donation when asked) and the provision of services to those who give the gift of life—areas in which psychologists likely have expertise.

There are two ways in which organs become available for transplantation: through cadaveric or live donation. In the case of cadaveric donation, a family has consented to donate the organs of a loved one who has suffered a severe head injury, for instance, and has been declared brain dead. There are many important factors that play a role in how family members decide whether to donate organs under such intensely traumatic circumstances (e.g., Siminoff, Gordon, Hewlett, & Arnold, 2001). Some of these factors include knowledge of the deceased's donation intentions, whether previous discussion about organ donation had occurred within the family, the quality of the interactions with hospital staff and organ requestors, and previous attitudes toward organ donation. Of particular relevance to pediatric psychologists is that these decisions occur in the context of an intensive care environment, acute affective distress, intense grief reactions, and a family system thrust unexpectedly into chaos.

Pediatric psychologists can play an important clinical role in cadaveric donation in at least three innovative ways. First, they can work collaboratively with organ procurement organizations in developing training programs for organ requestors. Such programs might involve providing educational programs on grief and bereavement, the impact of traumatic injury and brain death on families, and how best to approach families when requesting consent for organ donation. Second, the provision of support services for organ requestors is urgently needed. The burnout and turnover rates within the procurement profession are exceedingly high and attributed largely to the emotionally exhaustive nature of the job. Indeed, the stress associated with requesting organs likely parallels that of other trauma team members, such as intensive care nurses and emergency rescue personnel. Often cited as especially traumatic for requestors are those cases involving the brain death of young children and the grief reactions of their parents. Many pediatric psychologists have considerable experience working with health professionals in the critical care setting and can use their expertise and competencies in providing individual and group counseling services to organ requestors. These services could potentially reduce psychological distress, increase job satisfaction and retention, facilitate the acquisition and maintenance of effective coping strategies, foster empathic communication with families, and indirectly increase consent rates for organ donation. Third, our anecdotal experience suggests that organ donation helps to resolve the parents' grief. The provision of short-term psychological services immediately following donation decisions has the potential to further help family members through the immediate loss and to prevent complicated bereavement in the longer term.

In addition to cadaveric donation, children may also receive organs from living donors. Living donation has been a part of kidney transplantation since the first successful transplant surgery (Merrill, Murray, Harrison, & Guild, 1956) but has only recently become an option for liver, pancreas, lung, and heart transplantation (Cohen et al., 1994; Oaks et al., 1994; Sutherland, Goetz, & Najarian, 1984; Uemoto et al., 2000). Healthy individuals can now donate a kidney (the remaining kidney enlarges and assumes the function of the one donated), a liver segment (which regenerates in days), a portion of the pancreas, and a lobe of the lung (which does not regenerate). A patient who receives a domino (combined heart–lung) transplant can also become a living heart donor by donating his or her otherwise healthy heart to another patient awaiting transplantation. Once considered revolutionary, living donation has increased by over 150% in the past decade (as opposed to a 45% increase in cadaveric donation) and is expected to surge in the next several years.

Living donor transplants have several advantages over cadaveric donor transplants. Patient survival rates are comparable, and in some instances superior, to those of cadaveric donor transplants (UNOS, 2001), perhaps due to better human leukocyte antigen compatibility and lower ischemia time associated with living donor transplants. Also, living donor transplants can be scheduled at the convenience of both the donor and the patient to ensure optimal health status at the time of surgery and to allow for selection of a high-quality graft from a healthy individual. They may preempt more costly and debilitating medical or surgical interventions while awaiting cadaveric donor transplantation, may allow for the administration of immunosuppressant medications a few days before transplant surgery (thereby reducing the risk of rejection), and may yield psychological benefit for the recipient (Rodrigue, Bonk, & Jackson, 2001). Despite these advantages, living donation poses risks to otherwise healthy individuals. These risks include physical pain and discomfort, wound infections, significant bleeding, psychological trauma, the development of hypertension, proteinuria, or progressive organ failure, and death. Overall, however, the quality of life and psychological outcomes reported to date have been quite favorable for living donors (Switzer, Dew, & Twillman, 2000).

Because parents make-up a large percentage of those who opt to donate an organ to their child, it is imperative that pediatric psychologists consulting with transplant programs assume an active role in providing psychological services across the spectrum of living donation. The recently published *Consensus Statement on the Live Organ Donor* (Live Organ Donor Consensus Group, 2000) strongly emphasizes the need for careful psychosocial evaluation of the prospective donor. In particular, the psychologist should examine the donor's psychological stability, competence, and ability to provide informed consent and determine whether the donation decision is being made freely and without coercion. Significant depression, substance use or abuse, or behavioral health problems that may affect surgical risk or recovery (e.g., obesity, smoking) should be identified and treated prior to donation surgery. When a parent donates an organ to a child, two family members (parent and child) will be hospitalized and will need caregiving assistance simultaneously, thus necessitating the availability of other immediate or extended family members. Shifts in family responsibilities and roles can be expected during this time and may cause some degree of instability in the absence of extended support. Also, some donors may feel guilty because they are reluctant to undergo major surgery. Family tension may exist about who will be evaluated first for donation and how this decision is made. Some parents may have unrealistic expectations about how the parent–child relationship and other aspects of their lives might change following donation and transplantation. Anticipated donor responses to posttransplant nonadherence by the child or adolescent recipient is useful to assess as well, particularly in light of the high rate of nonadherence in this population (Streisand & Tercyak, 2001). These issues, as well as others noted in Table 25.1, warrant careful assessment by the pediatric psychologist before donor surgery occurs.

It is also recommended that psychologists conduct postdonation assessments at regular intervals (e.g., quarterly for the first year) to assess and monitor the donor's experience (Rodrigue et al., 2001). A few common themes that may surface during this time period include pain and discomfort (usually in the first 4 to 6 weeks after surgery), affective distress, and changes in the donor–recipient relationship. Moreover, assessing whether presurgery expectations about the donation experience have been met is important. In our donor program, we attend carefully to the degree to which presurgery expectations have not been met, because this factor appears to be associated with increased risk for affective distress within the first year after donation. It is also essential for the pediatric psychologist to attend to any changes in the child recipient's medical status. Any significant deterioration in the child's health or the death of the child should trigger an assessment of the donor parent's psychological adjustment. Even when faced with medical data suggesting otherwise, some parent donors may feel personally responsible for their child's poor health status or death due to rejection or other related complications. Carefully monitoring these issues in donors, as well as the more positive outcomes, allows immediate intervention when problems surface.

Adherence

Prior to transplantation, most children and adolescents have had to deal with a complex regimen of medications, surgery, frequent laboratory tests, clinic appointments, dietary restrictions or supplements, and activity limitations. These demands are not unlike those for children with chronic health conditions that do not lead to organ transplantation. Indeed, an assessment of adherence is a critical component of the pretransplant evaluation process

TABLE 25.1. Issues for the Pediatric Psychologist to Assess with Potential Living Organ Donors

Donor motives
Donor decision-making process
Prior attitudes and beliefs about organ donation
Ambivalence about donation
Cognitive functioning and ability to provide informed consent
Knowledge of surgical procedure and associated risks
Expectations about recovery, recipient morbidity and mortality, recipient compliance behaviors, and changes in the donor–recipient relationship
Overt or subtle coercion from within the family system
Nature and stability of donor–recipient relationship and other relationships within the family system
Coping resources
Past and current psychological disturbance and treatments
History of pain tolerance and management strategies
Spirituality and/or religious issues pertinent to donation
Past and current substance use history (e.g., tobacco, alcohol, illicit drugs, prescribed narcotics)
Current life stress (e.g., occupational, family, marital, financial)
Availability and stability of instrumental and affective support

for all children and adolescents. As noted by LaGreca and Bearman (Chapter 8, this volume), thorough examination of the individual and systemic barriers that may interfere with optimal adherence allows for the development and implementation of appropriate psychological interventions. For those awaiting transplantation, such interventions may improve health prior to transplant surgery and may increase the likelihood of improved adherence after transplantation.

Following transplantation, organ rejection is the primary impediment to continued survival and better quality of life. Consequently, transplant recipients must commit to lifelong adherence to immunosuppressant medications designed to prevent the occurrence of both acute and chronic rejection episodes. Acute rejection usually occurs during the first few months after transplant surgery and is treatable, whereas chronic rejection typically occurs after the first year, can last for months or years, and is difficult to treat. Rejection may be due to nonadherence with the medication regimen, or its etiology may be unknown. Regardless of its cause, however, rejection carries with it several serious implications. These include graft failure, a return to end-stage disease, significant decline in quality of life, retransplantation, and death.

Immunosuppression, although offering clear survival advantages, raises the risk for infections and necessitates hypervigilance in avoiding contact with other people or situations in which infectious conditions may exist. Frequent lab visits and follow-up clinic appointments are essential components of posttransplant care and monitoring of organ functioning. For adolescents in particular, there is an inherent tension between taking medications to maintain life and the desire to shed the sick role along with the diseased organ. In addition, many side effects are associated with immunosuppression: irritability, mood swings, changes in appearance, excessive hair growth, cognitive changes, sleep problems, headaches, diarrhea, and restlessness, among others.

Although there are variations in conceptualization, definition, and methodology, nonadherence with immunosuppression medication is a common problem among adolescents, and its prevalence is estimated at between 9 and 75% (Fennell, Tucker, & Pedersen, 2001; Lurie et al., 2000; Serrano-Ikkos, Lask, Whitehead, & Eisler, 1998). In addition to the health consequences noted previously, nonadherence with immunosuppression may lead to increased utilization of health services, higher medical costs, ethical dilemmas in clinical decision making (e.g., Should we offer a second transplant when the first graft was lost due to nonadherence?), and problems interpreting the results of clinical trials in which the relative effectiveness of different immunosuppressant regimens is being examined. A host of individual, family, systemic, and treatment-related factors may account for the high rate of nonadherence, including health-related attitudes and beliefs, cognitive problems, poor parental supervision or inadequate support, limited financial resources, regimen complexity, and side effects. In attending to these barriers to adherence, pediatric transplant programs tend to focus primarily on educating patients and their parents about the medication regimen, its associated side effects, and the deleterious consequences of nonadherence. However, research with various pediatric populations has consistently shown that education alone is not sufficient to improve adherence among children and adolescents (e.g., Rapoff, 1999). Behavioral interventions that focus on self-monitoring, reinforcement, and contracting, as well as more family-based interventions, hold some promise for use with pediatric patients, although few efforts have been made to evaluate their effectiveness in preventing organ rejection following transplantation. Moreover, these interventions may not attend completely to some of the unique barriers experienced by young transplant recipients and their families.

Long-Term Psychological Care

The vast majority of research on the psychological aspects of pediatric transplantation has occurred during the pretransplant period or within a few years after transplantation. Indeed, such research has identified a number of important clinical issues that warrant assessment and possible intervention by the pediatric psychologist. Unfortunately, the long-term psychological, developmental, academic, quality-of-life, and family-based outcomes of pediatric transplantation are not as well known. Some evidence suggests heightened behavioral problems and affective distress, lower self-esteem and psychosocial competencies, vulnerability to cognitive deficits, and more family stress in some pediatric transplant recipients long after surgery (e.g., DeBolt, Stewart, Kennard, Petrick, & Andrews, 1995; Demaso et al., 1995; Rodrigue et al., 1997; Schulz et al., 2001; Schwering et al., 1997; Stewart et al., 1994; Törnqvist et al., 1999; Uzark et al., 1992), although the clinical significance of these findings relative to healthy peers remains equivocal.

Although these studies offer important insights into the long-term adaptation of pediatric transplant recipients and their families, the research in this area is largely retrospective and unidimensional, relies predominantly on parental report, is site or program specific, and/or lacks appropriate comparison groups. More studies that are prospective and multisystemic in nature (i.e., simultaneously examining outcomes at the level of the child, parents, family, and school) and that include follow-up assessment points several years after transplant surgery are needed. Moreover, more interdisciplinary collaboration that cuts across multiple transplant programs would not only address the problem of small sample sizes but would also potentially enable greater generalization of findings. This latter objective could be accomplished with the establishment of a consortium of pediatric transplant programs, much like those in pediatric oncology, for the primary purpose of gathering the types of outcome data being described here. Pediatric psychologists can play a central role in the development, implementation, and monitoring of such consortia.

Clearly, there is a need within the field to enhance understanding of the physical and mental health outcomes and needs of child transplant recipients as they grow and age. Indeed, this need assumes heightened urgency as more children undergo transplantation and subsequently live longer lives. Some important questions include: What is the long-term (5 years) quality of life of pediatric transplant recipients? How do pediatric transplant patients transition from pediatric to adult medical services? What are the behavioral health practices of pediatric transplant recipients compared with those of otherwise healthy peers? Do the neurocognitive deficits observed pre- and posttransplant have long-term academic and/or occupational consequences for pediatric transplant recipients? What are the long-term physical and mental health outcomes for caregivers of pediatric transplant recipients?

We have previously called for pediatric transplant programs to develop and implement a continuum of psychological care (Rodrigue et al., in press), and we reiterate this position here. Ideally, such care would include psychological assessment of each child and his or her family at 6-month intervals during the pretransplant waiting period and in the first 2 years after transplant surgery, as well as annual evaluations in all subsequent years. Focusing on quality of life, developmental progress, cognitive functioning, academic achievement, behavioral and psychological adaptation, adherence behaviors, and family functioning during these evaluations would provide much needed information about the effects of transplantation (and its associated medical demands) and provide opportunities for immediate intervention to prevent poor health outcomes. In addition, close collaboration with schoolteachers, school nurses, and administrators is imperative to ensure successful integration of the child into the academic and social milieu. Teachers, school nurses, and guidance counselors who are knowledgeable about pediatric transplantation, its treatment demands, and its associated long-term outcomes may be more likely to facilitate peer understanding of the transplant process and to encourage positive interactions with the child, to implement curricular activities that consider the child's medical history and medication regimen (e.g., via Section 504 of the Rehabilitation Act of 1973), and to report any changes in child functioning to the transplant team.

EMERGING ETHICAL ISSUES

There is no shortage of ethical issues and dilemmas within the field of transplantation. In his recent book devoted entirely to the topic, Veatch (2000) discussed bioethical issues that range from defining death, the use of living donors for organs, and the emergence of xenografting to the way patient selection decisions are made, retransplantation, and broader organ allocation issues. Others have similarly written about transplantation ethics (Caplan & Coelho, 1998) and have facilitated a dialogue that is essential reading for pediatric psychologists interested in this area. In this section, we review a few ethical issues that may be of particular interest and importance for pediatric psychologists. For a more complete discussion of key ethics concepts that are pertinent to pediatric psychology, see Rae, Brunnquell, and Sullivan (Chapter 3, this volume).

Virtually all professional organizations, including the American Psychological Association (2002), have a specific code of conduct and ethics that help to guide professional actions. However, these codes often cannot keep pace with, nor anticipate in most instances, the many changes inherent in the field of transplantation. Indeed, these changes constantly challenge our individual and professional standards of conduct. Of course, there are numerous ethical questions that arise in the context of organ transplantation. Should society value the lives of children more than those of adults? Should psychological or behavioral health factors be used in the selection of children or adolescents for transplant listing? Should retransplantation ever be considered for adolescents who reject their first transplant graft due to nonadherence? Should children with severe cognitive impairments compete equally for transplantation? Should anencephalic infants be used as a source of tissues and organs? Is the decision of a parent to be a live organ donor for his or her child truly one that is free of influence or coercion? In light of the prevailing practice of living organ donation, is it ever acceptable for a parent to sacrifice his or her life by donating a heart to save a child's life? Should children or adolescents ever be considered as sources of live organ donation? Should complete strangers (i.e., purely altruistic live donors) be permitted to donate an organ for a child on the transplant waiting list? What if it means saving the life of a parent or sibling who would otherwise die? How should death be defined for purposes of cadaveric organ donation? Should the donation wishes of the deceased supersede those of the surviving family members? Should financial incentives be offered for organ donation? Should animal organs and tissues be transplanted into human beings, especially into children? Encompassing the full spectrum of life and death, these questions have stimulated spirited debate and controversy. Pediatric psychologists must decide if, when, and where to enter this professional exchange—both as individual psychologists and as a professional organization with fundamental interests in the lives of children and families.

For instance, consider the following case example. A 16-year-old girl who received a liver transplant 2 years earlier is discovered, via routine laboratory tests, to be showing signs of organ rejection. Subsequent discussions with her and her parents indicate poor adherence to the immunosuppressant medication regimen. She is referred to the pediatric psychologist and receives both individual and family-based intervention designed to enhance adherence. During treatment, the transplant team determines that she will need another transplant within the next several months but decides to pursue it only if the patient demonstrates adequate adherence. Without eventual retransplantation, the patient will most certainly die. The psychologist, in the course of treatment, becomes aware of occasional lapses in taking medication, despite overall improvement in adherence. Should the pediatric psychologist communicate this information to the transplant team, knowing that it may affect the patient's candidacy for retransplantation? What if the nonadherence was more pervasive and extended beyond "occasional lapses"—would this alter decision making? What are the health professionals' obligations to the patient, her family, the potential organ donor, and society? Should retransplantation be considered at all in this case (i.e., considering that she had her chance and that others are in need of this lifesaving intervention), or is a life of inherent value regardless of whether or not the person failed in his or her previous chance? Should this patient be offered lower priority for transplantation, as the outcomes for retransplantation are not as favorable as they are for first transplants?

These are but a few of the ethical questions and issues that surface in the lives of pediatric transplant professionals. For the most part, the ethical issues confronted by pediatric psychologists will revolve around organ procurement and organ allocation. Nevertheless, as Gillett (2000) has noted, health care professionals must scrutinize each issue as it surfaces, consider both reasoned arguments and intuitive associations, and be willing to examine the issue from all perspectives.

EMERGING RESEARCH ISSUES

The pace of psychological research on pediatric transplantation lags far behind that focused on adult transplantation (Engle, 2001). The extant literature, with a few notable exceptions, is limited largely to single-site retrospective studies with small sample sizes. Furthermore, intervention research is virtually nonexistent. What is needed now is a clear research agenda for pediatric psychologists with interests in transplantation.

Organ Donation

In light of the critical organ shortage, one of the most significant ways in which psychologists can advance the field of pediatric transplantation is by identifying the most effective strategies for increasing cadaveric organ donation. Until recently, behavioral scientists have been largely absent from efforts designed to alleviate the severe organ shortage (e.g., Siminoff et al., 2001). This is unfortunate when one considers that the interpersonal nature of the request process, the stress and grief associated with sudden loss, the cognitive decision-making processes underlying donation decisions, and the primary reasons for donation consent and refusal are largely psychological in nature. With an unsettling shortage of pediatric donors in particular, psychologists have a unique opportunity to lend scientific expertise to help increase the likelihood that parents confronted with the traumatic death of a child will consent to organ donation.

Theoretical models can guide research efforts in this area. For instance, Radecki and Jaccard (1997) proposed a conceptual model summarizing how family members make donation decisions. Their theoretical framework, solidly grounded in attitude–behavior models commonly applied to other health behaviors, proposes that beliefs (religious, cultural, altruistic, attributional), attitudes toward donation, perceptions about the medical profession, and grief coping mechanisms all potentially affect how organ donation requests are processed and decided on. Although intuitively appealing, this model lacks scientific scrutiny and validation, but it nevertheless produces multiple targets for intervention. On the other hand, Robbins (1998) examined the applicability of the transtheoretical model of change by retrospectively studying 154 families who either provided or refused consent for organ donation. He found that next of kin were more likely to consent to donation if they were in the action stage at the time of request compared with those in the precontemplation or contemplation stages. However, of the 85% who donated organs, only about 40% retrospectively reported being in the action stage at the time the request was made.

These models illuminate several possible research questions: Do children who participate in school-based programs designed to increase awareness and interest in organ donation discuss their perceptions with their parents? Do such programs have a direct impact on organ donation consent rates? Are there interactional strategies that psychologists could train organ requestors to use that would increase consent rates? Does a psychological intervention designed to assist families throughout the grieving process (i.e., from declaration of brain death to long-term loss adjustment) increase consent rates? How can we help organ requestors to identify processes of change and tailor their approach to making requests on the basis of this assessment?

It is also critically important that research addresses the psychological risks and benefits associated with cadaveric organ donation. Families who have donated the organs of their deceased loved ones have reported several important benefits. For instance, Batten and

Prottas (1987) found that family members reported feeling that their loved one could live on following organ donation and that the donation process allowed them to derive meaning from the death. In essence, donor families were able to use the donation experience to facilitate effective and adaptive coping. These family-based perceptions appear to hold for situations involving the death of either a child or an adult (Batten & Prottas, 1987; Finlay & Dallimore, 1991). Despite these benefits, however, a sizable proportion of families are often dissatisfied with the donation process. For instance, in the most comprehensive study of satisfaction among donor and nondonor families, Burroughs and colleagues found that 21% of families would not make the same donation decision again. These researchers found that higher satisfaction was associated with being married, having the request made in a community hospital, feeling comfortable with the request process, being less religious, having an understanding of brain death, and perceiving support from family, friends, and health providers (Burroughs, Hong, Kappel, & Freedman, 1998). In addition, DeJong et al. (1998) retrospectively examined donor and nondonor families and found that they differed significantly in knowledge, beliefs, and attitudes about organ donation. Specifically, family members who consented to donation were more knowledgeable about brain death, more likely to have previously discussed organ donation, and more apt to have favorable attitudes and beliefs about donation.

Unfortunately, the Burroughs et al. (1998) study notwithstanding, very little is known about the influence of family discussions and dynamics on the organ donation decision of the legal next of kin. It is likely, for instance, that family roles and alliances, the positions of leadership within the family, and the degree of emotional support are important process-level variables that factor into organ donation consent decisions.

Living organ donation represents another area in which pediatric psychology research can influence the field in a substantial way. Living organ donation has more than doubled in the past decade, while cadaveric donation has remained relatively stable (UNOS, 2001). As more parents pursue the option of living organ donation, we should examine closely its associated costs and outcomes. Research on the sequelae of living organ donation has focused predominantly on the surgical complications and mortality associated with donation surgery. Studies addressing other outcomes (e.g., psychological, interpersonal, social, financial) have not kept pace with research on surgical morbidity and mortality. Recent reviews by Rodrigue et al. (2001) and Switzer et al. (2000) indicated that research has focused predominantly on the psychological costs of living donation, with little empirical attention directed toward psychological benefits.

More focused research on the broad range of health-related outcomes for living organ donors is desperately needed for several reasons. First, information gleaned from such studies will enhance the informed consent process and will permit professionals to more accurately disclose the full range of outcomes that are possible for living donors. Second, with few exceptions, little prospective and longitudinal investigation has been conducted. Third, information about the broad range of *both* positive and negative outcomes may help current and future efforts to increase living organ donation. Fourth, little is known about the impact of living donation on the psychological functioning of parents, the impact of the donation on the parent–child relationship, health service utilization after donation, or the incidental costs to the donor and his or her family. Fifth, the short- and long-term health outcomes of living-parent donors have not been scrutinized as closely as those for recipients of their organs.

The health service utilization patterns among living organ donors has not been the focus of systematic investigation. Similarly, although all medical costs associated with donation are generally paid for by the recipient's insurance coverage, very little is known about the incidental expenses incurred by living organ donors. Trotter et al. (2001) found that 29% of living liver donors initiated medical evaluations for donation-related symptoms experienced in the months after donation surgery. In this same study, the mean financial burden for donors was $3,660 and included costs for transportation, lodging, medication, and lost wages. Most required some type of financial assistance, including short-term disability (or sick leave), long-term disability, leave without pay, leave with full salary, or financial assistance from family or friends. Kim-Schluger (2000) found that 33% of living liver donors reported unresolved insurance issues in the months following donation and that one-third of donors considered their experience to be financially burdensome. It is not known from this study what the nature of the insurance issues were for the donors or how the financial burden translated into actual costs for donors.

Other research questions relevant to parent and living organ donation include: What variables moderate outcomes for donor, donor–recipient relationship, and health service utilization and cost (e.g., demographic characteristics, graft/recipient function)? What similarities and differences are there in clinical outcomes across donors (e.g., biological parent, sibling, other relative) and organ types (e.g., kidney, liver)? What are the psychosocial needs of living organ donors and how are these needs best met by transplant programs? What are the psychological ramifications for living organ donors, especially parents and siblings, when the recipient rejects the organ due to poor behavioral health practices or nonadherence?

Clinical Outcomes

Health professionals in pediatric transplantation now recognize the importance of measuring clinical outcomes that extend beyond survival. Relevant outcomes for children have been discussed throughout this chapter and include those at the individual (developmental, cognitive, affective, quality of life), family (family stress, caregiver burden, sibling adjustment), school (academic functioning, peer relations), and health care system (transition from pediatric to adult medicine) levels. With longer survival times, it is imperative that psychologists systematically assess these clinical outcomes beyond the first few years after transplantation and into early adulthood. Longitudinal studies from the pretransplant evaluation through 10 or 15 years after transplant surgery would permit the disentangling of effects that are due to disease and those due to transplant surgery and the posttransplant regimen. Such research also would provide valuable insight into the full range of benefits associated with pediatric transplantation.

However, if pediatric psychologists are to advance understanding of outcomes, they must consider a few key methodological issues. First, multisite collaborations must be forged to obtain adequate and statistically meaningful sample sizes. Most transplant programs handle very few pediatric cases per year, and there is considerable heterogeneity in these samples, thus making it difficult to properly examine important variables that may mediate or moderate outcomes. Second, resources (e.g., expertise, funds) must be pooled to obtain a comprehensive assessment of the range of clinical outcomes. Too often, studies have focused on one primary outcome (e.g., cognitive function) while excluding others completely (e.g., family stress). Third, measures used to assess outcomes should be standardized, appropriate for the developmental range expected within pediatric transplant populations, and representative of both generic and illness-specific indices whenever possible. Fourth, researchers should make every effort to include multiple perspectives, including those of the child, parents, and teachers, when conducting assessments. Fifth, less reliance should be made on a measure's normative population as a comparison group and greater use should be made of more appropriate control groups. For instance, Stewart et al. (1994) recommended using multiple contrast groups that are matched on relevant sets of variables when examining the possible contributions to cognitive deficits. Patients with similar disease histories who have not yet received transplantation (i.e., wait-listed) may be an appropriate comparison group to study the effects of transplantation and the associated drug regimens. Similarly, a group of pediatric bone-marrow-transplant patients may be a useful comparison group for a sample of solid-organ-transplant recipients when the effect of transplant surgery itself is of primary interest (i.e., although bone marrow patients receive similar immunosuppressant medications, they do not have transplant surgery).

In addition to the foregoing, it would be helpful to identify the behavioral health factors that best predict posttransplant clinical outcomes. Despite the relative importance of a thorough psychological evaluation prior to transplantation, little is known about the relationship between intrapersonal, interpersonal, and familial variables and posttransplant health and well-being. In the adult transplant literature, evidence is mixed concerning the predictive utility of psychological factors (Levenson & Olbrisch, 2000), yet the use of such factors in the patient selection process continues to be widespread. This issue represents an important area of scientific inquiry in pediatric transplantation, especially if patient selection decisions are based, in part, on various components of the psychological evaluation. Moreover, if professionals can identify the most salient behavioral health predictors of posttransplant outcomes, then psychological interventions designed to enhance functioning in these areas can be implemented more expeditiously and effectively.

There is also a need for pediatric psychology researchers to demonstrate how psychological interventions can affect the range of health outcomes both before and after transplantation. Indeed, there is a dearth of behavioral health intervention studies in pediatric transplantation. Interventions promoting physical and mental health (e.g., higher quality of life, psychological adaptation, effective school reintegration), preventing negative health outcomes (e.g., organ rejection and death from nonadherence, posttraumatic stress, family conflict), and highlighting medical cost offsets (e.g., lower health care costs, staff time savings, less utilization of health care resources) are desperately needed. Also, little is known about the application of existing pediatric psychology interventions to the problems encountered in solid organ transplantation. For instance, it would be helpful to determine whether the stress inoculation and reduction strategies used in the bone-marrow-transplant setting (e.g., Streisand, Rodrigue, Houck, Graham-Pole, & Berlant, 2000) can be translated effectively to solid organ transplantation.

The human, financial, and societal costs associated with nonadherence following transplantation are substantial. Consequently, the development, implementation, and evaluation of services designed to promote posttransplant adherence among adolescents, in particular, would represent a major advancement in this field. Rapoff (1999) highlights many educational, organizational, and behavioral strategies designed to enhance adherence in pediatric patients, yet little effort has been made to evaluate their effectiveness with transplant-specific populations. The effectiveness of electronic monitoring devices (e.g., Cyclotech Cyclosporine Oral Solution Dispenser) that contain timers and prompts for ordering additional medication warrants investigation with adolescents. Studies that identify individual barriers to adherence and develop intervention strategies to target these barriers should be a top priority for researchers in the field of pediatric transplantation. Finally, the role that Web-based technologies might play in promoting adherence following pediatric transplantation is currently unknown but also warrants empirical attention in light of its apparent success with adult heart transplant recipients (Dew et al., 2002).

Health Policy

Finally, pediatric psychologists should team up with health policy experts and transplant program administrators to provide needed behavioral science expertise in evaluating the impact of transplant-related initiatives and policies. When new initiatives are proposed, pediatric psychologists can join the discussion and help to design strategies for assessing how they affect children and families. For instance, the use of minors as living organ donors, changes in the allocation of livers for transplantation, and the potential use of xenografts all have implications for the lives of children, yet the absence of pediatric psychologists in such policy discussions is striking. What impact do health policy changes have on children and families? What are the prevailing public attitudes and beliefs about new initiatives? What are the behavioral health consequences associated with changes in federal funding for pediatric transplantation?

SUMMARY AND CONCLUSIONS

In summary, pediatric transplantation offers children a chance at life extension and improved quality of life and affords many exciting opportunities for psychologists. The field is riddled with clinical, ethical, and scientific issues that potentially affect the physical and mental well-being of children and families. As the number of children who are affected by transplantation increases, so too does the expectation that pediatric psychologists will continue to play a vital role as integral members of transplant teams. Moreover, pediatric psychologists may be called on to assess the psychological strengths and liabilities of pediatric transplant candidates and their families; to design, implement, and evaluate interventions to reduce behavioral health liabilities and to promote positive adaptation; and to conduct behavioral health research. Pediatric psychologists may also be asked to educate other health professionals and health policy experts about behavioral health issues and their relevance to pediatric transplantation. Several pediatric psychologists have already made substantial contributions to advancing our understanding of the psychological and behavioral health concomitants of organ transplantation, and we should continue to build on and expand their efforts. In this chapter, we have attempted to highlight some of the emerging issues that warrant our attention and consideration as clinicians, scientists, and educators. We have no doubt that the horizons of pediatric transplantation will continue to expand over the next several years. Pediatric psychologists must be ready to embrace these challenges and to participate actively in the interdisciplinary dialogue that characterizes this field.

ACKNOWLEDGMENTS

Support for the preparation of this chapter was provided, in part, by grants from the National Institutes of Health (DK55706) and the Health Resources and Services Administration (H390T00115-01) to James R. Rodrigue.

REFERENCES

American Psychological Association. (2002). Ethical principles of psychologists and code of conduct. *American Psychologist, 57,* 1060–1073.

Batten, H.L., & Prottas, J. M. (1987). Kind strangers: The families of organ donors. *Health Affairs, 6,* 35–47.

Boucek, M. M., Faro, A., Novick, R. J., Bennett, L. E., Keck, B. M., & Hosenpud, J. D. (2001). The Registry of the International Society for Heart and Lung Transplantation: Fourth official pediatric report—2000. *Journal of Heart and Lung Transplantation, 20,* 39–52.

Burroughs, T. E., Hong, B. A., Kappel, D. F., & Freedman, B. K. (1998). The stability of family decisions to consent or refuse organ donation: Would you do it again? *Psychosomatic Medicine, 60,* 156–162.

Canning, R. D., & Stuber, M. L. (2000). Pediatric transplantation. In P. T. Trzepacz & A. F. DiMartini (Eds.), *The transplant patient: Biological, psychiatric, and ethical issues in organ transplantation* (pp. 275–286). Cambridge, UK: Cambridge University Press.

Caplan, A. L., & Coelho, D. H. (Eds.). (1998). *The ethics of organ transplants: The current debate.* Amherst, NY: Prometheus Books.

Cohen, R. G., Barr, M. L., Schenkel, F. A., DeMeester, T. R., Wells, W. J., & Starnes, V. A. (1994). Living-related donor lobectomy for bilateral lobar transplantation in patients with cystic fibrosis. *Annals of Thoracic Surgery, 57,* 1423–1427.

DeBolt, A. J., Stewart, S. M., Kennard, B. D., Petrik, K., & Andrews, W. S. (1995). A survey of psychosocial adaptation in longterm survivors of pediatric liver transplants. *Children's Health Care, 24,* 79 96.

DeJong, W., Franz, H. G., Wolfe, S. M., Nathan, H., Payne, D., Reitsma, W., & Beasley, C. (1998). Requesting organ donation: An interview study of donor and nondonor families. *American Journal of Critical Care, 7,* 13–23

Demaso, D. R., Twente, A. W., Spratt, E. G., & O'Brien, P. (1995). Impact of psychological functioning, medical severity, and family functioning in pediatric heart transplantation. *Journal of Heart and Lung Transplantation, 14,* 1102–1108.

Dew, M. A., Kormos, R. L., Goycoolea, J. M., Lee, A., Zomak, R., & Griffith, B. P. (2002). An Internet-based intervention to improve mental health and medical compliance in heart transplant recipients. *Journal of Heart and Lung Transplantation, 21,* 109.

Engle, D. (2001). Psychosocial aspects of the organ transplant experience: What has been established and what we need for the future. *Journal of Clinical Psychology, 57,* 521–549.

Fennell, R. S., Tucker, C., & Pedersen, T. (2001). Demographic and medical predictors of medication compliance among ethnically different pediatric renal transplant patients. *Pediatric Transplantation, 5,* 343–348.

Finlay, I., & Dallimore, D. (1991). Your child is dead. *British Medical Journal, 302,* 1524–1525.

Gillett, G. (2000). Ethics and images in organ transplantation. In P. T. Trzepacz & A. F. DiMartini (Eds.), *The transplant patient: Biological, psychiatric, and ethical issues in organ transplantation* (pp. 239–254). New York: Cambridge University Press.

Hobbs, S. A., & Sexson, S. B. (1993). Cognitive development and learning in the pediatric organ transplant recipient. *Journal of Learning Disabilities, 26,* 104–113.

Howard, R. J. (2001). Organ donation: Social policy, ethical, and legislative issues. In J. R. Rodrigue (Ed.), *Biopsychosocial perspectives on transplantation* (pp. 39–58). New York: Kluwer Academic/Plenum.

Kennard, B. D., Stewart, S. M., Phelan-McAuliffe, D., Waller, D. A., Bannister, M., Fioravani, V., & Andrews, W. S. (1999). Academic outcome in long-term survivors of pediatric liver transplantation. *Journal of Developmental and Behavioral Pediatrics, 20,* 17–23.

Kim-Schluger, L. (2000, December). *Psychological follow-up after liver donation.* Paper presented at the workshop on Living Donor Liver Transplantation, Washington, DC.

Levenson, J. L., & Olbrisch, M. E. (2000). Psychosocial screening and selection of candidates for organ transplantation. In P. T. Trzepacz & A. F. DiMartini (Eds.), *The transplant patient: Biological, psychiatric, and ethical issues in organ transplantation* (pp. 21–41). New York: Cambridge University Press.

Live Organ Donor Consensus Group. (2000). Consensus statement on the live organ donor. *Journal of the American Medical Association, 284,* 2919–2926.

Lurie, S., Shemesh, E., Sheiner, P. A., Emre, S., Tindle, H. L., Melchionna, L., & Shneider, B. L. (2000). Non-adherence in pediatric liver transplant recipients: An assessment of risk factors and natural history. *Pediatric Transplantation, 4,* 200–206.

Mendley, S. R., & Zelko, F. A. (1999). Improvement in specific aspects of neurocognitive performance in children after renal transplantation. *Kidney International, 56,* 318–323.

Merrill, J. P., Murray, J. E., Harrison, J. H., & Guild, W. R. (1956). Successful homotransplantation of the human kidney between identical twins. *Journal of the American Medical Association, 160,* 277–282.

Oaks, T. E., Aravot, D., Dennis, C., Wells, F. C., Large, S. R., & Wallwork, J. (1994). Domino heart transplantation: The Papworth experience. *Journal of Heart and Lung Transplantation, 13,* 433–437.

Radecki, C. M., & Jaccard, J. (1997). Psychological aspects of organ donation: A critical review and synthesis of individual and next-of-kin donation decisions. *Health Psychology, 16*, 183–195.

Rapoff, M. A. (1999). *Adherence to pediatric medical regimens*. New York: Plenum Press.

Robbins, M. L. (1998, April). *Processes of change and the stages of change model for family consent to cadaveric organ donation*. Paper presented at the U. S. Department of Health and Human Services meeting on Increasing Donation and Transplantation: The Challenge of Evaluation, Alexandria, VA.

Rodrigue, J. R., Bonk, V., & Jackson, S. (2001). Psychological considerations of living organ donation. In J. R. Rodrigue (Ed.), *Biopsychosocial perspectives on transplantation* (pp. 59–70). New York: Kluwer Academic/Plenum.

Rodrigue, J. R., Gonzalez, R., & Langham, M. (in press). Solid organ transplantation. In R. T. Brown (Ed.), *Handbook of pediatric psychology in school settings*. Mahwah, NJ: Erlbaum.

Rodrigue, J. R., MacNaughton, K., Hoffmann, R. G., Graham-Pole, J., Andres, J. M., Novak, D. A., & Fennell, R. S. (1997). Transplantation in children: A longitudinal assessment of mothers' stress, coping, and perceptions of family functioning. *Psychosomatics, 38*, 478–486.

Schulz, K. H., Hofmann, C., Sander, K., Edsen, S., Burdelski, M., & Rogiers, X. (2001). Comparison of quality of life and family stress in families of children with living-related liver transplants versus families of children who received a cadaveric liver. *Transplantation Proceedings, 33*, 1496–1497.

Schweitzer, J. B., & Hobbs, S. A. (1995). Renal and liver disease: End-stage and transplantation issues. In M. C. Roberts (Ed.), *Handbook of pediatric psychology* (2nd ed., pp. 425–445). New York: Guilford Press.

Schwering, K. L., Febo-Mandl, F., Finkenauer, C., Rime, B., Hayez, J. Y., & Otte, J. B. (1997). Psychological and social adjustment after pediatric liver transplantation as a function of age at surgery and of time elapsed since transplantation. *Pediatric Transplantation, 1*, 138–145.

Serrano-Ikkos, Lask, B., Whitehead, B., & Eisler, I. (1998). Incomplete adherence after pediatric heart and heart–lung transplantation. *Journal of Heart and Lung Transplantation, 17*, 1177–1183.

Sexson, S., & Rubenow, J. (1992). Transplant in children and adolescents. In J. Craven & G. M. Rodin (Eds.), *Psychiatric aspects of organ transplantation* (pp. 33–49). Oxford, UK: Oxford University Press.

Siminoff, L. A., Gordon, N., Hewlett, J., & Arnold, R. M. (2001). Factors influencing families' consent for donation of solid organs for transplantation. *Journal of the American Medical Association, 286*, 71–77.

Stewart, S. M., & Kennard, B. D. (1999). Organ transplantation. In R. T. Brown (Ed.), *Cognitive aspects of chronic illness in children* (pp. 220–237). New York: Guilford Press.

Stewart, S. M., Kennard, B. D., Waller, D. A., & Fixler, D. (1994). Cognitive function in children who receive organ transplantation. *Health Psychology, 13*, 3–13.

Streisand, R., Rodrigue, J. R., Houck, C., Graham-Pole, J., & Berlant, N. (2000). Parents of children undergoing bone marrow transplantation: Documenting stress and implementing a psychological intervention program. *Journal of Pediatric Psychology, 25*, 331–337.

Streisand, R. M., & Tercyak, K. P. (2001). Evaluating the pediatric transplant patient: General considerations. In J. R. Rodrigue (Ed.), *Biopsychosocial perspectives on transplantation* (pp. 71–92). New York: Kluwer Academic/Plenum.

Studies of Pediatric Liver Transplantation Research Group (2001). Studies of Pediatric Liver Transplantation Research Group (SPLIT): Year 2000 outcomes. *Transplantation, 72*, 463–476.

Sutherland, D. E. R., Goetz, F. C., & Najarian, J. S. (1984). Pancreas transplants from related donors. *Transplantation, 38*, 625–633.

Switzer, G. E., Dew, M. A., & Twillman, R. K. (2000). Psychosocial issues in living organ donation. In P. T. Trzepacz & A. F. DiMartini (Eds.), *The transplant patient: Biological, psychiatric, and ethical issues in organ transplantation* (pp. 42–66). New York: Cambridge University Press.

Tejani, A., Cortes, L., & Sullivan, E. K. (1996). A longitudinal study of the natural history of growth post-transplantation. *Kidney International, 49*(Suppl. 53), S103–S108.

Todaro, J. F., Fennell, E. B., Sears, S. F., Rodrigue, J. R., & Roche, A. K. (2000). A review of cognitive and psychological outcomes in pediatric heart transplant recipients. *Journal of Pediatric Psychology, 25*, 567–576.

Törnqvist, J., Van Broeck, N., Finkenauer, C., Rosati, R., Schwering, K. L., Hayez, J. Y., et al. (1999). Long-term psychosocial adjustment following pediatric liver transplantation. *Pediatric Transplantation, 3*, 115–125.

Trotter, J. F., Talamantes, M., McClure, M., Wachs, M., Bak, T., Trouillot, T., et al. (2001). Right hepatic lobe donation for living donor liver transplantation: Impact on donor quality of life. *Liver Transplantation, 7*, 485–493.

Uemoto, S., Inomata, Y., Sakurai, T., Egawa, H., Fujita, S., Kiuchi, T., et al. (2000). Living donor liver transplantation for fulminant hepatic failure. *Transplantation, 70*, 152–157.

United Network for Organ Sharing. (2001). *2000 Annual Report of the U. S. Scientific Registry for Transplant Recipients and the Organ Procurement and Transplantation Network: Transplant data: 1990–1999*. Rockville, MD: U.S. Department of Health and Human Services, Health Resources and Services Administration, Office of Special Programs, Division of Transplantation.

U.S. Department of Health and Human Services. (2001). *Gift of life donation initiative*. Available from *http://www.organdonor.gov/SecInitiative.htm*.

Uzark, K. C., Sauer, S. N., Lawrence, K. S., Miller, J., Addonizio, L., & Crowley, D. C. (1992). The psychosocial impact of pediatric heart transplantation. *Journal of Heart and Lung Transplantation*, *11*, 1160–1167.

Veatch, R. M. (2000). *Transplantation ethics*. Washington, DC: Georgetown University Press.

Walker, A. M., Harris, G., Baker, A., Kelly, D., & Houghton, J. (1999). Post-traumatic stress responses following liver transplantation in older children. *Journal of Child Psychology and Psychiatry*, *40*, 363–374.

Wijdicks, E. F. M. (Ed.). (1999). *Neurologic complications in organ transplant recipients*. Boston, MA: Butterworth-Heinemann.

Wong, M., Mallory, G. B., Jr., Goldstein, J., Goyal, M., & Yamada, K. A. (1999). Neurologic complications of pediatric lung transplantation. *Neurology*, *53*, 1542–1549.

26

Pediatric Burns

KENNETH J. TARNOWSKI
RONALD T. BROWN

Burn injuries are relatively common phenomena and are considered among the most serious of human injuries (McLoughlin & McGuire, 1990). Burns share several characteristics of chronic diseases and can result in serious long-term physical and psychosocial morbidity (Patterson et al., 1993; Tarnowski, 1994; Tarnowski, Rasnake, & Drabman, 1987). Early studies of the behavioral aspects of pediatric burns largely comprised anecdotal reports, and subjective clinical impressions formed the bases for conclusions about child and family adjustment. Unfortunately, the relative dearth of interest in the psychological aspects of pediatric burns has continued until the present. As in many areas of clinical psychology, the adult literature is better developed. However, a review of the adult literature by Patterson et al. (1993) documents that progress has been relatively slow in that area as well. The emergence of specialty journals in the area, including *Burns* and the *Journal of Burn Care and Rehabilitation*, has focused much needed attention on medical advances and the psychosocial plight of burn survivors.

In several respects, burns are unique injuries that present novel opportunities to examine child, parent, and family adjustment and adaptation to a significant stressor. Burn injuries often share characteristics of acute disorders, as well as those of chronic illness (e.g., short-term disruptive developmental effects, long-term medical and behavioral consequences), simultaneously affecting multiple members of the same family. Burns are relatively unique in that these injuries can be associated with losses not typically associated with other forms of chronic illness (e.g., loss of parents, siblings, possessions, pets). Burns often result in characteristic forms of permanent disfigurement, are often related to premorbid parent–child–family psychopathology, and are frequently associated with negative psychosocial sequelae that are disproportionate to the extent of physical or medical impairment. Burn injuries are associated with protracted periods of severe pain that, unfortunately, often prove to be recalcitrant to standard pharmacological management strategies. The multitude, severity, and interaction of the medical and psychological problems caused by pediatric burns makes apparent the ceiling of effectiveness of commonly used pediatric psychology treatment methods (e.g., pain management, coping).

This chapter provides an overview of pediatric burn epidemiology, medical treatment, acute- and rehabilitation-phase issues and considerations, and prevention strategies. The purpose of the chapter is to acquaint readers with the medical and surgical challenges and to highlight the multiple points of possible psychosocial interaction with this population from the time of injury through extended follow-up.

EPIDEMIOLOGICAL CONSIDERATIONS

Approximately 1.25 million individuals sustain burn injuries each year in the United States (Brigham & McLoughlin, 1996). Burn injuries remain the fourth leading cause of accidental death in children with 5,500 deaths per year (Brigham & McLoughlin, 1996). Approximately 70,000 individuals are hospitalized for such injuries, and approximately 50% of victims are children and adolescents. Thirty-eight percent of hospitalized patients are less than 15 years of age (Barrow & Herndon, 1990). Burn fatalities disproportionately affect children and adolescents, with two-thirds of all fatalities occurring in those less than 15 years of age, and with a male-to-female ratio of 2:1 (U.S. Fire Administration, 1978). For children and adolescents to age 19, fire and burn injuries are the third leading cause of death; they rank second to motor vehicle accidents for children 1–4 years (Guyer & Gallagher, 1985). House fires account for the majority of pediatric fire-related deaths, and the majority of such deaths are attributable to smoke inhalation as opposed to direct burn insult.

Children under 5 years of age account for more than 50% of all pediatric burn injuries. Expectedly, the manner in which children sustain injury varies as a function of developmental factors (McLoughlin & Crawford, 1985). For example, as motor capabilities increase, toddlers are at increased risk from liquid and food spills and from hot tap water. Preschool and school-age children often sustain injury in experimental play with lighters, matches, and kitchen devices. During adolescence, the majority (60%) of injuries occur outside the home, and 20% are due to scalding injuries within the home. Data indicate a gender discrepancy that increases with age, with a male-to-female ratio approaching 4:1 in older children. The scope of contextual factors in burn injuries is outlined in Stoddard and Saxe (2001).

MEDICAL CONSIDERATIONS

Nature of Burn Injuries

Burn injuries are typically described in terms of Total Burn Surface Area (TBSA) and burn type (degree). Burn injuries are categorized as thermal, radiation, chemical, or electrical. TBSA is calculated through the use of standard charts that display dorsal and ventral views of the body, categorized into discrete areas of known percentage of TBSA (Lund & Browder, 1944). Heat intensity and duration of skin contact determine the extent and depth of skin damage. Injury that is restricted to the epidermis is called a first-degree burn. More extensive injuries involving the dermis are called second-degree, or partial thickness, burns. The dermis or corium is composed of a vascular plexus containing arterioles, venules, and capillaries. Epidermal appendages (sweat glands, sebaceous glands, and hair follicles) are located in the dermis, along with nerve endings and connective tissue. Below this structural base lies the fatty tissue of the subcutaneous fascia, muscle, and bone. Full-thickness (third degree) burns are extensive injuries involving multiple skin layers, and they may include injury of subcutaneous tissue and peripheral nerve fibers. Burns are classified as minor, moderate, or severe, according to criteria published by the American Burn Association (1984).

Current Treatments

Burn treatment consists of three overlapping phases: emergency period, acute phase, and rehabilitation phase. The following overview of treatment is based on Dyer and Roberts (1990) and Fratianne and Brandt (1994). Emergency treatment at the scene of injury involves removing the source of heat from the injured person. Standard first-aid treatment is provided to ensure an unobstructed airway and to assess pulmonary, hematological, and shock status. Cardiopulmonary resuscitation may be required. The primary concern at this time involves continued evaluation and stabilization of respiration. Bronchoscopy may be required to evaluate inflammation, irritation, and the presence of carbonaceous deposits. For serious injuries, an endotracheal tube placement is required. Compromised extremities may require splinting, and the patient's level of consciousness is carefully monitored.

Burn injuries cause diffusion of the intravascular fluid, into the extravascular fluid resulting in electrolyte imbalance and decreased blood volume. Several fluid resuscitation formulae are available that rectify homeostatic imbalances. A central line allows for fluid infusion, and a Foley bladder catheter permits assessment of output. Capillary function increases over the first days following injury, and a "fluid shift" occurs that results in marked diuresis. Increased cardiac output is associated with the fluid shift, and complications, including pulmonary edema and congestive heart failure, may result. Vital signs, cardiac functions, temperature, and intravenous (IV) fluid titration are monitored closely. Gastrointestinal (GI) complications are common as the decreased blood volume shunts fluid away from the GI tract. GI functions decrease markedly or cease entirely, and abdominal distention is common. Patients with more than 20% TBSA burns or those who are unconscious may require a nasogastric tube and low suction to empty stomach contents and to decrease distention and the probability of aspiration.

Once the patient has stabilized, care shifts to the wound itself. During this phase, the patient is subjected to a variety of aversive procedures (e.g., IV placements, dressing changes, wound cleansing, grafting). A central concern during this phase of treatment is that of serious infection. Within 48 hours following injury, untreated wounds contain gram-positive organisms, and gram-negative bacteria are present by the fifth day. Sepsis represents a major threat to patient survival. Clinical indications of infection include altered mental status, hypo- or hyperthermia, GI disturbances, deterioration of grafted burn sites, and conversion of partial-thickness to full-thickness injuries. Required treatment includes aggressive parenteral administration of antibiotics, autografting (transplanting skin from undamaged areas of the patient's body to the site of the burn injury), and intensive nutritional support. Should such treatments prove unsuccessful, sepsis is typically fatal.

Eschar (burned tissue) combines with edema to produce circulatory compromise. Eschar must be surgically removed. Circumferential burns of the hands, arms, fingers, neck, trunk, and feet often require escharotomy. One to two times daily, debridement procedures are conducted that entail vigorous removal of necrotic tissue. Frequently, debridement is conducted in a hydrotherapy tub filled with a solution of hypochlorite. Minor debridement occurs at the time of admission, and efforts are made to ensure that blisters remain intact and serve a protective function for underlying tissue. Topical antimicrobial agents are applied to minimize wound infection. Partial-thickness burns heal in approximately 3–4 weeks, and full-thickness burns in 3–5 weeks. Physiological dressings (transplanted skin from cadavers [heterografts] or animals [xenografts] or artificial preparations) may be used. These dressings function as barriers to reduce heat and fluid loss. They are, however, temporary and will ultimately be biologically rejected. Autografting is used to treat severe burns. This procedure is usually conducted in phases, due to differential rates of wound healing and the limited availability of donor material. Patients wear pressure dressings and garments to maintain the integrity of autografted sites and to minimize scarring. Advances in biologically cultivated skin will hopefully eliminate the major limitations of traditional physiological dressing and autograft procedures. During the rehabilitation phase, medical, surgical, physical therapy, nutritional, and self-care procedures continue. Reconstructive surgeries often require repeated hospitalizations over a period of several years.

PSYCHOLOGICAL CONSIDERATIONS

The multiple psychological challenges posed by burns often severely tax and overwhelm the coping resources of children and their families. Psychological factors are of central importance to the comprehensive care of pediatric burn victims. However, the breadth of potential areas of psychological interaction may not be fully appreciated. To acquaint readers with the range of these issues, an overview of psychological considerations in the acute and rehabilitation phases of treatment and prevention follows.

ACUTE-PHASE CONSIDERATIONS

Premorbid Risk Factors

A number of premorbid risk factors have been posited for children who have sustained burn injuries. As suggested earlier, these factors include the psychological characteristics and stability of the child, that of the family, and demographic and environmental factors. Considerable evidence supports the existence of marked emotional and behavioral disturbances, parental marital discord, learning handicaps, and environmental stressors in the premorbid histories of a subset of burned children (i.e., Kaslow, Koon-Scott, & Dingle, 1994; Miller, Elliott, Funk, & Pruitt, 1988). In sum, a variety of individual, family, and community factors have been described that appear to be related to increased burn injury risk (Stoddard & Saxe, 2001).

Considerable difficulty is associated with the assessment of child and family premorbid psychopathology (Tarnowski, Rasnake, Gavaghan-Jones, & Smith, 1991). Many of the methods used to study pediatric burn victims have been extrapolated from the adult burn literature. Attempts to accurately characterize children's premorbid functioning will necessarily rely on a broad-spectrum assessment of their preaccident cognitive, emotional, and behavioral status. Such evaluation can be very informative in differentiating acute reactions from long-term sequelae that are unique to the burn injury from those patterns of responding that reflect continuity or exacerbations of preexisting conditions. Importantly, the identification of premorbid dysfunction or characteristics associated with injury risk may contribute to the development of preventive tactics.

Acute-Phase Consultation Issues

During the acute-phase period, those areas of greatest concern include the child's mental status; management of pain; management of symptoms related to the trauma of the burn experience; nutritional intake; adherence to treatment demands; body image, particularly on discharge from the hospital setting; intense itching associated with the healing process; management of behavior that is perceived to be difficult by the burn unit staff; and, finally, issues regarding caregiver and family adjustment to the recovery experience.

Mental Status

Frequently, significant central nervous system (CNS) alterations occur following a burn injury (Brown, Dingle, & Koon-Scott, 1994). CNS effects include anoxic and hypoxic conditions such as carbon monoxide inhalation, effects of electrical injuries that may result in cardiac disturbances, and delirium or intensive care unit (ICU) psychosis that may result from sleep and sensory deprivation associated with long stays in the ICU (Brown et al., 1994). Further, metabolic complications and infections that frequently result from the burn injury often result in altered mental status. Management of disorientation while the patient is in the burn unit typically includes correcting electrolyte imbalances that result from fluid loss following the burn injury, as well as ongoing reality orientation that includes the use of visual aids (e.g., clocks, calendars, orientation to time of day through the use of windows), as well as the child being assigned the same staff members over the course of several days.

Nutritional Intake

High caloric and fluid intake are critical during both the acute and recovery phases of the burn injury (Fratianne & Brandt, 1994). Inadequate caloric intake is a frequently encountered problem on the pediatric burn unit, and one for which staff often seek consultation with the pediatric psychologist. Frequently, behavioral approaches, including contingency management, have been demonstrated as efficacious in increasing caloric, as well as fluid, intake, thereby diminishing the need for tube and intravenous feedings (Garner & Desai, 2001). Because the physical task of eating may prove a formidable challenge for children and adolescents who may have burned their arms, hands, and faces, occupational therapists often can be helpful in assisting children with adaptive devices so that they may be self-sufficient in feeding routines.

Disturbances in Body Image

Burn disfigurement may influence a child's sense of self-competence, as well as relationships with peers. Frequently, the child who sustains a severe burn and subsequent disfigurement must endure the loss of identity and physical competence, as well as social stigmatization (Sheridan, Hinson, & Liang, 2000; Stoddard, 2002). Not surprisingly, issues of adjustment difficulties and peer relationships seem to heighten following the acute or recovery phase of the burn injury long after children have been discharged from the hospital and are away from the support of the hospital and clinic staff. Some research suggests that these adjustment difficulties are exacerbated at adolescence (Brown et al., 1994). Clearly, ongoing monitoring of adjustment is imperative over the course of the burn injury and following discharge from the hospital. Finally, some emerging evidence suggests that social skills training is a viable strategy for teaching children and adolescents who have sustained disfiguring burn injuries how to cope with the disfigurement and how to manage teasing and taunting from peers, as well as other reactions to the disfigurement when confronting strangers and meeting new people (Robinson, Rumsey, & Partridge, 1996).

Self Excoriation

Intense itching typically follows the healing of burned tissues. Behavioral approaches (e.g., response interruption and distraction) have generally proved effective for younger children.

Posttraumatic Stress Disorder

Some literature concerning children who have survived chronic or acute diseases suggests that they indeed suffer from symptoms associated with posttraumatic stress disorder (Barakat & Kazak, 1999). Because children and adolescents who have survived burns frequently have also endured a traumatic experience or accident, posttraumatic stress symptoms are often encountered among burn survivors, both in the acute phase and during the rehabilitation phase of recovery (Stoddard & Saxe, 2001). In fact, as Stoddard and Saxe (2001) have suggested, posttraumatic stress disorder represents a marked feature of a child's psychological response to a number of injuries, including burns. Symptoms of posttraumatic stress often include sleep disturbances, nightmares, symptoms of depression and anxiety, and cognitive blunting (American Psychiatric Association, 2000). In addition, some of the symptoms associated with posttraumatic stress disorder, including preoccupations with the trauma and extreme levels of arousal, may impede learning at school. Given professionals' increasing sophistication regarding posttraumatic stress disorder and children who have survived traumas, psychologists have become much more aware of the importance of early management of issues surrounding the trauma (Barakat & Kazak, 1999).

Adherence to Treatment Demands

Frequent procedures and therapies are needed during the acute phase of the burn injury; these include physical and occupational therapy, use of pressure garments, and pharmacotherapy (Brown et al., 1994). More recently, problem-solving approaches have proven particularly useful in the management of potential adherence problems for adults with chronic diseases, and their potential efficacy for children with burn injuries would seem to be particularly promising. In addition, the use of contingency management approaches has long been demonstrated to be effective in the management of problems associated with adherence to various procedures necessary for the management of burn injuries during both the acute and rehabilitative phases of treatment. As with all pediatric conditions, caregivers also must be involved when addressing adherence issues with children and adolescents.

Disruptive Behaviors

Hospital burn staff frequently consult with the pediatric psychologist regarding disruptive behavior problems that might be present when the child begins the transition from the intensive care unit to the hospital ward. Some experts have suggested that children with various chronic illnesses experience a phase of learned helplessness whereby behavioral disturbances increase in response to children's exposure to aversive procedures (Brown & Macias, 2000). In such an environment, painful procedures such as debridement and hydrotherapy may be perceived as occurring randomly just at the time that these children are dependent on others for emotional support and pain analgesia (Brown et al., 1994). As a result, it is recommended that the hospital environment be both predictable and consistent and that, whenever possible, children be empowered and provided with maximum control (e.g., allowing children to remove dressings and splints whenever possible and to have a choice regarding timc of hydrotherapy and dressing changes).

It also should be noted that many symptoms associated with posttraumatic stress disorder, including behavioral reenactments of the traumatic event, might mirror behavioral disturbances. In addition, children with trauma histories may also exhibit comorbid symptoms of posttraumatic stress disorder, including mood disturbances, anxiety disorders, conduct problems, elimination disorders (i.e., enuresis and encopresis), learning, and attentional problems (Stoddard & Saxe, 2001). Children who have premorbid psychiatric disorders or those who come from families characterized as chaotic are apt to have a greater frequency of comorbid diagnoses (Stoddard & Saxe, 2001).

Family Issues

A healthy family environment seems to be predictive of good adaptation to a significant stressor such as a chronic illness, as well as good adjustment following the illness (Barakat & Kazak, 1999). Other familial variables that have been demonstrated to predict good adjustment include familial cohesiveness, effective communication skills within the family system, skills in conflict resolution among family members, and social support networks available to the family. Such family characteristics lead to better attachment patterns within families and help to regulate the child's affect and trust in others, such as medical staff (Stoddard & Saxe, 2001). Caregiver variables that have been demonstrated to predict children's adjustment following the burn injury include age-appropriate independence for their children and realistic appraisals of their children's injury (for review, see Kaslow et al., 1994). Not surprisingly, availability of financial resources and environments that are characterized by adequate social resources appear to be predictive of postburn adjustment. The coping literature has generally suggested that families who support an active or "engagement" style of coping often have children who fare better in the area of adjustment and adaptation than do children from families who support a passive or "disengagement" style of coping (for review, see Thompson & Gustafson, 1996).

One variable that has been demonstrated to be highly predictive of children's adjustment following the injury, as well as that of their families, is premorbid adjustment (Kaslow et al., 1994). Time since the injury seems to be a stable predictor of adjustment in children, with longer time since the injury predicting better adaptation and adjustment (for review, see Brown et al., 1994; Kaslow et al., 1994; Tarnowski & Simonian, in press).

Finally, given that adaptation to the trauma and subsequent hospitalization are highly associated with familial functioning, it is imperative to address the needs and concerns of all family members, including siblings, throughout the course of hospitalization (for review, see Kaslow et al., 1994). Clinical trials that assess the efficacy of family intervention programs, either alone or in combination with other treatments, are a necessary direction for research efforts in this area.

Pain Management

Appropriate management of pain is a major task during the acute phase following the burn injury. In fact, some emerging literature suggests that adequate pain management diminishes later symptoms of posttraumatic stress disorder (for review, see Stoddard & Saxe, 2001). As Stoddard and Saxe (2001) have astutely observed, appropriate management of pain diminishes anxiety, fears, and confusion during the acute phase of the burn injury. In support of this notion, Saxe et al. (2001) have provided evidence to indicate that the higher the dose of pain analgesia for children who have been injured by burns during the acute phase of hospitalization, the fewer the number of symptoms of posttraumatic stress disorder 6 months following the injury. The task of pain management is particularly great during the acute phase of the burn injury, as children and adolescents often experience significant pain due to the burn itself, as well as to the combination of the various procedures (e.g., dressing changes, debridement) that are necessary throughout treatment during the acute phase of the injury.

Fortunately, a burgeoning body of research in the neural sciences has clarified the neural pathways responsible for understanding the mechanisms of endogenous opioids and, as a result, the specific pathways of these agents on the neurotransmitters in the management of pediatric pain. In addition, recent evidence suggests that specific memories of pain and painful events are permanently stored in memory; recent research also suggests that these memories result in marked neurophysiological damage, including reduced hippocampal size and amygdala-modulated fear conditioning (Sapolsky, 2000).

Fortunately, we now have a much more complete understanding of pain and its appropriate management than we had previously. For example, it is now fairly accepted knowledge that pain has affective, cognitive, cultural, and physiological components (for review, see Walco, Sterling, Conte, & Engel, 1999). Appropriate assessment of pain is critical, including anatomical assessment (e.g., types of tissue damage, nerve pathways), types of pain (e.g., acute), and procedural-related pain (e.g., debridement, physical therapy). Various assessment procedures are available to the pediatric psychologist, including the well-known Visual Analogue Scales (Tarnowski & Kaufman, 1988), and other self-report ratings and physiological instruments that have been widely utilized and have established empirical support concerning their use (for review, see Walco et al., 1999).

Because of the increasing recognition that the adequate management of pain is a standard of care in both the acute and rehabilitative phases of treatment for all individuals who have sustained burn injuries (Sheridan et al., 2000; Stoddard, 2002), numerous protocols are available for the sensible management of pain for children and adolescents with burn injuries (e.g., American Pain Society Quality of Care Committee, 1995). Comprehensive pain management of children and adolescents with burn injuries should include the numerous psychological therapies that have been demonstrated to be efficacious for the management of pain (e.g., cognitive therapies, relaxation, hypnosis; Walco et al., 1999), as well as the numerous pharmacotherapies that are available for management of pain (e.g., nonsteroidal anti-inflammatory drugs, morphine, synthetic opioids) that may be delivered by numerous venues (e.g., patient-controlled analgesia, regional blocks, intravenous, intramuscular, and oral routes). Findings have generally indicated that timely intervention for the management of pain has resulted in an increase in a sense of control over aversive procedures (e.g., dressing changes), a reduction in rates of postoperative morbidity, and in significant reductions in health utilization (e.g., frequency of days hospitalized; Saxe et al., 2001).

Regarding specific pharmacotherapies, opioids and short-acting benzodiazepines (e.g., muscle relaxants such as Valium) have received widespread support in the empirical literature regarding their efficacy and safety when used appropriately and with careful rigorous monitoring (Stoddard, Martyn, & Sheridan, 1997). More recently, some emerging literature suggests that adjunctive pharmacotherapies such as the use of stimulants (e.g., methylphenidate), tricyclic antidepressants, and anticonvulsants may provide additional pain analgesia and perhaps diminish the need for higher doses of analgesia (for review, see Stoddard & Saxe, 2001). More important, as with any pharmacotherapy, careful and ongoing assessment of adverse effects, including medication side effects, toxicity, and complications, is critical and cannot be overemphasized. Most important, the pediatric psychologist must work collaboratively in an interdisciplinary context to comprehensively assess pain and provide for appropriate psychological intervention in addition to pharmacotherapy.

REHABILITATION-PHASE CONSIDERATIONS

During the rehabilitation phase, children are required to engage in specific self-care practices, including physical therapy and the wearing of pressure garments. Repeated hospitalization may be required for staged reconstructive surgeries. It is at this point that a child and family may first confront the reality of recovery that is incomplete and begin to face issues related to permanent scarring and to compromise or loss of adaptive function. Family stress and difficulties with school reentry are common.

Psychological Adjustment

On discharge, many children experience significant difficulty adjusting to the return to home and school environments. Problems cited in the clinical literature include difficulties with self-esteem, body image, and peer relations, altered school and career trajectories, coping with negative societal reactions to disfigurement, and increased family stressors (Tarnowski, 1994). Posttraumatic stress disorder, as well as associated comorbid difficulties including mood, internalizing, and externalizing symptoms and syndromes, are commonly encountered (Stoddard & Saxe, 2001). Given the devastating nature of burn injuries, it might be assumed that most children fare poorly in intermediate to long-term prognostications. However, reviews of the outcome literature by Tarnowski and colleagues (Tarnowski & Rasnake, 1994; Tarnowski, Rasnake, et al., 1991) revealed little empirical evidence to suggest that the *majority* of burn victims exhibit poor postburn adjustment. This conclusion is reinforced by the results of recent reviews, which indicate that, although the recovery period is protracted for children, most youth are able to successfully accomplish such recovery (Blakeney & Meyer, 1996; Sheridan et al., 2000). Adjustment appears to be a complex function of several intertwined variables, including patient injury parameters, behavioral risk factors, and child and family resource variables. As in other conditions, risk and resource variables may differentially combine to predict outcome (Tarnowski, King, Pease, & Green, 1991). A risk–resource outcome model for pediatric burns is described in Tarnowski and Simonian (in press).

CONCLUSIONS

Burns can induce a wide array of devastating injuries that are often associated with lifelong physical disfigurement and disability. Recent medical and surgical advances have dramatically improved the survival rate for patients with such injuries. There continues to be a relative dearth of information concerning the acute and chronic psychological effects of pediatric burn injuries. Recent data suggest that the psychosocial outcomes for pediatric burn victims are more positive than that expected based on earlier anecdotal reports. Research has just begun to address the synergistic interaction of an array of risk and resource variables in mediating outcomes from such injuries. Estimates indicate that the majority of pediatric burn injuries are entirely preventable, and prevention remains a central priority for future work in this area.

REFERENCES

American Burn Association. (1984). Guidelines for service standards and severity classifications in the treatment of burn injuries. *Bulletin of the American College of Surgeons*, *69*, 24–28.

American Pain Society Quality of Care Committee. (1995). Quality improvement guidelines for the treatment of acute pain and cancer pain. *Journal of the American Medical Association, 274*, 1874–1880.

American Psychiatric Association. (2000). *Diagnostic and statistical manual of mental disorders* (4th ed., text rev.). Washington, DC: Author.

Barakat, L. P., & Kazak, A. E. (1999). Family issues. In R. T. Brown (Ed.), *Cognitive aspects of chronic illness* (pp. 333–354). New York: Guilford Press.

Barrow, R. E., & Herndon, D. N. (1990). Incidence of mortality in boys and girls after severe thermal burns. *Surgery, Gynecology, and Obstetrics*, *170*, 295–298.

Blakeney, P. E., & Meyer, W. J. (1996). Psychosocial recovery of burned patients and reintegration into society. In D. N. Herndon (Ed.), *Total burn care* (pp. 176–192). London: Saunders.

Brigham, P. A., & McLoughlin, E. (1996). Burn incidence and medical care in the United States: Estimates, trends, and data sources. *Journal of Burn Care and Rehabilitation*, *17*, 95–103.

Brown, R. T., Dingle, A. D., & Koon-Scott, K. (1994). Inpatient consultation and liaison. In K. Tarnowski (Ed.), *Behavioral aspects of pediatric burns* (pp. 119–146). New York: Plenum Press.

Brown, R. T., & Macias, M. (2000). Chronically ill children and adolescents. In J. N. Hughes, A. M. La Greca, & J. C. Conoley (Eds.), *Handbook of psychological services for children and adolescents* (pp. 353–372). New York: Oxford University Press.

Dyer, C., & Roberts, D. (1990). Thermal trauma. *Nursing Clinics of North America*, *25*, 85–117.

Fratianne, R. B., & Brandt, C. P. (1994). Medical management. In K. Tarnowski (Ed.), *Behavioral aspects of pediatric burns* (pp. 25–53). New York: Plenum Press.

Garner, D. M., & Desai, J. J. (2001). Eating disorders in children and adolescents. In J. N. Hughes, A. M. La Greca, & J. C. Conoley (Eds.), *Handbook of psychological services for children and adolescents* (pp. 399–419). New York: Oxford University Press.

Guyer, B., & Gallagher, S. S. (1985). An approach to the epidemiology of childhood injuries. *Pediatric Clinics of North America*, *32*, 5–15.

Kaslow, N. J., Koon-Scott, K., & Dingle, A. (1994). Family considerations and interventions. In K. Tarnowski (Ed.), *Behavioral aspects of pediatric burns* (pp. 193–215). New York: Plenum Press.

Lund, C. C., & Browder, J. R. (1944). An estimation of areas of burns. *Surgery, Gynecology, and Obstetrics*, *79*, 224–252.

McLoughlin, E., & Crawford, J. D. (1985). Types of burn injuries. *Pediatric Clinics of North America*, *32*, 61–75.

McLoughlin, E., & McGuire, A. (1990). The causes, cost, and prevention of childhood burn injuries. *American Journal of Diseases of Children*, *144*, 677–683.

Miller, M. D., Elliott, C. H., Funk, M., & Pruitt, S. (1988). Implications of children's burn injuries. In D. K. Routh (Ed.), *Handbook of pediatric psychology* (pp. 426–447). New York: Guilford Press.

Patterson, D. R., Everett, J. J., Bombardier, C. H., Questad, K. A., Lee, V. K., & Marvin, J. A. (1993). Psychological effects of severe burn injuries. *Psychological Bulletin*, *113*, 362–378.

Robinson, E., Rumsey, N., & Partridge, J. (1996). An evaluation of the impact of social interaction skills training for facially disfigured people. *British Journal of Plastic Surgery*, *49*, 281–289.

Sapolsky, R. M. (2000). Glucocorticoids and hippocampal atrophy in neuropsychiatric disorders. *Archives of General Psychiatry*, *57*, 925–935.

Saxe, G., Stoddard, F., Courtney, D., Cunningham, K., Chawla, N., Sheridan, R., et al. (2001). Relationship between acute morphine and the course of PTSD in children with burns. *Journal of the American Academy of Child and Adolescent Psychiatry*, *40*(8), 915–921.

Sheridan, R. L., Hinson, M. I., & Liang M. H. (2000). Long-term outcome of children surviving massive burns. *Journal of the American Medical Association, 283*, 69–73.

Stoddard, F. J. (2002). Care of infants, children and adolescents with burn injuries. In M. Lewis (Ed.), *Child and adolescent psychiatry: A comprehensive textbook* (3rd ed., pp. 1188–1208). Baltimore: Lippincott Williams & Wilkins.

Stoddard, F. J., Martyn, J., & Sheridan, R. (1997). Psychiatric issues in pain of burn injury. *Current Review of Pain, 1*, 130–136.

Stoddard, F. J., & Saxe, G. (2001). Ten-year research review of physical injuries. *Journal of the American Academy of Child and Adolescent Psychiatry, 40*, 1128–1145.

Tarnowski, K. J. (Ed.). (1994). *Behavioral aspects of pediatric burns*. New York: Plenum Press.

Tarnowski, K. J., & Kaufman, K. (1988). Behavioral assessment of pediatric pain. In R. J. Prinz (Ed.), *Advances in behavioral assessment of children and families* (Vol. 4, pp. 119–158). Greenwich, CT: JAI Press.

Tarnowski, K. J., King, D. R., Pease, M. G., & Green, L. (1991). Congenital gastrointestinal anomalies: Psychosocial functioning of children with imperforate anus, gastoschisis, and omphalocele. *Journal of Consulting and Clinical Psychology, 59*, 587–590.

Tarnowski, K. J., & Rasnake, L. K. (1994). Long-term psychosocial sequelae. In K. J. Tarnowski (Ed.), *Behavioral aspects of pediatric burns* (pp. 81–118). New York: Plenum Press.

Tarnowski, K. J., Rasnake, L. K., & Drabman, R. S. (1987). Behavioral assessment and treatment of pediatric burns: A review. *Behavior Therapy, 18*, 417–441.

Tarnowski, K. J., Rasnake, L. K., Gavaghan-Jones, M. P., & Smith, L. (1991). Psychosocial sequelae of pediatric burn injuries: A review. *Clinical Psychology Review, 11*, 371–398.

Tarnowski, K. J., & Simonian, S. J. (2003). Psychological aspects of catastrophic pediatric injury: Considerations in traumatic burn and head injuries. In K. Anchor, J. E. Shmerling, & J. M. Anchor (Eds.), *The handbook of catastrophic injury* (pp. 200–212). Dubuque, IA: Kendall/Hunt.

Thompson, R. J., Jr., & Gustafson, K. (1996). *Chronic illness in children*. Washington, DC: American Psychological Association.

U. S. Fire Administration. (1978). *Fires in the United States*. Washington, DC: U. S. Department of Commerce, National Fire Data Center.

Walco, G. A., Sterling, C. M., Conte, P. M., & Engel, R. G. (1999). Empirically supported treatments in pediatric psychology: Disease-related pain. *Journal of Pediatric Psychology, 24*, 155–167.

27

Pediatric Gastrointestinal Disorders

Recurrent Abdominal Pain, Inflammatory Bowel Disease, and Rumination Disorder/Cyclic Vomiting

GERARD A. BANEZ
CARIN CUNNINGHAM

The field of pediatric gastroenterology is a growing medical subspecialty that presents numerous opportunities for psychologists interested in consulting with pediatricians. The problems and disorders seen in a pediatric gastroenterology practice are clinically challenging and range from the primarily functional in nature, such as recurrent abdominal pain (RAP), to those reflecting organic disease, such as ulcerative colitis or Crohn's disease. In the functional disorders, psychological or psychosocial factors often play a primary role in the development, as well as the course, of the disorder. With organic disease, the psychological impact of the disorder, as well as the child's attempts to manage the disease and its treatment, are of paramount importance. Interactions between physiological and psychological factors often shape the nature and outcome of the child's gastrointestinal symptoms. The challenge facing pediatric psychologists is to sort through the reciprocal influences of biological, psychological, and social variables in an effort to better understand and treat these disorders. The purpose of this chapter is to provide overviews of the existing literature on several common problems or disorders seen in pediatric gastroenterology: RAP, inflammatory bowel disease (IBD), and rumination disorder/cyclic vomiting. Our goal for this chapter is to be practice oriented but empirically informed, with an emphasis on clinically relevant research findings that have emerged since the previous edition of this text.

RECURRENT ABDOMINAL PAIN

Descriptions, Definitions, and Associated Issues

The term "recurrent abdominal pain" (RAP) has been used and defined in various ways over time. Almost every paper or presentation on RAP, however, begins with a reference to

Apley's criteria (Apley, 1975; Apley & Hale, 1973). According to Apley, RAP is characterized by three or more episodes of abdominal pain that occur over at least 3 months and are severe enough to interfere with daily activities. These episodes are characterized by vague abdominal pain that is dull or crampy, is poorly localized or periumbilical, and persists for less than 1 hour (Frazer & Rappaport, 1999). The pain frequently presents with nausea, vomiting, and other signs of autonomic arousal (Apley, 1975).

Though the term RAP is most often used to refer to functional abdominal pain, Apley's original description is broad and does not have specific etiological implications. Most investigators report that only 5–10% of affected children show an organic cause for their pain (Apley, 1975; Apley & Hale, 1973). Advances in medical diagnostics, however, have led to an increase in the identification of organic causes (Hyams, Burke, Davis, Rzepsaki, & Andrulonis, 1996), suggesting that past figures may somewhat underestimate the prevalence of organically caused pain.

Apley's criteria have recently been criticized for being ambiguous and allowing for both nonorganic and organic causes (Von Baeyer & Walker, 1999), and their continued use has been discouraged. Acknowledging this, Von Baeyer and Walker (1999) proposed a two-stage approach to classification of RAP: (1) a decision as to whether a child meets Apley's criteria and (2) identification of RAP subgroups on the basis of medical findings and other symptoms (e.g., RAP with constipation, RAP with peptic ulcer, RAP without identified etiology, and RAP with constipation and depression). Another system for classifying functional (i.e., not organically caused) abdominal pain was proposed by the pediatric gastroenterology multinational Rome Working Team (Rasquin-Weber et al., 1999). They delineated five diagnostic categories, including functional dyspepsia, irritable bowel syndrome (IBS), functional abdominal pain, abdominal migraine, and aerophagia, and presented specific symptom-based criteria for each.

Clearly, an important priority for future investigations is examination of the reliability and validity of the aforementioned and other systems for classifying RAP. At present, the majority of RAP research tends to utilize Apley's criteria and to exclude children with a presumed organic basis for their pain. Unless otherwise specified, the references cited in the remainder of this section describe children who meet these criteria and show no physical or organic basis for their pain.

EPIDEMIOLOGY

Studies of the prevalence of RAP have found disparate results, with rates ranging from 9% to almost 25% (Apley & Naish, 1958; Oster, 1972). Inconsistent use of diagnostic criteria and characteristics of the population being sampled (e.g., age, gender) contribute to the conflicting findings. In general, population-based studies suggest that RAP is experienced by 10–15% of school-age children (Apley, 1975; Apley & Naish, 1958) and almost 20% of middle school and high school students (Hyams et al., 1996). As children grow older, the incidence of RAP appears to decrease in boys but not in girls (Stickler & Murphy, 1979; Apley & Naish, 1958).

Investigations of the prognosis for RAP have also yielded conflicting findings. Differences in the severity of symptoms, nature of treatment, and/or length of follow-up may explain these discrepancies. Though many children (as many as 76%) with RAP no longer exhibited symptoms at follow-up, almost one-half of these children manifested other psychosomatic or physical complaints (Stickler & Murphy, 1979; Apley & Hale, 1973). Long-term follow-up of children hospitalized for RAP (as late as 28–30 years after) has indicated that a smaller number, between 30 and 47%, will experience complete resolution of their symptoms (Apley, 1959; Christensen & Mortensen, 1975).

ETIOLOGY/CONCEPTUAL MODELS

In the four decades since Apley's seminal research, conceptual models of RAP have become more complex (Walker, 1999). Studies conducted before the 1980s were characterized by a dualistic view of abdominal pain. In the 1980s, the focus of research shifted to nonorganic causes of RAP, including a host of psychosocial factors. In the 1990s, the research focus shifted to the identification of individual differences among children with RAP and the interactive effects between contributing factors. At the start of the 21st century, conceptual models of RAP are multivariate and acknowledge the contributions of a variety of biological, psychological, and social factors. For example, the Rome Group proposed a broad biopsychosocial conceptualization for a wide range of functional gastrointestinal disorders, including childhood functional (recurrent) abdominal pain (Drossman, 2000). This model presumes that a child's condition is a function of multiple interacting determinants, including early life factors, physiological factors, psychosocial factors, and interactions between physiological and psychological factors via the central nervous system–enteric nervous system axis. According to this model, a child with abdominal pain but with no psychosocial problems, as well as with good coping skills and social support, will have a better outcome than the child with pain and coexisting emotional difficulties, high life stress, and limited support. The child's clinical outcome (e.g., daily functioning, quality of life) will, in turn, affect the severity of the disorder.

PHYSIOLOGICAL FEATURES

More than 100 organic causes of abdominal pain have been identified in children and adolescents (Levine & Rappaport, 1984). Cases with a specific etiology usually display "red flags" on history or examination that lead to the proper medical diagnosis (Frazer & Rappaport, 1999). As noted, a specific organic cause is identified in only a small number of children with RAP. As such, the majority of research on physical or organic features has centered on nonpathological biological mechanisms, such as various indices of autonomic nervous system (ANS) functioning, altered gastrointestinal motility, and abnormalities in visceral sensation. Of these, the role of visceral hypersensitivity receives the most empirical support. Specifically, existing studies suggest that children with RAP may have abnormal perception of gastrointestinal physiological events and a lower threshold for pain (Duarte, Goulart, & Penna, 2000).

PSYCHOLOGICAL FEATURES

Studies of the psychological features of childhood RAP have examined a broad range of factors, including life stress, psychological state (e.g., anxiety and depression), attention to pain, coping, and parental responses. We provide here a brief summary of this growing literature. For more detailed information, please refer to excellent reviews written by Compas & Boyer (2001), Scharff (1997), and Walker (1999).

Children with RAP do not experience significantly more major life stressors than healthy children (McGrath, Goodman, Firestone, Shipman, & Peters, 1983; Wasserman, Whitington, & Rivara, 1988) or children with organic abdominal pain (Walker, Garber, & Greene, 1993; Walker & Greene, 1991). Research on daily life events, however, suggests that daily stress, including events related to family illness, may have a more important role than major stressors in precipitating episodes of abdominal pain (Walker, Garber, Smith, Van Slyke, & Lewis Claar, 2001).

Children with RAP score significantly higher on measures of anxiety than children in a control group (Hodges, Kline, Barbero, & Woodruff, 1985). The results of comparisons between children with RAP and children with organic abdominal pain, however, have been inconsistent (Walker, Garber, & Greene, 1993; Walker & Greene, 1989). This finding suggests that, although anxiety-related symptoms are associated with RAP, they may be the result rather than the cause of pain in at least some children (Walker & Greene, 1989).

Studies that have examined depressive symptoms have not found consistent differences between children with RAP and children in a control group (Hodges, Kline, Barbero, & Flanery, 1985; McGrath et al., 1983). Depression does not appear to be prevalent in children with RAP, albeit familial depression may play a role in the development of children's abdominal pain (Hodges, Kline, Barbero, & Flanery, 1985). As with anxiety, depressive symptoms in children with RAP may be secondary to underlying chronic pain (Raymer, Weininger, & Hamilton, 1984).

Children with RAP have also been hypothesized to display an attentional bias toward pain stimuli (Compas & Boyer, 2001; Zeltzer, Bursch, & Walco, 1997). This bias may increase their focus on environmental pain cues and sensations of pain, increasing their anxiety and fear, which, in turn, exacerbates the pain. Consistent with this hypothesis, Thomsen, Compas, Colletti, and Stanger (2000) reported that problems in attentional focus were associated with increased physical symptoms in children with RAP.

With respect to coping, existing studies have found that accommodative or secondary control engagement coping (e.g., distraction, acceptance, positive thinking, cognitive restructuring) proves helpful and is related to less pain in children with RAP (Thomsen et al., 2002; Walker, Smith, Garber, & Van Slyke, 1997). Passive or disengagement coping strategies (e.g., denial, cognitive avoidance, behavioral avoidance, wishful thinking), on the other hand, have been associated with increased levels of pain. The results regarding active or primary control coping strategies (e.g., problem solving, emotional expression, emotional modulation, decision making) have been inconsistent.

Finally, parental reactions or responses to their children's pain may also play an important role in the course of RAP. Walker and Zeman (1992) found that parents encourage children to adopt the sick role for gastrointestinal symptoms more than for cold symptoms. Children with RAP, compared with well children, reported that their parents more frequently responded to symptom complaints with increased attention and special privileges (Walker et al., 1993).

Clinical Evaluation

Medical Evaluation

Initial medical evaluation of RAP includes a history and thorough physical examination. Limited laboratory screening may include a complete blood count and erythrocyte sedimentation rate, stool studies, and breath hydrogen testing. The goal of this evaluation is to rule out serious, life-threatening physical causes for abdominal pain (Mahajan & Wyllie, 1999; Frazer & Rappaport, 1999).

Psychological Assessment

The psychological assessment, particularly the pain history, is helpful for establishing the diagnosis of RAP and distinguishing among its particular subtypes. Assessment data that shed light on the behavioral processes that maintain a child's symptoms are important for treatment-planning purposes. The format of the psychological assessment of RAP follows from the biopsychosocial model and is highly consistent with the approach utilized in assessment of other recurrent pains, such as headache or chest pain (see Dahlquist & Switkin, Chapter 13, this volume). Attention is given to all psychological and social factors felt to influence the child's pain and functional status, including descriptions of the child's behaviors when experiencing pain, associated functional limitations, and reinforcing consequences that maintain pain behavior (Masek, Russo, & Varni, 1984). Other factors routinely assessed include the child's mental status, social history, medical history, and previous psychological treatment.

A variety of questionnaires and rating scales are available for psychological assessment of RAP. For example, the Varni-Thompson Pediatric Pain Questionnaire (PPQ; Varni, Thompson, & Hanson, 1987) and the Children's Comprehensive Pain Questionnaire (CCPQ; McGrath, 1990) are examples of comprehensive pain assessment tools that can be utilized. Measures such as the Child Behavior Checklist (CBCL; Achenbach, 1991) and Behavior Assessment System for Children (BASC; Reynolds & Kamphaus, 1998) can be useful for screening and evaluating emotional and behavioral difficulties associated with the child's abdominal pain. In addition, a number of questionnaires have been developed specifically for the purpose of assessing RAP and associated factors (e.g., Schwankovsky & Hyman, 1999; Walker, Caplan-Dover, & Rasquin-Weber, 2000). Finally, a pain diary provides a method of ongoing assessment, including pain severity and duration, medication use, and any antecedent events and consequences.

Treatment Avenues

Medical Management

Standard pediatric care for RAP typically consists of reassurance that there is no serious organic disease and general advice about learning to manage pain. When accepted, this reassurance concludes the search for a physical cause and allows the child and family to move into the stage of learning to cope. Although this knowledge is important and can be sufficient for some children, medication and psychological therapies are often necessary.

In some cases, symptom-based pharmacological therapies are helpful. For example, tricyclic antidepressants such as desipramine and amitriptyline may be used to target the child's visceral pain. Anticholinergic medications such as dicyclomine and hyoscyamine have been used for their antispasmodic properties. In those with constipation, targeted therapies (e.g., laxatives, stool softeners) may be a helpful adjunct.

Psychological Treatment

Much of the existing literature on psychological treatments for RAP was summarized in an excellent article by Janicke and Finney (1999). They reviewed the treatment literature available prior to February 1, 1998, and identified nine studies that examined three distinctive treatment approaches, including operant procedures (Miller & Kratochwill, 1979; Sank & Biglan, 1974), fiber treatments (Christensen, 1986; Edwards, Finney, & Bonner, 1991; Feldman, McGrath, Hodgeson, Ritter, & Shipman, 1985), and cognitive-behavioral procedures (Finney, Lemanek, Cataldo, Katz, & Fuqua, 1989; Linton, 1986; Sanders et al., 1989; Sanders, Shepherd, Cleghorn, & Woolford, 1994). Treatments were categorized as either well established, probably efficacious, or promising (Chambless et al., 1996). Cognitive-behavioral procedures emerged as a probably efficacious treatment. Fiber treatment for RAP with constipation emerged as a promising intervention. Operant procedures did not meet the most lenient category of empirically supported treatments, and no treatment approach met the criteria for a well-established intervention.

One particularly promising psychological treatment is the cognitive-behavioral family intervention by Sanders and his colleagues (Sanders et al., 1989; Sanders et al., 1994), which consists of three components: explanation of RAP and rationale for pain management procedures, contingency management training for parents, and self-management training for children. In their initial study, Sanders et al. (1989) found that the treatment group improved more quickly and was more pain free at 3 months than a wait-list control group. In a second study, Sanders et al. (1994) found that the treatment group was significantly more pain free at follow-up and had a lower rate of relapse than children who received standard pediatric care (reassurance and general advice).

Since the publication of Janicke and Finney's article (1999), at least two other psychological treatment studies have appeared in the literature. Humphreys and Gevirtz (2000) compared four behavioral treatment protocols for RAP. Sixty-four children and adolescents with RAP were randomly assigned into four groups: (1) fiber-only comparison group; (2) fiber and skin temperature biofeedback; (3) fiber, skin temperature biofeedback, and cognitive-behavioral procedures; and (4) fiber, skin temperature biofeedback, cognitive-behavioral procedures, and contingency management training for parents. All groups showed improvement in self-reported pain. The active treatment groups, however, showed significantly more improvement than the fiber-only comparison group. Anbar (2001) published a case series to demonstrate the utility of self-hypnosis for the treatment of childhood functional abdominal pain. In 4 of 5 patients, abdominal pain resolved within 3 weeks of a single session of instruction in self-hypnosis. In the absence of a prospective controlled design and objective measures of pain and associated factors, the generalizability of these findings is limited.

INFLAMMATORY BOWEL DISEASE: ULCERATIVE COLITIS AND CROHN'S DISEASE

Inflammatory bowel disease (IBD), which includes both ulcerative colitis (UC) and Crohn's disease (CD), is a category of conditions characterized by inflammation of the digestive tract. IBD is distinguished by a characteristic set of symptoms (e.g., abdominal pain, fatigue, weight loss, diarrhea, cramping, and joint pain) that interfere with daily living and can have long-term effects, such as delayed sexual maturity and growth retardation. In CD, the inflammation extends through the full thickness of the intestinal wall and may affect any part of the GI tract from the mouth to the skin around the anus. In UC, the inflammation is confined to the large intestine and is restricted to the inner lining of the colon.

Epidemiology

Approximately 2 million Americans have been diagnosed with IBD, 300,000 of whom are in the pediatric age group (Benkov & Winter, 1996). Males and females are equally affected. IBD is diagnosed during childhood or adolescence in 20 to 25% of patients (Griffiths et al., 1999). The incidence of UC for those 10–19 years of age is 2.3 per 100,000. It is rare for UC to be diagnosed before the age of 5. The incidence of CD is 5–10 per 100,000 people per year and has been increasing since 1960, particularly in the pediatric population (Gryboski, 1994). The peak frequency of new cases in the pediatric population occurs in the mid-to-late teens, with an age-specific incidence of approximately 16 per 100,000 (Hyams, 1996). For most children, the disease course of IBD is one of unpredictable exacerbation and remission. A small minority (5% of patients) have one period of symptoms at diagnosis followed by a prolonged remission. A smaller number (< 5%) have recalcitrant disease requiring aggressive medical therapy and numerous surgeries (Hyams, 1996).

Etiology

The etiology of IBD is unknown. Current theories propose a multifactorial theory; the pathogenesis of the illness proceeds from a genetic predisposition (susceptible host) coupled with specific triggers (bacteria, viruses) that interact with the body's immune system and trigger the disease (Czinn, 2001). Although a high percentage of patients with IBD are convinced that stress or their personalities are the principal cause of their disorder (Levenstein, 1996), existing data do not support a psychological etiology. Psychological factors may, however, affect the course of the illness, albeit the exact mechanism between stress, the immune system, and IBD flare-ups has not been identified. Psychological problems can also result from having IBD and dealing with the complicated aspects of the illness. Depression is now recognized as a possible reaction to the stress and disruptions of living with IBD (Drossman, Patrick, & Mitchell, 1989), and an increased prevalence of depression has been documented in children who have IBD (Rabbett et al., 1996; Engström, 1999). Similarly, Burke, Meyer, Kochoshis, Orenstein, and Sauer (1989) reported that obsessive–compulsive symptoms in pediatric patients with IBD were likely secondary to the demands of living with the illness.

Psychological Factors/Features

As with any chronic illness, a child's developmental level plays a significant role in their understanding of and coping with IBD. School-age children tend to focus on immediate issues, such as pain associated with injections, blood tests, and invasive procedures. They worry about nausea and public restroom use and are upset by dietary and activity restrictions. IBD clearly affects important adolescent issues, such as the need to be in control, peer pressure to conform, and body image. Existing research on the psychological aspects of pediatric IBD focuses on the emotional sequelae of the illness, as well as its impact on important domains of daily functioning. This literature is summarized here.

Emotional Symptoms

As noted, pediatric IBD is often associated with depression, anxiety, and lower self-esteem. In comparison with healthy controls and children with diabetes, patients with IBD had more depressive and anxiety disorders, were more pessimistic about the future, and had more difficulty discussing their illness (Engström, 1992). Moody, Eaden, and Mayberry (1999) reported that children with CD expressed fears and anxieties about their future and fears about participating in common childhood activities. Akobeng et al. (1999) found that children who were taking steroids exhibited more depressive symptoms than those who were not.

Academic and Social Functioning

In comparison with healthy children, Akobeng et al. (1999) found that children with Crohn's disease missed more school and participated less in sports and peer-related activities. Ferguson, Sedgwick, and Drummond (1994) reported significant social morbidity in young adults with juvenile onset IBD, reflected by (1) absences from school, (2) interference with examinations, and (3) difficulties in pursuit of higher education. Moody et al. (1999) found that 66% of patients ages 6–17 years with IBD had significant absences from school and that 80% felt that they had underachieved due to their ill health. Patient responses also indicated that (1) 67% reported a decrease in sports-related activities and (2) 50% reported being unable to play with friends because of their illness. Socially, MacPhee, Hoffenberg, and Feranchak (1988) reported that adolescents with IBD were more likely to rely on their families than their peers for emotional support, suggesting a possible developmental lag.

Family Functioning

Pediatric IBD has also been found to affect parents and siblings of the child. Researchers report that many parents worry about future issues and about their children having problems at school. Parents reported that their lives had changed due to a decrease in social activities and changes in financial resources (Engström, 1992; Cunningham, 1985).

Sibling research has found that healthy siblings of IBD patients were concerned that their parents were keeping them uninformed about the illness (Akobeng et al., 1999). Engström (1992) found no increase in psychopathology of siblings with IBD but did find a decrease in their self-esteem and their self-reliance. Healthy siblings also reported jealousy because of the special treatment and attention their sibling received.

Health-Related Quality of Life

Although the importance of the health-related quality of life (HRQL) of children and adolescents with IBD has been recognized, the research to date has been limited due to lack of control groups, small sample sizes, use of focus groups, and use of nonvalidated questionnaires. To address these methodological issues, we recently conducted a study using a controlled group matched for age, sex and race, validated HRQL measures, and a disease-specific measure. The results indicated that (1) in comparison with healthy controls, children and adolescents with IBD demonstrate a lower HRQL; (2) children with IBD who reported significant physical side effects from steroids reported a decrease in their perception of their general health status; and (3) children with IBD and their parents reported differences in HRQL, with parents reporting a greater decrease in HRQL (Cunningham, 2001b).

Clinical Evaluation

Medical Evaluation

Physical diagnosis of IBD includes information from (1) stool examinations, (2) blood and urine tests, (3) radiological procedures (barium enemas, upper and lower GI studies, CT scans and abdominal ultrasounds), and (4) endoscopic procedures (e.g., sigmoidoscopy, colonoscopy, and upper GI endoscopy). Weight and height gains, sexual maturation, and extraintestinal symptoms are also assessed. Because many patients with IBD are initially misdiagnosed with IBS and believe that their symptoms are due to psychological factors, distinguishing between IBD and IBS is important.

Psychosocial Assessment

Psychosocial assessment should evaluate both the patient's and the family's functioning. Age-related assessments are necessary because of the developmental changes the child goes through over time. The following questions can be used as a framework for psychological assessment:

Patient Functioning

- *Cognitive perceptions of IBD.* What is the child's or adolescent's medical understanding of IBD? Of the cause of IBD? Do they understand the proposed treatment regimen, including possible side effects of the medications? What are their biggest fears about having IBD? Do they think that IBD is life threatening?
- *Social functioning.* Are friends aware of the patient's IBD? Is the patient involved in any school-related or extracurricular activities? How does the illness interfere with socializing with his or her peers? What activities does he or she *not* participate in because of IBD?
- *School.* Has the child missed school days or had to repeat a grade because of IBD? Can he or she participate in a full academic schedule? Is there academic pressure because of missed school days? Is the school cooperative with special needs (e.g., bathroom privileges, the need for medicine)?
- *Family relationships.* Is the family supportive? Who is responsible for making sure medication is taken? Do parents constantly remind the child about diet and medication issues? Have parents become overprotective? What are the reactions of siblings and grandparents?
- *Family Functioning.* What is the family's knowledge of IBD, including their attributions of the etiology? What are the strengths and difficulties in the family system? Who manages patient care? Are there additional stresses in the family system?

Treatment Avenues

Medical Management

Medical management of IBD in children and adolescents is not standardized and can include medical, nutritional, and surgical interventions. The goal of medical therapy is to control symptoms, induce remission, prevent complications, and improve growth; it is not curative. Medical therapy includes the use of the following medications: corticosteroids, 5-amino salicylic acid preparations, 6-mercaptopurine, Metronidazole, and cyclosporine. Steroids are indicated in cases of acute disease that is unresponsive to other medications. The side effects of the steroids are significant and can include growth suppression, cataracts, glaucoma, osteoporosis, hypertension, and vascular necrosis. For adolescents, the cosmetic side effects (e.g., acne, cushingoid features, weight gain, hirsutism, and striae) are particularly difficult. Recent use of infliximab has shown encouraging results in the pediatric population (Kugathasan et al., 1999).

The goals of nutritional therapy are to correct nutritional deficiencies due to reduced appetite, poor absorption, and diarrhea and to promote catch-up growth. Nutritional therapy can include (1) dietary modification, (2) nutritional supplementation, and (3) total parenteral nutrition (TPN) therapy. Nutritional therapy can be either the or the primary or the supplemental therapy. There are no scientific data to support the efficacy of alternative diets or supplements.

Surgical treatment is necessary when (1) medication cannot control the symptoms, (2) there is an intestinal obstruction, or (3) there are other complications. Surgery on patients with UC removes the colon and rectum with the creation of an ileostomy, or external stoma, which is curative. New techniques have been developed to avoid an ileostomy by creating an internal pouch from the small bowel and attaching it to the anal sphincter muscle. In CD, the inflamed part of the intestine is removed (resection), and the two ends of the healthy bowel are joined together (anastomoses). This surgery may provide symptom-free years; however, it is not curative because the disease can recur in other parts of the intestinal tract.

Psychological Treatment

At Diagnosis. Psychological intervention at the time of diagnosis focuses on acknowledging the patient's relief that a physical problem has been identified, providing information, and supporting the patient. Although IBD patients must deal with the reality that they have a chronic illness, the diagnosis of IBD can be a relief for some patients whose symptoms had previously been misattributed to psychological diagnoses such as depression or anorexia nervosa. Providing information is important at diagnosis because many families have not heard of IBD prior to their child's diagnosis. In our practice, an IBD library was created to present information in innovative ways to patients and families. The library consists of patient-created books, videotapes of interviews with patients with IBD, and a listing of relevant Web sites. Feedback from patients, families, and medical staff indicates that it has been helpful (Cunningham, 2001a).

Patients with IBD may feel discouraged that their lives have been abruptly and seriously disrupted and replaced by periods of intense pain, doctor's visits, blood tests, school pressures, and isolation from friends. Support is needed for patients dealing with the extraordinary demands of the medical care that IBD can require, including nasogastric tubes and restricted food intake.

At Reoccurrence. A reoccurrence highlights one of the most stressful aspects of IBD: the unpredictable course of illness. Symptoms may reappear with no apparent precipitant, often following long periods of relative health. Reoccurrence is devastating psychologically and may stimulate depression, frustration, and fear. For some patients, a reoccurrence marks the point at which they must accept the chronic nature of their illness and the reality of resuming unpleasant medical interventions (e.g., steroids). Psychological interventions should focus on helping patients identify and express their fears and their feelings of powerlessness over their flare-up.

It is important to elicit the child's or the adolescent's cognitive understanding of the reoccurrence (Perrin & Gerrity, 1984). Some patients worry that a reoccurrence means the inevitability of stomach cancer or the need for a colostomy. Patients may not share their fears with their parents or with their gastroenterologists, and they silently live with misinformation and anxiety.

Noncompliance. Problems associated with the cosmetic side effects of the steroids (e.g., acne, cushingoid features) may be as difficult as, if not worse than, the actual illness. Therefore, patients, especially adolescents, often minimize their symptoms until the pain becomes overwhelming and cannot be ignored. In our practice, adherence to the medical treatment seems to follow a predictable pattern. Immediately after diagnosis, adherence is generally good. Many patients become increasingly noncompliant when physical symptoms decrease. To avoid side effects, many adolescents stop taking their medicine, lower the dosage, or use medication only reactively (e.g., when bleeding occurs), often without informing medical staff.

Noncompliance is a complicated issue, and psychological intervention involves the caregiver, as well as the patient. Specific areas of noncompliance need to be identified, as patients with IBD can be compliant with dietary restrictions or moderating activity level and noncompliant in another area, such as taking medication. Many parents struggle with finding the balance between vigilance and intrusiveness (Cunningham, 1985).

School-Related Problems. School can pose many problems for patients with IBD. Patients with IBD need to use the bathroom more often than other children and are often embarrassed to ask the teacher or obtain special permission. Children and adolescents are often teased at school about their appearance and may be singled out because they cannot participate in gym or other activities. Absenteeism has been identified as a problem for patients with IBD (Akobeng et al., 1999). School avoidance can become a problem due to abdominal pain, fatigue, increased frequency of bathroom use, and peer teasing. Therefore, the child or adolescent with IBD needs to be encouraged to attend school, even part time. Moody et al. (1999) found that many teachers knew little about Crohn's disease. Parents are encouraged to establish a 504 Plan, an educational plan for children with specific medical conditions, that identifies IBD as a medical problem. This plan can formalize helpful strategies, such as bathroom usage, and provides a unique opportunity to educate school personnel about IBD.

Guidelines for Psychological Intervention with Pediatric and Adolescent IBD Patients

1. Be knowledgeable about the medical aspects of IBD: presenting symptoms, diagnostic procedures, treatment modalities, and medication side effects.
2. Introduce the pediatric psychologist at the time of diagnosis or as early in the disease course as possible, as a primary prevention approach that includes education, anticipatory guidance, and multidisciplinary involvement is most effective.
3. Elicit the patient's and the family's understanding of IBD in order to clarify misconceptions about prognosis and misattributions regarding etiology.
4. Normalize reactions to IBD and its treatment regimen. For example, reassuring the child that fears about bathroom issues or medication side effects are common may help to decrease anxiety.

5. Teach patients and families skills to cope with the illness. For patients, these skills include relaxation techniques or cognitive strategies to cope with their negative cognitions about appearance. For parents, general parenting techniques, suggestions regarding medication compliance, and emotional support are helpful.

RUMINATION DISORDER/CYCLIC VOMITING

Rumination Disorder

Rumination is characterized by voluntary regurgitation of stomach contents into the mouth, which are either expectorated or rechewed and reswallowed. The regurgitation is not due to an associated gastrointestinal condition or other medical condition. It is a rare disorder but one that may lead to serious complications (e.g., malnutrition, weight loss, failure to make expected weight gains) if not appropriately diagnosed and treated.

Although there are no recent prevalence reports, existing studies suggest that rumination is not a common disorder (Singh, 1981; Whitehead & Schuster, 1985). The typical age of onset is between ages 3 and 12 months, except in individuals with mental retardation, in whom the disorder may occur later. The disorder frequently remits spontaneously, but, in severe cases, the course may be continuous. Rumination also occurs in developmentally normal and physically healthy older children and adults, but it is much less common in these groups.

Thumshirn et al. (1998) reported that rumination is characterized physiologically by higher gastric sensitivity and decreased threshold for lower esophageal sphincter relaxation during gastric distention. Kahn, Hyman, Cocjin, and DiLorenzo (2000) performed antroduodenal manometry on a series of older children with rumination and identified a characteristic postprandial pattern of brief, simultaneous pressure increases at all recording sites.

The purpose of rumination is commonly believed to be self-stimulation. Theories of the etiology of rumination have focused on problems in the parent–child relationship and/or pleasure associated with the ruminative act and the attention that the rumination elicits from others (Linscheid & Cunningham, 1977). In terms of the parent–child relationship, lack of stimulation, neglect, and stressful life situations are among the factors associated with rumination (American Psychiatric Association, 1994). Though traditional psychodynamic explanations focused on disturbed or faulty mothering (Linscheid, 1983; Lourie, 1955), the development of rumination may result from reciprocal interactions between the parent and child. For example, the caregiver may become discouraged and alienated because of unsuccessful feeding experiences or the aversive odor of regurgitated food. As a result, the appropriate nurturing and comfort are not provided. Behavioral theories center on the function that the rumination serves in eliciting attention from caregivers (Linscheid, 1983; Linscheid & Cunningham, 1977). Over time, the ruminative act may be maintained by its pleasant, self-stimulatory nature and become habitual.

The diagnosis of rumination is made only after all physical or organic causes for regurgitation have been ruled out. Observation of the ruminative act is essential. It is important to be aware, however, that rumination may cease the moment the infant or child notices the observer (Rasquin-Weber et al., 1999). Observation of aversive interactions between the infant and caregiver supports the diagnosis. Treatment efforts are typically directed toward enhancing the parent–child relationship. Improving the caregiver's ability to recognize and respond appropriately to the child's needs is often an important component of therapy. Behavioral treatments have typically utilized aversive techniques (e.g., electric shock contingent on rumination, lemon juice squirted into the child's mouth following the ruminative act) with good success (e.g., Lang & Melamed, 1969; Sajwaj, Libet, & Agras, 1974). Short-term follow-up of infants treated with aversive methods does not suggest adverse side effects (Linscheid, 1983). More recent reports suggest that techniques such as relaxation and biofeedback may be helpful to older ruminators (Kahn et al., 2000).

Cyclic Vomiting

Cyclic vomiting syndrome (CVS) is characterized by bouts or cycles of severe nausea and vomiting that last hours to days, separated by symptom-free intervals. Numerous stressors and events, physical and emotional, may trigger vomiting episodes, but there is no evidence of medical disease or psychiatric disorder. As many as 70 episodes are experienced per year, with an average of 9–12. Episodes usually last from 1–4 days but can last as long as 10 days.

Population-based studies suggest that the prevalence of CVS is approximately 2%, with equal numbers of males and females affected. CVS occurs from infancy through adulthood, but typical age of onset is between 2 and 7 years. Prakash, Staiano, Rothbaum, & Clouse (2001) reported that many of the characteristics of CVS are similar irrespective of age at onset. Duration of episodes, however, was reported to increase with age, up to age 20 years. In a study of the medium term prognosis of CVS, Dignan, Symon, Abu-Arafeh, & Russell (2001) found that 50% of affected individuals had continuing CVS and/or migraine headaches, whereas the remainder were currently asymptomatic.

The cause of CVS is not clear. Among the physiological factors under investigation are autonomic nervous system dysfunction (e.g., GI dysmotility, altered corticotropin-releasing factor and vasopressin release at the hypothalamic pituitary level) and disorders of fatty acid oxidation and mitochondrial metabolism (Li et al., 1999). Similarities between CVS and migraine headaches support the notion that CVS may be a variant of migraine.

The older psychological literature characterized individuals with CVS as manifesting a tendency toward anxiety and excitability and blamed the disorder on disturbed relationships with parents (Forbes, 1999). More recent research (Forbes, Withers, Silburn, & McKelvey, 1999) found that children with CVS had more clinically significant scores on the Child Behavior Checklist (CBCL) than healthy children. CVS can be incapacitating and result in considerable functional impairment, including poor school attendance.

Diagnosis of CVS is difficult and is made by review of history, physical examination, and studies to rule out other possible causes for vomiting. The numerous medical explanations for vomiting, as well as the complications associated with severe vomiting, underscore the importance of an accurate diagnosis (Rasquin-Weber et al., 1999). Medical management of CVS is individually tailored and guided by the phase of illness. During the prodrome, abortive medications (e.g., ibuprofen or another analgesic, ranitidine) can be tried. Once the episode begins, treatment is generally supportive. During the symptom-free interval, medications used for migraine prophylaxis, such as propranolol and cyproheptadine, may be helpful. The symptom-free interval is also appropriate for identification and treatment of factors that may predispose to or trigger attacks (e.g., family therapy to reduce emotional stress).

CONCLUSIONS

Gastrointestinal problems and disorders are frequently encountered in children's health care. These problems can be viewed as existing on a continuum, from those having a primarily psychosocial component to those having a primarily organic component (Friedrich & Jaworski, 1995). The appeal of this model is that no condition is viewed as totally psychosocial or totally organic. Interactions between biological and psychosocial variables result in varied clinical presentations that demand comprehensive evaluations and individualized treatment plans. Although a considerable amount of research has already been conducted, more needs to be accomplished to advance our understanding of these problems. Among the important areas for future research are the following: (1) examination and refinement of systems for categorizing RAP; (2) implementation and evaluation of empirically supported treatments for RAP in real-world settings; (3) examination of the psychological side effects of steroid use in children and adolescents with IBD; and (4) differences in psychological reactions of pediatric patients with CD as opposed to UC.

REFERENCES

Achenbach, T. M. (1991). *Manual of the Child Behavior Checklist/4–18 and 1991 Profile* (CBCL). Burlington, VT: University of Vermont.

Akobeng, A. K., Suresh-Babu, M. V., Firth, D., Miller, V., Mir, P., & Thomas, A. G. (1999). Quality-of-life in children with Crohn's disease: A pilot study. *Journal of Pediatric Gastroenterology and Nutrition, 4*, S37–39.

American Psychiatric Association. (1994). *Diagnostic and statistical manual of mental disorders* (4th ed.). Washington, DC: American Psychiatric Association.

Anbar, R. D. (2001). Self-hypnosis for the treatment of functional abdominal pain in childhood. *Clinical Pediatrics, 40*, 447–451.

Apley, J. (1959). *The child with abdominal pain*. London: Blackwell.

Apley, J. (1975). *The child with abdominal pains* (2nd ed.). London: Blackwell.

Apley, J., & Hale, B. (1973). Children with recurrent abdominal pain: How do they grow up? *British Medical Journal, 7*, 7–9.

Apley, J., & Naish, N. (1958). Recurrent abdominal pain: A field survey of 1,000 school children. *Archives of Diseases of Childhood, 33*, 165–170.

Benkov, K., & Winter, H. (1996). *Managing your child's Crohn's disease or ulcerative colitis*. New York: Crohn's and Colitis Foundation of America.

Burke, P., Meyer, V., Kochoshis, S., Orenstein, D., & Sauer, J. (1989). Obsessive-compulsive symptoms in childhood inflammatory bowel disease and cystic fibrosis. *Journal of the American Academy of Child and Adolescent Psychiatry, 4*, 525–527.

Chambless, D., Sanderson, W. C., Shoham, V., Johnson, S. B., Pope, K. S., Crits-Cristoph, P., et al. (1996). An update on empirically validated therapies. *Clinical Psychologist, 49*, 5–18.

Christensen, M. F. (1986). Recurrent abdominal pain and dietary fiber. *American Journal of Diseases in Children, 140*, 738–739.

Christensen, M. F., & Mortensen, O. (1975). Long-term prognosis in children with recurrent abdominal pain. *Archives of Diseases of Childhood, 50*, 110–115.

Compas, B. E., & Boyer, M. C. (2001). Coping and attention: Implications for child health and pediatric conditions. *Journal of Developmental and Behavioral Pediatrics*, 22, 323–333.

Cunningham, C. (1985). *A parent's group for pediatric patients with IBD*. Unpublished manuscript.

Cunningham, C. (2001a). A unique educational intervention for pediatric and adolescent patients with IBD. *Progress Notes, 25*, 4–5.

Cunningham, C. (2001b). *The health-related quality of life of pediatric and adolescent patients with IBD*. Manuscript submitted for publication.

Czinn, S. (2001). *Research in pediatric inflammatory bowel disease*. Paper presented at the Breaking the Silence Conference, Cleveland, OH.

Dignan, F., Symon, D. N., Abu-Arafeh, I., & Russell, G. (2001). The prognosis of cyclic vomiting syndrome. *Archives of Disease in Childhood, 84*, 55–57.

Drossman, D. A. (2000). The functional gastrointestinal disorders and the Rome II process. In D. A. Drossman, E. Corazziari, N. J. Talley, W. G. Thompson, & W. E. Whitehead (Eds.), *Rome II: The functional gastrointestinal disorders* (pp. 1–29). Lawrence, KS: Allen Press.

Drossman, D. A., Patrick, D. L., & Mitchell, C. M. (1989). Health-related quality of inflammatory bowel disease: Functional status and patient worries and concerns. *Digestive Diseases and Sciences, 34*, 1379–1386.

Duarte, M. A., Goulart, E. M., & Penna, F. J. (2000). Pressure pain threshold in children with recurrent abdominal pain. *Journal of Pediatric Gastroenterology and Nutrition, 31*, 280–285.

Edwards, M. C., Finney, J. W., & Bonner, M. (1991). Matching treatment with recurrent abdominal pain symptoms: An evaluation of dietary fiber and relaxation treatments. *Behavior Therapy, 20,* 283–291.

Engström, I. (1992). Mental health and psychological functioning in children and adolescents with inflammatory bowel disease: A comparison with children having other chronic illnesses and with healthy children. *Journal of Child Psychology and Psychiatry, 33,* 563–582.

Engström, I. (1999). Inflammatory bowel disease in children and adolescents: Mental health and family functioning. *Journal of Pediatric Gastroenterology and Nutrition, 28*(4), 528–533.

Feldman, W., McGrath, P., Hodgeson, C., Ritter, H., & Shipman, R. T. (1985). The use of dietary fiber in the management of simple, childhood, idiopathic, recurrent abdominal pain. *Archives of Diseases of Childhood, 139,* 1216–1218.

Ferguson, A., Sedgwick, D. M., & Drummond, J. (1994). Morbidity of juvenile onset inflammatory bowel disease: Effects on education and employment in early adult life. *Gut, 35,* 665–668.

Finney, J. W., Lemanek, K. L., Cataldo, M. F., Katz, H. P., & Fuqua, R. W. (1989). Pediatric psychology in primary health care: Brief targeted therapy for recurrent abdominal pain. *Behavior Therapy, 20,* 283–291.

Forbes, D. (1999). Cyclic vomiting syndrome. In P. E. Hyman (Ed.), *Pediatric functional gastrointestinal disorders* (pp. 5.1–5.12). New York: Academy Professional Information Services.

Forbes, D., Withers, G., Silburn, S., & McKelvey, R. (1999). Psychological and social characteristics and precipitants of vomiting in children with cyclic vomiting syndrome. *Digestive Diseases and Sciences, 44*(Suppl., August 1999), 19S–22S.

Frazer, C. H., & Rappaport, L. A. (1999). Recurrent pains. In M. D. Levine, W. B. Carey, & A. C. Crocker (Eds.), *Developmental-behavioral pediatrics* (pp. 357–364). Philadelphia, PA: Saunders.

Friedrich, W. N., & Jaworski, T. (1995). Pediatric abdominal disorders: Inflammatory bowel disease, rumination/vomiting, and recurrent abdominal pain. In M. C. Roberts (Ed.), *Handbook of pediatric psychology* (2nd ed., pp. 479–497). New York: Guilford Press.

Griffiths, A. M., Nicholas, D., Smith, C., Munk, M., Stephens, D., Durno, C., & Sherman, P. M. (1999). Development of a quality-of-life index for pediatric inflammatory bowel disease: Dealing with differences related to age and IBD type. *Journal of Pediatric Gastroenterology and Nutrition, 4,* S46–S52.

Gryboski, J. D. (1994). Crohn's disease in children 10 years old and younger: Comparison with ulcerative colitis. *Journal of Pediatric Gastroenterology and Nutrition, 18*, 174–182.

Hodges, K., Kline, J. J., Barbero, G., & Flanery, R. (1985). Depressive symptoms in children with recurrent abdominal pain and in their families. *Journal of Pediatrics, 107,* 622–626.

Hodges, K., Kline, J. J., Barbero, G., & Woodruff, C. (1985). Anxiety in children with recurrent abdominal pain and in their parents. *Psychosomatics, 26,* 859–866.

Humphreys, P. A., & Gervitz, R. N. (2000). Treatment of recurrent abdominal pain: Components analysis of four treatment protocols. *Journal of Pediatric Gastroenterology and Nutrition, 31*, 47–51.

Hyams, J. S. (1996). Crohn's disease in children. *Pediatric Clinics of North America, 43,* 255–277.

Hyams, J. S., Burke, G., Davis, P. M., Rzepsaki, B., & Andrulonis, P. A. (1996). Abdominal pain and irritable bowel syndrome in adolescents: A community-based study. *Journal of Pediatrics, 129,* 220–226.

Janicke, D. M., & Finney, J. W. (1999). Empirically supported treatments in pediatric psychology: Recurrent abdominal pain. *Journal of Pediatric Psychology, 24,* 115–127.

Kahn, S., Hyman, P. E., Cocjin, J., & DiLorenzo, C. (2000). Rumination syndrome in adolescents. *Journal of Pediatrics, 136,* 528–531.

Kugathasan, S., Levy, M. B., Saeian, K., Vasilopoulos, S., Kim, J. P., Prajapati, D., et al. (2002). Infliximab retreatment in adults and children with Crohn's disease: Risk factors for the development of delayed severe systemic reaction. *American Journal of Gastroenterology, 97,* 1408–1414.

Lang, P. J., & Melamed, B. G. (1969). Avoidance conditioning therapy of an infant with chronic ruminative vomiting. *Journal of Abnormal Psychology, 74,* 139–142.

Levenstein, S. (1996). Psychosocial issues in Crohn's disease. In C. Prantera & B. Korelitz (Eds.), *Crohn's disease* (pp. 429–443). New York: Marcel Dekker.

Levine, M. D., & Rappaport, L. A. (1984). Recurrent abdominal pain in school children: The loneliness of the long-distance physician. *Pediatric Clinics of North America, 31*, 969–991.

Li, B. U. K., Issenman, R. M., Sarna, S. K., & the Faculty of the Second International Scientific Symposium on Cyclic Vomiting Syndrome. (1999). Consensus statement: 2nd International Scientific Symposium on CVS. *Digestive Diseases and Sciences, 44*(Suppl., August 1999), 9S–11S.

Linscheid, T. R. (1983). Eating problems in children. In C. E. Walker & M. C. Roberts (Eds.), *Handbook of clinical child psychology* (pp. 616–639). New York: Wiley.

Linscheid, T. R., & Cunningham, C. E. (1977). A controlled demonstration of the effectiveness of electric shock in the elimination of chronic infant rumination. *Journal of Applied Behavior Analysis, 10,* 500.

Linton, S. J. (1986). A case study of the behavioural treatment of chronic stomach pain in a child. *Behaviour Change, 3,* 70–73.

Lourie, R. S. (1955). Treatment of psychosomatic problems in infants. *Clinical Procedures in Children's Hospitals, 2,* 142–151.

MacPhee, M., Hoffenberg, E. J., & Feranchak, A. (1988). Quality-of-life factors in adolescents' inflammatory bowel disease. *Inflammatory Bowel Disorder, 1,* 6–11.

Mahajan, L., & Wyllie, R. (1999). Chronic abdominal pain of childhood and adolescence. In R. Wyllie & J. S. Hyams (Eds.), *Pediatric gastrointestinal disease: Pathophysiology, diagnosis, and management* (pp. 3–13). Philadelphia, PA: Saunders.

Masek, B. J., Russo, D. C., & Varni, J. W. (1984). Behavioral approaches to the management of chronic pain in children. *Pediatric Clinics of North America, 31,* 1113–1131.

McGrath, P. A. (1990). *Pain in children: Nature, assessment, and treatment.* New York: Guilford Press.

McGrath, P. J., Goodman, J. T., Firestone, P., Shipman, R., & Peters, S. (1983). Recurrent abdominal pain: A psychogenic disorder? *Archives of Diseases in Childhood, 58,* 888–890.

Miller, A. J., & Kratochwill, T. R. (1979). Reduction of frequent stomach complaints by time out. *Behavior Therapy, 10,* 211–218.

Moody, G., Eaden, J., & Mayberry, J. (1999). Social implications of childhood Crohn's disease. *Journal of Pediatric Gastroenterology and Nutrition, 28,* S43–S45.

Oster, J. (1972). Recurrent abdominal pain, headache and limb pains in children and adolescents. *Pediatrics, 50,* 429–436.

Perrin, E. C., & Gerrity, P. S. (1984). Development of children with a chronic illness. *Pediatric Clinics of North America, 31,* 19–31.

Prakash, C., Staiano, A., Rothbaum, R. J., & Clouse, R. E. (2001). Similarities in cyclic vomiting syndrome across age groups. *American Journal of Gastroenterology, 96,* 684–688.

Rabbett, H., Elbadri, A., Thwaites, R., Northover, H., Dady, I., Firth, D., et al. (1996). Quality of life in children with Crohn's disease. *Journal of Pediatric Gastroenterology and Nutrition, 5,* 528–533.

Rasquin-Weber, A., Hyman, P. E., Cucchiara, S., Fleisher, D. R., Hyams, J. S., Milla, P. J., & Staiano, A. (1999). Childhood functional gastrointestinal disorders. *Gut, 45*(Suppl. 2), 1160–1168.

Raymer, D., Weininger, O., & Hamilton, J. R. (1984). Psychological problems in children with abdominal pain. *The Lancet, 1,* 439–440.

Reynolds, C. R., & Kamphaus, R. W. (1998). *Behavior Assessment System for Children: Manual.* Circle Pineas, MN: American Guidance Service.

Sajwaj, T., Libet, J., & Agras, S. (1974). Lemon juice therapy: The control of life-threatening rumination in a six-month-old infant. *Journal of Applied Behavior Analysis, 7,* 557–563.

Sanders, M. R. Rebgetz, M., Morrison, M. M., Bor, W., Gordon, A., Dadds, M. R., & Shepherd, R. (1989). Cognitive-behavioral treatment of recurrent non-specific abdominal pain in children: An analysis of generalization and maintenance side effects. *Journal of Consulting and Clinical Psychology, 57,* 294–300.

Sanders, M. R., Shepherd, R. W., Cleghorn, G., & Woolford, H. (1994). The treatment of recurrent abdominal pain in children: A controlled comparison of cognitive-behavioral family intervention and standard pediatric care. *Journal of Consulting and Clinical Psychology, 62,* 306–314.

Sank, L. I., & Biglan, A. (1974). Operant treatment of a case of recurrent abdominal pain in a 10-year-old boy. *Behavior Therapy, 5,* 677–681.

Scharff, L. (1997). Recurrent abdominal pain in children: A review of psychological factors and treatment. *Clinical Psychology Review, 17,* 145–166.

Schwankovsky, L., & Hyman, P. E. (1999). Pediatric Functional Gastrointestinal Disorders Diagnostic Questionnaire. In P. E. Hyman (Ed.), *Pediatric functional gastrointestinal disorders* (pp. A1–A8). New York: Academy Professional Information Services, Inc.

Singh, N. N. (1981). Rumination. *International Review of Research in Mental Retardation, 10,* 139–182.

Stickler, G. B., & Murphy, D. B. (1979). Recurrent abdominal pain. *American Journal of Diseases in Childhood, 133,* 486–489.

Thomsen, A. H., Compas, B. E., Colletti, R. B., & Stanger, C. (2000). *Self-report of coping and stress responses in adolescents with recurrent abdominal pain.* Manuscript submitted for publication.

Thomsen, A. H., Compas, B. E., Colletti, R. B., Stanger, C., Boyer, M. C., & Konik, B. S. (2002). Parent reports of coping and stress responses in children with recurrent abdominal pain. *Journal of Pediatric Psychology, 27,* 215–226.

Thumshirn, M., Camilleri, M., Hanson, R. B., Williams, D. E., Schei, A. J., & Kammer, P. P. (1998). Gastric mechanosensory and lower esophageal sphincter function in rumination syndrome. *American Journal of Physiology, 275*(2), G314–G321.

Varni, J. W., Thompson, K. L., & Hanson, V. (1987). The Varni/Thompson Pediatric Pain Questionnaire: I. Chronic musculoskeletal pain in juvenile rheumatoid arthritis. *Pain, 28,* 27–38.

Von Baeyer, C. L., & Walker, L. S. (1999). Children with recurrent abdominal pain: Issues in the selection and description of research participants. *Journal of Developmental and Behavioral Pediatrics, 20*, 307–313.

Walker, L. S. (1999). The evolution of research on recurrent abdominal pain: History, assumptions, and a conceptual model. In P. J. McGrath & G. A. Finley (Eds.), *Chronic and recurrent pain in children and adolescents* (pp. 141–172). Seattle, WA: International Association for the Study of Pain.

Walker, L. S., Caplan-Dover, A., & Rasquin-Weber, A. (2000). *Questionnaire on Gastrointestinal Symptoms for Children and Adolescents*. Unpublished manuscript.

Walker, L. S., Garber, J., & Greene, J. W. (1993). Psychosocial correlates of recurrent childhood pain: A comparison of pediatric patients with recurrent abdominal pain, organic illness, and psychiatric disorders. *Journal of Abnormal Psychology, 102*, 248–258.

Walker, L. S., Garber, J., Smith, C. A., Van Slyke, D. A., & Lewis Claar, R. (2001). The relation of daily stressors to somatic and emotional symptoms in children with and without recurrent abdominal pain. *Journal of Consulting and Clinical Psychology, 69*, 85–91.

Walker, L. S., & Greene, J. W. (1989). Children with recurrent abdominal pain and their parents: More somatic complaints, anxiety, and depression than other patient families? *Journal of Pediatric Psychology, 14*, 231–243.

Walker, L. S., & Greene, J. W. (1991). Negative life events and symptom resolution in pediatric abdominal pain patients. *Journal of Pediatric Psychology, 16*, 341–360.

Walker, L. S., Smith, C. A., Garber, J., & Van Slyke, D. A. (1997). Development and validation of the Pain Response Inventory for Children. *Psychological Assessment, 9*, 392–405.

Walker, L. S., & Zeman, J. L. (1992). Parental response to child illness behavior. *Journal of Pediatric Psychology, 17*, 49–71.

Wasserman, A. L., Whitington, P. F., & Rivara, F. P. (1988). Psychogenic basis for abdominal pain in children and adolescents. *Journal of the American Academy of Child and Adolescent Psychiatry, 27*, 179–184.

Whitehead, W. E., & Schuster, M. M. (1985). Rumination syndrome, vomiting, aerophagia, and belching. In W. E. Whitehead & M. M. Schuster (Eds.), *Gastrointestinal disorders: Behavioral and physiological basis for treatment* (pp. 67–90). Orlando, FL: Academic Press.

Zeltzer, L., Bursch, B., & Walco, G. (1997). Pain responsiveness and chronic pain: A psychobiological perspective. *Journal of Developmental and Behavioral Pediatrics, 18*, 413–422.

Part IV

DEVELOPMENTAL, BEHAVIORAL, AND COGNITIVE/ AFFECTIVE CONDITIONS

28

Pediatric Feeding Problems

THOMAS R. LINSCHEID
KAREN S. BUDD
L. KAYE RASNAKE

Feeding problems can occur in children with medical conditions, children with developmental disabilities, and in normally developing children. Several estimates of incidence of feeding problems have been offered, ranging from 25% (Manikam & Perman, 2000) to 45% (Bentovim, 1970) in normally developing children to 80% in developmentally disabled children (Manikam & Perman, 2000). With advances in medical techniques, children with prematurity or severe medical complications in infancy are now surviving. For the pediatric psychologist, these children represent a special challenge because they frequently have feeding problems either related to the medical condition or induced iatrogenically as a result of treatment (Ginsberg, 1988). The diagnosis and treatment of feeding problems is a common activity for pediatric psychologists, who often work collaboratively with other health professionals on feeding cases (Douglas & Harris, 2001; Kedesdy & Budd, 1998; Miller et al., 2001).

Notably, certain medical diagnoses inherently increase the risk of feeding problems. Among these are gastroesophageal reflux disease (GERD), bronchopulmonary displagia (BPD), congenital cardiac conditions, cystic fibrosis, neurological disorders, prematurity, HIV, cerebral palsy, and childhood cancers. For example, infants and children with GERD can develop esophagitis, a condition that can produce pain or discomfort both during and after eating. To compound the problem, one treatment for chronic GERD is a surgical procedure, Nissan Fundoplication, that tightens the gastroesophageal sphincter, preventing stomach contents from refluxing upward into the esophagus. The procedure requires the temporary placement of a gastrostomy tube (G-tube) for feeding until the surgical site is healed. Interruption of normal oral feeding, coupled with a history of physical discomfort during and following eating, increases the likelihood that these children will refuse or limit their oral intake (Mathisen, Worrall, Masel, Wall, & Shepherd, 1999). In addition, the surgical procedure, though successfully eliminating reflux, also prevents the normal functions of burping and vomiting and may produce bloating. GERD is noted here as an example of how a medical condition and its appropriate treatment can interact with the normal development of feeding to produce a feeding problem. The other aforementioned medical conditions and their treatments have similar interactive effects.

This chapter addresses the development of feeding practices and skills in the context of the overall development of the child, describes behavioral techniques and strategies for treating feeding problems, and reviews published accounts of the implementation of behavioral feeding treatments, including both inpatient and outpatient interventions. This *Handbook* contains a separate chapter on nonorganic failure to thrive (see Black, Chapter 29, this volume). To differentiate, the present chapter primarily addresses feeding problems that occur in conjunction with organic conditions. However, to the extent that certain forms of nonorganic failure to thrive relate to behavioral mismanagement during specific developmental periods (cf. Linscheid & Rasnake, 1985), the techniques described for organically based problems apply as well.

NORMAL DEVELOPMENT AND FEEDING

"The development of feeding skills is complex; it depends on the motor, emotional, and social maturation of the child as well as on the child's temperament and relationship with family members" (American Academy of Pediatrics, 1988, p. 125). The feeding situation requires action from both the parent and the child. The parent determines what, when, and where food is offered. The infant or child chooses what and how much is eaten. This division of responsibility becomes more complex as the child grows and matures.

In terms of feeding capabilities and the types of foods consumed, several stages of infant feeding have been identified (Satter, 1999). The first two stages occur during the first 6 months of life and include (1) early infancy (1 to 4 months of age), when breast milk or formula is the sole source of nutrients, and (2) later infancy (4 to 6 months of age), when semisolid foods are added to the diet. The third and fourth stages occur in the second half of the first year, when finger foods, liquid in a cup, and pieces of soft food are introduced. The final stage (12 months and beyond) represents the time at which children begin to eat the same foods as other members of the family and develop strong food preferences. Compared with infants, toddlers show a preference for greater texture complexity. However, early positive experiences with difficult-to-chew textures may facilitate an acceptance of complex textures (Lundy et al., 1998). During the final period, behavior problems in feeding are most likely to be identified (Linscheid & Rasnake, 1985); thus it is the period of primary concern here. In addition, appetite changes are expected. Normal infants show a fairly consistent appetite across feeding times and triple their weight in the first year of life. After 12 months, weight gain decreases, with gains of approximately 5 pounds a year expected for the next 3 to 4 years. Toddlers also typically show a decrease and a variability in appetite. A child may consume large quantities at one meal and very little at another meal. Thus, in a relatively short period, the infant or toddler and parent experience many changes in the feeding situation.

Importantly, these changes must be considered in relation to the ongoing social-emotional development of the child. During the toddler period, children begin to assert themselves in their quest for autonomy and must learn to adjust to socialization demands and adult limit setting (Satter, 1999). Often, as a result of this quest for autonomy, noncompliant behaviors emerge. In fact, some authors argue that these noncompliant behaviors give the child the opportunity to develop strategies to express their autonomy in socially acceptable ways (e.g., Kuczynski, Kochanski, Radke-Yarrow, & Girius-Brown, 1987). Thus noncompliant behaviors, in the feeding situation and other situations (e.g., dressing, toy cleanup), are not only expected but also represent an important opportunity for children to mature socially.

A parent's or caregiver's understanding of and response to these overlapping developments (i.e., changes in eating patterns and social-emotional maturation) can have a significant impact on the feeding situation. For example, at the same time that the quest for autonomy is emerging, the onset of self-feeding and establishment of food preferences are expected. Thus the feeding situation changes from one in which parents have primary control to one of required shared control between parent and child. The need to share control of the feeding situation (parent determines type of food, time of eating, etc.) may conflict with the child's efforts to establish social-emotional maturity. The toddler's food refusal and insistence of food preferences may represent a means of expressing autonomy and individuality.

The caregiver's response to these behaviors may lead to ongoing battles over eating and to the eventual development of serious feeding problems. Caregiver responses are often determined by the importance attached to feeding. One means (and often the primary means) of assessing one's success as a parent is through the child's eating. Many parents believe a good parent is one whose child eats well. When faced with a noncompliant child, the parent who defines his or her parenting success in this way may develop strategies to encourage compliance, such as bribing and cajoling. Such parental behavior results in significant attention given to food refusal behaviors. Thus the awareness of the concurrently emerging developments affecting the feeding situation and the sometimes conflicting nature of these developments (i.e., the development of motor skills enabling self-feeding and the social-emotional needs of autonomy that conflict with parental determination of nutritional needs) is essential for the development of prevention strategies. In addition, this awareness may help parents and caregivers better understand the dynamics of the feeding difficulties and respond to treatment interventions. For a comprehensive discussion of the developmental components of the feeding relationship, the reader is referred to Satter (1999).

Given that motor, sensory, behavioral, and social-emotional factors all play a role in the successful acquisition of feeding skills, it is easily seen how the existence of a medical condition can interfere with this progression. Patients whose medical conditions preclude oral feedings during infancy will not make the normal transition from liquid to solid foods. Children whose activities or diet are restricted or controlled may experience increased conflict during the process of gaining autonomy. Toddlers and preschoolers with diabetes mellitus, who must eat consistent quantities at set times during a period in which appetite and taste preference are highly variable, provide an excellent example of the clash between normal development and medical condition (Wysocki, Huxtable, Linscheid, & Wayne, 1989).

CLASSIFICATION

Feeding problems can be classified by type and cause (cf. Burklow, Phelps, Schultz, McConnell, & Rudolph, 1998; Kededsy & Budd, 1998). Generally, the type of problem relates to the developmental appropriateness of foods eaten (texture and variety), quantity consumed (over- or underconsumption), mealtime behaviors (tantrums, spitting food), or delays in self-feeding skills. Causes can most easily be classified as those related to medical condition (GERD, prematurity), those related to oral–motor delay or competencies (cerebral palsy), and those related to environmental experience, such as behavioral mismanagement or conditioned anxiety (i.e., choking phobia). In practice, children with feeding difficulties often have multiple types of problems with more than one cause. The relative contributions of medical condition, oral–motor dysfunction, and environment to the clinical problem are often difficult to sort out. Consider the case of a child with cystic fibrosis who has an increased need for calories due to the disease itself. In order to ensure that the child will get sufficient calories, parents may concede to the child's request for ice cream when vegetables are refused. As a result, the child eliminates nutritionally appropriate foods from his or her diet and may demonstrate mealtime behavior problems when parents attempt to introduce healthier foods. The interactive nature of these possible causes requires that treatment be undertaken in a setting in which each of the disciplines having expertise in the various areas can work together closely (cf. Miller et al., 2001).

ASSESSMENT

The purposes of a feeding assessment are to identify presenting problems, adaptive skills, and historical, as well as current, conditions related to feeding problems and to establish realistic treatment goals. Assessment is somewhat easier when children are inpatients than when they are outpatients. Many inpatients have long and well-documented feeding histories with readily available nutritional records. Parents, nurses, and other staff members who regularly feed the child are also available for interview, and the child can be observed several times a day during meals. In the assessment of outpatients, feeding professionals have access to the child only during scheduled sessions, rather than continuously on the hospital unit. Thus it is important to take maximum advantage of outpatient sessions for data gathering by directly observing ongoing interactions and using caregivers as informants. Feeding assessment includes a minimum of three components: (1) clinical interview with the major caregiver(s); (2) direct observation of feeder–child interactions during a simulated (outpatient) or actual (inpatient) meal; and (3) sample records of the child's food intake. Also, when developmental abnormalities are suspected, evaluation of the child's cognitive, adaptive, and behavioral repertoire often is informative. If family functioning or parenting competence is of concern, the assessment should identify major family stressors or parenting problems that are likely to have an impact on treatment planning. Information gathered by other professionals (e.g., oral–motor or dental evaluations, anthropometric measures, and medical test results) should also be reviewed.

Clinical Interview with Caregivers

Caregivers are a critical source of information about the child's feeding history, including the onset and nature of eating problems, feeding milestones, mealtime routines, current feeding concerns, and techniques that have been tried to get the child to eat (Babbitt et al., 1994). In outpatient assessment, parents often provide the sole or major source of information about the child's eating habits. Depending on the nature of the clinical setting, interviews may be conducted by an individual therapist or by representatives of a multidisciplinary team.

Caregivers provide information about their expectations of the child's eating, which may reveal cultural or family practices that have an impact on feeding problems (Birch, 1990). Parents often do not know the recommended ages for feeding and drinking milestones. They may not realize their child is out of phase and thus feel less urgency to intervene. Age, education, and ethnicity influence attitudes about how messy a child should be and how much independence a child should be given in food selection (Humphry & Thigpen-Beck, 1997). Finally, there is convincing evidence for a strong association between childhood feeding problems and maternal eating disorders (e.g., Whelan & Cooper, 2000). All of these factors should be kept in mind during the clinical interview with the parent(s), particularly if the parent is going to be expected to act as the primary therapist (as is typical in outpatient treatment).

Observation of Feeder–Child Interactions during Mealtimes

For successful treatment planning, whether treatment is to be conducted on an inpatient or an outpatient basis, direct observation of the current child–feeder interaction is crucial. This is especially true for outpatient treatment, in which parents or caregivers actually implement the treatment. Whereas their involvement optimizes treatment effectiveness in both modalities, caregiver participation is fundamental to outpatient treatment. Because parents are ultimately responsible for the child's intake, it is essential to see how they interact with the child in regard to eating. There is some evidence that dysfunctional interactional patterns (e.g., mothers who are less sensitive and less cooperative) may be present between caregivers and infants who show food refusal (Lindberg, Bohlin, Hagekull, & Palmerus, 1996). Because these patterns can help to maintain problematic feeding behaviors, it is essential to document any occurrences so that they can be considered in the treatment plan. Mealtime observations can take many forms, but for outpatient assessment, observations usually involve asking parents to simulate a typical home meal. To enhance the likelihood of hunger, parents should be notified in advance not to feed the child for at least 2 hours before an outpatient visit. When possible, parents are asked to bring a selection of foods (both preferred and nonpreferred) that the child is routinely served at home, as well as serving containers, utensils, and any other usual mealtime supplies. They are asked to present menu items and respond to the child as they do at home while the therapist watches, often from the corner of the room or from behind a one-way mirror.

During feeding, the clinician observes patterns of interactions and foods consumed. Pertinent child behaviors include the specific foods and liquids the child accepts or refuses, when and how the child communicates likes and dislikes, the extent to which the child is able to eat independently, and changes in eating patterns as the meal progresses. Pertinent feeder behaviors include how food is offered (e.g., spoon-fed vs. placed in front of child), the extent of structure imposed (e.g., child's positioning, access to food), verbal encouragement to eat, reactions to the child's acceptances and refusals, the relative frequency and timing of the feeder's positive and negative attention, and what determines the end of the meal.

The behavioral feeding literature provides several examples of observation methods for coding and analyzing feeder–child behaviors. They range from recording a few target behaviors (Luiselli, 1993) to more advanced systems designed for comprehensive evaluation (Babbitt et al., 1994; Werle, Murphy, & Budd, 1993, 1998). For clinical purposes, a therapist often tailors the behaviors recorded to the specific problems present in a particular case. Nevertheless, the use of explicit behavioral categories for documenting problems and adaptive skills is recommended, both to focus the clinician's attention during mealtime observations and to provide a means of documenting progress across treatment sessions.

When clinic simulation of feeding is not feasible but some direct representation of mealtimes is considered important, therapists may ask parents to audiotape (Madison & Adubato, 1984) or videotape home meals. These methods offer many of the advantages of live observation but are obviously limited to families with motivation and resources. Alternatively, therapists may conduct an occasional home visit in order to observe feeding in the natural environment. Budd, Chugh, and Berry (1998) describe a case in which the therapist scheduled two home visits to observe a toddler referred for restricted diet and mealtime fussiness whose behavior in an outpatient session was unusually cooperative. At the second home visit, the child was irritable and refused nearly all food offered, which gave the therapist an opportunity to see how the mother responded (making persistent food offers and allowing the child to sit on her lap and play during the meal). Based on this information, the therapist devised a treatment plan to rearrange the social contingencies of mealtime. As Budd and Li (1994) noted, interactions with other family members, distracting stimuli, or familiar surroundings may affect feeding at home in a manner that is not evident in a clinic analogue setting.

Sample Records of the Child's Food Intake

Records of the child's food intake provide a basis for estimating the nutritional adequacy of the child's diet. Many techniques are available for gathering this information (e.g., diaries, food frequency questionnaires, short-term recall methods), and all have advantages and disadvantages (Wolper, Heshka, & Heymsfield, 1995). In outpatient assessment, caregivers provide this information, usually in the form of 24-hour to 7-day food diaries (Stark et al., 1993). Parents are instructed to record everything the child eats and drinks on a written log (e.g., 3 ounces of whole milk, one-quarter of an apple). They may also be asked to record the time or location of meals, who else eats with the child, or (for children on artificial feeding regimens) oral versus nonoral intake. For inpatient cases, food intake records are most generally provided by nurses or by the caregiver. Nutritionists and dieticians are skilled in analyzing the records regarding nutrients, calories, and food variety. Alternatively, intake records can be summarized using a variety of dietary software programs (Food and Nutrition Information Center, 2002).

Other Child or Parent Measures

When the child's developmental or behavioral adjustment is in question, additional assessment of the child may be indicated. Assessment can clarify whether the child's feeding skills are consistent with other areas of functioning, whether global attentional or behavioral deficits exist that interfere with feeding, and whether the child has prerequisite skills for feeding (e.g., trunk stability, receptive language, fine motor coordination). Measures used in some feeding assessments include behavior problem checklists such the Child Behavior Checklist (Achenbach, 1991, 1992), developmental screening instruments, or standardized intelligence tests. When concern exists about marital difficulties, emotional disturbance, or other parenting stressors, inventories such as the Parenting Stress Index (Abidin, 1995) may be appropriate. Given that the primary referral questions relate to feeding problems, assessment of other issues is recommended on an individual case basis. Two parent-report questionnaire-format instruments to assess the extent of feeding and mealtime problems in children are available. The Children's Eating Behavior Inventory (CEBI; Archer, Rosenbaum, & Streiner, 1991) and the Behavioral Pediatrics Feeding Assessment Scale (BPFAS; Crist & Napier-Phillips, 2001) have been shown to be useful assessment tools. Also, given the frequency with which feeding problems are found in children with mental retardation, a screening tool designed specifically for use with persons with mental retardation (the Screening Tool of Feeding Problems [STEP]; Matson & Kuhn, 2001) has been shown to have good stability over time and raters.

BEHAVIORAL COMPONENTS OF FEEDING

To understand feeding as behavior, both instrumental (operant) and respondent (classical) conditioning models are necessary. Kedesdy and Budd (1998) provide a detailed overview of behavioral principles and procedures related to feeding problems. The feeding setting can be conceptualized in the traditional antecedent–behavior–consequence model, in which the presence of food, prompts to eat, location (e.g., high chair), and other stimuli serve as antecedents; behaviors such as food acceptance, refusal, tantrums, gagging, and others can be emitted; and these behaviors can have reinforcing or punishing consequences, which determine their future probability of occurrence. The role of respondent conditioning in the development of a feeding problem can best be understood in the case of a child who may gag, choke, or suffer pain on swallowing. Stimuli associated with the presentation of that food can acquire the ability to elicit the anxiety naturally associated with gagging or choking. Both respondent and operant conditioning combine in the classic two-factor model. The child who has conditioned anxiety and fear at the sight of food may engage in avoidance behaviors (e.g., pushing food away, having tantrums). If the behavior results in a withdrawal of the food or the demand to eat, the behavior is being negatively reinforced through anxiety reduction or escape. This process is most clearly seen in children who develop food refusal following an episode of choking (cf. Chatoor, Conley, & Dickson, 1988). The practice of forced feeding has also been associated with the development of anxiety related to food acceptance (Linscheid, Oliver, Blyler, & Palmer, 1978, Case 2), which can lead to a functional food phobia (Palmer, Thompson, & Linscheid, 1975).

Behavior management techniques are an integral part of inpatient and outpatient feeding interventions. Behavioral techniques are used to systematically modify environmental variables that affect children's feeding patterns. Four common ingredients of treatment are: (1) contingent social attention, (2) positive and negative tangible consequences, (3) appetite manipulation, and (4) stimulus control procedures.

Contingent Social Attention

Perhaps the most fundamental behavioral procedure used to enhance children's feeding is social approval contingent on desired feeding behavior. Both discrete praise and other forms of positive attention (e.g., hugs, pleasant conversation) appear to function as positive reinforcement for most children. Virtually all behavioral intervention programs include contingent positive social attention as a component of treatment (Kerwin, 1999). Positive social attention for cooperative behavior often is combined with "planned ignoring" (i.e., turning away and providing no attention for 5–15 seconds) following misbehavior such as tantrums or food refusal. This procedure is labeled "differential social attention," because it provides contrasting forms of social feedback following desired and undesired behaviors. Several feeding programs have employed differential social attention as a treatment component (Stark et al., 1996; Werle et al., 1993, 1998). However, ignoring is often difficult for caregivers to implement effectively, and thus care is needed in training lay feeders to use the procedure (Linscheid & Rasnake, 2001).

Other forms of contingent social attention also have been employed in outpatient interventions to modify feeding behaviors. Often, some physical control is applied along with social attention, thereby blurring the distinction between social and tangible consequences. For example, Madison and Adubato (1984) taught parents to use verbal disapproval and noise contingent on their child's ruminative vomiting, along with 10 seconds of attention withdrawal. A commonly used disciplinary technique is time out, in which a child is restricted from access to attention and other reinforcing stimuli for a brief period (5–60 seconds) contingent on inappropriate behaviors. Time out is distinguished from simple ignoring by physically moving the child, the caregiver, or available materials out of the area for the duration of time out.

Positive and Negative Tangible Consequences

In addition to social attention, tangible consequences often are provided contingently as part of behavioral feeding programs. The most common positive consequence for desired eating is offering one or more bites of preferred food (Palmer et al., 1975). Other incentives have included access to television, the opportunity to play with toys, or tokens redeemable for items of value (e.g., Linscheid, Tarnowski, Rasnake, & Brams, 1987; Stark, Bowen, Tyc, Evans, & Passero, 1990). These procedures employ the "Premack principle" (Premack, 1959), which states that access to a higher probability behavior serves to reinforce a lower probability behavior. Foods initially classified as nonpreferred often become preferred after treatment is under way (Thompson, Palmer, & Linscheid, 1977) and thus come to serve as positive reinforcers.

Negative consequences consist of either the removal of favored items or delivery of unpleasant stimuli contingent on dawdling, expelling food, or disruptive mealtime behavior. Various forms of physical control have been used to induce swallowing or restrict disruptive movements during mealtimes. These include touching the child's tongue to initiate a swallowing reflex (Hagopian, Farrell, & Amari, 1996; Lamm & Greer, 1988), brief interruption and redirection of hand movements contingent on self-stimulatory behavior (Luiselli, 1993), or physical guidance (Ahearn, Kerwin, Eicher, Shantz, & Swearingin, 1996). More intrusive forms of aversive consequences (such as overcorrection or forced feeding) rarely are included in outpatient feeding programs, due to the unpleasantness and potential health risks of the procedures. However, a few early studies (e.g., Ives, Harris, & Wolchik, 1978) reported use of negative consequences such as forced feeding as a component of outpatient treatment.

Appetite Manipulation

Appetite is presumed to be conditioned by a combination of biological and environmental variables (Birch, 1990). Manipulation of the feeding schedule can be effective in promoting appetite, particularly for children who have a history of unlimited or irregular access to food. Children fed via artificial means, such as a G-tube or total parenteral nutrition (TPN), may be receiving 100% of their daily nutritional needs via these methods. In addition, the method of infusing formula or TPN gradually across the day precludes the child's ever feeling anything but mild hunger. In order to induce hunger and establish a normal cyclical appetite, a substantial reduction in the calories provided artificially is necessary. A frequent practice during our inpatient treatment is to reduce artificial feeding to perhaps 30% of daily needs and to deliver these calories while the child is sleeping so that daytime hunger can be established. The extent of calorie reduction depends on the child's current weight and medical condition. On a daily basis, the percentage of daily calorie needs and fluids delivered artificially can be adjusted so as to balance daytime hunger against weight loss and hydration status. Children who are not fed artificially generally receive only water between meals. For toddlers and preschool children, it is common and normal to allow between-meal snacks; however, during feeding treatment the restriction on snacks ensures that the children come to the treatment meals feeling hungry. The ability to produce the greatest hunger while ensuring that the child is medically safe is one of the strongest reasons for treatment on an inpatient basis. Appetite manipulation is an important part of the treatment and needs to be carefully considered in the treatment planning phase and also carefully documented in empirical reports (Linscheid, 1999).

Whereas appetite manipulation is a core ingredient of most inpatient feeding regimens, the technique often needs to be modified for use by caregivers on an outpatient basis. Clinically, we often encounter parents who are unwilling to restrict their child's access to food, and indeed they fail to see the practice as credible in view of their child's chronic problems with under-consumption. Outpatient application of schedule interventions generally consist of offering meals and snacks on a consistent schedule from day to day and restricting intake between planned eating occasions (Thompson et al., 1977; Werle et al., 1998). Only a limited amount of favored food may be offered at a meal, at least until after nonpreferred foods are consumed.

Stimulus Control Procedures

Stimulus conditions that precede or occur concomitant with target responses acquire discriminative properties by virtue of the repeated pairing of the stimuli with positive or negative reinforcement for the behavior. Parents or caregivers may be trained to provide consistent verbal or physical prompts to eat (e.g., "take a bite") as part of the intervention program (Werle et al., 1993). When used systematically, the antecedent instruction appears to become a discriminative cue for appropriate eating. Other forms of discriminative stimuli in outpatient treatment include modeling of appropriate eating (Greer, Dorow, Williams, McCorkle, & Asnes, 1991) and visual cues of appropriate hand placement between bites (Luiselli, 1993).

Two stimulus control techniques, shaping and fading, involve progressive changes in the criteria for delivery of antecedent stimuli and consequences in relation to child feeding behavior. Both techniques are used extensively in feeding interventions, particularly with children who exhibit developmental delays relative to feeding. For example, to promote acceptance of a wider range of foods, a child might initially receive reinforcement for accepting any foods. The criteria for reinforcement are then altered in small steps to require intake of a small amount of new foods or items with different textures, based on the child's performance (Johnson & Babbitt, 1993; Linscheid et al., 1987). Fading involves the gradual removal of prompts, assistance, or reinforcement needed in order to establish independent performance of a behavior. Utensil use may be taught by progressively fading the extent of verbal and physical assistance a child is given as he or she develops more control over self-feeding (Luiselli, 1993).

This section has summarized the techniques most commonly employed in feeding interventions. Other procedures, such as desensitization of eating-related fears (Siegel, 1982) and relaxation to ease abdominal pain after food intake (Stark et al., 1993), have been reported in a few studies with specialized types of feeding problems.

CONSIDERATIONS FOR INPATIENT VERSUS OUTPATIENT TREATMENT

The use of brief inpatient admission to treat feeding problems was initially described by Linscheid and colleagues (Linscheid et al., 1978). These authors feel that inpatient admission for treatment is justified under the following circumstances: (1) a child's feeding problems are leading to excessive weight loss or nutritional status poor enough to interfere with adequate physical growth; (2) outpatient treatment has proven unsuccessful, and the child–parent interaction relating to the feeding problem has become sufficiently dysfunctional to preclude effective home-based or outpatient treatment; and (3) parents are willing to participate in the process, so that generalization to the home setting can be achieved. In addition to these criteria, treatments utilizing forced feeding or swallowing induction may require medical monitoring due to the possibility of aspiration (e.g., Hagopian et al., 1996). The advantages of inpatient treatment are numerous. It is possible to control and measure the patient's intake of solids and liquids precisely, and medical intervention is immediately available if needed. The patient's weight and hydration status can be more accurately measured and monitored than can be done in the home by parents. Restricting a child's access to food to induce hunger (appetite manipulation) is difficult for parents to do at home, because they may have understandable fears of their children losing too much weight or becoming dehydrated during the treatment process. Hospitalization also allows the use of frequent feeding sessions (three or four per day) and the consistency of having the same trainers involved in each meal. Parents are freed from normal home responsibilities that may distract them during home-based (outpatient) treatments.

Although inpatient treatment is medically necessary for some feeding problems, it has the disadvantages of high cost, extensive professional time involvement, and possible problems with generalization beyond the hospital environment. Outpatient treatment, by contrast, offers greater latitude for individualizing many clinical aspects to specific cases. For example, the frequency of outpatient sessions, the specific professionals involved, and methods of training parents or other caregivers can be tailored to the needs of individual children and families. Outpatient intervention frequently takes place at a hospital-based clinic or rehabilitation setting, which ideally provides access to the varied disciplines with expertise in feeding issues. A less common but promising alternative is home-based treatment, which allows intervention to be adapted to the child's natural feeding environment (Gutentag & Hammer, 2000; Werle et al., 1993, 1998). For children whose feeding problems are associated with developmental delays and/or physical handicaps, intervention often occurs at school as part of special education programming.

Douglas and Harris (2001) describe a unique behaviorally based, comprehensive day-center-based feeding program that differs from an inpatient program, a standard outpatient program, or home-based intervention. Children and families are seen for one morning every 2 weeks (with a maximum of 12 appointments). A standardized evaluation form is completed at the beginning and end of treatment by the clinicians and parents. Given the multiple components of the program (i.e., a playroom experience, individual consultation about eating behaviors, interactions with other families), it is impossible to identify the value of each feature. However, the data suggest that the program is an effective way to increase weight, reduce the need for tube feedings, and reduce food selectivity. The authors suggest that this type of program reduces the burden on families of making multiple, frequent trips to a treatment center and also allows therapists to treat a large number of cases (approximately 60–70 cases in a year).

Whether outpatient, home-based, or day-center program, there are three prerequisites for outpatient feeding intervention: (1) the child's medical status is stable; (2) one or more caregivers are available to participate in treatment; and (3) recommended treatment is acceptable to all caregivers. With regard to the first prerequisite, "medical stability" implies that the child consumes sufficient calories and nutrients to maintain minimum health requirements. Furthermore, it implies that, if the child has a life-threatening condition (e.g., respiratory or intestinal disorder, swallowing dysfunction), caregivers know how to respond appropriately and when to enlist professional assistance. Thus outpatient treatment may be precluded for children who are severely malnourished or have life-threatening medical conditions or for children whose parents are unable to provide a safe caretaking environment.

The second prerequisite of outpatient treatment is that a primary caregiver (usually one or both parents) participate to some extent in intervention. At a minimal level, the caregiver(s) must ensure that the child gets to therapeutic feeding sessions and must be informed about the basic goals and procedures of therapy. At a more extensive level, parents take part in feeding sessions and become proficient in implementing intervention procedures. The greater the caregivers' expected role in treatment, the more important is the third prerequisite: that the caregivers perceive the treatment recommendations as acceptable. If parents view the procedures as cumbersome, ineffective, or distressing, they are unlikely to apply them at home, even after receiving instruction (Ahearn et al., 1996; Hoch, Babbit, Coe, Krell, & Hackbert, 1994).

EXAMPLES OF BEHAVIORAL TREATMENT IN INPATIENT AND OUTPATIENT SETTINGS

Behavioral techniques have been utilized in inpatient settings to induce oral feeding in children whose medical conditions have necessitated feeding via artificial means (G-tube or TPN). Perhaps because they have missed a critical period for the introduction of oral solid foods or because of certain medical treatments (as described earlier in the case of GERD), many children fed exclusively via artificial methods develop a pronounced food phobia that leads to total food refusal. Physically forcing food into the child's mouth has been used in successful behavioral treatments for chronic food refusal. Ahearn and colleagues (1996) compared forced feeding, termed "physical guidance," with an escape-extinction procedure (nonremoval of spoon) in three children presenting with chronic food refusal. Although both treatments were effective, the forced feeding procedure produced fewer undesirable behaviors and shorter meal duration. In addition, parents preferred the forced feeding. Clearly, forced feeding procedures need to be conducted in a medical setting, as there is a slight but significant danger of the child's aspirating food into the lungs. Moreover, this is not a treatment that parents would be able to accomplish, because of the intense distress engendered in the child by the fear of the food and subsequent choking or gagging. To the extent that the child has a phobia of food, this procedure is analogous to "flooding" or implosion techniques used in the treatment of adults with phobias.

Other types of physical interventions have also been reported. Lamm and Greer (1988) described the use of a swallow-induction procedure to treat three infants with dysphagia. During treatment, positive contingent social interaction and a system of physical prompts ranging from least to most intrusive were used. The most intrusive physical prompt to swallow was the touching of the right posterior portion of the infant's tongue by the feeder. (This action produces a gag response with arching of the back of the tongue, followed by a swallow.) After food or liquid was placed in the infant's mouth, 3 seconds would elapse with no prompt; if a swallow did not occur, a verbal prompt to swallow was given. If the infant still did not swallow, the verbal prompt was repeated, with a physical touch to the infant's lip, then to the lower gum, and finally the swallow-eliciting touch. A combined reversal and changing criterion design was used to document the effects of the treatment package and demonstrated that other caregivers (nurses, parents) were not successful in producing the swallowing response until they were trained in the procedures. More recently, Hoch, Babbitt, Coe, Ducan, and Trusty (1995) used swallow induction to establish feeding in a 3½ year old child with severe mental retardation. Small amounts of pureed food were put on a rubber stimulator that was placed on the posterior portion of the child's tongue and gently depressed if the child did not voluntarily swallow.

Another treatment program utilizing both forced feeding and operant procedures was developed by Iwata and colleagues (Riordan, Iwata, Finney, Wohl, & Stanley, 1984). A modified graduated prompt system (cf. Lamm & Greer, 1988) was used. The spoon was placed in front of the child's mouth for approximately 2 seconds. If the child did not accept the food from the spoon, the food was placed in the child's mouth, forcibly if necessary. This created a situation in which the child's acceptance of the spoon prior to the food being forced into the mouth was negatively reinforced by escape from the assumed aversive forced feeding. In addition, positive reinforcement in the form of social praise and access to preferred foods was utilized.

Treatment of total food refusal or specific texture-related refusal has also been accomplished without forced feeding by using techniques consistent with the concept of systematic desensitization. Geertsma, Hyams, Pelletier, and Reiter (1985) reported the initiation of oral feeding in an infant who had been deprived of oral feeding due to the use of a G-tube. The process involved desensitization to oral area aversion by tactile stimulation while the trainer engaged the child in positive social interaction, the insertion of fingers and objects into the child's mouth, and the pairing of oral stimulation with infusion of formula via the G-tube. With this procedure, artificial feeding was discontinued after 6 months of treatment.

Utilizing purely operant-based techniques, Linscheid et al. (1978) treated solid food refusal in a severely delayed and medically involved 2-year-old child, who was accepting liquids only from a bottle. The treatment involved the systematic reinforcement of behaviors compatible with food acceptance (i.e., sitting quietly, allowing spoon into mouth, and taking food from spoon). Initially, mere presentation of the spoon resulted in tantrum behavior. Quiet behavior was taught by reinforcing successive approximations to the desired behavior. For example, initially the child was reinforced with social praise and access to the bottle if he allowed the spoon within 15 inches of his mouth without crying or kicking for 1 second.

The requirements for reinforcement were gradually changed so that the spoon was moved closer to the mouth and the time period extended. Later in treatment, acceptance of the spoon with formula, followed by acceptance of nonpreferred foods, was required before reinforcement was given. Treatment lasted for 15 days; the parents were trained as feeders during the last few days of the admission.

In the older child who has either dysphagia or food phobia, forced feeding techniques may not be possible because of the child's size and ability to resist. Inducing the gag reflex to induce swallowing in a resistant child with well-developed teeth can pose a danger to the feeder. Linscheid et al. (1987) treated food refusal in a 6-year-old child who had previously consumed only minimal quantities of liquid. The patient had a congenital malformation of the gut. Due to numerous surgeries, the patient had been hospitalized for the first 3 years of his life, with 38 readmissions for complications between ages 3 and 6 years. The child had been maintained on artificial feedings, including TPN and G-tube feedings. Whenever food was brought anywhere near his mouth, he displayed a phobic response, including trembling, crying, and verbalized fear of choking. The intensity of this response was so great that the use of forced feeding was ruled out. A program was developed to systematically reinforce approximations to eating and to punish refusals to comply with the successive and gradual steps in this process. Social praise and interaction was contingent on compliance during the time-limited meals, and a "hero" badge was given contingent on meeting the behavioral or intake criterion for each meal. The badge permitted access to hospital activities and to the playroom, as well as the right to have visitors. It also served as a discriminative stimulus for medical staff to verbally reinforce the patient for having met his goal at the last meal. Also, one body part of a "Mr. Potato Head" was earned for each successful meal; when all parts were earned, the patient was taken to the hospital gift shop and allowed to pick out a small toy of his choosing (token reinforcement). If the patient failed to complete the minimum requirements at a meal, the badge was withheld, he lost privileges, and he was required to spend the next 2 hours in his room alone. A multiple-baseline design across food types with a changing criterion component was employed. The patient moved from consumption of small quantities of liquids to acceptance of five different foods during the 6 weeks of treatment. The phobic-like emotional response decreased as new foods were introduced. A desensitization-like treatment can be successful if strong reinforcers and effective punishers are available to induce the child to attempt each gradual step toward the feared stimulus. The degree of control over behavioral contingencies needed, as in this case, coupled with the need for medical monitoring, requires that these treatments be conducted in hospital settings.

Several studies have described inpatient behavioral techniques designed to increase the variety of foods eaten or to increase the quantity consumed (Johnson & Babbitt, 1993; Larson, Ayllon, & Barrett, 1987; Rasnake & Linscheid, 1987). Similar techniques have been used to treat nonorganic failure to thrive in hospitalized children. Larson et al. (1987) used music to mask the introduction of the feeding time (presumably to reduce conditioned anxiety in the child) and trained mothers in the use of time-out procedures to reduce aversive mealtime interactions. All of the children treated with these procedures showed increases in food acceptance that were directly related to the presence or absence of music. Ramsey and Zelazo (1988) increased oral intake in five hospitalized infants by decreasing feeding aversion. They initially paired pleasant social interaction and auditory stimuli with nasogastric feeding; when distress related to feeding decreased, oral intake was reestablished.

Although reports of inpatient treatment are more numerous, applied research demonstrates that outpatient treatment has successfully altered a range of child feeding problems. Outpatient treatment utilizes many of the same techniques developed for inpatient treatment, with modifications for home use, and generally is conducted more by parents than by professionals. Several studies have targeted selective food refusal (e.g., Werle et al., 1993, 1998), often in conjunction with disruptive mealtime behavior (Thompson et al., 1977) or eating-related fears (Siegel, 1982). Gutentag and Hammer (2000) trained the parents of a tube-dependent child to increase acceptance of oral foods using positive attention and shaping procedures and demonstrated generalization to the school setting. In addition, outpatient methods have been effective in modifying chronic rumination (Madison & Adubato, 1984), insufficient total caloric intake (Stark et al., 1996), and dysphagia (Lamm & Greer, 1988, Patient 3; Greer et al., 1991). For children with developmental or physical impairments, outpatient intervention has focused on enhancing feeding skills in areas such as oral–motor coordination, independent use of utensils, and/or table manners (Lusielli, 1993). An outpatient mode is also recommended for providing preventive advice to parents regarding management of normal mealtime problems (Finney, 1986).

Various disciplines are often involved in outpatient feeding interventions. Nutritionists can provide age-appropriate menus, food preparation suggestions, or other nutritional tips to enhance children's intake of desired foods, and can prescribe dietary supplements (Satter, 1999). Speech and language, physical, or occupational therapists often are involved in treating children whose oral–motor, neuromuscular, or other developmental impairments interfere with acquisition of independent feeding skills. Therapy focuses on strengthening muscle tone, posture, or oral–motor coordination and on reducing sensitivity or oral contact through skills-oriented sessions. Overall, the applied literature suggests that outpatient, multidisciplinary interventions are a viable approach for many feeding problems.

CONCLUSIONS AND FUTURE RESEARCH RECOMMENDATIONS

Significant empirical support for behavioral interventions for treating pediatric feeding disorders exists. Kerwin (1999) identified a variety of intervention strategies for treating severe feeding problems (i.e., behavioral, interactional, hypnosis, family intervention). However, "when evaluated against stringent methodological criteria [as defined by the Task Force on Promotion and Dissemination of Psychological Procedures, 1995], behavioral interventions are the only documented effective or promising treatments for pediatric feeding problems" (Kerwin, 1999, p. 202). Although behavioral interventions are the only documented effective treatments, this does not mean that interventions based on other theoretical perspectives are not efficacious. For example, Turner, Sanders, and Wall (1994) conducted a controlled group comparison of outpatient behavioral treatment and nutritional education for children with chronic food refusal. They found that behavioral treatment was superior to nutritional education for improving parent–child interactions but that both approaches resulted in improvements in target feeding and nutritional behaviors.

Although behavioral techniques are known to be effective, a general critique of the behavioral feeding literature is that intervention techniques usually are implemented either in combination or sequentially, so little is known about the relative effectiveness of each component (Kerwin, 1999). Only one study to date has systematically evaluated a multicomponent treatment using additive introduction of treatment procedures (Hoch et al., 2001). Thus an important area for future research is to systematically evaluate the relative effectiveness of specific treatment modalities for subgroups of feeding problems. Further, most research has concentrated on child outcomes, with relatively little attention to parent–child interactions involved in child feeding patterns, the environmental context associated with eating, or techniques needed to adequately train caregivers to effectively implement treatment procedures (Black, 1999; Werle et al., 1993). Few studies have monitored the long-term effects of feeding treatment, although two studies (Lamm & Greer, 1988; Stark et al., 1993) offer exceptions by documenting maintenance of treatment gains at 2-year follow-up. Additionally, Stark (1999) emphasized the need to consider nutritional adequacy of children's diet, not simply amount or type of food accepted.

Finally, the viability of inpatient versus outpatient treatment, or perhaps some combination of the two approaches, is in need of systematic study. Because outpatient treatment emphasizes cost-effective, community-based health care, it is likely to play an increasingly important role in future service delivery. On the other hand, inpatient treatment allows for professional delivery of round-the-clock services that may produce quicker behavior change in a medically safe environment and therefore may be less emotionally distressing for parents.

The efficacy of behavioral interventions for treating pediatric feeding disorders is well established. The emphasis now necessarily shifts to finding efficient ways to implement these treatments in the applied setting. Across inpatient treatment programs, there appears to be wide variability in duration of treatment. For example, Babbitt et al. (1994) reported that the average length of admission for inpatients treated at the Kennedy Krieger Institute is 61 days. By contrast, in a follow-up study of patients treated at Columbus Children's Hospital, Cook, Linscheid, Rasnake, and Lukens (2000) reported an average length of stay of less than 10 days. Differential length of stay could be explained by differences in patient acuity but may also reveal differences in treatment efficiency. In light of managed care restrictions on inpatient admissions, research on treatment efficiency should be given priority.

REFERENCES

Abidin, R. R. (1995). *Parenting Stress Index: Professional manual* (3rd ed.) Odessa, FL: Psychological Assessment Resources.

Achenbach, T. M. (1991). *Manual for the Child Behavior Checklist/4–18 and 1991 Profile.* Burlington: University of Vermont, Department of Psychiatry.

Achenbach, T. M. (1992). *Manual for the Child Behavior Checklist/2–3 and 1992 Profile.* Burlington: University of Vermont, Department of Psychiatry.

Ahearn, W. H., Kerwin, M. E., Eicher, P. S., Shantz, J., & Swearingin, W. (1996). An alternating treatments comparison of two intensive interventions for food refusal. *Journal of Applied Behavior Analysis, 29,* 321–332.

American Academy of Pediatrics, Committee on Psychosocial Aspects of Child and Family Health. (1988). *Guidelines for health supervision: II.* Elk Grove Village, IL: American Academy of Pediatrics.

Archer, L. A., Rosenbaum, P. L., & Streiner, D. L. (1991). The Children's Eating Behavior Inventory: Reliability and validity results. *Journal of Pediatric Psychology, 16,* 629–642.

Babbitt, R. L., Hoch, T. A., Coe, D. A., Cataldo, M. F., Kelly, K. J., Stackhouse, C., & Perman, J. A. (1994). Behavioral assessment and treatment of pediatric feeding disorders. *Journal of Developmental and Behavioral Pediatrics, 15,* 248–291.

Bentovim, A. (1970). The clinical approach to feeding disorders in childhood. *Journal of Psychosomatic Research, 14,* 267–276.

Birch, L. L. (1990). The control of food intake by young children: The role of learning. In E. D. Capaldi & T. L. Powley (Eds.), *Taste, experience, and feeding* (pp. 116–135). Washington, DC: American Psychological Association.

Black, M. M. (1999). Feeding problems: An ecological perspective [Commentary]. *Journal of Pediatric Psychology, 24,* 217–219.

Budd, K. S., Chugh, C. S., & Berry, S. L. (1998). Parents as therapists for children's food refusal problems. In J. M.

Briesmeister & C. E. Schaefer (Eds.), *Handbook of parent training: Parents as co-therapists for children's behavior problems* (2nd ed., pp. 418–440). New York: Wiley.

Budd, K. S., & Li, N. L. (1994, May). *Ingredients of behavioral feeding assessment: What do we need to know?* Paper presented at the annual conference of the Association for Behavior Analysis, Atlanta, GA.

Burklow, K. A., Phelps, A., Schultz, J. R., McConnell, K., & Rudolph, C. (1998). Classifying complex pediatric feeding disorders. *Journal of Pediatric Gastroenterology and Nutrition, 27,* 143–147.

Chatoor, I., Conley, C., & Dickson, L. (1988). Food refusal after an incident of choking: A posttraumatic eating disorder. *Journal of the American Academy of Child and Adolescent Psychiatry, 27,* 105–110.

Cook, C., Linscheid, T. R., Rasnake, L. K., & Lukens, C. (2000). *Long-term follow-up of patients treated for feeding problems.* Paper presented at the Millennium Conference of the Great Lakes Society of Pediatric Psychology, Cleveland, OH.

Crist, W., & Napier-Phillips, A. (2001). Mealtime behaviors of young children: A comparison of normative and clinical data. *Journal of Developmental and Behavioral Pediatrics, 22,* 279–286.

Douglas, J., & Harris, B. (2001). Description and evaluation of a day-centre-based behavioural feeding programme for young children and their parents. *Clinical Child Psychology and Psychiatry, 6,* 241–256.

Finney, J. W. (1986). Preventing common feeding problems in infants and young children. *Pediatric Clinics of North America, 33,* 775–788.

Food and Nutrition Information Center. (2002). *FNIC databases.* Retrieved February 1, 2002, from *http://www.nal.usda.gov/fnic/databases.html*

Geertsma, M. A., Hyams, J. S., Pelletier, J. M., & Reiter, S. (1985). Feeding resistance after parenteral hyperalimentation. *American Journal of Diseases in Children, 140,* 52–54.

Ginsberg, A. (1988). Feeding disorders in the developmentally disordered population. In D. C. Russo & J. H. Kadesty (Eds.), *Behavioral medicine with the developmentally disabled* (pp. 21–39). New York: Plenum Press.

Greer, R. D., Dorow, L., Williams, G., McCorkle, N., & Asnes, R. (1991). Peer-mediated procedures to induce swallowing and food acceptance in young children. *Journal of Applied Behavior Analysis, 24,* 783–790.

Gutentag, S., & Hammer, D. (2000). Shaping oral feeding in a gastronomy tube-dependent child in natural settings. *Behavior Modification, 24,* 395–410.

Hagopian, L. P., Farrell, D. A., & Amari, A. (1996). Treating total liquid refusal with backward chaining and fading. *Journal of Applied Behavior Analysis, 29,* 573–575.

Hoch, T. A., Babbitt, R. L., Coe, D. A., Ducan, A., & Trusty, E. M. (1995). A swallow induction avoidance procedure to establish eating. *Journal of Behavior Therapy and Experimental Psychiatry, 26,* 41–50.

Hoch, T. A., Babbitt, R. L., Coe, D. A., Krell, D. M., & Hackbert, L. (1994). Contingency contacting: Combining positive reinforcement and escape extinction procedures to treat persistent food refusal. *Behavior Modification, 18,* 106–128.

Hoch, T. A., Babbitt, R. L., Farrar-Schneider, D., Berkowitz, M. J., Owens, J. C., Knight, T. L., et al. (2001). Empirical examination of a multicomponent treatment for pediatric food refusal. *Education and Treatment of Children, 24,* 176–198.

Humphry, R., & Thigpen-Beck, B. (1997). Caregiver role: Ideas about feeding infants and toddlers. *Occupational Therapy Journal of Research, 17,* 237–263.

Ives, C. C., Harris, S. L., & Wolchik, S. A. (1978). Food refusal in an autistic type child treated by a multi-component forced feeding procedure. *Journal of Behaviour Therapy and Experimental Psychiatry, 9,* 61–64.

Johnson, C. R., & Babbitt, R. L. (1993). Antecedent manipulation in the treatment of primary solid food refusal. *Behavior Modification, 17,* 510–521.

Kedesdy, J. H., & Budd, K. S. (1998). *Childhood feeding disorders: Biobehavioral assessment and intervention.* Baltimore: Brookes.

Kerwin, M. E. (1999). Empirically supported treatments in pediatric psychology: Severe feeding problems. *Journal of Pediatric Psychology, 24,* 193–214.

Kuczynski, L., Kochanski, G., Radke-Yarrow, M., & Girius-Brown, O. (1987). A developmental interpretation of young children's noncompliance. *Developmental Psychology, 23,* 799–806.

Lamm, N., & Greer, R. D. (1988). Induction and maintenance of swallowing responses in infants with dysphagia. *Journal of Applied Behavior Analysis, 21,* 143–156.

Larson, K. L., Ayllon, T., & Barrett, D. H. (1987). A behavioral feeding program for failure-to-thrive infants. *Behavior Research and Therapy, 25,* 39–47.

Lindberg, L., Bohlin, G., Hagekull, B., & Palmerus, K. (1996). Interactions between mothers and infants showing food refusal. *Infant Mental Health Journal, 17,* 334–347.

Linscheid, T. R. (1999). Responses to empirically supported treatments for feeding problems [Commentary]. *Journal of Pediatric Psychology, 24,* 215–216.

Linscheid, T. R., Oliver, J., Blyler, E., & Palmer, S. (1978). Brief hospitalization in the behavioral treatment of feeding problems in the developmentally disabled. *Journal of Pediatric Psychology, 3,* 72–76.

Linscheid, T. R., & Rasnake, L. K. (1985). Behavioral approaches to the treatment of failure to thrive. In D. Drotar (Ed.), *New directions in failure to thrive: Implications for research and practice* (pp. 279–294). New York: Plenum Press.

Linscheid, T. R., & Rasnake, L. K. (2001). Eating problems in children. In C. E. Walker & M. C. Roberts (Eds.), *Handbook of clinical child psychology* (3rd ed., pp. 523–541). New York: Wiley & Sons, Inc.

Linscheid, T. R., Tarnowski, K. J., Rasnake, L. K., & Brams, J. S. (1987). Behavioral treatment of food refusal in a child with short-gut syndrome. *Journal of Pediatric Psychology, 12,* 451–460.

Luiselli, J. K. (1993). Training self-feeding skills in children who are deaf and blind. *Behavior Modification, 17,* 457–473.

Lundy, B., Field, T., Carraway, K., Hart, S., Malphurs, J., Rosenstein, M., et al. (1998). Food texture preferences in infants versus toddlers. *Early Child Development and Care, 146,* 69–85.

Madison, L. S., & Adubato, S. A. (1984). The elimination of ruminative vomiting in a 15-month-old child with gastroesophageal reflux. *Journal of Pediatric Psychology, 9,* 231–239.

Manikam, R., & Perman, J. A. (2000). Pediatric feeding disorders. *Journal of Clinical Gastroenterology, 30,* 34–46.

Mathisen, B., Worrall, L., Masel, J., Wall, C., & Shepherd, R. W. (1999). Feeding problems in infants with gastroesophageal reflux disease: A controlled study. *Journal of Pediatrics and Child Health, 35,* 163–169.

Matson, J. L, & Kuhn, D. E. (2001). Identifying feeding problems in mentally retarded persons: Development and reliability of the screening tool of feeding problems (STEP). *Research in Developmental Disabilities, 21,* 165–172.

Miller, C. K., Burklow, K. A., Santoro, K., Kirby, E., Mason, D., & Rudolph, C. (2001). An interdisciplinary team approach to management of pediatric feeding and swallowing disorders. *Children's Health Care, 30,* 201–218.

Palmer, S., Thompson R. J., & Linscheid, T. R. (1975). Applied behavior analysis in the treatment of childhood feeding problems. *Developmental Medicine and Child Neurology, 17,* 333–339.

Premack, D. (1959). Toward empirical behavior laws. I. Positive reinforcement. *Psychological Review, 66,* 219–233.

Ramsey, M., & Zelazo, P. (1988). Food refusal in failure-to-thrive infants: Naso-gastric feeding combined with interactive-behavioral treatment. *Journal of Pediatric Psychology, 13,* 329–347.

Rasnake, L. K., & Linscheid, T. R. (1987). A behavioral approach to the treatment of pediatric feeding problems. *Journal of Pediatric and Perinatal Nutrition, 1,* 75–82.

Riordan, M. M., Iwata, B. A., Finney, J. W., Wohl, M. K., & Stanley, A. E. (1984). Behavioral assessment and treatment of food refusal by handicapped children. *Journal of Applied Behavior Analysis, 17,* 327–341.

Satter, E. (1999). The feeding relationship. In D. B. Kessler & P. Dawson (Eds.), *Failure to thrive and pediatric undernutrition: A transdisciplinary approach* (pp. 121–149). Baltimore: Brookes.

Siegel, L. J. (1982). Classical and operant procedures in the treatment of a case of food aversion in a young child. *Journal of Clinical Child Psychology, 11,* 167–172.

Stark, L. J. (1999). Beyond feeding problems: The challenge of meeting dietary recommendations in the treatment of chronic diseases in pediatrics [Commentary]. *Journal of Pediatric Psychology, 24,* 221–222.

Stark, L. J., Bowen, A. M., Tyc, V. L., Evans, S., & Passero, M. A. (1990). A behavioral approach to increasing calorie consumption in children with cystic fibrosis. *Journal of Pediatric Psychology, 15,* 309–326.

Stark, L. J., Knapp, L. G., Bowen, A. M., Powers, S. W., Jelalian, E., Evans, S., et al. (1993). Increasing calorie consumption in children with cystic fibrosis: Replication with 2-year follow-up. *Journal of Applied Behavior Analysis, 26* 435–450.

Stark, L. J., Mulvihill, M. M., Powers, S. W., Jelalian, E., Keating, K., Creveling, S., et al. (1996). Behavioral interventions to improve caloric intake of children with cystic fibrosis: Treatment versus wait list control. *Journal of Pediatric Gastroenterology and Nutrition, 22,* 240–253.

Task Force on Promotion and Dissemination of Psychological Procedures. (1995). Training in and dissemination of empirically validated psychological treatments: Report and recommendations. *Clinical Psychologist, 48,* 3–23.

Thompson, R. J., Palmer, S., & Linscheid, T. R. (1977). Single-subject design and interaction analysis in the behavioral treatment of a child with a feeding problem. *Child Psychiatry and Human Development, 8,* 43–53.

Turner, K. M. T., Sanders, M. R., & Wall, C. (1994). Behavioural parent training versus dietary education in the treatment of children with persistent feeding difficulties. *Behaviour Change, 11,* 244–258.

Werle, M. A., Murphy, T. B., & Budd, K. S. (1993). Treating chronic food refusal in young children: Home-based parent training. *Journal of Applied Behavior Analysis, 26,* 421–433.

Werle, M. A., Murphy, T. B., & Budd, K. S. (1998). Broadening the parameters of investigation in treating young children's chronic food refusal. *Behavior Therapy, 29,* 87–105.

Whelan, E., & Cooper, P. (2000). The association between childhood feeding problems and maternal eating disorder: A community study. *Psychological Medicine, 30,* 69–77.

Wolper, C., Heshka, S., & Heymsfield, S. B. (1995). Measuring food intake: An overview. In D. B. Allison (Ed.), *Handbook of assessment methods for eating behaviors and weight-related problems* (pp. 215–240). London: Sage.

Wysocki, T., Huxtable, K., Linscheid, T. R., & Wayne, W. (1989). Behavioral adjustment of diabetic preschoolers. *Diabetes Care, 12,* 524–529.

29

Failure to Thrive

MAUREEN M. BLACK

Growth serves as an objective measure of children's well-being during the first years of life when energy needs are high. Birthweight triples in the first year, and birth length increases by 50% over the first year and doubles by age 4 (Berhane & Dietz, 1999). "Failure to thrive" (FTT) is a term used to describe children whose growth falls below expected patterns, based on age and gender-specific growth charts from the National Center for Health Statistics (NCHS, 2000). This chapter reviews the definition of FTT, including parameters used to measure growth, and recommendations for evaluation and management of children with FTT.

DEFINITION OF FTT

Multiple terms are used almost interchangeably to describe the condition that occurs when children's weight gain is below expectations, including pediatric undernutrition, malnutrition, poor growth, growth deficiency, growth delay, growth failure, and FTT. The most common term, FTT, is often seen as pejorative, and some clinicians rely on descriptive terms such as "growth delay." FTT is used throughout this chapter to be consistent with the primary term in the literature. Confusion also arises because some clinicians base their diagnosis of FTT on a single measure of weight-for-age or weight-for-height below the 5th or 3rd percentile, with little attention to the child's growth history, and others base their diagnosis on a deceleration in growth over time (Wright, 2000). A child who is proportional (weight-for-height approximates the 50th percentile) and is gaining weight along the 5th percentile, with no health or nutritional problems, may be small but normal. In contrast, a child whose rate of growth is below expectations may be of concern, even if none of the growth indices has dropped below the 5th percentile. Deceleration in the rate of growth is a good indicator of growth problems but requires multiple measures over time and relatively sophisticated interpretation (Wright, Matthews, Waterson, & Aynsley-Green, 1994). With no universally agreed-on criteria to determine when FTT has occurred or even the index that should be used to assess growth, FTT can be an imprecise diagnosis (Casey, 1992).

ANTHROPOMETRIC INDICES

Weight-for-age is commonly used in pediatric clinics to track children's growth and is an excellent indicator of changes in weight over time. However, weight-for-age is difficult to interpret because it does not account for variations in height (Waterlow et al., 1977). When a child's weight-for-age is low, it is not clear whether the primary problem is low weight, short stature, or a combination of the two. Weight-for-height (weight plotted by height regardless of age) reflects body proportionality. The recent update of the growth charts (NCHS, 2000) includes body mass index (BMI) for children over 2 years of age (BMI = weight in kg/height in m^2).

Low weight-for-height, or wasting, is often an early sign of malnutrition and may reflect low caloric intake. Chronic malnutrition may result in decelerated skeletal growth, indicated by low height-for-age, or stunting. Thus weight-for-height and height-for-age provide a nonredundant, comprehensive picture of growth (Waterlow et al., 1977; Sherry, 1999). Because children's height also reflects genetic contributions from their parents, height-for-age should be adjusted by a formula using the mean height of their parents (Himes, Roche, Thissen, & Moore, 1985). Growth of premature infants may be plotted on special charts (Casey, Kraemer, Bernbaum, Yogman, & Sells, 1991) or on standard growth charts adjusted for prematurity. Recommendations are to adjust for gestational age up to 24 months on weight, 40 months on height, and 36 months on head circumference (Cunningham & McLaughlin, 1999).

Weight-for-age, weight-for-height, and height-for-age can be expressed as percentile scores, percent of median scores, or standard deviation scores. Percentile scores are commonly used clinically because they are relatively easy to interpret, but they are less useful when describing variations at the extremes (e.g., < 5th percentile). Percent of median scores are often used to describe change and are calculated by dividing the child's weight (or height) by the median expected weight (or height; 50th percentile) based on the child's chronological age. Standard deviation scores (*z* scores) are commonly used for analyses because they can be used to characterize extremes and to facilitate comparisons across ages (Waterlow et al., 1977).

PREVALENCE

Based on national surveys, the prevalence rates of height-for-age and weight-for-height below the 5th percentile are consistent with expectations of 5% (National Center for Health Statistics, 2003). Surveys conducted among young children from low-income families have found growth deficiency severe enough to jeopardize children's linear growth. For example, in a survey conducted in 1983 among 1,429 children from low-income families in Massachusetts, 10.4% had height-for-age below the 5th percentile (Guyer et al., 1986). Up to 50% of children with FTT are never identified (Wright, 2000), suggesting an even higher prevalence. Although FTT is more common among infants from low-income families with limited resources, it can be found in all segments of the population (Karp, 1993).

CONSEQUENCES OF FTT

Little reliable information is available on the long-term consequences of FTT. However, FTT is widely recognized as a serious pediatric problem (Frank, Drotar, Cook, Bleiker, & Kasper, 2001). The long-term consequences of FTT are thought to include growth deficits, decreased immunological resistance, diminished physical activity, depressed performance in assessments of cognitive development, and poor academic performance (Frank et al., 2001). The relationship between nutritional status and consequences is often mediated by family, environmental, and cultural variables (Black, 1995; Drotar, 1991; Frank et al., 2001), making the family an ideal context for prevention of the negative consequences of FTT.

Evidence from community-based studies suggests that growth improves and that by 6–9 years of age, most children with FTT have experienced growth recovery (Black & Krishnakumar, 1999; Drewett, Corbett, & Wright, 1999). Although they are shorter and thinner than peers who did not experience FTT, their growth parameters no longer indicate wasting or stunting. Children with FTT who received intervention showed better growth than those who did not (Wright, Callum, Birks, & Jarvis, 1998). In addition, evidence suggests that by school age, children with a history of FTT do not have lower cognitive skills than children without a history of FTT when comparison groups are matched for socioeconomic variables (Boddy, Skuse, & Andrews, 2000; Kerr, Black & Krishnakumar, 2000; Mackner, Black, & Starr, 2003). However, there is some evidence that children with a history of FTT experience more academic problems than do adequately nourished peers (Black et al., 2002; Drewett et al., 1999).

Some caution is recommended in reading the existing literature on FTT, because much of the information has been derived from hospitalized children in academic, referral centers. Because most children with FTT are treated on an outpatient basis, studies that rely on hospitalized patients are likely to represent extreme and complex cases of FTT (Wright et al., 1998). In addition, many studies of FTT feature small samples, a lack of appropriately matched comparison groups, unstandardized assessments, evaluators who are aware of group assignment, inattention to differences in age or nutritional status, and cross-sectional, rather than longitudinal, research designs (Drotar, 1990; Drotar & Robinson, 1999).

EVALUATION AND MANAGEMENT

Because FTT is a complex, multifaceted problem with medical, nutritional, and psychosocial issues, an interdisciplinary approach is optimal to ensure that children and families receive a comprehensive evaluation and an integrated set of recommendations (Kessler, 1999). Children with FTT who receive care in interdisciplinary growth and nutrition clinics achieve better growth than children served through primary care clinics (Bithoney et al., 1991). Interdisciplinary teams often include medical, nutritional, and psychological clinicians.

Medical Considerations

Although some medical conditions can undermine children's growth (e.g., cystic fibrosis, HIV infection), most cases of FTT have no clear medical explanations (Sills, 1978). Until recently, FTT was divided into organic or nonorganic types, based on etiological factors. Organic FTT was determined by specific medical problems. When no organic cause could be identified, children's poor growth was attributed to dysfunctional psychosocial variables.

This distinction is artificial because both groups of children may experience malnutrition and may be at risk for diminished growth potential, immunological, and psychosocial consequences. Regardless of the etiology, when a child does not eat or grow at a rate consistent with age expectations, most families are concerned and at risk for conflict over mealtime choices and behaviors. The dichotomy between organic and nonorganic FTT has been replaced by a conceptualization that incorporates medical, psychological, interpersonal, family, ecological, and cultural factors into the evaluation and intervention strategies (Drotar, 1991).

Children with FTT require a careful perinatal and early medical history. Low birthweight, particularly small-for-gestational-age, is a common cause for growth delay during infancy and early childhood. Children with low birthweight remain behind their peers until approximately 5 years of age (Yip & Mei, 1996). Children with FTT are more likely to have recurring illnesses, particularly respiratory (including otitis media) and gastrointestinal problems (Rider & Bithoney, 1999).

Nutritional Considerations

A feeding interview, or diet history, is often used to evaluate children's nutritional intake. A common strategy is to ask parents to recall and report the food offered and consumed during a 24-hour period. Information from the dietary history is used to calculate the adequacy of the child's diet and to identify family mealtime patterns. In addition to questions regarding feeding practices, the clinician asks about the introduction of solid food, the child's acceptance of new foods, and the child's method of expressing pleasure or displeasure with food (Cunningham & McLaughlin, 1999).

Psychological and Developmental Considerations

Evaluations of children include their growth and feeding history; mealtime behavior; temperament; cognitive, motor, language, and social-emotional development; and parent–child interaction (Black, 1995). Oral–motor and physical problems, such as cerebral palsy, may be present in children with FTT. If the parent provides a history that includes choking or difficulty with foods of varying texture, the child's oral–motor development should be examined by an occupational therapist or another professional with training in feeding disorders (Sullivan & Rosenbloom, 1996). Children's mealtime behavior should also be assessed, including questions about where the meal takes place, availability of child-sized equipment (e.g., high chair), involvement of other family members, and competing activities (e.g., television). Parents should also be asked about feeding-behavior problems, including refusal, negativism, appetite, and pica.

Behavior Problems

Children with FTT often display difficult behavior in other settings, measured through both observation and maternal report (Black, Hutcheson, Dubowitz, Berenson- Howard, & Starr, 1996). Among some children, the behavior problems associated with feeding are part of their overall temperament, including irritability, apathy, and generalized inactivity or overactivity (Singer, Song, Hill, & Jaffee, 1990; Wolke, Skuse, & Mathiesen, 1990). Temperament refers to children's responses to their physical and social environment. A child with a passive temperament who does not demand food may be forgotten or neglected and not fed, particularly in a chaotic family. In contrast, a child with a very active temperament may be very reactive to environmental events and have difficulty maintaining the attention and focus necessary for successful feeding (Chatoor, Hirch, & Persinger, 1997). In either case, the relationship between feeding and the temperamental characteristics of the child cannot be understood without examining family dynamics and the relationship between the parent and the child. Temperament can be assessed directly through observations of the child during feeding and indirectly through questions to the parent regarding the child's adjustment to daily routines such as feeding, bedtime, bathing, dressing, and social interactions. Children who are temperamentally difficult are often resistant to changes, such as new foods.

An optimal way to evaluate children's feeding skills and temperament is to videotape parents and children having a meal. Parents may bring food or the clinic may provide food (e.g., baby food, microwavable meals, applesauce, pudding, crackers, and milk). Feeding occurs in a room equipped with a high chair, child's table and chair, and adult chairs. Rating systems, such as the Behavioral Pediatrics Mealtime Observation Scale, are useful in characterizing the interaction between the parent and child (Crist & Napier-Phillips, 2001)

Cognitive, Motor, Language, and Socioemotional Development

Standardized, norm-referenced assessments, such as the Bayley Scales of Infant Development—II (BSID-II; Bayley, 1993), the Receptive Expressive Emergent Language Scale (Bzoch & League, 1971), and the Temperamental and Atypical Behavior Scale (Neisworth, Bagnato, Salvia, & Hunt, 1999) are often used to determine children's cognitive, motor, language, and socioemotional development, because children with FTT often have developmental delays (Black, Hutcheson, Dubowitz, & Berenson-Howard, 1994).

Parent–Child Interaction

Caregivers help their children build expectations about food and mealtimes. Children, in turn, learn to interpret and satisfy feelings of hunger and satiety through feeding. A partnership develops whereby children and caregivers communicate with one another, forming a basis for the emotional attachment that is essential to healthy social functioning (Ainsworth & Bell, 1974; Satter, 1987). Parents are responsible for feeding their children healthy food on a predictable schedule in a nurturant, developmentally appropriate setting, and children are responsible for determining how much they will eat (Satter, 1987). If there is a disruption in the communication between children and parents, feeding may become an occasion for counterproductive battles over food. Although it may appear to be paradoxical, children who refuse to eat often gain power and control over their parents. Thus, when mealtimes become stressful or confrontational, children may be denied both the nutrients they require and healthy, responsive interactions with parents.

Interactional problems, such as low maternal responsivity, insensitivity to cues, and poor problem-solving skills, have been reported between children with FTT and their mothers who were observed during mealtime and playtime (Hutcheson, Black, & Starr, 1993; Robinson, Drotar, & Boutry, 2001). Under optimal circumstances, the communication between parents and children is clear because each adapts to the signals of the other and to the demands of the situation. Parent–child interaction breaks down if communication is distorted and marked by signals that lack clarity, misperceptions of signals, inconsistent responses, or responses that are not in keeping with the signal. Children vary in their capacity to communicate with their parents, and children who are ill, premature, or temperamentally challenging may be less able to initiate or sustain clear communication (Goldberg, 1977). Parents also vary in their ability to interpret their children's signals and to respond to them. For example, during the second 6 months of life children become more aware of their surroundings and may pause during feeding to look at something in their environment. A parent who interprets the pause as meaning that the child is no longer hungry may terminate the meal prematurely, leaving both parent and child frustrated. Distorted parent–child communication can contribute to higher rates of insecure attachment found among children with FTT (Brinich, Drotar, & Brinich, 1989).

Maternal Depression

Early clinical descriptions of FTT suggested an association with maternal depression (Elmer, 1960). However, controlled studies have reported no differences in psychopathology between mothers of children with FTT and mothers of adequately growing children from similar socioeconomic backgrounds (Singer et al., 1990; Benoit, Zeanah, & Barton, 1989). Nevertheless, maternal depression has a negative impact on children's behavior and development (Teti & Gelfand, 1990) and dampens the benefits of early intervention on the behavior and development of children with FTT (Hutcheson et al., 1997). Children who received home intervention early in life showed better cognitive development and more interactive behavior at age 4, but only if their mothers were not depressed

Neglect

In the past, FTT was sometimes considered to be a form of neglect. Although FTT often occurs with neglect, FTT also occurs in the absence of neglect. When neglect and FTT co-occur, children are at increased risk for cognitive delays during infancy (Mackner, Starr, & Black, 1997) and for cognitive, academic, and behavioral problems at age 6 (Kerr et al., 2000).

Beliefs about Food and Growth

Parental beliefs regarding children's size and health, nutritional needs, access to food, and family mealtime patterns contribute to children's growth by influencing the availability of foods and the feeding atmosphere (Birch & Johnson, 1994; Costanzo & Woody, 1985; Sturm, Drotar, Laing, & Zimet, 1997). Approximately one-third of families of children with FTT do not recognize that their child has a growth problem (Ayoub & Milner, 1985). If parents do not believe that their child is small or experiencing a growth problem, they may be unlikely to adhere to recommendations.

Poverty and Resources for Food Acquisition, Storage, and Preparation

Poverty can affect children directly through lack of food, health care, and adequate educational opportunities and indirectly through increased family stress, which may interfere with parents' ability to provide nutritious meals on a regular basis or in a nurturant context that facilitates eating. A family's ability to purchase healthy food may be hampered by the lack of supermarkets in low-income neighborhoods, by transportation, or by economics (Wiecha & Palombo, 1989). For families with limited financial resources, the clinician should ask about access to public assistance programs, such as food stamps, WIC (Special Supplemental Nutrition Program for Women, Infants, and Children), and TANF (Temporary Assistance to Needy Families).

Home visits provide an ideal opportunity to assess family interactions, mealtime behavior, and facilities for food preparation and storage (Black, Berenson-Howard, & Cureton, 1999). Observing the child and family in their natural environment enables clinicians to consider the contextual variables that may influence meals, including the physical environment and the presence of other family members.

TREATMENT OF CHILDREN WITH FTT

In the past, FTT was often conceptualized as a child issue, with little attention directed to families. However, with the recognition that feeding occurs within a social context (Drotar, 1991), effective interventions are interdisciplinary and involve the family and broader culture.

Nutrition

The food guide pyramid, developed by the U.S. Department of Agriculture, serves as a useful guide to ensure that children are receiving an adequate variety of foods. A daily vitamin ensures that children receive the required vitamins and minerals for their age. Nutritional recommendations should be consistent with the child's feeding skills and with the family's cultural preferences, financial limitations, and access to food stores. Children require extra calories to achieve catch-up growth or to improve their relative position on the growth charts. Families are encouraged to increase the fat content of foods and limit intake of nonnutritious foods, including juice and other sweetened drinks that provide a sense of satiety and lack of hunger at mealtimes (Cunningham & McLaughlin, 1999).

Feeding Behavior

Feeding habits and a consistent daily structure are important components of the intervention. Children need to develop expectations about when mealtimes will occur, with about 2 hours between meals and snacks. They need to eat frequently but should not "graze" or eat continuously throughout the day. Parents are responsible for establishing mealtime routines and determining what food will be offered at what times (Satter, 1987). Children are responsible for determining how much they will eat. When children refuse to eat, parents should terminate the meal, rather than engaging in conflict, bribery, or force feeding.

Parent–Child Interaction

Effective interventions focus on children within their families (Black, Dubowitz, Hutcheson, Berenson-Howard, & Starr, 1995; Wright et al., 1998). Videotapes made by families during mealtimes can be an effective part of the intervention. By watching themselves with their children, parents serve as their own models and identify strategies that promote better feeding. They practice newly acquired skills through repeated videotaped observations, analyze interaction patterns, and identify aspects of their own behavior that contribute to feeding problems or success in their children. The therapeutic use of videotaped interactions has been effective in promoting interactive behavior with adolescent mothers (Black & Teti, 1997) and caregivers who are intellectually limited or burdened with multiple stressors (McDonough, 1995; Koniak-Griffin, Verzememnieks, & Cahill, 1992). Repeated videotaping becomes familiar to families if it is incorporated into routine clinical evaluation and intervention procedures.

Parent Behavior

Viewing a mealtime videotape can help parents recognize how important they are to their child. Parents of children with FTT may feel frustrated, guilty, and disappointed with their child's poor growth. These feelings can be exacerbated by clinicians who either encourage parents to get more calories into their children without addressing the problems associated with low weight gain or blame parents when their children do not gain weight. Effective clinicians look for examples of the strength of the parent–child relationship, such as the child looking to the parent for guidance, cues, or reactions. This strategy emphasizes the parent's importance in the partnership and helps the parent develop a sense of efficacy in improving the relationship. Screening for common mental health problems, such as depression, can identify parents who may benefit from a therapeutic intervention for their own mental health needs.

Child's Behavior

Viewing a mealtime videotape can help parents see the relationship from the child's perspective. They see how the child communicates hunger and satiety and reacts to smiles or criticisms from parents. For example, children may signal satiety by upsetting their bowls. Recognizing the child's perspective is a critical step in intervention because it helps parents understand the importance of their own behavior in influencing their child's actions.

By watching themselves with their child, parents learn to differentiate successful from unsuccessful strategies. Parents serve as their own models and are empowered by identifying strategies that work for them and their child. By practicing newly acquired skills through repeated videotaped observations, parents learn to analyze interaction patterns and to identify aspects of their own behavior that contribute to feeding problems or success in their children. Clinicians do not teach parents how to interact with their children, but help parents gain a better understanding of the feeding partnership and how behavior in either partner influences the entire interaction.

Behavioral Principles

Behavioral strategies, such as modeling and natural consequences, are important components of interventions to encourage children to eat during mealtimes (Birch, 1980). Although behavioral principles form the basis of many interventions that are used to eliminate severe feeding behavior problems (Linscheid, Budd, & Rasnake, Chapter 27, this volume), there has been little research in which behavioral principles have been integrated into a social context or used with children who are living with their families and exhibit milder forms of feeding problems. In some situations, external behavioral controls may contribute to feeding problems by interfering with internal regulatory mechanisms regarding hunger and satiety (Birch & Fisher, 2000).

CONCLUSION

Recent evidence suggests that by school age, children with a history of FTT often experience recovery of BMI, though they remain shorter than their peers and may be at risk for academic problems. Children benefit from interdisciplinary services that include attention to their health, nutrition, development, and behavior, as well as to the family's beliefs toward feeding, household routines, access to food, and mealtime interactions.

REFERENCES

Ainsworth, M., &Bell, S. (1974). Mother–infant interaction and the development of competence. In K. Connolly & J. Bruner (Eds.), *The growth of competence* (pp. 97–118). New York: Academic Press.

Ayoub, C., & Milner, J. (1985). Failure to thrive: Parental indicators, types, and outcomes. *Child Abuse and Neglect, 9,* 491–499.

Bayley, N. (1993). *The Bayley scales of infant development.* San Antonio, TX: Psychological Corporation.

Benoit, D., Zeanah, C. H., & Barton, M. L. (1989). Maternal attachment disturbance in failure to thrive. *Infant Mental Health Journal, 10,* 185–202.

Berhane, R., & Dietz, W. H. (1999). Clinical assessment of growth. In D. B. Kessler & P. Dawson (Eds.), *Failure to thrive and pediatric undernutrition* (pp. 195–214). Baltimore: Brookes.

Birch, L. L. (1980). Effects of peer models' food choices and eating behaviors on preschoolers' food preferences. *Child Development, 51,* 489–496.

Birch, L. L., & Fisher, J. O. (2000). Mothers' child-feeding practices influence daughters' eating and weight. *American Journal of Clinical Nutrition, 71,* 1054–1061.

Birch, L. L., & Johnson, S. L. (1994). Appetite control in children. In J. D. Fernstrom & G. D. Miller (Eds.), *Appetite and body weight regulation* (pp. 5–15). New York: CRC Press.

Bithoney, W. G., McJunkin, J., Michalek, J., Snyder, J., Egan, H., & Epstein, D. (1991). The effect of a multidisciplinary team approach on weight gain in nonorganic failure-to-thrive children. *Journal of Developmental and Behavioral Pediatrics, 12,* 254–258.

Black, M. M. (1995). Failure to thrive: Strategies for evaluation and intervention. *School Psychology Review, 24,* 171–185.

Black, M. M., Berenson-Howard, J., & Cureton, P. L. (1999). Home-visiting intervention for families of children who experience growth delay. In D. B. Kessler & P. Dawson (Eds.), *Failure to thrive and pediatric undernutrition* (pp. 385–394). Baltimore: Brookes.

Black, M. M., Dubowitz, H., Hutcheson, J., Berenson-Howard, J., & Starr, R. H. (1995). A randomized clinical trial of home intervention for children with failure to thrive. *Pediatrics, 95,* 807–814.

Black, M. M., Dubowitz, H., Starr, R. H., Le, K. Y., Papas, M. A., & Pitts, S. (2002). Randomized trial of early home intervention among children with failure-to-thrive: Findings at age 8. Paper presented at the annual meeting of the Pediatric Academic Societies, Baltimore, MD.

Black, M. M., Hutcheson, J., Dubowitz, H., & Berenson-Howard, J. (1994). Parenting style and developmental status among children with non-organic failure to thrive. *Journal of Pediatric Psychology, 19,* 689–707.

Black, M. M., Hutcheson, J., Dubowitz, H., Berenson-Howard J., & Starr, R. H. (1996). The roots of competence: Mother–infant interaction among low-income, African-American families. *Applied Developmental Psychology, 17,* 367–391.

Black, M. M., & Krishnakumar, A. (1999). Predicting height and weight longitudinal growth curves using ecological factors among children with and without early growth deficiency. *Journal of Nutrition, 129,* 539S–543S.

Black, M. M., & Teti, L. (1997). A culturally sensitive strategy to promote communication and healthy nutrition among adolescent mothers and their infants [Videotape]. *Pediatrics, 99,* 432–437.

Boddy, J., Skuse, D., & Andrews, B. (2000). The developmental sequelae of nonorganic failure to thrive. *Journal of Child Psychology and Psychiatry, 41,* 1003–1014.

Brinich, E., Drotar, D., & Brinich, P. (1989). Security of attachment and outcome of preschoolers with histories of nonorganic failure to thrive. *Journal of Clinical Child Psychology, 18,* 142–152.

Bzoch, K. R., & League, R. (1971). *Assessing language skills in infancy: A handbook for the multidimensional analysis of language.* Baltimore: University Park Press.

Casey, P. H. (1992). Failure to thrive. In M. D. Levine, W. B. Carey, & A. C. Crocker (Eds.), *Developmental behavioral pediatrics* (2nd ed., pp. 375–383). Philadelphia: Saunders.

Casey, P. H., Kraemer, H. C., Bernbaum, J., Yogman, M. W., & Sells, J. C. (1991). Growth status and growth rates of a varied sample of low birth weight, premature infants: A longitudinal cohort from birth to three years. *Journal of Pediatrics, 119*, 599–605.

Chatoor, I., Hirch, R., & Persinger, M. (1997). Facilitating internal regulation of eating: A treatment model for infantile anorexia. *Infants and Young Children, 9*, 12–22.

Costanzo, P. R., & Woody, E. Z. (1985). Domain-specific parenting styles and their impact on the child's development of particular deviance: The example of obesity proneness. *Journal of Social and Clinical Psychology, 3*, 425–445.

Crist, W., & Napier-Phillips, A. (2001). Mealtime behaviors of young children: A comparison of normative and clinical data. *Journal of Developmental and Behavioral Pediatrics, 22*, 279–286.

Cunningham, C. F., & McLaughlin, M. (1999). Nutrition. In D. B. Kessler & P. Dawson (Eds.), *Failure to thrive and pediatric undernutrition* (pp. 99–119). Baltimore: Brookes.

Drewett, R. F., Corbett, S. S., & Wright, C. W. (1999). Cognitive and educational attainment at school age of children who failed to thrive in infancy: A population-based study. *Journal of Child Psychology and Psychiatry, 40*, 551–561.

Drotar, D. (1990). Sampling issues in research with nonorganic failure-to-thrive children. *Journal of Pediatric Psychology, 15*, 255–273.

Drotar, D. (1991). The family context of nonorganic failure to thrive. *American Journal of Orthopsychiatry, 61*, 23–34.

Drotar, D., & Robinson, J. (1999). Researching failure to thrive: Progress, problems, and recommendations. In D. B. Kessler & P. Dawson (Eds.), *Failure to thrive and pediatric undernutrition* (pp. 77–98). Baltimore: Brookes.

Elmer, E. (1960). Failure to thrive: Role of the mother. *Pediatrics, 25*, 717–725.

Frank, D. A., Drotar, D., Cook, J. T., Bleiker, J. S., & Kasper, D. (2001). Failure to thrive. In R. M. Reece & S. Ludwig (Eds.), *Child abuse: Medical diagnosis and management* (2nd ed,, pp. 307–338). Philadelphia: Lea & Feiber,

Goldberg, S. (1977). Social competence in infancy: A model of parent–infant interaction. *Merrill–Palmer Quarterly, 23*, 163–177.

Guyer, B., Wehler, C. A., Anderka, M. T., Friede, A. M., Bithoney, W., Frank, D. A., & Fogerty, S. A. (1986). Anthropometric evidence of malnutrition among low income children in Massachusetts. *Massachusetts Journal of Community Health, 1*, 3–9.

Himes, J. H., Roche, A. F., Thissen, D., & Moore, W. M. (1985). Parent-specific adjustments for evaluation of recumbent length and stature of children. *Pediatrics, 75*, 304–313.

Hutcheson, J., Black, M., & Starr, R. (1993). Developmental changes in interactional characteristics of mothers and their children with failure to thrive. *Journal of Pediatric Psychology, 18*, 453–466.

Hutcheson, J. J., Black, M. M., Talley, M., Dubowitz, H., Berenson-Howard, J., Starr, R. H., & Thompson, B. S. (1997). Risk status and home intervention among children with failure to thrive: Follow-up at age 4. *Journal of Pediatric Psychology*, 22, 651–668.

Karp, R. J. (1993). *Malnourished children in the United States: Caught in the cycle of poverty.* New York: Springer.

Kerr, M., Black, M. M., & Krishnakumar, A. (2000). Failure-to-thrive, maltreatment and the behavior and development of 6–year-old children from low-income urban families: A cumulative risk model. *Journal of Child Abuse and Neglect, 24*, 587–598.

Kessler, D. B. (1999). Failure to thrive and pediatric undernutrition: Historical and theoretical context. In D. B. Kessler & P. Dawson (Eds.), *Failure to thrive and pediatric undernutrition* (pp. 3–18). Baltimore: Brookes.

Koniak-Griffin, D., Verzememnieks, I., & Cahill, D. (1992). Using videotape instruction and feedback to improve adolescents' mothering behaviors. *Journal of Adolescent Health, 13*, 570–575.

Mackner, L., Black, M. M., & Starr, R. H. (2003). Cognitive development of children with failure to thrive: A prospective study through age 6. *Journal of Child Psychology and Psychiatry and Allied Disciplines, 44*, 518–523.

Mackner, L., Starr, R. H., & Black, M. M. (1997). The cumulative effect of neglect and failure to thrive on cognitive functioning. *Journal of Child Abuse and Neglect, 21*, 691–700.

McDonough, S. C. (1995). Promoting positive early parent–infant relationships through interaction guidance. *Child and Adolescent Psychiatric Clinics of North America*, 4, 661–672.

National Center for Health Statistics. (2000). *2000 CDC growth charts: United States*. Retrieved February 24, 2003, from *http://www.cdc.gov/growthcharts/*

National Center for Health Statistics. (2003). *National Health and Nutrition Examination Survey.* Retrieved February 24, 2003, from *http://www.cdc.gov/nchs/nhanes.htm*

Neisworth, J. T., Bagnato, S. J., Salvia, J., & Hunt, F. M. (1999). *TABS Manual for the Temperament and Atypical Behavior Scale.* Baltimore: Brookes.

Rider, E. A., & Bithoney, W. G. (1999). Medical assessment and management and the organization of medical services. In D. B. Kessler & P. Dawson (Eds.), *Failure to thrive and pediatric undernutrition* (pp. 173–193). Baltimore: Brookes.

Robinson, J. R., Drotar, D., & Boutry, M. (2001). Problem-solving abilities among mothers of infants with failure to thrive. *Journal of Pediatric Psychology, 26*, 21–32.

Satter, E. (1987). *How to get your kid to eat . . . but not too much*. New York: Bull.

Sherry, B. (1999). Epidemiology of inadequate growth. In D. B. Kessler & P. Dawson (Eds.), *Failure to thrive and pediatric undernutrition* (pp. 19–36). Baltimore: Brookes.

Sills, R. H. (1978). Failure to thrive: The role of clinical and laboratory evaluation. *American Journal of Diseases of Childhood, 32*, 967–969.

Singer, L. T., Song, L., Hill, B. P., & Jaffee, A. C. (1990). Stress and depression in mothers of failure to thrive children. *Journal of Pediatric Psychology, 15*, 711–720.

Sturm, L. A., Drotar, D., Laing, K., & Zimet, G. D. (1997). Mothers' beliefs about the causes of infant growth deficiency: Is there attributional bias? *Journal of Pediatric Psychology, 22*, 329–344.

Sullivan, P. B., & Rosenbloom, L. (1996). An overview of the feeding difficulties experienced by disabled children. In P. B. Sullivan & L. Rosenbloom (Eds.), *Feeding the disabled child* (pp. 1–10). London: MacKeith Press.

Teti, D., & Gelfand, D. (1990). The effects of maternal depression on children. *Clinical Psychology Review, 10*, 329–353.

Waterlow, J. C., Buzina, R., Keller, W., Lane, J. M., Nichaman, M. Z., & Tanner, J. M. (1977). The presentation and use of height and weight data for comparing the nutritional status of groups of children under 10 years. *Bulletin of the World Health Organization, 55*, 489–498.

Wiecha, J., & Palombo, R. (1989). Multiple program participation: Comparison of nutrition and food assistance program benefits with food costs in Boston, Massachusetts. *American Journal of Public Health, 9*, 591–594.

Wolke, D., Skuse, D., & Mathiesen, B. (1990). Behavioral style in failure to thrive infants: A preliminary communication. *Journal of Pediatric Psychology, 15*, 237–243.

Wright, C. M. (2000). Identification and management of failure to thrive: A community perspective. *Archives of Disease in Childhood, 82*, 5–9.

Wright, C. M., Callum, J., Birks, E., & Jarvis, S. (1998). Effect of community based management in failure to thrive: Randomized trial. *British Medical Journal, 317*, 571–574.

Wright, C. M., Matthews, J. N. S., Waterson, A., & Aynsley-Green, A. (1994). What is the normal rate of growth in infancy? *Acta Pediatrica, 83*, 351–356.

Yip, R., & Mei, Z. (1996). Variation of infant and childhood growth. In F. Battaglia, G. Pedraz, & F. Sawatzki (Eds.), *Maternal and extrauterine nutritional factors: Their influence on fetal and infant growth* (pp. 77–84). Madrid, Spain: Ediciones Ergon, S.A.

30

Autism and Mental Retardation

SAM B. MORGAN
JONATHAN M. CAMPBELL
JENNIE N. JACKSON

Pediatric psychologists have a history of strong involvement in clinical work and research with children who have developmental disorders such as autism and mental retardation (MR). Although pediatric psychology today deals with a diverse array of problems, many psychologists working in pediatric settings still provide clinical services to children with developmental disorders and also conduct research on these disorders. This chapter presents a current overview of defining characteristics, proposed causal mechanisms, diagnosis and assessment, treatment, and outcomes for children with autism and children with MR. The literature on these disorders is both voluminous and complex, so our presentation selectively focuses on material that we consider most relevant to professionals and students in pediatric psychology.

AUTISM

Definition and Demographics of Autism and Pervasive Developmental Disorders

The essential features of autism, as first described by Kanner (1943), have survived in fairly intact form in the current criteria set forth in the text revision of the fourth edition of the *Diagnostic and Statistical Manual of Mental Disorders* (DSM-IV-TR), which refers to autism as "autistic disorder" and classifies it as a pervasive developmental disorder (PDD; American Psychiatric Association [APA], 2000). These criteria specify three categories of symptoms that the child typically shows before 3 years of age, often referred to as the "autistic triad": (1) qualitative impairments in social interaction, (2) qualitative impairments in communication, and (3) restricted, repetitive, stereotyped behavior, interests, and activities. The core features represented by these criteria are shown in different degrees and combinations in persons with autism, and they also vary with age and level of cognitive functioning (Stone, MacLean, & Hogan, 1995).

Qualitative Impairments in Social Interaction

Autistic children show marked deficits in nonverbal behaviors that regulate social interaction, such as eye contact, facial expression, body postures, and gestures. They fail to develop normal peer relationships, to spontaneously share enjoyment and interests with other people, or to engage in social and emotional "give-and-take" with others (APA, 2000).

Qualitative Impairments in Communication

Children with autism are usually delayed in speaking or do not develop speech at all. Those who do speak may show salient problems in initiating or sustaining conversation with others, and their speech may be stereotyped, repetitive, or idiosyncratic. They typically exhibit marked deficits in engaging in varied, spontaneous make-believe play or social imitative play (APA, 2000).

Restricted, Repetitive, Stereotyped Behavior, Interests, and Activities

Children with autism may abnormally preoccupy themselves with stereotyped and restricted interests and with parts of objects. They inflexibly adhere to specific routines or rituals that have no apparent function and/or engage in stereotyped and repetitive motor mannerisms, such as hand flapping and rocking (APA, 2000).

The incidence of reported cases of autism and related PDD appears to have risen in recent years, with some prevalence estimates as high as 6 in 1,000 (Chakrabarti & Fombonne, 2001). Whether this reported increase reflects an actual rise in the number of cases, rather than wider recognition of the disorder or changes in diagnostic criteria, is still the subject of debate. Autism appears in boys about 4 times more often than in girls, although girls with autism tend to be more severely impaired (Lord & Schopler, 1987).

Other Pervasive Developmental Disorders

In addition to autism or "autistic disorder," DSM-IV-TR describes three additional subtypes of PDD: Asperger's disorder, Rett's disorder, and childhood disintegrative disorder (APA, 2000; Van Acker, 1997; Volkmar, Klin, Marans, & Cohen, 1997). These disorders, along with autistic disorder, are increasingly known as "autism spectrum disorders." All children with PDD show severe impairments, typically in communication and social interactions, that emerge in early childhood and deviate from their overall developmental level (Towbin, 1997). They usually engage in repetitious, stereotyped behaviors, interests, and activities, such as those described with autistic children. Most children with PDD (except those with Asperger's disorder) function within the mentally retarded range and are most often male (except for those with Rett's disorder, which has been reported only in females).

Asperger's disorder is the PDD category most related to autism, both historically and in common features (Klin, Volkmar, & Sparrow, 2000). It was first described by Asperger in 1944, one year after Kanner first defined infantile autism as a clinical disorder (Asperger, 1944). Asperger's disorder has only recently been recognized in the United States as a distinct syndrome, and some controversy exists as to whether individuals with Asperger's disorder show meaningful differences from high-functioning individuals with autism (Campbell & Morgan, 1998; Schopler, Mesibov, & Kunce, 1998). It appears to be more common than autism, with prevalence estimates as high as 3–4 children in 1,000, and is found about 2–4 times more frequently in boys than in girls.

The symptoms of Asperger's disorder are less evident than those of typical autism and may not become apparent until the child reaches 3 or 4 years of age or older. The two essential features are: (1) *qualitative impairments in social interaction*, such as gaze aversion, failure to develop normal peer relations, and lack of social or emotional reciprocity; and (2) *restricted and stereotyped patterns of behavior*, such as intense, persistent preoccupations with narrow interests or objects, rigid adherence to nonfunctional routines, and/or stereotyped motor mannerisms (APA, 2000). Unlike children with autism, children with Asperger's disorder typically show no significant delay in language and cognitive development. The long-term prognosis for individuals with Asperger's disorder is better than that for most individuals with autism. Most can achieve independent adjustment in adulthood, although problems in social interaction often persist (Klin et al., 2000).

Many children fail to fully meet the diagnostic criteria for a specific PDD, so the DSM-IV-TR includes the category of "PDD not otherwise specified" (PDD-NOS; APA, 2000). These children show severe impairment in reciprocal social interaction along with impairment in communication skills or the presence of stereotypic behaviors, interests, and activities (Towbin, 1997).

Biological Factors in Autism

No consistent cause of autism has been determined, but considerable evidence points to biological factors. Twin studies reveal a substantial genetic predisposition toward idiopathic autism, with concordance rates ranging from 36 to 91% for identical twins as compared with 0% for fraternal twins in general-population-based studies (Bailey et al., 1995). The heritability for an underlying risk for autism, estimated to be 90–93%, is considered to be due to polygenic influences rather than to a single gene operating in Mendelian fashion (Bailey et al., 1995).

Autism is also associated with a number of diverse neuropathological medical conditions, including phenylketonuria, congenital rubella, tuberous sclerosis, lead intoxication, congenital syphilis, fragile X, and epilepsy (Dykens & Volkmar, 1997). However, most children with autism fail to show the clear anomalies of brain structure or physiology found in many severely retarded children. Research on possible neurochemical and neuroanatomical abnormalities specific to autism has yielded few consistent findings. Perhaps the most noteworthy of the neuroimaging findings have involved anomalies in the limbic system and in the cerebellum (Courchesne, 1995; Minshew, Sweeney, & Bauman, 1997). The consensus from available genetic and neurobiological evidence is that autism is the behavioral end product of central nervous system dysfunction that may be related to a variety of prenatal, perinatal, and postnatal causal mechanisms (Dykens & Volkmar, 1997).

Intellectual, Adaptive, and Language Impairment in Autism

Although level of intelligence varies widely in children with autism, most function within the retarded range and continue to do so throughout their lives. Research indicates that only 23% of individuals with autism have IQs of 70 or higher, whereas 50% have IQs between 50 and 70 and 27% have IQs below 50 (Gillberg, 1984). Their everyday adaptive functioning is typically more impaired than their intellectual functioning and lower than that of nonautistic children of comparable developmental level (Carpentieri & Morgan, 1996). On the Vineland Adaptive Behavior Scales, children with autism show a characteristic profile, with socialization skills being lowest and communication skills next lowest (Kraijer, 2000; Rodrigue, Morgan, & Geffken, 1991).

Speech delay often represents the earliest problem noted by parents of children with autism. At least 35 to 40% fail to develop functional or communicative language at all during their lifetimes (Mesibov, Adams, & Klinger, 1997). Those who develop speech show a wide range of individual differences in ability to communicate, with most demonstrating substantial difficulty in pragmatics and semantics. On intelligence measures, they typically perform higher on nonverbal tests than on verbal comprehension tests, on which they usually show lower scores than nonautistic children of comparable age and IQ (Carpentieri & Morgan, 1994; Dennis et al., 1999). Cognitive functioning in children with autism is sometimes complicated by the presence of "splinter" skills. These isolated abilities, which may be strikingly higher than the child's general level of functioning, include motor and spatial skills, rote memory, and hyperlexia (Treffert, 1988). Savant skills occur more rarely (in only about 10% of persons with autism) and may include uncanny numerical or calendar skills or exceptional talents in music or art; in most cases these skills are demonstrated in individuals who are otherwise impaired in general intellectual and adaptive functioning.

Hypotheses Addressing the Basic Deficit in Autism

Most individuals with autism are mentally retarded, but most individuals with mental retardation are not autistic. Persons with autism appear to have peculiar deficits that go beyond those associated with typical mental retardation—deficits that impair not only cognitive functioning but also social and affective responsiveness and other reactions to the world (Bieberich & Morgan, 1998). A number of hypotheses have addressed the question of what cognitive defects account for the features of autism. As early as 1971, Lovaas and his colleagues proposed that a basic feature in autism is "stimulus overselectivity," due to an inability to shift attention (Lovaas, Schreibman, Koegel, & Rehm, 1971). Based on findings indicating cerebellar and parietal anomalies in autism, Courchesne (1995) has proposed that individuals with autism exhibit deficits in regulation of three attention operations: orienting, shifting, and distributing attention to, between, and across locations of potential importance. Another hypothesis that has received some empirical support suggests that autism may involve a deficit in executive functioning as mediated by the frontal lobes, resulting in deficiencies in flexibility and planning (e.g., Ozonoff & McEvoy, 1994). Research has also provided some support for the hypothesis that children with autism show "theory of mind" deficits; that is, they show specific difficulty in inferring that others have beliefs or intentions that differ from their own (Baron-Cohen, Leslie, & Frith, 1985; Kleinman, Marciano, & Ault, 2001).).

Early Detection and Diagnostic Assessment of Autism

With the increasing emphasis on early intervention with autistic children, the past decade has seen the development of useful tools for early detection of autism and PDD (Klinger & Renner, 2000). The Checklist for Autism in Toddlers (CHAT; Baron-Cohen, Allen, & Gillberg, 1992) and the Screening Tool for Autism in Two-Year-Olds (STAT; Stone, Coonrod, & Ousley, 2000) are designed to screen very young children for symptoms of autism. The CHAT, which includes parent report and performance-based observations, and its modified version (the M-CHAT; Robins, Fein, Barton, & Green, 2001) have been shown to be effective in screening children as young as 18 months for autism. The recently developed STAT, designed for children between 2 and 3 years of age and based on performance observations, also appears to be a promising screening tool.

The Childhood Autism Rating Scale (CARS; Schopler, Reichler, & Renner, 1988; Morgan, 1988a) and the Autism Diagnostic Observation Schedule—Generic (ADOS-G; Lord et al., 2000) represent two observational measures with strong psychometric properties. The CARS is designed as a screening measure for children 3 years of age or older, whereas the ADOS-G is a performance-based measure designed for diagnosis of autism and PDD-NOS in children 2½ years of age or older. The Autism Diagnostic Interview-Revised (ADI-R; Lord, Rutter, & Le Couteur, 1994) and the Parent Interview for Autism (PIA; Stone & Hogan, 1993) are two useful techniques based on parent interviews. (For a special issue on diagnostic assessment of autism spectrum disorders, see the *Journal of Autism and Developmental Disorders*, *29*, No. 6, 1999.)

Cognitive and Psychoeducational Assessment

Once the diagnosis of autism is made, professionals should help parents to understand what the disorder means for their child and make recommendations for further assessment (Morgan, 1984). To aid in developing treatment and educational programs, many instruments are available to assess cognitive functioning, developmental attainment, patterns of abilities and deficits, academic achievement, and adaptive skills. For very young or very low functioning children, infant scales, such as the Bayley Scales of Infant Development—Second Edition (Bayley, 1993), can yield reliable and valid measures of developmental level. Other cognitive instruments suitable for younger children include the Stanford-Binet Intelligence Scales (Thorndike, Hagen, & Sattler, 1986) and the Mullen Scales of Early Learning (Mullen, 1997), as well as the Leiter International Performance Scale—Revised (Roid & Miller, 1997) and the Merrill–Palmer Scale (Stutsman, 1948) for nonverbal, severely verbally impaired children. For older and higher functioning children, the Wechsler Intelligence Scale for Children—Third Edition (WISC-III; Wechsler, 1991) can be used.

In assessing the adaptive skills of children with autism, the Vineland Adaptive Behavior Scales (Sparrow, Balla, & Cicchetti, 1984) are quite useful, especially with the recent publication of supplementary norms for individuals with autism (Carter et al., 1998). Because the Vineland yields an overall score and specific domain scores, the child's general adaptive level can be determined, as well as a profile of adaptive functioning that can be used in treatment and educational programs.

The Psychoeducational Profile—Revised (PEP-R; Schopler, Reichler, Bashford, Lansing, & Marcus, 1990) is a measure designed to gain developmental, cognitive, and behavioral information for use in individualized education and treatment of children with autism. An adolescent and adult form of the PEP, the AAPEP, has also been developed to assess vocational and work-related behaviors and skills, as well as leisure activities (Mesibov, Schopler, Schaffer, & Landrus, 1988).

Intervention, Treatment, and Long-Term Outcome

Despite claims by ardent proponents of certain treatments for autism, no treatment has yielded a "cure," although certain interventions have been shown to be more effective than others in helping autistic persons adapt. (For a recent series of articles on pharmacological, psychoeducational, and behavioral treatments, see the *Journal of Autism and Developmental Disorders*, *30*, No. 5, 2000.)

Pharmacological Treatments

Although a number of drugs have been tried, none has been successful in significantly reducing the core symptoms of autism (Volkmar, 2001). For example, neuroleptics (e.g., haloperidol), beta blockers, clonidine, tricyclic antidepressants (e.g., clomipramine), opiate antagonists (e.g., naltrexone), and stimulants (e.g., methylphenidate) have been reported to be useful in reducing secondary symptoms, such as self-injury, stereotypic behavior, aggression, hyperactivity, and sleep disturbances (Volkmar, 2001).

Psychosocial Interventions

Children with autism spectrum disorders represent a highly heterogeneous group who respond differentially to behavioral and educational interventions, with some children showing substantial gains and others making very slow progress (Lord & McGee, 2001). The behavioral treatment program that has reported the highest success rates for children with autism is that developed by Lovaas (1987). Children began the program at about age 3 and continued for 3 years. Well-trained therapists worked with each child for an average of 40 hours per week in the child's home, school, and community. Parents were thoroughly trained in treatment procedures so that intervention took place for most of the child's waking hours. Of the 19 children in the intensive behavioral treatment group, 9 performed at normal intellectual and educational levels by first grade, whereas only 1 child in the control group achieved this level. By late childhood and adolescence, 9 of the original sample of children in the intensive-treatment group continued to be in regular educational placements with no evidence of learning problems, whereas all of the children in the control group were in special educational placements (McEachin, Smith, & Lovaas, 1993).

Although the research of Lovaas and colleagues has been generally viewed as promising, it has not escaped criticism regarding certain aspects of the design and the need for replication (e.g., Kazdin, 1993). In an evaluation of behavioral treatments based on published studies, Rogers (1998) noted that all programs reported positive results, although not as positive as those of Lovaas. She specified several variables related to treatment outcome. First, younger children (i.e., less than 5 years of age) respond more positively than older children. Second, children with higher pretreatment IQs and language skills show a better response. Third, all of the treatment studies involved 20 or more hours of therapy, with the best results coming from the program offering the most hours of treatment.

Parents should be involved as much as possible in treatment because treatments that employ parents as therapists are superior to those taking place only in the clinic (Schreibman, 2000). One obvious advantage of incorporating the parents into treatment is that it greatly enhances generalization. Although parent training is often included in treatment, an important but often neglected aspect of intervention concerns the impact children with autism have on parents and family members. Parents and siblings of autistic children may experience special stressors, and an autistic child may have a disruptive influence on the family system (Morgan, 1988b; Sanders & Morgan, 1997). To address these concerns, supportive counseling for individual family members and family therapy may be needed, as well as respite care services (Marcus, Kunce, & Schopler, 1997).

As a part of any comprehensive treatment program, a well-structured special education program is essential for the vast majority of children with autism. Such a program should begin as soon as a child is suspected of having autism and should be based on a set of individualized objectives and plans (Lord & McGee, 2001). Many children with autism and other types of PDD are now being integrated as much as possible into regular classroom programs, but most still require extensive special educational services. As the individual with autism approaches adulthood, increased emphasis should be given to assessment and training of vocational skills that will allow the individual better adjustment as an adult. A related concern is the development of community group homes that can serve as an alternative to institutional placement for adults with autism. The most effective intervention programs for children with autism and their families are broad-based and extend into the home, school, and community. The *T*reatment and *E*ducation of *A*utistic and Related *C*ommunication Handicapped *CH*ildren (TEACCH) program in North Carolina represents a model community approach that provides comprehensive, long-term treatment, educational, and vocational services to children with autism and their families (Schopler, 1997).

For a recent, comprehensive set of recommendations for interventions with children with autism spectrum disorders, see Lord and McGee (2001).

Long-Term Outcome

Any conclusions drawn from outcome studies must be tentative and subject to ongoing revision for several reasons. First, inclusion criteria have varied from study to study over the years. Second, many of the individuals studied, especially those who are now adults, did not have the benefit of programs for early diagnosis and intervention, of well-structured special education, and of vocational training that are now available in many communities. Third, adolescents and adults with autism now have more employment opportunities because of recent legal mandates (such as the Americans with Disabilities Act).

Perhaps for these reasons, the earlier studies generally presented a more dismal picture than the more recent ones, which show more variable outcomes (Stone et al., 1995). Nevertheless, as many as 66–75% of children with autism continue to function within the mentally retarded range as adults, being generally unable to lead fully independent lives (Lotter, 1978; Rumsey, Rapoport, & Sceery, 1985; Gillberg, 1991). Only 10 to 20% show relatively good outcomes in adolescence and early adulthood; that is, they show adequate social adjustment and may hold independent jobs. As adults, most retain at least some of their autistic characteristics, although these features may vary from individual to individual; most do not develop new psychiatric syndromes, but 25 to 30% develop seizures before age 30, with the typical onset in adolescence or early adulthood (Gillberg, 1991; Rumsey et al., 1985)

Research has consistently shown that the strongest predictor of positive outcome is onset of meaningful speech before age 5 or 6 (e.g., Lotter, 1978; Rumsey et al., 1985). The child who develops functional speech by this age has a much better chance of attaining marginal or good adjustment than the child with no communicative speech. Level of measured intelligence also serves as a potent predictor of eventual level of adaptation. Individuals with IQs above 60 or 70 have a much better chance of educational progress and relatively independent social and vocational adjustment than do individuals with lower IQs, who typically end up in highly sheltered settings or residential facilities (Rumsey et al, 1985; Stein et al., 2001). Other factors related to later adjustment include degree of neuropathology, presence of seizures, severity of early symptoms, and appropriateness of early play behavior (Rumsey et al., 1985). Finally, and most important from an intervention standpoint, if parents are willing to commit themselves to a structured behavioral and educational program for the child at an early age, then chances of later adaptation are increased (Lord & McGee, 2001; Schreibman, 2000).

MENTAL RETARDATION

Definitions and Classification Systems

Diagnostic guidelines published by the DSM-IV-TR (APA, 2000) and the American Association for Mental Retardation (AAMR; Luckasson et al., 1992) define MR as the presence of significantly subaverage intellectual functioning and concurrent delays in adaptive skills, with onset prior to the age of 18. Within each diagnostic system, adaptive skills include a wide range of areas such as communication, self-help, social skills, work and home living, functional academics, and self-direction. The DSM-IV-TR delineates four subcategories of MR that describe an individual's level of impairment based on intellectual functioning: mild (IQ of 50–55 to about 70), moderate (IQ of 35–40 to 50–55), severe (IQ of 20–25 to 35–40), and profound (IQ < 20–25; APA, 2000).

In contrast to the DSM-IV-TR subcategories, the 1992 AAMR guidelines introduced a level-of-supports model to describe an individual's need for intervention services within areas of delay (i.e., intermittent, limited, extensive, and pervasive). The AAMR subcategories were proposed in order to reduce reliance on IQ for classifying disability level, as well as to provide descriptions of an individual's needs for intervention services. Perhaps due to ongoing debate, the 1992 AAMR levels-of-support model has not been included in state guidelines for classification of children with MR (Denning, Chamberlain, & Polloway, 2000).

Prevalence rates of MR are frequently reported to range from 1–3% for school-age children, although rates vary considerably depending on definitions of MR, on the methods used to detect individuals with MR, and on the size of the study population. In a recent review, the average reported prevalence rate for severe MR (i.e., IQ < 50) was 3.8 per 1,000 and for mild MR (i.e., IQ from 50–70) was 29.8 per 1,000, or roughly 3% (Roelveld, Zielhuis, & Gabreëls, 1997). Males are more frequently diagnosed with MR than females, at a rate of approximately 1.2:1 in the severe range of MR and 1.4:1 in the mild range of MR (Roelveld et al., 1997).

Etiology and Causal Mechanisms

MR is associated with a large number of conditions, including genetic disorders (e.g., Down syndrome, fragile-X syndrome, tuberous sclerosis), prenatal or early environmental insults (e.g., fetal alcohol syndrome, lead poisoning), and PDD (e.g., autism, Rett's disorder; Murphy, Boyle, Schendel, Decoufle, & Yeargin-Allsop, 1998). More than 500 genetic disorders have been identified that are associated with MR, with Down syndrome and fragile-X syndrome often reported as the two most frequent genetic causes (Flint & Wilkie, 1996; Moldavsky, Lev, & Lerman-Sagie, 2001). Down syndrome occurs in about 1 in every 800–1,000 births (Ramirez & Morgan, 1998), whereas fragile-X syndrome occurs in approximately 1 in 1,000 males and 1 in 2,000 females (Murphy et al., 1998). Outside of genetic etiology, fetal alcohol syndrome is considered to be one of the leading causes of MR in the United States, occurring in about 1 per 1,000 births (Murphy et al., 1998). In approximately 30 to 40% of all individuals diagnosed with MR, no etiology can be determined (APA, 2000). In individuals with IQ scores of less than 50, approximately 40–70% receive a medical diagnosis; however, in individuals with IQ scores in the mild range of MR (50–70), a medical diagnosis is rendered in only about 20–24% of cases (Flint & Wilkie, 1996; Murphy et al., 1998). In cases in which no clear etiology exists, MR is typically thought to be the result of multiple causal factors, such as polygenic inheritance and environmental risks (e.g., Flint & Wilkie, 1996; Roelveld et al., 1997).

Characteristics

Although all individuals with MR show intellectual and adaptive deficits, they vary widely in level of intellectual functioning and present unique patterns of strengths and liabilities in adaptive skills (Luckasson et al., 1992). For example, one individual with mild MR may exhibit impaired adaptive skills in the areas of functional academics and self-care, whereas another individual with severe MR may show impairments across the entire range of adaptive areas. As noted previously, MR is associated with varied etiologies and behavioral phenotypes (Moldavsky et al., 2001). In this section, three of the most common syndromes associated with MR, Down, fragile-X, and fetal alcohol syndromes, are briefly described to illustrate the heterogeneity of cognitive and behavioral phenotypes present across individuals with MR.

Down Syndrome

Down syndrome is caused by the presence of extra genetic material from chromosome 21. Approximately 95% of individuals with Down syndrome have an extra chromosome 21 and are identified as having the "trisomy 21" subtype (Ramirez & Morgan, 1998). Approximately 3–4% of individuals with Down syndrome are classified as "translocation" subtypes due to a portion of chromosome 21 being attached to other chromosomes. The "mosaicism" subtype of Down syndrome refers to the presence of normal and trisomic cells within the individual and occurs in about 1–2% of cases. Among others, common physical characteristics associated with Down syndrome include muscle hypotonia, flat facial profile, an upward slant to the eyes (i.e., oblique palpebral fissures), and hyperflexibility (Moldavsky et al., 2001; Ramirez & Morgan, 1998). Individuals with Down syndrome often show moderate to severe MR, expressive language delays with relative strengths in pragmatical versus grammatical language abilities, and relative strengths in visual over auditory/verbal short-term memory (Chapman & Hesketh, 2000).

Persons with Down syndrome show a greater risk for a range of serious health problems, such as heart defects, leukemia, hypothyroidism, and gastrointestinal disorders (Ramirez & Morgan, 1998); therefore, increased screening for medical problems and congenital anomalies is recommended. Down syndrome is also associated with an increased risk of developing Alzheimer's-type dementia. Up to 25% of individuals with Down syndrome develop Alzheimer's-type dementia by the age of 35, and more than 50% over the age of 50 develop dementia (Chapman & Hesketh, 2000; Ramirez & Morgan, 1998). Postmortem brain studies have consistently documented the presence of the characteristic senile plaques and tangles associated with Alzheimer's-type dementia in individuals with Down syndrome over the age of 40 (Chapman & Hesketh, 2000).

In general, individuals with Down syndrome show lower levels of maladaptive behaviors and psychiatric disorders when compared with peers with MR (Chapman & Heseketh, 2000). However, parents and teachers have reported higher rates of depression when compared with peers with MR and more behavioral problems when compared with the general population (Chapman & Hesketh, 2000; Ramirez & Morgan, 1998).

Fragile-X Syndrome

Fragile-X syndrome, the most common form of inherited MR, is caused by an expanded repetition of the normally occurring CGG (cytosine/guanine/guanine) genetic sequence on the long arm of the X chromosome (Mazzocco, 2000). The abnormal genetic repetition inhibits the fragile X MR-1 (FMR-1) gene from producing a protein and results in the cognitive, affective, physical, and behavioral difficulties observed in the syndrome (Moldavsky et al., 2001). Full mutation (CGG repetitions of greater than 200) and premutation (CGG repetitions of about 50 to about 200) subtypes have been identified, with the premutation subtype generally resulting in less severe symptoms. Although significant phenotypic variability exists within each group, females are typically less severely affected than males (Mazzocco, 2000). The majority of males with fragile-X syndrome meet criteria for MR, as compared to only 50% of females with the full mutation (Klaiman & Phelps, 1998). Characteristic physical features in boys with fragile X include hyperextensible finger joints, flat feet, large ears, narrow face, and macroorchidism (i.e., enlarged testicles; Moldavsky et al., 2001). In general, the presence of physical characteristics is less prevalent in girls with fragile X (Klaiman & Phelps, 1998).

Males with fragile-X syndrome frequently exhibit social deficits, including autistic-like features (such as poor eye contact, stereotyped behavior, and perseverative speech), pragmatic language deficits, and social anxiety. Approximately 7–25% of children with fragile-X syndrome also meet criteria for autistic disorder (Mazzocco, 2000; Moldavsky et al., 2001). In contrast to males with autism, however, males with fragile-X syndrome tend to use more repetitive speech and tangential language, possibly due to increased difficulties with social anxiety, hypersensitivity, and behavioral inhibition (Belser & Sudhalter, 2001; Sudhalter & Belser, 2001). Boys with fragile-X syndrome frequently show sensory hypersensitivity across tactile, visual, and auditory channels. Hyperactivity and distractibility are also common, with up to 70% of boys meeting full criteria for attention-deficit/hyperactivity disorder (Moldavsky et al., 2001). Females with fragile-X syndrome often show a pattern of shyness, social anxiety, poor eye contact, and social avoidance, but they may also exhibit hyperactivity, inattention, and distractibility (Klaiman & Phelps, 1998).

Fetal Alcohol Syndromes

Prenatal exposure to alcohol can result in fetal alcohol syndrome or other disorders of less severity, such as partial fetal alcohol syndrome and alcohol-related neurodevelopmental disorder (Hagerman, 1999). Fetal alcohol syndrome is characterized by prenatal and/or postnatal growth delay, abnormalities of the face and head (e.g., microcephaly), and central nervous system dysfunction (Astley & Clarren, 2001). The characteristic facial phenotype includes small eyes, smooth philtrum (i.e., indistinct groove between upper lip and nose), and a thin upper lip. In addition to these physical features, children with fetal alcohol syndrome are more likely to suffer from chronic otitis media, visual problems (e.g., strabismus), cardiac problems, skeletal malformations, and immune system deficits (Smith & Graden, 1998). In addition to MR, children with fetal alcohol syndrome often exhibit problems with sustained attention, overactivity, and deficient social skills. Their conversational style has been characterized as active, over-inquisitive, and intrusive (Smith & Graden, 1998). Adults with fetal alcohol syndrome show an increased risk for psychopathology and social problems, such as incarceration, attention-deficit disorders, depression, alcohol and drug dependence, and suicide (Hagerman, 1999). It is unclear what contribution social factors play in these outcomes, as children with fetal alcohol syndrome may reside with parents who continue to abuse alcohol.

Assessment

Intelligence and Adaptive Behavior

As specified in the definition of MR, diagnosis requires documentation of significant subaverage performance on an individually administered test of intellectual ability, such as the WISC-III (Wechsler, 1991). Significant delays in adaptive behavior must also be documented across several domains. As with autism, the Vineland scales are widely used to measure adaptive behavior in individuals with MR, allowing for the assessment of adaptive functioning within the home (Sparrow et al., 1984) and classroom environments (Sparrow, Balla, & Cicchetti, 1985). Other frequently used measures of adaptive behavior include the American Association on Mental Retardation (AAMR) Adaptive Behavior Scales (Nihira, Leland, & Lambert, 1993) and the Scales of Independent Behavior, Revised (Bruininks, Woodcock, Weatherman, & Hill, 1996). The 1992 AAMR guidelines describe diagnosis of MR as the first step in a three-step process of appropriate assessment of an individual with MR. In addition to the measurement of intellectual and adaptive functioning, the AAMR recommends assessment of the individual's psychological functioning, physical health, and current environmental placement so that the most appropriate level of support and intervention can be provided (Luckasson et al., 1992).

Psychological and Emotional Assessment

Individuals with MR can suffer from the full range of psychopathology, often at rates higher than reported in the general population (Luckasson et al., 1992; Szymanski & King, 1999); therefore, assessment of emotional functioning is essential. Historically, psychological disorders appear to have been underdiagnosed in individuals with MR because the presence of MR tended to eclipse other psychopathology (Luckasson et al., 1992). Psychological and emotional assessment of individuals with MR presents problems due to their cognitive limitations and associated language delays; therefore, a focus on behavioral signs of mental illness as opposed to verbally reported symptoms is recommended. Recently published standards of practice recommend that emotional assessment should comprise a parent or caregiver interview, an interview with the individual with MR, and appropriate behavioral rating scales (Szymanski & King, 1999). A few measures of psychopathology exist for the specific purpose of assessing the psychological functioning of individuals with MR, such as the Reiss Scales (Reiss & Valenti-Hein, 1994).

Health, Physical, and Etiological Considerations

As illustrated earlier in the chapter, when contrasted with the general population, individuals with MR are at greater risk for developing a host of physical problems, such as epilepsy, cerebral palsy, and cardiac abnormalities. The AAMR guidelines and recently published practice parameters also assert that the assessment of physical health is important to establish the etiology of MR, if possible (Szymanski & King, 1999). Etiological information is important because it (1) increases professionals' awareness of associated health problems, (2) suggests possible prescriptive interventions (e.g., dietary restriction for PKU), (3) helps to guide prevention efforts, and (4) allows for individuals to be grouped together for research, administrative, and clinical purposes (Luckasson et al., 1992).

Environmental Considerations

Environmental factors significantly influence behavioral adaptation through facilitating or hindering independence, community integration, and overall well-being. For example, providing access to medical services improves an individual's physical health, and allowing an individual control of possessions improves independence and self-efficacy. For these reasons, the AAMR provides recommendations for the analysis of environments across educational programs, living environments, and employment settings (Luckasson et al., 1992). The analysis identifies factors within each environment that facilitate or inhibit adaptation and allows for the most appropriate recommendations for support systems and intervention.

Prevention and Intervention

Prevention

The last four decades have seen an increase in research on prevention of MR, resulting in the discovery of new causes of MR, new methods of early diagnosis, and new modes of prevention (Alexander, 1998). Prevention of MR can now begin before conception. For example, new technology allows parents to be tested to determine if they are carrying a gene that might indicate a higher risk for their child developing MR or another developmental disability. There are several ways that pregnant women can help prevent MR. Dietary supplementation of folic acid prior to and during pregnancy lowers, by 50–75%, the risk for neural tube defects, a cause of MR. Early diagnosis with screening techniques, such as ultrasound imaging, amniocentesis, and maternal serum alpha-fetoprotein screening, allows parents more time to prepare for rearing a child with a disability or to consider experimental treatment. Blood tests conducted in the first few days after birth can detect metabolic disorders such as PKU and congenital hypothyroidism, both of which lead to MR if left untreated. Regular immunizations for newborns and infants also have been associated with reduced prevalence rates of MR (Alexander, 1998).

When compared with medical risk factors, environmental and sociocultural contributions to MR are often more complex and difficult to alter, and successful prevention efforts have been grounded in legal mandates and social policy. For example, a 98% decrease in rates of MR due to lead poisoning has been associated with legislation limiting the use of lead in materials such as paint and gasoline (Alexander, 1998). Legislation requiring seat belt use, airbags, and bike helmets also has been associated with reductions in the incidence of MR due to head injury (Alexander, 1998).

Lack of stimulation contributes to diminished brain development and poor cognitive functioning in some individuals (Alexander, 1998). Based on such findings, early intervention programs have been implemented to improve the cognitive development of infants, toddlers, and young children identified with developmental delays. Provision of an enriched and stimulating environment has been shown to reduce the risk of poor cognitive development, particularly within the first 5 years of life, a crucial developmental period for children

(Alexander, 1998; Guralnick, 1998). Research suggests that intervention programs that provide greater amounts of intensive and direct individualized services to children appear to have the greatest benefits in altering the child's earlier experiences (Ramey & Ramey, 1999).

Behavioral Intervention

The predominant approach to treating children and adults with MR employs behavioral methods to increase adaptive skills and decrease maladaptive behaviors. Behavioral techniques, such as task analysis, shaping, chaining, and prompting, are frequently used in combination to teach adaptive skills in a systematic manner (Miltenberger, 2001). Once adaptive skills are reliably performed within one setting, intervention focuses on teaching the individual to generalize the skills to other settings. Numerous single-subject research studies have documented the efficacy of behavioral training to improve self-care, social, academic, and vocational skills (e.g., Garff & Storey, 1998; LeBlanc, Hagopian, & Maglieri, 2000; McDougall & Brady, 1998).

Within educational and health-care settings, up to 15% of individuals with MR exhibit problem behaviors such as self-injury, self-stimulation, and/or aggression (Emerson et al., 2001). Extensive reviews have indicated that problem behaviors can be reduced significantly through behavioral intervention, with positive and punishment-based interventions producing equivalent results (Carr et al., 1999; Scotti, Evans, Meyer, & Walker, 1991). Behavioral interventions that include a functional analysis and attempt to generalize behavioral changes typically result in improved treatment outcomes (e.g., Scotti et al., 1991). Carr et al. (1999) recommended that service providers reduce problem behaviors through the use of positive behavior support techniques, such as curricular modification and functional communication training, that are grounded in knowledge about the functional relationship between the individual's environment and his or her skill deficits.

Psychopharmacological Intervention

As with autism, a variety of drugs has been used to manage cognitive, behavioral, and psychiatric difficulties in individuals with MR (Szymanski & King, 1999). In the case of fragile X, for example, stimulants, selective serotonin reuptake inhibitors (SSRIs), mood stabilizers, and atypical antipsychotics have been used to treat symptoms of hyperactivity, anxiety, agitation, and aggression (Hagerman, 1999). Similar guidelines have been offered in the management of behavioral difficulties in individuals with other causes of MR, such as fetal alcohol syndrome. At present, significant overlap exists in the psychopharmacological treatment recommendations across syndromes; however, identification of "psychopharmacological phenotypes" has been identified as a future goal within psychiatry (Hagerman, 1999). Successful psychopharmacological phenotyping would lead to the use of medications that work best for various syndromes. Controlled research on the clinical efficacy of psychotropic medication in treating individuals with MR is lacking (e.g., Hagerman, 1999) and has resulted in criticisms regarding the use of psychotropic medications with individuals with MR (e.g., Matson et al., 2000).

Special Education and Inclusion

The reauthorization of the Individuals with Disabilities Education Act (IDEA; 1997) continued legal mandates designed to improve education for children with disabilities, such as

MR. IDEA requires educational systems to educate children with MR in the least restrictive environment with appropriate educational supports. The least restrictive environment for some children with MR constitutes full inclusion, that is, the practice of educating children with special needs within general classroom settings. Inclusion is a controversial educational practice, as evidenced by research reports and expert opinions that differ regarding the benefits and risks associated with educating children with special needs alongside typically developing peers. Chesley and Calaluce (1997), for example, argued that inclusive educational practices may not focus on teaching necessary functional and vocational skills to individuals with MR. This position is countered by recent research findings that demonstrate the social and academic benefits of inclusion (e.g., Freeman & Alkin, 2000). The controversy points to the need for research on the question of whether inclusion is equally applicable to all children with MR.

Outcomes

Employment

Employment opportunities for individuals with MR have grown in the past few decades due to federal policies, such as the Americans With Disabilities Act (ADA), that promote employment for individuals with disabilities and prohibit discrimination (McDermott, Martin, & Butkus, 1999). After the ADA was passed, the employment rate for individuals with MR rose 2% from 1986 to 1991, and approximately 30–40% of adults with MR were employed in 1994 and 1995 (Blanck, 1998). McDermott et al. (1999) found that 10% of individuals with MR were employed, working in grocery stores, fast-food restaurants, large department stores, and other service settings, earning about $105 per week, on average. In the past, individuals with MR typically began working in sheltered workshops soon after high school, learning skills consistent with remaining on task and maintaining stamina. Although sheltered workshops may be appropriate for certain individuals with MR, they are highly structured and overprotective, and skills that are learned show little transfer to other job situations (Kiernan, 2000). There is limited opportunity for the worker to become self-sufficient or develop peer networks with people other than those with disabilities. These restrictions associated with sheltered workshops have led to the development of supported employment programs that place individuals with MR in real job settings with a range of supports, such as on-site training (McDermott et al., 1999). Recent research suggests that 70% of the individuals in supported employment settings have been diagnosed with MR (Mank, Cioffi, & Yovanoff, 1997).

Living

In 1998, there were approximately 3.24 million people with MR and other developmental disabilities living in the United States, about 1.2% of the population (Braddock, Emerson, Felce, & Stancliffe, 2001). Of this population, 13% were living in supervised residential services, 60% were living with family caregivers, 13% were living on their own, and 15% were living with a spouse (Braddock et al., 2001). The deinstitutionalization movement, which advocated the closing of numerous state-funded mental hospitals in order to integrate patients into the community, resulted in an expansion of community-based services. Lakin, Prouty, Polister, and Anderson (2000) found that, as of June 1999, three-fourths of individuals with MR and other developmental disorders were living in residential facilities of 15 or fewer occupants. The Independent Living Movement (ILM) has also had an impact on the living situations of individuals with MR (Keigher, 2000). The goal of the ILM movement is to maximize independence and self-sufficiency for individuals with MR and other disabilities (Keigher, 2000).

Mortality

Researchers have found that mortality rates among individuals with MR increase with the severity of their disabilities and disabling conditions (Hayden, 1998). Respiratory diseases are among the most common causes of death for people with MR and are best predicted by nonambulation (Chaney & Eyman, 2000; Hayden, 1998). Other common causes of death among individuals with MR are cardiovascular disease and neoplasms (i.e., a new growth of tissue serving no physiological function), which affect men and women equally (Patja, Molsa, & Iivanainen, 2001). Researchers have concluded that health promotion in the community to fight and prevent infections and cardiac disease is crucial in reducing these causes of death for people with MR. Suicide has been found to be a rare occurrence among people with MR in comparison with the general population, On average, individuals with MR commit suicide at a rate that is 33% lower than that of the general population; however, the risk factors are similar for both groups. As with adults in the general population who commit suicide, most individuals with MR who commit suicide suffer from untreated depression and poor social support (Patja, Iivanainen, Raitasuo, & Lonnqvist, 2001).

SUMMARY AND CONCLUSIONS

This chapter has selectively reviewed current topics in research and practice concerning autism and mental retardation. Pediatric psychologists should continue to play a substantive role in the early identification and assessment of children with these disorders, as well as in the development and implementation of effective intervention programs. Such programs should include individualized treatment and educational services that begin as early in the child's life as possible and that actively involve the parents and family. Pediatric psychologists should also continue to make contributions through research that provides not only a better understanding of autism and mental retardation but that also yields information that benefits the lives of children and families affected by these disorders.

REFERENCES

Alexander, D. (1998). Prevention of mental retardation: Four decades of research. *Mental Retardation and Developmental Disabilities, 4,* 50–58.

American Psychiatric Association. (2000). *Diagnostic and statistical manual of mental disorders* (4th ed., text rev.). Washington, DC: Author.

Asperger, H. (1944). Die "autistichen psychopathen" in Kindesalter. *Archiv fur Psychiatrie and Nervenkrankheiten, 117*, 76–136.

Astley, S. J., & Clarren, S. K. (2001). Measuring the facial phenotype of individuals with prenatal alcohol exposures: Correlations with brain dysfunction [Electronic version]. *Alcohol and Alcoholism, 36,* 147–159.

Bailey, A., Le Couteur, A., Gottesman, I., Bolton, P., Simonoff, E., Yuzda, E., et al. (1995). Autism as a strongly genetic disorder: Evidence from a British twin study. *Psychological Medicine, 25*, 63–77.

Baron-Cohen, S., Allen, C., & Gillberg, C. (1992). Can autism be diagnosed at 18 months? The needle, the haystack, and the CHAT. *British Journal of Psychiatry, 161*, 839–843.

Baron-Cohen, S., Leslie, A.M., & Frith, U. (1985). Does the autistic child have a theory of mind? *Cognition, 21,* 37–46.

Bayley, N. (1993). *Bayley Scales of Infant Development—Second Edition.* San Antonio, TX: Psychological Corporation.

Belser, R. C., & Sudhalter, V. (2001). Conversational characteristics of children with Fragile X syndrome: Repetitive speech. *American Journal on Mental Retardation, 106,* 28–38.

Bieberich, A., & Morgan, S. B. (1998). Affective expression in children with autism or Down syndrome. *Journal of Autism and Developmental Disorders, 28,* 333–338.

Blanck, P. (1998). *The Americans With Disabilities Act and the emerging workforce: Employment of people with mental retardation.* Washington DC: American Association on Mental Retardation.

Braddock, D., Emerson, E., Felce, D., & Stancliffe, R. J. (2001). Living circumstances of children and adults with mental retardation or developmental disabilities in the United States, Canada, England, and Wales, and Australia. *Mental Retardation and Developmental Disabilities, 7,* 115–121.

Bruininks, R. H., Woodcock, R. W., Weatherman, R. F., & Hill, B. K. (1996). *Scales of Independent Behavior, Revised.* Chicago, IL: Riverside.

Campbell, J. M., & Morgan, S. B. (1998). Asperger's disorder. In L. Phelps (Ed.), *Health-related disorders in children and adolescents* (pp. 68–73). Washington, DC: American Psychological Association.

Carpentieri, S., & Morgan, S. B. (1994). Brief report: Patterns of cognitive functioning on the Stanford-Binet, Fourth Edition: A comparison of autistic and retarded children. *Journal of Autism and Developmental Disorders, 24,* 215–223.

Carpentieri, S., & Morgan, S. B. (1996). Adaptive and intellectual functioning in autistic and non-autistic retarded children. *Journal of Autism and Developmental Disorders, 26,* 611–620.

Carr, E. G., Horner, R. H., Turnbull, A. P., Marquis, J. G., McLaughlin, D. M., McAtee, M. L., et al. (1999). *Positive behavior support for people with developmental disabilities: A research synthesis.* Washington, DC: American Association on Mental Retardation.

Carter, A. S., Volkmar, F. R., Sparrow, S. S., Wang, J., Lord, C., Dawson, G., et al. (1998). The Vineland Adaptive Behavior Scales: Supplementary norms for individuals with autism. *Journal of Autism and Developmental Disorders, 28,* 287–302.

Chakrabarti, S., & Fombonne, E. (2001). Pervasive developmental disorders in preschool children. *Journal of the American Medical Association, 285,* 3093–3099.

Chaney, R. H., & Eyman, R. K. (2000). Patterns of mortality over 60 years among persons with mental retardation in a residential facility. *Mental Retardation, 38,* 289–293.

Chapman, R. S., & Hesketh, L. J. (2000). Behavioral phenotype of individuals with Down syndrome. *Mental Retardation and Developmental Disabilities Research Reviews, 6,* 84–95.

Chesley, G. M., & Calaluce, P. D. (1997). The deception of inclusion. *Mental Retardation, 35,* 488–490.

Courchesne, E. (1995). Infantile autism: Part 1. MR imaging abnormalities and their neurobehavioral correlates. *International Pediatrics, 10,* 141–154.

Denning, C. B., Chamberlain, J. A., & Polloway, E. A. (2000). An evaluation of state guidelines for mental retardation: Focus on definition and classification practices. *Education and Training in Mental Retardation and Developmental Disabilities, 35,* 226–236.

Dennis, M., Lockyer, L., Lazenby, A. L., Donnelly, R. E., Wilkinson, M., & Schoonheyt, W. (1999). Intelligence patterns among children with high-functioning autism, phenylketonuria, and childhood head injury. *Journal of Autism and Developmental Disorders, 29,* 5–17.

Dykens, E. M., & Volkmar, F. R. (1997). Medical conditions associated with autism. In D. J. Cohen & F. R. Volkmar (Eds.), *Handbook of autism and pervasive developmental disorders* (2nd ed., pp. 388–410). New York: Wiley.

Emerson, E., Kiernan, C., Alborz, A., Reeves, D., Mason, H., Swarbrick, R., et al. (2001). The prevalence of challenging behaviors: A total population study. *Research in Developmental Disabilities, 22,* 77–93.

Flint, J., & Wilkie, A. O. M. (1996). The genetics of mental retardation. *British Medical Bulletin, 52,* 453–464.

Freeman, S. F., & Alkin, M. C. (2000). Academic and social attainment of children with mental retardation in general education and special education settings. *Remedial and Special Education, 21,* 3–18.

Garff, J. T., & Storey, K. (1998). The use of self-management strategies for increasing the appropriate hygiene of persons with disabilities in supported employment settings. *Education and Training in Mental Retardation and Developmental Disabilities, 33,* 179–188.

Gillberg, C. (1984). Infantile autism and other childhood psychoses in a Swedish urban region: Epidemiological aspects. *Journal of Child Psychology and Psychiatry, 25,* 35–43.

Gillberg, C. (1991). Outcome in autism and autistic-like conditions. *Journal of the American Academy of Child and Adolescent Psychiatry, 30,* 375–382.

Guralnick, M. J. (1998). Effectiveness of early intervention for vulnerable children: A developmental perspective. *American Journal on Mental Retardation, 102,* 319–345.

Hagerman, R. J. (1999). Psychopharmacological interventions in fragile X syndrome, fetal alcohol syndrome, Prader-Willi syndrome, Angelman syndrome, Smith-Magenis syndrome, and velocariofacial syndrome. *Mental Retardation and Developmental Disabilities Research Reviews, 5,* 305–313.

Hayden, M. F. (1998). Mortality among people with mental retardation living in the United States: Research review and policy application. *Mental Retardation, 36,* 345–359.

Individuals with Disabilities Education Act Amendments of 1997, Public Law No. 105–17, 20 U.S.C. Chapter 33, Section 1415 *et seq.* (EDLAW, 1997).

Kanner, L. (1943). Autistic disturbances of affective contact. *Nervous Child, 2,* 217–250.

Kazdin, A. E. (1993). Replication and extension of behavioral treatment of autistic disorder. *American Journal on Mental Retardation, 97,* 375–376.

Keigher, S. (2000). Emerging issues in mental retardation: Self-determination versus self-interest. *Health and Social Work, 25,* 163–168.

Kiernan, W. (2000). Where we are now: Perspectives on employment of persons with mental retardation. *Focus on Autism and Other Developmental Disabilities, 15,* 90–96.

Klaiman, R. S., & Phelps, L. (1998). Fragile X syndrome. In L. Phelps (Ed.), *Health-related disorders in children and adolescents* (pp. 299–308). Washington, DC: American Psychological Association.

Kleinman, J., Marciano, P. L., & Ault, R. L. (2001). Advanced theory of mind in high-functioning adults with autism. *Journal of Autism and Developmental Disorders, 31,* 29–36.

Klin, A., Volkmar, F. R., & Sparrow, S. S. (Eds.). (2000). *Asperger syndrome.* New York: Guilford Press.

Klinger, L. G., & Renner, P. (2000). Performance-based measures in autism: Implications for diagnosis, early detection, and identification of cognitive profiles. *Journal of Clinical Child Psychology, 29,* 479–492.

Kraijer, D. (2000). Review of adaptive behavior studies in mentally retarded persons with autism/pervasive developmental disorder. *Journal of Autism and Developmental Disorders, 30,* 39–47.

Lakin, K. C., Prouty, R., Polister, B., & Anderson, L. (2000). Over three quarters of all residential service recipients in community settings as of June 1999. *Mental Retardation, 38,* 378–379.

LeBlanc, L. A., Hagopian, L. P., & Maglieri, K. A. (2000). Use of a token economy to eliminate excessive inappropriate social behavior in an adult with developmental disabilities. *Behavioral Interventions, 15,* 135–143.

Lord, C., & McGee, J. P. (Eds.). (2001). *Educating children with autism.* Washington, DC: National Academy Press.

Lord, C., Risi, S., Lambrecht, L., Cook, E. H., Leventhal, B. L., DiLavore, P. C., et al. (2000). The Autism Diagnostic Observation Schedule—Generic: A standard measure of social and communication deficits associated with the spectrum of autism. *Journal of Autism and Developmental Disorders, 30,* 205–223.

Lord, C., Rutter, M., & Le Couteur, A. (1994). Autism Diagnostic Interview—Revised: A revised version of a diagnostic interview for caregivers of individuals with possible pervasive developmental disorders. *Journal of Autism and Developmental Disorders, 24,* 659–685.

Lord, C., & Schopler, E. (1987). Neurobiological implications of sex differences in autism. In E. Schopler & G. B. Mesibov (Eds.), *Neurobiological issues in autism* (pp. 191–211). New York: Plenum Press.

Lotter, V. (1978). Follow-up studies. In M. Rutter & E. Schopler (Eds.), *Autism: A reappraisal of concepts and treatment* (pp. 475–505). New York: Plenum Press.

Lovaas, O. I. (1987). Behavioral treatment and normal educational and intellectual functioning in young autistic children. *Journal of Consulting and Clinical Psychology, 55,* 3–9.

Lovaas, O. I., Schreibman, L., Koegel, R., & Rehm, R. (1971). Selective responding by autistic children to multiple sensory input. *Journal of Abnormal Psychology, 77,* 211–222.

Luckasson, R., Coulter, D. L., Polloway, E. A., Reiss, S., Schalock, R. L., Snell, M. E., et al. (Eds.). (1992). *Mental retardation: Definitions, classification, and systems of support.* Washington, DC: Author.

Mank, D., Cioffi, A., & Yovanoff, P. (1997). Analysis of the typicalness of supported employment jobs, natural supports, and wage and integration outcomes. *Mental Retardation, 35,* 185–197.

Marcus, L. M., Kunce, L. J., & Schopler, E. (1997). Working with families. In D. J. Cohen & F. R. Volkmar (Eds.), *Handbook of autism and pervasive developmental disorders* (2nd ed., pp. 631–649). New York: Wiley.

Matson, J. L., Bamburg, J. W., Mayville, E. A., Pinkston, J., Bielecki, J., Kuhn, D., et al. (2000). Psychopharmacology and mental retardation: A 10-year review (1990–1999). *Research in Developmental Disabilities, 21,* 263–296.

Mazzocco, M. M. (2000). Advances in research on the fragile X syndrome. *Mental Retardation and Developmental Disabilities Research Reviews, 6,* 96–106.

McDermott, S., Martin, M., & Butkus, S. (1999). What individual, provider, and community characteristics predict employment of individuals with mental retardation? *American Journal on Mental Retardation, 104,* 346–355.

McDougall, D., & Brady, M. P. (1998). Initiating and fading self-management interventions to increase math fluency in general education classes. *Exceptional Children, 64,* 151–166.

McEachin, J. J., Smith, T., & Lovaas, O. I. (1993). Long-term outcome for children with autism who received early intensive behavioral treatment. *American Journal on Mental Retardation, 97,* 359–372.

Mesibov, G., Schopler, E., Schaffer, B., & Landrus, R. (1988). *Individualized assessment and treatment for autistic and developmentally disabled children: Vol. 4. The Adolescent and Adult Psychoeducational Profile (AAPEP).* Austin, TX: Pro-Ed.

Mesibov, G. B., Adams, L. W., & Klinger, L. G. (1997). *Autism: Understanding the disorder.* New York: Plenum Press.

Miltenberger, R. C. (2001). *Behavior modification: Principles and procedures* (2nd ed.). Belmont, CA: Wadsworth/Thomson Learning.

Minshew, N. J., Sweeney, J. A., & Bauman, M. L. (1997). Neurological aspects of autism. In D. J. Cohen & F. R. Volkmar (Eds.), *Handbook of autism and pervasive developmental disorders* (2nd ed., pp. 344–369). New York: Wiley.

Moldavsky, M., Lev, D., & Lerman-Sagie, T. (2001). Behavioral phenotypes of genetic syndromes: A reference guide for psychiatrists. *Journal of the American Academy of Child and Adolescent Psychiatry, 40,* 749–761.

Morgan, S. (1988a). Diagnostic assessment of autism: A review of objective scales. *Journal of Psychoeducational Assessment, 6,* 139–151.

Morgan, S. B. (1984). Helping parents understand the diagnosis of autism. *Journal of Developmental and Behavioral Pediatrics, 5,* 78–85.

Morgan, S. B. (1988b). The autistic child and family functioning: A developmental–family systems perspective. *Journal of Autism and Developmental Disorders, 18,* 263–280.

Mullen, E. M. (1997). *Mullen Scales of Early Learning.* Los Angeles: Western Psychological Services.

Murphy, C. C., Boyle, C., Schendel, D., Decoufle, P., & Yeargin-Allsopp, M. (1998). Epidemiology of mental retardation in children. *Mental Retardation and Developmental Disabilities Research Reviews, 4,* 6–13.

Nihira, K., Leland, H., & Lambert, N. (1993). *AAMR Adaptive Behavior Scale, Residential and Community* (2nd ed.). Austin, TX: Pro-Ed.

Ozonoff, S., & McEvoy, R. (1994). A longitudinal study of executive function and theory of mind development in autism. *Development and Psychopathology, 6,* 415–431.

Patja, K., Iivanainen, M., Raitasuo, S., & Lonnqvist, J. (2001). Suicide mortality in mental retardation: A 35-year follow-up study. *Acta Psychiatrica Scandinavica, 103,* 307–311.

Patja, K., Molsa, P., & Iivanainen, M. (2001). Cause-specific mortality of people with intellectual disability in a population-based, 35-year follow-up study. *Journal of Intellectual Disability Research, 45,* 30–40.

Ramey, S. L., & Ramey, C. T. (1999). Early experience and early intervention for children "at risk" for developmental delay and mental retardation. *Mental Retardation and Developmental Disabilities, 5,* 1–10.

Ramirez, S. Z., & Morgan, V. (1998). Down syndrome. In L. Phelps (Ed.), *Health-related disorders in children and adolescents* (pp. 68–73). Washington, DC: American Psychological Association.

Reiss, S., & Valenti-Hein, D. (1994). Development of a psychopathology rating scale for children with mental retardation. *Journal of Consulting and Clinical Psychology, 62,* 28–33.

Robins, D. L., Fein, D., Barton, M. L., & Green, J. A. (2001). The Modified Checklist for Autism in Toddlers: An initial study investigating the early detection of autism and pervasive developmental disorder. *Journal of Autism and Developmental Disorders, 31,* 131–144.

Rodrigue, J. R., Morgan, S. B., & Geffken, G. R. (1991). A comparative evaluation of adaptive behavior in children and adolescents with autism, Down syndrome, and normal development. *Journal of Autism and Developmental Disorders, 21,* 187–196.

Roelveld, N., Zielhuis, G. A., & Gabreëls, F. (1997). The prevalence of mental retardation: A critical review of recent literature. *Developmental Medicine and Child Neurology, 39,* 125–132.

Rogers, S. J. (1998). Empirically supported comprehensive treatments for young children with autism. *Journal of Clinical Child Psychology, 27,* 168–179.

Roid, G., & Miller, L. (1997). *Leiter International Performance Scale—Revised.* Wood Dale, IL: Stoelting.

Rumsey, J. M., Rapoport, J. L., & Sceery, W. R. (1985). Autistic children as adults: Psychiatric, social, and behavioral outcomes. *Journal of the American Academy of Child Psychiatry, 24,* 465–473.

Sanders, J. L., & Morgan, S. B. (1997). Family stress and adjustment as perceived by parents of children with autism or Down syndrome: Implications for intervention. *Child and Family Behavior Therapy, 19,* 15–32.

Schopler, E. (1997). Implementation of TEACCH philosophy. In D. J. Cohen & F. R. Volkmar (Eds.), *Handbook of autism and pervasive developmental disorders* (2nd ed., pp. 767–795). New York: Wiley.

Schopler, E., Mesibov, G., & Kunce, L. J. (Eds.). (1998). *Asperger syndrome or high-functioning autism?* New York: Plenum Press.

Schopler, E., Reichler, R. J., Bashford, A., Lansing, M., & Marcus, L.(1990). *Individualized assessment and treatment for autistic and developmentally disabled children: Vol. 1. The Psychoeducational Profile—Revised (PEP-R).* Austin, TX: Pro-Ed.

Schopler, E., Reichler, R. J., & Renner, B. R. (1988). *The Childhood Autism Rating Scale (CARS).* Los Angeles: Western Psychological Services.

Schreibman, L. (2000). Intensive behavioral/psychoeducational treatments for autism: Research needs and future directions. *Journal of Autism and Developmental Disorders, 30*, 373–378.

Scotti, J. R., Evans, I. M., Meyer, L. H., & Walker, P. (1991). A meta-analysis of intervention research with problem behavior: Treatment validity and standards of practice. *American Journal of Mental Retardation, 96*, 233–256.

Smith, J. J., & Graden, J. L. (1998). Fetal alcohol syndrome. In L. Phelps (Ed.), *Health-related disorders in children and adolescents* (pp. 68–73). Washington, DC: American Psychological Association.

Sparrow, S. S., Balla, D. A., & Cicchetti, D. V. (1984). *Vineland Adaptive Behavior Scales, Interview Edition, Survey Form Manual.* Circle Pines, MN: American Guidance Service.

Sparrow, S. S., Balla, D. A., & Cicchetti, D. V. (1985). *Vineland Adaptive Behavior Scales, Classroom Edition Manual.* Circle Pines, MN: American Guidance Service.

Stein, D., Ring, A., Shulman, C., Meir, D., Holan, A., Weizman, A., & Barak, Y. (2001). Children with autism as they grow up: Description of adult inpatients with severe autism. *Journal of Autism and Developmental Disorders, 31*, 355–360.

Stone, W. L., Coonrod, E. E., & Ousley, O. Y. (2000). Screening tool for autism in two-year-olds (STAT): Development and preliminary data. *Journal of Autism and Developmental Disorders, 30*, 607–612.

Stone, W. L., & Hogan, K. L. (1993). A structured parent interview for identifying young children with autism. *Journal of Autism and Developmental Disorders, 23*, 639–652.

Stone, W. L., MacLean, W. E., & Hogan, K. L. (1995). Autism and mental retardation. In M. C. Roberts (Ed.), *Handbook of pediatric psychology* (2nd ed., pp. 655–675). New York: Guilford Press.

Stutsman, R. (1948). *The Merrill–Palmer Scale of Mental Tests.* Chicago, IL: Stoelting.

Sudhalter, V., & Belser, R. C. (2001). Conversational characteristics of children with Fragile X syndrome: Tangential language. *American Journal on Mental Retardation, 106*, 389–400.

Szymanski, L., & King, B. H. (1999). Practice parameters for the assessment and treatment of children, adolescents, and adults with mental retardation and comorbid mental disorders. *Journal of the American Academy of Child and Adolescent Psychiatry, 38*(Suppl.), 5S–31S.

Thorndike, R. L., Hagen, E. P., & Sattler, J. M. (1986). *Guide for administering and scoring for the Stanford-Binet Intelligence Scale* (4th ed.). Chicago: Riverside.

Towbin, K. F. (1997). Pervasive Developmental Disorder Not Otherwise Specified. In D. J. Cohen & F. R. Volkmar (Eds.), *Handbook of autism and pervasive developmental disorders* (2nd ed., pp. 123–147). New York: Wiley.

Treffert, D. A. (1988). The idiot savant: A review of the syndrome. *American Journal of Psychiatry, 145*, 563–572.

Van Acker, R. (1997). Rett's syndrome: A pervasive developmental disorder. In D. J. Cohen & F. R. Volkmar (Eds.), *Handbook of autism and pervasive developmental disorders* (2nd ed., pp. 60–93). New York: Wiley.

Volkmar, F. R. (2001). Pharmacological interventions in autism: Theoretical and practical issues. *Journal of Clinical Child Psychology, 30*, 80–87.

Volkmar, F., Klin, A., Marans, W., & Cohen, D. J. (1997). Childhood disintegrative disorder. In D. J. Cohen & F. R. Volkmar (Eds.), *Handbook of autism and pervasive developmental disorders* (2nd ed., pp. 47–59). New York: Wiley.

Wechsler, D. (1991). *Manual for the Wechsler Intelligence Scale for Children—Third Edition.* San Antonio, TX: Psychological Corporation.

31

Pediatric Obesity

ELISSA JELALIAN
ROBYN MEHLENBECK

PREVALENCE OF PEDIATRIC OBESITY

Pediatric obesity is a significant public health concern. The U.S. Surgeon General issued a "Call to Action to Prevent and Decrease Overweight and Obesity" in December of 2001, which noted that "overweight and obesity may soon cause as much preventable disease and death as smoking" (U.S. Department of Health and Human Services, 2001). The prevalence of overweight and obesity in children, adolescents, and adults has increased dramatically during the past two decades. Data from the recent National Health and Nutrition Examination Survey (NHANES III) indicate that approximately 11% of children and adolescents are overweight as defined by criteria of body mass index (BMI; weight in kilograms/height in meters^2) greater than the 95th percentile (Troiano & Flegal, 1998). The rates increase to almost 22% of children and adolescents when the 85th percentile BMI is used as a cutoff (Troiano & Flegal, 1998). Although the rates of obesity have increased for all pediatric populations, the prevalence is particularly high for minority populations.

HEALTH CONSEQUENCES

The rise in prevalence of pediatric obesity has been associated with a number of health consequences, including increased rates of type 2 diabetes (Pinhas-Hamiel et al., 1996), as well as risk factors for heart disease (Freedman, Dietz, Srinivasan, & Berenson, 1999). Body fatness assessed by triceps and subscapular skinfold thickness has been associated with risk for elevated blood pressure, total cholesterol, and serum lipoprotein ratios (Berenson, Srinivasan, Wattigney, & Harsha, 1993; Dwyer et al., 1998; Williams et al., 1992). Furthermore, overweight children and adolescents are almost 10 times more likely than nonoverweight peers to have two or more risk factors for cardiovascular disease (Freedman et al., 1999). A recent report presented at the meeting of the American College of Cardiology indicated a high prevalence of ventricular hypertrophy in healthy young women, the majority of whom were overweight (Winslow, 2002). Recent studies also documented increased rates of impaired glucose tolerance in obese children and adolescents (Sinha et al., 2002), as well as a positive relationship between BMI and insulin resistance in adolescents (Sinaiko, Donahuem, Jacobs, & Prineas, 1999), both of which are probable precursors to type 2 diabetes. Although childhood and adolescent obesity pose multiple health concerns, weight loss may lead to improvement in health outcomes (Epstein, Kuller, Wing, Valoski, & McCurley, 1989).

Childhood and adolescent obesity are significant predictors of overweight status in adulthood (Charney, Goodman, McBride, Lyon, & Pratt, 1976; Guo, Roche, Chumlea, Gardner, & Siervogel, 1994). For example, young adolescents at the 95th percentile for BMI are at much greater risk for becoming overweight in adulthood, and this risk increases with the age of the child (Guo et al., 1994). As early as preadolescence, a child's weight is a stronger predictor of adult overweight status than parent weight (Whitaker, Wright, Pepe, Seidel, & Dietz, 1997). Furthermore, both childhood and adolescent obesity pose a risk factor for adult morbidity and mortality, particularly for males (Gunell, Frankel, Nanchahal, Peters, & Davey-Smith, 1998; Must, Jacques, Dallal, Bajema, & Dietz, 1992).

PSYCHOSOCIAL CORRELATES

Being overweight during childhood and adolescence is potentially associated with a number of negative psychosocial outcomes. Studies of overweight children seeking weight-loss treatment have found global deficits in parent ratings of social competence compared with normal-weight controls (Braet, Mervielde, & Vandereycken, 1997) or a community sample (Banis et al., 1988; Wallander & Varni, 1989). Estimates of the prevalence of social problems in children who are overweight and present for treatment vary, ranging from 11% (Epstein, Wisniewski, & Wing, 1994) to 45% of boys and 28% of girls with elevated scores on the Social Problems subscale of the Child Behavior Checklist (CBCL; Epstein, Myers, & Anderson, 1996).

A second dimension of psychosocial functioning that has been evaluated in samples of overweight children and adolescents is that of self-perception or self-esteem. There is some evidence of diminished self-esteem in overweight school-age children. Children seeking weight-loss treatment, as well as a nonclinical sample of overweight children between the ages of 9 and 12 years, were found to have lower scores than normal-weight controls on dimensions of physical and general self-worth (Braet et al., 1997). Children seeking weight-loss treatment also had higher scores on the Total Problem scale of the CBCL. Furthermore, a recent longitudinal study demonstrated decreases in self-esteem in obese children between school age and adolescence (Strauss, 2000). Findings from other studies do not indicate deficits in global self-worth in overweight children but do support the finding of decreased body esteem or physical appearance self-worth (French, Story, & Perry, 1995). Furthermore, cross-sectional studies consistently demonstrate an inverse relationship between self-esteem and BMI in adolescents, and there is some evidence for an inverse relationship between self-esteem and weight gain in prospective studies (French et al., 1995). In a related area, overweight children and adolescents may be particularly vulnerable to diminished self-efficacy related to physical activity. Findings from a recent study indicated that children who are obese endorsed significantly lower levels of physical-activity-related self-efficacy compared with normal-weight peers (Trost, Kerr, Ward, & Pate, 2001).

Another area of psychosocial functioning that has been evaluated in children who are overweight is the relationship between weight and depressive symptoms. In a large-scale study conducted with a cohort of third graders, BMI was positively related to depressive symptoms in girls but not in boys (Erickson, Robinson, Haydel, & Killen, 2000). However, this relationship did not hold after accounting for the effects of concern about overweight, indicating that such concerns might be the link to depressive symptoms in school-age girls. A study of adolescent girls also documented increased body and weight dissatisfaction, but no increased risk for depressive symptoms, in girls who were obese relative to normal weight peers (Wadden, Foster, Stunkard, & Linowitz, 1989).

In summary, empirical findings suggest that children and adolescents who are overweight are not systematically at risk for increased psychological distress. However, there appear to be higher rates of difficulty in social functioning among overweight children presenting for weight-loss treatment. Furthermore, both children and adolescents who are overweight are at increased risk for diminished self-esteem, particularly in the area of physical appearance. Practical implications of these findings include the importance of assessing dimensions of social functioning, self-concept, and mood in children and adolescents presenting for weight-loss treatment. Conversely, it may be important to evaluate weight concerns in overweight children and adolescents presenting with emotional or behavioral problems to determine the extent to which concerns with weight contribute to psychological difficulties.

VARIABLES CONTRIBUTING TO THE DEVELOPMENT OF OBESITY

Familial Variables/Genetics

There is general consensus that genetic variables play a role regarding whether or not a given individual is at risk for development of obesity (Myer & Stunkard, 1993). Considerable research has been conducted during the past decade to identify genetic markers or genes associated with obesity phenotypes, as well as to find specific chromosomal abnormalities, such as that observed in Prader-Willi syndrome, that lead to development of obesity. Identification of genetic markers related to obesity is an area of significance and promise for development of future interventions targeting obesity. For a recent review of work on the "obesity gene map," see Rankinen and colleagues (2002).

Familial Variables/Shared Environment

Parents influence children's weight status through genetic makeup, as well as a shared environment related to physical activity and eating. Attention to the family environment related to eating is one avenue for understanding the familial clustering of obesity (Birch & Fisher, 1998). For infants and young children, parents play a central role in food and activity choices available within the home. With increased autonomy associated with later school age and adolescence, children have more choices related to nutrition and physical activity. A programmatic line of research suggests a relationship between parental variables and development of eating patterns and regulation of hunger and satiety cues in preschool and young school-age children (Birch & Fisher, 1998). In one such study, mothers who described themselves as more controlling of their young child's food intake had children who demonstrated less evidence of ability to regulate their own energy intake (Johnson & Birch, 1994). In the same study, parental control over dietary intake was related to child adiposity for girls. In a related study of children ages 3 to 6 years, maternal restriction of snack foods was associated with greater intake of these foods in a free-access situation for girls (Fisher & Birch, 1999). Maternal restriction was also positively related to children's adiposity. In another study, mother's disinhibition related to her own eating was positively related to her daughter's overweight status, as well as to greater caloric intake by daughters during a situation in which they were given free access to palatable snacks following consumption of a meal (Cutting, Fisher, Grimm-Thomas, & Birch, 1999). Findings from this study suggest that maternal disinhibition may mediate the relationship between mother and daughter weight status.

Another dimension that has been assessed with regard to parental influence on children's eating habits is the relationship between parent and child food preferences and weight status. Fisher and Birch (1995) found that children's preferences for and consumption of dietary fat were related to parental BMI, suggesting the possibility that preference for certain foods may in some way mediate the relationship between parent and child weight status. Research has also shown a specific positive relationship between parental obesity status and the percentage of energy from fat in children's diets (Eck, Klesges, Hanson, & Slawson, 1991; Nguyen, Larson, Johnson, & Goran, 1996). In one study, this relationship held only for maternal obesity and was not significant for fathers (Nguyen et al., 1996). Although the majority of these studies are cross-sectional and do not provide direct information regarding the "causes" of obesity, this line of research highlights patterns of family interaction that might support the development of eating habits consistent with the development of obesity. See Birch and Fisher (1998) for an extensive review of this literature.

Cultural Variables

On a more global level than immediate family are the cultural variables that may relate to increased rates of pediatric obesity. Several dimensions specific to industrialized societies have been identified as contributing to the increased prevalence of obesity in the United States. These include decreased access to physical activity, increased involvement with sedentary activities, and increased access to high-fat, high-calorie foods. There is a clear trend toward increased sedentary activities in both children and adolescents, including television viewing and computer use. According to the American Academy of Pediatrics (2001), the average child spends 3 hours per day watching television. Several studies examine the relationship between hours of television viewing and obesity in children. Recently, Gordon-Larsen, Adair, and Popkin (2002) found that the probability of being overweight for teenagers was nearly 50% higher with high rates of television or video viewing (> 35 hours per week). Other studies have also documented that the probability of being overweight increases in relation to amount of television viewing (Anderson, Crespo, Bartlett, Cheskin, & Pratt, 1998; Dietz & Gortmaker, 1985; Robinson, 1999).

Paralleling increased involvement in sedentary activity is reduction in frequency of physical activity, both within and outside of the school setting. Studies have shown that significant predictors of increase in BMI include lack of participation in sports teams and exercise programs (Dowda, Ainsworth, Addy, Saunders, & Riner, 2001), playing video games daily, and overall low rate of physical activity (O'Loughlin, Gray-Donald, Paradis, & Meshefedjian, 2000). Schools have reduced physical education requirements such that the modal number of physical education (PE) periods may be two per week, and even less at the high school level (Neergaard, 2002). Outside of school, children are participating in fewer physical activities for many reasons, including perceived or real safety concerns, limited supervised opportunities (especially for children and adolescents who are not competitive athletes), and structure of the environment (e.g. neighborhoods without sidewalks; Nestle & Jacobson, 2000). Data from the 1997 Youth Risk Behavior Survey indicate that, during high school, there is a decline in participation in both school sports and organized sports unrelated to school, especially for girls (Kann et al., 1998).

Finally, prevalence and accessibility of high-calorie foods have been identified as a culturally based contributor to both pediatric and adult obesity. One study estimated that up to 40% of children's meals come from fast-food chains, convenience stores, and restaurants and that there are fast-food franchise outlets in up to 13% of schools nationwide (Murphy, 2000). Overall, Americans spend nearly half of their food budget on and obtain approximately one-third of their daily energy from meals and drinks consumed outside the home (Lin, Frazao, & Guthrie, 1999).

PREVENTIVE INTERVENTIONS/HEALTH PROMOTION

Efforts to regulate weight in children and adolescents range from primary prevention, typically targeting large groups of children, to tertiary interventions focused on individual overweight children and their families. We review intervention and prevention efforts separately, as these involve fairly distinct strategies and are targeted at different populations, with our primary focus on intervention approaches with overweight pediatric populations.

Preventive interventions related to obesity are typically geared at changing dietary and/or physical activity patterns of large groups of children or decreasing risk factors for children who are considered to be at increased risk for obesity. Children and adolescents spend at least 30 hours per week in school, making it an ideal place to target the health behaviors of large samples of children. However, schools appear to be sending conflicting messages to children about the importance of healthy eating and activity habits. First, as mentioned, required physical education is less common, especially at the high school level. In addition, many schools have stores that are supplied with high-calorie and high-fat snack choices and soda machines that help generate revenue for schools, use candy as frequent fundraisers, and serve lunch options that are high in fat and total calories.

Several studies conducted within the school setting target health risk behaviors related to obesity, including primary prevention of cardiovascular disease (Project CATCH; Luepker et al., 1996) and increasing physical fitness (Sallis et al., 1997). One study that targeted prevention of obesity directly provided a 2-year intervention for all students in grades 6 to 8, with sessions aimed at decreasing television viewing, decreasing consumption of high-fat foods, increasing fruit and vegetable consumption, and increasing moderate physical activity (Planet Health; Gortmaker et al., 1999). Findings from this intervention indicated a decrease in obesity in girls, as well as a decrease in television viewing for both boys and girls. Decreases in hours of television viewing were directly related to decreases in obesity for both boys and girls. A second study also documented intervention-related decreases in television viewing and associated decreases in weight. Two other school-based interventions targeting modification of school lunch programs did not have a significant effect on weight status (Leupker et al., 1996; Sahota et al., 2001).

A more proximal approach to prevention of obesity is identification of specific children who are at risk for overweight status: specifically, normal-weight children of an obese parent. In one such intervention, parents who were instructed to increase fruit and vegetable consumption showed greater decreases in percent overweight than parents who were instructed to decrease high-fat and high-sugar foods. Participants who received the intervention to increase fruit and vegetable intake also decreased high-fat, high-sugar foods, although this result was not specifically targeted (Epstein, Gordy, et al., 2001). Additional research needs to be conducted to determine the long-term efficacy of interventions that promote healthy practices without specifically targeting restriction of less healthy behaviors.

WEIGHT MANAGEMENT INTERVENTIONS

Interventions with children and adolescents who are overweight are typically delivered in a group setting and include several common components. These include dietary restriction, physical activity prescription, common behavior modification components, including self-monitoring of diet and physical activity, stimulus control strategies, and contingency management, as well as varying levels of parent involvement. Considerable empirical support documents the efficacy of comprehensive behavioral weight-management interventions with school-age children, whereas fewer studies have been conducted on the efficacy of interventions with adolescents (Jelalian & Saelens, 1999). Decreases of approximately 5% to 20% overweight have been observed in treatment studies with children between the ages of 8 and 12 years immediately following intervention. Furthermore, at least one research group has demonstrated the long-term efficacy of family-based behavioral interventions at 5- and 10-year follow-up (Epstein, McCurley, Wing, & Valoski, 1990; Epstein, Valoski, Wing, & McCurley, 1994).

Dietary Interventions

A dietary intervention that has been effective in comprehensive programs with children is the "Traffic Light Diet" (Epstein, Wing, & Valoski, 1985), which categorizes food into the colors of a stoplight based on caloric density and nutrient content. Children and parents are asked to limit consumption of "red" foods that are high in dietary fat, consume moderate numbers of "yellow" foods, and eat "green" foods freely. A major strength of this dietary plan is that it involves concepts that are easily understood by school-age children. Other common dietary interventions are based on the food pyramid and prescribe consumption of specific numbers of foods from each of the six categories, including grains, fruits, vegetables, dairy products, protein, and fat. Such prescriptions may be accompanied by particular calorie restrictions. A more restrictive dietary intervention that has been used with adolescents is the protein-sparing modified fast or very low calorie diet (VLCD). Data suggest that VLCDs, when implemented in a closely supervised setting, can result in significant reductions in percent overweight for adolescents (e.g. Stallings, Archibald, Pencharz, Harrison, & Bell, 1988).

Few studies have evaluated the efficacy of specific dietary prescriptions in pediatric weight-loss programs. One dimension that has been manipulated is the level of caloric restriction prescribed. In a randomized group intervention with children ages 10–12 years in which calorie restriction was manipulated, children who received the more restrictive calorie intervention demonstrated greater weight loss (Amador, Ramos, Morono, & Hermelo, 1990). Similar findings were reported in a study of children and adolescents comparing a hypocaloric diet to protein-sparing modified fast, with participants who were prescribed protein-sparing modified fast, followed by balanced deficit diet, demonstrating greater decrease in percent overweight at the end of the initial treatment period than those prescribed a hypocaloric diet (Figueroa-Colon, von Almen, Franklin, Schuftan, & Suskind, 1993). However, at follow-up, the groups were comparable and demonstrated a decrease of approximately 20% overweight. In one of the few specific comparisons of dietary prescriptions, a low-glycemic-index (GI) diet was compared with a reduced-fat diet in a sample of children presenting to an outpatient obesity treatment program (Spieth et al., 2000). Glycemic index refers to the increase in blood glucose that follows consumption of a standard amount of carbohydrate, with a low-GI diet tending to include liberal amounts of legumes, fruits, and vegetables and limited amounts of refined grain products and sugars. In this retrospective study, results suggested a greater average decrease in BMI for children prescribed the low-glycemic-index diet. However, we are unaware of published *randomized* studies comparing a low-glycemic-index diet with a low-fat diet in pediatric populations.

Physical Activity Interventions

Physical activity prescriptions are commonly included in pediatric weight-management interventions. Effective physical activity interventions include increasing lifestyle physical activity, as well as decreasing sedentary behaviors (Epstein, Paluch, Gordy, & Dorn, 2000). Findings from investigations assessing the benefit of adding an exercise component to weight-loss interventions for school-age children provide mixed results when weight loss is the targeted outcome. Diet combined with aerobic exercise led to greater reductions in percent overweight than diet alone on a short-term basis (Epstein, Wing, Penner, & Kress, 1985). However, in a second study, diet alone led to weight losses comparable with combined diet and lifestyle physical activity at the end of treatment, as well as 5 and 10 years from the start of treatment (Epstein, Valoski, et al., 1994).

Two treatment studies conducted with children between the ages of 10 and 16 years compared dietary intervention and behavior modification with the same program plus an exercise component that included on-site physical activity three times per week (Rocchini et al., 1988; Rocchini, Katch, Schork, & Kelch, 1987). Both groups demonstrated comparable modest weight losses (approximately 2.5 kg) at the end of treatment. In a study targeting adolescents, an intervention that included gradual increase in frequency of exercise from one to three times per week resulted in nearly twice the decrease in percent overweight as one that began with five times per week of exercise and decreased to three (Emes, Velde, Moreau, Murdoch, & Trussell, 1990).

A series of studies conducted with school-age children compares the efficacy of different physical activity interventions in pediatric weight-loss interventions. Diet and lifestyle exercise was compared with diet and programmed exercise, lifestyle exercise alone, and programmed exercise alone (Epstein, Wing, Koeske, Osspi, & Beck, 1982). Lifestyle exercise refers to physical activity that can be incorporated into one's daily routine, such as using stairs instead of the elevator or parking further from a destination. This is distinguished from programmed aerobic exercise, participation in a specific physical activity to increase heart rate for a designated period of time. At the end of treatment, all groups demonstrated similar weight losses; however the lifestyle activity interventions were found to be superior to programmed exercise at 11-month follow-up. A subsequent study compared diet and aerobic exercise with diet and lifestyle activity and diet and calisthenics (Epstein, Wing, Koeske, & Valoski, 1985). All groups demonstrated comparable decreases in percent overweight at the end of treatment. The diet and lifestyle intervention was superior to diet and calisthenics at

5 years posttreatment (Epstein et al., 1990), and both lifestyle and aerobics were superior to calisthenics at 10-year follow-up (Epstein, Valoski, et al., 1994).

An innovative development in physical activity interventions for pediatric weight management involves prescription of decreased sedentary activity as an alternative to increased exercise. Epstein and colleagues observed that reducing access to sedentary activities was associated with increases in physical activity in a laboratory setting (Epstein, Saelens, Myers, & Vito, 1997). Clinical studies of overweight children provide mixed findings with regard to the effectiveness of decreasing sedentary behavior relative to increasing physical activity. In the first such study, participants were randomly assigned to conditions of diet and reinforcement for decreased sedentary activity, diet and reinforcement for increased physical activity, or a combination of these two conditions (Epstein et al., 1995). The group that was reinforced for decreased sedentary activity demonstrated greater decreases in percent overweight than the group reinforced for increased physical activity at the end of treatment, as well as 12 months from the start of treatment. In a more recent study, children were randomly assigned to one of four treatment groups that crossed decreasing sedentary behavior and increasing physical activity with high and low doses of each of these conditions (Epstein, Paluch, Gordy, & Dorn, 2000). Overall, decreases of approximately 25% overweight were observed at the end of treatment, with comparable reductions in percent overweight and improvements in physical work capacity in both the increased physical activity and reduced sedentary behavior conditions.

Interventions that include exercise in the treatment of pediatric obesity provide mixed support for the addition of a physical activity component for decreasing percent overweight. However, there are potential fitness benefits associated with exercise that are not assessed by change in percent overweight, leading Epstein and colleagues to conclude that exercise provides benefits beyond that of diet alone in the short-term treatment of pediatric obesity (Epstein & Goldfield, 1999). Additionally, studies of maintenance of weight loss in adults indicate a primary role for physical activity in the long-term maintenance of weight loss (Klem, Wing, McGuire, Seagle, & Hill, 1997).

Behavioral Interventions

Behavioral strategies, including self-monitoring of dietary intake and physical activity, stimulus control, and contingency management, are common components of pediatric weight-management interventions. Self-monitoring of diet and physical activity are the cornerstones of behavioral weight-management interventions. Stimulus control strategies refer to manipulations to assist in managing the environment related to eating and physical activity, and contingency management involves providing positive contingencies for adherence to dietary and physical activity interventions. Research supports the overall effectiveness of behavioral intervention relative to education alone (Epstein, Wing, Steranchak, Dickson, & Michelson, 1980). Although a small number of investigations manipulate specific behavior modification interventions, treatment tends to include multiple variables, and it is difficult to identify which particular components are effective.

A small number of studies focus on manipulation of specific behavioral components. In one such study, children ages 7 to 13 years of age were randomized to diet with stimulus control plus reinforcement plus monitoring of food and activity plus relaxation training, or all of these with cognitive restructuring, problem solving, and self-reinforcement instead of relaxation training (Duffy & Spence, 1993). The two groups demonstrated comparable decreases in percent overweight, indicating no specific advantage to relaxation training. Findings are mixed with regard to the benefits of problem-solving interventions in behavioral pediatric weight-management programs. In one study, a greater reduction in percent overweight was observed in children who received problem-solving compared with standard behavioral intervention (Graves, Meyers, & Clark, 1988), whereas in a second, there was no advantage to adding a problem-solving intervention to standard behavioral treatment (Epstein, Paluch, Gordy, Saelens, & Ernst, 2000).

A final behavioral component that has been evaluated in weight-management interventions is positive reinforcement. In one study, adolescents between the ages of 13 and 17 years were provided with nutrition education, caloric restriction, and behavioral intervention (Coates, Jeffery, Slinkard, Killen, & Danaher, 1982). In addition, frequency of contact and reinforcement were manipulated such that participants were seen for either 1 or 5 days per week, and monetary reward was provided for weight loss versus achieving calorie goals. At the end of treatment, as well as at 6-month follow-up, only the group who received contact 5 times per week and monetary reward for weight loss demonstrated a significant decrease in percent overweight.

Role of Parents

Determining the appropriate target for intervention is another key component of pediatric weight management interventions. Depending on the age of the child, treatment efforts may most appropriately be geared toward parent, child, or a combination of parent and child. Studies conducted both with children (Kirschenbaum, Harris, & Tomarken, 1984) and with adolescents (Brownell, Kelman, & Stunkard, 1983; Coates, Killen, & Slinkard, 1982) provide mixed results with regard to the relative advantage of including parents in pediatric weight-management interventions. Nonetheless, parental involvement is an integral component of the most effective short- and long-term pediatric weight-management programs. Furthermore, evidence from long-term follow-up studies indicates that there is a clear advantage to parental involvement in which both parent and child are specifically aiming for weight loss (Epstein et al., 1990; Epstein, Valoski, et al., 1994). More recently, parents have been effectively used as the exclusive facilitators of weight-management interventions for children (Golan, Weizman, Apter, & Fainaru, 1998). Based on this evidence, there appears to be an advantage to including parents in weight-loss interventions with children and to targeting parent weight loss or weight management as a specific treatment strategy. The data with regard to the role of parents in adolescent weight-management interventions is more equivocal.

Role of Peers

One promising area for weight-management interventions with adolescent populations is the peer context. Although behavioral weight-control programs for adolescents are conducted in a group setting, they do not include peers as active components of the intervention. Preliminary findings from a small sample of adolescents suggest that a cognitive-behavioral weight management intervention enhanced by peer group activities may be a useful treatment modality (Jelalian & Mehlenbeck, 2002). Enhancing further understanding of the potential role of peers in adolescent weight-management intervention is an area for future research.

PHARMACOLOGICAL INTERVENTIONS

An area that is likely to receive more attention in the next decade is using pharmacological interventions to aid in pediatric weight management. Increasingly, medications such as orlistat and sibutramine have been used independently or as adjuncts to behavioral weight treatment in adults. Preliminary medication trials to address adolescent obesity have been conducted. A recent study combining ephedrine and caffeine led to significant weight loss for adolescents during a 20-week period (Molnar, Torok, Erhard, & Jeges, 2000); however, there are potential side effects, and the intervention is not well suited for long-term maintenance. Although ongoing clinical trials are evaluating the efficacy of medications such as sibutramine and orlistat with adolescents (Yanovski, 2001), there is continued need for innovative behavioral and psychosocial interventions in this area. Weight-loss medications await FDA approval for use with pediatric populations.

APPLICATION OF WEIGHT-MANAGEMENT INTERVENTIONS TO PEDIATRIC SETTINGS

Effective multicomponent interventions are available to facilitate weight control in children. The majority of these treatments have been developed and implemented as part of group-based clinical trials. A major challenge facing pediatric psychologists is the application of existing interventions to pediatric settings, in which the potential is high for reaching greater numbers of children. There are at least two documented examples of initiatives in the primary care setting. In a nonrandomized study, children and adolescents ranging from 6 to 16 years were consecutively assigned to one of three interventions: (1) monthly physician visits for 1 year, followed by two visits during the second year, five meetings with a nutritionist, and caloric restriction; (2) monthly physician visits for 1 year, followed by two visits during the second year and seven separate child and parent group sessions that included the involvement of a nutritionist; or (3) monthly school nurse visits for 1 year, followed by two visits during the second year. After the first year of intervention, the two groups that received physician intervention demonstrated significant decreases in percent overweight from pretreatment, whereas the group receiving school-based intervention did not (Nuutinen, 1991).

A recent application to the primary care setting compared one session of physician weight counseling with a behavioral weight-management intervention that included initial interview, didactic written information, and scheduled telephone counseling. BMI z scores increased for adolescents who were randomized to one session of physician counseling, but a slight decrease was shown in BMI for adolescents who received the behavioral intervention (Saelens et al., 2002). A recent publication by Epstein and colleagues reviewed practical considerations in implementing obesity treatment for children and in translating information from empirical studies into pediatric and clinical practice (Epstein, Roemmich, & Raynor, 2001).

PRACTICAL RECOMMENDATIONS

Pediatric psychologists may be presented with a number of opportunities to help address weight concerns with children and adolescents, even when obesity is not the presenting problem. One mechanism for influencing weight is to routinely address eating and physical activity patterns with all patients, as these habits can have an effect on a number of medical conditions. For example, physical activity has a positive effect on depression, a common comorbid condition with many medical issues (Dunn, Trivedi, & O'Neal, 2001). In addition, nutrition plays a key role in a number of chronic illnesses (e.g., diabetes) and may also have implications for both physical and mental health functioning.

Two distinct circumstances may be addressed when considering intervention with an overweight child. The first involves initial presentation of concerns to the family and/or child, particularly when weight is not the presenting problem. Practitioners may have concern that identifying weight as a problem will damage a child's self-esteem or embarrass a child. This

TABLE 31.1. Practical Recommendations for Practitioners

I. General considerations

Assess the child's or adolescent's motivation for weight loss. For example, does the child have concerns about weight? Does she or he get teased? Is it important for the child to be able to keep up in physical activities with friends? If motivation for weight loss comes primarily from the parent, focus on family interventions to improve habits. This approach allows for addressing physical activity and eating patterns without discounting a child's or adolescent's opinions. If the child is interested in weight loss, specific encouragement can be provided for adapting healthier behaviors.

II. Family-based interventions

A. Engage the entire family as opposed to just the "problem" overweight child. This involvement will facilitate normalization of healthy habits and decrease arguments related to restricting food.

B. Promote the idea that healthy habits may benefit all family members. Research demonstrates that healthy eating and physical activity patterns play a role in decreasing risk of cardiovascular disease and certain types of cancer, regardless of weight status (Kohl, 2001).

C. Encourage parents to assume responsibility for the foods available within the home. Parents have some control regarding foods purchased for the home regardless of the child's age.

D. Promote activities unrelated to eating to mark special events such as birthdays. Parents can have a significant impact on determining family activities, particularly for younger children.

E. Encourage parents to find motivators other than food to reinforce positive behaviors. For example, good behavior or grades can be rewarded with activity or time motivators rather than food.

F. Encourage parents to monitor frequency of television viewing. Increasing evidence suggests a relationship between sedentary behavior and obesity. Parents can limit the amount of television viewing and other sedentary activities, such as video games, to less than 2 hours per day (American Academy of Pediatrics, 2001), and this rule should be implemented for all children.

III. Individually-based interventions

A. Encourage children and adolescents to self-monitor physical activity and eating habits. Self-recording helps to increase awareness of behaviors that may be targeted for intervention.

B. Set reasonable and behaviorally oriented goals. If a child makes healthy changes in his or her eating and physical activity habits, weight loss or a decline in accelerated weight gain is likely to follow. It is helpful to provide developmentally appropriate positive rewards for accomplishment of behavioral goals.

C. Encourage healthier eating behaviors, such as avoiding situations in which overeating occurs, planning ahead, bringing lunch from home rather than buying at school, taking smaller portions, and eating out less often.

D. Encourage increase in physical activity and decrease in sedentary behavior. Lifestyle activities, such as using the stairs instead of the elevator, are effective ways to increase physical activity.

E. Finally, if the child is invested in weight regulation, weekly monitoring of weight may be beneficial. It is important to tie weight decrease or stabilization to behavior changes made by the child.

concern needs to be balanced with the finding that the self-esteem of children and adolescents who are overweight may be at risk due to weight status. Helping a child may mean addressing healthy eating and physical activity patterns on a family level while the child is young and before the more consistent impact on self-esteem is observed. If presented in a sensitive manner as part of an overall initiative to promote healthy habits, weight can be addressed effectively.

The second circumstance is that in which a family or child may specifically be seeking weight-management intervention. Particularly for preschool and school-age children, it is important to include the entire family in recommended changes to physical activity and eating patterns. Even with adolescents, some empirical support exists for recommending involvement of parents. In addition, because parents have continued responsibility for availability of food within the home, their cooperation is critical. Table 31.1 outlines practical considerations for practitioners providing weight-management interventions.

CONCLUSIONS

Pediatric obesity is a serious concern that affects a significant number of children and families. The increasing prevalence of overweight children and adolescents appears to be contributing to the onset of chronic medical conditions, such as Type II diabetes, previously observed almost exclusively in adults. To the extent that cultural variables play a role in the increased rates of pediatric obesity, broad "upstream" interventions such as food taxes and reintroduction of school-based physical activity programs may be necessary to have significant impact. In addition, long-term obesity prevention studies are needed to identify effective strategies that can be implemented with large numbers of children. Although the school setting has been the exclusive focus of such trials, other community venues, such as churches and supermarkets, may also be explored. At the level of individual children and families, effective weight-management interventions are available for school-age children. A major challenge for pediatric psychologists is dissemination of such comprehensive interventions to primary care and other pediatric settings. Future research efforts should focus on development and implementation of interventions that can be delivered within existing primary care settings.

REFERENCES

Amador, M., Ramos, L. T., Morono, M., & Hermelo, M. P. (1990). Growth rate reduction during energy restriction in obese adolescents. *Experimental and Clinical Endocrinology, 96*, 73–82.

American Academy of Pediatrics. (2001). Children, adolescents and television: A policy statement. *Pediatrics, 107*, 423–426.

Anderson, R. E., Crespo, C. J., Bartlett, S. J., Cheskin, L. J., & Pratt, M. (1998). Relationship of physical activity and television watching with body weight and level of fatness among children: Results from the Third National Health and Nutrition Examination study. *Journal of the American Medical Association, 279*, 938–942.

Banis, H. T., Varni, J. W., Wallander, J. L., Korsch, B. M., Jay, S. M. Adler, R., et al. (1988). Psychological and social adjustment of obese children and their families. *Child: Care, Health, and Development, 14*, 157–173.

Berenson, G. S., Srinivasan, S. R., Wattigney, W. A., & Harsha, D. W. (1993). Obesity and cardiovascular risk in children. *Annals of the New York Academy of Sciences, 699*, 93–103.

Birch, L. L., & Fisher, J. O. (1998). Development of eating behaviors among children and adolescents. *Pediatrics, 111*, 539–549.

Braet, C., Mervielde, J., & Vandereycken, W. (1997). Psychological aspects of childhood obesity: A controlled study in a clinical and non-clinical sample. *Journal of Pediatric Psychology, 22*, 59–71.

Brownell, K. D., Kelman, J. H., & Stunkard, A. J. (1983). Treatment of obese children with and without their mothers: Changes in weight and blood pressure. *Pediatrics, 71*, 515–523.

Charney, M., Goodman, H. C., McBride, M., Lyon, B., & Pratt, R. (1976). Childhood antecedents of adult obesity: Do chubby infants become obese adults? *New England Journal of Medicine, 295*, 6–9.

Coates, T. J., Jeffery, R. W., Slinkard, L. A., Killen, J. D., & Danaher, B. G. (1982). Frequency of contact and monetary reward in weight loss, lipid change, and blood pressure reduction with adolescents. *Behavior Therapy, 13*, 175–185.

Coates, T. J., Killen, J. D., & Slinkard, L. A. (1982). Parent participation in a treatment program for overweight adolescents. *International Journal of Eating Disorders, 1*, 37–48.

Cutting, T. M., Fisher, J. O., Grimm-Thomas, K., & Birch, L. L. (1999). Like mother, like daughter: Familial patterns of overweight are mediated by mothers' dietary disinhibition. *American Journal of Clinical Nutrition, 69*, 608–613.

Dietz, W. H., & Gortmaker, S. L. (1985). Do we fatten our children at the TV set? Obesity and television viewing in children and adolescents. *Pediatrics, 75*, 807–812.

Dowda, M., Ainsworth, B. E., Addy, C. L., Saunders, R., & Riner, W. (2001). Environmental influences, physical activity, and weight status in 8- to 16-year-olds. *Archives of Pediatric Adolescent Medicine, 155*, 711–717.

Duffy, G., & Spence, S. H. (1993). The effectiveness of cognitive self-management as an adjunct to a behavioral intervention for childhood obesity: A research note. *Journal of Child Psychology and Psychiatry, 34*, 1043–1050.

Dunn, A. L., Trivedi, M. H., & O'Neal, H. A. (2001). Physical activity dose-response effects on outcomes of depression and anxiety. *Medicine and Science in Sports and Exercise, 33*(6, Suppl.), S587–S597.

Dwyer, J. T., Stone, E. J., Yang, M., Feldman, H., Webber, L. S., Must, A., et al. (1998). Predictors of overweight and overfatness in a multiethnic pediatric population: Child and Adolescent Trial for Cardiovascular Health Collaborative Research Group. *American Journal of Clinical Nutrition, 67*, 602–610.

Eck, L. H., Klesges, R. C., Hanson, C. L., & Slawson, D. (1991). Children at familial risk for obesity: An examination of dietary intake, physical activity, and weight status. *International Journal of Obesity, 16*, 71–78.

Emes, C., Velde, B., Moreau, M., Murdoch, D. D., & Trussell, R. (1990). An activity based weight control program. *Adapted Physical Activity Quarterly, 7*, 314–324.

Epstein, L. H., & Goldfield, G. S. (1999). Physical activity in the treatment of childhood overweight and obesity: Current evidence and research issues. *Medicine and Science in Sports and Exercise, 31*, S553–S559.

Epstein, L. H., Gordy, C. C., Raynor, H. A., Beddome, M., Kilanowski, C. K., & Paluch, R. (2001). Increasing fruit and vegetable intake and decreasing fat and sugar intake in families at risk for childhood obesity. *Obesity Research, 9*, 171–178.

Epstein, L. H., Kuller, L. H., Wing, R. R., Valoski, A., & McCurley, J. (1989). The effect of weight control on lipid changes in obese children. *American Journal of Diseases of Children, 143*, 454–457.

Epstein, L. H., McCurley, J., Wing, R. R., & Valoski, A. (1990). Five-year follow-up of family-based behavioral treatments for childhood obesity. *Journal of Consulting and Clinical Psychology, 58*, 661–664.

Epstein, L. H., Myers, M. D., & Anderson, K. (1996). The association of maternal psychopathology and family socioeconomic status with psychological problems in obese children. *Obesity Research, 4*, 65–74.

Epstein, L. H., Paluch, R. A., Gordy, C. C., & Dorn, J. (2000). Decreasing sedentary behaviors in treating pediatric obesity. *Archives of Pediatric and Adolescent Medicine, 154*, 220–226.

Epstein, L. H., Paluch, R. A., Gordy, C. C., Saelens, B. E., & Ernst, M. M. (2000). Problem solving in the treatment of childhood obesity. *Journal of Consulting and Clinical Psychology, 68*, 717–721.

Epstein, L. H., Roemmich, J. N., & Raynor, H. A. (2001). Behavioral therapy in the treatment of pediatric obesity. *Pediatric Clinics of North America, 48*, 981–993.

Epstein, L. H., Saelens, B. E., Myers, M. D., & Vito, D. (1997). Effects of decreasing sedentary behaviors on activity choice in obese children. *Health Psychology, 16*, 107–113.

Epstein L. H., Valoski, A., Wing, R. R., & McCurley, J. (1994). Ten-year outcomes of behavioral family-based treatment for childhood obesity. *Healthy Psychology, 13*, 373–383.

Epstein, L. H., Valoski, A. M., Vara, L., McCurley, J., Wisniewski, L., Kalarchian, M. A., et al. (1995). Effects of decreasing sedentary behavior and increasing activity on weight change in obese children. *Health Psychology, 14*, 109–115.

Epstein, L. H., Wing, R. R., Koeske, R., Osspi, D., & Beck, S. (1982). A comparison of life-style change and programmed aerobic exercise on weight and fitness changes in obese children. *Behavior Therapy, 13*, 651–665.

Epstein, L. H., Wing, R. R., Koeske, R., & Valoski, A. (1985). A comparison of lifestyle exercise, aerobic exercise, and calisthenics on weight loss in obese children. *Behavior Therapy, 16*, 345–356.

Epstein, L. H., Wing, R. R., Penner, B. C., & Kress, M. J. (1985). The effect of diet and controlled exercise on weight loss in obese children. *Journal of Pediatrics, 107*, 358–361.

Epstein, L. H., Wing, R. R., Steranchak, L., Dickson, B., & Michelson, J. (1980). Comparison of family-based behavior modification and nutrition education for childhood obesity. *Journal of Pediatric Psychology, 5*, 25–36.

Epstein, L. H., Wing, R. R., & Valoski, A. (1985). Childhood obesity. *Pediatric Clinics of North America, 32*, 363–379.

Epstein, L. H., Wisniewski, L., & Wing, R. (1994). Child and parent psychological problems influence child weight control. *Obesity Research, 2*, 509–515.

Erickson, S. J., Robinson, T. N., Haydel, K. F., & Killen, J. D. (2000). Are overweight children unhappy? Body mass index, depressive symptoms, and overweight concerns in elementary school children. *Archives of Pediatrics and Adolescent Medicine, 154*, 931–935.

Figueroa-Colon, R., von Almen, T. K., Franklin, F. A, Schuftan, C., & Suskind, R. M. (1993). Comparison of two hypocaloric diets in obese children. *American Journal of Disease in Children, 147*, 160–166.

Fisher, J. O., & Birch, L. L. (1995). Fat preferences and fat consumption of 3– to 5–year-old children are related to parental adiposity. *Journal of the American Dietetic Association, 95*, 759–764.

Fisher, J. O., & Birch, L. L. (1999). Restricting access to foods and children's eating. *Appetite, 32*, 405–419.

Freedman, D. S., Dietz, W. H., Srinivasan, S. R., & Berenson, G. S. (1999). The relation of overweight to cardiovascular risk factors among children and adolescents: The Bogalusa heart study. *Pediatrics, 103*, 1175–1182.

French, S. A., Story, M., & Perry, C. L. (1995). Self-esteem and obesity in children and adolescents: A literature review. *Obesity Research, 3*, 479–490.

Golan, M., Weizman, A., Apter, A., & Fainaru, M. (1998). Parents as the exclusive agents of change in the treatment of childhood obesity. *American Journal of Clinical Nutrition, 67*, 1130–1135.

Gordon-Larsen, P., Adair, L. S., & Popkin, B. M. (2002). Ethnic differences in physical activity and inactivity patterns and overweight status. *Obesity Research, 10*, 141–149.

Gortmaker, S. L., Peterson, K., Wiecha, J., Sobol, A. M., Dixit, S., Fox, M. K., et al. (1999). Reducing obesity via a school-based interdisciplinary intervention among youth: Planet Health. *Archives of Pediatric Adolescent Medicine, 153*, 409–418.

Graves, T., Meyers, A. W., & Clark, L. (1988). An evaluation of parental problem-solving training in the behavioral treatment of childhood obesity. *Journal of Consulting and Clinical Psychology, 56*, 246–250.

Gunell, D. J., Frankel, S. J., Nanchahal, K., Peters, T. J., & Davey-Smith, G. (1998). Childhood obesity and adult cardiovascular mortality: A 57-year follow-up study based on the Boyd Orr cohort. *American Journal of Clinical Nutrition, 67*, 1111–1118.

Guo, S. S., Roche, A. F., Chumlea, W. C., Gardner, J. D., & Siervogel, R. M. (1994). The predictive value of childhood body mass index values for overweight at age 35 years. *American Journal of Clinical Nutrition, 59*, 810–819.

Jelalian, E., & Mehlenbeck, R. (2002). Peer-enhanced weight management treatment for overweight adolescents: Some preliminary findings. *Journal of Clinical Psychology in Medical Settings, 9*, 15–23.

Jelalian, E., & Saelens, B. (1999). Empirically supported treatment in pediatric psychology: Pediatric obesity. *Journal of Pediatric Psychology, 24*, 223–248.

Johnson, S. L., & Birch, L. L. (1994). Parents' and children's adiposity and eating style. *Pediatrics, 94*, 653–661.

Kann, L., Kinchen, S. A., Williams, B. I., Ross, J. G., Lowry, R., Hill, C. V., et al. (1998). Youth Risk Behaviors Surveillance—United States, 1997. *Journal of School Health, 68*, 355–369.

Kirschenbaum, D. S., Harris, E. S., & Tomarken, A. J. (1984). Effects of parental involvement in behavioral weight loss therapy for preadolescents. *Behavior Therapy, 15*, 485–500.

Klem, M. L., Wing, R. R., McGuire, M. T., Seagle, H. M., & Hill, J. O. (1997). A descriptive study of individuals successful at long-term maintenance of substantial weight loss. *American Journal of Clinical Nutrition, 66*, 239–246.

Kohl, H. W., III. (2001). Physical activity and cardiovascular disease: Evidence for a dose response. *Medicine and Science in Sports and Exercise, 33*, S472–S483.

Lin, B. H., Frazao, E., & Guthrie, J. (1999). Away-from-home foods increasingly important to quality of American diet. *Agricultural Information Bulletin No. 749*. Washington, DC: U.S. Department of Agriculture.

Luepker, R. V., Perry, C. L., McKinlay, S. M., Nader, P. R., Parcel, G. S., Stone, E. J., et al. (1996). Outcomes of a field trial to improve children's dietary patterns and physical activity: The Child and Adolescent Trial for Cardiovascular Health. *Journal of American Medical Association, 275*, 768–776.

Molnar, D., Torok, K., Erhard, E., & Jeges, S. (2000). Safety and efficacy of treatment with an ephedrine/caffeine mixture: The first double-blind placebo-controlled pilot study in adolescents. *International Journal of Obesity, 24*, 1573–1578.

Murphy, J. (2000). *The super-sizing of America: Are fast food chains to blame for the nation's obesity?* Retrieved January 21, 2002, from www.speakout.com.

Must, A., Jacques, P. F., Dallal, G. E., Bajema, C. J., & Dietz, W. H. (1992). Long-term morbidity and mortality of overweight adolescents: A follow-up of the Harvard Growth Study of 1922 to 1935. *New England Journal of Medicine, 327*, 1350–1355.

Myer, J. M., & Stunkard, A. J. (1993). Genetics and human obesity. In A. J. Stunkard & T. A. Wadden (Eds.), *Obesity: Theory and therapy* (2nd ed., pp. 137–149). New York: Raven Press.

Neergaard, L. (2002). *Surgeon General warns obesity may overtake tobacco as leading preventable killer.* Retrieved January 21, 2002, from *www.nandotimes.com.*

Nestle, M., & Jacobson, M. (2000). Halting the obesity epidemic: A public health policy approach. *Public Health Reports, 115*, 12.

Nguyen, V. T., Larson, D. E., Johnson, R. K., & Goran, M. I. (1996). Fat intake and adiposity in children of lean and obese parents. *American Journal of Clinical Nutrition, 63*, 507–513.

Nuutinen, O. (1991). Long-term effects of dietary counseling on nutrient intake and weight loss in obese children. *European Journal of Clinical Nutrition, 45*, 287–297.

O'Loughlin, J., Gray-Donald, K., Paradis, G., & Meshefedjian, G. (2000). One- and two-year predictors of excess weight gain among elementary schoolchildren in multiethnic, low-income, inner-city neighborhoods. *American Journal of Epidemiology, 152*, 739–746.

Pinhas-Hamiel, H. O., Dolan, C. M., Daniels, S. R., Standiford, D., Khoury, P. R., & Zeitler, P. (1996). Increased incidence of non-insulin-dependent diabetes mellitus among adolescents. *Journal of Pediatrics, 128*, 608–615.

Rankinen, T., Perusse, L., Weisnagel, S. J., Snyder, E. E., Chagnon, Y. C., & Bouchard, C. (2002). The human obesity gene map: The 2001 update. *Obesity Research, 10*, 196–243.

Robinson, T. N. (1999). Reducing children's television viewing to prevent obesity: A randomized controlled trial. *Journal of the American Medical Association, 282*, 1561–1567.

Rocchini, A. P., Katch, V., Anderson, J., Hinderlite, J., Becque, D., Martin, M., et al. (1988). Blood pressure in obese adolescents: Effect of weight loss. *Pediatrics, 82*, 16–23.

Rocchini, A. P., Katch, V., Schork, A., & Kelch, R. P. (1987). Insulin and blood pressure during weight loss in obese adolescents. *Hypertension, 10*, 267–273.

Saelens, B. E., Sallis, J. F., Wilfley, D. E., Patrick, K., Cella, J. A., & Buchta, R. (2002). Behavioral weight control for overweight adolescents initiated in primary care. *Obesity Research, 10*, 22–32.

Sahota, P., Rudolf, M. C., Dixey, R., Hill, A. J., Barth, J. H., & Cade, J. (2001). Randomized controlled trial of primary school based intervention to reduce risk factors for obesity. *British Medical Journal, 323*, 1029–1032.

Sallis, J. F., McKenzie, T. L., Alcaraz, J. E., Kolody, B., Faucette, N., & Hovell, M. F. (1997). The effects of a 2–year physical education program (SPARK) on physical activity and fitness in elementary school students. *American Journal of Public Health, 87*, 1328–1334.

Sinaiko, A. R., Donahuem, R. P., Jacobs, D. R., & Prineas, R. J. (1999). Relation of weight and rate of increase in weight during childhood and adolescence to body size, blood pressure, fasting insulin, and lipids in young adults: The Minneapolis Children's Blood Pressure Study. *Circulation, 99*, 1471–1476.

Sinha, R., Fisch, G., Teague, B., Tamborlane, W. V., Banyas, B., Allen, K., et al. (2002). Prevalence of impaired glucose tolerance among children and adolescents with marked obesity. *New England Journal of Medicine, 346*, 802–810.

Spieth, L. E., Harnish, J. D., Lenders, C. M., Raezer, L. B., Pereira, M. A., Hangen, J., et al. (2000). A low-glycemic index diet in the treatment of pediatric obesity. *Archives of Pediatric Adolescent Medicine 154*, 947–951.

Stallings, V. A., Archibald, E. H., Pencharz, P. B., Harrison, J. E., & Bell, L. E. (1988). One-year follow-up of weight, total body potassium, and total body nitrogen in obese adolescents treated with the protein-sparing modified fast. *American Journal of Clinical Nutrition, 48*, 91–94.

Strauss, R. S. (2000). Childhood obesity and self-esteem. *Pediatrics, 105*, e15–e19.

Troiano, R. P., & Flegal, K. M. (1998). Overweight children and adolescents: Description, epidemiology, and demographics. *Pediatrics, 101*, 497S–504S.

Trost, S. G., Kerr, L. M., Ward, D. S., & Pate, R. R. (2001). Physical activity and determinants of physical activity in obese and non-obese children. *International Journal of Obesity and Related Metabolic Disorders, 25*, 822–829.

U.S. Department of Health and Human Services. (2001). *The Surgeon General's call to action to prevent and decrease overweight and obesity.* Rockville, MD: U. S. Department of Health and Human Services, Public Health Service, Office of the Surgeon General.

Wadden, T. A., Foster, G. D., Stunkard, A. J., & Linowitz, J. R. (1989). Dissatisfaction with weight and figure in obese girls: Discontent but not depression. *International Journal of Obesity, 13*, 89–97.

Wallander, J. L., & Varni, J. W. (1989). Social support and adjustment in chronically ill and handicapped children. *American Journal of Community Psychology, 17*, 185–201.

Whitaker, R. C., Wright, J. A., Pepe, M. S., Seidel, K. D., & Dietz, W. H. (1997). Predicting obesity in young adulthood from childhood and parental obesity. *New England Journal of Medicine, 337*, 869–873.

Williams, D. P., Going, S. B., Lohman, T. G., Harsha, D. W., Srinivasan, S. R., Webber, L. S., et al. (1992). Body fatness and risk for elevated blood pressure, total cholesterol, and serum lipoprotein ratios in children and adolescents. *American Journal of Public Health, 82*, 358–363.

Winslow, R. (2002, March 20). Obese youth face heart problems, new study finds. *The Wall Street Journal*, pp. B1, B4.

Yanovski, J. A. (2001). Intensive therapies for pediatric obesity. *Pediatric Clinics of North America, 48*, 1041–1049.

32

Elimination Disorders

Enuresis and Encopresis

C. EUGENE WALKER

ENURESIS

Definition

The essential feature of enuresis is that the child repeatedly voids urine inappropriately, such as wetting his or her clothes during the day or wetting the bed at night. Criteria included in the *Diagnostic and Statistical Manual of Mental Disorders* (DSM-IV; American Psychiatric Association, 1994) state that it (1) may be involuntary or intentional; (2) requires a chronological or developmentally equivalent age of 5 years; (3) must be clinically significant in terms of a frequency of twice a week for at least 3 consecutive months or associated with distress or impairment in social, academic (occupational), or other important areas; and (4) is functional in etiology. Whether the wetting is diurnal, nocturnal, or both should be specified. Also of interest is whether it is primary and continuous, referring to wetting accidents from birth, or secondary, defined as enuresis following a period of urinary continence lasting at least 6 months.

Prevalence

By definition, enuresis does not exist until age 5 (even though girls mature a year sooner than boys, no distinction is made between males and females in DSM-IV). At age 5, 7% of males and 3% of females have enuresis; by age 10 the percentages are 3% and 2%, respectively; by age 18, 1% for males and less than 1% for females. Diurnal enuresis along with nocturnal enuresis and diurnal enuresis alone are much less frequent than nocturnal enuresis alone. Approximately 85% of all cases of enuresis are primary. Secondary enuresis generally appears between the ages of 5 to 8 (American Psychiatric Association, 1994).

Theories of Etiology

There are three general approaches to understanding the etiology of enuresis: biological, emotional, and learning.

Biological Variables

Urinary incontinence can be caused by numerous organic factors, ranging from anomalies of the spinal cord or bladder to bladder infections, as well as secondary effects from various chronic diseases such as diabetes. However, enuresis is, by definition, a functional disorder and therefore not the result of organic dysfunction. Nevertheless, numerous ideas regarding the etiology of enuresis presuppose some biological contribution to the problem. Some of these appear to have merit. Others are currently without substantiation, though additional research may lend support to some of them. Two biological theories that have received a reasonable amount of support from research literature are those involving genetics and those involving developmental delay. It has often been noted that enuresis runs in families and shows the same general trends of occurrence in immediate family and relatives that is characteristic of many genetically determined disorders (e.g., Elian, 1991). However, no specific mechanism has been determined to explain the inheritance of enuresis, and genetic factors appear to be insufficient to account for the total incidence of the problem.

With respect to developmental delay, although some studies do show children with enuresis to be delayed in reaching certain milestones in development, others do not (MacKeith, 1972). In addition, the developmental delays that are occasionally noted are very mild. Given that children are generally considered to have sufficient developmental maturity by the age of 2 to develop control, the presence of a mild delay at age 5 or 6 would not seem to be sufficient to totally account for the problem.

Food allergies have occasionally been proposed as a biological factor contributing to the problem of enuresis (e.g., Egger, Carter, Soothill, & Wilson, 1992), but more research is needed to determine whether such allergies are involved and to develop a valid list of foods to avoid.

The possibility that decreased production of antidiuretic hormone (ADH) by some children at night may result in overproduction of urine and consequent wetting of the bed has led to the use of desmopressin (DDAVP), a vasopressin analogue, as a treatment to decrease the volume of urine produced. Unfortunately, the link between ADH levels and bedwetting, as well as response to DDAVP treatment, has not been clear-cut (Evans & Meadow, 1992). More research is needed on this.

Emotional Variables

At one time mental health workers generally assumed that enuresis was primarily a symptom of emotional disorder. Thus enuresis was sometimes thought of as related to depression and representing "weeping through the bladder" (Imhof, 1956), or it was associated with sexual conflict in which urination was symbolic of suppressed sexual urges and related to ejaculation or lubrication (Fenichel, 1946). It was also thought that hostility toward the mother might be the main motivation (Solomon & Patch, 1969). However, several large sample studies comparing children who have enuresis with children who do not have failed to find significant emotional disturbance in the majority of children with enuresis (Cullen, 1966; Tapia, Jekel, & Domke, 1960).

Learning Variables

The third, and most widely accepted, view regarding the etiology of enuresis assumes a problem in learning to be the major cause. This approach has the advantage of fitting well with all known information regarding enuresis and child development. In addition, it can easily incorporate important features of the biological and emotional theories. At birth, the process of urination is governed by reflex action. Adults learn to delay the reflexive behavior of urination for relatively long periods of time. Children during their developmental years are attempting to master the learning task of controlling a reflexive behavior. Children with enuresis have difficulty in learning this control.

Associated Features

Several variables related to enuresis have attracted considerable attention and research over the years.

Intelligence

Some studies report a slightly lower than average level of intellectual functioning for children with enuresis (e.g., Iester et al., 1991). However, other studies have not found this relationship (e.g., Steinhausen, & Gobel, 1989). The majority of children with enuresis probably fall within the normal range of intelligence. Many children of superior intelligence also have enuresis.

Emotional Adjustment

Available data are not sufficient to completely understand the relationship between emotional problems and enuresis. However, the following statements appear to be supported by the bulk of the literature:

1. The majority of children with enuresis are not emotionally disturbed.
2. Most emotionally disturbed children do not suffer from enuresis.
3. There is, nevertheless, a higher incidence of enuresis among emotionally disturbed children than among the general population. This area of overlap might be expected because stress tends to increase the frequency of urination and might also distract the young child from the vigilance necessary to control urine and attend to proper toileting.
4. No specific diagnosis or emotional condition is associated with enuresis. The most commonly noted problems are anxiety, family conflict, and immaturity (Douglas, 1973; Foxman, Valdez, & Brook, 1986).
5. Although the data are somewhat conflicting, the likelihood that emotional disturbance will be present along with enuresis appears to increase if the child is female and older and if daytime wetting is present (e.g., Wagner, Smith, & Norris, 1988).
6. Although clinical lore has it that secondary enuresis is more likely than primary enuresis to be associated with emotional disturbance, research has failed to conclusively confirm this (e.g., Cho, 1984).

Socioeconomic and Ethnic Variables

Enuresis has been found to be more prevalent in lower socioeconomic groups, in larger families, and in families in which the mother has less education (Bakwin & Bakwin, 1972; MacKeith, Meadow, & Turner, 1973). It also varies from country to country and among ethnic and racial groups (de Jonge, 1973). These differences have not been researched sufficiently but are no doubt related to attitudes about toilet training and the amount of energy devoted to the process in different groups.

Toilet Training

Enuresis is thought by some to be related to excessively early, late, strict, or lax training methods (e.g., Bakwin & Bakwin, 1972). However, due to a lack of research in this area, no firm conclusion can be drawn at this time.

Sleep

One of the most common reports from parents who bring their child for treatment of enuresis is that their child is an exceedingly deep sleeper. However, historically the majority of the better controlled studies have failed to demonstrate any relationship between depth of sleep or stage of sleep and enuresis (e.g., Mikkelsen et al., 1980). Two recent studies (Neveus et al., 1999; Wolfish, 1999) suggest that children with enuresis may indeed be more difficult to arouse. It is to be hoped that, as data accumulate, a definitive answer will be given on this issue.

Enuresis, Fire Setting, and Cruelty to Animals Triad

Some years ago MacDonald (1963), following an impressionistic study involving interviews with 100 highly aggressive criminals, stated that there appeared to be a triad in their childhoods involving the presence of enuresis, fire setting, and cruelty to animals. Although this intriguing observation has become part of clinical folklore, studies have failed to validate this triad (e.g., Heller, Ehrlich, & Lester, 1984). In particular, enuresis does not seem hold up as a precursor of later aggressive behavior. On the other hand, fire setting and cruelty to animals are frequently associated with conduct disorder, which may well be a precursor of later criminal behavior (Jacobson, 1984).

Treatment

In considering possible treatments for enuresis, one would be well advised to consider the discomfort of the problem versus the danger and possible consequences of the attempted cure. Humane, conservative, and gentle approaches to treatment, along with a significant measure of patience, would appear to be most appropriate.

When to Treat

Because there is a steady progression in "spontaneous" remission each year and because the incidence of enuresis persisting into adulthood is very low, there is some question as to whether or not enuresis should be treated at all and, if so, at what age. However, there are good reasons for treatment. Sanitation problems leading to bladder and kidney infections need to be considered, particularly in the case of females. The degree of family conflict and parent–child antagonism that occurs in connection with the problem can have significant and long-lasting effects on the personality of the child and the relationship between parent and child. The embarrassment, teasing, and ostracism of the child by other children has significant effects on the child's emotional well-being and self-esteem. Considerable evidence shows that successful treatment results in an improvement in these areas and has an overall beneficial effect on self-esteem (Moffatt, 1989). Care should be taken to advise parents that many children have difficulty succeeding in enuresis treatment programs and that relapses are frequent (Van Londen, Van Londen-Barentsen, Van Son, & Mulder, 1995).

Urine Alarm Treatment

One of the most effective treatments for enuresis is a system in which an alarm is sounded when the child wets. Originally, these devices used a pad that the child slept on, which was attached to a bell (and sometimes a light). Current versions use an electrode that is inserted in the child's underclothes rather than a pad and a small buzzer that is attached by Velcro to the top of the underwear at the shoulder. Over a period of five decades, there have been dozens of demonstrations of the effectiveness of urine alarm training (Scott, Barclay, & Houts, 1992). Application of the alarm for a period of 8 to 12 weeks can be expected to result in between a 75 to 90% success rate in initial arrest of bedwetting. Urine alarms have been compared with every other form of treatment, including medication, in research studies and have consistently demonstrated equal or superior effectiveness (Iester et al., 1991). Reliable and reasonably inexpensive equipment can be obtained from numerous sources (see *www.bedwettingstore.com*). Best success is achieved when these devices are used under professional supervision. A recent and very interesting development in this area is the invention of a miniature ultrasonic sensor that is worn on a belt around the abdomen. This sensor determines urine volume in the bladder and sounds an alarm at a predetermined point (Petrican & Swan, 1998).

Although the underlying conditioning principle accounting for the effectiveness of this approach to treatment is not completely understood, it appears that the bell (and in some cases the light that accompanies the bell) is a mildly annoying stimulus because it awakens the child. As a result, the child usually learns to awaken in time to go to the bathroom or simply retains urine until morning in order to avoid the aversive stimulus.

Relapse rates with the urine alarm are substantial, generally in the neighborhood of 40% (Doleys, 1977). The simplest procedure for dealing with relapse is to use a second course of treatment; generally, success is quicker with the second course. Seldom is a third or fourth course required. Other approaches to dealing with the relapse problem have been the use of overlearning (Young & Morgan, 1972) and intermittent schedules of reinforcement (Finley, Rainwater, & Johnson, 1982).

Retention Control and Sphincter Exercises

Numerous studies have indicated that many children with enuresis have small functional bladder capacity. The actual physical size of their bladders is within normal limits; however, they appear to respond with the urge to urinate with much smaller volumes of urine than other children do. These children are noted to urinate frequently during the day and have a great deal of urgency when they need to urinate (Sorotzkin, 1984; Starfield, 1967). Obviously, the length of time they are in bed sleeping at night exceeds their limit for retaining urine. Observations of this sort led to employment of two approaches to treatment based on training and exercises (Miller, 1973). Retention control training involves having the child practice refraining from urination, after the urge develops, for longer and longer periods of time. The strategy in this technique is to increase the tolerance of the bladder for larger and larger volumes of urine. Sphincter control exercises involve starting and stopping the stream of urine once urination begins. The rationale for this approach is that it may increase the voluntary control of the sphincter, thus preventing unwanted urination. Early studies suggested that these methods might have considerable usefulness (Starfield & Mellits, 1968; Paschalis, Kimmel, & Kimmel, 1972). Later studies were disappointing in outcome (e.g., Harris & Purohit, 1977). Ronen and Abraham (1996)reported success with these methods for younger children but not for older ones. Although neither of these treatments can be regarded as producing firm experimental evidence of success, I have used a protocol involving retention control training followed by sphincter exercises, along with potent reinforcers for practicing these skills assiduously. This protocol has been described elsewhere (Walker, Milling, & Bonner, 1988), and in clinical practice it appears to work well.

Multiple Intervention Package Programs

Various programs have been developed over the years that incorporate multiple components in the treatment of enuresis. Two of the better known and more carefully researched programs of this sort are dry-bed training (Azrin, Sneed, & Foxx, 1973) and full-spectrum home training (Houts, Liebert, & Padawer, 1983). Dry-bed training involves the following components: urine alarm, potty alert device that makes a sound when the toilet is used, hourly awakenings, reinforcement for proper toileting, and reprimands and positive practice following accidents. The initial report indicated a success rate of 100% for this program (Azrin, Sneed, & Foxx, 1973). Later reports failed to replicate that level of success, but success rates of 85 to 95% are common (Bollard, Nettelbeck, & Roxbee, 1982).

Full-spectrum home training, developed by Houts and his associates, employs urine alarm, retention control training, and overlearning. A detailed description of this approach is available in *Bedwetting: A Guide for Parents and Children* (Houts & Liebert, 1984). Success rates for this method have been reported to be approximately 80% (Bollard & Nettelbeck, 1982; Houts, Peterson, & Whelan, 1986).

Medication

Three medications are currently prescribed with some frequency for enuresis. The most commonly prescribed medication is imipramine (Tofranil). Research has indicated that this medication has some usefulness and success in treatment of enuresis. Unfortunately, less than 50% of children treated with this become completely dry. The remainder show a reduction in frequency or no effect. When the medication is terminated, most children who have been treated with imipramine relapse. The percentage of those who do not relapse is about equivalent to the spontaneous remission rate (Blackwell & Currah, 1973). Another medication that is increasing in popularity is desmopressin acetate (DDAVP). This is a synthetic form of the vasopressin hormone that stimulates the kidneys to concentrate urine. Concentration of urine reduces the volume of urine produced during the night and enables some individuals to sleep through the night without wetting. A number of studies have shown a modest success rate for desmopressin (e.g., Klauber, 1989). Others have found little usefulness for it (e.g., Morton, Uling, & Williams, 1996). All studies indicate that it is effective only during use. On termination of the treatment, wetting returns to its previous level in the overwhelming majority of cases. DDAVP appears to be safe and has relatively few if any side effects but its modest improvement rate makes it of limited value (Djurhuus, Norgaard, Hjalmas, & Wille, 1992). In a comparison of DDAVP with the urine alarm, the alarm was found to be more effective (Wille, 1986).

Some clinicians and researchers have used oxybutynin chloride (Ditropan) to treat bedwetting (Buttarazzi, 1977). This drug reduces spasms of the bladder and appears to increase bladder capacity. Very limited research has been done on this drug to date. What research has been accomplished indicates modest effectiveness (e.g., Lovering, Tallett, & McKendry, 1988). Oxybutynin is often used if imipramine fails.

Hypnosis

Some studies have indicated that hypnosis and similar procedures are effective in the treatment of enuresis. The procedures generally involve having the child visualize the urinary system, along with the muscles and nerves. The child is then given suggestions for controlling the sphincters or awakening if such control is no longer possible. Karen Olness is noted for classic work in this area (Olness, 1975; Olness & Gardner, 1978). Her success rate was around 75%.

Other Treatment Approaches

A wide variety of other approaches to treatment have been employed. Some of these are known to be ineffective; others simply have not been studied sufficiently. Such measures as restriction of fluids before bed, urinating immediately before retiring, and reassurance and encouragement from the pediatrician have all been used extensively but are helpful in only a very small number of mild cases. Awakening the child before the wetting has occurred and gradually moving the time backward appears to help some children (Creer & Davis, 1975). Older children can even do this themselves with an alarm clock (Walker, 1978).

Ronen, Rahav, and Wozner (1995) reported very promising results using a cognitive therapy approach in which children were given self-control training to recognize a full bladder to increase their belief that they could change their behavior, and to motivate them to change the behavior. The researchers reported that follow-up data indicated that results improved with time using this approach, whereas they tended to decrease with time when other methods (e.g., urine alarm or token economy) were used. If their results hold up well on replication, this will be one of the more exciting developments in treatment in this area in some time.

A number of reports involving family therapy (and related approaches such as neurolinguistic reprogramming and metaphors) have appeared in the literature (e.g., Selig, 1982; Wood, 1988). However, these are, to date, mostly case studies or anecdotal reports recommending a wide variety of interventions. There is no uniformity in the literature regarding family therapy for enuresis, nor are there sufficient data to verify effectiveness.

ENCOPRESIS

Definition

The essential feature of encopresis is that the child repeatedly passes feces in inappropriate places, such as in clothing or on the floor. The passage of feces can be involuntary or intentional. The DSM-IV definition (American Psychiatric Association, 1994) requires a chronological or developmental age of at least 4 years and inappropriate passage of feces at least once a month for a minimum of 3 months. Because this is, by definition, a functional disorder, DSM-IV specifies that the condition not be due to a physiological or general medical problem. DSM-IV further stipulates that constipation and resultant overflow incontinence be indicated as present or absent.

The general term for fecal soiling or loss of control of the bowels is "fecal incontinence." When the incontinence cannot be accounted for by organic medical conditions and appears to be psychogenic, it is referred to as "functional encopresis." Even though this distinction tends to be blurred in the literature, it is wise to be precise in use of the two terms. Additional descriptive terms regarding encopresis involve the time, frequency, and history of the disorder. In contrast to enuresis, most cases of encopresis occur during the day and are therefore termed diurnal. However, nocturnal encopresis is not unknown. Encopresis may be characterized as continuous or intermittent. Some children soil virtually every day, whereas other children alternate between periods of soiling and continence. Finally, in terms of history, some children have never been toilet trained. This situation is referred to as "primary encopresis." Others have had a period of at least 6 months during which they were free of soiling before the problem began. This case is referred to as "secondary encopresis." Walker (1978), following an extensive review of the literature, concluded that three subtypes of encopresis could be identified. First, some children can be described as manipulative soilers. These children soil for some secondary benefit, such as passively expressing anger toward their parents, avoiding a test at school, or some similar social stimulus. The soiling appears to be at least partially under voluntary control and deliberate. Although older psychiatric literature suggested that this was the main etiology for soiling, more recent data indicate that this is really a relatively rare occurrence. The older impression was, no doubt, based on selective referrals to mental health professionals. Second, some cases of soiling appear to be due to stress-induced diarrhea and loose bowels. Careful history taking in these cases will usually show a parallel between life stress and bouts of soiling. A possibly related disorder is recurrent abdominal pain, which sometimes includes diarrhea and is thought to be a precursor of irritable bowel syndrome in adults. The third category of encopresis is the most common. This is retentive encopresis, or encopresis based on chronic constipation. It has estimated that between 80 to 95% of the cases fall in this category (Levine, 1975). Some explanation may be in order to describe how fecal soiling can be related to constipation, which would appear to be the exact opposite.

Numerous variables can result in a child becoming constipated. Such variables include a hereditary tendency toward constipation, unfortunate dietary choices, withholding stools, and emotional factors, among others. Whatever the initial cause, constipation can easily become chronic in children. This results because children do not pay much attention to their defecation frequency, and failure by the child to have a bowel movement is not immediately apparent to the parents in the way that bedwetting accidents are. The soiling then occurs in the following manner. As fecal material builds up in the intestine it creates a blockage of the intestine and eventually enlargement of the intestine. This is referred to as "psychogenic megacolon." In this condition, the walls of the intestine are stretched, become thin, and lose muscle tone. As a result, they are not able to move the impacted material along through the normal peristaltic movement. In the impacted colon, the fluid material from the stomach and small intestine forms a pool above the point of impaction. Liquid from this pool eventually seeps down around the impacted mass and out the anus. This produces a pasty stain on the clothing. When such soiling occurs, children state that they were unaware of the need to defecate. Although parents generally regard this as highly questionable, it is entirely accurate. The seepage is a passive process and not accompanied by the normal contractions and sensations of defecation. Occasionally, large portions of the impacted material may loosen and be evacuated. Parents are frequently amazed by the amount of material expelled at these times and by the diameter of the stools. There are numerous reports of stools so large that they had to broken into smaller pieces for the plumbing to accommodate them. Instances in which the impaction was so severe that manual removal was required have also been reported (Hatch, 1988).

Prevalence

By definition, functional encopresis does not begin before the age of 4. Estimates of the occurrence of functional encopresis have ranged from 1.5 to 7.5% of children (Doleys, Schwartz, & Ciminero, 1981). Encopresis is four or five times more common in males than in females and tends to decrease with age (Levine, 1975). Encopresis becomes infrequent in adolescence and rare in adulthood. Approximately 30% of children with encopresis simultaneously have problems with enuresis (Levine, 1975).

Theories of Etiology

As with enuresis, there are three general approaches to understanding the etiology of encopresis: biological, emotional, and learning.

Biological Variables

Encopresis by definition is fecal incontinence based on a functional disorder and not the result of organic dysfunction. Nevertheless, some notions regarding the etiology of encopresis involve a biological or physiological underlay. For one, the tendency to develop diarrhea or constipation may be greater in some individuals because of hereditary predisposition (Pettei & Davidson, 1991). Second, some form of subtle developmental delay has been proposed as a possible basis for encopresis (Pawl, 1988). However, it is unlikely that such variables play a significant role in most cases of encopresis (Bellman, 1966). Finally, one biological condition that definitely requires medical evaluation prior to treatment for encopresis is Hirschsprung's disease, or aganglionic megacolon. In this condition, there is insufficient nerve innervation in a section of the colon to produce sufficient peristalsis to move material through the tract. As a result, impaction develops at this site. In severe cases, this condition is discovered shortly after birth and is corrected by surgery. The surgical procedure involves removal of the section of intestine that does not have sufficient nerve innervation and reconnecting the two functional sections. However, mild cases of Hirschsprung's can go undetected and cause elimination problems later in life. Investigation generally involves a barium enema and should be performed by a gastroenterologist (Kirschner, 1991).

Emotional Variables

Early mental health literature on encopresis often assumed a psychodynamic etiology to the problem. Thus this symptom was sometimes thought of as a sign of unconscious conflict. Various personality profiles were proposed with respect to this disorder. Children with encopresis were, for example, considered to be immature, passive–aggressive, angry, insecure, anally fixated, negative, anxious, and low in self-esteem (Bemporad, Kresch, Asnes, & Wilson, 1978; Hoag, Norriss, Himeno, & Jacobs, 1971). Their mothers have been depicted as rigid and masochistic; their fathers as weak, ineffectual, and uninvolved (Bemporad et al., 1978). However, other studies have generally failed to replicate such results (Levine, 1975; Fritz & Armbrust, 1982). In addition, psychotherapy has a very modest success rate (if any) with children who have encopresis. Thus, although emotional factors may be involved in some children who have encopresis, this notion does not satisfactorily account for the etiology of the problem. This topic is discussed further later in the chapter.

Learning Variables

The third, and definitely the most useful, view of the etiology of encopresis is that it is based on principles of learning. Consideration of the three subcategories of encopresis within a learning theory framework suggests several possible explanations for the behavior. First, manipulative soiling appears to follow a reinforcement model. Use of soiling to successfully manipulate the environment serves to reinforce the child's soiling behavior. For example, the child may learn that complaints about abdominal pain or actual soiling episodes result in being permitted to leave school, in which an exam or some other stressful performance activity is imminent, and return to the safety of mother, home, and an afternoon of TV viewing. Chronic diarrhea and irritable bowel syndrome can be understood as symptoms in children in whom stress and anxiety lead to impaired bowel control and loss of successful performance of previously learned toileting behaviors. Associated with this might well be an inherited predisposition to react with intestinal distress in difficult situations, along with a failure to learn effective coping behaviors to reduce stress. Finally, the most common form of encopresis involves constipation. Poor dietary choices and failure to establish good toilet habits, both of which are learned, play a role in development of this disorder. In addition, children may learn to voluntarily withhold stools for various reasons. This withholding can readily precipitate constipation. Children, for example, may withhold stools while outside playing because they do not wish to take time to return to the house to go to the bathroom. Removal of the doors in the stalls of the bathrooms at a school or unsanitary conditions in school bathrooms have been known to precipitate epidemics of encopresis.

Associated Features

Encopresis has received much less research attention than has enuresis. This may be due to the fact that only in recent times has our diet and lifestyle been one that favored constipation.

Intelligence

There are conflicting reports regarding intelligence and encopresis. Some studies have reported slightly lower IQs than normal in children with the disorder (Olatawura, 1973);

others have reported essentially normal IQs (Bellman, 1966). There is certainly no intrinsic relationship between intellectual ability and constipation. Most children with encopresis are within the normal range of intelligence.

Emotional Adjustment

The general statements about emotional factors made with respect to enuresis apply equally well to encopresis. That is, most emotionally disturbed children do not have encopresis. Most children with encopresis are not emotionally disturbed. However, there does tend to be a higher rate of emotional disturbance among these children than among the general population. For example, Gabel, Hegedus, Wald, Chandra, and Chiponis (1986), in a study of children with encopresis, found that more of these children had signs of emotional disturbance that went beyond what would be expected for other children their age but had less emotional disturbance than children referred for psychotherapy or mental health care. There is no consistency in the type of emotional problem that these children appear to suffer. However, a fairly common observation is that there is frequently a great deal of turmoil and conflict within the family. It is possible that turmoil and conflict in the family interfere with proper toilet training. Conversely, it has been observed that the presence of encopresis can increase family conflict and is associated with feelings of distress and low self-esteem in the child with encopresis (Landman, Rappaport, Fenton, & Levine, 1986). These feelings appear to improve following successful treatment of the problem (Young, Brennen, Baker, & Baker, 1995).

Socioeconomic and Ethnic Variables

Very limited data are available with respect to socioeconomic and ethnic factors related to encopresis. There is some evidence that encopresis is more common in lower socioeconomic groups (Wolters, 1974). Given the differences in diet and in toilet training practices from one ethnic group to another, it is almost certain that investigation would uncover differences in rates of encopresis.

Child Abuse

The relationship between soiling and child abuse is somewhat puzzling. Literature from gastroenterologists and pediatricians seldom mentions this as an issue. However, reports have appeared in the child abuse literature suggesting a possible connection (Herbert, 1987). There appear to be two rationales for a possible connection. One is that sexual abuse involving anal penetration or stimulation might produce sufficient emotional conflict surrounding that part of the body to result in incontinence (Krisch, 1980). The other is that repeated anal intercourse might damage or weaken the anal sphincters to the extent that incontinence occurs (Krisch, 1980). Although both of these are possible, each would require fairly severe child abuse involving anal sex. A cautionary note is sounded by Clayden (1988), who studied 129 children with chronic constipation. He noted that chronic constipation itself can produce anal dilation, which could easily lead to an erroneous diagnosis of sexual abuse. There is no evidence that the majority of children with encopresis have been subjected to child abuse. Thus one should be alert to the possibility of sexual abuse (or even physical abuse based on the conflict over the problem) in children with encopresis. However, one should keep firmly in mind that such an association is probably the exception rather than the rule and that errors can readily be made unless a thorough evaluation is done (Brayden & Altemeier, 1989).

Treatment

Consideration of the three categories of encopresis described earlier suggests that different treatments would be advisable for the different etiologies.

Manipulative Soiling

In those relatively infrequent cases in which the child is using soiling as a way of manipulating the environment, a combination of behavioral and family therapy is indicated. Efforts should be made to teach the child more effective ways of coping with the environment, and the parents should be taught ways to communicate with and respond appropriately to their child. Sources of reinforcement that support the soiling behavior should be removed and more appropriate behavior rewarded. Family counseling and intervention may be necessary to accomplish these goals. Basic principles involved in this form of treatment have been described by Gurman and Kniskern (1981) and by Henggeler and Borduin (1990), as well as by many others. Behavioral treatment programs also have been discussed extensively in the literature (e.g., Walker, Hedberg, Clement, & Wright, 1981).

Chronic Diarrhea or Irritable Bowel Syndrome

Because the effects of stress and anxiety play a major role in the development of this problem, stress reduction and learning effective coping skills are crucial parts of treatment of this difficulty. In addition, supportive psychotherapy, as well as certain medications, are sometimes useful. Antidiarrhea medications are often used by physicians (see Angelides & Fitzgerald, 1981, for a review). Although some practitioners might prescribe antianxiety or antidepressant medications for children experiencing these symptoms, long-term use of psychotropic medication is not a recommended practice. Long-term effective control of these symptoms depends more on psychological intervention. Chronic diarrhea has been successfully treated with systematic desensitization (Hedberg, 1973) and hypnosis (Byrne, 1973). In addition, a variety of approaches, such as relaxation training, stress inoculation training, assertiveness training, and general stress management procedures, may be effective in managing diarrhea in these patients.

Retentive Encopresis

Because 80 to 95% of children with encopresis fall in the category of retentive or constipation-based encopresis, a number of treatments have been developed for dealing with these cases.

The standard medical treatment for constipation-based encopresis involves thorough evacuation of the bowel through laxatives and/or enemas followed by oral administration of 1 to 3 teaspoons of mineral oil two to three times a day for a period of 3 months to a year. A very thorough position statement on the medical treatment of this disorder has been prepared by the North American Society for Pediatric Gastroenterology and Nutrition (Baker et al., 1999). Laxatives, enemas, and mineral oil are available without prescription in any pharmacy. Because mineral oil has a tendency to retard the absorption of certain fat-soluble vitamins, most practitioners administer the mineral oil 1 to 2 hours after a meal and recommend that multiple-vitamin tablets be taken along with the mineral oil. Mineral oil acts as a gentle laxative and lubricant to enhance production of regular and soft stools. Once regular bowel habits are established using mineral oil, the mineral oil is phased out. Initial success with this type of treatment is fairly good. Generally around 80% of children become continent during active employment of this protocol. Unfortunately, when the child is removed from the regimen, relapse tends to occur. Stark, Spirito, Lewis, and Hart (1990) found that a substantial number of children, especially those with behavioral problems, are unsuccessful on such programs. Referral to a psychologist may be necessary for a treatment program that incorporates psychological intervention and careful behavioral management when the patient fails with simple medical management (Stark et al., 1997).

Although there have been occasional reports of the treatment of encopresis with psychotherapy, no systematic research has been done in this area (Thapar, Davies, Jones, & Rivett, 1992). Reviews of the area have generally concluded that psychotherapy is ineffective as a specific treatment for encopresis (e.g., Achenbach & Lewis, 1971). Reports have appeared involving the treatment of encopresis using family therapy or a systems approach (e.g., Wells & Hinkle, 1990). These reports have generally been case studies or anecdotal reports. There are no controlled studies with adequate follow-up to indicate that family therapy is effective in dealing with the problem of encopresis.

Numerous case studies and research reports have indicated a very high level of effectiveness for behavioral treatment of encopresis (for a review, see Christophersen & Mortweet, 2001). Most effective are package programs involving a combination of procedures. For example, Wright and Walker (1978) reported virtually 100% effectiveness for a treatment program involving medical procedures such as enemas and suppositories along with positive reinforcement for bowel movements and mild aversive consequences for soiled underclothing. Houts (Houts, Mellon, & Whelan, 1988) has described an excellent program that is very similar to the aforementioned and that adds an additional emphasis on diet manipulation (a high-fiber diet with restrictions on milk and cheese). The preponderance of evidence supports the efficacy of such combined programs. Useful clinical protocols for the application of these procedures may be found in Houts and Abramson 1990, and Howe and Walker, 1992. Variations of these programs have been successfully employed with children with mental retardation and other handicapping conditions (e.g., see Richmond, 1983).

Numerous reports have appeared involving the use of biofeedback for bowel problems (Whitehead, 1992). Biofeedback procedures are used to evaluate functioning of the sphincters and in training children to synchronize and control these muscles for effective elimination.

ACKNOWLEDGMENTS

Sincere appreciation is expressed to Mindy Thomas and Carolyn Drake who provided invaluable assistance in the preparation of the original draft of this chapter.

REFERENCES

Achenbach, T. M., & Lewis, M. (1971). A proposed model for clinical research and its application for encopresis and enuresis. *Journal of the American Academy of Child Psychiatry, 10*, 535–554.

American Psychiatric Association. (1994). *Diagnostic and statistical manual of mental disorders* (4th ed., rev.). Washington, DC: Author.

Angelides, A., & Fitzgerald, J. F. (1981). Pharmacologic advances in the treatment of gastrointestinal diseases. *Pediatric Clinics of North America, 28*, 95–112.

Azrin, N. H., Sneed, T. J., & Foxx, R. M. (1973). Dry bed: A rapid method of eliminating bedwetting (enuresis) of the retarded. *Behaviour Research and Therapy, 11*, 427–434.

Baker, S. S., Liptak, G. S., Colletti, R. B., Croffie, J. M., DiLorenzo, C., Ector, W., & Nurko, S. (1999). Constipation in infants and children: Evaluation and treatment. *Journal of Pediatric Gastroenterology and Nutrition, 29*, 612–626.

Bakwin, H., & Bakwin, R. M. (1972). *Behavior disorders in children*. Philadelphia: Saunders.

Bath, R., Morton, R., Uing, A., & Williams, C. (1996). Nocturnal enuresis and the use of desmopression: Is it helpful? *Child: Care Health and Development, 22*(2), 73–84.

Bellman, M. (1966). Studies on encopresis. *Acta Paediatrica Scandinavica, 170*(Suppl.), 1–137.

Bemporad, J. R., Kresch, R. A., Asnes, R., & Wilson, A. (1978). Chronic neurotic encopresis as a paradigm of a multifactorial psychiatric disorder. *Journal of Nervous and Mental Disease, 166*, 472–479.

Blackwell, B., & Currah, J. (1973). The psychopharmacology of nocturnal enuresis. In I. Kolvin, R. C. MacKeith, & S. R. Meadow (Eds.), *Bladder control and enuresis* (pp. 231–257). Philadelphia: Lippincott.

Bollard, J., & Nettelbeck, T. (1982). A component analysis of dry- bed training for treatment for bedwetting. *Behaviour Research and Therapy, 20*, 383–390.

Bollard, J., Nettelbeck, T., & Roxbee, L. (1982). Dry-bed training for childhood bedwetting: A comparison of group with individually administered parent instruction. *Behaviour Research and Therapy, 20*, 209–217.

Brayden, R., & Altemeier, W. A. (1989). Encopresis and child sexual abuse. *Journal of the American Medical Association, 262*(17), 2446.

Buttarazzi, P. J. (1977). Oxybutynin Chloride (Ditropan) in enuresis. *Journal of Urology, 118*, 46.

Byrne, S. (1973). Hypnosis and the irritable bowel: Case histories, methods and speculation. *American Journal of Clinical Hypnosis, 15*, 263–265.

Cho, S. C. (1984). Clinical study on childhood enuresis. *Seoul Journal of Medicine, 25*, 599–608.

Christophersen, E. R., & Mortweet, S. L. (2001). *Treatments that work with children*. Washington, DC: American Psychological Association.

Clayden, G. S. (1988). Reflex anal dilatation associated with severe chronic constipation in children. *Archives of Disease in Childhood, 63*, 832–836.

Creer, T. L., & Davis, M. H. (1975). Using a staggered-wakening procedure with enuretic children in an institutional setting. *Journal of Behavior Therapy and Experimental Psychiatry, 6*, 23–25.

Cullen, K. J. (1966). Clinical observations concerning behavior disorders in children. *Medical Journal of Australia, 1*, 712–715.

de Jonge, G. A. (1973). Epidemiology of enuresis: A survey of the literature. In I. Kolvin, R. C. MacKeith, & S. R. Meadow (Eds.), *Bladder control and enuresis* (pp. 39–46). Philadelphia: Lippincott.

Djurhuus, J. C., Norgaard, J. P., Hjalmas, K., & Wille, S. (1992). Nocturnal enuresis. *Scandinavian Journal of Urology and Nephrology, 143*(Suppl.), 3–29.

Doleys, D. M. (1977). Behavioral treatments for nocturnal enuresis in children: A review of the recent literature. *Psychological Bulletin, 84*(1), 30–54.

Doleys, D. M., Schwartz, M. S., & Ciminero, A. R. (1981). Elimination problems: Enuresis and encopresis. In E. J. Mash & L. G. Terdal (Eds.), *Behavioral assessment of childhood disorders* (pp. 679–710). New York: Guilford Press.

Douglas, J. W. B. (1973). Early disturbing events and later enuresis. In I. Kolvin, R. C. MacKeith, & S. R. Meadow (Eds.), *Bladder control and enuresis* (pp. 109–117). Philadelphia: Lippincott.

Egger, J., Carter, C. H., Soothill, J. F., & Wilson, J. (1992). Effect of diet treatment on enuresis in children with migraine or hyperkinetic behavior. *Clinical Pediatrics, 31*(5), 302–307.

Elian, M. (1991). Treating bed wetting. *British Medical Journal, 302*(6778), 729.

Evans, J. H. C., & Meadow, S. R. (1992). Desmopressin for bed wetting: Length of treatment, vasopressin secretion, and response. *Archives of Disease in Childhood, 67*, 184–188.

Fenichel, O. (1946). *The psychoanalytic theory of neurosis*. London: Routledge & Kegan Paul.

Finley, W. W., Rainwater, A. J., & Johnson, G. (1982). Effect of varying alarm schedules on acquisition and relapse parameters in the conditioning treatment of enuresis. *Behaviour Research and Therapy, 20*, 69–80.

Foxman, B., Valdez, R. B., & Brook, R. H. (1986). Childhood enuresis: Prevalence, perceived impact, and prescribed treatments. *Pediatrics, 77*(4), 482–487.

Fritz, G. K., & Armbrust, J. (1982). Enuresis and encopresis. *Pediatric Clinics of North America, 5*, 283–296.

Gabel, S., Hegedus, A. M., Wald, A., Chandra, R., & Chiponis, D. (1986). Prevalence of behavior problems and mental health utilization among encopretic children: Implications for behavioral pediatrics. *Developmental and Behavioral Pediatrics, 7*(5), 293–297.

Gurman, A. S., & Kniskern, D. P. (Eds.). (1981). *Handbook of family therapy*. New York: Brunner/Mazel.

Harris, L. S., & Purohit, A. P. (1977). Bladder training and enuresis: A controlled trial. *Behaviour Research and Therapy, 15*, 485–490.

Hatch, T. F. (1988). Encopresis and constipation in children. *Pediatric Clinics of North America, 35*(2), 257–280.

Hedberg, A. G. (1973). The treatment of chronic diarrhea by systematic desensitization: A case report. *Journal of Behavior Therapy and Experimental Psychiatry, 4*, 67–68.

Heller, M. S., Ehrlich, S. M., & Lester, D. (1984). Childhood cruelty to animals, firesetting and enuresis as correlates of competence to stand trial. *Journal of General Psychology, 110*, 151–153.

Henggeler, S. W., & Borduin, C. M. (1990). *Family therapy and beyond*. Pacific Grove, CA: Brooks/Cole.

Herbert, C. P. (1987). Expert medical assessment in determining probability of alleged child sexual abuse. *Child Abuse and Neglect, 11*, 213–221.

Hoag, J. M., Norriss, N. G., Himeno, E. T., & Jacobs, J. (1971). The encopretic child and his family. *Journal of the American Academy of Child Psychiatry, 10*, 242–256.

Houts, A. C., & Abramson (1990). Assessment and treatment for functional childhood enuresis and encopresis: Toward a partnership between health psychologists and physicians. In S. B. Morgan & T. M. Okwumabua (Eds.), *Child and adolescent disorders: Developmental and health psychology perspectives* (pp. 47–103). Hillsdale, NJ: Erlbaum.

Houts, A. C., & Liebert, R. M. (1984). *Bedwetting: A guide for parents and children*. Springfield, IL: Thomas Books.

Houts, A. C., Liebert, R. M., & Padawer, W. (1983). A delivery system for the treatment of primary enuresis. *Journal of Abnormal Psychology, 11*, 513–520.

Houts, A. C., Mellon, M. W., & Whelan, J. P. (1988). Use of dietary fiber and stimulus control to treat retentive encopresis: A multiple baseline investigation. *Journal of Pediatric Psychology, 13*(3), 435–445.

Houts, A. C., Peterson, J. K., & Whelan, J. P. (1986). Prevention of relapse in full-spectrum home training for primary enuresis: A components analysis. *Behavior Therapy, 17*, 462–469.

Howe, A. C., & Walker, C. E. (1992). Behavioral management of toilet training, enuresis, and encopresis. *Pediatric Clinics of North America, 39*(3), 413–432.

Iester, A., Marchesi, A., Cohen, A., Iester, M., Bagnasco, F., & Bonelli, R. (1991). Functional enuresis: Pharmacological versus behavioral treatment. *Child's Nervous System, 7*, 106– 108.

Imhof, B. (1956). Bettwasser in der erziehungsberatung. *Heilpaedagogische Werkblaetter, 25*, 122–127.

Jacobson, R. R. (1984). Child firesetters: A clinical investigation. *Journal of Child Psychology and Psychiatry, 26*(5), 759–768.

Kirschner, B. S. (1991). Hirschsprung's disease. In W. A. Walker, P. R. Durie, J. R. Hamilton, J. H. Walker-Smith, & J. B. Watkins (Eds.), *Pediatric gastrointestinal disease: Vol. 1. Pathophysiology, diagnosis, management* (pp. 829–832). Philadelphia: Decker.

Klauber, G. T. (1989). Clinical efficacy and safety of desmopressin in the treatment of nocturnal enuresis. *Journal of Pediatrics, 114*, 719–722.

Krisch, K. (1980). Encopresis as protection from homosexual annoyance. *Praxis der Kinderpsychologie und Kinderpsychiatrie, 37*, 260–265.

Landman, G. B., Rappaport, L., Fenton, T., & Levine, M. D. (1986). Locus of control and self-esteem in children with encopresis. *Developmental and Behavioral Pediatrics, 7*(2), 111–113.

Levine, M. D. (1975). Children with encopresis: A descriptive analysis. *Pediatrics, 56*(3), 412–416.

Lovering, J. S., Tallett, S. E., & McKendry, B. J. (1988). Oxybutinin efficacy in the treatment of primary enuresis. *Pediatrics, 82*, 104–106.

MacDonald, J. (1963). The threat to kill. *American Journal of Psychiatry, 120*, 125–130.

MacKeith, R. C. (1972). Is maturation delay a frequent factor in the origins of primary nocturnal enuresis? *Developmental Medicine and Child Neurology, 14*, 217–223.

MacKeith, R. C., Meadow, R., & Turner, R. K. (1973). How children become dry. In. I. Kolvin, R. C. MacKeith, & S. R. Meadow (Eds.), *Bladder control and enuresis* (pp. 3– 21). Philadelphia: Lippincott.

Mikkelsen, E. J., Rapoport, J. L., Nee, L., Gruenau,C., Mendelson, W., & Gillin, J. C. (1980). Childhood enuresis: I. Sleep patterns and psychopathology. *Archives of General Psychiatry, 37*, 1139– 1144.

Miller, P. M. (1973). An experimental analysis of retention control training in the treatment of nocturnal enuresis in two institutionalized adolescents. *Behavior Therapy, 4*, 288–294.

Moffatt, M. E. K. (1989). Nocturnal enuresis: Psychologic implications of treatment and nontreatment. *Journal of Pediatrics, 114*(4),697–704.

Neveus, T., Hetta, J., Cnattingius, S., Tuvemo, T., Lackgren, G., Olsson, U., & Stenberg, A. (1999). Depth of sleep and sleep habits among enuretic and incontinent children. *Acta Paediatrica, 88*(7), 748–752.

Olatawura, M. O. (1973). Encopresis: A review of thirty-two cases. *Acta Paediatrica Scandinavica, 62*, 358–364.

Olness, K. (1975). The use of self-hypnosis in the treatment of childhood nocturnal enuresis: A report on forty patients. *Clinical Paediatrics, 14*, 273–279.

Olness, K., & Gardner, G. G. (1978). Some guidelines for uses of hypnotherapy in pediatrics. *Pediatrics, 62*, 228–233.

Paschalis, A. P., Kimmel, H. D., & Kimmel, E. (1972). Further study of diurnal instrumental conditioning in the treatment of enuresis nocturna. *Journal of Behavior Therapy and Experimental Psychiatry, 3*, 253–256.

Pawl, G. A. (1988). Encopresis. In C. J. Kestenbaum & D. T. Williams (Eds.), *Handbook of clinical assessment of children and adolescents* (Vol. II, pp. 711–721). New York: New York University Press.

Petrican, P., & Swan, M. A. (1998). Design of a miniaturized ultrasonic bladder volume monitor and subsequent preliminary evaluation on 41 enuretic patients. *Transactions on Rehabilitation Engineering, 6*(1), 66–74.

Pettei, M. J., & Davidson, M. (1991). Idiopathic constipation. In W. A. Walker, P. R. Durie, J. R. Hamilton, J. H. Walker-Smith, & J. B. Watkins (Eds.), *Pediatric gastrointestinal disease: Vol. 1. Pathophysiology, diagnosis, management* (pp. 818–829). Philadelphia: Decker.

Richmond, G. (1983). Shaping bladder and bowel continence in developmentally retarded preschool children. *Journal of Autism and Developmental Disorders, 13*(2), 197–204.

Ronen, T., & Abraham, Y. (1996). Retention control training in the treatment of younger versus older enuretic children. *Nursing Research, 45*(2), 78–82.

Ronen, T., Rahav, G., & Wozner, Y. (1995). Self-control and enuresis. *Journal of Cognitive Psychotherapy: An International Quarterly, 9*(4), 249–258.

Scott, M. A., Barclay, D. R., & Houts, A. C. (1992). Childhood enuresis: Etiology, assessment, and current behavioral treatment. In M. Hersen, R. M. Eisler, & P. M. Miller (Eds.), *Progress in behavior modification* (Vol. 28, pp. 83–117). Sycamore, IL: Sycamore.

Selig, A. L. (1982). Treating nocturnal enuresis in one session of family therapy: A case study. *Journal of Clinical Child Psychology, 11*(3), 234–237.

Solomon, P., & Patch, V. D. (1969). *Handbook of psychiatry.* Los Altos, CA: Lange Medical.

Sorotzkin, B. (1984). Nocturnal enuresis: Current perspectives. *Clinical Psychology Review, 4*, 293–315.

Starfield, B. (1967). Functional bladder capacity in enuretic and nonenuretic children. *Journal of Pediatrics, 70*, 777–781.

Starfield, B., & Mellits, E. D. (1968). Increase in functional bladder capacity and improvements in enuresis. *Journal of Pediatrics, 72*, 483–487.

Stark, L. J., Opipari, L. C., Donaldson, D. L., Danovsky, M. B., Rasile, D. A., & DelSanto, A. F. (1997). Evaluation of a standard protocol for retentive encopresis: A replication. *Journal of Pediatric Psychology, 22*(5), 619–633.

Stark, L. J., Spirito, A., Lewis, A. V., & Hart, K. J. (1990). Encopresis: Behavioral parameters associated with children who fail medical management. *Child Psychiatry and Human Development, 20*(3), 169–179.

Steinhausen, H.-C., & Gobel, D. (1989). Enuresis in child psychiatric clinic patients. *Journal of the American Academy of Child and Adolescent Psychiatry, 28*(2), 279–281.

Tapia, F., Jekel, J., & Domke, H. R. (1960). Enuresis: An emotional symptom? *Journal of Nervous and Mental Disease, 130*, 61–66.

Thapar, A., Davies, G., Jones, T., & Rivett, M. (1992). Treatment of childhood encopresis: A review. *Child: Care, Health and Development, 18*, 343–353.

Van Londen, A., Van Londen-Barentsen, M. W. M., Van Son, M. J. M., Mulder, G. A. L. A. (1995). Relapse rate and subsequent parental reaction after successful treatment of children suffering from nocturnal enuresis: A 2½ year follow-up of bibliotherapy. *Behavior Research Therapy, 33*(3), 309–311.

Wagner, W. G., Smith, D., & Norris, W. R. (1988). The psychological adjustment of enuretic children: A comparison of two types. *Journal of Pediatric Psychology, 13*(1), 33–38.

Walker, C. E. (1978). Toilet training, enuresis, and encopresis. In P. Magrab (Ed.), *Psychological management of pediatric problems* (Vol. 1, pp. 129–189). Baltimore: University Park Press.

Walker, C. E., Hedberg, A. G., Clement, P. W., & Wright, L. (1981). *Clinical procedures for behavior therapy.* Englewood Cliffs, NJ: Prentice-Hall.

Walker, C. E., Milling, L. S., & Bonner, B. L. (1988). Incontinence disorders: Enuresis and encopresis. In D. K. Routh (Ed.), *Handbook of pediatric psychology* (pp. 363–397). New York: Guilford Press.

Wells, M. E., & Hinkle, J. S. (1990). Elimination of childhood encopresis: A family systems approach. *Journal of Mental Health Counseling, 12*(4), 520–526.

Whitehead, W. E. (1992). Biofeedback treatment of gastrointestinal disorders. *Biofeedback and Self-Regulation, 17*(1), 59–76.

Wille, S. (1986). Comparison of desmopressin and enuresis alarm for nocturnal enuresis. *Archives of Disease in Childhood, 61*, 30–33.

Wolfish, N. (1999). Sleep arousal function in enuretic males. *Scandinavian Journal of Urology and Nephrology Supplementum, 202*, 24–26.

Wolters, W. H. G. (1974). A comparative study of behavioural aspects in encopretic children. *Psychotherapy and Psychosomatics, 24*, 86–97.

Wood, A. (1988). King tiger and the roaring tummies: A novel way of helping young children and their families change. *Journal of Family Therapy, 10*, 49–63.

Wright, L., & Walker, C. E. (1978). A simple behavioral treatment program for psychogenic encopresis. *Behaviour Research and Therapy, 16*, 209–212.

Young, G. C., & Morgan, R. T. T. (1972). Overlearning in the conditioning treatment of enuresis: A long-term follow-up study. *Behaviour Research and Therapy, 10*, 419–420.

Young, M. H., Brennen, L. C., Baker, R. D., & Baker, S. S. (1995). Functional encopresis: Symptom reduction and behavioral improvement. *Developmental and Behavioral Pediatrics, 16*(4), 226–232.

33

Habit Disorders
Bruxism, Trichotillomania, and Tics

ALAN G. GLAROS
CATHERINE C. EPKINS

In this chapter, we discuss three common habit disorders in children: bruxism, trichotillomania (TTM), and tics. Each is characterized by behaviors that are nonfunctional. Each is common in children, at least in their milder forms, and each may occur in adults, as well as in children. However, there are considerable differences between the disorders. TTM and tics are listed as mental disorders in the *Diagnostic and Statistical Manual of Mental Disorders* (DSM-IV; American Psychiatric Association [APA], 1994), whereas bruxism is not. Drugs are more frequently used to treat TTM and tics, and dental techniques are commonly used to treat bruxism. A considerable proportion of knowledge regarding the etiology and treatment of these conditions comes from studies on adults with these conditions. Where there are gaps in our knowledge of these disorders in children, we turn to data based on studies with adults.

BRUXISM

Bruxism is the nonfunctional contact of the teeth. When measured by recordings from the masseter muscles, at least two distinctly different behaviors can be discerned: (1) high amplitude, brief rhythmic EMG bursts that can vary in total duration, and (2) arrhythmic, high amplitude activity, typically of short duration (Wruble, Lumley, & McGlynn, 1989). The first behavior is associated with grinding, gnashing, or tapping behaviors of the teeth, and the second is associated with teeth clenching. In the neurologically intact individual, grinding most commonly occurs at night, whereas clenching can occur both at night and during the day. However, the bite forces exerted during sleep may be greater than the forces created voluntarily (Nishigawa, Bando, & Nakano, 2001). Both self-report data and sleep studies suggest that bruxists can engage in both clenching and grinding behaviors, although the ratio between the behaviors differs among individual bruxists. Furthermore, at least some parafunctional tooth contact appears to be normal during sleep.

Bruxism can have a variety of symptomatic effects. These include abnormal wear on the teeth (atypical wear facets), tooth mobility, changes in gingival tissues and resorption of the alveolar bone, hypertrophy or tenderness in the masticatory muscles, and facial/temporomandibular joint (TMJ) pain (see Glaros & Rao, 1977b; Vanderas, 1994, for reviews; Molina, dos Santos, Nelson, & Nowlin, 2000). The severity of bruxing is positively associated with muscular and joint disorders (Molina, dos Santos, Nelson, & Nowlin, 1999). Atypical wear facets are a poor diagnostic indicator of ongoing teeth grinding, as they may reflect a prior history of grinding. Studies indicate that approximately 30 to 50% of children show atypical facets (Lindqvist, 1971), but only half of these children are identified as bruxers by parental report alone. Clenching, on the other hand, is not as easily detected by dental examinations. Instead, the usual correlates of clenching are self-reported pain in the TMJ, in the musculature of the face, neck, or shoulders, or in the teeth directly or reports of headache or other facial pain.

Reported prevalence rates of bruxism in children and adolescents vary widely, ranging from 6 to 90% (American Academy of Pediatric Dentistry [AAPD], 1990; Bayardo, Mejia, Orozco, & Montoya, 1996; Kaidonis, Richards, & Townsend, 1993; Widmalm, Christiansen, & Gunn, 1995). The rates vary so dramatically because of disparities in defining the condition, the diagnostic signs and symptoms for the behaviors involved, and the failure to separate bruxism from other oral habits and parafunctions. Bruxism can occur as soon as teeth erupt (Arnold, 1981). A considerable proportion of children experience intermittent and temporary bruxing, whereas bruxing will continue into adolescence and adulthood for a smaller proportion (Egermark, Carlsson, & Magnusson, 2001; Magnusson, Egermark, & Carlsson, 2000). There is little evidence of gender differences in those who brux, at least among adolescents (Koidis, Zarifi, Grigoriadou, & Garefis, 1993). In the United States, the prevalence of both parafunctions and pain may be higher in African American children (Widmalm, Gunn, Christiansen, & Hawley, 1995) than in white children. Western cultures appear to have lower levels of bruxism than non-Western cultures (Johansson et al., 1993); in non-Western societies, high rates of dental wear facets may be more attributable to diet, harsh environmental and climatic conditions, and other factors than to bruxism. A familial predisposition to bruxism, as suggested in twin studies, may also indicate a biological component to the disorder (Lindqvist, 1974). Children of bruxing parents exhibit teeth grinding significantly more often than children of parents who were not, or had not, been bruxists (Abe & Shimakawa, 1966). Within an individual, bruxing behaviors are highly variable, even over the course of a few nights.

Bruxism has been linked to a variety of physical, behavioral, and psychological disorders. Bruxism is a common correlate of Rett's disorder and various dystonias (FitzGerald, Jankovic, & Percy, 1990; Watts, Tan, & Jankovic, 1999). The presence of oral tori (rounded bony protuberances), particularly on the mandible, is associated with increased clenching and grinding (Clifford, Lamey, & Fartash, 1996). Nutritional deficiencies, histamine release associated with allergies, colds, and stress (Marks, 1980), and hyperthyroidism have been linked to bruxism (see Ahmad, 1986; Cash, 1988, for reviews). Mental retardation, especially Down syndrome, is consistently associated with bruxism (Lindqvist & Heijbel, 1974). Patients with headaches, tinnitus, vertigo, facial muscle soreness or pain, tooth pain, or juvenile rheumatoid arthritis may also report symptoms associated with bruxism (Rubinstein,

Axelsson, & Carlsson, 1990; Tanchyk, 1991). Various drugs can also trigger or exacerbate bruxism. Amphetamines and other stimulant medications, alone or in combination with other substances, may produce bruxism (Gara & Roberts, 2000). Thus children who receive these drugs for attention-deficit/hyperactivity disorder (ADHD) may be at high risk for bruxism.

There is strong evidence that bruxism is a disorder of sleep (Wruble et al., 1989). Comparisons of "normal" sleepers with those exhibiting "violent behaviors" during sleep showed that bruxism was significantly more common in the sleep-disordered groups (Ohayon, Caulet, & Priest, 1997). Among adults, nocturnal bruxers report more snoring, breathing pauses during sleep, symptoms of obstructive sleep apnea, and a variety of other parasomnias (Ohayon, Li, & Guilleminault, 2001). The sleep microstructure of bruxists contains more sleep instability and "arousal oscillations" in delta sleep than among nonbruxists (Zucconi, Oldani, Ferini-Strambi, & Smirne, 1995). Gross bodily movements and changes in EEG activity, heart rate, respiratory rhythms, and digital vasoconstriction also occur during nocturnal bruxism (see reviews by Glaros & Rao, 1977a; Wruble et al., 1989). Between 14.5 and 17.3% of adult participants who reported restless leg syndrome also reported bruxism, and the risk of bruxism was about twice as high among those with restless legs. Other studies suggest that bruxers have more generalized disturbances of autonomic control (Sjoholm, Piha, & Lehtinen, 1995). Most parasomnias decrease throughout childhood, but sleep bruxism, leg restlessness and somniloquy continue to be relatively more common from early adolescence through adulthood (Laberge, Tremblay, Vitaro, & Montplaisir, 2000). Broadly summarized, these findings support the hypothesis advanced by Broughton (1968) that bruxism is a sleep-related disorder of arousal (Kato, Rompré, Montplaisir, Sessle, & Lavigne, 2001).

Stress may also play a role in bruxism (Hicks, Conti, & Bragg, 1990; Pierce, Chrisman, Bennett, & Close, 1995). Children who brux display more stress symptoms and nervous disorders than nonbruxists (Lindqvist, 1972). Children who experience "unpleasant life events" show more grinding, clenching, and lip/cheek biting (Vanderas, 1995). The temporal relationship between bruxism and stress is less clear, although some research suggests that the anticipation of stress may be a better predictor of the relationship between stressors and bruxism, at least in an adult population (Hopper, Gevirtz, Nigl, & Taddey, 1992). Follow-up examination of urinary catecholamine levels in children showed that higher levels of epinephrine and dopamine were significantly predictive of bruxism (Vanderas, Menenakou, Kouimtzis, & Papagiannoulis, 1999). The pain reported by bruxers diminishes quality of life, as it does for other individuals with pain (Dao, Lund, & Lavigne, 1994). Finally, case studies have suggested that childhood sexual abuse may be associated with bruxism.

The role of occlusion ("bite") in bruxism and TMJ dysfunction has received considerable attention in the dental literature. Some studies suggest that occlusal problems are a major etiological factor in bruxism whereas others do not. Occlusal defects are very common in children, even among children who have received occlusal treatments (Kirveskari, Alanen, & Jämsa, 1992). Most children adapt without difficulty to ongoing changes in their occlusion. Perhaps children who are generally more irritable and less adaptable are also those more likely to be affected by occlusal changes. The evidence of a relationship between malocclusion and bruxism is weak and does not justify the use of irreversible treatment of occlusal conditions to prevent or treat bruxism (Vanderas & Manetas, 1995).

The treatment literature on bruxism in children is very sparse. In adults, one commonly used dental technique is the fabrication and use of an interocclusal appliance. This device is usually constructed of hard acrylic, and it functions as a mouth guard or splint to cover either the maxillary or mandibular teeth. When worn at night, the device prevents the teeth from contacting each other, thereby preventing damage from grinding. It may also reduce pain and soreness in the TMJ and masticatory muscles that can be a consequence of bruxism (Sheikholeslam, Holmgren, & Riise, 1993). There is, however, little evidence that these appliances actually prevent bruxism. Unfortunately, the therapeutic effect appears to last only as long as the individual uses the device (Sheikholeslam et al., 1993). The continued growth and development of the mandible and cranial structures make hard acrylic splints a poor choice for children. In addition, children may not be particularly cooperative in the processes involved in making, fitting, or wearing an acrylic appliance. As an alternative, they may be given soft splints, which are easier and less expensive to fabricate. However, children using soft splints should be monitored closely because the devices may increase parafunctional habits and associated symptomatology (Okeson, 1987). Children, like adults, may not tolerate the device in their mouths during sleep and may be unable to adapt to its presence.

Nocturnal alarms have also been used to treat bruxism in adults. Typically, the alarm monitors EMG activity of a masticatory muscle (usually the masseter or temporalis) during sleep. The alarm sounds when EMG activity exceeds a threshold for some period of time or when a certain number of suprathreshold EMG events occur within a brief period of time. If awakening is then combined with an arousal task, the therapeutic effect (i.e., reduction in bruxing duration and frequency) is enhanced (Cassisi, McGlynn, & Belles, 1987). Nocturnal alarms appear to be similar to bell-and-pad systems for nocturnal enuresis. The short-term follow-up data show a varied pattern. Some studies indicate at least some maintenance of gains following treatment (e.g., Cassisi & McGlynn, 1988), whereas some studies have reported increases in bruxing activity following treatment (e.g., Funch & Gale, 1980). The procedural or subject variables that account for these reported differences are not well known. We do not know whether nocturnal alarms are more efficacious for grinding or clenching. Nonetheless, the technique is sufficiently promising to warrant further studies, especially with children (Glaros & Melamed, 1992).

EMG biofeedback is commonly used to treat symptoms of facial pain, which is a common correlate of bruxism. Although the technique appears to be efficacious and competitive with dental techniques (see Crider & Glaros, 1999, for a meta-analytic review), there is little agreement on the mechanisms of change. Furthermore, biofeedback's utility with children has not been explored. Other techniques that may be used to treat bruxism include massed practice (satiation; Pierce & Gale, 1988), stress management, and psychotherapy. Massed practice may cause structural damage to the teeth and should not be used without a mouth guard in place. One study compared "directed muscular relaxation" (similar to progressive muscle relaxation training) with a "competency reaction technique" emphasizing parental and teacher habits that produced anxious reactions. The study was conducted on 33 children, ages 3 to 6 years, with signs of bruxism, high anxiety levels, and temporomandibular disorders (TMD). Both treatments were reportedly successful in reducing the frequency of signs of TMD and reducing anxiety (Restrepo, Alvarez, Jaramillo, Velez, & Valencia, 2001). Unfortunately, it is not clear whether the treatments had a specific effect on bruxism. Tranquilizers have been used to treat facial pain in bruxing and clenching adults, but they do not appear to have any therapeutic advantage over occlusal appliance treatment (Nemcovsky, Gazit, Serfati, & Gross, 1992). Because these medications have significant side effects, and because a number of conservative, reversible treatments are available, they cannot be recommended for routine use in children.

TRICHOTILLOMANIA

In DSM-IV, trichotillomania (TTM) is defined as "recurrent pulling out of one's hair resulting in noticeable hair loss" (APA, 1994, p. 621). Common sites of pulling are the scalp, eyelashes, and eyebrows. Other conditions, including alopecia areata, tinea capitis (ringworm), and other less common fungal infections can cause hair loss. In some cases, a scalp biopsy is required to rule out other pathological conditions, and children may admit to pulling out their hair only when they are confronted with biopsy results (Swedo & Rapoport, 1991).

The most medically serious consequence of TTM, although uncommon, is the development of trichobezoars, hairballs that form in the stomach when patients eat the hair. These individuals can present with anemia, loss of appetite, abdominal pain, diarrhea or constipation, nausea, vomiting, and hematemesis (blood-stained vomit; Slagle & Martin, 1991). Bezoars can cause intestinal obstruction, gastrointestinal bleeding, bowel perforation, acute pancreatitis, and obstructive jaundice.

Hair pulling can occur in brief sessions, resulting in the loss of just a few hairs, to sessions lasting several hours during which hundreds of hairs are pulled (Swedo & Rapoport, 1991). Hair pulling usually occurs in solitude, although very young children will pull hair in the presence of family members. Increased pulling can occur during periods of stress and during periods of relaxation and distraction (e.g., watching television or reading). Often, patients are not aware of their hair pulling (Christenson, Mackenzie, & Mitchell, 1991).

For diagnosis, the DSM-IV requires an increasing tension before pulling or when attempting to resist the behavior and a sense of relief or gratification when pulling out the hair. However, most child hair pullers do not report any urge to pull, rising tension, or relief after pulling (King, Scahill, et al., 1995; King, Zohar, et al., 1995; Reeve, Bernstein, & Christenson, 1992). Thus this tension requirement in DSM-IV may not be applicable for diagnosing TTM in children. In addition, DSM-IV requires the condition be associated with significant distress and social or other impairments. Research is beginning to document the negative social and interpersonal effects of hair pulling in youth (Boudjouk, Woods, Miltenberger, & Long, 2000).

TTM is found in less than 1% of clinic samples of children (Mannino & Delgado, 1969), and lifetime prevalence rates are 1% in nonreferred adolescents (King, Zohar, et al., 1995). In college student samples, 1–2% have a past or current history of TTM (APA, 1994). Yet an estimated 4% of the population are hair pullers, and roughly 10% have had the habit at some time (Azrin & Nunn, 1977). It usually begins in childhood (Swedo & Rapoport, 1991). TTM is more common in children than adults, yet it is frequently found in adult females. The incidence rates are not influenced by socioeconomic status or ethnicity (Krishnan, Davidson, & Guajardo, 1985).

There are both chronic and remitting forms, which seem to differ in age of onset and sex distribution (Swedo & Rapoport, 1991). When TTM begins before age 6, it is usually mild, lasting several weeks to months, even without treatment. Frequency among boys and girls is similar among children with TTM (APA, 1994). Later onset TTM, developing after 6 but typically around age 13, is mainly seen in females. In this group, TTM tends to be more severe, difficult to treat, and chronic, lasting up to decades (Swedo & Rapoport, 1991). The relationship of the child and adolescent forms of the disorder to the adult form is unclear (Vitulano, King, Scahill, & Cohen, 1992), yet most adults with TTM report that their symptoms began in childhood or adolescence (Christenson et al., 1991).

Mood and anxiety disorders, as well as alcohol and drug abuse, are common in adult TTM patients, and they have greater lifetime prevalence of these disorders than is noted in the general population (Christenson et al., 1991). The degree of psychopathology among children with TTM is much less than in older, adult populations. However, TTM is frequently associated with anxiety and affective disorders (Reeve et al., 1992), and it is associated with more internalizing than externalizing problems (Hanna, 1997). However, some studies note high rates of disruptive behavior disorders in youth with TTM (King, Scahill, et al., 1995).

Hair pulling may be a developmentally appropriate "habit" in preschool-age children who exhibit no other problems, and many have described TTM in children beginning as a "habit disorder." Perhaps, as Reeve et al. (1992) suggest, cases in which hair pulling exists as an isolated symptom should be diagnosed as a stereotypy or habit disorder. On the other hand, hair pulling in some children may exist in association with anxiety or depressive disorders. Indeed, screening for associated depression and anxiety symptoms should be conducted with children who present with hair pulling. Longitudinal studies of TTM in children are needed to clarify the natural history of the disorder, identify the mechanisms that initiate and sustain hair pulling, and understand the connections and relationship of TTM to other forms of psychopathology.

The specific causes of TTM are unknown, and it is generally assumed to be multidetermined. A triggering event may be the hospitalization of the child, school difficulties, or a disrupted mother–child relationship. Predisposing factors may include excessive concern about weight, severe medical illness, and previous scalp surgery or trauma. Environmental factors such as stress at school may play a role in the onset and clinical course of hair pulling (Hanna, 1997; Reeve et al., 1992). Family dynamics have also been implicated as a possible initiating and maintaining factor of hair pulling. A consistent pattern seen in families of female adolescents with TTM involves a passive, detached, or ineffectual father and an ambivalent, double-binding, hostile, and critical mother (Greenberg & Sarner, 1965). Children with TTM may regard their families as less cohesive and less expressive than they would like them to be (Reeve et al., 1992). Although TTM is not more prevalent in bulimic females than in nonbulimic females (Christenson & Mitchell, 1991), it has been suggested that a common etiological factor might be unresolved sexual conflicts that are suppressed through repetitive disordered patterns of eating, hair pulling, or both (Tattersall, 1992).

Increased familial rates of affective disorders, obsessive–compulsive disorder (OCD), and TTM have been found in TTM patients (Greenberg & Sarner, 1965). First-degree relatives of patients with TTM have a greater frequency of OCD than the general population and than relatives of a psychiatric control group (Lenane et al., 1992). Increased frequency of OCD and OCD-like symptoms is also found in parents of children with TTM (King, Scahill, et al., 1995).

Some suggest that TTM may be a subset of OCD, rather than an impulse control disorder or a manifestation of depression or anxiety (Swedo & Rapoport, 1991). Findings from family history data, neuropharmacological evidence in treatment studies (discussed later), the apparent similarities of the symptoms of OCD and TTM, and similar neuropsychological test patterns reported for TTM and OCD patient groups (Rettew et al., 1991; Swedo et al., 1989) have been put forth in support of this hypothesis. However, studies of adults and children with TTM report lower rates of OCD (13–25%) than one might predict if TTM were a variant of OCD (Christenson et al., 1991; King, Scahill, et al., 1995; King, Zohar, et al., 1995), and comparisons of the clinical features of TTM and OCD groups find important differences that call this hypothesis into question (e.g., Stanley, Swann, Bowers, Davis, & Taylor, 1992). Furthermore, childhood TTM can occur in the absence of obsessive or compulsive symptomatology, and many children with TTM fail to meet diagnostic criteria for

OCD, although many do have significant OCD symptoms (King, Zohar, et al., 1995; Reeve et al., 1992; Riddle et al., 1990). However, as Reeve et al. (1992) suggest, TTM may represent monosymptomatic OCD, or a form of TTM may be related to OCD. Additional research is necessary to delineate the possible etiological connections between affective disorders, OCD, and TTM.

The incidence of TTM in TTM patients' relatives ranges from 5–8% (Christenson, Mackenzie, & Reeve, 1992; Lenane et al., 1992). Such findings may reflect not only genetic tendencies toward the disorder but also the impact of environmental modeling (Christenson, Mackenzie, & Mitchell, 1992). To what degree the familial patterns reflect genetic mediation is unknown, as genetic studies of TTM have yet to be conducted.

With respect to treatment, psychodynamic therapy and hypnosis have been reported to be useful but have not been studied with large samples of children and have not included follow-up and objective measures of improvement. Behavioral methods can be effective in reducing both the urge and frequency of hair pulling (Friman, Finney, & Christophersen, 1984). Behavioral treatments have included self-monitoring, aversion therapy, habit reversal, covert desensitization, relaxation training, competing response training, overcorrection, and negative practice training (see Friman et al., 1984, for a review, and Mansueto, Golomb, Thomas, & Townsley Stemberger, 1999, for a comprehensive behavioral treatment model). Habit reversal appears superior to other behavioral methods (Azrin, Nunn, & Frantz, 1980). Modified habit reversal has been effective with adolescents (Rapp, Miltenberger, Long, Elliott, & Lumley, 1998).

Treatment programs that combine multiple behavioral treatments appear promising (cf. Mansueto et al., 1999). Rothbaum's (1992) nine-session cognitive-behavioral treatment consists of self-monitoring, habit reversal, stimulus control, and stress management techniques such as relaxation, thought stopping, and cognitive restructuring. This general protocol, conducted with a sample comprising both children and adults, is reported to be relatively effective; 86% of treatment completers were classified as responders, yet only 31% met responder criterion at long-term follow-up (Lerner, Franklin, Meadows, Hembree, & Foa, 1998). Vitulano et al.' s (1992) six-session program involves self-monitoring, relaxation, habit interruption, prevention training, and competing reaction training. In addition, overcorrection, or positive practice, was employed, as well as annoyance review, in which children detail the reasons they want to stop pulling their hair. Future work should evaluate the relative or differential efficacy of the individual components with both larger samples of children and longer follow-ups.

Drug therapies have been used infrequently as treatment for children with TTM, and data on the pharmacological treatment of youths with TTM are sparse. The adult literature indicates that serotonin reuptake inhibitors such as fluoxetine and clomipramine are helpful in some patients with TTM (see Hollander & Allen, 2001, for a review). The literature on the use of medication for the treatment of TTM in children includes only case reports. Clearly the role of clomipramine or other serotonin reuptake inhibitors, such as fluoxetine, in the treatment of childhood TTM remains to be examined in controlled studies. However, the potential side effects of these drugs in youths merits caution (Riddle et al., 1991). The side effects include insomnia, self-destructive and dangerous behavior, sudden death, increased blood pressure, and increased heart rate.

Systematic research is needed on the relative merits of behavioral and pharmacological treatments, alone or in combination with each other. In addition, controlled comparisons between different treatments for children are needed. Furthermore, follow-up studies are greatly needed regarding the longitudinal course of treatment outcome for youth with TTM.

How treatment choice and outcome are related to patterns of psychiatric comorbidity and genetic vulnerability should be clarified with systematic research.

TICS

Tics represent the most common involuntary movement disorder of childhood. Tics are defined as sudden, brief, involuntary, rapid, nonrhythmic, repetitive movements or utterances that are purposeless and stereotypic (Singer & Walkup, 1991). A tic is neither a habit nor a spasm. The old term, "habit spasm," reflects previous concerns with bad habits, as well as lack of clarity regarding the voluntary or involuntary origin of the movements (Leung & Fagan, 1989). Tic disorders are classified into three main categories in the DSM-IV (APA, 1994), based on the duration of symptoms and the composition of movements or vocalizations: (1) transient tic disorder (TTD), (2) chronic motor or vocal tic disorder (CTD), and (3) Tourette's disorders (TD).

Common transient motor tics include eye blinking, facial grimacing, nose puckering, head turning, and shoulder shrugging. Transient vocal tics consist of throat clearing, coughing, hissing, or other distracting noises. A transient tic may be especially noticeable with heightened excitement or fatigue. It typically increases with emotional stress, diminishes with distraction and concentration, and decreases during sleep (Leung & Fagan, 1989). Transient tics usually last from a few weeks to a few months, and by DSM-IV definition, transient tic disorder does not persist for more than 1 year. However, it is common for a child to have a series of transient tics over the course of a few years. Diagnosis is strictly retrospective, as there is no way to predict whether an individual who develops a single tic will develop others and whether the tics will persist and become chronic.

CTD is differentiated from TTD by the duration and consistency of the tics. For diagnosis, there must be single or multiple chronic tics, either motor or vocal, but not both, for at least 1 year. Chronic motor tics are more common than chronic vocal tics. On the other hand, TD involves multiple motor tics and one or more vocal tics that occur every day or intermittently for more than 1 year. Over time the tics may change in location, number, frequency, and complexity (APA, 1994). Like all tics, the movements and sounds are involuntary, but voluntary suppression is possible for brief periods. An outburst of tics often occurs when the individual no longer tries to suppress them. The vocalizations, of which there must be at least one, may begin with such ordinary sounds as sniffing or throat clearing, and they are not recognized as repetitions until later. Coprolalia, repeating unacceptable words and obscenities, may begin years after onset and occurs in less than one-third of individuals with TD (Cohen, Riddle, & Leckman, 1992).

It is important to distinguish tics from other involuntary stereotypic movements, such as myoclonus, tremor, and dystonia (Leung & Fagan, 1989). The differential diagnosis of chronic complex tics also includes hyperthyroidism, Wilson's disease, choreiform syndromes (cerebral palsy, Huntington's, Sydenham's), encephalitis, focal seizures, head trauma, drug effects, and carbon monoxide intoxication (Lacey, 1986; Leung & Fagan, 1989).

Epidemiological studies find that transient tics occur in about 18% of children under 10 years old, with decreasing prevalence rates (2–3%) found in these youths when they reach adolescence (Peterson, Pine, Cohen, & Brook, 2001). Thus the majority of transient tics remit by adolescence. Boys are affected 2 to 3 times more often than girls, and age of onset varies between 4 and 12 years, with a mean onset at age 7 (Lacey, 1986). Onset is usually sudden and may follow a particularly disturbing event. Chronic tics have been estimated to occur in about 1.6% of the United States population (Shapiro, Shapiro, Young, & Feinberg, 1988). Age of onset is typically during childhood or adolescence, and boys are affected 3 to 4 times more often than girls.

The mean age of onset in TD is 6.5 years, with most patients being affected before age 13. TD is more prevalent in Caucasians than in blacks or Hispanics (Singer & Walkup, 1991). TD is found in every country, ethnic group, and social class (Cohen, Bruun, & Leckman, 1988). Recent epidemiological studies on TD in youths have reported prevalence rates ranging from 0.15% to 1.1% (Kadesjo & Gillberg, 2000; Peterson et al., 2001), a higher rate among school children than previously noted (Caine et al., 1988). A substantial proportion (41%) of children identified with TD have not sought medical help (Caine et al., 1988). Although children in specialized programs for TD and those with TD in other clinical settings are similar in terms of tic severity and duration, age of onset, and patterns of comorbidity (Coffey, Biederman, Spencer et al., 2000), the applicability of these findings to nonreferred youths with TD is unknown.

The natural history of tics and tic disorders is unclear. Approximately 5–24% of children with TTD may develop CTD (found in 1–2% of adults), followed by the emergence of TD (Cohen et al., 1992). However, no longitudinal follow-up studies have been conducted to document this progression. It has been estimated, however, that in 30 to 40% of children with TD, all tic symptoms will disappear by late adolescence, and in an additional 30%, tics will diminish markedly. The remaining patients will have symptoms that persist into adulthood (Erenberg, Cruse, & Rothner, 1987). Characteristics that predict whether tics will improve or persist have yet to be identified.

Whereas transient tics are not usually associated with learning or behavioral disorders (Lerer, 1987), TD may be associated with severe behavioral, emotional, social, and academic dysfunction. Interestingly, the severity of tic symptoms is not significantly related to dysfunction, adjustment, or psychiatric comorbidity in youths with TD (Carter et al., 2000; Coffey, Biederman, Geller, et al., 2000). However, non-OCD anxiety disorders, particularly separation anxiety disorder, are associated with tic severity (Coffey, Biederman, Smoller, et al., 2000). Research indicates that much of the behavioral and social dysfunction in youths with TD is related to the co-occurrence of other disorders. In clinical samples, for example, 50 to 64% of children with TD also meet diagnostic criteria for ADHD (Kadesjo & Gillberg, 2000), with ADHD usually preceding the onset of tic disorders (Spencer, Biederman, Coffey, et al., 1999). However, ADHD in early adolescence weakly predicts tics in later adolescence (Peterson et al., 2001). The co-occurrence of ADHD and TD is more likely when TD is severe (Comings & Comings, 1988), but others find that the presence of ADHD is not related to TD severity (Coffey, Biederman, Smoller, et al., 2000). Children with both TD and ADHD have been found to have more social problems and more externalizing and internalizing behavior problems than children with TD only and/or ADHD only (Carter et al., 2000). Thus, much of the dysfunction in youths with TD appears to be associated with ADHD and not the TD alone.

However, it is important to note that youths with TD, with or without ADHD, have significantly elevated levels of internalizing problems and social withdrawal in comparison with control groups (Carter et al., 2000). Comorbid mood disorders have been found to be the best predictors of hospitalization and impaired functioning in youth with TD (Coffey, Biederman, Geller, et al., 2000). Many children with TD also have learning disabilities (Golden, 1990).

A number of studies have reported high rates of OCD in patients with TD, usually around 50% or above (Pauls, Towbin, Leckman, Zahner, & Cohen, 1986; Peterson et al.,

2001), although many studies report far lower proportions (ranges between 10 and 28%; cf. Caine et al., 1988; Carter et al., 2000). A recent prospective study found that tics in childhood and early adolescence predicted an increase in OCD symptoms in late adolescence and early adulthood (Peterson et al., 2001). Studies of children and adolescents with OCD find that 30–32% have tics, chronic motor tics, or TD (Rapoport, Swedo, & Leonard, 1992). Those with TD and OCD tend to have higher levels of impairment than those without comorbid OCD (Coffey et al., 1998). Clearly, the developmental, descriptive, and potential etiological (to be discussed later) relationships among TD, ADHD, and OCD will be of continuing research and clinical interest.

TD and CTD appear to show a familial concentration with genetic transmission (Cohen & Leckman, 1994). In families with TD, CTD may be a milder manifestation of the same disorder. A major advance in understanding TD has emerged from family genetic studies that have demonstrated that TD appears to be the result of a single, dominant autosomal gene (Cohen & Leckman, 1994). Some have proposed that TTD and CTD/TD represent an expression of the same genetic defect (Kurlan, Behr, Medved, & Como, 1988), whereas others have shown that CTD tends to be a mild form of TD and that both are transmitted as inherited traits in the same families (Pauls, Towbin et al., 1986; Pauls et al., 1990). Twin studies also support a genetic factor in the etiology of TD and CTD (Pauls & Leckman, 1988). However, the incomplete concordance in monozygotic twins (77% or higher) implies that other nongenetic factors may also play a role (see Cohen & Leckman, 1994).

In addition, segregation analyses of family study data support a sex-influenced autosomal dominant mode of inheritance with variable expressivity as either TD, CTD, or OCD (Pauls, Towbin, et al., 1986; Pauls et al., 1990), suggesting that OCD is etiologically and genetically related to TD. This TD gene has a high degree of penetrance in males, with almost all males who carry the gene having CTD or TD, yet the penetrance in females is somewhat lower, with females more likely to manifest OCD, as well as tics (Pauls & Leckman, 1988). It remains uncertain however, how to determine which cases of tics and of OCD are part of TD and which are not.

A hypothesized genetic relationship between TD and ADHD is at present controversial. Some studies support such a relationship (Comings & Comings, 1984), whereas others find that the two disorders are genetically separate and transmitted independently in families at risk (Pauls, Hurst, et al., 1986) and that the two disorders have distinct courses (Spencer, Biederman, Coffey, et al., 1999). The high incidence of ADHD in TD patients may be due to an ascertainment bias, whereby the child with both TD and ADHD is more likely to come to the attention of physicians and/or health care professionals for diagnosis and treatment.

There has been little evidence regarding environmental factors that may influence the onset of TD, although some data support a stress–diathesis model of TD (Bornstein, Stefl, & Hammond, 1990). Nongenetic factors are likely to mediate the form or severity of the expression or phenotype of the TD diathesis among vulnerable individuals (Leckman et al., 1987). Perinatal factors, such as severity of maternal life stress during pregnancy and severe nausea and/or vomiting during the first trimester, are associated with current tic severity (Leckman et al., 1990). Future longitudinal studies of high-risk individuals (offspring or siblings of TD probands) are needed to confirm these findings.

The exact neurological and neurochemical processes involved in tics are not known. The basal ganglia, frontal cortex, and limbic system have been frequently mentioned as sites of pathology (see Cohen & Leckman, 1994). A dysfunction of central neurotransmitter systems has been suggested in TD. The dopaminergic, serotonergic, nonadrenergic, cholinergic,

GABAergic, and opioid systems have shown abnormalities, but which, if any, represent the main pathophysiological factor(s) remains to be delineated (see Hollander & Allen, 2001).

Drug therapy for tic disorders should be considered only if the symptoms are disabling and adversely affect the child's academic and psychosocial development or interpersonal relationships and if the symptoms do not respond to nondrug interventions (Cohen et al., 1992). Dopamine-receptor-blocking neuroleptics appear to be the most effective. Haloperidol reduces or eliminates tics in about 80% of children. However, only 20–30% continue to use and benefit from haloperidol for an extended period of time because of the high incidence of unacceptable side effects. Some reports suggest that other neuroleptic drugs, such as pimozide and fluphenazine, are about as effective in reducing tics as haloperidol, with fewer adverse side effects (Cohen et al., 1992; Golden, 1990).

Clonidine, a centrally active α-adrenergic agonist, may be more effective than placebo in patients with TD (Leckman et al., 1991), and it is often helpful in patients with milder TD symptoms, as well as in improving attentional and behavioral problems (Golden, 1990). Clonidine thus may be especially effective in treating children with both TD and ADHD, as all of the stimulant drugs commonly used to treat ADHD have been reported to increase tic response (Golden, 1988). Although some reports suggest that stimulant medications either can suppress or have no effect on tics or tic disorders in many ADHD youths (e.g., Gadow, Sverd, Sprafkin, Nolan, & Grossman, 1999), others feel that this group of children requires cautious use of stimulants if ADHD and TD symptoms do not respond to clonidine (Cohen et al., 1992). Interestingly, children with ADHD and comorbid tic disorders showed a better behavioral response to clonidine than did children with ADHD without tic disorders (96% vs. 53%; Steingard, Biederman, Spencer, Wilens, & Gonzalez, 1993). Open or retrospective trials suggest desipramine (Spencer, Biederman, Kerman, Steingard, & Wilens, 1993) and nortriptyline (Spencer, Biederman, Wilens, Steingard, & Geist, 1993) are therapeutic for children with ADHD and tic disorders.

Alternative treatments for children with tic disorders are important to consider, particularly because 15–20% of children with TD do not respond to medication and others may not tolerate the side effects of the medications. Major sources of dysfunction in many children with TD are the coexisting symptoms of ADHD, OCD, and learning disabilities and/or the social and developmental consequences of TD and these other symptoms. Nonpharmacological treatments are often effective in the management of tics and these associated symptoms.

Several behavioral treatment approaches to TD show promise as alternatives to drug treatment. These include massed negative practice, contingency management, relaxation training, self-monitoring, and habit reversal (see Azrin & Peterson, 1988, for a review). Habit reversal is a multicomponent program that incorporates self-monitoring, relaxation training, contingency management, and competing response training. In a wait-list controlled study with 10 patients with TD, habit reversal yielded a 93% tic reduction at home and in the clinic (Azrin & Peterson, 1990). An examination of the effectiveness of three of the most promising behavioral treatments in a counterbalanced design revealed that tics were reduced an average of 55% with habit reversal, 44% with self-monitoring, and 32% with relaxation training (Peterson & Azrin, 1992). Thus all three approaches may be potentially useful in treating TD.

Children with TD, particularly those with ADHD, learning disabilities, and school problems, may benefit from educational interventions (see Carter et al., 1999, for classroom suggestions). Significant others from the child's social system and educational environment should be included in interventions, as these systems have a direct impact on the child and can assist in improving or preventing the social, behavioral, and educational problems that are associated with tic disorders.

SUMMARY

The disorders described here form a heterogeneous collection. Fortunately, the most prevalent forms of these disorders tend to be both mild and transient. Only when the problems are persistent and severe is intervention necessary. Behavioral techniques appear to have the greatest utility in managing these disorders, although medications may be of benefit for TTM and tics.

There are several gaps in our knowledge of these disorders. In all three, the neurological basis for the behaviors is unclear. Although stress may play a role in these disorders, the processes by which stressors influence motor functioning are not well understood. And although all three involve motor activity, the role that cognitive factors play in each has not been adequately addressed. In short, although researchers and clinicians have made considerable progress in understanding and managing bruxism, TTM, and tics, there is a need for continuing work on these disorders.

ACKNOWLEDGMENTS

Preparation of this chapter was supported by Grant No. DE13563 to the first author.

REFERENCES

Abe, K., & Shimakawa, M. (1966). Genetic and developmental aspects of sleep-talking and teeth-grinding. *Acta Paedopsychiatrica, 33,* 339–344.

Ahmad, R. (1986). Bruxism in children. *Journal of Pedodontics, 10,* 105–126.

American Academy of Pediatric Dentistry. (1990). Treatment of temporomandibular disorders in children: Summary statements and recommendations. *Journal of the American Dental Association, 120,* 265–269.

American Psychiatric Association. (1994). *Diagnostic and statistical manual of mental disorders* (4th ed.). Washington, DC: Author.

Arnold, M. (1981). Bruxism and the occlusion. *Dental Clinics of North America, 25,* 395–407.

Azrin, N. H., & Nunn, R. G. (1977). *Habit control in a day.* New York: Simon & Schuster.

Azrin, N. H., Nunn, R. G., & Frantz, S. E. (1980). Treatment of hair pulling: A comparative study of habit reversal and negative practice training. *Journal of Behavior Therapy and Experimental Psychiatry, 11,* 13–20.

Azrin, N. H., & Peterson, A. L. (1988). Behavior therapy for Tourette's syndrome and tic disorders. In D. J. Cohen, R. D. Bruun, & J. F. Leckman (Eds.), *Tourette's syndrome and tic disorders: Clinical understanding and treatment* (pp. 237–255). New York: Wiley.

Azrin, N. H., & Peterson, A. L. (1990). Treatment of Tourette syndrome by habit reversal: A waiting-list control group comparison. *Behavior Therapy, 21,* 305–318.

Bayardo, R. E., Mejia, J. J., Orozco, S., & Montoya, K. (1996). Etiology of oral habits. *Journal of Dentistry for Children, 63,* 350–353.

Bornstein, R. A., Stefl, M. E., & Hammond, L. (1990). A survey of Tourette syndrome patients and their families: The 1987 Ohio Tourette survey. *Journal of Neuropsychiatry, 2,* 275–281.

Boudjouk, P. J., Woods, D. W., Miltenberger, R. G., & Long, E. S. (2000). Negative peer evaluation in adolescents: Effects of tic disorders and trichotillomania. *Child and Family Behavior Therapy, 22,* 17–29.

Broughton, R. J. (1968). Sleep disorders: Disorders of arousal? *Science, 159,* 1070–1078.

Caine, E. D., McBride, M. C., Chiverton, P., Bamford, K. A., Rediess, S., & Shiao, J. (1988). Tourette's syndrome in Monroe County school children. *Neurology, 38,* 472–475.

Carter, A. S., Fredine, N. J., Findley, D., Scahill, L., Zimmerman, L. & Sparrow, S. S. (1999). Recommendations for teachers. In J. F. Leckman & D. J. Cohen (Eds.), *Tourette's syndrome—Tics, obsessions, compulsions: Developmental psychopathology and clinical care* (pp. 360–369). New York: Wiley.

Carter, A. S., O'Donnell, D. A., Schultz, R. T., Scahill, L., Leckman, J. F., & Pauls, D. L. (2000). Social and emotional adjustment in children affected with Gilles de la Tourette's syndrome: Associations with ADHD and family functioning. *Journal of Child Psychology and Psychiatry, 41,* 215–223.

Cash, R. G. (1988). Bruxism in children: Review of the literature. *Journal of Pedodontics, 12,* 107–127.

Cassisi, J. E., & McGlynn, F. D. (1988). Effects of EMG-activated alarms on nocturnal bruxism. *Behavior Therapy, 19,* 133–142.

Cassisi, J. E., McGlynn, F. D., & Belles, D. R. (1987). EMG-activated feedback alarms for the treatment of nocturnal bruxism: Current status and future directions. *Biofeedback and Self-Regulation, 12,* 13–30.

Christenson, G. A., Mackenzie, T. B., & Mitchell, J. E. (1991). Characteristics of 60 adult chronic hair pullers. *American Journal of Psychiatry, 148,* 365–370.

Christenson, G. A., Mackenzie, T. B., & Mitchell, J. E. (1992). Further comments on trichotillomania. *American Journal of Psychiatry, 149,* 284–285.

Christenson, G. A., Mackenzie, T. B., & Reeve, E. A. (1992). Familial trichotillomania. *American Journal of Psychiatry, 149,* 283.

Christenson, G. A., & Mitchell, J. E. (1991). Trichotillomania and repetitive behavior in bulimia nervosa. *International Journal of Eating Disorders, 10,* 593–598.

Clifford, T., Lamey, P. J., & Fartash, L. (1996). Mandibular tori, migraine and temporomandibular disorders. *British Dental Journal, 180,* 382–384.

Coffey, B. J., Biederman, J., Geller, D. A., Spencer, T. J., Kim, G. S., Bellordre, C. A., et al. (2000). Distinguishing illness severity from tic severity in children and adolescents with Tourette's disorder. *Journal of the American Academy of Child and Adolescent Psychiatry, 39,* 556–561.

Coffey, B. J., Biederman, J., Smoller, J. W., Geller, D. A., Sarin, P., Schwartz, S., & Kim, G. S. (2000). Anxiety disorders and tic severity in juveniles with Tourette's disorder. *Journal of the American Academy of Child and Adolescent Psychiatry, 39,* 562–568.

Coffey, B. J., Biederman, J., Spencer, T., Geller, D. A., Faraone, S. V., & Bellordre, C. A. (2000). Informativeness of structured diagnostic interviews in the identification of Tourette's disorder in referred youth. *Journal of Nervous and Mental Disease, 188,* 583–588.

Coffey, B., Miguel, E., Biederman, J., Baer, L., Rauch, S. L., O'Sullivan, R. L., et al. (1998). Tourette's disorder with and without obsessive–compulsive disorder in adults: Are they different? *Journal of Nervous and Mental Disease, 186,* 201–206.

Cohen, D. J., Bruun, R. D., & Leckman, J. F. (Eds.). (1988). *Tourette's syndrome and tic disorders: Clinical understanding and treatment.* New York: Wiley.

Cohen, D. J., & Leckman, J. F. (1994). Developmental psychopathology and neurobiology of Tourette's syndrome. *Journal of the American Academy of Child and Adolescent Psychiatry, 33,* 2–15.

Cohen, D. J., Riddle, M. A., & Leckman, J. F. (1992). Pharmacotherapy of Tourette's syndrome and associated disorders. *Psychiatric Clinics of North America, 15,* 109–129.

Comings, D. E., & Comings, B. G. (1984). Tourette's syndrome and attention deficit disorder with hyperactivity: Are they genetically related? *Journal of the American Academy of Child and Adolescent Psychiatry, 23,* 138–146.

Comings, D. E., & Comings, B. G. (1988). Tourette's syndrome and attention deficit disorder. In D. J. Cohen, R. D. Bruun, & J. F. Leckman (Eds.), *Tourette's syndrome and tic disorders: Clinical understanding and treatment* (pp. 119–135). New York: Wiley.

Crider, A. B., & Glaros, A. G. (1999). A meta-analysis of EMG biofeedback treatment of temporomandibular disorders. *Journal of Orofacial Pain, 13,* 29–37.

Dao, T. T., Lund, J. P., & Lavigne, G. J. (1994). Comparison of pain and quality of life in bruxers and patients with myofascial pain of the masticatory muscles. *Journal of Orofacial Pain, 8,* 350–356.

Egermark, I., Carlsson, G. E., & Magnusson, T. (2001). A 20-year longitudinal study of subjective symptoms of temporomandibular disorders from childhood to adulthood. *Acta Odontologica Scandinavica, 59,* 40–48.

Erenberg, G., Cruse, R. P., & Rothner, A. D. (1987). The natural history of Tourette syndrome: A follow-up study. *Annals in Neurology, 22,* 383–385.

FitzGerald, P. M., Jankovic, J., & Percy, A. K. (1990). Rett syndrome and associated movement disorders. *Movement Disorders, 5,* 195–202.

Friman, P. C., Finney, J. W., & Christophersen, E. R. (1984). Behavioral treatment of trichotillomania: An evaluative review. *Behavior Therapy, 15,* 249–265.

Funch, D. P., & Gale, E. N. (1980). Factors associated with nocturnal bruxism and its treatment. *Journal of Behavioral Medicine, 3,* 385–397.

Gadow, K. D., Sverd, J., Sprafkin, J., Nolan, E. E., & Grossman, S. (1999). Long-term methylphenidate therapy in children with comorbid attention-deficit hyperactivity disorder and chronic multiple tic disorder. *Archives of General Psychiatry, 56,* 330–336.

Gara, L., & Roberts, W. (2000). Adverse response to methylphenidate in combination with valproic acid. *Journal of Child and Adolescent Psychopharmacology, 10,* 39–43.

Glaros, A. G., & Melamed, B. G. (1992). Bruxism in children: Etiology and treatment. *Applied and Preventive Psychology, 1,* 191–199.

Glaros, A. G., & Rao, S. M. (1977a). Bruxism: A critical review. *Psychological Bulletin, 84,* 767–781.

Glaros, A. G., & Rao, S. M. (1977b). Effects of bruxism: A review of the literature. *Journal of Prosthetic Dentistry, 38,* 149–157.

Golden, G. S. (1988). The relationship between stimulant medication and tics. *Psychiatric Annals, 18,* 409–413.

Golden, G. S. (1990). Tourette syndrome: Recent advances. *Pediatric Neurology, 8,* 705–714.

Greenberg, H. R., & Sarner, C. A. (1965). Trichotillomania, symptom and syndrome. *Archives of General Psychiatry, 12,* 482–489.

Hanna, G. L. (1997). Trichotillomania and related disorders in children and adolescents. *Child Psychiatry and Human Development, 27,* 255–268.

Hicks, R. A., Conti, R. A., & Bragg, H. R. (1990). Increases in nocturnal bruxism among college students implicate stress. *Medical Hypotheses, 33,* 230–240.

Hollander, E., & Allen, A. (2001). Serotonergic drugs and the treatment of disorders related to obsessive-compulsive disorder. In M. T. Pato & J. Zohar (Eds.), *Current treatments of obsessive–compulsive disorder* (2nd ed., pp. 193–220). Washington, DC: American Psychiatric Association.

Hopper, D. K., Gevirtz, R. N., Nigl, A. J., & Taddey, J. (1992). Relationship between daily stress and nocturnal bruxism. *Biofeedback and Self-Regulation, 17,* 309.

Johansson, A., Omar, R., Fareed, K., Haraldson, T., Kiliaridis, S., & Carlsson, G. E. (1993). Comparison of the prevalence, severity and possible causes of occlusal tooth wear in two young adult populations. *Journal of Oral Rehabilitation, 20,* 463–471.

Kadesjo, B., & Gillberg, C. (2000). Tourette's disorder: Epidemiology and comorbidity in primary school children. *Journal of the American Academy of Child and Adolescent Psychiatry, 39,* 548–555.

Kaidonis, J. A., Richards, L. C., & Townsend, G. C. (1993). Nature and frequency of dental wear facets in an Australian aboriginal population. *Journal of Oral Rehabilitation, 20,* 333–340.

Kato, T., Rompré, P., Montplaisir, J. Y., Sessle, B. J., & Lavigne, G. J. (2001). Sleep bruxism: An oromotor activity secondary to micro-arousal. *Journal of Dental Research, 80,* 1940–1944.

King, R. A., Scahill, L., Vitulano, L. A., Schwab-Stone, M., Tercyak, K. P., & Riddle, M. A. (1995). Childhood trichotillomania: Clinical phenomenology, comorbidity, and family genetics. *Journal of the American Academy of Child and Adolescent Psychiatry, 34,* 1451–1459.

King, R. A., Zohar, A. H., Ratzoni, G., Binder, M., Kron, S., Dycian, A., et al. (1995). An epidemiological study of trichotillomania in Israeli adolescents. *Journal of the American Academy of Child and Adolescent Psychiatry, 34,* 1212–1215.

Kirveskari, P., Alanen, P., & Jämsa, T. (1992). Association between craniomandibular disorders and occlusal interferences. *Journal of Prosthetic Dentistry, 67,* 692–696.

Koidis, P. T., Zarifi, A., Grigoriadou, E., & Garefis, P. (1993). Effect of age and sex on craniomandibular disorders. *Journal of Prosthetic Dentistry, 69,* 93–101.

Krishnan, K. R., Davidson, J. R. T., & Guajardo, C. (1985). Trichotillomania: A review. *Comprehensive Psychiatry, 26,* 123–128.

Kurlan, R., Behr, J., Medved, L., & Como, P. (1988). Transient tic disorder and the clinical spectrum of Tourette's syndrome. *Archives of Neurology, 45,* 1200–1201.

Laberge, L., Tremblay, R. E., Vitaro, F., & Montplaisir, J. (2000). Development of parasomnias from childhood to early adolescence. *Pediatrics, 106,* 67–74.

Lacey, D. J. (1986). Diagnosis of Tourette syndrome in childhood: The need for heightened awareness. *Clinical Pediatrics, 25,* 433–435.

Leckman, J. F., Dolnansky, E. S., Hardin, M. T., Clubb, M., Walkup, J. T., Stevenson, J., & Pauls, D. L. (1990). Perinatal factors in the expression of Tourette's syndrome: An exploratory study. *Journal of the American Academy of Child and Adolescent Psychiatry, 29,* 220–226.

Leckman. J. F., Hardin, M. T., Riddle, M. A., Stevenson, J., Ort, S., & Cohen, D. J. (1991). Clonidine treatment of Gilles de la Tourette's syndrome. *Archives of General Psychiatry, 48,* 324–328.

Leckman, J. F., Price, R. A., Walkup, J. T., Ort, S., Pauls, D. L., & Cohen, D. J. (1987). Non-genetic factors in Gilles de la Tourette's syndrome. *Archives of General Psychiatry, 44,* 100.

Lenane, M. C., Swedo, S. E., Rapoport, J. L., Leonard, H., Sceery, W., & Guroff, J. J. (1992). Rates of obsessive–compulsive disorder in first-degree relatives of patients with trichotillomania: A research note. *Journal of Child Psychology and Psychiatry, 33,* 925–933.

Lerer, R. J. (1987). Motor tics, Tourette syndrome, and learning disabilities. *Journal of Learning Disabilities, 20,* 266–267.

Lerner, J., Franklin, M. E., Meadows, E. A., Hembree, E., & Foa, E. B. (1998). Effectiveness of a cognitive behavioral treatment program for trichotillomania: An uncontrolled evaluation. *Behavior Therapy, 29,* 157–171.

Leung, A. K. C., & Fagan, J. E. (1989). Tic disorders in childhood (and beyond). *Postgraduate Medicine, 86,* 251–261.

Lindqvist, B. (1971). Bruxism in children. *Odontologisk Revy, 22,* 413–424.

Lindqvist, B. (1972). Bruxism and emotional disturbance. *Odontologisk Revy, 23,* 231–242.

Lindqvist, B. (1974). Bruxism in twins. *Acta Odontologica Scandinavica, 32,* 177–187.

Lindqvist, B., & Heijbel, J. (1974). Bruxism in children with brain damage. *Acta Odontologica Scandinavica, 32,* 313–319.

Magnusson, T., Egermark, I., & Carlsson, G. E. (2000). A longitudinal epidemiologic study of signs and symptoms of temporomandibular disorders from 15 to 35 years of age. *Journal of Orofacial Pain, 14,* 310–319.

Mannino, F. V., & Delgado, R. A. (1969). Trichotillomania in children: A review. *American Journal of Psychiatry, 126,* 505–511.

Mansueto, C. S., Golomb, R. G., Thomas, A. M., & Townsley Stemberger, R. M. (1999). A comprehensive model for behavioral treatment of trichotillomania. *Cognitive and Behavioral Practice, 6,* 23–43.

Marks, M. B. (1980). Bruxism in allergic children. *American Journal of Orthodontics, 77,* 48–59.

Molina, O. F., dos Santos, J., Nelson, S. J., & Nowlin, T. (1999). A clinical study of specific signs and symptoms of CMD in bruxers classified by the degree of severity. *Journal of Craniomandibular Practice, 17,* 268–279.

Molina, O. F., dos Santos, J., Jr., Nelson, S. J., & Nowlin, T. (2000). Profile of TMD and bruxer compared to TMD and nonbruxer patients regarding chief complaint, previous consultations, modes of therapy, and chronicity. *Journal of Craniomandibular Practice, 18,* 205–219.

Nemcovsky, C. E., Gazit, E., Serfati, V., & Gross, M. (1992). A comparative study of three therapeutic modalities in a temporomandibular disorder (TMD) population. *Journal of Craniomandibular Practice, 10,* 148–157.

Nishigawa, K., Bando, E., & Nakano, M. (2001). Quantitative study of bite force during sleep-associated bruxism. *Journal of Oral Rehabilitation, 28,* 485–491.

Ohayon, M. M., Caulet, M., & Priest, R. G. (1997). Violent behavior during sleep. *Journal of Clinical Psychiatry, 58,* 369–376.

Ohayon, M. M., Li, K. K., & Guilleminault, C. (2001). Risk factors for sleep bruxism in the general population. *Chest, 119,* 53–61.

Okeson, J. P. (1987). The effects of hard and soft occlusal splints on nocturnal bruxism. *Journal of the American Dental Association, 114,* 788–791.

Pauls, D. L., Hurst, C. R., Kruger, S. D., Leckman, J. F., Kidd, K. K., & Cohen, D. J. (1986). Gilles de la Tourette's syndrome and attention-deficit disorder with hyperactivity: Evidence against a genetic relationship. *Archives of General Psychiatry, 43,* 1177–1179.

Pauls, D. L., & Leckman, J. F. (1988). The genetics of Tourette's syndrome. In D. J. Cohen, R. D. Bruun, & J. F. Leckman (Eds.), *Tourette's syndrome and tic disorders: Clinical understanding and treatment* (pp. 91–101). New York: Wiley.

Pauls, D. L., Pakstis, A. J., Kurlan, R., Kidd, K. K., Leckman, J. F., Cohen, D. J., et al. (1990). Segregation and linkage analysis of Tourette's syndrome and related disorders. *Journal of the American Academy of Child and Adolescent Psychiatry, 29,* 195–203.

Pauls, D. L., Towbin, K. E., Leckman, J. F., Zahner, G. E. P., & Cohen, D. J. (1986). Gilles de la Tourette's syndrome and obsessive–compulsive disorder: Evidence supporting a genetic relationship. *Archives of General Psychiatry, 43,* 1180–1182.

Peterson, A. L., & Azrin, N. H. (1992). An evaluation of behavioral treatments for Tourette syndrome. *Behaviour Research and Therapy, 30,* 167–174.

Peterson, B. S., Pine, D. S., Cohen, P., & Brook, J. S. (2001). Prospective, longitudinal study of tic, obsessive–compulsive, and attention-deficit/hyperactivity disorders in an epidemiological sample. *Journal of the American Academy of Child and Adolescent Psychiatry, 40,* 685–695.

Pierce, C. J., Chrisman, K., Bennett, M. E., & Close, J. M. (1995). Stress, anticipatory stress, and psychologic measures related to sleep bruxism. *Journal of Orofacial Pain, 9,* 51–56.

Pierce, C. J., & Gale, E. N. (1988). A comparison of different treatments for nocturnal bruxism. *Journal of Dental Research, 67,* 597–601.

Rapoport, J. L., Swedo, S. E., & Leonard, H. L. (1992). Childhood obsessive compulsive disorder. *Journal of Clinical Psychiatry, 53,* 11–16.

Rapp, J. T., Miltenberger, R. G., Long, E. S., Elliott, A. J., & Lumley, V. A. (1998). Simplified habit reversal treatment for chronic hair pulling in three adolescents: A clinical replication with direct observation. *Journal of Applied Behavior Analysis, 31,* 299–302.

Reeve, E. A., Bernstein, G. A., & Christenson, G. A. (1992). Clinical characteristics and psychiatric comorbidity in children with trichotillomania. *Journal of the American Academy of Child and Adolescent Psychiatry, 31,* 132–138.

Restrepo, C. C., Alvarez, E., Jaramillo, C., Velez, C., & Valencia, I. (2001). Effects of psychological techniques on bruxism in children with primary teeth. *Journal of Oral Rehabilitation, 28,* 354–360.

Rettew, D. C., Cheslow, D. L., Rapoport, J. L., Leonard, H. L., Lenane, M. C., Black, B., & Swedo, S. E. (1991). Neuropsychological test performance in trichotillomania: A further link with obsessive–compulsive disorder. *Journal of Anxiety Disorders, 5,* 225–235.

Riddle, M. A., King, R. A., Hardin, M. T., Scahill, L., Ort, S. I., & Leckman, J. F. (1991). Behavioral side effects of fluoxetine. *Journal of Child Psychopharmacology, 3,* 193–198.

Riddle, M. A., Scahill, L., King, R., Hardin, M. T., Towbin, K. E., Ort, S. I., et al. (1990). Obsessive compulsive disorder in children and adolescents: Phenomenology and family history. *Journal of the American Academy of Child and Adolescent Psychiatry, 29,* 766–772.

Rothbaum, B. O. (1992). The behavioral treatment of trichotillomania. *Behavioural Psychotherapy, 20,* 85–90.

Rubinstein, B., Axelsson, A., & Carlsson, G. E. (1990). Prevalence of signs and symptoms of craniomandibular disorders in tinnitus patients. *Journal of Craniomandibular Disorders: Facial & Oral Pain, 4,* 186–192.

Shapiro, A. K., Shapiro, E. S., Young, J. G., & Feinberg, T. E. (1988). *Gilles de la Tourette syndrome* (2nd ed.). New York: Raven Press.

Sheikholeslam, A., Holmgren, K., & Riise, C. (1993). Therapeutic effects of the plane occlusal splint on signs and symptoms of craniomandibular disorders in patients with nocturnal bruxism. *Journal of Oral Rehabilitation, 20,* 473–482.

Singer, H. S., & Walkup, J. T. (1991). Tourette syndrome and other tic disorders: Diagnosis, pathophysiology, and treatment. *Medicine, 70,* 15–32.

Sjoholm, T. T., Piha, S. J., & Lehtinen, I. (1995). Cardiovascular autonomic control is disturbed in nocturnal teethgrinders. *Clinical Physiology, 15,* 349–354.

Slagle, D. A., & Martin, T. A. (1991). Trichotillomania. *American Family Physician, 43,* 2019–2024.

Spencer, T., Biederman, J., Coffey, B., Geller, D., Wilens, T., & Faraone, S. (1999). The 4-year course of tic disorders in boys with attention-deficit/hyperactivity disorder. *Archives of General Psychiatry, 56,* 842–847.

Spencer, T., Biederman, J., Kerman, K., Steingard, R., & Wilens, T. (1993). Desipramine treatment with attention-deficit hyperactivity disorder and tic disorder or Tourette's syndrome. *Journal of the American Academy of Child and Adolescent Psychiatry, 32,* 354–360.

Spencer, T., Biederman, J., Wilens, T., Steingard, R., & Geist, D. (1993). Nortriptyline treatment of children with attention-deficit hyperactivity disorder and tic disorder or Tourette's syndrome. *Journal of the American Academy of Child and Adolescent Psychiatry, 32,* 205–210.

Stanley, M. A., Swann, A. C., Bowers, T. C., Davis, M. L., & Taylor, D. J. (1992). A comparison of clinical features in trichotillomania and obsessive compulsive disorder. *Behavioural Research and Therapy, 30,* 39–44.

Steingard, R., Biederman, J., Spencer, T., Wilens, T., & Gonzalez, A. (1993). Comparison of clonidine response in the treatment of attention-deficit hyperactivity disorder with and without comorbid tic disorders. *Journal of the American Academy of Child and Adolescent Psychiatry, 32,* 350–353.

Swedo, S. E., Leonard, H. L., Rapoport, J. L., Lenane, M. C., Goldberger, E. L., & Cheslow, D. L. (1989). A double-blind comparison of clomipramine and desipramine in the treatment of trichotillomania (hair pulling). *New England Journal of Medicine, 321,* 497–501.

Swedo, S. E., & Rapoport, J. L. (1991). Annotation: Trichotillomania. *Journal of Child Psychology and Psychiatry, 32,* 401–409.

Tanchyk, A. P. (1991). Dental considerations for the patient with juvenile rheumatoid arthritis. *General Dentistry, 39,* 330–332.

Tattersall, M. L. (1992). Further comments on trichotillomania. *American Journal of Psychiatry, 149,* 284.

Vanderas, A. P. (1994). Relationship between oral parafunctions and craniomandibular dysfunction in children and adolescents: A review. *Journal of Dentistry for Children, 61*(5–6), 378–381.

Vanderas, A. P. (1995). Relationship between craniomandibular dysfunction and oral parafunctions in Caucasian children with and without unpleasant life events. *Journal of Oral Rehabilitation, 22,* 289–294.

Vanderas, A. P., & Manetas, K. J. (1995). Relationship between malocclusion and bruxism in children and adolescents: A review. *Pediatric Dentistry, 17,* 7–12.

Vanderas, A. P., Menenakou, M., Kouimtzis, T., & Papagiannoulis, L. (1999). Urinary catecholamine levels and bruxism in children. *Journal of Oral Rehabilitation, 26,* 103–110.

Vitulano, L. A., King, R. A., Scahill, L., & Cohen, D. J. (1992). Behavioral treatment of children and adolescents with trichotillomania. *Journal of the American Academy of Child and Adolescent Psychiatry, 31,* 139–146.

Watts, M. W., Tan, E. K., & Jankovic, J. (1999). Bruxism and cranial–cervical dystonia: Is there a relationship? *Journal of Craniomandibular Practice, 17,* 196–201.

Widmalm, S. E., Christiansen, R. L., & Gunn, S. M. (1995). Oral parafunctions as temporomandibular disorder risk factors in children. *Journal of Craniomandibular Practice, 13,* 242–246.

Widmalm, S. E., Gunn, S. M., Christiansen, R. L., & Hawley, L. M. (1995). Association between CMD signs and symptoms, oral parafunctions, race and sex, in 4–6-year-old African-American and Caucasian children. *Journal of Oral Rehabilitation, 22,* 95–100.

Wruble, M. K., Lumley, M. A., & McGlynn, F. D. (1989). Sleep-related bruxism and sleep variables: A critical review. *Journal of Craniomandibular Disorders: Facial and Oral Pain, 3,* 152–158.

Zucconi, M., Oldani, A., Ferini-Strambi, L., & Smirne, S. (1995). Arousal fluctuations in non-rapid eye movement parasomnias: The role of cyclic alternating pattern as a measure of sleep instability. *Journal of Clinical Neurophysiology, 12,* 147–154.

34

Pediatric Sleep Disorders

RANDI STREISAND
LISA A. EFRON

Sleep is a complex process required by all human beings and animals. Although the exact purpose of sleep remains somewhat elusive, it has been theorized that the functions of sleep include physical restoration, brain development, and memory consolidation (Rechtschaffen, 1998). More clear, however, is the evidence that without adequate sleep, cognitive and physical impairments are likely to ensue in both children and adults. Sleep is therefore an important consideration throughout the lifespan. Issues pertaining to children's sleep are among the most common types of behavioral concerns raised during pediatric visits. The reason is that sleep not only affects the child's daytime functioning but also has significant implications for the well-being of parents and the family system (Chavin & Tinson, 1980). Given that sleep is a necessary function for all children and that its regulation can affect and be affected by medical and psychiatric conditions, concepts related to sleep are far-reaching within pediatric psychology.

Sleep problems during childhood and adolescence are relatively common, with prevalence rates reported to be approximately 10–20% throughout childhood (Lozoff, Wolf, & Davis, 1985; Stein, Mendelsohn, Obermeyer, Amromin, & Benca, 2001). Sleep is a particularly important topic for health care professionals to be familiar with given the interplay between sleeping and medical and psychiatric phenomena. However, sleep is not a topic regularly covered during professional training. Several studies conducted by Mindell and colleagues (1994) indicated substantial variability in medical residency instruction related to sleep, with few programs offering didactics about specific sleep disorders. Although data on the number of doctoral programs in pediatric psychology offering sleep instruction are unavailable, it is likely that relatively few offer formal training in sleep. In light of the fact that many of the underlying causes of, as well as treatments for, pediatric sleep disorders are behavioral rather than pharmacological or physiological in nature, this chapter focuses on sleep disorders during childhood and the role of pediatric psychology in addressing them. Specific disorders and their etiology are reviewed, and the relationship between sleep disorders and medical and psychiatric problems is discussed. We then describe relevant assessment and treatment strategies.

STAGES OF SLEEP

A detailed understanding of sleep architecture and related physiological systems is paramount to evaluating several sleep disturbances. In fact, books and chapters are dedicated to the description of the phenomenon of sleep (see Culebras, 1996; see also Kryger, Roth, & Dement, 2000). For the purposes of this chapter, however, we offer a more general description of the process of sleep to provide a working framework for understanding the underlying mechanisms for several of the disorders.

Sleep is divided into two states: rapid-eye-movement (REM) and non-rapid-eye-movement (NREM) sleep. Electroencephalograph (EEG; an apparatus for detecting and recording brain waves) can distinguish REM from NREM sleep, and an individual's response to the environment can also provide information as to the current sleep stage (Lin-Dyken & Dyken, 1996). NREM sleep usually occurs first, and it is further divided into four stages. Stage 1 occurs just as an individual transitions into sleep, and little activity can be observed on EEG recordings. Stage 2 marks the beginning of increased EEG activity, or the appearance of "spindles," followed by Stages 3 and 4, which are considered "deep" sleep and are evidenced by delta slow wave patterns on EEG. Arousal during Stages 3 and 4 is difficult, and when awakened during this stage, children may be disoriented or confused.

Following the initial NREM cycle, REM occurs. REM includes both deep and light sleep. In addition to the occurrence of rapid eye movements, muscle tone is decreased, blood pressure becomes more variable, and heart rate and respiration are increased (Culebras, 1996). Dreaming occurs during REM sleep, and children will usually become alert rather quickly when awakened during this stage. The first REM period is brief (approximately 10 minutes), with later REM periods lasting for longer periods of time. Following REM, NREM stages repeat, occurring in cycles of 60 to 90 minutes in adults and longer in children and adolescents (80 to 120 minutes). These REM cycles repeat throughout the night, and their duration also increases as the night progresses, with the longest cycle usually occurring just prior to waking.

The regulation of sleep depends on the individual's homeostatic process and circadian system, with age playing a large role in regulation. For example, the newborn has more REM versus NREM sleep, and sleep onset usually occurs with REM sleep; this proportion of REM versus NREM sleep slowly decreases during childhood, with REM sleep accounting for 20 to 25% of sleep in adulthood (Mindell, Owens, & Carskadon, 1999). Arousals during sleep are common and occur throughout the night. In fact, children typically awaken an average of five times per sleep period, returning to sleep with little difficulty and without recall of the awakening.

SLEEP REQUIREMENTS

The nature, quality, and duration of sleep changes throughout the lifespan, with the most significant changes occurring during the first few years of life. Given the wide variations in total sleep time of children within given age groups, it is difficult to consider an ideal amount of sleep for a child of a particular age. That being said, it is still important to understand the individual child's amount of sleep in comparison with same-aged peers, and several guidelines exist for determining average sleep time across ages to assist clinicians when working with these children (e.g., Ferber, 1985). Newborns spend approximately 16 hours a day sleeping, and 1-year-olds sleep an average of 13 hours per day (including naps totaling 2 to 2½ hours). By 4 years of age, sleep may decrease to 11 hours, and most children ages 5 and older have given up daytime naps. Sleep time further decreases to 9 or 10 hours by ages 6 to 10 years. Adolescence through adulthood is marked by further decrease in total sleep time, usually to 8 to 9 hours.

PREVALENCE OF SLEEP DISORDERS ACROSS CHILDHOOD

Infancy and Early Childhood

Sleep problems within the first few years of life are most often related to night awakenings and refusal to go to sleep, with one study finding 6 to 10% of children 1 to 2 years old illustrating sleep related symptoms (Richman, 1981). Night waking was studied prospectively in a sample of children and found that parents of 21.5% of 5-month-olds reported night waking problems (Zuckerman, Stevenson, & Bailey, 1987). Difficulties did not decrease significantly over time, with 21.8% of parents reporting similar difficulties when children were 20 months of age. By 4½ years of age, 13.3% of parents reported continued difficulties with their youngsters waking during the night.

Later Childhood

Sleep continues to be an important issue for parents of older children, with one study finding that 43% of children 8 to 10 years of age experienced difficulty sleeping over at least 6 months' duration, per their parents' report (Kahn et al., 1989). The most commonly reported disturbances were parasomnias (e.g., disorders that interrupt sleep and often the sleep of family members, as well), including nighttime fears, sleepwalking, and enuresis. Blader, Koplewicz, Abikoff, and Foley (1997) administered a parent report survey to a large community sample and found similar results. Twenty-seven percent of parents of children ages 5 to 12 years (mean age of 7 years) reported that their children demonstrated bedtime resistance at least three times each week. Other common disturbances included sleep-onset delays, night waking, morning wake-up problems, and complaints of fatigue.

Adolescence

Although sleep time typically decreases during adolescence, researchers have suggested that there is a physiological need for more rather than less sleep during this time (Carskadon & Dement, 1987). Common sleep problems for adolescents include insomnia, delayed sleep phase, and insufficient sleep (Carskadon, 1992). One large study indicated that 33% of adolescents (ages 13 to 15 years) reported having sleep difficulties, with 25% acknowledging a need for attaining more sleep (Morrison, McGee, & Stanton, 1992).

PEDIATRIC SLEEP DISORDERS

Classification Systems

Prior to discussing various types of sleep disorders, a brief mention of sleep classification systems is necessary. In the fourth edition of the *Diagnostic and Statistical Manual of Mental Disorders* (DSM-IV), sleep problems are classified in the following four categories: (1) primary sleep disorders, (2) sleep disorder related to another mental disorder, (3) sleep disorder due to a general medical condition, and (4) substance-induced sleep disorder (American Psychiatric Association, 1994). The International Classification of Sleep Disorders—Revised (ICSD-R) describes more than 80 sleep problems, which are categorized as (1) dyssomnias; (2) parasomnias; (3) sleep disorders associated with mental, neurological, or other medical disorders; and (4) proposed sleep disorders (American Sleep Disorders Association [ASDA], 1997). The ICSD-R is more comprehensive and logically structured than both the DSM-IV and previous ICD sleep classification schemes. However, as Stores (2001) suggested, similar to the other classification systems described here, the ICSD-R is adult oriented and therefore requires some modifications when used with children and adolescents. The discussion of sleep disorders that follows will be structured according to the ICSD-R classification system.

Dyssomnias

As described by the ICSD-R, the dyssomnias are sleep disorders that involve difficulty initiating or maintaining sleep or those that cause excessive sleepiness during the day. They are subdivided into either intrinsic sleep disorders, which originate from within the body, extrinsic sleep disorders, which are caused by factors external to the individual, and circadian rhythm sleep disorders, which involve the inappropriate timing of the sleep phase within a 24-hour day.

Obstructive Sleep Apnea (OSA)

OSA is an intrinsic dyssomnia characterized by repetitive episodes of complete (apnea) or partial (hypopnea) cessation of airflow, which generally result in lowered blood oxygen levels and/or increased CO_2 levels (Mindell et al., 1999). Each episode is associated with a brief arousal in order to restore ventilation and oxygenation (Anders & Eiben, 1997). Such arousals may occur many times in a night, resulting in fragmented and insufficient sleep and, not surprisingly, also daytime fatigue and inattention. Common symptoms of OSA during sleep include heavy snoring, irregular breathing, mouth breathing, and restless sleep. In toddlers and young children, OSA is most often the result of enlarged tonsils and adenoids, whereas in adults OSA is most often associated with obesity. Congenital malformations of the mouth, palate, and oropharynx are also linked to OSA in children (Anders & Eiben, 1997). OSA is estimated to occur in 1–3% of children, with onset most often between the ages of 2 and 6 years (Mindell et al., 1999).

Narcolepsy

Narcolepsy is an intrinsic dyssomnia and is the only dyssomnia of REM sleep. The initial symptom of narcolepsy is often daytime sleepiness, frequently presenting as irresistible sleep attacks that occur throughout the day. Sleep attacks are episodes of REM sleep, generally lasting between 20 and 40 minutes (Anders & Eiben, 1997). Following each sleep attack the individual feels alert and refreshed until the next episode. Other characteristics of the disorder include cataplexy (sudden and reversible loss of muscle tone), hypnogogic hallucinations (vivid, visual hallucinations that occur at sleep onset), and sleep paralysis (inability to move voluntary muscles at sleep onset). It is estimated that 1 in 10,000 individuals have narcolepsy (Dahl, Holttum, & Trubnick, 1994). Onset occurs most frequently during adolescence or early adulthood; 25% of adults with narcolepsy report having experienced symptoms in adolescence (Adair & Bauchner, 1993). Polysomnography is necessary to confirm the diagnosis. The disorder appears to be genetically determined, although the precise etiology is unknown. Narcolepsy is a chronic condition with potentially disabling effects in terms of education, career, and overall well-being (Broughton & Broughton, 1994; Thiedke, 2001).

Restless Leg Syndrome

Restless leg syndrome and periodic limb movement disorder are categorized as intrinsic dyssomnias. Restless leg syndrome is characterized by uncomfortable sensations in the legs and an irresistible urge to move the legs. Symptoms are typically at their worst during periods of inactivity and at night; movement of the legs tends to provide relief. Periodic limb movements (PLMs) in sleep often accompany restless leg syndrome. Such movements during sleep are brief contractions that occur in NREM sleep, last approximately 2 seconds, and affect primarily toes, knees, and hips at intervals of 5 to 90 seconds (Mindell et al., 1999). PLMs result in multiple wakenings during the night, as well as in fragmented sleep, causing daytime fatigue. PLMs have been associated with impairment in the dopamine system, with metabolic disorders, and with use of antidepressants and other medications that affect the central nervous system (Montplaisir, Michaud, Denesle, & Gosselin, 2000; Stores, 2001). It is interesting to note that the sleep disruption caused by PLMs in sleep and restless leg syndrome can result in symptoms of attention-deficit/hyperactivity disorder (ADHD; Picchietti, England, Walters, Willis, & Verrico, 1998).

The extrinsic dyssomnias, which are quite common during childhood and amenable to treatment, involve delayed sleep onset and/or nighttime wakenings that occur as a function of the external environment. In terms of the developmental progression of such problems, difficulties with nighttime wakening typically precede difficulties falling asleep, which generally precede difficulties settling to bed (Anders, Halpern, & Hua, 1992).

Sleep-Onset Association Disorder

Sleep-onset association disorder occurs when the child goes to sleep requiring certain conditions that cannot be reproduced by the child him- or herself during the night (e.g., parent singing, parent lying in bed with child). If the child has grown accustomed to falling asleep while interacting with the parent in some way, the child will be likely to require that same interaction when he or she awakens during the night. According to Ferber (1987, p. 644), the core of the problem is the child's "lack of individual control over the conditions associated with sleep." Thus, for most children with sleep-onset association disorder, a significant level of involvement by parents is required both at bedtime and during nighttime wakenings. According to Stores (1996), sleep-onset association disorder accounts for the majority of settling and nighttime waking problems experienced by children. Treatment of this disorder focuses on encouraging the child to fall asleep independently, without the involvement of the parent (Ferber, 1987).

Excessive Nighttime Feedings

Excessive nighttime feedings may lead to sleeplessness in infants and children, resulting in a diagnosis of nocturnal eating (drinking) disorder. This disorder is characterized by the infant or child waking at night and requiring food or drink prior to returning to sleep. By 6 months of age, an infant should be able to obtain all of his or her nutrition during the day; after 6 months of age, eating or drinking at night is considered a habit, although an infant or child may appear to be hungry or thirsty (Schmitt, 1985). Parents often continue nighttime feedings when they are no longer necessary; thus nocturnal eating (drinking) disorder emerges from normal infant feeding habits. Excessive nighttime feedings lead not only to the development of sleep associations whereby the child learns to require feeding in order to resume sleep but also to excessive nighttime feedings that result in increased urine output, requiring additional diaper changes (hence additional and prolonged wakenings) during the night. Consequently, excessive nighttime feedings often result in sleep fragmentation and insufficient sleep. The estimated prevalence of nocturnal eating (drinking) disorder is 5% in infants and children between the ages of 6 months and 3 years (Adair & Bauchner, 1993).

Limit Setting

Poor limit setting may lead to sleeplessness in infants, toddlers, and school-age children, resulting in limit-setting sleep disorder. Specifically, when parents are unable or unwilling to establish and enforce rules pertaining to sleep, children are likely to have poor sleep hygiene (e.g., inconsistent bedtime, inappropriate evening routines) and, consequently, sleeplessness. There are many reasons for lack of limit setting. Many parents are inconsistent in setting limits pertaining to bedtime when a child resists going to bed, as it is emotionally difficult to separate from a distressed child. Inconsistent limit setting pertaining to bedtime also occurs if parents make other evening activities a priority over bedtime and the evening routine; in this situation bedtimes are often variable, and evening routines are often truncated. As Stores (1996) suggests, if a child is able to settle to sleep with some adults (presumably those who set limits) but not with others (presumably those who do not set limits), it is likely that the child has a limit-setting sleep disorder. Limit-setting sleep disorder is most common in children between the ages of 2 and 6 years old (Adair & Bauchner, 1993). The goal of treatment is to have the caretakers identify and enforce reasonable rules pertaining to sleep on a consistent basis.

Delayed Sleep Phase Syndrome (DSPS)

DSPS is a circadian rhythm sleep disorder (Weitzman et al., 1981) with symptoms that include sleep-onset insomnia and morning hypersomnolence. These symptoms typically occur as a result of sleep deprivation and poor sleep hygiene and ultimately cause the biological clock to be disrupted (Anders & Eiben, 1997). DSPS is most common among adolescents; estimated prevalence in adolescents is 7% (Mindell et al., 1999). During adolescence, parental control decreases and academic and social demands increase, often resulting in late bedtimes and insufficient amounts of sleep for adolescents. In order to compensate for this "sleep debt," adolescents tend to wake up late in the morning and take naps in the afternoon, when possible. On weekends and vacations they are likely to sleep longer than the 8 or 9 hours per night that they require, with no difficulty falling asleep or staying asleep; however, sleep onset generally occurs later than during the week, or at a delayed time. As a result of the continual sleep deprivation and persistent irregularities in sleep hygiene that they experience, the biological clock is altered and the entire sleep phase shifts forward (Anders & Eiben, 1997). Consequently, when an attempt is made to go to sleep at a reasonable time, the adolescent is likely to experience severe insomnia; there is a significant disconnection between the time at which he or she attempts to sleep and the time at which the body is ready to sleep (Carskadon, 1992). Therefore, the adolescent frequently has difficulty waking up in the morning to attend school or work and experiences daytime fatigue, as well. With DSPS, even adolescents who are extremely motivated will have difficulty shifting their sleep back to a more normal time frame without assistance.

Parasomnias

The parasomnias are disorders that interfere with the sleep process; they rarely involve complaints of insomnia or excessive sleepiness. Parasomnias are categorized in the ICSD-R according to the phase of sleep in which they occur, as follows: (1) arousal disorders, which occur during NREM sleep; (2) sleep–wake transition disorders; (3) parasomnias usually associated with REM sleep; and (4) other parasomnias that do not fall into any of the three aforementioned categories (ASDA, 1997). Males generally exhibit parasomnias more often than do females, and individuals who experience one type of parasomnia are likely to exhibit symptoms of other parasomnias, as well (Anders & Eiben, 1997). Several of the most common parasomnias are reviewed in this section.

Sleep Terror Disorder and Sleepwalking Disorder (Somnambulism)

Sleep terror disorder and somnambulism are both categorized as arousal disorders. As such, they generally occur within the first 3 hours of sleep, during a transition from NREM Stage 4 sleep to REM sleep (Anders & Eiben, 1997). Sleep terror disorder is characterized by episodes in which the child sits up in bed, stares into space, and screams as if in intense distress. The child often experiences palpitations and profuse sweating and is generally inconsolable. Episodes typically last only a few minutes, at which point the child generally calms down and resumes sleep. Sleep terrors occur in approximately 3% of children (Adair & Bauchner, 1993). Onset can be as early as 18 months of age (Anders & Eiben, 1997), and terrors occur most frequently in children between the ages of 3 and 8 years (Thiedke, 2001). It has been suggested that sleep terrors beginning before the age of 7 continue, on average, for an additional 4 years; sleep terrors beginning after the age of 7 tend to last considerably longer (DiMario & Emery, 1987).

Sleepwalking disorder is more common than sleep terrors, occurring in up to 17% of children (Stores, 2001). Onset is most frequently between the ages of 4 and 8 (Adair & Bauchner, 1993). During an episode of sleepwalking, children generally walk purposelessly around their room or home in an uncoordinated manner, with their eyes open in a glassy stare. Polysomnography has demonstrated that sleepwalkers experience slow-wave sleep while somnambulating (Mahowald & Rosen, 1990). Sleepwalking disorder can be dangerous, as there is a risk of accidental injury. Sleepwalking episodes can last up to 10 minutes (Stores, 1996). Because slow-wave sleep decreases with age, arousal disorders become less common as children grow older. In fact, sleep terrors and sleepwalking generally remit spontaneously by adolescence (Adair & Bauchner, 1993). Other similarities between sleep terrors and sleepwalking include the following: (1) the individual appears confused and disoriented; (2) the individual remains asleep throughout the episode; (3) the individual is unresponsive to environmental cues during the episode; and (4) the individual has no recollection of the episode on awakening. These disorders are believed to have a hereditary basis (Thiedke, 2001), although they tend to be triggered by excessive fatigue or stress (Adair & Bauchner, 1993).

Rhythmic Movement Disorder

Rhythmic movement disorder is a sleep–wake transition disorder and is characterized by rhythmic movements (i.e., head banging, head rolling, body rocking) that occur at sleep onset, during nocturnal wakenings, and occasionally at the end of a sleep period (Stores, 1996). Head banging is the most common of these behaviors, involving banging the head into the pillow, mattress, or some other object (i.e., wall) in a forward–backward motion. Head rolling involves rolling the head from side to side, and body rocking generally involves moving the body back and forth while on one's hands and knees. Episodes typically occur nightly and last up to 15 minutes, with movements often occurring at a rate of 45 per minute (Horne, 1992). Movements can occur in combination and may be accompanied by vocalizations (Stores, 2001). Rhythmic movement disorder is common in young children and is generally considered a variant of normal behavior rather than pathological; many children exhibit some form of rhythmic movement disorder during the first year of life, but the behavior generally spontaneously remits by age 4 (Stores, 1996). It is thought that such movements likely have a neurophysiological rather than a psychological basis; the activity may be a form of vestibular stimulation that the child finds soothing (Horne, 1992).

Nightmares

Nightmares, or frightening dreams, are the most common REM parasomnia, occurring in the latter part of sleep when REM predominates (Stores, 2001). Children generally wake from nightmares, recalling dream content in vivid detail. Common themes of nightmares involve fear of attack, falling, and death (Kales et al., 1980). The distress of a nightmare is manifested after the child wakes up rather than during the episode itself. Nightmares are quite common during childhood, with prevalence rates ranging from 10 to 50% (Anders & Eiben, 1997). They tend to decrease in frequency over time; only a small proportion of adolescents and adults experience nightmares (Mindell et al., 1999). Although nightmares are normative, recurring nightmares may be indicative of daytime distress (Adair & Bauchner, 1993). In addition, the frequency and severity of nightmares may be increased by certain medications, including B-adrenergic blockers and antidepressants (Mindell et al., 1999). The terms nightmare and sleep terror (i.e., night terror) are often mistakenly used interchangeably. As can be seen in Table 34.1, the distinctions between these two parasomnias are actually quite clear.

Sleep Enuresis

Recurrent, involuntary bedwetting is a parasomnia that is not consistently associated with a particular stage of sleep (Adair & Bauchner, 1993). Enuresis is one of the most common and

TABLE 34.1. Comparison of Nightmares and Sleep (Night) Terrors

	Nightmare	Sleep terror
Time of night	Latter part of night	First 3 hours of sleep
Stage of sleep	REM	NREM
Experience of distress	After event	During event
Recall of event	Yes	No

persistent sleep problems experienced by children (Thiedke, 2001), and the incidence is higher in males than in females (Adair & Bauchner, 1993). For a detailed review of enuresis, see Walker, Chapter 32, this volume.

Sleep Bruxism

Another parasomnia that is not consistently associated with a particular sleep stage is sleep bruxism, which refers to stereotypic movements of the mouth, resulting in teeth clenching and grinding during sleep. Bruxism typically occurs in individuals between the ages of 10 and 20, although it is also often observed in infants who are teething (Anders & Eiben, 1997). Episodes of bruxism last up to 10 seconds, and over time, can result in a variety of problems, such as tooth wear and facial muscle and joint pain and dysfunction (Adair & Bauchner, 1993). For a detailed review of bruxism, see Glaros and Epkins, Chapter 33, this volume.

SLEEP PROBLEMS OCCURRING WITH PSYCHIATRIC AND MEDICAL DISORDERS

Although sleep problems are rather common throughout childhood, children with a medical or psychiatric disorder may be at greater risk for sleep disturbance. In addition to the importance of considering sleep function in children with a known medical or psychiatric diagnosis, it is also imperative to consider medical or psychiatric etiologies in children presenting with sleep problems. For example, neurological disorders should be ruled out in youngsters who appear to have immediate sleep onset or violent movements during sleep. Similarly, insomnia or difficulty with sleep onset may be a sign of depression or anxiety, and bedtime resistance could stem from a larger behavioral disorder.

Distinguishing between differential diagnoses can be complicated, given that sleep problems have been found to result in a variety of changes in children's mood and behavior (Ali, Pitson, & Stradling, 1993), and disturbances of mood and behavior can certainly alter sleep. Although sleep problems are typically associated with decreased quality and quantity of sleep, children with sleep problems may appear to be overactive or irritable, behaving similarly to a child with ADHD. Most research on the impact of sleep problems has been conducted with adults, with studies most often reporting symptoms of depression and diminished cognitive function (Alapin et al., 2000). However, similar findings have emerged in studies of children with OSA, suggesting that children with sleep problems may have associated neuropsychological difficulties related to attention, reaction time, and executive function (Hansen & Vandenberg, 1997).

PSYCHIATRIC ISSUES

Developmental Disorders, Behavior, and ADHD

Sleep problems have been associated with pervasive developmental disorders, with difficulties estimated to occur in approximately 75% of children with autism (Richdale, 1999). Children with mental retardation have also been found to experience sleep disturbance (Stores, 1992). Sleep problems are comorbid with behavioral problems in preschool children (Minde et al., 1993) and in older children, as well. In a study examining the relationship between sleep and behavioral problems in children ages 4 to 12 years, Stein and colleagues (2001) found a significant positive association between sleep and behavioral concerns in parents of non-clinic-referred children. Changes in sleep have also been seen in children with conduct disorder (Coble et al., 1984). Specific differences detected by EEG included less sleep time and increased arousals. The underlying mechanism for these sleep difficulties is unclear, and sleep problems can further complicate children's daytime functioning or interfere with ongoing treatment of the developmental or behavioral concerns.

Several studies have explored sleep in children with ADHD, both on and off stimulant medication. Although parents of children with ADHD generally report significantly greater sleep problems in their children than do parents of children who do not have ADHD (Ball, Tiernan, Janusz, & Furr, 1997), studies that rely on objective measures of sleep have not resulted in clear evidence to support reports of increased disturbance (Greenhill, Puig-Antich, Goetz, Hanlon, & Davies, 1983; Khan, 1982). However, in contrast to earlier reports, one recent objective study did find increased variability with respect to sleep onset, duration, and total sleep time in children with ADHD (Gruber, Sadeh, & Raviv, 2000). Studies of children with ADHD on stimulant medication suggest slightly greater difficulties with sleep onset as compared with nonmedicated children (Dahl & Puig-Antich, 1990), yet specific effects of varying dosages are unknown (Stein & Pao, 2000). In addition to reports of delayed sleep onset, ADHD has also been associated with sleep movement disorders (Picchietti et al., 1998) and OSA (Chervin, Dillon, Bassetti, Ganoczy, & Pituch, 1997). Despite the relative lack of objectively measured differences within the literature, several researchers have found that reported sleep disturbances may be associated with increased ADHD symptomatology (Dahl, Pelham, & Wierson, 1991).

Depression

Sleep disturbance is one hallmark symptom of major depressive disorder (MDD), with the majority of children and adolescents with depression reporting insomnia (Ryan et al., 1987). Although EEGs of adults in a depressive episode differ significantly from EEGs of healthy adults, these same sleep abnormalities may not be seen in children. Dahl and Puig-Antich (1990) reviewed studies of objective sleep measurements in children and adolescents with MDD and found inconsistent results across the literature, with some studies citing short latencies to the first REM period, delayed sleep onset, and increased awake time. For children or adolescents with bipolar disorder, sleep may be affected by a significantly decreased need for sleep during a manic episode.

Anxiety

Nightmares or nighttime fears are the most common sleep difficulties associated with anxiety in children. Children experiencing trauma, including those diagnosed with posttraumatic stress disorder, may exhibit delayed sleep onset and recurrent nightmares (Sadeh, 1996) and increased nighttime waking, parasomnias, and enuresis (Udwin, 1993). Although the initial occurrence of nightmares or sleep terrors is often unrelated to level of anxiety, stress or worries may increase their frequency.

Taken together, many psychiatric conditions affecting children and adolescents are associated with sleep difficulties. By considering the impact of these difficulties on the child and family, the health care professional may gain insight in case conceptualization. Although it is not recommended to treat the sleep disturbance in absence of treating the psychiatric issue, it is possible that treatment of the psychiatric issue could be assisted by concomitant treatment for sleep. Similarly, treatment of the psychiatric issue, in particular for depression and anxiety, often relieves some of the sleep difficulty.

MEDICAL ISSUES

Sleep difficulties are associated with a variety of pediatric conditions and are thought to result from both physiological processes of medications and the illness itself, as well as from changes in the child's routine as a function of the illness or medical treatment. This section highlights issues related to sleep in several populations often encountered in the pediatric setting.

Neurological Disorders

It has been estimated that sleep-related epilepsy accounts for 30% of seizure disorders in childhood (Kohrman & Carney, 2000). In sleep-related epilepsy, the majority of seizures occur during sleep. Nocturnal seizures lead to fragmented sleep, which typically affects daytime functioning, and inadequate sleep can also trigger seizures. Poor sleep may be one reason that children with epilepsy perform worse on achievement testing than do healthy peers (Kohrman & Carney, 2000). Children with Tourette's disorder often report sleep difficulties, and tics have been found to occur throughout the sleep period (Burd & Kerbeshian, 1988; Nee, Caine, Polinsky, Eldridge, & Ebert, 1980). Children with Tourette's disorder have increased partial arousals, placing them at risk for parasomnias such as sleep terrors, sleepwalking, and enuresis. Blindness is also associated with sleep problems. Children who are blind are unable to rely on external cues to regulate their sleep–wake cycle, and delayed sleep onset, awakenings, and fatigue are often the result (Mindell et al., 1999). These sleep disturbances are thought to be caused by a circadian rhythm disturbance. The reason is that circadian rhythms are based on a 25-hour sleep cycle, and without external cues, children who are blind are likely to have a continuous 1- to 2-hour delay in their sleep phase. Headaches are another neurological disorder often associated with sleep problems. For individuals experiencing headaches during the sleep period, the headaches typically occur within the first 2 hours after sleep onset (Kohrman & Carney, 2000). One self-report study found that children with both tension and migraine headaches reported increased sleep problems, as compared with healthy peers (Bruni et al., 1997). Finally, OSA has also been associated with headaches.

Chronic Illness

Children with respiratory illnesses such as asthma and cystic fibrosis (CF) are at increased risk for sleep problems, and sleep-disordered breathing in particular. Compared with healthy children, children with asthma have been found to experience increased nighttime awakenings and arousals (Kales et al., 1970). Sleep problems in children with CF include decreased sleep efficiency, increased awakenings, and decreased REM sleep (Mindell et al., 1999). Endocrine disorders are also associated with sleep difficulties. In a study of 25 children with Type 1 diabetes and age-matched peers, children with diabetes were found to have an increased incidence of apneaic episodes of longer duration. Medical control of diabetes was also associated with sleep difficulties, with children with poorly controlled diabetes having more apneaic episodes than children with better controlled diabetes (Villa et al., 2000). Increased nighttime wakings as evidenced by polysomnography have also been demonstrated in children with diabetes (Matyka, Crawford, Wiggs, Dunger, & Stores, 2000). Research with this population has not suggested an association between hypoglycemia and sleep problems, despite the fact that hypoglycemia often occurs during the sleep period. Although data on sleep problems in children with Type 2 diabetes are not available, it is likely that these youngsters will be at risk for experiencing sleep-related breathing difficulties, such as OSA, given the relationship between obesity and Type 2 diabetes and the increased prevalence of OSA in obese children (Silvestri et al., 1993).

Although adults with rheumatoid arthritis have been found to have fragmented sleep with frequent wakings, likely a result of muscular stiffness and joint pain, less is known about children with juvenile rheumatoid arthritis (JRA). In one study comparing the sleep patterns of 16 children with JRA to age-matched controls, children with JRA had 90% more arousals and less REM sleep (Zamir, Press, Tal, & Tarasiuk, 1998). Children with JRA also reported taking more afternoon naps than peers. Despite these objective measurements, children with JRA did not differ from peers on self-reported sleep disturbances.

Pain and Hospitalization

Children with a variety of acute and chronic illnesses encounter pain, and the effects of pain and sleep are thought to be bidirectional. Obtaining sufficient sleep is necessary for ameliorating or coping with the pain, yet experiencing pain frequently negatively affects one's sleep. Lewin and Dahl (1999) cited several connections between pain management and sleep issues that are particularly relevant to pediatric psychology: (1) insufficient sleep can interfere with coping skills by negatively affecting daytime functioning, (2) fear and anxiety have a negative impact on sleep and pain, and (3) adequate sleep can promote physiological and psychological processes inherent in recovery from the pain or illness. Although the issues relevant to pediatric pain are often present for hospitalized children, hospitalized children without acute or chronic pain experiences may encounter additional difficulties related to sleep. Being separated from parents and familiar settings, the absence of routines or limits, and being awakened during the night by hospital staff all contribute to sleep difficulties for the hospitalized child. One study of hospitalized young children found that up to 25% of total sleep time was lost as a result of delayed sleep onset (Hagemann, 1981). Unfortunately, sleep problems may not be eliminated after discharge (Reid, Hebb, McGrath, Finley, & Forward, 1995).

Medication

The use of medications to treat these pediatric conditions may also contribute to sleep disturbance. Research suggests that medications used for the management of asthma and seizure disorders negatively affect children's sleep (Mindell et al., 1999); however, children without a chronic condition may also be affected by the use of medication. For example, antihistamines may contribute to drowsiness or may have a paradoxical effect on the child.

ASSESSMENT OF SLEEP DISORDERS

Clinical Interview

As with any other pediatric condition, the assessment of the child presenting with sleep problems begins with a detailed clinical interview. Sleep problems may be the concern of the parent and not the child or may be concerning to the child and not the parent. It is therefore essential to elicit information from both parent and child whenever possible. In order to differentiate between sleep problems and other pediatric or psychiatric conditions, a thorough history, including developmental, school, family (including history of sleep problems), and psychiatric functioning, must be included. Interview topics specifically related to sleep are described later in this section (see Figure 34.1 for an example of an intake form). A detailed account of the presenting sleep problems must be obtained. It is helpful for the clinician to know how long sleep problems have been present and whether other sleep problems have occurred and remitted. Children's and parents' past attempts to treat the problem should be elicited, including use of any prescribed or over-the-counter medications. In order to estimate children's sleep period and to determine whether they are receiving an adequate amount of sleep, a thorough report of the child's sleep schedule should be obtained. This includes bedtime and waking time for both weekdays and weekends, estimated length of time to sleep onset, and number and length of nighttime awakenings. Children and parents should also be asked about the frequency and duration of naps. Total sleep time for weekdays and total sleep time for weekends can then be calculated and can be compared with average sleep time for same-age children (Ferber, 1985).

Sleep Behavior

The child's sleep behaviors should also be assessed. These include any activity that occurs during the child's sleep and that is usually noticed by parents, siblings, or friends who may share a room with the child. Sleep behaviors to inquire about include rhythmic movements (e.g., head banging, rocking, leg moving), snoring, interrupted breathing, talking, walking, bruxism, and enuresis.

Sleep Habits

Children and parents should be asked about sleep habits and hygiene, and to describe the child's typical bedtime routine. Inquiring about where the routine takes place, which parent participates in the routine, and specifically where the child is put to bed are essential. Asking these questions will help answer such questions as whether the child shares a room with a sibling, sleeps in the parents' bed, or even falls asleep on the couch and is later moved to his or her bed. Another issue to consider is the comfort level of the child's room (i.e., comfortable bed, quiet and dark room that is not used for time out, comfortable temperature).

Sleep Hygiene

Assessing sleep hygiene also includes inquiring about activities aside from sleep that the child does on his or her bed (e.g., eating, telephone, television, homework, reading), the regularity of the child's meals and other activities such as exercise, and use of caffeine, alcohol, and tobacco. Children having difficulty falling asleep or returning to sleep after awakening should be asked about what they do when unable to sleep (e.g., stay in bed, watch television, etc.).

Daytime Sleepiness

Clinicians should also inquire about the child's daytime sleepiness and whether functioning seems to improve following nights of better sleep. Also, does the child fall asleep during sed-

Name: ______________________________ Date: ______________________________
Date of Birth: ______________________ Grade: ______________________________

CHIEF COMPLAINT:

HISTORY OF PRESENTING PROBLEM: (Include duration, change from previous pattern, anything that improves or worsens problem, previously tried treatments [e.g., medication or behavioral treatment].)

____

PREVIOUS PSYCHIATRIC TREATMENT: [ ] None

Date	Provider/Agency	Reason	Modality/Frequency	Disposition

If currently in outpatient treatment, frequency: ______________________
Date last seen: ______________________
Current psychological functioning (recent stressors): ______________________

DEVELOPMENTAL SCREEN: (Any Problems with . . . :)

[ ] No [ ] Yes Motor ______________ [ ] No [ ] Yes Toileting ______________
[ ] No [ ] Yes Language ______________ [ ] No [ ] Yes Socialization ______________
[ ] No [ ] Yes Feeding ______________

SLEEP PATTERN:

Bedtime (weekdays): ______________ (weekends): ______________
Sleep onset latency: ______________
Wakenings after sleep onset: ______________ Terror/nightmare: ______________
Early morning awakenings: ______________
Wake time (weekdays): ______________ (weekends): ______________
Total sleep time (bad night): ______________ (good night): ______________

NIGHTTIME ROUTINE:

After-dinner activities: [ ] Bath [ ] Television [ ] Computer [ ] Game with parent/sibling [ ] Very active play [ ] Other
Bedtime ritual: [ ] Book [ ] Snack [ ] Other Who puts child to bed? ______________
Sleep location (share room, bed, etc.): ______________
What strategies do parents currently use to get the child back to bed/sleep? ______________

PROBLEMS WITH DAYTIME FUNCTIONING: [ ] None

[ ] No [ ] Yes Fatigue ______________
[ ] No [ ] Yes Mood changes: ____Depressed ____Anxious ____Irritable
[ ] No [ ] Yes Decreased concentration ______________
[ ] No [ ] Yes Sad ______________
[ ] No [ ] Yes Falls asleep during focused activities ______________
[ ] No [ ] Yes Falls asleep during sedentary activities ______________
[ ] No [ ] Yes Needs to nap: When______________ How long______________
[ ] No [ ] Yes Functioning improves with better sleep______________

SLEEP-INCOMPATIBLE BEHAVIORS: [ ] None

[ ] No [ ] Yes Remains in bed without sleep? ______________
[ ] No [ ] Yes Worries about sleep? Other: ______________
[ ] No [ ] Yes Watches television in bed ______________
[ ] No [ ] Yes Reads in bed ______________
[ ] No [ ] Yes Listens to music in bed ______________
[ ] No [ ] Yes Talks on telephone in bed ______________
[ ] No [ ] Yes Eats in bed: What? ______________
[ ] No [ ] Yes School work ______________
[ ] No [ ] Yes Other ______________

(continued on next page)

ACTIVITIES WHEN UNABLE TO SLEEP: [ ] None

[ ] TV [ ] Reading [ ] Eating [ ] Schoolwork [ ] Other ______________________

SLEEP HABITS:

[ ] No [ ] Yes Irregular meals; Dinner time ______________________

[ ] No [ ] Yes Hungry after dinner; Time and content of snack ______________________

[ ] No [ ] Yes Caffeinated beverages; What and how much?____________ Latest? ________

[ ] No [ ] Yes Chocolate; How much?____________ Latest? ______________

[ ] No [ ] Yes Use of other substances; What and when? ______________________

[ ] No [ ] Yes Lack of exercise; Type?________________ Time? ____________

MEDICAL HISTORY:

Growth and development:________________ Medications: ______________________

Allergies/medical disorders:________________ Family history (medical, psychiatric, sleep):________

Hospitalizations/surgeries: ________________

REVIEW OF SYSTEMS:

[ ] No [ ] Yes Sleep attacks: ______________________

[ ] No [ ] Yes Cataplexy: ______________________

[ ] No [ ] Yes Sleep paralysis: ______________________

[ ] No [ ] Yes Hypnogogic hallucinations: ______________________

PHYSICAL EXAMINATION:

____

____

IMPRESSIONS AND PLANS:

____

____

____

Note. Adapted from Adult Sleep Assessment Form, by Donn Posner, PhD, Insomnia Program, Sleep Disorders Center of Lifespan Hospitals. Adapted by permission.

FIGURE 34.1. Pediatric Sleep Assessment Form

entary or even more active activities? Although gathering information about each of the aforementioned areas will be helpful in conceptualizing the child's case, clinicians are likely to focus more on certain areas once the presenting problem is clear. For example, if the clinician suspects a limit-setting sleep disorder, additional information related to sleep behaviors and the sleep schedule will likely be assessed, such as how the parent responds to nighttime awakenings (e.g., bringing the child back to his or her room, allowing the child to stay in the parents' room).

Self-Report Measures

Sleep diaries are the most common self-report tool used in sleep assessment. Sleep diaries of at least 3 nights' duration are suggested, but data from a greater number of nights will likely lead to a clearer conceptualization of the sleep difficulties. With the exception of adolescents, parents are usually asked to complete their child's sleep diary. Bedtime, waking time, and the time and duration of any nighttime awakenings, as well as naps, are recorded. Other self-report questionnaires can also be utilized in the sleep assessment. These are particularly helpful for understanding how much of an impact the sleep difficulties have on the child and the family. Self-report measures can also provide clinicians with specific information about the child's sleep schedule or habits and can be used to guide the clinical interview. Unfortunately, most research with large samples of children have included measures designed only for that particular study, making it difficult to draw conclusions about the psychometric properties of assessment tools. An exception is the Children's Sleep Habits Questionnaire, a well-validated measure that has successfully distinguished between children from clinical and normal samples (Owens, Spirito, & McGuinn, 2000).

Actigraphy

Over the past several years, actigraphs, or miniaturized sensors of physical motion, have been increasingly utilized in research with both children and adults with sleep difficulties. Children wear the actigraph on their wrists or ankles for up to 1 week, after which time the data are downloaded. Studies have evaluated the reliability of actigraphs in a variety of sleep disorders. Although actigraphs may not be adequate to diagnose a specific sleep disorder in the absence of other assessment tools, they can provide a cost-effective means for assessing a child's sleep–wake pattern (Sadeh, Hauri, Kripke, & Lavie, 1995).

Sleep Studies

When the clinical interview does not provide enough information to account for symptoms, a sleep study or polysomnography (PSG) may be warranted. PSG consists of an overnight sleep study in a laboratory, in which EEG and other physiological measurements are taken throughout the night. PSG may be particularly helpful in assessing breathing-related sleep disorders. A specific type of sleep study that may be useful when working with adolescents presenting with hypersomnolence is the multiple sleep latency test (MSLT; Carskadon, 1992). During an MSLT, the child is given the opportunity to take a series of at least four naps at 2-hour intervals across the day. Sleepiness and the presence of narcolepsy are assessed by the recording of sleep latency and sleep state for each nap.

Physical Examination

As with any other pediatric condition, underlying physical causes must also be considered when evaluating children with sleep difficulties. Many pediatric sleep clinics include assessment by both a mental health professional and a physician. The physical examination may be particularly important for cases involving disrupted breathing and hypersomnolence.

TREATMENT

Treatment of pediatric sleep disorders is multifaceted and frequently involves using a variety of approaches. Although clear treatment implications exist for several disorders, such as OSA, other disorders have less well-studied treatment strategies. In this section we describe different treatment approaches commonly used in pediatric sleep disorders and provide examples of disorders treated with each approach. These examples should not be considered to be exhaustive, as several different treatment modalities may apply to a single disorder. Similarly, as noted previously, treatment of many disorders requires utilizing techniques from more than one type of approach.

Education

Education is typically the first step in treatment of pediatric sleep disorders. Simply by understanding that sleep problems are quite common in childhood, children and parents can begin to cope with the sleep disorder. By providing education to parents and child, the family can gain a better understanding of the cause of the disorder and may also be more willing to adhere to subsequent treatment recommendations. Education is particularly helpful for families of children with parasomnias. It is most important that children are kept safe when awakened and do not injure themselves during sleep terrors or while sleepwalking. Parents of children with sleep terrors can be educated about how to keep their child safe, such as removing sharp furniture or objects from near the child's bed. For children who sleepwalk, parents are instructed to keep the child's bedroom floor clear and to secure all windows, doors, and stairways. In addition to educating families, treatment of sleep disorders involving hypersomnolence may include educating teachers about the cause of the child's sleepiness in school.

Behavioral/Psychological

Most children with a pediatric sleep disorder can benefit from some type of behavioral intervention, and, as with behavioral interventions for other pediatric disorders, treatment of sleep disorders usually requires participation from both parent and child. Behavioral interventions for sleep disorders include typical behavioral treatments such as using behavioral contracts or positive reinforcement. Types of interventions also include improving the child's sleep habits, schedule, and hygiene. For example, disorders related to inadequate sleep can often be improved by helping children stick to a strict sleep schedule, and improvements in sleep habits and hygiene can assist children with narcolepsy, movement disorders, and nightmares. For children who have difficulty falling asleep on their own, extinction approaches have been found to be effective. When compared with standard ignoring, gradual-ignoring procedures have been associated with higher rates of adherence and less parental stress (Reid, Walter, & O'Leary, 1999). Gradual-ignoring procedures instruct parents to wait progressively longer periods of time prior to checking on their child, both at bedtime and during nighttime awakenings (Ferber, 1987). For example, on the first night of treatment, parents will briefly check on the child after 5 minutes of crying. Parents are instructed to then wait an additional 10 minutes of crying prior to their next check. All subsequent checks are at 15-minute intervals on the first evening. On each successive night of treatment, checking intervals are lengthened by 5 minutes.

Scheduled awakenings are another behavioral technique that have been successful in working with children with parasomonias, as well as with other types of nighttime awakenings (Frank, Spirito, Stark, & Owens-Stively, 1997; Rickert & Johnson, 1988). For example, after determining the typical timing of their child's awakening, parents may purposefully wake up the child 15 to 60 minutes prior to that time in order to reset the child's sleep cycle. In a sample of 33 infants and toddlers with nighttime awakenings, Rickert and Johnson (1988) examined the use of scheduled awakenings as compared with systematic ignoring and a control condition. Children in both treatment conditions showed improved sleep, or decreased awakenings during and following treatment, yet the sleep of children in the systematic-ignoring condition improved more quickly.

For adolescents with a delayed sleep phase, gradually shifting their bedtime backward in 15-minute increments can assist them in obtaining a more reasonable bedtime. Sometimes, however, adolescents cannot fall asleep until much past midnight, necessitating several weeks or even months for gradual shifting to reach an optimal bedtime. Another approach that has been found successful with these adolescents is chronotherapy, or shifting the child's bedtime forward rather than backward (Czeisler et al., 1981). This shift is achieved by delaying the child's bedtime by approximately 3 hours each night and requiring the child to wake after 8 hours of sleep (waking time is 3 hours later each day of treatment). Using this approach, bedtime can be moved around the clock and can be maintained at the desired hour so long as strict sleep schedule, habits, and hygiene are followed.

Psychotherapy has also been found effective for some sleep disturbances, and in particular for treating children with nightmares. Treatment success is most likely when the nightmares are closely linked to some type of anxiety-provoking event (Cavior & Deutsch, 1975) and when systematic desensitization is a component of the therapy.

Medical

Relatively little research supports the use of medication in pediatric sleep disorders, and its use is generally reserved as a last attempt at treatment, given potential side effects or the likelihood of the sleep problem returning following withdrawal of the medication. Despite the lack of empirical evidence for its use, stimulant medications have been used to treat children with narcolepsy and hypersomnolence. Medications have also been used in severe cases of partial arousal disorders, such as sleep terrors, particularly when the child is at risk for harming him- or herself (Popoviciu & Corfariu, 1983). In such cases, benzodiazepines or tricyclic antidepressants have been used with some success, although the arousals may return once the child is weaned from the medication. Other uses of medication include clonidine for sleep disturbances in children with ADHD (Prince et al., 1996) and melatonin for various sleep problems in children with developmental disabilities (Dodge & Wilson, 2001). OSA is the one pediatric sleep disorder most often treated by surgical intervention. A tonsillectomy and/or adenoidectomy is the treatment of choice for most children with OSA, with the majority of children who undergo surgery experiencing symptom relief (Gozal, 2000; Nieminen, Tolonen, & Lopponen, 2000). Continuous positive airway pressure (CPAP), a device frequently used in treating adults with OSA, can also be used in children. CPAP can be particularly useful for treating children who are inappropriate candidates for surgery or for whom surgery was minimally successful (Gozal, 2000). In addition, for the obese youngster with OSA, weight loss may be the first line of treatment.

Other Interventions

Light therapy is another potential approach to treatment of pediatric sleep disorders. In an adult sample with delayed sleep phase disorders, 2 hours of bright light exposure, coupled with light restriction in the evening, was successful in altering the sleep phase (Rosenthal et al., 1990). Data on the utility of light therapy with children are unavailable, yet some clinicians consider its use with children with hypersomnolence, such as in Klein-Levin or chronic fatigue syndrome.

CONCLUDING REMARKS

Although the literature on adult sleep disorders far surpasses that in the field of pediatric sleep disorders, much information has been gained in the past 20 years in the area of children's sleep. Research has demonstrated that, despite advances in treatment strategies, sleep disturbances continue to be problematic for a large number of children. Sleep issues are relevant to many individuals working with children, and children's sleep should therefore be assessed, and if necessary, treated, whenever children present with psychiatric or medical conditions.

REFERENCES

Adair, R. H., & Bauchner, H. (1993). Sleep problems in childhood. *Current Problems in Pediatrics, 23,* 147–170.

Alapin, I., Fichten, C. S., Libman, E., Creti, L., Bailes, S., & Wright, J. (2000). How is good and poor sleep in older adults and college students related to daytime sleepiness, fatigue, and ability to concentrate? *Journal of Psychosomatic Research, 49,* 381–390.

Ali, N. J., Pitson, D. J., & Stradling, J. R. (1993). Snoring, sleep disturbance, and behaviour in 4–5 year olds. *Archives of Disease in Childhood, 68,* 360–366.

American Psychiatric Association. (1994). *Diagnostic and statistical manual of mental disorders* (4th ed.). Washington, DC: Author.

American Sleep Disorders Association. (1997). *The international classification of sleep disorders, revised: Diagnostic and coding manual.* Rochester, MN: Author.

Anders, T. F., & Eiben, L. A. (1997). Pediatric sleep disorders: A review of the past 10 years. *Journal of the American Academy of Child and Adolescent Psychiatry, 36,* 9–20.

Anders, T. F., Halpern, L. F., & Hua, J. (1992). Sleeping through the night: A developmental perspective. *Pediatrics, 90,* 554–560.

Ball, J. D., Tiernan, M., Janusz, J., & Furr, A. (1997). Sleep patterns among children with attention-deficit hyperactivity disorder: A reexamination of parent perceptions. *Journal of Pediatric Psychology, 22,* 389–398.

Blader, J. C., Koplewicz, H. S., Abikoff, H., & Foley, C. (1997). Sleep problems of elementary school children. A community survey. *Archives of Pediatrics and Adolescent Medicine, 151,* 473–480.

Broughton, W. A., & Broughton, R. J. (1994). Psychosocial impact of narcolepsy. *Sleep, 17,* S45–S49.

Bruni, O., Fabrizi, P., Ottaviano, S., Cortesi, F., Giannotti, F., & Guidetti, V. (1997). Prevalence of sleep disorders in childhood and adolescence with headache: A case-control study. *Cephalalgia: An International Journal of Headache, 17,* 492–498.

Burd, L., & Kerbeshian, J. (1988). Nocturnal coprolalia and phonic tics. *American Journal of Psychiatry, 145,* 132.

Carskadon, M. A. (1992). Sleep disturbances. In S. B. Friedman, M. Fisher, & S. K. Schonberg (Eds.), *Comprehensive adolescent health care* (pp. 747–754). St. Louis, MO: Quality Medical Publishing.

Carskadon, M. A., & Dement, W. C. (1987). Sleepiness in the normal adolescent. In C. Guilleminault (Ed.), *Sleep and its disorders in children* (pp. 53–66). New York: Raven Press.

Cavior, N., & Deutsch, A. M. (1975). Systematic desensitization to reduce dream-induced anxiety. *Journal of Nervous and Mental Disease, 161,* 433–435.

Chavin, W., & Tinson, S. (1980). The developing child: Children with sleep difficulties. *Health Visitor, 53,* 477–480.

Chervin, R. D., Dillon, J. E., Bassetti, C., Ganoczy, D. A., & Pituch, K. J. (1997). Symptoms of sleep disorders, inattention, and hyperactivity in children. *Sleep, 20,* 1185–1192.

Coble, P. A., Taska, L. S., Kupfer, D. J., Kazdin, A. E., Unis, A., & French, N. (1984). EEG sleep "abnormalities" in preadolescent boys with a diagnosis of conduct disorder. *Journal of the American Academy of Child Psychiatry, 23,* 438–447.

Culebras, A. (1996). *Clinical handbook of sleep disorders.* Boston: Butterworth-Heinemann.

Czeisler, C. A., Richardson, G. S., Coleman, R. M., Zimmerman, J. C., Moore-Ede, M. C., Dement, W. C., & Weitzman, E. D. (1981). Chronotherapy: Resetting the circadian clocks of patients with delayed sleep phase insomnia. *Sleep, 4,* 1–21.

Dahl, R. E., Holttum, J., & Trubnick, L. (1994). A clinical picture of child and adolescent narcolepsy. *Journal of the American Academy of Child and Adolescent Psychiatry, 33,* 834–841.

Dahl, R. E., Pelham, W. E., & Wierson, M. (1991). The role of sleep disturbances in attention deficit disorder symptoms: A case study. *Journal of Pediatric Psychology, 16,* 229–239.

DiMario, F. J., & Emery, E. S. (1987). The natural history of night terrors. *Clinical Pediatrics, 26,* 505–511.

Dahl, R. E., & Puig-Antich, J. (1990). Sleep disturbances in child and adolescent psychiatric disorders. *Pediatrician, 17,* 32–37.

Dodge, N. N., & Wilson, G. A. (2001). Melatonin for treatment of sleep disorders in children with developmental disabilities. *Journal of Child Neurology, 16,* 581–584.

Ferber, R. (1985). *Solve your child's sleep problems.* New York: Simon & Schuster.

Ferber, R. A. (1987). Behavioral "insomnia" in the child. *Psychiatric Clinics of North America, 10,* 641–653.

Frank, N. C., Spirito, A., Stark, L., & Owens-Stively, J. (1997). The use of scheduled awakenings to eliminate childhood sleepwalking. *Journal of Pediatric Psychology, 22,* 345–353.

Gozal, D. (2000). Obstructive sleep apnea in children. *Minerva Pediatrica, 52,* 629–639.

Greenhill, L., Puig-Antich, J., Goetz, R., Hanlon, C., & Davies, M. (1983). Sleep architecture and REM sleep measures in prepubertal children with attention deficit disorder with hyperactivity. *Sleep, 6,* 91–101.

Gruber, R., Sadeh, A., & Raviv, A. (2000). Instability of sleep patterns in children with attention-deficit/hyperactivity disorder. *Journal of the American Academy of Child Psychiatry, 39,* 495–501.

Hagemann, V. (1981). Night sleep of children in a hospital: Sleep duration. *Maternal–Child Nursing Journal, 10,* 1–13.

Hansen, D. E., & Vandenberg, B. (1997). Neuropsychological features and differential diagnosis of sleep apnea syndrome in children. *Journal of Clinical Child Psychology, 26,* 304–310.

Horne, J. (1992). Sleep and its disorders in children. *Journal of Child Psychology and Psychiatry, and Allied Disciplines, 33,* 473–487.

Kahn, A., Van de Merckt, C., Rebuffat, E., Mozin, M. J., Sottiaux, M., Blum, D., & Hennart, P. (1989). Sleep problems in healthy preadolescents. *Pediatrics, 84,* 542–546.

Kales, A., Kales, J. D., Sly, R. M., Scharf, M. B., Tan, T. L., & Preston, T. A. (1970). Sleep patterns of asthmatic children: All-night electroencephalographic studies. *Journal of Allergy, 46,* 300–308.

Kales, A., Soldatos, C. R., Caldwell, A. B., Charney, D. S., Kales, J. D., Markel, D., & Cadieux, R. (1980). Nightmares: Clinical characteristics and personality patterns. *American Journal of Psychiatry, 137,* 1197–1201.

Khan, A. U. (1982). Sleep REM latency in hyperkinetic boys. *American Journal of Psychiatry, 139,* 1358–1360.

Kohrman, M. H., & Carney, P. R. (2000). Sleep-related disorders in neurologic disease during childhood. *Pediatric Neurology, 23,* 107–113.

Kryger, M. H., Roth, T., & Dement, W. C. (Eds.). (2000). *Principles and practice of sleep medicine* (3rd ed). Philadelphia: Saunders.

Lewin, D. S., & Dahl, R. E. (1999). Importance of sleep in the management of pediatric pain. *Journal of Developmental and Behavioral Pediatrics, 20,* 244–252.

Lin-Dyken, D. C., & Dyken, M. E. (1996). Sleep in infancy, childhood, and youth. In A. Culebras (Ed.), *Clinical handbook of sleep disorders* (pp. 345–374). Boston: Butterworth-Heinemann.

Lozoff, B., Wolf, A. W., & Davis, N. S. (1985). Sleep problems seen in pediatric practice. *Pediatrics, 75,* 477–483.

Mahowald, M. W., & Rosen, G. M. (1990). Parasomnias in children. *Pediatrician, 17,* 21–31.

Matyka, K. A., Crawford, C., Wiggs, L., Dunger, D. B., & Stores, G. (2000). Alterations in sleep physiology in young children with insulin-dependent diabetes mellitus: Relationship to nocturnal hypoglycemia. *Journal of Pediatrics, 137,* 233–238.

Minde, K., Popiel, K., Leos, N., Falkner, S., Parker, K., & Handley-Derry, M. (1993). The evaluation and treatment of sleep disturbances in young children. *Journal of Child Psychology and Psychiatry, and Allied Disciplines, 34,* 521–533.

Mindell, J. A., Moline, M. L., Zendell, S. M., Brown, L. W., & Fry, J. M. (1994). Pediatricians and sleep disorders: Training and practice. *Pediatrics, 94,* 194–200.

Mindell, J. A., Owens, J. A., & Carskadon, M. A. (1999). Developmental features of sleep. *Child and Adolescent Psychiatric Clinics of North America, 8,* 695–725.

Montplaisir, J., Michaud, M., Denesle, R., & Gosselin, A. (2000). Periodic leg movements are not more prevalent in insomnia or hypersomnia but are specifically associated with sleep disorders involving a dopaminergic impairment. *Sleep Medicine, 1,* 163–167.

Morrison, D. N., McGee, R., & Stanton, W. R. (1992). Sleep problems in adolescence. *Journal of the American Academy of Child and Adolescent Psychiatry, 31,* 94–99.

Nee, L. E., Caine, E. D., Polinsky, R. J., Eldridge, R., & Ebert, M. H. (1980). Gilles de la Tourette syndrome: Clinical and family study of 50 cases. *Annals of Neurology, 7,* 41–49.

Nieminen, P., Tolonen, U., & Lopponen, H. (2000). Snoring and obstructive sleep apnea in children: A 6–month follow-up study. *Archives of Otolaryngology–Head and Neck Surgery, 126,* 481–486.

Owens, J. A., Spirito, A., & McGuinn, M. (2000). The Children's Sleep Habits Questionnaire (CSHQ): Psychometric properties of a survey instrument for school-aged children. *Sleep, 23,* 1043–1051.

Picchietti, D. L., England, S. L., Walters, A. S., Willis, K., & Verrico, T. (1998). Periodic limb movement disorder and restless legs syndrome in children with attention-deficit hyperactivity disorder. *Journal of Child Neurology, 13,* 588–594.

Popoviciu, L., & Corfariu, O. (1983). Efficacy and safety of midazolam in the treatment of night terrors in children. *British Journal of Clinical Pharmacology, 16*(Suppl. 1), 97S–102S.

Prince, J. B., Wilens, T. E., Biederman, J., Spencer, T. J., & Wozniak, J. R. (1996). Clonidine for sleep disturbances associated with attention-deficit hyperactivity disorder: A systematic chart review of 62 cases. *Journal of the American Academy of Child and Adolescent Psychiatry, 35,* 599–605.

Rechtschaffen, A. (1998). Current perspectives on the function of sleep. *Perspectives in Biology and Medicine, 41,* 359–390.

Reid, G. J., Hebb, J. P., McGrath, P. J., Finley, G. A., & Forward, S. P. (1995). Cues parents use to assess postoperative pain in their children. *Clinical Journal of Pain, 11,* 229–235.

Reid, M. J., Walter, A. L., & O'Leary, S. G. (1999). Treatment of young children's bedtime refusal and nighttime wakings: A comparison of "standard" and graduated ignoring procedures. *Journal of Abnormal Child Psychology, 27,* 5–16.

Richdale, A. L. (1999). Sleep problems in autism: Prevalence, cause, and intervention. *Developmental Medicine and Child Neurology, 41,* 60–66.

Richman, N. (1981). A community survey of characteristics of one- to two-year-olds with sleep disruptions. *Journal of the American Academy of Child Psychiatry, 20,* 281–291.

Rickert, V. I., & Johnson, C. M (1988). Reducing nocturnal awakening and crying episodes in infants and young children: A comparison between scheduled awakenings and systematic ignoring. *Pediatrics, 81,* 203–212.

Rosenthal, N. E., Joseph-Vanderpool, J. R., Levendosky, A. A., Johnston, S. H., Allen, R., Kelly, K. A., et al. (1990). Phase-shifting effects of bright morning light as treatment for delayed sleep phase syndrome. *Sleep, 13,* 354–361.

Ryan, N. D., Puig-Antich, J., Ambrosini, P., Rabinovich, H., Robinson, D., Nelson, B., et al. (1987). The clinical picture of major depression in children and adolescents. *Archives of General Psychiatry, 44,* 854–861.

Sadeh, A. (1996). Stress, trauma, and sleep in children. *Child and Adolescent Psychiatric Clinics of North America, 5,* 685–700.

Sadeh, A., Hauri, P. J., Kripke, D. F., & Lavie, P. (1995). The role of actigraphy in the evaluation of sleep disorders. *Sleep, 18,* 288–302.

Schmitt, B. D. (1985). When baby just won't sleep. *Contemporary Pediatrics, 2,* 38–52.

Silvestri, J. M., Weese-Mayer, D. E., Bass, M. T., Kenny, A. S., Hauptman, S. A., & Pearsall, S. M. (1993). Polysomnography in obese children with a history of sleep-associated breathing disorders. *Pediatric Pulmonology, 16,* 124–129.

Stein, M. A., Mendelsohn, J., Obermeyer, W. H., Amromin, J., & Benca, R. (2001). Sleep and behavior problems in school-aged children. *Pediatrics, 107,* E60.

Stein, M. A., & Pao, M. (2000). Attention deficit hyperactivity disorder and Ritalin side effects: Is sleep delayed, disrupted, or disturbed? In L. L. Greenhill & B. B. Osman (Eds.), *Ritalin: Theory and practice* (2nd ed., pp. 287–299). Larchmont, NY: Liebert.

Stores, G. (1992). Sleep studies in children with a mental handicap. *Journal of Child Psychology and Psychiatry, and Allied Disciplines, 33,* 1303–1317.

Stores, G. (1996). Practitioner review: Assessment and treatment of sleep disorders in children and adolescents. *Journal of Child Psychology and Psychiatry, and Allied Disciplines, 37,* 907–925.

Stores, G. (2001). *A clinical guide to sleep disorders in children and adolescents.* Cambridge, UK: Cambridge University Press.

Thiedke, C. C. (2001). Sleep disorders and sleep problems in childhood. *American Family Physician, 63,* 277–284.

Udwin, O. (1993). Children's reactions to traumatic events. *Journal of Child Psychology and Psychiatry, and Allied Disciplines, 34,* 115–127.

Villa, M. P., Multari, G., Montesano, M., Pagani, J., Cervoni, M., Midulla, F., et al. (2000). Sleep apnoea in children with diabetes mellitus: Effect of glycaemic control. *Diabetologia, 43,* 696–702.

Weitzman, E. D., Czeisler, C. A., Coleman, R. M., Spielman, A. J., Zimmerman, J. C., Dement, W., et al. (1981). Delayed sleep phase syndrome. A chronobiological disorder with sleep-onset insomnia. *Archives of General Psychiatry, 38,* 737–746.

Zamir, G., Press, J., Tal, A., & Tarasiuk, A. (1998). Sleep fragmentation in children with juvenile rheumatoid arthritis. *Journal of Rheumatology, 25,* 1191–1197.

Zuckerman, B., Stevenson, J., & Bailey, V. (1987). Sleep problems in early childhood: Continuities, predictive factors, and behavioral correlates. *Pediatrics, 80,* 664–671.

35

Behavior Problems in a Pediatric Context

SUSAN L. MORTWEET
EDWARD R. CHRISTOPHERSEN

Problem behaviors in children, especially externalizing behaviors, are a common referral issue for pediatric psychologists (Sobel, Roberts, Rayfield, Barnard & Rapoff, 2001). Regardless of whether the child has a medical condition or developmental disruptions, behavior problems, including opposition and noncompliance, are a trademark of childhood. Many children come to the attention of the practitioner when such negative and noncompliant behaviors reach a level of concern for the parent or the child's medical care providers or when the child receives a medical diagnosis, either due to illness or trauma, that demands compliance with a medical regimen. Often, these general behavior problems must be addressed before interventions for a pediatric or developmental problem can be successful. Thus the initial step in addressing many referral questions is often to improve or manage the child's ability to behave appropriately and to comply with daily demands of the environment. Of course, internalizing behaviors such as anxiety and depression also come to the attention of the pediatric psychologist and can affect how successfully developmental or medical conditions are managed by the child and caregivers. The reader is referred to other resources for information on how to assess and treat internalizing disorders that can affect the child's health and development (e.g., Hibbs & Jensen, 1996; March, 1995).

The purpose of this chapter is to provide the practitioner with suggestions on how to assess and manage behavior problems, including noncompliance, in children. These suggestions are applicable to the typically developing child, as well as to the child with a presenting medical condition. Recommendations are made for assessing key characteristics of the child and the environment, including parenting techniques, which may influence the child's behavior and compliance. Information on empirically supported interventions for behavior problems are presented if available. Suggestions specific to addressing adherence issues related to medical regimens are found elsewhere in this *Handbook* (see La Greca & Bearman,

Chapter 8). Also, behavior management issues related to attention-deficit/hyperactivity disorder (ADHD) are discussed by Shelton (Chapter 36, this volume).

ASSESSMENT OF BEHAVIOR PROBLEMS IN CHILDREN

In order to provide appropriate and effective treatment for a child's behavior problems, a targeted assessment is critical. Adequate assessment requires knowledge of typical child development, the relationship between parent and child temperaments, and genetic influences on behavior, as well as knowledge of the characteristics, prevalence, and impact of problematic behaviors (Mash & Terdal, 1988; Sattler, 1998). Such information is vital for identifying the target behaviors of concern, for formulating a treatment plan, and for evaluating treatment effectiveness. As treatment progresses, reassessment of key areas, such as the current impact of the problematic behavior, is often necessary to identify further intervention goals or to document treatment outcome.

The most useful assessment tools for evaluating any child behavior problem are those that will accurately describe the characteristics and impact of the behaviors of concern. For most childhood behavior problems, a multimethod assessment, which considers information obtained from at least two different assessment methods, is usually necessary to provide the most accurate description of the concerning situation (Eyberg, 1985; Morrison & Anders, 1999). Examples of assessment methods include caregiver and child interviews; standardized rating scales from parents, teachers, and the child; and direct observations in the office or the child's home or school setting. A description of these assessment methods related to the evaluation of behavioral problems and noncompliance are presented in the following sections.

Caregiver and Child Interviews

A clinical interview with the caregiver and child is often the first step in collecting vital historical information related to the referral issue. Typically, this initial contact with the family begins the process of identifying characteristics of the child, parent, and environment that may be contributing to the behavior problems in the child (Patterson, 1982). An interview by telephone or in person with the child's teacher, school nurse, or medical care provider may also be necessary depending on the behaviors of concern. For example, if a parent reports that the child is well behaved at home but is having behavior problems at school (e.g., not coming to the nurse's office to have his blood sugar levels checked), an interview with the school nurse, teacher, or both may be required. Telephone or personal interviews can also clarify information reported by the informants on standardized rating scales that they have been asked to complete. Standardized interview formats are available to the practitioner, although they can be time-consuming to complete. Two examples of such interviews include the Diagnostic Interview Schedule for Children (DISC-IV; Shaffer, Fisher, Lucas, Dulcan, & Schwab-Stone, 2000) and the Children's Interview for Psychiatric Syndromes (ChIPS; Weller, Weller, Fristad, Rooney, & Schecter, 2000). Both tools are useful for the school-age child. Nonstandardized interviews should include a thorough family history with an emphasis on problematic situations, child characteristics, and environmental factors, including parent characteristics and family mental health history of disruptive or mood disorders (La Greca, 1983). More specific suggestions for caregiver and child interview content are described later.

For children with medical conditions, especially those conditions with acute onset, such as burns, it is important to begin an assessment as soon as possible after diagnosis to establish baseline behavior before the injury or illness occurred. A child who presented with significant compliance problems prior to the injury or illness is much more likely to exhibit behavior problems and to be more difficult to treat than a child without behavior problems. Such information can guide the treatment plan to address preexisting behavioral or mood disturbances, in addition to goals related to the medical condition. In the authors' experience, it is all too common for practitioners to determine that behavior problems are the result of being diagnosed with a chronic illness, such as diabetes, when the problems were actually abundantly present prior to onset of the illness or trauma. The practitioner who addresses such problems as though they are a result of the illness or trauma is usually unproductive due to a lack of intervention related to problems that the parents and the child had prior to the medical problem. Disruptive children who are required to follow complicated medical regimens provide additional challenges. If premorbid functioning is not assessed thoroughly, the practitioner may focus on helping the child understand or structure the regimen, even though the real issue is the parent's lack of limit setting for illness- and non-illness-related matters. In summary, the importance of collecting premorbid functioning data is vital. Such timely interviews with children with acute medical conditions are often possible only for the practitioner who serves on an inpatient consultation and liaison service. For an outpatient practitioner, however, preincident indicators of functioning, such as grade cards or interviews with past teachers, may be useful.

Another important assessment issue for all children, including those with pediatric conditions, is to obtain data from multiple informants. Some caregivers may have better success in getting the child to comply with the demands of his or her medical care. Such variability can give insights into treatment areas, as well as possible interventions to try. For example, if the child shows fewer disruptive behaviors toward his grandmother who allows him to play video games after taking his shot, it may be useful to train the child's mother in how to use meaningful positive consequences to improve compliance with her, as well. Significant differences in parenting styles and resulting behaviors on the part of the child will most likely require a more comprehensive intervention than that needed for a family with only one caregiver or with similar parenting strategies.

Caregiver Interview

Many important areas of information related to the child's functioning should be addressed in the caregiver interview. For children with pediatric issues, a history of general behavioral functioning, as well as adherence to the prescribed medical regimen, is important. When possible, other members of the family should be interviewed to obtain another perspective on the way the parents and the child functioned prior to the trauma or illness. A grandparent or an aunt or uncle who is not as close to the child may willingly admit that the child or the parent had significant problems prior to the trauma or illness. Following are some key topics to assess during the caregiver interview.

Presenting Problem. In order to obtain a complete understanding of the parent's concern, several questions must be asked related to the presenting problem. These questions can serve as the foundation for a functional analysis of the problematic behavior. First, ask the parents to clearly define what behaviors concern them. A statement that the child has a "bad attitude" or "never listens" is not sufficient to address the problem. Parents should be asked to describe the behaviors of concern, as well as the behaviors they want their child to demonstrate. Information on the course of the problematic behavior should also be solicited. How long has the behavior been exhibited? What is the frequency of its occurrence, and has that changed over time? How intense is the behavior, and how much disruption does it cause the child or others? Are there factors such as hunger, fatigue, or being in a public setting that seem to increase the frequency or intensity of the problem? For example, a child who will not take her medication on the weekends at her grandmother's house but who does so willingly during the week at home will most likely require a different intervention than a child who will not take her medication at all.

Once the problem is defined, it is important to assess the antecedents and consequences of the behavior. First, where does the behavior occur and with whom? What is the child typically doing before exhibiting the problematic behavior? What does the parent say when asking the child to perform a behavior that is currently not being performed to the parent's satisfaction? These questions can establish the conditions under which the child is having difficulty behaving or complying, and they provide targets for intervention. The consequences of the child's misbehavior are also important. Is the child praised, rewarded, or ignored for positive behavior or compliance? Is the child sent to time out, reasoned with, or begged to comply when refusing to complete a task? Does the parent simply complete the task instead of asking the child to comply yet again? Similar to analyzing the antecedents of behavior, parent and child behaviors that can be targeted for intervention can be found by assessing the consequences of the child's problematic behavior. If parents have a difficult time answering some of these questions, it may be useful to have them keep a diary of their concerns for a week or two to provide documentation. The parents could simply list in columns the antecedents, behavior, and consequences as an initial attempt to clarify the nature of the behavior problems.

Level of General Compliance. Of course, if the referral issue were that of assisting with negative behavior, the preceding assessment questions would represent the majority of the interview. If the presenting problem is related to the child's developmental or pediatric condition, however, it is equally as important to question parents about the child's general level of compliance with non-medical-related tasks. For example, if the parent is seeking help for toileting refusal, the practitioner must assess how well the child follows instructions that are not related to the toileting issue. Similarly, if the reported problem is that of nonadherence to an aspect of a medical regimen, such as wearing a splint, a thorough discussion of how well the child complies with other tasks is important. Questions in this area should assess how well the child follows the parent's commands to complete tasks, how many instructions the child can follow through with at a time, and what type of consequences result from not completing the task.

Child Characteristics. A thorough developmental history for the child should be obtained. Parents should be asked about prenatal care, pregnancy complications, and postnatal course. Was the child premature or of low birthweight? Was the child routinely discharged with the mother? What type of sleep and eating habits did he or she exhibit as an infant? Was he or she as an infant easy to soothe or difficult to quiet? Questions about any serious illnesses, injuries, or hospitalizations should be asked. Has the child had a recent physical exam? What types of medications does the child take, if any? Does the child have any frequent somatic complaints? If so, is there a pattern to the complaints? Are the complaints related to an identifiable medical condition? Do physiological conditions such as fatigue or pain accompany the child's pediatric condition? Children with a complicated medical course may require more extensive questioning in the areas of health issues and their impact on their developmental course. For example, a child with gastrointestinal problems since birth may have oppositional behaviors related to food textures and eating that may be different from those of a child who is simply described by her parents as a "picky eater."

Other questions should be asked of the child's developmental progression. Is the child meeting expected milestones in the areas of gross motor, fine motor, and language skills? Has the child demonstrated any learning problems? Does he or she seem to be motivated to learn new things or participate in novel situations? If applicable, how has the child's pediatric condition interfered with meeting developmental milestones? In addition to physical development questions, it is also important to ask about the child's social development. Does the child seem to take interest in other people? Does he or she interact appropriately with adults and children? How successful is the child in making and keeping friends? Does he or she get invited to birthday parties? Does the child have any extracurricular interests or hobbies? What types of social skills deficits can the parent identify? For example, the parent may state that the child seems to be able to make friends but cannot keep them. How does the child's pediatric condition affect his or her social life? For example, does the child complain that her meal plan for her diabetes care interferes with her ability to interact "normally" with her friends?

Comorbid Disorders. It is important to assess for comorbid disruptive and mood disorders, as the prevalence of such conditions can be significant. Kazdin (1996) found that a significant number of children (45–70%) diagnosed with either ADHD or conduct disorder also met criteria for the other disorder. Children with disruptive behavior disorders are also at risk for comorbid mood disorders, such as depression and anxiety (Kazdin, 1996; Vitiello & Jensen, 1995). The prevalence of comorbid mental health problems in children with a medical condition is difficult to establish. Literature reviews of emotional and behavioral adjustment of children with chronic illness show variable ranges of dysfunction, from minimal to significant, when compared with their healthy peers (e.g., Bachanas et al., 2001; Noll et al., 1997; Sullivan & Chang, 1999; Todaro, Fennell, Sears, Rodrigue, & Roche, 2000). As a more specific example, some studies show that adolescents with Type 1 diabetes (insulin dependent) demonstrate a higher prevalence of eating disorders than peers without diabetes (Engstrom, Kroon, Arvidsson, Segnestam, & Aman, 1999; Rodin, Johnson, Garfinkel, Daneman & Kenshole, 1986), whereas other studies report no significant differences (Birk & Spencer, 1989; Byrden et al., 1999; Meltzer et al., 2001). The demands of many chronic illnesses can be great and can have a negative impact on the adjustment of the child and family. This impact, however, is quite individualized to the child, family, and pediatric condition. Thus a screen for comorbid disorders for the child with chronic illness who also demonstrates disruptive behaviors is crucial. Mood disorders or other psychiatric conditions, if left untreated, can interfere with progress in managing the disruptive behavior, as well as managing the child's illness.

Environmental Factors. One of the most important environmental factors to assess is parenting techniques and stressors. In order to effectively address behavioral problems in a child, the practitioner must have some sense of the parent's beliefs about appropriate and inappropriate behavior, about how they view discipline and what strategies they use to manage behavior, and about how much stress parenting issues cause them. Parents of children with disruptive disorders such as ADHD, for example, when compared with parents of children without ADHD, report more parenting-related stressors, such as dissatisfaction with the parenting role and greater personal distress (Barkley, Anastopoulos, Guevremont & Fletcher, 1992; Podolski & Nigg, 2001). Many parents of children with a chronic illness also suffer from parenting stress and psychological distress (Hilbert, Walker, & Rinehart, 2000; Ievers & Drotar, 1996; Wiener, Vasquez, & Battles, 2001). A discussion about how their parenting has changed since diagnosis is vital. For example, many well-meaning parents will relax their limits on their child after diagnosis out of guilt, fear, or sadness for the new stressors in the child's life. It may be at this point that the child's noncompliant behavior begins to increase. Questions about global family stressors are also important, including any marital or vocational problems, financial strains, and major life changes in the previous year, such as deaths, births, moves, and so on.

Parents should also be asked about the mental health history of immediate and extended family. Are there family members with a history of learning or attention problems, regardless of whether the problems were formally diagnosed? Does anyone suffer from depression or anxiety symptoms? Is there a history of substance abuse? These questions are especially relevant to the parent's mental health. As mentioned previously, a disruptive child can increase parental stress. A child with a pediatric condition can also stress a parent's coping skills, possibly influencing mood or other disturbances. Thus a thorough assessment of mental health problems for parents and a possible referral for the parent to seek treatment for these problems is vital.

Child Interview

An interview with the child can provide valuable information, as well as an opportunity to observe his or her behavior. Observing the child actually interacting with the parent, particularly when the parent makes reasonable demands on the child, can also yield valuable information. Most interviews will include a combination of questions that require a knowledge base (e.g., what she understands about her illness and behavioral difficulties), the way the child relates to his or her parents and any siblings, and open-ended questions that do not have any right or wrong answers. It is important to verify what the child understands about the illness. Oftentimes, oppositional behavior may be based on a misinterpretation by the child (or parent) that can be rectified with the help of the child's medical providers. For example, a child who is "sneaking" food may simply need a new meal plan to accommodate an increase in hunger. The child's responses to any self-report measures, including those assessing for depression or anxiety, can also be discussed during the child interview. More information about how to interview a child can be found in the pediatric literature (e.g., Bierman, 1983; Boggs & Eyberg, 1988; Schroeder & Gordon, 1991), including structured interviews (e.g., Hodges, Kline, Stern, Cytryn, & McKnew, 1982; McConaughy & Achenbach, 1990).

Standardized Behavior Rating Scales

Standardized behavior rating scales are a useful way to obtain input from multiple informants, including parents, teachers, and the child. Such rating scales provide a current indication of how parents, teachers, and the child perceive the child's conduct and emotional state. When data are collected from more than one informant, the practitioner can ascertain how consistently or inconsistently the child is perceived in the environment (Achenbach & McConaughy, 1996). The use of rating scales can also provide a way to repeat assessment during and after treatment and before and after medication changes to monitor progress. Some commonly used behavior rating scales for assessing problematic behavior and comorbid disorders are described here. Each measure asks the informant to rate the extent to which the child is demonstrating various behaviors related to internalizing and externalizing disorders.

Child Behavior Checklist

The Child Behavior Checklist (CBCL; Achenbach, 1991) is a commonly used behavior rating scale designed to assess for externalizing and internalizing problems in children. CBCL forms are available for parents, teachers, and the adolescent to complete. Norms are available by age and gender for children ages 2 to 17. Scores are available for both internalizing and externalizing behavior syndromes such as "anxious/depressed" and "aggressive behavior." Scoring may be completed manually or via a computerized program. The CBCL has been documented to discriminate effectively between normal children and those referred to mental health clinics (Achenbach, 1991). The practitioner should be cautious, however, about interpreting the results of the CBCL for the child with medical problems (Mathews, Spieth, & Christophersen, 1995). For example, items related to physical symptoms may artificially inflate subscale scores for the pediatric patient and thus should be analyzed carefully. Of course, the CBCL is best used as only one part of a comprehensive assessment and thus should be interpreted in the context of the information obtained from other sources as well. The publisher of the CBCL (Achenbach System of Empirically Based Assessment) reports the availability of a revised version of the CBCL as of November 2001. The revised scale has updated norms and new scales oriented toward the *Diagnostic and Statistical Manual of Mental Disorders* (4th ed., DSM-IV; American Psychiatric Association, 1994) criteria. The interested reader is referred to the organization's website for information on the most current edition of the CBCL at *www.aseba.org*.

Behavior Assessment System for Children

The Behavior Assessment System for Children (BASC; Reynolds & Kamphaus, 1992) is available in Parent Rating Scales (PRS), Teacher Rating Scales (TRS), and Self-Report of Personality (SRP). Norms are available by age and gender for children ranging in age from 2 years 6 months to 18 years 11 months. SRP data are available for adolescents ages 12 to 18 years old. Scores are reported for overall number of behavioral symptoms, externalizing problems, internalizing problems, school problems, adaptive skills, and atypicality. The adaptive-skills scores provide information about the child's functioning related to social skills, study skills, and leadership. A computer scoring program is available from the publisher that provides extensive information, including T-scores, score narrative, and item content for each of the subscales. Similar to other rating scales, the BASC was normed on children both with and without a mental health diagnosis. Norms specific to children with pediatric conditions are not available, and thus the BASC should be interpreted with other measures from multiple informants. Further information about the BASC is available from their website at *www.agsnet.com*.

Conners Rating Scale

The Conners Rating Scales—Revised (CRS-R; Conners, 1997) are also available for assessing problematic behavior in children, especially those with suspected ADHD. Similar to other rating scales, a parent, teacher and adolescent self-report measure is available. Both long and short versions of each informant's scale can be used in an assessment. Examples of subscale scores for the long parent version (CPRS-R:L) include Oppositional, Cognitive Problems/Inattention, Hyperactivity, Anxious–Shy, Perfectionism, Social Problems, and Psychosomatic. The teacher long version (CTRS-R:L) includes the same scales with the exception of the Psychosomatic scale. Both of these versions also include a DSM-IV (American Psychiatric Association, 1994) symptom subscale to screen for ADHD. The short version of the parent and teacher scales screen for oppositional behavior and cognitive problems, including inattention and hyperactivity. The adolescent self-report measure also has both a long and short version that assess conduct problems, cognitive problems, and hyperactivity. The long version also has scales that assess family, emotional, and anger-control problems. Forms are sent to the practitioner using a "quick score" method on NCR ("no carbon required") forms.

The parent and teacher rating forms are normed for children ages 3 to 17. The self-report form is for adolescents ages 12 to 17 years. The Conners Rating Scales—Revised were normed based on standardized scores from children with ADHD and without identified mental health or medical problems. Thus, as with the other rating scales discussed previously, it is important to use clinical discretion when interpreting the results of these assessment tools for children with pediatric conditions. Further information on the Conners Rating Scales is available at the ADD Warehouse website: *http://addwarehouse.com*.

Behavioral Observations

The practitioner may be able to obtain useful information about a child by conducting a behavioral observation in the office or other natural settings such as home or school. Typically, an observer will conduct a formal observation on the patient in question and at least one peer in the classroom. The inclusion of a nonclinical peer helps to control for the classroom atmosphere and the behavior of other classmates at the time of the observation. These observations are usually conducted in 5- or 10-second increments, and the observer notes the time the children spend on task, moving about the classroom, following directions, and making noises. Such observations are usually easier to conduct if the observer is someone from the school who is known to the classroom as opposed to an outsider who just happens to enter the classroom and begin recording observations. In some cases a much more formal functional analysis of behavior (FAB) may be necessary. For the FAB, the observer would record antecedent events, the child's behavior, and any consequences of that behavior, either planned or unplanned. The FAB is used to determine the extent to which the contingencies in the classroom may be maintaining or encouraging inappropriate or aberrant behavior. The fact that a child does or does not exhibit a particular behavior during an observation, however, cannot solely determine a diagnosis. This is especially true of observations in the practitioner's office, during which many different contingencies, such as novel toys and individual attention, can influence the child's behavior. Consequently, multimethod assessment is important for this reason as well.

Diagnostic Issues

Once assessment data are collected, it is usually necessary to indicate a diagnosis for the child. Oftentimes this can be difficult if the child does not meet DSM-IV (American Psychiatric Association, 1994) diagnostic criteria. Some children who display significantly disruptive behaviors may meet criteria for ADHD, oppositional defiant disorder or conduct disorder. Others may be demonstrating an adjustment disorder, with a disturbance in their mood or conduct as a result of a new medical diagnosis or a change in family functioning. Psychological factors such as depression and anxiety may also negatively affect the child's medical condition; these factors can also be coded using the DSM-IV.

The requirement of a diagnosis for insurance payment or other purposes can be problematic when the child has behavioral problems that do not extend to the point of clinically significant impairment. This may be especially true for the pediatric patient. In such cases, the practitioner should consult with colleagues about standard practice for generating an accurate diagnosis. New current procedural terminology (CPT) codes are available for mental health services rendered associated with the evaluation and treatment of behavioral and emotional issues related to a medical condition in cases in which the child does not meet criteria for a mental health diagnosis. The pediatric psychologist can use the medical diagnosis instead of a mental health diagnosis for treatment and billing purposes. These codes have been developed specifically for the nonphysician and, in fact, cannot be used by physicians. Once again, the practitioner should consult with colleagues and insurance companies for a better understanding of these codes and how they may apply to an individual practice or case.

EMPIRICALLY SUPPORTED INTERVENTIONS

Empirically supported interventions are available for addressing behavior problems in children. At the base of many of these treatments are strategies for improving behavioral compliance. Christophersen and Mortweet (2001) conducted a review of empirically supported interventions for childhood behavior problems. They found that behavioral parent training and cognitive behavior therapy, mainly in the form of problem-solving skills training, had the most support as effective interventions for common behavior problems in children. Preliminary support was also found for structural family therapy (e.g., Barkley, Guevremont, Anastopoulos, & Fletcher, 1992). Each of these treatments is discussed in this section, and, as mentioned earlier in this chapter, focuses on externalizing disorders that are disruptive to developmental or medical outcomes for the child.

The review by Christophersen and Mortweet (2001) supported the need for early intervention for children with behavior problems. For example, Campbell and Ewing (1990) found that 67% of 3-year-old children who were hard to manage and who did not receive any type of intervention were still exhibiting externalizing behavior disorders at age 9. In contrast, a 14-year postintervention follow-up study demonstrated that adolescents who had participated in a parent training program with their mothers when they were young were rated as similar to a matched community sample (a nonclinic population) on various measures of delinquency and emotional adjustment (Long, Forehand, Wierson & Morgan, 1994). Thus early intervention for children with behavior problems can promote more appropriate behaviors and decrease the likelihood that the negative behaviors will continue. This point is especially relevant to the pediatric patient if the problematic behaviors are interfering with medical care.

Parent Training

One of the primary interventions for managing disruptive behaviors in children is to train parents in improved behavior management techniques and is based on the pioneering work of Patterson (1982) and his colleagues (Webster-Stratton, 1996). Sheila Eyberg and her colleagues have also developed a comprehensive parent–child interaction therapy program that is often used in pediatric settings (see Hembree-Kigin & McNeil, 1995). Parent training techniques have been carefully documented and have significant empirical support in the literature as an intervention for behavior problems in children (Brestan & Eyberg, 1998; Fleischman, 1981; Forehand & Long, 1996; Long et al., 1994; Patterson, 1974). There are some key components to most parent training programs, including teaching parents how to provide differential attention to behaviors, how to provide effective instructions, how to use consequences such as rewards and time out appropriately, and how to integrate these skills into a comprehensive behavior management plan. Parent training programs are typically offered in 8- to 12-session formats, often introducing skills in a "stepwise" manner (e.g., Forehand & Long, 1996; Long et al., 1994). Each skill is taught using didactic information, as well as modeling and role playing with the parent and child in the office. Recommendations for the parent to structure practice times for each skill are also given. Webster-Stratton (1996) also used videotaped "vignettes" of problematic parent–child interactions to generate group discussions with parents on how to best intervene with disruptive behaviors. More information on these typical parent training components is provided here; more extensive information can be found in the treatment manuals by Barkley and Benton (1998), Forehand and Long (1996), Kazdin (1996), and Patterson (1971). Christophersen and Mortweet (2002) also provide information on important parent skills in a format designed for the parent to use alone or in conjunction with strategies offered by the practitioner.

Differential Attention

One purpose of teaching parents how to use differential attention with their children is to increase their likelihood of recognizing positive behaviors when they do occur. Oftentimes, by the time parents are seeking mental health help, they may have a difficult time even noticing when their child is complying or behaving appropriately. Thus, one step in parent training is to teach them to be aware of and acknowledge the child's compliant and positive behaviors. The second step is to teach them how to ignore minor misbehaviors or to use time out to remove the child from the parent's attention or from a preferred activity (cf. Christophersen, 1994, 1998).

In our Developmental and Behavioral Sciences clinic at Children's Mercy Hospital in Kansas City, Missouri, we teach parents the concept of "time in" as a means of helping them recognize appropriate behaviors in their children. Time in is described to the parent as the use of frequent, consistent physical contact with the child when he or she is engaged in appropriate behavior. Examples include patting the child's arm when he is riding in the car, rubbing the child's back briefly as she plays independently with her dolls, or briefly squeezing the child's hand as she stands by patiently waiting for her mother to finish a conversation with a friend.

Once parents have mastered the technique of enriching the environment through time in, or the rewarding of appropriate behavior, strategies such as ignoring or time out can become much more effective (Solnick, Rincover, & Peterson, 1977). Specific instructions on what types of behaviors to ignore, such as whining, should be provided by the practitioner. Parents will often state that "time out does not work." Once parents are provided with a complete description of how time out works most effectively, they may find that the strategy that "didn't work" was not time out at all, as they continued to talk to or yell at the child while he or she was supposed to be in time out. Parents should be informed that the child's behavior might become more disruptive before it improves once parents begin to effectively ignore minor misbehaviors. This can be especially upsetting for the parent of a child with a pediatric condition. Children with medical conditions may need more supervision during a time out episode, but in general they can still be managed effectively with differential reinforcement strategies. Further suggestions for consequences are provided later.

Effective Instruction Giving

Another skill for parents to develop to manage a child with behavior problems is providing effective instruction (Anastopoulos, Barkley, & Shelton, 1996; Forehand & McMahon, 1981). The instruction that a parent provides serves as an important antecedent to the desired (or undesired) behavior. Parents should be taught to reduce ineffective strategies such as nagging, giving too many commands at once, and ignoring their child when he or she does comply. More effective techniques should be discussed, such as being close to the child, making eye contact, giving a brief, specific, and positive command, and allowing the child time to complete the task before issuing another command. Parents should also focus on praising their child once she does comply within a reasonable time frame. A parent's ability to provide effective instructions can be especially important for children with pediatric conditions who are demonstrating problematic behaviors. Many medical regimens, such as those required to manage diabetes, ask the child to follow numerous and complicated instructions. Thus asking the child to follow yet another command, whether it is related to medical care or not, can be frustrating or can at least provide the setting for oppositional behavior. Effective instruction giving can reduce the number of ineffective requests and increase the likelihood that the child will comply.

Using Appropriate Consequences

One way to provide structure to the differential attention parents provide is to organize a reinforcement system of rewards and response costs. A token economy can offer such structure for the parent and the child (Christophersen, 1994). A token economy refers to an exchange system in which conditioned reinforcers are earned and lost based on whether the child does or does not perform defined behaviors. The use of a token or "conditioned reinforcer," often a poker chip, point, or sticker, is paired with a preferred item or activity, increasing the reinforcing properties of the conditioned object. If a child performs a desirable behavior, the token provides a bridge between the time at which the child performs the behavior and the time at which he or she is able to earn the reward. If he performs an undesirable behavior, the token serves as an immediate consequence in the form of a "fine" for the problem behavior.

The types of behaviors targeted for the token system, as well as the rewards and fines, should be individualized for each child. For example, targeted behaviors may include completing tasks, such as feeding the dog, or adequately performing a component of a medical regimen, such as checking blood sugar level. Social behaviors, such as sharing or tolerating frustration, and compliance with practicing desired skills, such as progressive muscle relaxation for anger management, can also be targeted for rewards. Examples of rewards include opportunities to play a video game, have a pizza party, spend the night with a friend, or play a game for 30 minutes with a parent. These rewards are typically not available immediately at the completion of the task; thus the token can provide immediate positive feedback to the child until he or she can "cash in" on his or her appropriate behavior.

The benefits of a token economy for managing behavior problems have been demonstrated for numerous child populations (Barnard, Christophersen, & Wolf, 1977; Bushell, 1978; Christophersen, Arnold, Hill, & Quilitch, 1972), including those with medical problems (Lowe & Lutzker, 1979; Rapoff, Lindsley, & Christophersen, 1984; Wolf, Kirigan, Fixsen, Blasé, & Braukmann, 1995). Kazdin (1977, 1982) provides excellent reviews of the early use of token economies. An example of a treatment manual for a token system, the home chip system for children ages 3 to 7 years, can be found in Christophersen and Mortweet (2001). Other examples of token systems are given by Barkley and colleagues (Barkley & Benton, 1998; Barkley, Guevremont, et al., 1992), and by Kazdin, Siegel, and Bass (1992).

Comprehensive Behavior Management Plan

Once parents are taught these techniques in a systematic manner, it is important to help them to recognize how each strategy interplays with the others and that each must be maintained for the best behavioral outcome for their child. The practitioner should also recommend to the parent that babysitters and other caregivers receive instruction in the behavior management plan to improve consistency and thus effectiveness for addressing the child's behavior problems. For example, if the child receives a sticker for taking his medication when Mom asks him to, he should receive a sticker from Grandmother if he complies for her as well. Parents should also be given suggestions on how to use these techniques in public places and during high-stress events, such as family gatherings.

Group Parent Training

Webster-Stratton and her colleagues have conducted numerous, well-designed studies of group parent training for families with a disruptive child (Webster-Stratton, 1990, 1996; Webster-Stratton & Hammond, 1997). A major component in the Webster-Stratton therapy is the use of videotapes to document situations such as the child being cooperative and parents dealing with various child-related events. The natural situations depicted in the videotapes of parents' modeling of effective and ineffective behavior management strategies can be a very useful teaching tool. Webster-Stratton and Hammond (1997) reported an example of Webster-Stratton's therapy for children with conduct disorder. The authors compared group child therapy alone, group parent training alone, a combination of group child and parent therapy, and a wait-list control group for children ages 4 to 8 years diagnosed with conduct disorder. The results showed that child therapy alone and in combination with parent training significantly improved the child's problem-solving and conflict-resolution skills with a peer. The combined therapy also resulted in maintained improvements in functioning at 1-year follow-up. A comprehensive description of Webster-Stratton's video-based course for parents, teachers, and other caregivers working with young children with conduct problems can be found in her *Parents and Children Series* (Webster-Stratton, n.d.). This publication offers one of the most systematic attempts to distribute a type of "treatment manual" for intervening with children with conduct problems.

Cognitive-Behavioral Therapy

Cognitive-behavioral therapy, often in the form of problem-solving skills training, has been used as an effective strategy for managing disruptive behaviors in children. An example of a problem-solving skills training (PSST) program is offered by Kazdin, Bass, Siegel, and Thomas (1989). The training used structured games and stories to depict common interpersonal situations that may be encountered on a daily basis. Children were taught how to use a step-by-step approach, using both cognitive and behavioral techniques, to effectively manage interactions with peers, parents, teachers, and others. For example, in this program, children are taught to ask themselves questions about what they are supposed to do, what all of the possibilities are, what the best choice is, and what could be done to improve the outcome the next time. The skills are taught using practice, modeling, role playing, and social and token reinforcement during the sessions.

Such problem-solving skills training is often compared with parent training to determine treatment effectiveness or is used in combination with parent training strategies. For example, Kazdin et al. (1992) conducted a large prospective study with random assignment to treatment groups to compare the effectiveness of problem-solving skills training (PSST) alone, PSST with a parent training program, and the parent training program alone. The parent training program, Parent Management Training (PMT), was based on procedures described by Patterson, Reid, Jones, and Conger (1975) and included many of the components discussed earlier in this chapter, such as the use of differential attention, effective instruction, and appropriate consequences. The results of the study showed that the children in all three groups improved with treatment with respect to overall functioning, prosocial skills, and reduced negative behaviors such as aggression. The combined PSST and PMT training resulted in the best outcomes. Another large prospective study by Kazdin and Wassell (2000) also provides support for PSST as an effective treatment option for children with conduct problems. Kazdin and his colleagues have conducted rigorous scientific evaluation of their model and offer the practitioner a promising intervention for managing difficult behaviors in children.

Structural Family Therapy

Structural family therapy has also been investigated as an intervention for addressing behavior problems in children and may have benefits for family functioning. Minuchin's (1974) structural family therapy program provides key principles for helping families identify and change their maladaptive interactions. Barkley, Guevremont, et al. (1992) compared structural family therapy with behavior management training and problem-solving and communication training. The authors reported that all three interventions significantly reduced conflicts, anger, negative communications, and symptoms of internalizing and externalizing disorders. Improvements were also noted in ratings of school adjustment and maternal depression. Szapocznik et al. (1989) also found that structural family therapy improved behavioral problems in children, as well as family functioning. The authors compared structural family therapy with psychodynamic child therapy and found that the families receiving family therapy maintained the most gains in positive family functioning. These examples of family therapy demonstrate the most efficacy in the literature. Further comparisons of structural family therapy with both parent training and cognitive-behavioral therapy are now needed to determine the role of this therapy as an intervention for children with disruptive behaviors and their families.

Improving Adherence to Treatment Suggestions

Although the focus of this chapter is on strategies to improve a child's behavioral compliance with the demands of their day, it is also useful for the practitioner to be aware of strategies to improve a caregiver's adherence with treatment recommendations as well. These suggestions are adapted from the adherence literature related to medical regimens and are certainly applicable to interventions for managing childhood disruptive disorders. Most strategies to improve adherence involve addressing the educational, organizational, and behavioral components of the treatment program (Lemanek, Kamps, & Chung, 2001). Examples of educational strategies to improve parent adherence to treatment suggestions would be to provide verbal and written information that is tailored to the cognitive level, literacy level, and learning style of the caregiver. Most word-processing programs have readability tools that can facilitate the development of written handouts at an appropriate grade level. Other examples of how to develop easy-to-read materials can be found in Stanley (1999). Effective organizational strategies for improving adherence include increased follow-up by telephone or more frequent appointments. Other strategies include designing the treatment regimen to meet the logistical needs of the family and incorporating treatment aspects into existing household routines. Finally, behavioral strategies include helping the family set up self-monitoring systems with cues and reminders to help them adhere to treatment components. For example, a parent might hang a data collection sheet for recording toileting habits and outcomes in the bathroom for the child with encopresis. Further suggestions on improving adherence to medical regimens that can be applied to improving adherence to treatment recommendations for managing disruptive behaviors can be found in Christophersen and Mortweet (2001) and Rapoff (1999).

SUMMARY AND CONCLUSIONS

One of the primary roles of the pediatric psychologist is to teach parents what to expect about childhood behaviors, about how children learn, and how to encourage consistent, cooperative, and compliant behaviors from them. In fact, general behavioral compliance is the cornerstone for assisting children in developing the skills they will need to be happy and productive adults. For example, oppositional behavior that undermines a child's willingness to sit and complete a preacademic task may have a negative impact on that child's progress once he enters school. Disruptive behaviors that annoy peers may earn a child the label of an unlikeable peer throughout elementary school. Children with medical conditions may suffer equal or even more serious consequences of noncompliant behaviors by interfering with their medical care and health outcomes. Thus, addressing behavioral compliance issues, preferably early in a child's life, is necessary to maintain that child's intended developmental trajectory and, for the pediatric patient, her physical well-being. For the pediatric psychologist, treating general behavioral compliance issues is often necessary to improve intervention efforts for the more specific developmental or pediatric problem.

In order to effectively assist parents in managing the disruptive child, with or without a medical condition, a targeted assessment of child and family functioning is necessary. Information should be collected from multiple informants, including parents, teachers, medical care providers if appropriate, and the child him- or herself. Interviews, rating scales, and behavioral observations provide methods for collecting data on global mental health functioning, as well as on issues specific to the child and his pediatric condition. Careful attention should also be paid to how the child and family functioned before the diagnosis of an acute or chronic illness was made. In order to design an effective treatment, the practitioner must have a clear understanding of the behavior and parenting challenges present before the medical diagnosis. Otherwise, it can be deceptively easy to focus on what appears to be illness-related disruptive behaviors instead of a long-standing lack of parental limit setting.

Effective treatments for managing disruptive behaviors in children are available to the practitioner. Parent training is a mainstay for addressing negative behavior and noncompliance. Parents are typically taught how to pay attention to the positive behaviors of their child, how to provide the child with effective commands, and how to structure a consequence system that will encourage cooperative, pleasant behavior. Token economies are often used to develop desired behaviors related to general functioning, as well as performance related to managing a pediatric condition. Older children may benefit from cognitive-behavioral treatment that teaches problem-solving strategies. Finally, preliminary evidence supports structural family therapy as another option for improving child behavior and family functioning.

REFERENCES

Achenbach, T. M. (1991). *Manual for the Child Behavior Checklist/4–18 and 1991 Profile.* Burlington, VT: University of Vermont, Department of Psychiatry.

Achenbach, T. M., & McConaughy, S. H. (1996). Relations between DSM-IV and empirically based assessment. *School Psychology Review, 25*, 329–341.

American Psychiatric Association. (1994). *Diagnostic and statistical manual of mental disorders* (4th ed.). Washington, DC: Author.

Anastopoulos, A. D., Barkley, R. A., & Shelton, T. L. (1996). Family-based treatment: Psychosocial intervention for children and adolescents with attention deficit hyperactivity disorder. In E. D. Hibbs & P. S. Jensen (Eds.), *Psychosocial treatments for child and adolescent disorders: Empirically based strategies for clinical practice* (pp. 267–309). Washington, DC: American Psychological Association.

Bachanas, P. J., Kullgren, K. A., Schwartz, K. S., Lanier, B., McDaniel, J. S., Simth, J., & Nesheim, S. (2001). Predictors of psychological adjustment in school-aged children infected with HIV. *Journal of Pediatric Psychology, 26*, 343–352.

Barkley, R. A., Anastopoulos, A. D., Guevremont, D. C., & Fletcher, K. E. (1992). Adolescents with attention deficit hyperactivity disorder: Mother–adolescent interactions, family beliefs and conflicts, and maternal psychopathology. *Journal of Abnormal Child Psychology, 20*, 263–288.

Barkley, R. A., & Benton, C. M. (1998). *Your defiant child: Eight steps to better behavior.* New York: Guilford Press.

Barkley, R. A., Guevremont, D. C., Anastopoulos, A. D., & Fletcher, K. E. (1992). A comparison of three family therapy programs for treating family conflicts in adolescents with attention-deficit hyperactivity disorder. *Journal of Consulting and Clinical Psychology, 60*, 450–462.

Barnard, J. D., Christophersen, E. R., & Wolf, M. M. (1977). Teaching children appropriate shopping behavior through parent training in the supermarket setting. *Journal of Applied Behavior Analysis, 10*, 49–59.

Bierman, K. L. (1983). Cognitive development and clinical interviews with children. In B. B. Lahey & A. E. Kazdin (Eds.), *Advances in clinical child psychology* (Vol. 6, pp. 217–251). New York: Plenum Press.

Birk, R., & Spencer, M. L. (1989). The prevalence of anorexia nervosa, bulimia, and induced glycosuria in IDDM females. *Diabetes Education, 15*, 336–341.

Boggs, S. R., & Eyberg, S. M. (1988). Interviewing techniques and establishing rapport. In A. La Greca (Ed.), *Childhood assessment: Through the eyes of a child* (pp. 85–108). Newton, MA: Allyn & Bacon.

Brestan, E. V., & Eyberg, S. M. (1998). Effective psychosocial treatments of conduct-disordered children and adolescents: 29 years, 82 studies, and 5,272 kids. *Journal of Clinical Child Psychology, 27*, 180–189.

Bushell, D. (1978). An engineering approach to the elementary classroom: The behavior analysis follow-through project. In A. C. Catania & T. A. Brigham (Eds.), *Handbook of applied behavior analysis: Social and instructional processes* (pp. 525–563). New York: Irvington.

Byrden, K. S., Neil, A., Mayou, R. A., Peveler, R. C., Fairburn, C. G., & Dunger, D. (1999). Eating habits, body weight, and insulin misuse. *Diabetes Care, 22*, 1956–1960.

Campbell, S. B., & Ewing, L. J. (1990). Follow-up of hard-to-manage preschoolers: Adjustment at age 9 and predictors of continuing symptoms. *Journal of Child Psychology and Psychiatry, 31*, 871–889.

Christophersen, E. R. (1994). *Pediatric compliance: A guide for the primary care physician.* New York: Plenum Press.

Christophersen, E. R. (1998). *Beyond discipline: Parenting that lasts a lifetime* (2nd Ed.). Shawnee Mission, KS: Overland Press, 1998.

Christophersen, E. R., Arnold, C. M., Hill, D. W., & Quilitch, H. R. (1972). The home point system: Token reinforcement procedures for application by parents of children with behavior problems. *Journal of Applied Behavior Analysis, 5*, 485–497.

Christophersen, E. R., & Mortweet, S. L. (2001). *Treatments that work with children: Empirically supported strategies for managing childhood problems*. Washington, DC: American Psychological Association.

Christophersen, E. R., & Mortweet, S. L. (2002). *Parenting that works: Building skills that last a lifetime*. Washington, DC: American Psychological Association.

Conners, C. K. (1997). *Conners' Rating Scales—Revised: Technical manual*. North Tonawanda, NY: Multi-Health Systems.

Engstrom, I., Kroon, M., Arvidsson, C. G., Segnestam, K., & Aman, J. (1999). Eating disorders in adolescent girls with insulin-dependent diabetes mellitus: A population-based case-control study. *Acta Paediatrica, 88*, 175–180.

Eyberg, S. M. (1985). Behavioral assessment: Advancing methodology in pediatric psychology. *Journal of Pediatric Psychology, 10*, 123–139.

Fleischman, M. J. (1981). A replication of Patterson's "Intervention for boys with conduct problems." *Journal of Consulting and Clinical Psychology, 49*, 342–351.

Forehand, R. L., & Long, N. (1996). *Parenting the strong-willed child*. Chicago: Contemporary Books.

Forehand, R. L., & McMahon, R. J. (1981). *Helping the noncompliant child: A clinician's guide to parent training*. New York: Guilford Press.

Hembree-Kigin, T. L., & McNeil, C. B. (1995). *Parent–child interaction therapy*. New York: Plenum Press.

Hibbs, E. D., & Jensen, P. S. (1996). *Psychosocial treatments for child and adolescent disorders: Empirically based strategies for clinical practice*. Washington, DC: American Psychological Association.

Hilbert, G. A., Walker, M. B., & Rinehart, J. (2000). "In for the long haul": Responses of parents caring for children with Sturge-Weber syndrome. *Journal of Family Nursing, 6*, 157–179.

Hodges, K., Kline, L., Stern, L., Cytryn, L., & McKnew, D. (1982). The development of a child assessment interview for research and clinical use. *Journal of Abnormal Child Psychology, 10*, 173–189.

Ievers, C. E., & Drotar, D. (1996). Family and parental functioning in cystic fibrosis. *Journal of Developmental and Behavioral Pediatrics, 17*, 48–55.

Kazdin, A. E. (1977). *The token economy: A review and evaluation*. New York: Plenum Press.

Kazdin, A. E. (1982). The token economy: A decade later. *Journal of Applied Behavior Analysis, 15*, 431–445.

Kazdin, A. E. (1996). Problem solving and parent management in treating aggressive and antisocial behavior. In E. D. Hibbs & P. S. Jensen (Eds.), *Psychosocial treatments for child and adolescent disorders: Empirically based strategies for clinical practice* (pp. 377–408). Washington, DC: American Psychological Association.

Kazdin, A. E., Bass, D., Siegel, T., & Thomas, C. (1989). Cognitive-behavioral therapy and relationship therapy in the treatment of children referred for antisocial behavior. *Journal of Consulting and Clinical Psychology, 57*, 522–535.

Kazdin, A. E., Siegel, T. C., & Bass, D. (1992). Cognitive problem-solving skills training and parent management training in the treatment of antisocial behavior in children. *Journal of Consulting and Clinical Psychology, 60*, 733–747.

Kazdin, A. E., & Wassell, G. (2000). Therapeutic changes in children, parents, and families resulting from treatment of children with conduct problems. *Journal of American Academy of Child and Adolescent Psychiatry, 39*, 414–420.

La Greca, A. M. (1983). Interviewing and behavioral observations. In C. E. Walker & M. C. Roberts (Eds.), *Handbook of clinical child psychology* (pp. 109–131). New York: Wiley.

Lemanek, K. L., Kamps, J., & Chung, N. B. (2001). Empirically supported treatments in pediatric psychology: Regimen adherence. *Journal of Pediatric Psychology, 26*, 253–276.

Long, P., Forehand, R., Wierson, M., & Morgan, A. (1994). Does parent training with young noncompliant children have long term effects? *Behavior Research and Therapy, 32*, 101–107.

Lowe, K., & Lutzker, J. R. (1979). Increasing compliance to a medical regimen with a juvenile diabetic. *Behavior Therapy, 10*, 57–64.

March, J. S. (Ed.). (1995). *Anxiety disorders in children and adolescents*. New York: Guilford Press.

Mash, E. J., & Terdal, L. G. (1988). Behavioral assessment of child and family disturbance. In E. J. Mash & L. G. Terdal (Eds.), *Behavioral assessment of childhood disorders* (2nd ed., pp. 3–65). New York: Guilford Press.

Mathews, J. R., Spieth, L. E., & Christophersen, E. R. (1995). Behavioral compliance in a pediatric context. In M. C. Roberts (Ed.), *Handbook of pediatric psychology* (2nd ed., pp. 617–632). New York: Guilford Press.

McConaughy, S. H., & Achenbach, T. M. (1990). *Guide for the semistructured clinical interview for children aged 6–11*. Burlington, VT: University Associates in Psychiatry.

Meltzer, L. J., Bennett-Johnson, S., Prine, J. M., Banks, R. A., Desrosiers, P. M., & Silverstein, J. H. (2001). Disordered eating, body mass, and glycemic control in adolescents with type 1 diabetes. *Diabetes Care, 24*, 678–682.

Minuchin, S. (1974). *Families and family therapy*. Cambridge, MA: Harvard University Press.

Morrison, J., & Anders, T. F. (1999). *Interviewing children and adolescents: Skills and strategies for effective DSM-IV diagnosis*. New York: Guilford Press.

Noll, R. B., MacLean, W. E., Whitt, J. K., Kaleita, T. A., Stehbens, J. A., Waskerwitz, M. J., et al. (1997). Behavioral adjustment and social functioning of long-term survivors of childhood leukemia: Parent and teacher reports. *Journal of Pediatric Psychology*, 22, 827–841.

Patterson, G. R. (1971). *Families: Application of social learning to family life*. Champaign, IL: Research Press.

Patterson, G. R. (1974). Interventions for boys with conduct problems: Multiple settings, treatments, and criteria. *Journal of Consulting and Clinical Psychology*, 42, 471–481.

Patterson, G. R. (1982). *Coercive family process*. Eugene, OR: Castalia.

Patterson, G. R., Reid, J. B., Jones, R. R., & Conger, R. W. (1975). *A social learning approach to family intervention* (Vol. 1). Eugene, OR: Castalia.

Podolski, C. L., & Nigg, J. T. (2001). Parent stress and coping in relation to child ADHD severity and associated child disruptive behavior problems. *Journal of Clinical Child Psychology, 30*, 503–513.

Rapoff, M. A. (1999). *Adherence to pediatric medical regimens*. New York: Kluwer Academic/Plenum.

Rapoff, M. A., Lindsley, C. B., & Christophersen, E. R. (1984). Improving compliance with medical regimens: Case study with juvenile rheumatoid arthritis. *Archives of Physical Medicine and Rehabilitation, 65*, 267–269.

Reynolds, C. R., & Kamphaus, R. W. (1998). *BASC: Behavior Assessment System for Children: Manual including preschool norms for ages 2–6 though 3–11*. Circle Pines, MN: American Guidance Service.

Rodin, G. M., Johnson, L. E., Garfinkel, P. E., Daneman, D., & Kenshole, A. B. (1986). Eating disorders in female adolescents with insulin-dependent diabetes mellitus. *International Journal of Psychiatry in Medicine, 16*, 49–57.

Sattler, J. M. (1998). *Clinical and forensic interviewing of children and families: Guidelines for the mental health, education, pediatric, and child maltreatment fields*. San Diego, CA: Author. (Available from *http://www.sattlerpublisher.com*)

Schroeder, C. S., & Gordon, B. N. (1991). *Assessment and treatment of childhood problems: A clinician's guide*. New York: Guilford Press.

Shaffer, D., Fisher, P., Lucas, C. P., Dulcan, M. K., & Schwab-Stone, M. E. (2000). NIMH Diagnostic Interview Schedule for Children—Version IV (NIMH DISC-IV): Description, differences from previous versions, and reliability of some common diagnoses. *Journal of the American Academy of Child and Adolescent Psychiatry, 39*, 28–38.

Sobel, A. B., Roberts, M. C., Rayfield, A. D., Barnard, M. U., & Rapoff, M. A. (2001). Evaluating outpatient pediatric psychology services in a primary care setting. *Journal of Pediatric Psychology, 26*, 395–405.

Solnick, J. V., Rincover, A., & Peterson, C. P. (1977). Some determinants of the reinforcing and punishing effects of time-out. *Journal of Applied Behavior Analysis, 10*, 415–424.

Stanley, K. (1999). Low-literacy materials for diabetes nutrition education. *Practical Diabetology, 18*, 36–44.

Sullivan, J. E., & Chang, P. (1999). Emotional and behavioral functioning in phenylketonuria [Review]. *Journal of Pediatric Psychology, 24*, 281–299.

Szapocznik, J., Rio, A., Murray, E., Cohen, R., Scopetta, M., Rivas-Vazquez, A., et al. (1989). Structural family therapy versus psychodynamic child therapy for problematic Hispanic boys. *Journal of Consulting and Clinical Psychology, 57*, 571–578.

Todaro, J. F., Fennell, E. B., Sears, S. F., Rodrigue, J. R., & Roche, A. K. (2000). Cognitive and psychological outcomes in pediatric heart transplantation [Review]. *Journal of Pediatric Psychology, 25*, 567–576.

Vitiello, B., & Jensen, P. (1995). Disruptive behavior disorders. In H. I. Kaplan & B. J. Sadock (Eds.), *Comprehensive textbook of psychiatry* (6th ed., pp. 2311–2319). Baltimore: Williams & Wilkins.

Webster-Stratton, C. H. (n.d.). *The parents and children series: A comprehensive course divided into four programs*. Seattle, WA: Author. (Available from Incredible Years, 1411 8th Avenue West, Seattle, WA 98119, or *http://www.incredibleyears.com*)

Webster-Stratton, C. H. (1990). Long-term follow-up of families with young conduct problem children: From preschool to grade school. *Journal of Clinical Child Psychology, 19*, 144–149.

Webster-Stratton, C. H. (1996). Early intervention with videotaped modeling: Programs for families of children with oppositional defiant disorder or conduct disorder. In E. D. Hibbs & P. S. Jensen (Eds.), *Psychosocial treatments for child and adolescent disorders: Empirically based strategies for clinical practice* (pp. 435–474). Washington, DC: American Psychological Association.

Webster-Stratton, C. H., & Hammond, M. (1997). Treating children with early-onset conduct problems: A comparison of child and parent training interventions. *Journal of Consulting and Clinical Psychology, 65*, 93–109.

Weller, E. B., Weller, R. A., Fristad, M. A., Rooney, M. T., & Schecter, J. (2000). Children's Interview for Psychiatric Syndromes (ChIPS). *Journal of the American Academy of Child and Adolescent Psychiatry, 39*, 76–84.

Wiener, L. S., Vasquez, M. P., & Battles, H. B. (2001). Fathering a child living with HIV/AIDS: Psychosocial adjustment and parenting stress. *Journal of Pediatric Psychology, 26*, 353–358.

Wolf, M. M., Kirigan, K. A., Fixsen, D. G., Blasé, K. A., & Braukmann, C. J. (1995). The teaching-family model: A case study in data-based program development and refinement (and dragon wrestling). *Journal of Organizational Behavior Management, 15*, 11–68.

36

Attention-Deficit/Hyperactivity Disorder

TERRI L. SHELTON

Attention-deficit/hyperactivity disorder (AD/HD) is not a new clinical phenomenon. Descriptions of children exhibiting AD/HD-type difficulties appeared as early as the middle of the 19th century. Since then, however, what is now called AD/HD has had a variety of diagnostic labels, symptoms, and etiological explanations. In this chapter, current diagnostic criteria, symptoms, prevalence, and etiology of AD/HD are reviewed. The potential impact on child and family functioning is also addressed, and implications of these variables for assessment and treatment are briefly noted.

DIAGNOSTIC DESCRIPTION

In what is thought to be one of the first formal diagnostic descriptions of AD/HD, Still (1902) talked about "volitional inhibition" of behavior, as well as "defects in moral control," to describe children having significant difficulties with inattention and overactivity that began in early childhood, persisted over time, and were not due to poor parenting or other environmental factors but rather to underlying neurological factors. With the large-scale outbreak of encephalitis around World War I, descriptions of AD/HD began to highlight the presumed role of some type of organic damage. Because many of the children who survived the epidemic displayed behavioral, emotional, or cognitive difficulties, including impaired attention span, impulse control, and regulation of motor activity, *etiologically based descriptions* (Ebaugh, 1923) such as postencephalitic behavior disorder (Hohman, 1922) and organic driveness (Kahn & Cohen, 1934; Strauss & Kephart, 1955; Strauss & Lehtinen, 1947) began to emerge. Based on research showing that inattention, impulsivity, and hyperactivity appeared more often among children having brain damage than among those diagnosed with mental retardation without such damage, Strauss and colleagues reasoned that any child exhibiting such behavioral difficulties very likely suffered from brain damage. Hence, the concept of the brain-injured child syndrome came into usage, which later evolved into what was known as minimal brain damage syndrome.

During the middle of the 1930's, *symptom-based descriptions* began to emerge. For example, Childers (1935) emphasized the hyperactivity symptoms. So did Levin (1938), who coined the phrase "restlessness syndrome," as well as Laufer and his associates, who used terms such as "hyperkinetic impulse disorder" (Laufer, Denhoff, & Solomons, 1957) and Hyperkinetic Behavior Syndrome (Laufer & Denhoff, 1957). This emphasis on hyperactivity was also apparent in Chess's (1960) symptom-based description of the condition, the hyperactive child syndrome.

These symptom-based descriptions set the stage for current diagnostic guidelines found in formal diagnostic classification systems such as the American Psychiatric Association's (APA) *Diagnostic and Statistical Manual of Mental Disorders* (DSM). The DSM criteria also have undergone numerous transformations. What began as a simple description in DSM-II (hyperkinetic reaction of childhood; APA, 1968), the essential features of which were hyperactivity and inattention, has now evolved into a rather complex, multifaceted set of diagnostic criteria. Each iteration of the DSM has reflected our evolving understanding of the disorder, its etiology, and its accompanying features. (See Anastopoulos & Shelton, 2001, for a review of the changing DSM diagnostic criteria).

Current diagnostic criteria for AD/HD encompass three primary symptoms—inattention, impulsivity, and hyperactivity—subdivided into two distinct groups of nine inattention symptoms and nine hyperactivity–impulsivity symptoms. A diagnosis of AD/HD under DSM-IV (APA, 1994) requires:

- Six or more of the nine symptoms of inattention and/or six or more of the nine hyperactivity–impulsivity symptoms to be present.
- Symptoms to have persisted for at least 6 months.
- Symptoms to be at a level that is greater than would be expected for the individual's developmental level.
- Some symptoms to be present before the age of 7.
- Symptoms that result in impairment to be present in two or more settings.
- That there be functional impairment in social, academic, or occupational domains.
- That the symptoms not occur exclusively during the course of pervasive developmental disorder, schizophrenia, or other psychotic disorder.
- That the symptoms not be better accounted for by another mental disorder (e.g., mood disorder, anxiety disorder, dissociative disorder, or a personality disorder).

One of the most important changes in DSM-IV is that *all* AD/HD diagnoses must include subtype distinctions. If six or more symptoms from both lists are present, and if all other AD/HD criteria are met, AD/HD, combined type (Code 314.01) is the appropriate diagnosis. This seems to be DSM-IV's version of what had been ADHD in DSM-III-R (APA, 1987). If six or more inattention symptoms but less than six hyperactivity–impulsivity symptoms present, the subtype is AD/HD, predominantly inattentive type (314.00), which appears conceptually related to what DSM-III-R had termed UADD. Conversely, if six or more hyperactivity–impulsivity symptoms but less than six inattention symptoms are present, a diagnosis of AD/HD, predominantly hyperactive–impulsive type (314.01), is given. This is a completely new subtype category, with support coming from numerous factor analytic studies (DuPaul, 1991; Lahey et al., 1988), as well as various clinical investigations (Barkley, Fischer, Edelbrock, & Smallish, 1990; Loeber, Keenan, Lahey, Green, & Thomas, 1993).

Two additional subtype categories are AD/HD, in partial remission, and AD/HD, not otherwise specified. The first most often applies to those adolescents and adults who, as children, very likely met criteria for one of the three major AD/HD subtypes but who no longer do. This is similar to ADD-RT in DSM-III but differs in that it includes the option to identify the three major subtypes described earlier. The other new category is intended for adolescents and adults who present with clinically significant symptoms that do not meet criteria for any of the three major AD/HD subtypes and in cases in which there is uncertainty regarding the onset of AD/HD symptoms.

Other changes in the criteria include: (1) evidence of symptomatology in at least two settings; (2) evidence of functional impairment in social, academic, or occupational domains; and (3) expanded listing of exclusionary conditions (see the preceding list). Some symptom descriptions have been revised to be developmentally more appropriate for adolescents and adults, although there is still concern that the wording, number, and onset of symptoms may not be developmentally sensitive, either for adolescents and adults (e.g., Barkley & Murphy, 1995; DuPaul, 1991) or for preschoolers (e.g., Campbell, 1987).

CLINICAL PRESENTATION OF PRIMARY SYMPTOMS

The current diagnostic classification highlights the key features of AD/HD as developmentally inappropriate levels of inattention, impulsivity, and hyperactivity. It is important to be familiar with the way in which DSM-IV describes these symptoms. But more important, one needs to be aware of the differing ways in which symptoms may be expressed in everyday situations, across different ages.

Inattention

Clinical descriptions of children with AD/HD frequently include complaints of "not listening to instructions," "not finishing assigned work," "daydreaming," "becoming bored easily," and having difficulty sustaining attention to tasks (Douglas, 1983). Such problems are more likely to occur during dull, boring, or repetitive tasks (Milich, Loney, & Landau, 1982), in which children with AD/HD are more likely to shift "off task" to engage in competing activities that provide relatively more immediate and meaningful gratification. Although such off-task behavior may stem from heightened distractibility, it may also result from a diminished persistence in responding to tasks that have little intrinsic appeal and/or relatively delayed consequences for completion (Barkley, 1990).

The exact manner in which inattentiveness is expressed can vary a great deal, in part as a function of age. For example, preschoolers may have difficulty attending for more than a few minutes to even a favorite television program or videotape or in day care settings. Older children might start an activity, such as getting dressed, but then stop before the task is completed, due to being distracted by something of greater interest. During the middle and high school years, many students with AD/HD have a great deal of difficulty remembering to bring books home or to turn in homework assignments, particularly when the tasks are long term in nature and require careful planning and organization.

Impulsivity

Sometimes defined as rapid, inaccurate responding (Brown & Quay, 1977), impulsivity may also refer to poor sustained inhibition of responding (Gordon, 1979), poor delay of gratification (Rapport, Tucker, DuPaul, Merlo, & Stoner, 1986), and/or impaired adherence to commands requiring inhibition of behavior in social contexts (Kendall & Wilcox, 1979). As with inattention, the exact manner in which impulsivity is expressed is subject to developmental influences.

Preschoolers with AD/HD may be more likely to knock down several children en route to get a preferred toy, not because they are aggressive but rather because of an inability to wait to walk across the room or to wait for the other child to finish using it. When at home, elementary school-age children have an especially difficult time refraining from interrupting a parent who is on the phone, making dinner, or visiting with company. At school, teachers frequently complain of careless mistakes that reflect the impulse to be finished. In adolescence, impulsivity might be seen in terms of various risk-taking behaviors, including sexual indiscretions and reckless experimentation with alcohol or illicit drugs (Mannuzza, Gittelman-Klein, Bessler, Malloy, & LaPadula, 1993).

Hyperactivity

Symptoms of hyperactivity are most often displayed through physical activity, but they can sometimes be expressed through increased verbalizations, as well. Whether physical or verbal, research suggests that individuals with AD/HD often fail to regulate their motor activity in response to situational demands (Porrino et al., 1983; Routh, 1978; Taylor, 1986). Once again, developmental factors exert a powerful influence over the manner in which hyperactivity symptoms appear. Even as toddlers or preschoolers, these children are described as being into everything and requiring constant monitoring. Having difficulty sitting in one place, settling to take a nap, or refraining from running when asked to walk in line are often mentioned. For elementary school-age children with AD/HD, remaining seated at a desk or on the bus can be challenging. Even when able to remain seated, many children continue to exhibit hyperactivity, such as noisily tapping fingers on a desk or rocking a chair back and forth. At home, elementary school-age children may have difficulty sitting anywhere, including the dinner table, during religious services, or at movie theaters. In addition to physical restlessness, many children with AD/HD exhibit what might be termed verbal hyperactivity, which can be just as disruptive and annoying.

For a variety of reasons, such as developmental maturity, most adolescents with AD/HD do not display as many of these physical features of hyperactivity as do younger children. When such symptoms are present, they typically appear in the form of restless leg movements or finger tapping or in subjective feelings of restlessness, often described in terms of racing thoughts. They are also more likely to exhibit verbal forms of hyperactivity, such as incessant talking in class and not letting others get a word in during social conversations.

Situational Variability

In addition to variations in symptoms due to the age of the individual, symptoms can vary in response to different situational demands (Zentall, 1985). AD/HD symptomatology is more likely to be evident in situations that are highly repetitive, boring, or familiar than in those that are novel or stimulating (Barkley, 1977); in situations in which others place demands or set rules versus free play or low-demand settings (Luk, 1985); or in group settings versus one-on-one situations. There is also an increased likelihood for AD/HD symptoms to arise in situations in which feedback is dispensed infrequently or on a delayed basis (Douglas, 1983). As a result, children with AD/HD often display tremendous inconsistency in their task performance, in terms of both their productivity and accuracy. As a result, it is not uncommon for parental perceptions to differ from what teachers observe in the classroom. Furthermore, parents or other family members may disagree with each other and teachers may disagree with other teachers from one grade to the next, or possibly within the same academic year.

ETIOLOGY

The current data suggest that there are multiple pathways that lead to AD/HD. Although psychosocial explanations have been suggested (e.g., poor parenting, chaotic home environments), they have not been supported, as these studies do not control for the role of biology in explaining the influence of environment. Although these factors certainly can contribute to the exacerbation of AD/HD symptoms and the increased likelihood of comorbid features, various biological explanations, with a few psychological conceptualizations, seem more promising.

Biological Explanations

Neurochemistry

Although many assume that AD/HD is caused by chemical imbalances in the brain, relatively few investigations have directly addressed this matter. Among those that have, inconsistent findings have emerged. Some studies have reported abnormalities in one of the monoaminergic systems involving either dopamine (Raskin, Shaywitz, Shaywitz, Anderson, & Cohen, 1984) or norepinephrine (Arnsten, Steere, & Hunt, 1996). In others, serotonin deficiencies have been implicated (Nemzer, Arnold, Votolato, & McConnell, 1986). These inconsistencies may be due to the variable manner in which AD/HD was defined (Halperin, Nercorn, Koda, et al., 1997), to various subtype differences, or to comorbid features. For example, Pliszka, McCracken, and Maas (1996) proposed that norepinephrine dysregulation might be expected in cases in which the primary difficulties are attentional in nature, whereas dopamine deficiencies would be predicted in cases in which hyperactivity and impulsivity are prominent. Halperin and his associates (Halperin, Newcorn, Kopstein, et al., 1997) detected serotonin abnormalities in an AD/HD sample but only when co-occurring aggressive features were present.

Neuroanatomical Structures

In addition to neurochemical deficiencies, structural abnormalities in the brain have been cited as causing AD/HD (Zametkin & Rapoport, 1987). There are inconsistencies in this research as well. In studies using coaxial tomographic (CT) scans, structural differences between children with AD/HD and those without have not usually been detected (Shaywitz, Shaywitz, Byrne, Cohen, & Rothman, 1983). In studies using higher resolution magnetic resonance imaging (MRI) devices, differences in brain structure have emerged, but not in any consistent fashion. More specifically, some have found that children with AD/HD have a smaller corpus callosum than do normal children (Baumgardner et al., 1996; Hynd et al., 1991), but others have not (Castellanos et al., 1996). Data from MRI studies have suggested that the caudate nucleus and other prefrontostriatal areas may be smaller among children with AD/HD (Castellanos et al., 1996; Filipek et al., 1997; Hynd et al., 1993). Whether or not these anatomical differences are functionally important has not been adequately addressed. Preliminary findings suggest that they probably are, given that the size of the prefrontostriatal area has been shown to be significantly correlated with performance on a psychological test of behavioral inhibition (Casey et al., 1997).

Neurophysiological Functioning

Brain functioning of children with AD/HD has been addressed primarily through cerebral blood flow (CBF) and positron emission tomography (PET) studies. CBF investigations have consistently found decreased blood flow in the prefrontal regions of the brain and in the various pathways connecting these regions to the limbic system, including the caudate nucleus (Lou, Henriksen, & Bruhn, 1984; Sieg, Gaffney, Preston, & Hellings, 1995). These deficits were reversed when stimulant medication was administered. PET scans with adults have shown evidence of diminished cerebral glucose metabolism in the prefrontal and cingulate regions, as well as in the caudate and in other subcortical structures (Zametkin et al., 1990). Similar PET results were initially reported for adolescent girls with AD/HD (Ernst et al., 1994; Zametkin et al., 1993), but recent efforts to replicate this finding have not been successful (Ernst, Cohen, Liebenauer, Jons, & Zametkin, 1997). Likewise, PET scan abnormalities have yet to be found among adolescent boys (Zametkin et al., 1993).

Genetics

Findings supporting a genetic link have emerged from comparisons between biological and adoptive relatives of children with AD/HD (Deutsch, 1987; Morrison & Stewart, 1973). High rates of AD/HD have also been detected among the immediate and extended biological relatives of children with AD/HD (Biederman et al., 1987). Among biological siblings, anywhere from 11 to 32% may have this disorder as well (Biederman et al., 1992; Levy, Hay, McStephen, Wood, & Waldman, 1997). An even higher degree of concordance exists for twins, with rates ranging from 29 to 38% for dizygotic pairs and 51 to 82% for monozygotic pairs (Gilger, Pennington, & DeFries, 1992; Levy et al., 1997). Further analyses of these twin data have yielded consistently high heritability estimates, ranging from .64 to .91 (Edelbrock, Rende, Plomin, & Thompson, 1995; Gillis, Gilger, Pennington, & DeFries, 1992; Goodman & Stevenson, 1989; Levy et al., 1997; Zahn-Waxler, Schmitz, Fulker, Robinson, & Emde, 1996). Additional genetic support comes from research that indicates that when one parent has AD/HD, there is a 50% chance that at least one of the offspring will also have this condition (Biederman et al., 1995).

These findings suggest that some type of genetic connection exists. Some speculate that a single gene may account for the expression of this disorder (Faraone et al., 1992) but with different locations implicated, including a dopamine transporter gene on chromosome 5 (Cook et al., 1995), a dopamine D4 receptor gene on chromosome 11 (Lahoste et al., 1996), or the HLA site on chromosome 6 (Cardon et al.,1994). These variations may be due to differences in procedure but may also be an indication that multiple genes are involved, with different genes or combinations of genes leading to the expression of different AD/HD subtypes.

Some of these more recent genetic findings suggest that these dopamine gene defects may help to tie together findings from the other biological studies. More specifically, the dopamine gene defects may be precursors to the dopamine deficiencies that have been reported in the neurochemical literature. These deficiencies, in turn, may be linked to some of the structural and functional abnormalities that have been reported.

Prenatal Complications

Certainly anoxia, as well as excessive maternal consumption of alcohol and/or nicotine, have been associated with increased risk of AD/HD (e.g., Streissguth, Bookstein, Sampson, & Barr, 1995). However, the specific nature by which these factors increase the risk for AD/HD is not clear. These results tend to be highly correlational in nature and complicated by other competing explanations. For example, many studies do not control for maternal AD/HD so as to rule out genetic influences as a possible explanation for the child's AD/HD, nor do they directly link specific amounts of maternal alcohol or nicotine consumption to abnormal brain development in the fetus. Only one study has attempted to address these factors (Milberger, Biederman, Faraone, Chen, & Jones, 1996). In that investigation, the risk for AD/HD remained high for children prenatally exposed to maternal nicotine, independent of whether or not maternal AD/HD was present.

Other Biological Factors

There have been reports that damage to certain parts of the brain, such as the prefrontal-limbic areas, can lead to AD/HD (Heilman & Valenstein, 1979). Because less than 5% of the population with AD/HD is likely to have a history of this type of problem (Rutter, 1983), brain damage is generally not considered to be a major cause of this disorder. Investigators have also found a relatively higher incidence of AD/HD among children with elevated lead levels (Gittelman & Eskinazi, 1983). Unfortunately, the physiological mechanisms responsible for this association have yet to be identified. Moreover, most children with AD/HD do not have histories of lead poisoning, suggesting that elevated lead levels are at best a minor cause of this disorder. Despite their widespread public appeal, there is also little support for the assertions of Feingold (1975) and others that the ingestion of sugar or various other food substances directly causes AD/HD (Wolraich, Wilson, & White, 1995).

Biological Variation

Periodically, the notion of biological variation has been put forth as an explanation for AD/HD (Chess, 1960; Kinsbourne, 1977). This view suggests that AD/HD characteristics, like those of intelligence, are distributed in a normal or bell-shaped manner within the general population. Thus children with AD/HD are labeled as such simply because their levels of inattention, impulsivity, and hyperactivity lie at the extreme ends of the normal continuum. Most experts today would certainly agree with that children with AD/HD display behavioral features that lie at the extreme ends of the normal continuum (Levy et al., 1997). Many would not, however, attribute these behaviors to normal biological variation (Barkley, 1997).

Psychological Conceptualizations

Over the years numerous psychological theories have also been put forth to explain the manner in which AD/HD affects psychosocial functioning. Many have focused on the attentional aspects, suggesting that poor executive functioning may be at the core of some of the difficulties evident in AD/HD. These explanations include core deficiencies in the regulation of behavior to situational demands (Routh, 1978), in self-directed instruction (Kendall & Braswell, 1993), in the self-regulation of arousal to environmental demands (Douglas, 1983), and in rule-governed behavior (Barkley, 1981). Building on what is now known about the biology of AD/HD, more recent theories have emphasized neuropsychological explanations for the impulsivity features of this disorder. In an elaboration of Quay's (1997) view of a neurologically based behavioral inhibition system, Barkley (1998) suggests that a deficit in behavioral inhibition leads to impairment in four major areas of executive functioning, which in turn sets the stage for the cognitive, behavioral, and social deficits that occur within AD/HD populations. These recent conceptualizations represent an important attempt to integrate biological theories with the more overt expression of AD/HD.

EPIDEMIOLOGY AND DEVELOPMENTAL CONSIDERATIONS

Prevalence

As with any prevalence data, the percentages reported in various studies are affected by the composition of the sample and the manner in which it is diagnosed (e.g., symptom cutpoints, assessment procedures, definition of developmental deviance). As a result, it is not surprising that there has been great variability in the AD/HD prevalence estimates. According to the DSM-IV itself, the overall prevalence of AD/HD among children—that is, the sum total of all subtyping categories—is 3–5% (APA, 1994). As might be expected, higher global estimates have been reported for community samples, ranging from 7.5% in a large, nationwide sampling of parent ratings of children and adolescents from 5 to 18 years of age using symptom frequency alone (DuPaul et al., 1998) to 11.4 to 21.6% in three investigations using teacher report (Baumgaertel, Wolraich, & Dietrich, 1995; DuPaul et al., 1997; Wolraich, Hannah, Pinnock, Baumgaertel, & Brown, 1996).

In terms of subtypes, the combined category was the most prevalent in the DSM-IV clinical field trials, outnumbering the inattentive and hyperactive–impulsive subgroups on the order of 2:1 and 3:1, respectively (Lahey et al., 1994). Community-based studies report somewhat different results, with the inattentive subtype most prevalent (DuPaul et al., 1998; DuPaul et al., 1997; Gaub & Carlson, 1997a; Wolraich et al., 1996). Among studies using teachers as informants, prevalence rates have ranged from 4.5 to 10% for the inattentive type, from 1.7 to 3.2% for the hyperactive–impulsive type, and from 1.9 to 8.4% for the combined type. When parents served as informants, rates of 3.2%, 2.1%, and 2.2% were reported for the inattentive, hyperactive–impulsive, and combined types, respectively (DuPaul et al., 1998).

Age and Gender Considerations

Of the many individual difference variables that might be considered when examining prevalence, age and gender are certainly among the most important. In their analysis of their teacher-generated data, DuPaul and his associates found overall prevalence rates of 25.3% for children 5–7 years of age, 23.8% for 8- to 10-year-old children, 21.5% for the 11- to 13-year-olds, and 15.0% for those 14–18 years of age (DuPaul et al., 1997). When parents served as informants, the overall prevalence rates were 9.1% for 5- to 7-year-old children, 6.4% for 8- to 10-year-old children, 8.3% for 11- to 13-year-old children, and 5.8% for adolescents between 14 and 18 years of age (DuPaul et al., 1998). These results raise the possibility that the overall prevalence of AD/HD, as defined by DSM-IV symptom frequency criteria, declines with age.

These trends appear to be true for the subtypes as well. Children 5 to 10 years of age are much more likely to be identified with the combined subtype by teachers, followed in order by the inattentive and hyperactive–impulsive subtypes (DuPaul et al., 1997). For students 11 to 18 years of age, the inattentive subtype becomes the most prevalent, followed in order by the combined and hyperactive–impulsive classifications. In parent ratings, the hyperactive–impulsive subtype appears to occur more often than the other two major subtyping categories among children 5–7 years of age (DuPaul et al., 1998) and in clinical samples (Lahey et al., 1994; McBurnett, Pfiffner, Tamm, & Capasso, 1996). In contrast, it decreased dramatically among children 8 years of age and older, making it the least likely subtype to occur among this age group (DuPaul et al., 1998). For this same age group, the prevalence of the inattentive category increases, thereby making it the most frequently encountered subtyping classification (DuPaul et al., 1998). Whether or not these same developmental trends would be evident in longitudinal studies is unknown. Until research of this sort is completed, these cross-sectional data raise the possibility that developmental trends may exist.

Gender differences have also been noted (Gaub & Carlson, 1997b). The overall prevalence of AD/HD is consistently reported as being substantially higher among boys than girls (APA, 1994; Arnold, 1996; Lahey et al., 1994). According to DSM-IV, the ratio of AD/HD in boys versus girls ranges from 4:1 to 9:1 (APA, 1994). Substantially lower ratios have been reported in community-based investigations, with boys outnumbering girls 2.2:1 in parent-generated samples (DuPaul et al., 1998) and 2.3:1 in samples based on teacher input (DuPaul et al., 1997). Boys also outnumber girls across all three major subtyping categories (Lahey et al., 1994), but the exact magnitude of these differences seems to depend on both the informant and the subtype. In one study, the ratio of boys to girls was 1.4:1 for the inattentive type, 3.1:1 for the hyperactive–impulsive type, and 3.3:1 for the combined type, using parent ratings (DuPaul et al., 1998). A similar pattern emerged from teacher ratings, with ratios of 2:1 for the inattentive type, 3.2:1 for the hyperactive–impulsive type, and 2.6:1 for the combined type (DuPaul et al., 1997).

Socioeconomic Status

To date, researchers have not yet systematically addressed the impact that socioeconomic status might have on the prevalence of AD/HD, defined in accordance with DSM-IV. Thus whether or not it will be the same as that found for earlier versions of AD/HD remains to be determined. To the extent that the results of earlier research are indicative of what might be found in future research, one would expect to find AD/HD occurring across the entire socioeconomic spectrum (Barkley, 1990). Although there have been some indications that AD/HD appears more often among lower socioeconomic backgrounds (Szatmari, 1992), the exact distribution of this disorder is not well understood. Furthermore, the degree to which any higher incidence might be due to other factors, such as the relationship between minority status and economic status or any variation in identification and assessment among children or color, has yet to be examined fully.

Ethnic and Cultural Diversity

In the DSM-IV clinical field trials, ethnicity was not a major factor influencing the prevalence of AD/HD (Lahey et al., 1994). It also did not seem to have a significant impact on the prevalence rates that were reported in the community-based study conducted by Gaub and Carlson (1997a), in which 92% of their sample came from minority backgrounds. In contrast, DuPaul and his associates reported ethnic differences in a community-based study. Approximately 6.3% of the Caucasian children and adolescents were identified via teacher ratings as having one of the three major subtypes of AD/HD versus a rate of 12.3% among children and adolescents from minority backgrounds (DuPaul et al., 1997). With regard to the total number of children and adolescents identified with any type of AD/HD, 43.4% were from minority backgrounds, even though minority children and adolescents made up only 34.8% of the total teacher-generated sample. Similar findings emerged from the parallel investigation in which parent-generated data were employed (DuPaul et al., 1998). Little of the AD/HD research that has been published to date has addressed ethnic diversity issues, and additional research of this type is clearly needed to establish a more definitive connection between ethnicity and the prevalence of AD/HD.

In one study that examined prevalence rates using DSM-IV outside of North America, Baumgaertal et al. (1995) reported an overall prevalence rate of 17.8% based on teacher ratings in Germany. Although these results are clearly discrepant with the findings reported in one North American–based study (Gaub & Carlson, 1997a), they are consistent with those of another (DuPaul et al., 1997). In another community-based study using public school teachers in Puerto Rico as informants, approximately 16% of the Spanish-speaking students were identified as having AD/HD (Bauermeister, Berrios, Jimenez, Acevedo, & Gordon, 1990). A relatively lower rate of 9.9% was reported in another community-based study, in which estimates were based on teacher ratings of Chinese students attending public schools in Taiwan (Wang, Chong, Chou, & Yang, 1993). Whether these discrepancies reflect real cross-cultural differences in the prevalence of AD/HD, in expectations for behavior, or perhaps just differences in scientific methodology is not known at this time. What is readily apparent from this line of research is that AD/HD can be found throughout the world and therefore is not just an artifact of the American lifestyle and culture.

Onset

Current findings suggest that most individuals with AD/HD begin to display their symptoms in early childhood, with hyperactive–impulsive difficulties typically preceding inattention. Most often such symptoms appear around 3 to 4 years, but they can also surface during infancy or on school entrance (Barkley et al., 1990; Green, Loeber, & Lahey, 1991; McGee, Williams, & Feehan, 1992). According to some researchers, the earlier the onset, the more likely it is that the child will have secondary or comorbid conditions and an overall higher degree of psychosocial impairment (McGee et al., 1992). At face value, these findings suggest that AD/HD symptoms do indeed arise in early childhood, thereby justifying DSM's requirement of an onset prior to 7 years of age. Although long-standing and widely held, such an assumption has recently been challenged (Barkley & Biederman, 1997).

Another question relates to whether onset of symptoms should be identified as the point at which they are first noticed or at which they result in some degree of functional impairment, as required by DSM-IV. Based on further analyses of the DSM-IV field trial data, Applegate et al. (1997) noted that nearly all children with AD/HD diagnoses had been reported by parents as showing onset of their symptoms prior to 7 years. However, many of these same children did not show any evidence of functional impairment stemming from these symptoms until after 7 years. On average, there was a 2-year difference between the time parents first noticed any AD/HD symptoms and the time when they labeled such symptoms problematic. On the basis of these and related findings, Applegate and associates suggest either retaining 7 years as the cutoff for detecting the presence of any AD/HD symptoms or increasing the cutoff to 9 years and requiring that there be evidence of functional impairment associated with these symptoms.

Developmental Course

According to most experts in the field, AD/HD is a chronic condition that persists across the lifespan (Barkley, 1998; Weiss & Hechtman, 1993). Although this might suggest constancy in its clinical presentation, long-term follow-up studies have consistently shown that no more than 50 to 80% of the children identified as having AD/HD will continue to meet full diagnostic criteria for this condition as adolescents (e.g., Barkley et al., 1990). This may be due to the decreased frequency of parent- and teacher-reported hyperactive–impulsive symptoms over this time period (see the earlier prevalence discussion), resulting in an decreased likelihood that adolescents will receive either the combined subtype or the hyperactive–impulsive subtype classification (DuPaul et al., 1997; DuPaul et al., 1998).

In comparison with AD/HD in childhood, little is known about how AD/HD unfolds from adolescence into adulthood. Available evidence suggests that no more than 30% of those individuals who were identified as children or adolescents with AD/HD will continue to meet diagnostic criteria as adults (Gittelman, Mannuzza, Shenker, & Bonagura, 1985; Mannuzza et al., 1993). Up to 50% of these individuals continue to exhibit subclinical levels of these symptoms, which interfere with daily functioning (Weiss & Hechtman, 1993). The overall frequency of AD/HD symptoms appears to decline across adulthood for both hyperactive–impulsive and inattention symptoms. Some investigators suggest that the overall incidence of AD/HD in adults is probably less than 1% in a clinical population (Shaffer, 1994), with a somewhat higher overall prevalence rate of 4.7% (1.3% for inattentive; 2.5% for hyperactive–impulsive; 0.9% for combined) from a local community sample (Murphy & Barkley, 1996).

PSYCHOSOCIAL IMPACT AND COMORBIDITY

Having AD/HD does not automatically lead to psychosocial difficulties. It does, however, place an individual at higher risk for such problems to occur. The "goodness of fit" model provides a useful framework for understanding how this disorder can disrupt normal functioning. According to this model, when there is a poor match between the challenges of a particular developmental period and an individual's abilities to meet those challenges, psychosocial difficulties will arise. Thus it is not just AD/HD that determines the types of problems that an individual might experience. It is the manner in which AD/HD interacts with the developmental challenges at a particular age that may increase the risk for psychosocial difficulties in various domains.

Behavioral Functioning

As outlined earlier, one of the ways in which AD/HD might be evident is in the difficulty many children have in completing tasks, following rules, or complying with requests. This failure to follow through or attempts to avoid failure or activities they perceive as boring may be the reason that so many children with AD/HD exhibit defiance or noncompliance.

More specifically, in clinic-referred samples of children with AD/HD, up to 60% will meet criteria for a secondary diagnosis of oppositional–defiant disorder (ODD), with another 25% meeting criteria for conduct disorder (CD; Barkley, 1990; Jensen, Martin, & Cantwell, 1997; Pelham, Gnagy, Greenslade, & Milich, 1992). Somewhat lower rates have been noted in community samples, with ODD and CD occurring up to 32% and 12% of the time, respectively (August, Realmuto, MacDonald, Nugent, & Crosby, 1996). The risk for ODD and CD also seems to be greater when hyperactive–impulsive features are prominent (Eiraldi, Power, & Nezu, 1997; Gaub & Carlson, 1997a) or during developmental periods such as adolescence when even those without AD/HD often demonstrate defiance and noncompliance with rules (Barkley, Anastopoulos, Guevremont, & Fletcher, 1991).

Emotional Functioning

Because children with AD/HD are at increased risk for various behavioral and academic problems, as well as difficulties in their peer and family relations, they tend to have fewer success opportunities and to receive more negative feedback than do most other children. Such circumstances may explain findings that as many as 13 to 51% of the children with AD/HD may have secondary emotional disorders (Jensen et al., 1997). In both clinic-referred and community samples, up to 30% of the children with AD/HD have been found to have a secondary mood disorder, with major depression and dysthymic disorder occurring most often (August et al., 1996; Biederman, Newcorn, & Sprich, 1991). Co-occurring anxiety disorders are common as well, affecting as many as 34% of the AD/HD population (August et al. 1996). There have also been reports, albeit controversial, that up to 11% of the children with AD/HD may be diagnosed with bipolar disorder (Biederman et al., 1996). This risk may be increased among those adolescents who also have long-standing histories of repeated academic failure, requiring often ineffective special education assistance (Barkley et al., 1990).

Family Functioning

For many parents of children with AD/HD, typical developmental separation and striving for independence very often become an intense battle for control. Daily self-care activities, following household rules, completing homework, and the like can become a test of wills because of the AD/HD symptoms. In response to these more frequent displays of negative and noncompliant behavior, many children with AD/HD and their parents report increased interpersonal conflict (Barkley, Anastopoulos, Guevremont, & Fletcher, 1992), as well as increased use of aversive, coercive, and controlling strategies to keep things in check (e.g., Campbell, 1995; Cunningham & Barkley, 1979; Mash & Johnston, 1982; Pisterman et al., 1992). Over time, such battles often contribute to increased parenting stress and marital discord (Barkley, Shelton et al., 1996; Shelton et al., 1998). Not being able to control their child's behavior may lead many parents to the conclusion that they are less skilled and less knowledgeable in their parenting roles (Mash & Johnston, 1990). For similar reasons, they may experience considerable stress in their parenting roles, especially when comorbid oppositional–defiant features are present (Anastopoulos, Guevremont, Shelton, & DuPaul, 1992; Johnston, 1996). Of additional clinical concern is that many parents of children with AD/HD report higher rates of depression, alcohol abuse, and marital difficulties (Cunningham, Benness, & Siegel, 1988; Lahey et al., 1988; Pelham & Lang, 1993).

Academic Functioning

Given the nature of AD/HD symptoms, it is not surprising that many children with AD/HD are at increased risk for difficulties in academic functioning. Whether because of their difficulty completing assignments (e.g., Hooks, Milich, & Lorch, 1994), organizing complex materials (e.g., Douglas & Benezra, 1990), decreased productivity (e.g., DuPaul & Stoner, 2003), or some other expression of AD/HD symptoms, children and adolescents with AD/HD are consistently identified as having an increased risk for academic difficulties. Anywhere from 18 to 53% of the population will perform significantly below what one would predict based on their intelligence (Barkley, 1990; Frick et al., 1991). Some children with AD/HD may also have comorbid learning disorders. The reported incidence of such difficulties within the AD/HD population has ranged from 10 to 50%, depending on the type of learning disorder under consideration and the manner in which it is defined (e.g., August & Garfinkel, 1990; Frick et al., 1991; Tannock & Schachar, 1996). As a group, children with AD/HD score slightly lower on standardized intelligence tests than do children without AD/HD (McGee, Williams, Moffitt, & Anderson, 1989). Studies suggest that many adolescents with AD/HD experience significant difficulties in school, including lower grades and greater utilization of special education services (Barkley, Guevremont, Anastopoulos, & Fletcher, 1992). They are more likely to repeat a grade, to be suspended from school, to drop out of high school, and to become employed after graduating from high school rather than attending college (Klein & Mannuzza, 1991). Whether these findings represent real differences in intellectual functioning, differences in achievement, or just differences in test-taking behavior is unclear. But what is clear is that without supportive educational environments, many children and adolescents with AD/HD may not be performing up to their full capability in this domain.

Social Functioning

As with academics, many of the core symptoms of AD/HD place a child with this disorder at risk for less-than-successful social interactions. As mentioned, there is an increased risk for more conflict within their families, but this risk also may extend to peer relationships. It is certainly not the case that children with AD/HD are doomed to a life without friends. Their energy, as well as their creative and funny behavior, can be assets. But all too often, some of the symptoms interfere with establishing good friendships. Children and adolescents with AD/HD seem to have more difficulty regulating their behavior. They are more likely to interrupt and to have trouble taking turns, and they may seemingly not be concerned about the perspectives of others (e.g., Lahey, Carlson, & Frick, 1997; Pelham & Bender, 1982). When AD/HD is accompanied by other externalizing behaviors, such as aggression, this too increases the chance for peer rejection (e.g., Campbell, 1995). These behaviors not only complicate the process of establishing new friendships (Grenell, Glass, & Katz, 1987) but may also result in the alienation of existing friends and acquaintances, who in turn respond with social rejection or avoidance (Barkley, Anastopoulos, et al., 1991; Taylor, Chadwick, Heptinstall, & Danckaerts, 1996).

IMPLICATIONS FOR ASSESSMENT AND TREATMENT

It is clear from the preceding discussion that no one procedure by itself can provide all the assessment data needed to address the complete DSM-IV criteria for AD/HD, all aspects of psychosocial functioning, and the possible comorbid conditions that one might find with AD/HD. Although single measures can be very helpful in screening, a more comprehensive multimethod assessment approach is needed. Clinical interviews, rating scales from multiple informants, and direct observations that are integrated with the individual's history are more likely to yield the type of information that is needed not only for accurate diagnosis but also for designing treatments (see Anastopoulos & Shelton, 2001, for a discussion of assessment approaches).

Clarifying the diagnostic picture is important in and of itself, but knowledge of how AD/HD plays out in a particular individual is critical for treatment. Gathering information about a child's strengths and needs at school, home, and with friends not only helps in making an accurate determination of severity and cross-situational pervasiveness but also sheds light on where intervention is needed. Just as it is unlikely that a single assessment measure is sufficient given the complexity of AD/HD, so to is it unlikely that any single treatment approach will meet all the needs of children with AD/HD and their families. Fortunately, there is a growing body of literature on empirically supported treatments not only for AD/HD (see Jensen & Members of the MTA Cooperative Group, 2002) but also for comorbid conditions (see *www.samhsa.gov* for information on system of care and other empirically supported treatments, especially for reduction of violence). There are several excellent articles about the state of empirically supported treatments for children with AD/HD and other disorders, including the efficacy of pharmacotherapy, parent training, classroom interventions, cognitive-behavioral therapy, and combined interventions (see *Clinical Psychology Science and Practice*, 2002, Vol. 9, No. 2; *Journal of Clinical Child Psychology*, 1998, Vol. 27, No. 2). Although the exact details of what causes AD/HD are still not well understood, future advances in our understanding of the etiology of AD/HD, as well as the development of empirically supported prevention and intervention approaches, can be helpful in limiting the negative impact of this disorder.

REFERENCES

American Psychiatric Association. (1968). *Diagnostic and statistical manual of mental disorders* (2nd ed.). Washington, DC: Author.

American Psychiatric Association. (1987). *Diagnostic and statistical manual of mental disorders* (3rd ed., rev.). Washington, DC: Author.

American Psychiatric Association. (1994). *Diagnostic and statistical manual of mental disorders* (4th ed.). Washington, DC: Author.

Anastopoulos, A. D., Guevremont, D. C., Shelton, T. L., & DuPaul, G. J. (1992). Parenting stress among families of children with attention deficit hyperactivity disorder. *Journal of Abnormal Child Psychology, 20*, 503–520.

Anastopoulos, A. D., & Shelton, T. L. (2001). *Assessing attention-deficit/hyperactivity disorder.* New York: Kluwer.

Applegate, B., Lahey, B. B., Hart, E. L., Waldman, I., Biederman, J., Hynd, G. W., et al. (1997). Validity of the age of onset criterion for ADHD: A report from the DSM-IV field trials. *Journal of the American Academy of Child and Adolescent Psychiatry, 36*, 1211–1221.

Arnold, L. E. (1996). Sex differences in ADHD: Conference summary. *Journal of Abnormal Child Psychology, 24*, 555–570.

Arnsten, A. F. T., Steere, J. C., & Hunt, R. D. (1996). The contribution of 2 noradrenergic mechanism to prefrontal cortical cognitive function. *Archives of General Psychiatry, 53*, 448–455.

August, G. H., & Garfinkel, G. D. (1990). Comorbidity of ADHD and reading disability among clinic-referred children. *Journal of Abnormal Child Psychology, 18*, 29–45.

August, G. J., Realmuto, G. M., MacDonald, A. W., Nugent, S. M., & Crosby, R. (1996). Prevalence of ADHD and comorbid disorders among elementary school children screened for disruptive behavior. *Journal of Abnormal Child Psychology, 24*, 571–595.

Barkley, R. A. (1977). The effects of methylphenidate on various measures of activity level and attention in hyperkinetic children. *Journal of Abnormal Child Psychology, 5*, 351–369.

Barkley, R. A. (1981). *Hyperactive children: A handbook for diagnosis and treatment.* New York: Guilford Press.

Barkley, R. A. (1990). *Attention-deficit hyperactivity disorder: A handbook for diagnosis and treatment.* New York: Guilford Press.

Barkley, R. A. (1997). *ADHD and the nature of self-control.* New York: Guilford Press.

Barkley, R. A. (1998). *Attention-Deficit Hyperactivity Disorder—A handbook for diagnosis and treatment* (2nd ed.). New York: Guilford Press.

Barkley, R. A., Anastopoulos, A. D., Guevremont, D. C., & Fletcher, K. E. (1991). Adolescents with attention deficit hyperactivity disorder: Patterns of behavioral adjustment, academic functioning, and treatment utilization. *Journal of the American Academy of Child and Adolescent Psychiatry, 30*, 752–761.

Barkley, R. A., Anastopoulos, A. D., Guevremont, D. C., & Fletcher, K. E. (1992). Adolescents with attention deficit hyperactivity disorder: Mother–adolescent interactions, family beliefs and conflicts, and maternal psychopathology. *Journal of Abnormal Child Psychology, 20*, 263–288.

Barkley, R. A., & Biederman, J. (1997). Towards a broader definition of the age of onset criterion for attention deficit hyperactivity disorder. *Journal of the American Academy of Child and Adolescent Psychiatry, 36*, 1204–1210.

Barkley, R. A., Fischer, M., Edelbrock, C. S., & Smallish, L. (1990). The adolescent outcome of hyperactive children diagnosed by research criteria: 1. An 8-year prospective follow-up study. *Journal of the American Academy of Child and Adolescent Psychiatry, 29*, 546–557.

Barkley, R. A., Guevremont, D. C., Anastopoulos, A. D., & Fletcher, K. E. (1992). A comparison of three family therapy programs for treating family conflicts in adolescents with attention deficit hyperactivity disorder. *Journal of Consulting and Clinical Psychology, 60*, 450–462.

Barkley, R. A., & Murphy, K. R. (1995). *An examination of ADHD symptomatology in an adult community sample.* Unpublished manuscript.

Barkley, R. A., Shelton, T. L., Crosswait, C. R., Moorehouse, M., Fletcher, K., Barrett, S., et al. (1996). Preliminary findings of an early intervention program with aggressive hyperactive children. In C. F. Ferris & T. Grisso (Eds.), *Annals of the New York Academy of Sciences, 794*, 277–289.

Baumgardner, T. L., Singer, H. S., Denckla, M. B., Rubin, M. A., Abrams, M. T., Colli, M. J., & Reiss, A. L. (1996). Corpus callosum morphology in children with Tourette syndrome and attention deficit hyperactivity disorder. *Neurology, 47*, 477–482.

Baumgaertel, A., Wolraich, M. L., & Dietrich, M. (1995). Attention deficit disorders in a German elementary school-aged sample. *Journal of the American Academy of Child and Adolescent Psychiatry, 34*, 629–638.

Bauermeister, J. J., Berrios, V., Jimenez, A. L., Acevedo, L., & Gordon, M. (1990). Some issues and instruments for the assessment of attention-deficit hyperactivity disorder in Puerto Rican children. *Journal of Clinical Child Psychology, 19*, 9–16.

Biederman, J., Faraone, S. V., Keenan, K., Benjamin, J. Kritcher, B., Moore, C., et al. (1992). Further evidence for family-genetic risk factors in attention deficit hyperactivity disorder: Patterns of comorbidity in probands and relatives in psychiatrically and pediatrically referred samples. *Archives of General Psychiatry, 49*, 728–738.

Biederman, J., Faraone, S. V., Mick, E., Spencer, T., Wilens, T., Kiely, K., et al. (1995). High risk for attention deficit hyperactivity disorder among children of parents with childhood onset of the disorder: A pilot study. *American Journal of Psychiatry, 152*, 431–435.

Biederman, J., Faraone, S. V., Milberger, S., Curtis, S., Chen, L., Marrs, A., et al. (1996). Predictors of persistence and remission of ADHD into adolescence: Results from a four-year prospective follow-up study. *Journal of the American Academy of Child and Adolescent Psychiatry, 35*, 343–351.

Biederman, J., Munir, K., Knee, D., Armentano, M., Autor, S., Waternaux, C., & Tsuang, M. (1987). High rate of affective disorders in probands with attention deficit disorders and in their relatives: A controlled family study. *American Journal of Psychiatry, 144*, 330–333.

Biederman, J., Newcorn, J., & Sprich, S. (1991). Comorbidity of attention deficit hyperactivity disorder with conduct, depressive, anxiety, and other disorders. *American Journal of Psychiatry, 152*, 1652–1658.

Brown, R. T., & Quay, L. C. (1977). Reflection-impulsivity of normal and behavior disordered children. *Journal of Abnormal Child Psychology, 5*, 457–462.

Campbell, S. B. (1987). Parent-referred problem three-year-olds: Developmental changes in symptoms. *Journal of Child Psychology and Psychiatry, 28*, 835–846.

Campbell, S. B. (1995). Behavior problems in preschool children: A review of recent research. *Journal of Child Psychology and Psychiatry, 36*, 113–149.

Cardon, L. R., Smith, S. D., Fulker, D. W., Kimberling, W. J., Pennington, B. F., & DeFries, J. C. (1994). Quantitative trait locus for reading disability in chromosome 6. *Science, 266*, 276–279.

Casey, B. J., Castellanos, F. X., Giedd, J. N., Marsh, W. L., Hamburger, S. D., Schubert, A. B., et al. (1997). Implication of right frontostriatal circuitry in response inhibition and attention-deficit/hyperactivity disorder. *Journal of the American Academy of Child and Adolescent Psychiatry, 36*, 374–383.

Castellanos, F. X., Giedd, J. N., Marsh, W. L., Hamburger, S. D., Vaituzis, A. D., Dickstein, D. P., et al. (1996). Quantitative brain magnetic resonance imaging in attention-deficit hyperactivity disorder. *Archives of General Psychiatry, 53*, 607–616.

Chess, S. (1960). Diagnosis and treatment of the hyperactive child. *New York State Journal of Medicine, 60*, 2379–2385.

Childers, A. T. (1935). Hyperactivity in children having behavior disorders. *American Journal of Orthopsychiatry, 5*, 227–243.

Cook, E. H., Stein, M. A., Krasowski, M. D., Cox, N. J., Olkon, D. M., Kieffer, J. E., & Leventhal, B. L. (1995). Association of attention deficit disorder and the dopamine transporter gene. *American Journal of Human Genetics, 56*, 993–998.

Cunningham, C. E., & Barkley, R. A. (1979). The interactions of hyperactive and normal children with their mothers during free play and structured task. *Child Development, 50*, 217–224.

Cunningham, C. E., Benness, B. B., & Siegel, L. S. (1988). Family functioning, time allocation, and prenatal depression in the families of normal and ADDH children. *Journal of Clinical Child Psychology, 17*, 169–177.

Deutsch, K. (1987). *Genetic factors in attention deficit disorders*. Paper presented at the Symposium on Disorders of Brain and Development and Cognition, Boston, MA.

Douglas, V. I. (1983). Attention and cognitive problems. In M. Rutter (Ed.), *Developmental neuropsychiatry* (pp. 280–329). New York: Guilford Press.

Douglas, V. I., & Benezra, E. (1990). Supraspan verbal memory in attention deficit disorder with hyperactivity, normal, and reading disabled boys. *Journal of Abnormal Child Psychology, 18*, 617–638.

DuPaul, G. J. (1991). Parent and teacher ratings of ADHD symptoms: Psychometric properties in a community-based sample. *Journal of Clinical Child Psychology, 20*, 245–253.

DuPaul, G. J., Anastopoulos, A. D., Power, T. J., Reid, R., Ikeda, M. J., & McGoey, K. E. (1998). Parent ratings of attention-deficit/hyperactivity disorder symptoms: Factor structure and normative data. *Journal of Psychopathology and Behavioral Assessment,* 20, 83–102.

DuPaul, G. J., Power, T. J., Anastopoulos, A. D., Reid, R., McGoey, K. E. & Ikeda, M. J. (1997). Teacher ratings of attention-deficit/hyperactivity disorder symptoms: Factor structure and normative data. *Psychological Assessment, 9*, 436–444.

DuPaul, G. J., & Stoner, G. (2003). *ADHD in the schools: Assessment and intervention strategies* (2nd ed.). New York: Guilford Press.

Ebaugh, F. G. (1923). Neuropsychiatric sequelae of acute epidemic encephalitis in children. *American Journal of Diseases of Children, 25*, 89–97.

Edelbrock, C. S., Rende, R., Plomin, R., & Thompson, L. (1995). A twin study of competence and problem behavior in childhood and early adolescence. *Journal of Child Psychology and Psychiatry, 36*, 775–786.

Eiraldi, R. B., Power, T. J., & Nezu, C. M. (1997). Patterns of comorbidity associated with subtypes of attention-deficit/hyperactivity disorder among 6- to 12-year-old children. *Journal of the American Academy of Child and Adolescent Psychiatry, 36*, 503–514.

Ernst, M., Cohen, R. M., Liebenauer, L. L., Jons, P. H., & Zametkin, A. J. (1997). Cerebral glucose metabolism in adolescent girls with attention-deficit/hyperactivity disorder. *Journal of the American Academy of Child and Adolescent Psychiatry, 36*, 1399–1406.

Ernst, M., Liebenauer, L. L., King, A. C., Fitzgerald, G. A., Cohen, R. M., & Zametkin, A. J. (1994). Reduced brain metabolism in hyperactive girls. *Journal of the American Academy of Child and Adolescent Psychiatry, 33*, 858–868.

Faraone, S. V., Biederman, J., Chen, W. J., Krifcher, B., Keenan, K., Moore, C., et al. (1992). Segregation analysis of attention deficit hyperactivity disorder. *Psychiatric Genetics,* 2, 257–275.

Feingold, B. (1975). *Why your child is hyperactive*. New York: Random House.

Filipek, P. A., Semrud-Clikeman, M., Steingrad, R. J., Renshaw, P. F., Kennedy, D. N., & Biederman, J. (1997). Volumetric MRI analysis comparing subjects having attention-deficit hyperactivity disorder with normal controls. *Neurology, 48*, 589–601.

Frick, P. J., Kamphaus, R. W., Lahey, B. B., Loeber, R., Christ, M. A., Hart, E. L., et al. (1991). Academic underachievement and the disruptive behavior disorders. *Journal of Consulting and Clinical Psychology, 59*, 289–294.

Gaub, M., & Carlson, C. (1997a). Behavioral characteristics of DSM-IV AD/HD subtypes in a school-based population. *Journal of Abnormal Child Psychology, 25*, 103–111.

Gaub, M., & Carlson, C. (1997b). Gender differences in ADHD: A meta-analysis and critical review. *Journal of the American Academy of Child and Adolescent Psychiatry, 36*, 1036–1045.

Gilger, J. W., Pennington, B. F., & DeFries, J. C. (1992). A twin study of the etiology of comorbidity: Attention-deficit hyperactivity disorder and dyslexia. *Journal of the American Academy of Child and Adolescent Psychiatry, 31*, 343–348.

Gillis, J. J., Gilger, J. W., Pennington, B. F., & DeFries, J. C. (1992). Attention deficit disorder in reading-disabled twins: Evidence for a genetic etiology. *Journal of Abnormal Child Psychology, 20,* 303–315.

Gittelman, R., & Eskinazi, B. (1983). Lead and hyperactivity revisited. *Archives of General Psychiatry, 40,* 827–833.

Gittelman, R., Mannuzza, S., Shenker, R., & Bonagura, N. (1985). Hyperactive boys almost grown up: 1. Psychiatric status. *Archives of General Psychiatry, 42,* 937–947.

Goodman, R., & Stevenson, J. (1989). A twin study of hyperactivity: I. An examination of hyperactivity scores and categories derived from Rutter teacher and parent questionnaires. *Journal of Child Psychology and Psychiatry, 30*(5), 671–689.

Gordon, M. (1979). The assessment of impulsivity and mediating behaviors in hyperactive and nonhyperactive children. *Journal of Abnormal Child Psychology, 7,* 317–326.

Green, S. M., Loeber, R., & Lahey, B. B. (1991). Stability of mothers' recall of the age of onset of their child's attention and hyperactivity problems. *Journal of the American Academy of Child and Adolescent Psychiatry, 30,* 131–137.

Grenell, M. M., Glass, C. R., & Katz, K. S. (1987). Hyperactive children and peer interaction: Knowledge and performance of social skills. *Journal of Abnormal Child Psychology, 15,* 1–13.

Halperin, J. M., Newcorn, J. H., Koda, V. H., Pick. L., McKay, K. E., & Knott, P. (1997). Noradrenergic mechanisms in ADHD children with and without reading disabilities: A replication and extension. *Journal of the American Academy of Child and Adolescent Psychiatry, 36,* 1688–1697.

Halperin, J. M., Newcorn, J. H., Kopstein, I., McKay, K. E., Schwartz, S. T., Siever, L. J., & Sharma, V. (1997). Serotonin, aggression, and parental psychopathology in children with attention-deficit hyperactivity disorder. *Journal of the American Academy of Child and Adolescent Psychiatry, 36,* 1391–1398.

Heilman, K. M., & Valenstein, E. (1979). *Clinical neuropsychology.* New York: Oxford University Press.

Hohman, L. B. (1922). Post-encephalitic behavior disorders in children. *Johns Hopkins Hospital Bulletin, 33,* 372–375.

Hooks, K., Milich, R., & Lorch, E. P. (1994). Sustained and selective attention in boys with attention deficit hyperactivity disorder. *Journal of Clinical Child Psychology, 23,* 69–77.

Hynd, G. W., Hern, K. L., Novey, E. S., Eliopulos, D., Marshall, R., Gonzalez, J. J., & Voeller, K. K. (1993). Attention-deficit hyperactivity disorder and asymmetry of the caudate nucleus. *Journal of Child Neurology, 8, 339–347.*

Hynd, G. W., Semrud-Clikeman, M., Lorys, A. R., Novey, E. S., Eliopulos, D., & Lytinen, H. (1991). Corpus callosum morphology in attention deficit-hyperactivity disorder: Morphometric analysis of MRI. *Journal of Learning Disabilities, 24,* 141–146.

Jensen, P. S., Martin, D., & Cantwell, D. P. (1997). Comorbidity of ADHD: Implications for research, practice, and DSM-V. *Journal of the American Academy of Child and Adolescent Psychiatry, 36,* 1065–1079.

Jensen, P. S., & Members of the MTA Cooperative Group. (2002). ADHD comorbidity findings from the MTA study: New diagnostic subtypes and their optimal treatments. In J. E. Helzer & J. U. Hudziak (Eds.). *Defining psychopathology in the 21st century: DSM-V and beyond* (pp. 169–192). Washington, DC: American Psychiatric Publishing.

Johnston, C. (1996). Parent characteristics and parent–child interactions in families of nonproblem children and ADHD children with higher and lower levels of oppositional-defiant behavior. *Journal of Abnormal Child Psychology, 24,* 85–104.

Kahn, E., & Cohen, L. H. (1934). Organic driveness; A brain stem syndrome and an experience. *New England Journal of Medicine, 210,* 748–756.

Kendall, P. C., & Braswell, L. (1993). *Cognitive-behavioral therapy for impulsive children* (2nd ed.). New York: Guilford Press.

Kendall, P. C., & Wilcox, L. E. (1979). Self-control in children: Development of a rating scale. *Journal of Consulting and Clinical Psychology, 47,* 1020–1029.

Kinsbourne, M. (1977). The mechanism of hyperactivity. In M. Blau, I. Rapin, & M. Kinsbourne (Eds.), *Topics in child neurology.* New York: Spectrum.

Klein, R. G., & Mannuzza, S. (1991). Long-term outcome of hyperactive children: A review. *Journal of American Academy of Child and Adolescent Psychiatry, 30,* 383–387.

Lahey, B. B., Applegate, B., McBurnett, K., Biederman, J., Greenhill, L., Hynd, G. W., et al. (1994). DSM-IV field trials for attention deficit/hyperactivity disorder in children and adolescents. *American Journal of Psychiatry, 151,* 1673–1685.

Lahey, B. B., Carlson, C. L., & Frick, P. J. (1997). Attention deficit disorder without hyperactivity: A review of research relevant to DSM-IV. In T. A. Wideger, A. J. Frances, H. A. Pincus, R. Ross, M. B. First, & W. Davis (Eds.), *DSM-IV Sourcebook* (Vol. 3, pp. 189–209). Washington, DC: American Psychiatric Association.

Lahey, B. B., Pelham, W. E., Schaughency, E. A., Atkins, M. S., Murphy, H. A., Hynd, G. W., et al. (1988). Dimensions and types of attention deficit disorder with hyperactivity in children: A factor and cluster-analytic approach. *Journal of the American Academy of Child and Adolescent Psychiatry, 27,* 330–335.

Lahoste, G. J., Swanson, J. M., Wigal, S. B., Glabe, C., Wigal, T., King, N., & Kennedy, J. L. (1996). Dopamine D4 receptor gene polymorphism is associated with attention deficit hyperactivity disorder. *Molecular Psychiatry, 1,* 121–124.

Laufer, M., & Denhoff, E. (1957). Hyperkinetic behavior syndrome in children. *Journal of Pediatrics, 50,* 463–474.

Laufer, M., Denhoff, E., & Solomons, G. (1957). Hyperkinetic impulse disorder in children's behavior problems. *Psychosomatic Medicine, 19,* 38–49.

Levin, P. M. (1938). Restlessness in children. *Archives of Neurology and Psychiatry, 39,* 764–770.

Levy, F., Hay, D. A., McStephen, M., Wood, C., & Waldman, I. (1997). Attention-deficit hyperactivity disorder: A category or a continuum? *Journal of the American Academy of Child and Adolescent Psychiatry, 36*(6), 737–744.

Loeber, R., Keenan, K., Lahey, B. B., Green, S. M., & Thomas, C. (1993). Evidence for developmentally based diagnoses in oppositional defiant disorder and conduct disorder. *Journal of Abnormal Child Psychology, 21,* 377–410.

Lou, H. C., Henriksen, L, & Bruhn, P. (1984). Focal cerebral hypoperfusion in children with dysphasia and/or attention deficit disorder. *Archives of Neurology, 41,* 825–829.

Luk, S. (1985). Direct observation studies of hyperactive studies of hyperactive behaviors. *Journal of the American Academy of Child Psychiatry, 24,* 338–344.

Mannuzza, S., Gittelman-Klein, R., Bessler, A., Malloy, P., & LaPadula, M. (1993). Adult outcome of hyperactive boys: Educational achievement, occupational rank, and psychiatric status. *Archives of General Psychiatry, 50, 565–576.*

Mash, E. J., & Johnston, C. (1982). A comparison of mother–child interactions of younger and older hyperactive and normal children. *Child Development, 53,* 1371–1381.

Mash, E. J., & Johnston, C. (1990). Determinants of parenting stress: Illustrations from families of hyperactive children and families of physically abused children. *Journal of Clinical Child Psychology, 19,* 313–328.

McBurnett, K., Pfiffner, L. J., Tamm, L., & Capasso, L. (1996). *Clinical correlates of children experimentally classified by DSM-IV attention-deficit/hyperactivity disorder subtypes: Cross-validation of field trials impairment patterns.* Paper presented at the meeting of the Society for Research in Child and Adolescent Psychopathology, Santa Monica, CA.

McGee, R., Williams, S., & Feehan, M. (1992). Attention deficit disorder and age of onset of problem behaviors. *Journal of Abnormal Child Psychology, 20,* 487–502.

McGee, R., Williams, S., Moffitt, T., & Anderson, J. (1989). A comparison of 13-year-old boys with attention deficit and or reading disorder on neuropsychological measures. *Journal of Abnormal Child Psychology, 17,* 37–53.

Milberger, S., Biederman, J., Faraone, S. V., Chen, L., & Jones, J. (1996). Is maternal smoking during pregnancy a risk factor of attention deficit hyperactivity disorder in children? *American Journal of Psychiatry, 153,* 1138–1142.

Milich, R., Loney, J., & Landau, S. (1982). The independent dimensions of hyperactivity and aggression: A validation with playroom observation data. *Journal of Abnormal Psychology, 91,* 183–198.

Morrison, J., & Stewart, M. (1973). The psychiatric status of the legal families of adopted hyperactive children. *Archives of General Psychiatry, 28,* 888–891.

Murphy, K., & Barkley, R. A. (1996). Prevalence of DSM-IV symptoms of ADHD in adult licensed drivers: Implication for clinical diagnosis. *Journal of Attention Disorders, 1,* 147–161.

Nemzer, E. D., Arnold, L. E., Votolato, N. A., & McConnell, H. (1986). Amino acid supplementation as therapy for attention deficit disorder. *Journal of the American Academy of Child Psychiatry, 25,* 509–513.

Pelham, W. E., & Bender, M. E. (1982). Relationships in hyperactive children: Description and treatment. *Advances in Learning and Behavioral Disabilities, 1,* 365–436.

Pelham, W. E., Gnagy, E. M., Greenslade, K. E., & Milich, R. (1992). Teacher ratings of DSM-III-R symptoms for the disruptive behavior disorders. *Journal of the American Academy of Child and Adolescent Psychiatry, 31,* 210–218.

Pelham, W. E., & Lang, A. R. (1993). Parental alcohol consumption and deviant child behavior: Laboratory studies of reciprocal effects. *Clinical Psychology Review, 13,* 763–784.

Pisterman, S., Firestone, P., McGrath, P., Goodman, J., Webster, I., & Mallory, R. (1992). The role of parent training in the treatment of preschoolers with attention deficit disorder with hyperactivity. *American Journal of Orthopsychiatry, 62,* 397–408.

Pliszka, S. R., McCracken, J. T., & Maas, J. W. (1996). Catecholamines in attention-deficit hyperactivity disorder: Current perspectives. *Journal of the American Academy of Child and Adolescent Psychiatry, 35,* 264–272.

Porrino, L. J., Rapoport, J. L., Behar, D., Sceery, W., Ismond, D. R., & Bunney, W. E. (1983). A naturalistic assessment of motor activity of hyperactive boys. *Archives of General Psychiatry, 40,* 681–687.

Quay, H. C. (1997). Inhibition and attention deficit hyperactivity disorder. *Journal of Abnormal Child Psychology, 25,* 7–13.

Rapport, M. D., Tucker, S. B., DuPaul, G. J., Merlo, M., & Stoner, G. (1986). Hyperactivity and frustration: The influence of size and control over rewards in delaying gratification. *Journal of Abnormal Child Psychology, 14,* 191–204.

Raskin, L. A., Shaywitz, S. E., Shaywitz, B. A., Anderson, G. M., & Cohen, D. J. (1984). Neurochemical correlates of attention deficit disorder. *Pediatric Clinics of North America, 31,* 387–396.

Routh, D. K. (1978). Hyperactivity. In P. Magrab (Ed.), *Psychological management of pediatric problems* (pp. 3–48). Baltimore, MD: University Park Press.

Rutter, M. (1983). Introduction: Concepts of brain dysfunction syndromes. In M. Rutter (Ed.), *Developmental neuropsychiatry* (pp. 1–14). New York: Guilford Press.

Shaffer, D. (1994). Attention-deficit hyperactivity disorder in adults. *American Journal of Psychiatry, 151,* 633–638.

Shaywitz, B. A., Shaywitz, S. E., Byrne, T., Cohen, D. J., & Rothman, S. (1983). Attention deficit disorder: Quantitative analysis of CT. *Neurology, 33,* 1500–1503.

Shelton, T., Barkley, R., Crosswait, C., Moorehouse, M., Fletcher, K., Barrett, S., et al. (1998). Psychiatric and psychological morbidity as a function of adaptive disability in preschool children with aggressive and hyperactive–impulsive–inattentive behavior. *Journal of Abnormal Child Psychology, 26,* 475–494.

Sieg, K. G., Gaffney, G. R., Preston, D. F., & Hellings, J. A. (1995). SPECT brain imaging abnormalities in attention deficit hyperactivity disorder. *Clinical Nuclear Medicine, 20,* 55–60.

Still, G. F. (1902). Some abnormal physical conditions in children. *Lancet, 1,* 1008–1012, 1077–1082, 1163–1168.

Strauss, A. A., & Kephart, N. C. (1955). *Psychopathology and education of the brain-injured child: Vol. 2. Progress in theory and clinic.* New York: Grune & Stratton.

Strauss, A. A., & Lehtinen, L. E. (1947). *Psychopathology and education of the brain-injured child.* New York: Grune & Stratton.

Streissguth, A. P., Bookstein, F. L., Sampson, P. D., & Barr, H. M. (1995). Attention: Prenatal alcohol and continuities of vigilance and attentional problems from 4 through 14 years. *Development and Psychopathology, 7,* 419–446.

Szatmari, P. (1992). The epidemiology of attention-deficit hyperactivity disorders. In G. Weiss (Ed.), *Child and adolescent psychiatric clinics of North America: Attention-deficit hyperactivity disorder* (pp. 361–372). Philadelphia: Saunders.

Tannock, R., & Schachar, R. (1996). Executive dysfunction as an underlying mechanism of behavior and language problems in attention deficit hyperactivity disorder. In J. H. Beitchman, N. J. Cohen, M. M. Konstantareas, & R. Tannock (Eds.), *Language, learning and behavior disorders: Developmental, biological, and clinical perspectives* (pp. 128–155). New York: Cambridge University Press.

Taylor, E., Chadwick, O., Heptinstall, E., & Danckaerts, M. (1996). Hyperactivity and conduct problems as risk factors for adolescent development. *Journal of the American Academy of Child and Adolescent Psychiatry, 35,* 1213–1226.

Taylor, E. A. (1986). Childhood hyperactivity. *British Journal of Psychiatry, 149,* 562–573.

Wang, Y. C., Chong, M. Y., Chou, W. J., & Yang, J. L. (1993). Prevalence of attention deficit hyperactivity disorder in primary school children in Taiwan. *Journal of Formosa Medical Association, 92,* 133–138.

Weiss, G., & Hechtman, L. (1993). *Hyperactive children grown up* (2nd ed.). New York: Guilford Press.

Wolraich, M. L, Hannah, J. N., Pinnock, T. Y., Baumgaertel, A., & Brown, J. (1996). Comparison of diagnostic criteria for attention-deficit hyperactivity disorder in a county-wide sample. *Journal of the American Academy of Child and Adolescent Psychiatry, 35,* 319–324.

Wolraich, M. L., Wilson, D. B., & White, J. W. (1995). The effect of sugar on behavior or cognition in children: A meta-analysis. *Journal of the American Medical Association, 274,* 1617–1621.

Zahn-Waxler, C., Schmitz, S., Fulker, D., Robinson, J., & Emde, R. (1996). Behavior problems in 5-year-old monozygotic and dizygotic twins: Genetic and environmental influences, patterns of regulation, and internalization of control. *Development and Psychopathology, 8,* 103–122.

Zametkin, A. J., Liebenauer, L. L., Fitzgerald, G. A., King, A. C., Minkunas, D. V., Herscovitch, P., et al. (1993). Brain metabolism in teenagers with attention-deficit hyperactivity disorder. *Archives of General Psychiatry, 50,* 333–340.

Zametkin, A. J., Nordahl, T. E., Gross, M., King, A. C., Semple, W. E., Rumsey, J., et al. (1990). Cerebral glucose metabolism in adults with hyperactivity of childhood onset. *New England Journal of Medicine, 323,* 1361–1366.

Zametkin, A. J., & Rapoport, J. L. (1987). Neurobiology of attention deficit disorder with hyperactivity: Where have we come in 50 years? *Journal of the American Academy of Child and Adolescent Psychiatry, 26,* 676–686.

Zentall, S. (1985). A context for hyperactivity. In K. D. Gadox & I. Bialer (Eds.), *Advances in learning and behavioral disabilities* (Vol. 4, pp. 273–343). Greenwich, CT: JAI Press.

37

Anorexia Nervosa and Bulimia Nervosa

THOMAS R. LINSCHEID
CATHERINE BUTZ

Pediatric psychologists have become more involved in the treatment of anorexia nervosa and bulimia nervosa over the past 20 years for several reasons. These include the onset of these disorders in the pediatric age range, the increased use of behavioral and cognitive behavioral techniques to treat these conditions, and the increasing trend toward treating the medical complications of anorexia nervosa and bulimia nervosa on medical rather than on psychiatric units (Linscheid, 1994). The onset of eating disorders can occur from early childhood through late adolescence, and therefore the initial diagnosis is often suspected or made by pediatricians or family physicians. Generally, hospital admissions to medical units are shorter and are designed to treat or prevent medical complications associated with eating disorder diagnoses. Psychotherapy is increasingly conducted on an outpatient basis in community settings. This chapter reviews the diagnostic criteria, etiology, and treatment of eating disorders, with attention given to the role of the pediatric psychologist in the interdisciplinary management of these disorders. Because of the similarities and contrasting differences, these disorders are discussed in common sections.

DIAGNOSTIC CRITERIA

Anorexia Nervosa

The DSM-IV (American Psychiatric Association [APA], 1994) diagnostic criteria for anorexia nervosa defines the disorder. There must be actual weight loss to below 85% of expected weight for height or, of significance to pediatric psychologists, a failure to make expected gains during periods of normal weight gain (early adolescence). In addition, there must be a fear of weight gain that does not subside as weight loss progresses. Denial of the seriousness of the disorder or related medical complications and an overemphasis on body shape and weight for self-evaluation are also present. The final diagnostic criterion is the absence of three consecutive menstrual periods in women who have passed menarche. The most significant change in diagnostic criteria in DSM-IV was the addition of two subtypes of anorexia nervosa, namely, binge-eating/purging type and restricting type. The binge-eating/purging subtype includes those who engage in binge eating, with weight loss caused by excessive purging (self-induced vomiting, laxative or diuretic abuse). Individuals in the restricting subtype utilize excessive calorie restriction and/or exercise to produce weight loss. The inclusion of the two subtypes follows a consensus by researchers and clinicians (Steiger, Liquornik, Chapman, & Hussain, 1991) who suggested etiological and outcome differences for the subtypes. Some individuals may move from the restricting category to the binge-eating/purging category as the disease progresses or following initial treatment.

Bulimia Nervosa

The DSM-IV diagnostic criteria for bulimia nervosa require the presence of a binge/purge cycle. Binges are defined as the consumption of large quantities of food in a discrete period of time (less than 2 hours) accompanied by a feeling of lack of control over eating. Purging occurs to prevent weight gain from the binge and can take several forms, as described in the disorder's subtypes. The binge/purge cycle occurs twice per week for 3 months, and there must be an overemphasis on body shape and weight for self-evaluation. Additionally, the disorder cannot occur with anorexia nervosa. As with anorexia nervosa, there are two subtypes of bulimia nervosa. The purging subtype refers to the use of vomiting, laxatives or diuretic, and the nonpurging subtype includes those individuals who use severe calorie restriction or excessive exercise to control weight gain following binges.

EPIDEMIOLOGY

Studies that have used inpatient admission rates have been biased toward only severe cases. Studies that have used questionnaire and self-report methods probably overestimate the prevalence of eating disorders, as questionnaires identify individuals who have attitudes or behaviors that resemble those of eating-disordered patients but may not meet diagnostic criteria. The best estimates come from studies in which a two-stage process is used: administration of a questionnaire to large numbers of individuals and then subsequent face-to-face interviews with those whose scores are consistent with those of individuals known to have eating disorders (Hsu, 1990). Unfortunately, there have been few such studies.

Anorexia Nervosa

In 1983, the U.S. Government published a pamphlet entitled *Facts about Anorexia Nervosa* (U.S. Department of Health and Human Services, 1983) suggesting that 1 out of every 200 American females between the ages of 12 and 18 will develop anorexia nervosa. Prevalence rates are much lower in males, with a male-to-female ratio of about 1 to 10. However, in patients in early to middle adolescence, the ratio is thought to be as high as 3 to 10 (APA, 2000). Crisp, Palmer, and Kalucy (1976) found prevalence rates as high as 1 in 100 females over the age of 16 who attended private schools in Great Britain. Halmi, Casper, Eckert, Goldberg, and Davis (1979) reported a bimodal distribution in the age of onset for anorexia, with peaks at 14 and 18 years of age. Lask and Bryant-Waugh (1992) concluded that the number of children below age 14 with eating disorders was low compared with late adolescent and early adulthood ages, but that there has been an increase in the number of cases in this age range. Whether this is a true increase in incidence or simply an increase in cases referred and reported is unclear. Bunnell, Shenker, Nussbaum, Jacobson, and Cooper (1990) suggested that the use of DSM-III-R criteria may have underestimated the incidence of anorexia nervosa in the younger population due to the requirement of three consecutive missed menstrual cycles. Preadolescent or early adolescent female patients may not have experienced menarche or may have delayed menarche, making it impossible to meet the criteria. Partial support for this comes from their study of clinic patients, ages 13–22 years, in which those who did not meet the full DSM-III-R diagnostic criteria were younger than those who did. Similar problems exist in the DSM-IV criteria, contributing to possible underestimation of the incidence of the disorder in younger patients. Recent reports have questioned the amenorrhea requirement and suggest lifetime rates of anorexia nervosa as high as 3.7% using a broader definition of the disorder (Garfinkel et al., 1996).

Bulimia Nervosa

Early studies of the prevalence of bulimia nervosa suggested rates in the 12 to 19% range for high school and college students (Pope, Hudson, Yurgelun-Todd, & Hudson, 1984). Studies that suggested very high rates of bulimia nervosa often utilized self-report measures and are now considered to be overestimates. Recent reviews of the literature have suggested a prevalence rate of 0.9 % for adolescents and young adults (Fairburn & Beglin, 1994; Hoek, 1993). Lask and Bryant-Waugh (1992) reviewed studies of adolescents and found prevalence rates ranging from 0.7% to as high as 2.5%. Changes in the diagnostic criteria in DSM-III-R from DSM-III resulted in a lowered diagnostic rate for bulimia nervosa (Ledoux, Choquet, & Flament, 1991). Hsu (1990) concluded that with the stricter DSM-III-R criteria the prevalence of bulimia nervosa is probably between 2% and 4.5%.

PSYCHOLOGICAL ASSESSMENT

Psychological instruments developed for the assessment of eating disorders can be helpful as aids in the diagnostic process, for use as screening instruments, and for treatment planning. These instruments should not be solely relied on for diagnoses, as eating disorders are best diagnosed by actual observed behaviors and outcomes (e.g., weight loss) and self-report of the patient. For the pediatric psychologist, the usefulness of some measures is limited because they were originally developed for a late adolescent or young adult population. The most well-known self-report instrument, the Eating Attitudes Test (EAT; Garner, Olmstead, Bohr, & Garfinkel, 1982) has been found to overestimate the number of respondents who meet diagnosis for eating disorders (Lask & Bryant-Waugh, 1992). Maloney, McGuire, and Daniels (1988) developed the Children's Eating Attitudes Test (ChEAT), which is based on the EAT but with questions designed to be understandable to children ages 8 to 13 years. It appears that the ChEAT identifies about the same proportion of individuals with eating disorder–related attitudes as does the EAT, again overestimating the prevalence of the disorder. Another widely used self-report instrument is the Eating Disorders Inventory (EDI), originally developed by Garner, Olmstead and Polivy (1983). A more recent version, the EDI-2 (Garner, 1991), comprises the original eight subscales with three additional scales. In addition, it contains a four-page symptom checklist that allows assessment of specific behaviors and their frequency. Semistructured interview instruments are available and are generally accepted to be more valid for diagnosis than self-report measures, as they provide an assessment of the individual's actual behaviors rather than only attitudes and beliefs. The most commonly used measures in this category are the Eating Disorders Examination (EDE; Fairburn & Cooper, 1993) and the Yale–Brown–Cornell Eating Disorders Scale (Mazure, Halmi, Sunday, Romano, & Einhorn, 1994).

ETIOLOGY

Anorexia Nervosa

Whereas some of the initial conceptualizations of anorexia nervosa described a purely psychological disorder, more recent conceptualizations characterize the disorder as multifactorial in nature and note that the disorder may begin for reasons different from those that maintain it. To understand anorexia nervosa, cultural/environmental, personality, psychological, physiological, and genetic factors must all be considered. Hsu (1990) believes that adolescent dieting often provides the entree to an eating disorder. This dieting becomes abnormal due to factors such as adolescent turmoil, poor self-esteem and body image, and poor identity formation. Hsu also considers other factors, such as family history and comorbidity.

In recent years, American society has embraced the concept of a slim body type as the ideal. Maloney, McGuire, Daniels, and Specker (1989) surveyed children in grades 3 through 6 and found that 86% of sixth-grade girls wanted to be thinner, with 60% reporting that they had been on at least one diet. The results of this study and others (Childress, Brewerton, Hodges, & Jarrell, 1993) suggest that cultural emphasis on thinness and dieting, particularly in girls, begins very early and may well contribute to the onset of eating disorders.

Developmental factors in adolescence have also been associated with the onset of anorexia nervosa. Attie and Brooks-Gunn (1989) found that bodily changes were better predictors of onset in early adolescence, whereas social-emotional and family factors were associated with onset in later adolescence. Gowers, Crisp, Joughlin, and Bhat (1991) found that anxiety over impending menarche was a factor in the onset of anorexia nervosa in premenarcheal females, and this group was premorbidly shorter and lighter than a group of patients who were postmenarcheal but matched for age of illness onset. The premenarcheal patients tended to come from intact families and were less likely to use laxatives or other dramatic measures to produce weight loss.

The personality of the patient with anorexia nervosa is often described as rigid, with a concrete cognitive style (Garner, 1993). These patients use weight, body shape, and thinness as the single reference for self-worth and personal value. They seem to be constantly striving to avoid or manage anxiety and in some cases show the anxiety-based symptoms of obsessive–compulsive disorder (Mills & Medlicott, 1992). Overachievement in academic areas has been documented (Dura & Bornstein, 1989), and Halmi et al. (2000) found convincing evidence that perfectionism is a strong and discriminating characteristic of the "anorexic personality."

The role of depression in the onset of anorexia nervosa is an unresolved issue. Halmi et al. (1991) observed that nearly 70% of anorexia nervosa patients in a follow-up study displayed major depression. However, there is evidence that comorbid depression in patients with eating disorders at the time of diagnosis has little, if any, predictive value for treatment outcome (Keel & Mitchell, 1997). The difficulty in assessing the role of depression in the patient with anorexia nervosa is, of course, whether or not the depressive symptomatology is the result of starvation and malnutrition or whether it is a predisposing factor.

It has also been hypothesized that family structure and family functioning is a predisposing variable in anorexia nervosa. Minuchin and colleagues (Minuchin, Rossman, & Baker, 1978) viewed family dysfunction within a homeostatic framework wherein one family member has an identified problem that serves the function of distracting attention from different and more deep-seated family issues. Enmeshment and overprotectiveness, excessive concern with physical appearance, and the avoidance of family conflict have been identified as characteristic of families of patients with anorexia nervosa (Garner, 1993). There may also be a genetic–familial pattern that precipitates the onset of anorexia nervosa. Holland, Sicotte, and Treasure (1988) found a concordance rate for monozygotic twins of over 50% and a corresponding concordance rate of only 10% for dizygotic twins. Other studies have shown that female first-degree relatives of anorexia nervosa patients have a significantly higher risk of exhibiting an eating disorder than a control population (Strober, Lampert, Morrell, Burroughs, & Jacob, 1990). More recently, Wade, Bulik, Neale, and Kendler (2000) found a heritability of 58% for anorexia nervosa in a population-based sample of 2,163 twins. With advances in genetic research, it is expected that the role of genetics in eating disorders will be found to be stronger than originally assumed.

In short, current theories of the etiology of anorexia nervosa postulate cultural, personality, and family variables, including genetic predispositions, as collectively contributing to the development of anorexia nervosa. It has been difficult to isolate the etiological variables of anorexia nervosa because the disease is usually studied only after its onset. Biological and emotional variables noted in patients with anorexia nervosa are increasingly being recognized as secondary to malnutrition and other components of the disease. It is very important not to judge these variables as causative when observed in these patients. Many patients function very well prior to the onset of anorexia nervosa (Lask & Bryant-Waugh, 1992).

Bulimia Nervosa

Recent research has indicated a significant genetic component to the etiology of bulimia (Bulik, Sullivan, Wade, & Kendler, 2000). However, most speculation as to the cause of bulimia nervosa has focused on personality characteristics, comorbidity of this disorder with other affective and addictive disorders, and the continuum of bulimia nervosa with normal eating and exercise practices.

Patients with bulimia nervosa appear to share some of the personal characteristics of those with anorexia nervosa but differ on several dimensions. Soukup, Beiler, and Terrell (1990) found that patients with anorexia and bulimia reported higher levels of stress, lowered self-confidence in their ability to solve problems, a style of avoidance when confronted with problems, a reluctance to share personal problems, and feelings of being driven when compared with non-eating-disordered controls. However, patients with bulimia reported a greater incidence of negative life events and increased feelings of being pressured than did a non-eating-disordered group. In contrast to the restrictive eating patterns of anorexia, individuals with bulimia nervosa are characterized as being impulsive, socially outgoing, aware that their pattern of eating and purging is abnormal, and self-conscious in regard to this pattern (Herzog, Keller, Sacks, Yeh, & Lavori, 1992). Investigation of dependency factors suggests that symptoms of anorexia are a means of resolving dependency while asserting one's individualism. In contrast, patients with bulimia express dependency in their attempt to manage low self-esteem that comes from the failure to meet cultural ideals of being thin (Rogers & Petrie, 2001). Low self-esteem has been reported in patients with bulimia but has been shown to be independent of depression (Silverstone, 1990). Other research reports that depression serves as a contributing factor to the maintenance of body dissatisfaction (Keel, Mitchell, Davis, & Crow, 2001), which has been shown to be a prognostic indicator of the development of bulimic eating patterns (Keel, Fulkerson, & Leon, 1997). Similarly, body dissatisfaction and pressure to be thin have been shown to be risk factors for dieting, depression, and consequent bulimic symptoms (Stice, Mazotti, Krebs, & Martin, 1998). Shisslak, Pazda, and Crago (1990) studied women with bulimia who were underweight, normal weight, and overweight and compared them with patients with anorexia, normal controls, and obese patients. Using a variety of personality inventories, they concluded that the highest psychopathology, lowest self-esteem, and highest level of external locus of control were found in the underweight women with bulimia.

Studies have also shown comorbid psychiatric diagnoses in patients with bulimia nervosa. Herzog et al. (1992) found that 60% of bulimia nervosa patients had current comorbid Axis I diagnoses, with major depression as the most commonly diagnosed disorder. Again, depending on the nutritional status of the patient, depression may be a side effect of the eating disorder rather than part of the etiology. Other studies have reported high comorbidity of obsessive–compulsive disorder (Braun, Sunday, & Halmi, 1994). A higher incidence of personality disorders has been found in eating-disordered patients, with a highest prevalence of borderline personality disorder found in patients with bulimia nervosa (Kennedy, McVey, & Katz, 1990). Herzog et al. (1992) also found a higher incidence of personality disorders in their bulimia nervosa and mixed bulimia nervosa–anorexia nervosa subgroups than in their anorexia nervosa group in a sample of women seeking treatment, with the greatest frequency of comorbid personality disorders occurring in the anorexia nervosa–bulimia nervosa mixed group. This subgroup showed a longer duration of symptoms and much greater comorbid Axis I psychopathology compared with the other groups in their sample. In addition, patients with bulimia are prone to other addictions, especially alcoholism (Lilenfeld et al., 1997). Hudson, Weiss, Pope, and Harrison (1992) found that 15% of 143 women hospitalized for substance abuse had a lifetime diagnosis of anorexia or bulimia nervosa, whereas only 1% of men had such a history. They found that women with eating disorders had higher rates of stimulant abuse and lower rates of opiate abuse than substance-abusing women without eating disorders.

Sexual abuse has been reported to occur at high rates in women with eating disorders (Vize & Cooper, 1995). Although sexual abuse has been reported for both patients with anorexia and those with bulimia, research suggests a higher likelihood of a history of unwanted sexual experience in patients with bulimia than in those with anorexia (Wonderlich, Brewerton, Jocic, Dansky, & Abbott, 1997). DeGroot, Kennedy, Rodin, and McVey (1992) found sexual abuse in the histories of 25% of patients with anorexia nervosa and bulimia and reported that previous sexual abuse was associated with greater psychological disturbance. Folsom et al. (1993) did not find this relationship between sexual abuse and eating-disorder symptoms. However, within their eating-disorder group, sexually abused participants exhibited more intense psychiatric disturbances, specifically of an obsessive or phobic nature, than did other patients. These authors concluded that sexual abuse in the history of eating-disordered patients might be related to premorbid distress but did not predict severity of eating-disorder symptomatology.

Family factors have also been shown to differentiate between bulimia and anorexia nervosa. Shisslak, McKeon, and Crago (1990) studied normal-weight patients with bulimia and patients with anorexia nervosa, bulimic subtype. Both groups perceived their families as more dysfunctional than did a normal control group. The dimensions of cohesion, expressiveness, conflict, recreational orientation, emotional support, and communication differed between the bulimia and control groups. Moreno, Selby, Aved, and Besse (2000) also reported that patients with bulimia had more family disturbances, such as greater rigidity and more difficulty communicating with mothers, when compared with patients with anorexia.

Biological variables have also been considered in the etiology of bulimia. The excessive quantity of food consumed during a binge suggests the possibility of abnormal appetite control mechanisms. Recently, the role of the gastrointestinal tract itself and gastric-inhibitory polypeptides, specifically cholecystokinin (CCK), have been implicated (Lask & Bryant-Waugh, 1992). The role of CCK is of special interest in that there are hypothalamic receptors that are sensitive to CCK, and therefore abnormalities in this region may contribute to cognitive distortions, appetite regulation disturbances, and delayed or abnormal gastrointestinal functioning.

The relationship between eating disorders and insulin-dependent diabetes mellitus (IDDM) has been the focus of research. Stancin, Link, and Reuter (1989) reported that nearly 40% of female diabetics underdose insulin as a means of weight control, perhaps similar to purging in bulimia. Although some early reports (e.g., La Greca, Schwarz, & Satin, 1987) suggested a high incidence of eating disorders in females with IDDM, these studies suffer from use of clinical and small samples. In recent reports (e.g., Crow, Keel, & Kendall, 1998), there does not appear to be an increased incidence of eating-disorder symptomatology in IDDM patients compared with norms.

At present, no agreed-upon single etiology exists for bulimia nervosa. Factors related to personality, family characteristics, and possible biochemical abnormalities have been postulated. Clinically, many therapists report that the binge/purge eating practice is described by patients as providing a coping strategy or a means for them to express anger, frustration, or self-deprecation. The personality similarities between the patient with anorexia nervosa, bulimic subtype and those with bulimia nervosa are strikingly similar. This similarity suggests an interplay of the etiological factors between the major eating disorders.

One final note about etiology is needed. Eating disorders are more common among athletes than in age-matched controls (Powers & Johnson, 1997). Certain sports that emphasize a thin body or small stature, such as ballet, gymnastics, and figure skating, place participants at risk for developing eating disorders. Recently, a "female athlete triad" has been proposed that includes disordered eating, amenorrhea, and osteoporosis (Nattiv, Agostini, Drinkwater, & Yeager, 1994). In males, body building and wrestling are related to developing eating disorders. The recent national emphasis on wellness, exercise, and weight reduction may actually result in an increase in eating disorders. As such, it will be important to design health-promoting programs for athletes and for the general public that take into account the susceptibility of certain younger females and males to restricting their eating patterns while striving for ideal body types.

TREATMENT

Intervention for anorexia and bulimia nervosa has changed over the past 20 years. Early therapeutic modalities were primarily psychodynamically oriented and relied a great deal on patient insight. More behaviorally based and cognitive-behavioral approaches have been utilized, and advances in psychopharmacological treatment have been helpful in some cases.

Anorexia Nervosa

The treatment of anorexia nervosa involves two phases, refeeding (i.e., medically supervised weight restoration) and psychotherapy. Refeeding is best thought of as nutritional rehabilitation and is accomplished under medical supervision, generally on an inpatient medical or psychiatric hospital unit. Various forms of psychotherapy are utilized in treatment as well. The type of psychotherapy selected depends on the patient's nutritional status, the duration of the illness, the settings available in the community, and family and personality factors. The value of psychotherapy during the acute refeeding phase is uncertain, and group therapy as a modality during the refeeding phase may be contraindicated (Maher, 1980).

As a result of managed care and insurance limitations on inpatient length of stay and lifetime limits for mental disorders, it has been estimated that 75% of the nation's top eating-disorder programs have closed (Fox, 1997). With fewer traditional inpatient psychiatric programs as options, and with the recognition that the first stage of treatment for anorexia nervosa is refeeding, hospitalization on medical units is a logical and often preferred alternative to psychiatric hospitalization. Utilizing hospitalization on medical units for the refeeding process preserves the patient's limited mental health insurance benefits for the psychotherapy phase of treatment. Practice guidelines for patients with eating disorders issued by the American Psychiatric Association (APA, 2000) recommend that the decision to treat in a medical versus psychiatric unit be based on factors such as the patient's medical status, the skills and experiences of local medical or psychiatric staff, and the availability of suitable services. The involvement of the pediatrician or family practice physician in the management of the refeeding process has led to an expanded role for the pediatric psychologist in the management of these patients. Although many pediatric psychologists do not have expertise in traditional psychotherapeutic systems for patients with anorexia nervosa, they are skilled in behavior-based, shorter term therapeutic interventions designed to increase compliance, decrease fear, and so forth. In this model, during refeeding, physicians, nurses and dieticians monitor medical and nutritional status while the pediatric psychologist develops and implements behaviorally based procedures designed to increase the patient's caloric intake and address fears or cognitive distortions that may be influencing the patient's behavior. Medical management of refeeding using a team that includes a behavioral psychologist, a nutritionist, and others can be very effective.

Treatment guidelines for anorexia nervosa (APA, 2000) provide specific medical criteria for determining when patients with anorexia nervosa need to be hospitalized. For children and adolescents, these include a heart rate in the 40s and orthostatic instability as evidenced by increases in pulse of 20 beats or more and a 10–20 mm Hg drop in blood pressure. Pulse and blood pressure readings are taken after the patient has been lying down for 10 minutes and then repeated after 2 minutes of standing. In addition, admission is indicated if blood pressure is below 80/50 or if the patient has hypokalemia or hypophosphatemia.

In the initial stages of refeeding, patients with anorexia may not be able to eat normal quantities on a daily basis. Comerci (1993) recommends requiring about 250 calories above patient's own baseline and increasing by 200 to 300 calories per week until the daily intake of about 2,500 calories is achieved. APA (2000) guidelines recommend starting with the requirement for 30–40 calories per kilogram per day (approximately 1,000–1,600 calories) and advancing the intake as high as 70–100 calories per kilogram. In the program described by Linscheid (1994), the patient is presented with four 1,000-calorie meals a day but told that she may eat as much or as little as she wishes. This allows the patients to set their own pace of caloric increase. In extreme cases of emaciation, refeeding the patient too rapidly could result in fluid retention and place undue stress on cardiac function. Pediatric psychologists are encouraged to obtain descriptions of specific treatment programs for greater detail in developing or modifying inpatient treatment of anorexia nervosa.

Traditional insight-based psychotherapies are often not offered during the refeeding phase, because their utility has been questioned. Danziger, Carel, Tyano, and Mimouni (1989) described the treatment of anorexia nervosa on a pediatric day-care unit by a multidisciplinary team. Although the program recommends family psychotherapy for all patients, the authors reported on 45 patients. Twenty-four did not enter psychotherapy during the first 2 months of the refeeding period, and the remaining 21 did start psychotherapy during that period. The researchers found that weight gain was greater in the group that postponed formal psychotherapy. The authors concluded that formal psychotherapy was not necessary or mandatory during the initial refeeding period. In fact, they suggested that resistance and negativeness could serve to hinder rather than to help the psychotherapy process. To underscore the need for refeeding as the first stage of treatment, Garner and Bemis (1985) suggest that outpatient therapy should proceed only if the patient's weight remains above a predetermined level based on the patient's menstrual threshold.

Behavioral techniques have been very effective during the initial phase of refeeding. Although those with psychodynamic orientations initially rejected behavioral approaches, Halmi (1985) points out that many "nonbehavioral" approaches to the management of anorexia nervosa actually utilize behavioral techniques that are not labeled as such. For example, the practices of granting privileges or simply providing social reinforcement for weight gain are behavioral in nature. These techniques are based on operant conditioning and are widely used. Behavioral weight-gain programs have been shown to produce very good short-term results (Agras, 1987), and a body of evidence suggests that they are superior to medication treatments in producing weight gain and shorter hospital stays (Johnson & Conners, 1987). In one program (Linscheid, 1994), initial assessment of the patient involves determining whether medical criteria for hospital admission are met (see earlier in the chapter). The patient is admitted to the hospital and remains there until the acute medical conditions resolve through weight restoration. During the admission, common hospital activities and privileges are withheld and can be earned by the patient based on weight gain. Some treatment programs utilize contingency contracting, in which an agreement about privileges or rate of weight gain is reached with the patient. In other programs, the goal weight and specific privileges are imposed on the patient.

Surprisingly, little formal research has been done on the effectiveness of psychotherapy, despite general clinical consensus that it is useful in the treatment of anorexia nervosa. Psychotherapy appears most useful in assisting the patient to understand what she has experienced, what antecedents may have led to the development of the disorder, the function of the disorder, and how to avoid relapse (APA, 2000). Halmi (1985) believes that the four goals in the treatment of anorexia nervosa are: (1) to return the patient to a normal medical condition, (2) to get the patient to resume normal eating patterns, (3) to assess and treat relevant psychological issues, and (4) to work with the patient's family to assist them in understanding their role in the maintenance of anorexia nervosa and how to develop methods to promote normal functioning in the patient. Behavioral management is especially important in the first two of these goals (i.e., refeeding) but can also be helpful in the latter goals. For example, assertiveness and social skills training, as well as a variety of cognitive-behavioral techniques, are used in therapy (Garner & Garfinkel, 1985). In addition, if anorexia nervosa can be conceptualized as a fear of weight gain, forcing a patient to face the fear and to maintain a healthy weight should serve to decrease the anxiety associated with the fear of uncontrolled weight gain (Linscheid, Tarnowski, & Richmond, 1988). Behavioral techniques can also be useful in helping the family adjust to having a child with anorexia nervosa. The requirement of rehospitalization if weight is not maintained takes the responsibility of daily monitoring of food intake away from the family, thereby decreasing a major source of family stress. Educating the family as to the phobic nature of the disorder changes the perception of the patient from an uncooperative adolescent into one whose fear is understood in a much different light.

Cognitive-behavioral therapy (CBT) for anorexia nervosa has grown in popularity since it was developed in the early 1980s (Garner & Bemis, 1982). CBT is based on the premise that patients with anorexia nervosa show distorted thought processes, stereotypical distorted beliefs, reasoning errors, deficits in self-esteem, and deficits in the identification and expression of affect (Garner, 1993). Garner and Bemis (1985) discuss the role of both positive and negative reinforcement in the development and maintenance of anorexia nervosa. Negative reinforcement, in the form of escape from or avoidance of anxiety based on anorexic behavior (e.g., dieting, exercise), serves to maintain those behaviors through anxiety reduction. It is well known that avoidance behaviors are highly resistant to extinction, because exposure to the feared stimulus is prevented by the behavior itself. Positive reinforcement takes the form of social praise from peers in the early stages of weight loss, but in later stages it appears to come from feelings of accomplishment of a difficult task (i.e., denial of food) that others are not able to do.

Anorexia nervosa patients show two main areas of distorted thinking. First is the belief that they are evaluated on their size or shape. The thinking goes: "if it is good to be thin, then you are the best if you are the thinnest." Second is the belief that if they begin eating or gain weight (i.e., let go), they will not be able to stop and will become obese. Garner and Bemis (1985) describe other reasoning errors, including personalization, superstitious thinking, magnification, selective abstraction, and overgeneralization. Standard cognitive therapy techniques are used to address these reasoning errors. Despite the popularity of CBT for anorexia nervosa, little research is available at present to verify its superiority over other approaches such as family therapy or operant-based behavior therapy. For example, Channon, deSilva, Hensley, and Perkins (1989) found no differences between a CBT group and a standard behavioral treatment group on measures of weight, depression, and a self-report eating questionnaire. They did report that patients in the CBT group attended more sessions and concluded that this form of treatment was more acceptable to the patients. The popularity of CBT in the absence of definitive research findings is probably due to its straightforward focus on the central cognitive distortions characteristic of patients with anorexia nervosa and its shorter term treatment orientation.

Group therapy for anorexia nervosa has little research evidence to suggest its efficacy. Patients' social interaction difficulties and preoccupation with weight do not make them good candidates for this approach. However, Hall (1985) feels that groups can be helpful for patients with anorexia nervosa if they are carefully selected. She suggests two criteria: (1) patients must be either restored to a healthy weight or very near such a weight, and (2) patients must acknowledge that they are ill and need help. Denial of illness by the anorexic patient is the biggest obstacle to therapy, whatever the modality.

The role of various therapy approaches in treating anorexia nervosa is difficult to determine. Most patients are treated with weight-restoring approaches initially and then switched to more traditional psychotherapeutic approaches. Such strong clinical consensus supports this approach that few outcome studies have compared one specific modality with another. Although the conventional wisdom is that behavioral approaches work for weight restoration and that more dynamically oriented therapies are effective in increasing patient insight and preventing relapse, this model does not have the empirical support that is often assumed. Although weight restoration is a necessary condition for recovery from anorexia nervosa, the need for psychotherapy in all cases has not been empirically established.

The use of psychopharmacological agents in the treatment of anorexia nervosa is questionable (Comerci, 1993). Many of the physiological effects of malnutrition resolve with refeeding and therefore should not be seen as symptoms indicating the need for pharmacological interventions. For example, refeeding often leads to decreases in obsessional thinking and depressive symptomatology. Antianxiety medications (i.e., anxiolytics) may be somewhat helpful for brief periods in helping the patient control the anxiety and panic felt toward eating (Wells & Logan, 1987). There is, however, little indication for the use of antidepressants or antipsychotics in patients with anorexia nervosa until they have achieved a healthy nutritional state (APA, 2000). There is some indication that opiate blockers (e.g., Naltrexone) may be helpful in the treatment of anorexia nervosa, as it has been shown that endogenous opiates are elevated in the underweight patient with anorexia nervosa (Kaye, Pickar, Naber, & Ebert, 1982). A feeling of euphoria that patients with anorexia nervosa may induce through starvation and excessive exercise can be blocked by these medications, rendering these behaviors less "reinforcing." Because starvation-induced delayed gastric emptying leads to feelings of fullness and bloating early in the refeeding process, medications that promote gastric emptying (e.g., Reglan) can be helpful in allowing the patient to eat without physical discomfort (Comerci, 1993). Multivitamins and minerals should also be routinely used.

Bulimia Nervosa

Unlike anorexia nervosa, most patients with bulimia nervosa do not have the health risks associated with malnutrition that demand close medical supervision and can therefore be successfully treated as outpatients (Fichter & Quadflieg, 1997). Hsu (1990) estimates that about 10% will need inpatient treatment, indicated when the patient shows advanced medical complications, is suicidal, or has not responded to outpatient treatment. Also, unlike anorexia nervosa, patients presenting for treatment of bulimia nervosa most often do so voluntarily and with the realization that they have a problem.

As discussed earlier, patients show both the habit pattern of binge/purge and various personality, cognitive, and psychopathological components of the disorder. Although some feel that underlying factors must be addressed first, the most common course of treatment is to address the abnormal eating patterns first. Hsu (1990) describes four goals of treatment, which include: (1) establishing a regular eating pattern designed to reduce or eliminate the binge/purge cycle; (2) changing the thoughts and belief patterns that drive the binge/purge cycle; (3) addressing medical complications and coexisting psychiatric disorders; and (4) preventing relapse. Nutrition education and straightforward behavioral strategies are used.

CBT is often used to address distorted thoughts and extreme concerns about eating, weight, and shape. Fairburn, Marcus, and Wilson (1993) provide the most detailed description of one such cognitive-behavioral treatment for bulimia nervosa. This treatment package is divided into three stages that last a total of 18 weeks and involve 19 appointments. The goal of the first stage, which lasts 4 weeks, is the restoration of normal eating patterns, reduction of purging, education about the health risks of bulimia, and the initiation of self-monitoring. During Stage 1, appointments may be scheduled more frequently than once per week. During Stage 2, appointments are held once per week, and treatment is more cognitively oriented. Emphasis is placed on identifying the circumstances that lead to binge eating, helping the patient cope with such circumstances, and reducing the frequency of their occurrence. The therapist assists the patient in identifying thoughts, beliefs, and values that serve to perpetuate the problem and helps the patient deal with body image distortions. In Stage 3, appointments occur every 2 weeks, and the goal becomes termination and relapse prevention.

Another form of treatment, exposure plus response prevention, is based on an anxiety reduction model of bulimia nervosa (Mizes & Lohr, 1983). Unlike the eating habit or cognitive model of bulimia, the anxiety reduction model focuses on purging as the maintaining cause of the disorder. After either bingeing or eating normally, anxiety about weight gain builds, and the purge process eliminates or reduces the anxiety. Anxiety reduction becomes conditioned to purging, and patients may binge just so they can experience the relief of purging. In this mode, the possibility of purging serves as a trigger to binge. Indeed, patients with bulimia nervosa report a reduction in feelings of anger, inadequacy, and lack of control after bingeing (Johnson & Larson, 1982) and increases in anxiety when asked to eat a large meal knowing they will not be allowed to vomit afterward (Leitenberg, Gross, Peterson, & McGrath, 1984). Treatment involves having patients eat an amount of food that would normally result in their feeling a need to purge. They are not allowed to vomit, and they experience increased anxiety. Ultimately, anxiety dissipates, and the patient is taught that it is not necessary to purge in order to control the anxiety. The concept is very similar to "flooding" or implosion techniques used in the treatment of phobias.

Reviews of treatment effectiveness studies suggest that both behavioral and cognitive-behavioral treatments can result in rather dramatic reductions in bingeing and vomiting. Rosen (1987) concluded that, on average, there was a 70% reduction in vomiting, with 44% of patients completely abstinent at the end of behavioral treatments. Others note abstinence from binge/purging behavior 7–10 years later (Herzog et al., 1999). Moreover, CBT has also been found to be effective in improving distorted attitudes about shape (Stice, 1999) and restrictive dieting (Fairburn et al., 1993; Wilson & Fairburn, 1998). However, Garner, Fairburn, and Davis (1987), although concluding that there is adequate evidence for the effectiveness of CBT, point out several concerns about the studies they reviewed. First, there was a great deal of variability in results, probably attributable to lack of detail in consistency in how treatment was done. Some studies have used clinic patients as participants, whereas others have recruited from the general population. The use of self-monitoring and self-report of binges and purges (i.e., vomiting) has its inherent validity concerns. In addition, follow-up periods have been relatively brief (Mitchell, Raymond, & Specker, 1993). In a controlled study, Jones, Peveler, Hope, and Fairburn (1993) compared CBT with behavioral therapy and interpersonal therapy. All three approaches produced immediate reductions in bingeing and purging, with the effect lasting 8 weeks for individuals in the behavioral and CBT conditions and only 4 weeks in the interpersonal therapy condition. All participants improved on measures of depression, self-esteem, and eating-disordered attitudes. The authors concluded that patients with bulimia nervosa are likely to show nonspecific treatment effects and that behavioral therapy and CBT may have an immediate influence over and above the nonspecific effects.

Pharmacological treatment has been more successful with bulimia nervosa than with anorexia nervosa, especially the use of antidepressants (Fichter, Krueger, Rief, Holland, & Dohne, 1996). Although the use of medication has been shown to reduce bingeing and purging, maintenance of change with antidepressants is low (Goldstein, Wilson, & Thompson, 1995).

After reviewing controlled studies on the treatment of bulimia nervosa, Mitchell et al. (1993) drew several conclusions. Outpatient treatment of bulimia can be successful, and both individual and group approaches seem to work. Antidepressants can be helpful, but their addition to cognitive-behavior therapies did not produce results superior to either treatment alone. The authors suggest that future research should investigate matching subject to treatment, isolating the effective components of multicomponent treatments, and utilizing longer follow-up programs.

SUMMARY

The treatment of eating disorders has changed significantly over the past 20 years. Specifically, there has been movement away from a psychodynamically based model to one based on a recognition that cognitive and behavioral factors are major contributors to these disorders. Because of the serious medical complications that can arise, the decrease in long-term treatment facilities and approaches, and the increase in the number of pediatric psychologists employing behavioral-cognitive approaches, treatment is now increasingly conducted in medical units with outpatient psychotherapy as needed. There is increasing evidence of genetic and physiological components to these disorders, and the next decade will, no doubt, bring major advances in medical and psychological treatments for these multifaceted and complex disorders. There is a major need for more effective prevention programs, which must be carefully crafted so as to promote healthy eating behaviors but not place undue emphasis on thinness or nutritional perfection, factors that often lead to the onset of either anorexia nervosa or bulimia nervosa.

REFERENCES

Agras, W. S. (1987). *Eating disorders: Management of obesity, bulimia and anorexia nervosa.* Oxford, UK: Pergamon Press.

American Psychiatric Association. (1994). Diagnostic and statistical manual of mental disorders (4th ed.). Washington, DC: Author.

American Psychiatric Association. (2000). Practice guidelines for the treatment of patients with eating disorders (Rev ed.). *American Journal of Psychiatry, 157,* 1–39.

Attie, I., & Brooks-Gunn, J. (1989). Development of eating problems in adolescent girls: A longitudinal study. *Developmental Psychology, 25,* 70–79.

Braun, D. L., Sunday, S. R., & Halmi, K. A. (1994). Psychiatric comorbidity of bulimia nervosa in patients: Relationship to clinical variables and treatment outcome. *European Psychiatry, 8,* 15–23.

Bulik, C. M., Sullivan, P. F., Wade, T. D., & Kendler, K. S. (2000). Twin studies of eating disorders: A review. *International Journal of Eating Disorders, 27,* 1–20.

Bunnell, D. W., Shenker, I. R., Nussbaum, M. P., Jacobson, M. S., & Cooper, P. (1990). Subclinical versus formal eating disorders: Differentiating psychological features. *International Journal of Eating Disorders, 9,* 357–362.

Channon, S., deSilva, P., Hensley, P., & Perkins, R. E. (1989). A controlled trial of cognitive-behavioural and behavioural treatment for anorexia nervosa. *Behavior Research and Therapy, 27,* 529–535.

Childress, A. C., Brewerton, T. D., Hodges, E. L., & Jarrell, M. P. (1993). The Kids' Eating Disorder Survey (KEDS): A study of middle school students. *Journal of the American Academy of Child and Adolescent Psychiatry, 32,* 843–850.

Comerci, G. D. (1993). Special problems in the adolescent: Eating disorders. In F. D. Burg, J. R. Inglefinger, & E. R. Ward (Eds.), *Gellis and Kagan's current pediatric therapy* (pp. 818–826). Philadelphia: Saunders.

Crisp, A. H., Palmer, R. L., & Kalucy, R. S. (1976). How common is anorexia nervosa?: A prevalence survey. *British Journal of Psychiatry, 128,* 549–554.

Crow, S. J., Keel, P. K., & Kendall, D. (1998). Eating disorders and insulin-dependent diabetes mellitus. *Psychosomatics, 39,* 233–243.

Danziger, Y., Carel, C. A., Tyano, S., & Mimouni, M. (1989). Is psychotherapy mandatory during the acute refeeding period in the treatment of anorexia nervosa? *Journal of Adolescent Health Care, 10,* 328–331.

deGroot, J., Kennedy, S., Rodin, G., & McVey, G. (1992). Correlates of sexual abuse in women with anorexia nervosa and bulimia nervosa. *Canadian Journal of Psychiatry, 37,* 516–518.

Dura, J. R., & Bornstein, R. A. (1989). Differences between IQ and school achievement in anorexia nervosa. *Journal of Clinical Psychology, 45,* 433–435.

Fairburn, C. G., & Beglin, S. J. (1994). Assessment of eating disorders: Interview or self-report questionnaire? *International Journal of Eating Disorders, 16,* 363–370.

Fairburn, C. G., & Cooper, Z. (1993). The Eating Disorders Examination (12th ed.). In C. G. Fairburn & G. T. Wilson (Eds.), *Binge eating: Nature, assessment and treatment* (pp. 317–360). New York: Guilford Press.

Fairburn, C. G., Marcus, M. D., & Wilson, G. T. (1993). Cognitive-behavioral therapy for binge eating and bulimia nervosa: A comprehensive treatment manual. In C. G. Fairburn & G. T. Wilson (Eds.), *Binge eating: Nature, assessment, and treatment* (pp. 361–404). New York: Guilford Press.

Fichter, M. M., Krueger, R., Rief, W., Holland, R., & Dohne, J. (1996). Fluvoxamine in prevention of relapse in bulimia nervosa: Effects on eating-specific psychopathology. *Journal of Clinical Psychopharmacology, 16,* 9–18.

Fichter, M. M., & Quadflieg, N. (1997). Six-year course of bulimia nervosa. *International Journal of Eating Disorders, 22,* 361–384

Folsom, V., Krahn, D., Nairn, K., Gold, L., Demitrack, M. A., & Silk, K. R. (1993). The impact of sexual and physical abuse on eating disordered and psychiatric symptoms: A comparison of eating disordered and psychiatric inpatients. *International Journal of Eating Disorders, 13,* 249–257.

Fox, C. (1997). Starved out. *Life, 20,* 78–88.

Garfinkel, P. E., Lin, E., Goering, P., Spegg, C., Goldbloom, D., Kennedy, S., et al. (1996). Should amenorrhea be necessary for the diagnosis of anorexia nervosa? *British Journal of Psychiatry, 168,* 500–506.

Garner, D. M. (1991). *The Eating Disorder Inventory—2: Professional Manual.* Odessa, FL: Psychological Assessment Resources.

Garner, D. M. (1993). Pathogenesis of anorexia nervosa. *Lancet, 341,* 1631–1640.

Garner, D. M., & Bemis, K. M. (1982). A cognitive-behavioral approach to anorexia nervosa. *Cognitive Therapy and Research, 6,* 123–150.

Garner, D. M., & Bemis, K. M. (1985). Cognitive therapy for anorexia nervosa. In D. M. Garner & P. E. Garfinkel (Eds.), *Handbook of psychotherapy for anorexia nervosa and bulimia* (pp. 107–146). New York: Guilford Press.

Garner, D. M., Fairburn, C. G., & Davis, R. (1987). Cognitive-behavioral treatment for bulimia nervosa. *Behavior Modification, 11,* 398–431.

Garner, D. M., & Garfinkel, P. E. (1985). *Handbook of psychotherapy for anorexia nervosa and bulimia.* New York: Guilford Press.

Garner, D. M., Olmstead, M. P., Bohr, Y., & Garfinkel, P. E. (1982). The eating attitudes test: Psychometric features and clinical correlates. *Psychological Medicine, 12,* 871–878.

Garner, D. M., Olmstead, M. P., & Polivy, J. (1983). Development and validation of a multidimensional eating disorder inventory for anorexia nervosa and bulimia. *International Journal of Eating Disorders, 2,* 15–34.

Goldstein, D. J., Wilson, M. G., & Thompson, V. L. (1995). Long-term fluoxetine treatment of bulimia nervosa. *British Journal of Psychiatry, 166,* 660–666.

Gowers, S. C., Crisp, A. H., Joughin, N., & Bhat, A. (1991). Premenarchial anorexia nervosa. *Journal of Child Psychology and Psychiatry, 32,* 515–524.

Hall, A. (1985). Group psychotherapy for anorexia nervosa. In D. M. Garner & P. E. Garfinkel (Eds.), *Handbook of psychotherapy for anorexia nervosa and bulimia* (pp. 213–239). New York: Guilford Press.

Halmi, K. A. (1985). Behavioral management for anorexia nervosa. In D. M. Garner & P. E. Garfinkel (Eds.) *Handbook of psychotherapy for anorexia nervosa and bulimia* (pp. 147–159). New York: Guilford Press.

Halmi, K. A., Casper, R., Eckert, E. D., Goldberg, S. C., & Davis, J. M. (1979). Unique features associated with the age of onset of anorexia nervosa. *Psychiatric Research, 1,* 209–215.

Halmi, K. A., Eckert, E., Marchi, P., Sampagnaro, V., Apple, R., & Cohen, J. (1991). Comorbidity of psychiatric diagnoses in anorexia nervosa. *Archives of General Psychiatry, 48,* 712–718.

Halmi, K. A., Sunday, S. R., Strober, M., Kaplan, A., Woodside, D. B., Fichter, M., et al. (2000). Perfectionism in anorexia nervosa: Variation by clinical subtype, obsessionality, and pathological eating behavior. *American Journal of Psychiatry, 157,* 1799–1805.

Herzog, D. B., Dorer, D. J., Keel, P. K., Selwyn, S. E., Ekeblad, E. R., Flores, A. T., et al. (1999). Recovery and relapse in anorexia and bulimia nervosa: A 7.5–year follow-up study. *Journal of the American Academy of Child and Adolescent Psychiatry, 38,* 829–837.

Herzog, D. B., Keller, M. B., Sacks, N. R., Yeh, C. J., & Lavori, P. W. (1992). Psychiatric comorbidity in treatment-seeking anorexics and bulimics. *Journal of the American Academy of Child and Adolescent Psychiatry, 31,* 810–818.

Hoek, H. W. (1993). Review of the epidemiological studies of eating disorders. *International Review of Psychiatry, 5,* 61–74.

Holland, A. J., Sicotte, N., & Treasure, J. (1988). Anorexia nervosa: Evidence for a genetic basis. *Journal of Psychosomatic Research, 32,* 561–571.

Hsu, L. K. G. (1990). *Eating disorders.* New York: Guilford Press.

Hudson, J. I., Weiss, R. D., Pope, H. G., & Harrison, G. (1992). Eating disorders in hospitalized substance abusers. *American Journal of Drug and Alcohol Abuse, 18,* 75–85.

Johnson, C., & Conners, M. E. (1987). *The etiology and treatment of bulimia nervosa.* New York: Basic Books.

Johnson, C., & Larson, R. (1982). Bulimia: An analysis of moods and behavior. *Psychosomatic Medicine, 44,* 341–351.

Jones, R., Peveler, R. C., Hope, R. A., & Fairburn, C. G. (1993). Changes during treatment for bulimia nervosa: A comparison of three psychological treatments. *Behaviour Research and Therapy, 31,* 479–486.

Kaye, W. H., Pickar, D., Naber, D., & Ebert, M. N. (1982). Cerebrospinal fluid opiod activity in anorexia nervosa. *American Journal of Psychiatry, 139,* 643–645.

Keel, P. K., Fulkerson, J. A., & Leon, G. R. (1997). Disordered eating precursors in pre- and early adolescent girls. *Journal of Youth and Adolescence, 26,* 203–216.

Keel, P. K., & Mitchell, J. E. (1997). Outcome in bulimia nervosa. *American Journal of Psychiatry, 154,* 313–321.

Keel, P. K., Mitchell, J. E., Davis, T. L., & Crow, S. J. (2001). Relationship between depression and body dissatisfaction in women diagnosed with bulimia nervosa. *International Journal of Eating Disorders, 30,* 48–56.

Kennedy, S. H., McVey, G., & Katz, R. (1990). Personality disorders in anorexia nervosa and bulimia nervosa. *Journal of Psychiatric Research, 24,* 259–269.

La Greca, A. M., Schwarz, L. T., & Satin, W. (1987). Eating patterns in young women with IDDM: Another look. *Diabetes Care, 10,* 59–66.

Lask, B., & Bryant-Waugh, R. (1992). Early-onset anorexia nervosa and related eating disorders. *Journal of Child Psychology and Psychiatry, 33,* 281–300.

Ledoux, S., Choquet, M., & Flament, M. (1991). Eating disorders among adolescents in an unselected French population. *International Journal of Eating Disorders, 10,* 81–89.

Leitenberg, H., Gross, J., Peterson, J., & McGrath, P. (1984). Analysis of an anxiety model and the process of change during exposure plus response prevention treatment of bulimia nervosa. *Behavior Therapy, 15,* 3–20.

Lilenfeld, L., Kaye, W., Greeno, C., Merikangas, K. R., Plotnicov, K. H., Pollice, C., et al. (1997). Psychiatric disorders in women with bulimia nervosa and their first-degree relatives: Effects of comorbid substance dependence. *International Journal of Eating Disorders, 22,* 253–264.

Linscheid, T. R. (1994). Anorexia nervosa: Psychological issues. In R. A. Olson, L. L. Mullins, J. B. Gillman, & J. M. Chaney (Eds.), *The sourcebook of pediatric psychology* (pp. 322–345). Boston: Allyn & Bacon.

Linscheid, T. R., Tarnowski, K. J., & Richmond, D. A. (1988). Behavioral approaches to anorexia nervosa, bulimia and obesity. In D. K. Routh (Ed.), *Handbook of pediatric psychology* (pp. 332–362), New York: Guilford Press.

Maher, M. S. (1980). Group psychotherapy for anorexia nervosa. In P. S. Powers & R. C. Fernandez (Eds.), *Current treatment for anorexia nervosa and bulimia* (pp. 265–276). Basel, Switzerland: Karger.

Maloney, M. J., McGuire, J., & Daniels, S. R. (1988). Reliability testing of a children's version of the Eating Attitudes Test. *Journal of the American Academy of Child and Adolescent Psychiatry, 27,* 541–543.

Maloney, M. J., McGuire, J., Daniels, S. R., & Specker, B. (1989). Dieting behavior and eating attitudes in children. *Pediatrics, 84,* 482–489.

Mazure, C. M., Halmi, K. A., Sunday, S. R., Romano, S. J., & Einhorn, A. N. (1994). Yale–Brown–Cornell Eating Disorder Scale: Development, use, reliability and validity. *Journal of Psychiatric Research, 28,* 425–445.

Mills, I. H., & Medlicott, L. (1992). Anorexia nervosa as a compulsive behaviour disease. *Quarterly Journal of Medicine, 83,* 507–522.

Minuchin, S., Rossman, B. L., & Baker, L. (1978). *Psychosomatic families: Anorexia nervosa in context.* Cambridge, MA: Harvard University Press.

Mitchell, J. E., Raymond, N., & Specker, S. (1993). A review of the controlled trials of pharmacotherapy and psychotherapy in the treatment of bulimia nervosa. *International Journal of Eating Disorders, 14,* 229–247.

Mizes, J. S., & Lohr, J. M. (1983). The treatment of bulimia (binge-eating and self-induced vomiting): A quasi-experimental investigation of the effects of stimulus narrowing, self-reinforcement and self-control relaxation. *International Journal of Eating Disorders, 2,* 59–65.

Moreno, J. K., Selby, M. J., Aved, K., & Besse, C. (2000). Differences in family dynamics among anorexic, bulimic, obese and normal women. *Journal of Psychotherapy in Independent Practice, 1,* 75–87.

Nattiv, A., Agostini, R., Drinkwater, B., & Yeager, K. K. (1994). The female athlete triad: The inter-relatedness of disordered eating, amenorrhea, and osteoporosis. *Clinical Sports Medicine, 13,* 405–418.

Pope, H. G., Hudson, J. I., Yurgelun-Todd, D., & Hudson, M. S. (1984). Prevalence of anorexia nervosa and bulimia in three student populations. *International Journal of Eating Disorders, 3,* 45–51.

Powers, P. S., & Johnson, C. (1997). Small victories: Prevention of eating disorders among athletes. *Eating Disorders: Journal of Treatment and Prevention, 4,* 364–377.

Rogers, R. L., & Petrie, T. A. (2001). Psychological correlates of anorexia and bulimic symptomatology. *Journal of Counseling and Development, 79,* 178–187.

Rosen, J. C. (1987). A review of behavioral treatments for bulimia nervosa. *Behavior Modification, 11,* 464–486.

Shisslak, C. M., McKeon, R. T., & Crago, M. (1990). Family dysfunction in normal weight bulimic and bulimia nervosa families. *Journal of Clinical Psychology, 46,* 185–189.

Shisslak, C. M., Pazda, S. L., & Crago, M. (1990). Body weight and bulimia as discriminators of psychological characteristics among anorexic, bulimic, and obese women. *Journal of Abnormal Psychology, 99,* 380–384.

Silverstone, P. H. (1990). Low self-esteem in eating disordered patients in the absence of depression. *Psychological Reports, 67,* 276–278.

Soukup, V. M., Beiler, M. E., & Terrell, F. (1990). Stress, coping style, and problem solving ability among eating disordered patients. *Journal of Clinical Psychology, 46,* 592–599.

Stancin, T., Link, D. L., & Reuter, J. M. (1989). Binge eating and purging in young women with IDDM. *Diabetes Care, 12,* 601–603.

Steiger, H., Liquornik, K., Chapman, J., & Hussain, N. (1991). Personality and family disturbances in eating-disordered patients: Comparison of "restricters" and "bingers" to normal controls. *International Journal of Eating Disorders, 10,* 501–512.

Stice, E. (1999). Clinical implications of psychosocial research on bulimia nervosa and binge-eating disorder. *Journal of Clinical Psychology, 55,* 675–683.

Stice, E., Mazotti, L., Krebs, M., & Martin, S. (1998). *Predictors of adolescent dieting behaviors: A longitudinal study. Psychology of Addictive Behaviors, 12,* 195–205.

Strober, M., Lampert, C., Morrell, W., Burroughs, J., & Jacobs, C. (1990). A controlled family study of anorexia nervosa. *International Journal of Eating Disorders, 9,* 239–253.

U.S. Department of Health and Human Services. (1983). *Facts about anorexia nervosa.* Washington, DC: U.S. Government Printing Office.

Vize, C., & Cooper, P. (1995). Sexual abuse in patients with eating disorders, patients with depression and normal controls: A comparative study. *British Journal of Psychiatry, 167,* 80–85.

Wade, T., Bulik, C., Neale, M., & Kendler, K. (2000). Anorexia nervosa and major depression: Shared genetic and environmental risk factors. *American Journal of Psychiatry, 157,* 469–471.

Wells, L. A., & Logan, K. M. (1987). Pharmocologic treatment of eating disorders: A review of selected literature and recommendations. *Psychosomatics, 28,* 470–479.

Wilson, G. T., & Fairburn, C. G. (1998). Treatments for eating disorders. In P. E. Nathan, & J. M. Gorman (Eds.), *A guide to treatments that work* (pp. 501–530). New York: Oxford University Press.

Wonderlich, S. A., Brewerton, T. D., Jocic, Z., Dansky, B. S., & Abbott, D. W. (1997). Relationship of childhood sexual abuse and eating disorders. *Journal of the American Academy of Child and Adolescent Psychiatry, 36,* 1107–1115.

38

Child Maltreatment

BARBARA L. BONNER
MARY BETH LOGUE
MICHELLE KEES

Child maltreatment is now recognized as a major psychological, medical, and social problem by professionals and the general public in the United States and throughout the world. Over the past 15 years, several major events have occurred that have positively affected the interventions of psychologists and other professionals on behalf of maltreated children. Several of these have had a direct impact on psychologists and other mental health professionals who are providing services to abused children and their families. These include: (1) the establishment of two important professional organizations, the Section on Child Maltreatment by Division 37 of the American Psychological Association and the American Professional Society on the Abuse of Children (APSAC; *www.APSAC.org*), an interdisciplinary professional society; (2) the use of multidisciplinary teams and children's advocacy centers to improve the investigation, prosecution, and case management of child abuse cases; (3) an increase in research, with several hundred articles being published annually since 1990; (4) an increased focus on the prevention of child maltreatment at the local, state, and national levels; and (5) the establishment of child death review boards to review cases of suspected abuse and neglect (in many states all child deaths) and to make recommendations to improve the systems investigating child deaths.

Child abuse was initially brought to the attention of the medical profession in 1962 through the publication of an article describing "the battered child syndrome" by Henry Kempe and his colleagues (Kempe, Silverman, Steele, Droegemuller, & Silver, 1962). Since that time, the fields of medicine, law, psychology, social work, and law enforcement have expanded their knowledge and focus on the identification, protection, prosecution, and prevention of child maltreatment. This increased focus has resulted in a higher number of reported and confirmed cases of abuse and neglect across the United States.

SCOPE OF THE PROBLEM

The actual incidence and prevalence of child maltreatment is difficult to state accurately for a number of reasons. There is a lack of standard definitions of maltreatment applied across professions and across state, federal, and tribal laws. Maltreatment can be defined differently depending on the purpose of the definition (e.g., for investigation vs. treatment vs. research). Professionals from law enforcement, medicine, law, psychology, and social services may also have different interpretations of which acts constitute abuse and neglect because of differences in their professional training or roles. These differences in definitions can dramatically affect substantiated rates of maltreatment.

Furthermore, methods and standards of collecting data vary considerably. In 1993, the National Research Council reviewed the data-gathering process and made numerous recommendations to improve the methodology and reduce the disparity in the epidemiological reports from the states. However, few changes have been made at the state or national levels to standardize the data-gathering process. Reporting or referral bias may also skew the rates of maltreatment in certain ethnic and socioeconomic groups. For example, African American children and children living in poverty are more often reported and found to be maltreated than are children from other ethnic and economic groups (U.S. Department of Health and Human Services [USDHHS], 2002). Whether this is an artifact of bias in reporting or referral or an actual subpopulation-based variance in rates is unknown at this time.

Thus it is with the foregoing caveats that the following data are presented. In the most recent national data from 2000, almost 3 million reports of suspected abuse were received by state child protective service (CPS) agencies, 62% of which were referred for investigation or assessment (USDHHS, 2002). As in previous years, about 32% of the investigated cases resulted in a finding of indicated or substantiated maltreatment. The national rate of child maltreatment in 2000 was 12.2 per 1,000 children under age 18 in the U.S. population (USDHHS, 2002). The highest rate of maltreatment was 15.3 child victims per 1,000 in 1993, and the rate has continued to drop since that time.

The officially documented percentages of physical abuse, sexual abuse, and neglect have remained relatively consistent over the past 10 years. In 2000, approximately 63% of the cases involved neglect, 20% physical abuse, 10% sexual abuse, and 7% psychological maltreatment (USDHHS, 2002). An additional 17% were associated with "other types" of maltreatment. These percentages total greater than 100 because children, may be classified as the recipient of more than one type of abuse. The highest rate of victimization was for children 0–3 (15.7 per 1,000 children), and the rates declined as the age increased (USDHHS, 2002). Boys and girls were equally vulnerable to physical abuse and neglect, but girls were sexually abused at a rate 4 times that of boys (1.7 vs. 0.4 per 1,000). African American children were at the highest risk for abuse, with a rate of 24.7 per 1,000 children.

Despite the fact that neglect has consistently been the most prevalent type of child maltreatment, it has received the least attention by professionals, the media, and the general public. Child sexual abuse has clearly dominated the field in research, treatment interventions, and prevention programs since the mid-1980s. The rates of child sexual abuse have shown the greatest fluctuation over the past 10 to 15 years. The substantiated cases of child sexual abuse decreased by nearly one-third, from a peak of 149,800 cases in 1992 to 103,600 cases in 1998 (Jones & Finkelhor, 2001). Several possible reasons for the decline are suggested, including an actual decline in the rates of child sexual abuse; a decline in the reporting of suspected sexual abuse; and changes in attitudes, standards, and policies for confirmation in these cases (Jones & Finkelhor, 2001).

TYPES OF CHILD ABUSE

Physical Abuse

A 16-year-old girl with no previous psychiatric history presented to the emergency room following an overdose of aspirin. A consultation was requested to assess suicidality and her affective state. In the psychologist's assessment, the girl continued to express suicidal ideation and was unable to contract for safety. She was admitted to an inpatient psychiatric unit. During the course of admission, the girl disclosed that her stepfather had hit her repeatedly on her bare buttocks as discipline for a curfew violation. A physical exam showed multiple bruises and infected welts on her buttocks in varying stages of healing, suggesting that the beatings occurred across an extended time span. The girl's depressed mood and suicidality appeared to be directly related to the history of physical abuse and her fear of future abuse.

Physical abuse is generally defined as an act of commission by a parent or caretaker involving beatings, excessive discipline, or some other form of physical violence that results in fractures, bruises, burns, lacerations, or internal injuries (National Center on Child Abuse and Neglect, 1981). Children of all ages, including adolescents, are physically abused, with children under age 5 being at highest risk for serious injury and death due to physical abuse. Boys are more likely to be the victims of physical abuse and specifically more likely to be severely abused.

The effects of physical abuse on children can vary by the level of severity and intensity of the abuse and by the child's age and developmental stage. The effects can include medical and health problems, difficulties in academic performance, cognitive/perceptual and attributional problems, aggressive and other behavior disorders, internalizing problems, posttraumatic stress disorder (PTSD), and interpersonal and relationship problems (Kolko, 2002). Several well-designed longitudinal studies have documented the long-term effects of physical abuse. One study found that physically abused children had twice the risk for being arrested for a violent crime than well-matched controls (Widom, 1989). Another study showed, over a 17-year follow-up period, that, when compared with nonabused cases, physically abused children were significantly more impaired in adolescence and young adulthood, having more symptoms of anxiety and depression, emotional and behavioral problems, and suicidal ideation and attempts (Silverman, Reinherz, & Giaconia, 1996).

Munchausen by proxy syndrome (MBPS, or factitious disorder by proxy) is a specific and rare type of maltreatment that may be particularly relevant to pediatric psychology practice, as it is described in the DSM-IV-TR (American Psychiatric Association, 2000). This form of maltreatment is most often classified as physical abuse because it involves a caregiver, usually the mother, manufacturing, inducing, or simulating symptoms in the child (e.g., feeding toxic substances to induce vomiting or nausea; inducing seizures by suffocation) and then bringing the child for medical treatment (Parnell, 2002). However, it is not unusual for MBPS to co-occur with other forms of maltreatment, such as neglect or psychological maltreatment, and to continue for months or years before it is detected. MBPS is now recognized as an unusual form of abuse that can be detected conclusively only by observing the event surreptitiously (Ware, Orr, & Bond, 2001).

Sexual Abuse

A 7-year-old girl presented to a general pediatric clinic with a severely impacted bowel. She had been seen the year before with the same problem, at which time the problem was viewed as a medical issue (i.e., her bowel was cleaned out, she was given a diet with increased fiber, and appropriate medications were prescribed). With the recurrence of the problem, the girl was hospitalized, as anesthesia was necessary to evacuate the bowel, and a pediatric psychologist was asked to evaluate the girl and her family. In the initial interview with the girl, she revealed that she had difficulty using the toilet at home because her father had drilled holes in the bathroom door and peeked in at her when she attempted to use the toilet. The hospital social services department and law enforcement were notified, and within a week of the girl's disclosure, it was established that the father had also been having sexual intercourse with the girl's two teenage sisters for several years.

Child sexual abuse is broadly defined as any sexual activity with a child in which consent cannot be or is not given (Berliner, 2000). The definition includes touching and fondling, kissing of the genital areas, and digital or penile penetration of the mouth, vagina, or anus, as well as noncontact abuse, such as voyeurism and exhibitionism. It further includes sexual contact by actual force or threat of force, regardless of the ages of the participants, and all sexual activity between a child and an adult, regardless of physical contact (Berliner & Elliott, 2002). The definition often takes several factors into account, including the age of the child (17 to 18 or younger); the relationship of the child to the perpetrator (intrafamilial vs. extrafamilial); the difference in age, developmental level, or power status between the child and the offender; and the type of abuse (i.e. physical contact with the child vs. no contact; Wyatt & Peters, 1986).

Children of all ages, including young infants, are sexually abused. Girls are approximately 3 to 4 times more likely to be abused than boys, and disproportionate numbers of sexually abused children are reported from low-income families (Sedlak & Broadhurst, 1996). A wide array of symptoms has been documented in children and adolescents who have experienced sexual abuse, ranging from minimal symptoms to significant levels of disturbance. In general, symptoms in sexually abused children have been found to be more severe than in nonabused children but less severe than the symptoms of other child outpatient mental health populations (Cosentino & Collins, 1996; Kilpatrick & Saunders, 1999). One study documented that up to 49% of sexually abused children appeared to have none of the expected abuse-related problems (Kendall-Tackett, Williams, & Finkelhor, 1993).

The most frequently reported symptoms in sexually abused children include fearfulness of abuse stimuli and other symptoms of PTSD, inappropriate sexual behavior, nightmares and sleep disorders, depression, repressed anger and hostility, behavior problems, and somatic complaints (Berliner & Elliott, 2002; Conte & Schuerman, 1988). It should be noted, however, that inappropriate or aggressive sexual behavior should not be used as a definitive indicator of a history of sexual abuse, because studies have documented highly inappropriate and aggressive sexual behavior in children with no known history of sexual abuse (Bonner, Walker, & Berliner, 1999). In addition, all of these symptoms can appear in children and adolescents who have not been sexually abused.

It is not possible to list a set of symptoms that are exclusively associated with child sexual abuse. However, based on the presentations of children, clinicians should consider that a child might have experienced sexual abuse when he or she presents the following symptoms. In preschool and school-age children, one would be concerned if a child had symptoms of PTSD with no known antecedent event, high levels of anxiety or restlessness, sleep disorders, aggressive behavior, depression, or inappropriate sexual behavior or knowledge. In adolescents, the symptoms can include low self-esteem, depression, suicidal ideation or behavior, eating disorders, problems at school, substance abuse, and conflicts with authority figures (Hecht, Chaffin, Bonner, Worley, & Lawson, 2002). Generally, symptoms in adolescents are more closely related to those seen in adult survivors of childhood sexual abuse (for a recent review of child sexual abuse, see Berliner & Elliott, 2002).

Neglect

> Two boys, ages 7 and 14 years old, presented to the sleep disorders clinic with their mother for evaluation of sleep apnea. Both boys were morbidly obese, as was their mother. The boys were referred to a nutrition clinic to address the obesity and put on a regimen to treat the sleep disorder. The family failed to keep multiple appointments, and the older brother was brought to the emergency department on two occasions when he had stopped breathing. Both boys continued to show weight gain and had missed many days of school. The psychologist in the sleep disorders clinic contacted child protective services and made a report of suspected medical and educational neglect.

Although neglect accounts for the majority of maltreatment cases referred to CPS, researchers and clinicians have paid significantly less attention to neglect than to physical and sexual abuse (Cantwell, 1977). In 2000, almost 63% of substantiated maltreatment cases involved child neglect (USDHHS, 2002). Infants and toddlers made up the most at-risk developmental group, with a significant decline in neglect cases as children entered their teen years (USDHHS, 2002). Equally concerning are the very high rates of recurrence for child neglect. In comparison with children who experienced physical abuse, children who were neglected were 27% more likely to experience recurrence (USDHHS, 2002).

Neglect differs from other forms of child maltreatment in that it typically represents a chronic omission on the part of the caregiver rather than an identifiable act, such as a blow to the head. Neglect also differs from physical and sexual abuse in that it is often an ongoing and enduring pattern rather than an episodic event (Bonner, Logue, Kaufman, & Niec, 2001). Despite the pervasiveness of neglect, identification is frequently missed, because physical evidence is rare unless neglect is severe enough to lead to medical problems, as in cases of failure to thrive or an exacerbation of a chronic illness such as asthma or cystic fibrosis.

Neglect is defined as a caregiver's failure to provide for a child's basic needs, which can lead to potential or actual harm to the child (Garbarino & Collins, 1999). The basic needs of children generally include adequate shelter, food, clothing, hygiene, medical care, educational opportunity, protection, affection, and supervision. The various subtypes of neglect include physical, medical, educational, and emotional (a subtype of psychological maltreatment, discussed in a later section), as follows:

- *Physical neglect.* A caregiver's failure to provide for a child's basic physical needs, such as adequate housing, safety, nutrition, hygiene, supervision, and clothing, as well as exposure to domestic violence, prenatal substance use, or exposure to substance use.
- *Medical neglect.* A caregiver's failure to provide necessary medical treatment or a delay in seeking health care, including mental health care; this can also include noncompliance with medical recommendations, medication regimens, or required immunizations or even refusal of medical treatment for religious reasons (e.g., Jehovah's Witnesses refusing blood transfusions).

- *Educational neglect.* A caregiver's failure to comply with state statutes on educational attendance for their children, including not enrolling children in school, excessive truancy, or failure to address a child's special education needs.

Research focusing exclusively on neglected children suggests that neglect has more severe, long-lasting developmental consequences than either physical or sexual abuse (Gaudin, 1999). For example, studies with neglected infants show significant neurological and brain development changes, including reduced brain wave activity (Dawson, Klinger, & Panagiotides, 1997) and enlarged ventricles due to limited brain growth (Perry, 1997). Neglected children exhibit higher rates of behavior problems (Williamson, Borduin, & Howe, 1991), fewer social interactions (Bousha & Twentyman, 1984), poor peer and teacher relationships (Rohrbeck & Twentyman 1986), and more academic problems (Kendall-Tackett & Eckenrode, 1996). Longitudinal research has documented the long-term negative effects of neglect. Egeland and Erickson (1987) found that neglected children were more likely to experience learning problems, peer difficulties, and social rejection over the course of their lifetimes.

Psychological Maltreatment

A 7-year-old boy was referred to the neurology clinic for evaluation of recurrent headaches, staring spells, and depressed affect lasting about 1 year. Other than some notable gross and fine motor delays, the neurological and physical exams were normal, and no biological cause for the symptoms could be identified. A clinical interview revealed that the child was depressed about having been forced by his parents to participate in soccer since the age of 5. The patient described himself as "the worst kid on the team." He reported that the other children made fun of him, and he often was in tears at soccer practice. During the assessment, the boy was tearful and anxious when he described his father's method of coaching to help improve his physical skills: early morning and late afternoon practice sessions, in addition to daily team practice; a strict regimen of calisthenics, during which the father yelled at him; restriction of social activities to only soccer practice; and belittling him at practice and in games when he made errors. His mother reported that the other children in the family, both members of their school's varsity soccer teams, were also encouraged to join in the father's coaching of the patient.

Psychological maltreatment has been viewed as the "embedded psychological context behind other forms of abuse and neglect" (Hart, Brassard, Binggeli, & Davidson, 2002, p. 79). It is generally defined as a repeated pattern or extreme instances by a parent or caretaker that express to a child or adolescent that he or she is worthless, unloved, unwanted, endangered, or of value only in meeting someone else's needs (American Professional Society on the Abuse of Children, 1995 [APSAC]; Brassard, Hart, & Hardy, 1991). Psychological maltreatment involves acts of omission and commission by a caregiver and yields effects on a continuum from mild to very severe. Whether or not a caregiver's behavior constitutes psychological maltreatment or results in identifiable harm to a child is difficult to demonstrate empirically or legally.

The most commonly defined subtypes of psychological maltreatment include spurning, terrorizing, exploiting/corrupting, isolating, denying emotional responsiveness, and unwarranted denial of mental health care, medical care, or education (APSAC, 1995; Brassard & Hardy, 1997; Hart et al., 2002):

- *Spurning*. Verbal or nonverbal behaviors that reject and degrade a child, such as belittling, shaming, ridiculing, humiliating in public, or singling out one child to criticize or punish.
- *Terrorizing*. Threatening to harm the child, their loved ones, or their possessions or potentially harmful behaviors that put a child in an unpredictable, chaotic, or dangerous situation.
- *Exploiting/corrupting*. Encouraging the child to engage in inappropriate behaviors through modeling, permitting, or encouraging antisocial behaviors, such as prostitution, pornography, substance use, and shoplifting.
- *Isolating*. Excessive confinement or unreasonable limits on freedom or socialization.
- *Denying emotional responsiveness*. Parental ignoring, uninvolvement, or withdrawal from the child; a lack of appropriate expressions of affection, caring, or love.
- *Unwarranted denial of mental health care, medical care, or education*.

Prevalence rates of psychological maltreatment are difficult to determine because it can occur alone or in conjunction with other forms of abuse or neglect. In 2000, approximately 8% of substantiated child maltreatment cases exclusively involved psychological maltreatment (USDHHS, 2002). This figure does not include psychological maltreatment that occurs with other forms of maltreatment and is likely an underestimate of the prevalence (Hart et al., 2002). Additionally, because psychological maltreatment rarely shows physical evidence and is oftentimes difficult to prove, it is likely to be the least reported and prosecuted form of child maltreatment. Little is known about the specific effects of each of the subtypes of psychological maltreatment or about the comorbid overlap of the subtypes with one another (i.e., a child is spurned and terrorized). It is believed, however, that the psychological unavailability of the parent (i.e., denying emotional responsiveness) may be the most damaging to children (Egeland & Erickson, 1987).

Research examining the effects of psychological maltreatment on children and adolescents has found a wide range of negative outcomes, including poor peer relationships (Brassard, Hart & Hardy, 1991; Claussen & Crittenden, 1991), higher rates of peer aggression (Erickson, Egeland, & Pianta, 1989), and more academic difficulties (Erickson & Egeland, 1987). In cases of multiple forms of abuse, the presence and severity of psychological maltreatment may represent one of the most significant causes of problematic adjustment (Claussen & Crittenden, 1991; Hart et al., 2002).

ASSESSMENT AND TREATMENT

The clinical assessment and treatment aspects of child maltreatment should be kept separate from the forensic aspects (i.e., reporting and investigating allegations of abuse). The clinical approach to child maltreatment should follow a developmental psychopathology model (Friedrich, 2002), taking into consideration the child's developmental functioning and abilities. The goal of the clinical assessment is to determine the child's and caregivers' overall functioning, adaptation, and level of symptomatology. As a first step, a thorough assessment of the family's strengths and problems should be conducted, including the types of problems that need to be addressed at the parental, child, family, and social systems levels (Kolko, 2002). Assessments may include interviews, paper-and-pencil measures, or structured observations with the child, siblings, and caregivers. In addition to the standard measures to assess cognitive functioning and general behavior (e.g., Wechsler Intelligence Scale for

Children—IV, Behavior Assessment System for Children, Child Depression Inventory, Minnesota Multiphasic Personality Inventory—Adolescent), several specific measures have been developed and standardized that can be used to evaluate the child's symptoms associated with the abuse. These measures include general assessments of trauma symptoms, such as the Trauma Symptom Checklist for Children (TSC-C; Briere, 1996), and a measurement of sexual behavior problems, such as the Child Sexual Behavior Inventory (CSBI-II; Friedrich, 1997). To assess psychological maltreatment, the Psychological Maltreatment Rating Scales (Brassard, Hart, & Hardy, 1993) provide an observational structure to evaluate mother–child interactions. (For a complete review of assessment, see Bonner et al., 2001).

Various treatment approaches for abused children and adolescents have been developed, and empirical evaluations of treatment interventions are increasing. Treatment interventions for abused children have been conducted in therapeutic nurseries, day treatment centers, psychiatric or residential settings, and outpatient clinics. Clinicians should rely on techniques and approaches that are appropriate for the child's cognitive and developmental level of functioning and that have documented effectiveness in reducing the child's targeted symptoms. Reviews of the current treatment outcome literature indicate that abuse-specific cognitive-behavioral therapy (CBT) is effective in reducing symptoms of PTSD (Cohen, Berliner, & Mannarino, 2000). The treatment components include anxiety management techniques, exposure, psychoeducation, and cognitive therapy. Treatment for families in which physical abuse has occurred has typically focused on the abusive parents and has only more recently addressed the symptoms in the child victims (see Azar & Wolfe, 1998; Oates & Bross, 1995; Wolfe, 1999). For some forms of neglect, research has shown promising results for interventions that include home visitation as a primary approach (see Lutzker, 1990; Lutzker, Bigelow, Doctor, Gershater, & Greene, 1998; Olds et al., 1997).

CURRENT TRENDS IN RESPONDING TO CHILD MALTREATMENT

Multidisciplinary Teams

A major development in the field of child maltreatment occurred in the mid-1980s with the establishment of children's advocacy centers (CAC), staffed by personnel from CPS, law enforcement, medicine, mental health, and the legal system. The centers were developed primarily in response to cases of child sexual abuse to streamline and more comprehensively address child maltreatment. CACs are community- or hospital-based in child-friendly settings in which the child can be interviewed, medically examined, and triaged or treated for mental health problems, thereby reducing the number of places and times a child is interviewed. There are currently 234 centers operating nationally, and the National Children's Alliance (*www.nnac.org*) has been organized to set criteria for team structure and provide ongoing training and technical support. A study conducted in California (California Attorney General's Office, 1994) has documented the effectiveness of the centers in reducing the number of child interviews. Pediatric psychologists may serve as members of these multidisciplinary teams, particularly when the advocacy center is located in a hospital.

Pediatric Psychology and Child Maltreatment

The role of the pediatric psychologist in child maltreatment is varied and multifocal. Pediatric psychologists may be involved in identifying, reporting, treating, or collaborating with other professionals in addressing cases of child maltreatment. Child maltreatment is a complex problem, made more so by problems in definition, by the different roles of the professionals involved, and by the involvement of the legal system. The combination of these elements creates highly complex situations for pediatric psychologists and other professionals who work to protect children.

Pediatric psychologists work in several settings in which child maltreatment may be an issue. Both in inpatient medical hospital settings and outpatient clinics, there is a high likelihood of seeing children who have been maltreated. In some cases, the psychologist may be the first to suspect or identify maltreatment and will then be responsible for reporting the suspected abuse. Psychologists may serve on multidisciplinary review teams and provide consultation on evaluating and planning the disposition of cases of suspected maltreatment. They may also be involved in the treatment of abused or neglected children who present to the hospital or clinic. Furthermore, it is the experience of one of us (MBL) that the members of the hospital treatment team frequently consult the psychologist seeking some understanding or rationale for the caregiver's behavior.

Reporting

The immediate issues for pediatric psychologists in medical settings are to report suspected abuse and ascertain the child's safety. All 50 states have mandatory child abuse and neglect reporting laws; however, individual states vary in the implementation of these laws. All states require certain individuals to report suspected child abuse, and psychologists are more often than not included in this mandate. State requirements vary about what must be reported: Some require reporting when there is merely a suspicion of maltreatment; others require a higher degree of knowledge or certainty that maltreatment has occurred. Failure to report suspected child abuse can result in civil or criminal liability, typically a misdemeanor punishable by a fine. In most states, a person who reports suspected maltreatment in good faith is immune from criminal and civil liability, even if the maltreatment is not substantiated. Some states also have statutes that allow the prosecution of individuals who purposefully make false allegations of child maltreatment. (See Zellman & Fair, 2002, for a recent review.) In addition, professional organizations (e.g., American Psychological Association, state psychological associations) have ethical standards and practices that require reporting suspected child maltreatment.

In cases in which a pediatric psychologist is the first professional to suspect or identify maltreatment, it is rarely his or her role to investigate or assess the validity of the allegations. This function is the role of child protective service (CPS) or law enforcement professionals who are trained and responsible for conducting an investigation and determining whether a child should be removed from the home. In many hospitals, the social services department has trained personnel who conduct forensic interviews with suspected victims and who work closely with CPS and law enforcement. If a pediatric psychologist suspects child maltreatment, it is essential to obtain accurate, complete documentation of the allegations and the circumstances of the disclosure of suspicious events and to document the course of action taken by the psychologist, including contacts with CPS, other professionals, or other agencies. This attention to detail can be useful in reporting and in the investigation of the allegations, as well as in any subsequent legal or court involvement. To maintain the validity of a child's report, the psychologist should be aware of one's role in the reporting and investigative process and to gain initial information necessary for reporting without contaminating the child's report for the subsequent investigation.

Consulting

Many hospitals have child protection teams or similar groups that review cases of suspected abuse that are reported through the hospital. These multidisciplinary teams typically include psychologists, along with physicians, nurses, social workers, CPS staff, and representatives from law enforcement and the prosecutor's office. These professionals meet on a regular basis to discuss and provide follow-up on abuse-related cases. Sometimes the multidisciplinary team, rather than any one individual, makes recommendations to report suspected maltreatment to CPS or law enforcement. Pediatric psychologists may contribute valuable information to the team about child development, children's emotional and behavioral functioning, and family dynamics. They may be more knowledgeable about these variables than other team members and may assist the team in differentiating normal from abnormal behaviors or situations.

Treatment

Maltreatment may be a central or peripheral treatment focus with children who are seen in medical settings. Certainly some injuries due to maltreatment require medical intervention (e.g., extensive or severe physical abuse, neglect, or sexual abuse that results in sexually transmitted diseases or physical injury), and a psychologist may be asked to evaluate and address the psychological sequelae of the abuse. In other cases, a medical illness (rather than injury due to maltreatment) may be the primary presenting complaint (e.g., diabetes mellitus or renal failure), but maltreatment plays a role in the course and prognosis for the child. For example, a young child with diabetes mellitus may require close monitoring to adhere to diet and insulin protocols. A parent's failure to implement the regimen can lead to acute and critical problems, such as diabetic ketoacidosis (DKA). Repeated episodes of DKA can be indicators of medical neglect, and the pediatric psychologist may work with the family to increase the parents' and child's adherence to the regimen.

CONCLUSIONS

Child maltreatment is clearly recognized as a major social, medical, and psychological problem. As maltreated children present in emergency rooms or hospital clinics, pediatric psychologists are in an excellent position to provide consultation to other professionals involved in these cases or to serve as members of hospital-based child protection teams. Studies on both the short- and long-term consequences have documented the negative effects of abuse and neglect, and recent research has reported the effectiveness of some treatment interventions. Advances have been made in the field over the past 10 years, but continued research is necessary to identify effective methods in the intervention and prevention of child maltreatment.

REFERENCES

American Professional Society on the Abuse of Children. (1995). *Guidelines for the psychosocial evaluation of suspected psychological maltreatment in children and adolescents*. Chicago: Author.

American Psychiatric Association. (2000). *Diagnostic and statistical manual of mental disorders* (4th ed., text rev.). Washington, DC: Author.

Azar, S. T., & Wolfe, D. A. (1998). Child physical abuse and neglect. In E. J. Mash & R. A. Barkley (Eds.), *Treatment of childhood disorders* (2nd ed., pp. 501–544). New York: Guilford Press.

Berliner, L. (2000). What is sexual abuse? In H. Dubowitz & D. DePanfilis (Eds.), *Handbook for child protection* (pp. 18–22). Thousand Oaks, CA: Sage.

Berliner, L., & Elliott, D. M. (2002). Sexual abuse of children. In J. E. B. Myers, L. Berliner, J. Briere, C. T. Hendrix, C. Jenny, & T. A. Reid (Eds.), *The APSAC handbook on child maltreatment* (2nd ed., pp. 55–78). Thousand Oaks, CA: Sage.

Bonner, B. L., Logue, M. B., Kaufman, K. L., & Niec, L. N. (2001). Child maltreatment. In C. E. Walker & M. C. Roberts (Eds.), *Handbook of clinical child psychology* (3rd ed., pp. 989–1030). New York: Wiley.

Bonner, B. L., Walker, C. E., & Berliner, L. (1999). *Children with sexual behavior problems: Assessment and treatment (Final report).* Washington, DC: Office of Child Abuse and Neglect.

Bousha, D. M., & Twentyman, C. T. (1984). Mother–child interactional style in abuse, neglect, and control groups: Natural observations in the home. *Journal of Abnormal Psychology, 93,* 106–114.

Brassard, M. R., & Hardy, D. B. (1997). Psychological maltreatment. In M. E. Helfer, R. S. Kempe, & R. D. Krugman (Eds.), *The battered child* (5th ed., pp. 392–412). Chicago: University of Chicago Press.

Brassard, M. R., Hart, S. N., & Hardy, D. B. (1991). Psychological and emotional abuse of children. In T. Ammerman & M. Hersen (Eds.), *Case studies in treating family violence* (pp. 255–270). Boston: Allyn & Bacon.

Brassard, M. R., Hart, S. N., & Hardy, D. B. (1993). The psychological maltreatment rating scales. *Child Abuse and Neglect, 17,* 715–729.

Briere, J. (1996). *Trauma Symptom Checklist for Children (TSCC): Professional manual.* Odessa, FL: Psychological Assessment Resources.

California Attorney General's Office. (1994). *Child victim witness investigative pilot projects: Research and evaluation final report.* Sacramento, CA: State of California.

Cantwell, H. B. (1977). The neglect of child neglect. In M. E. Helfer, R. S. Kemp, & R. D. Krugman (Eds.), *The battered child* (5th ed, pp. 347–373). Chicago: University of Chicago Press.

Claussen, A. H., & Crittenden, P. M. (1991). Physical and psychological maltreatment: Relations among the types of maltreatment. *Child Abuse and Neglect, 15,* 5–18.

Cohen, J. A., Berliner, L., & Mannarino, A. P. (2000). Treating traumatized children: A research review and synthesis. *Trauma, Violence, and Abuse, 1,* 29–46.

Conte, J. R., & Schuerman, J. R. (l988). The effects of sexual abuse on children: A multidimensional view. In G. E. Wyatt & G. J. Powell (Eds.), *Lasting effects of child sexual abuse* (pp. 157–170). Newbury Park, CA: Sage.

Cosentino, C., & Collins, M. (1996). Sexual abuse of children: Prevalence, effects, and treatment. In J. A. Sechzer, S. M. Pfafflin, F. L. Denmark, & S. J. Blumenthal (Eds.), *Women and mental health* (pp. 45–65). New York: New York Academy of Sciences.

Dawson, G., Klinger, L., & Panagiotides, H. (1997). Infants of depressed mothers exhibit atypical frontal brain activity during the expression of negative emotions. *Developmental Psychology, 33,* 650–656.

Egeland, B., & Erickson, M. F. (1987). Psychologically unavailable caregiving. In M. Brassard, B. Germain, & S. Hart (Eds.), *Psychological maltreatment of children and youth* (pp. 110–120). Elmsford, NY: Pergamon.

Erickson, M. F., & Egeland, B. (1987). A developmental view of the psychological consequences of maltreatment. *School Psychology Review, 16,* 156–168.

Erickson, M. F., Egeland, B., & Pianta, R. C. (1989). The effects of maltreatment on the development of young children. In C. Cicchetti & V. Carlson (Eds.), *Child maltreatment: Theory and research on the causes and consequences of child abuse and neglect* (pp. 647–684). New York: Cambridge University Press.

Friedrich, W. N. (1997). *Child Sexual Behavior Inventory: Professional manual.* Odessa, FL: Psychological Assessment Resources.

Friedrich, W. N. (2002). An integrated model of psychotherapy for abused children. In J. E. B. Myers, L. Berliner, J. Briere, C. T. Hendrix, C. Jenny, & T. A. Reid (Eds.), *The APSAC handbook on child maltreatment* (2nd ed., pp. 141–158). Thousand Oaks, CA: Sage.

Garbarino, J., & Collins, C. C. (1999). Child neglect: The family with a hole in the middle. In H. Dubowitz (Ed.), *Neglected children: Research, practice, and policy* (pp. 1–23). Thousand Oaks, CA: Sage.

Gaudin, J. M. (1999). Child neglect: Short-term and long-term consequences. In H. Dubowitz (Ed.), *Neglected children: Research, practice, and policy* (pp. 89–108). Thousand Oaks, CA: Sage.

Hart, S. N., Brassard, M. R., Binggeli, N. J., & Davidson, H. A. (2002). Psychological maltreatment. In J. E. B. Myers, L. Berliner, J. Briere, C. T. Hendrix, C. Jenny, & T. A. Reid (Eds.), *The APSAC handbook on child maltreatment* (2nd ed., pp. 79–104). Thousand Oaks, CA: Sage.

Hecht, D. B., Chaffin, M., Bonner, B. L., Worley, K. B., & Lawson, L. (2002). Treating sexually abused adolescents. In J. E. B. Myers, L. Berliner, J. Briere, C. T. Hendrix, C. Jenny, & T. A. Reid (Eds.), *The APSAC handbook on child maltreatment* (2nd ed., pp. 159–174). Thousand Oaks, CA: Sage.

Jones, L., & Finkelhor, D. (2001, January). The decline in child sexual abuse cases. *Juvenile Justice Bulletin* (No.

NCJ 184741). Washington, DC: U.S. Department of Justice, Office of Juvenile Justice and Delinquency Prevention.

Kempe, C. H., Silverman, F. N., Steele, B. F., Droegemuller, W., & Silver, H. K. (1962). The battered-child syndrome. *Journal of the American Medical Association, 181*(17), 17–24.

Kendall-Tackett, K. A., & Eckenrode, J. (1996). The effects of neglect on academic achievement and disciplinary problems: A developmental perspective. *Child Abuse and Neglect, 20*, 161–169.

Kendall-Tackett, K. A., Williams, L. M., & Finkelhor, D. (l993). Impact of sexual abuse on children: A review and synthesis of recent empirical studies. *Psychological Bulletin, 113*, 164–180.

Kilpatrick, D. G., & Saunders, B. E. (1999). *Prevalence and consequences of child victimization: Results from the national survey of adolescents* (Report No. 93-IJ-CX-0023). Charleston, SC: Medical University of South Carolina, Department of Psychiatry & Behavioral Sciences, National Crime Victims Research and Treatment Center.

Kolko, D. J. (2002). Child physical abuse. In J. E. B. Myers, L. Berliner, J. Briere, C. T. Hendrix, C. Jenny, & T. A. Reid (Eds.), *The APSAC handbook on child maltreatment* (2nd ed., pp. 21–54). Thousand Oaks, CA: Sage.

Lutzker, J. R. (1990). Behavioral treatment of child neglect. *Behavior Modification, 14*, 301–315.

Lutzker, J. R., Bigelow, K. M., Doctor, R. M., Gershater, R. M., & Greene, B. F. (1998). An ecobehavioral model for the prevention and treatment of child abuse and neglect. In J. R. Lutzker (Ed.), *Handbook of child abuse research and treatment* (pp. 239–266). New York: Plenum Press.

National Center on Child Abuse and Neglect. (1981). *Study findings: National study of the incidence and severity of child abuse and neglect* (Publication No. OHDS 81-30325). Washington, DC: U. S. Department of Health and Human Services.

National Research Council (1993). *Understanding child abuse and neglect.* Washington, DC: National Academy Press.

Oates, R. K., & Bross, D. C. (1995). What have we learned about treating physical abuse? A literature review of the last decade. *Child Abuse and Neglect, 19*, 463–473.

Olds, D. L., Eckenrode, J., Henderson, C. R., Kitzman, H., Powers, J., Cole, R., et al. (1997). Long-term effects of home visitation on maternal life course and child abuse and neglect. *Journal of the American Medical Association, 278*, 637–643.

Parnell, T. F. (2002). Munchausen by proxy syndrome. In J. E. B. Myers, L. Berliner, J. Briere, C. T. Hendrix, C. Jenny, & T. A. Reid (Eds.), *The APSAC handbook on child maltreatment* (2nd ed., pp. 131–138). Thousand Oaks, CA: Sage.

Perry, B. (1997). Incubated in terror: Neurodevelopmental factors in the "cycle of violence. " In J. D. Osofsky (Ed.), *Children in a violent society* (pp. 124–149). New York: Guilford Press.

Rohrbeck, C. A., & Twentyman, C. T. (1986). Multimodal assessment of impulsiveness in abusing, neglectful, and nonmaltreating mothers and their preschool children. *Journal of Consulting and Clinical Psychology, 54*, 231–236.

Sedlak, A. J., & Broadhurst, D. D. (1996). *Executive summary of the Third National Incidence Study of Child Abuse and Neglect* (DHHS Pub. No. ACF-105-94-1840). Washington, DC: Government Printing Office.

Silverman, A. B., Reinherz, H. Z., & Giaconia, R. M. (1996). The long-term sequelae of child and adolescent abuse: A longitudinal community study. *Child Abuse and Neglect, 8*, 709–723.

U.S. Department of Health and Human Services, Administration on Children, Youth and Families. (2002). *11 years of reporting: Child maltreatment 2000*. Washington, DC: U.S. Government Printing Office.

Ware, J. C., Orr, W. C., & Bond, T. (2001). Evaluation and treatment of sleep disorders in children. In C. E. Walker & M. C. Roberts (Eds.), *Handbook of clinical child psychology* (3rd ed., pp. 317–337). New York: Wiley.

Widom, C. S. (1989). Does violence beget violence? A critical examination of the literature. *Psychological Bulletin, 106*, 3–28.

Williamson, J. M., Borduin, C. M., & Howe, B. A. (1991). The ecology of adolescent maltreatment: A multilevel examination of adolescent physical abuse, sexual abuse, and neglect. *Journal of Consulting and Clinical Psychology, 59*, 449–457.

Wolfe, D. (1999). *Child abuse: Implications for child development and psychopathology* (2nd ed.). Thousand Oaks, CA: Sage.

Wyatt, G. E., & Peters, S. D. (1986). Issues in the definition of child sexual abuse in prevalence research. *Child Abuse and Neglect, 10*, 231–240.

Zellman, G. L., & Fair, C. C. (2002). Preventing and reporting abuse. In J. E. B. Myers, L. Berliner, J. Briere, C. T. Hendrix, C. Jenny, & T. A. Reid (Eds.), *The APSAC handbook on child maltreatment* (2nd ed., pp. 449–475). Thousand Oaks, CA: Sage.

39

Sexual Behaviors and Problems of Adolescents

HEATHER HUSZTI
AHNA HOFF
CHRISTA JOHNSON

Although the spread of sexually transmitted diseases among adolescents has long been a concern, increased attention to this problem was paid with the advent of human immunodeficiency virus (HIV) in the late 1980s. The problem of HIV infection grew over the late 1980s into the early 1990s, and by 1993 acquired immune deficiency syndrome (AIDS) was the fourth leading cause of death among 15- to 24-year-olds (Centers for Disease Control and Prevention [CDC], 1993). However, several positive trends have also been reported in the past 10 years regarding adolescent sexual behavior, including record low pregnancy rates, decreases in sexual activity, and increased use of contraceptives among sexually active youth (CDC, 1998; Kirby, 2001; National Campaign to Prevent Teen Pregnancy, 2002; Santelli, Lindberg, Abma, McNeely, & Resnick, 2000). Although these findings are certainly encouraging, a number of problems remain related to teenage sexuality. Despite the decreases in pregnancy rates, the United States remains near the top of industrialized nations in adolescent pregnancies. Four out of 10 girls in the United States still become pregnant before age 20, which translates into nearly 1 million teenage pregnancies per year, most (78%) of which are unintended (National Campaign to Prevent Teen Pregnancy, 2002). Adolescents also continue to be at high risk for contracting human immunodeficiency virus (HIV) and other sexually transmitted diseases (STDs). For example, in 1999, people ages 13 to 24 years accounted for 13% of the cases of HIV infection (CDC, 2002). Additionally, of teens who are sexually active, up to one-fourth contract STDs each year (Kirby, 2001). Consequently, efforts to assess adolescent sexual behavior and promote safer sex behaviors among teens continues to be an area of national concern, particularly in the public health arena (Santelli, Lindberg, et al., 2000).

In order to outline the issues involved with the sexual behavior of adolescents, this chapter is divided into three sections. The first section reviews sexual behaviors, the incidence and prevalence of STDs and pregnancy, and the use of contraceptives in adolescence. The second section of the chapter reviews factors contributing to adolescent sexual behavior. The final section reviews prevention and intervention programs for HIV, STDs, and unplanned pregnancy, as well as future goals.

SEXUAL BEHAVIORS, SEXUALLY TRANSMITTED DISEASES, PREGNANCY, AND CONTRACEPTIVE USE IN ADOLESCENCE

Several national reports indicate a decrease in teen sexual behavior over the past 10 years (Abma, Chancra, Mosher, Peterson, & Piccinino, 1997; CDC, 1998; National Campaign to Prevent Teen Pregnancy, 2002). However, the age of first intercourse continues to decrease. In 1995, a national school-based survey of high school students indicated that 51% of the students reported having had sexual intercourse in their lifetimes, and 9.0% of these students report initiating sexual intercourse before the age of 13 (CDC, 1996). Males initiated sexual activity prior to age 13 more often than females and reported a higher number of lifetime sexual partners than females. Also, African American students (20.5%) were more likely than Caucasian (5.5%) and Hispanic (9.2%) students to initiate sexual activity prior to age 13 (CDC, 1996).

Female teenagers have the highest rates of many STDs, including chlamydia and gonorrhea (CDC, 2000). This high rate is due to numerous factors, including a higher likelihood of having multiple sexual partners and engaging in unprotected sex, selection of high-risk partners, and a physiological susceptibility to infection in females during pubertal development (CDC, 2000).

Adolescents are also at high risk for contracting HIV. One-fifth of all cases of AIDS are in the 20- to 29-year-old age group. Given the latency period from time of infection with HIV to time of diagnosis of AIDS (6 months to 10 years), many of these individuals were probably infected during adolescence but did not develop AIDS until early adulthood.

Pregnancy rates among adolescents increased throughout the late 1980s and into the early 1990s. However, since 1991, adolescent pregnancy rates in the United States have declined 22%, to 48.5 pregnancies per 1,000 females ages 15–19 years (CDC, 2002). Even with the decline, the pregnancy rate in the United States remains high as compared with other developed countries (Alan Guttmacher Institute [AGI], 2002). It is estimated that more than three-fourths of teen pregnancies are unintended (National Campaign to Prevent Teen Pregnancy, 2002).

The impact of pregnancy on teenagers, as well as on the society at large, can be profound. Teenage parents are more likely to drop out of school, to require public assistance, or to be able to hold only menial jobs with little hope of advancement. The societal price of teenage pregnancy includes public funding for housing, food, health care, and special education for teenage mothers and their children. These consequences can lead to an ongoing cycle of poverty and teenage pregnancy within generations of families (Koyle, Jensen, Olsen, & Cundick, 1989).

A teenage girl who does not use any form of contraception will have a 90% chance of becoming pregnant within a year (Harlap, Kost, & Forrest, 1991). The use of contraception at first intercourse has increased during the 1980s, climbing from 48% to 78% in 1995 (Moore et al., 1998). The majority of this increase appears to be due to an increase in condom use (AGI, 2000). Although male condoms are most likely to be used at first intercourse, over the course of the relationship oral contraceptives become more frequently used (AGI, 2000).

Although these increases are certainly encouraging, there are also some disturbing trends. Although increasing percentages of adolescents report using contraception at first intercourse, a study of patterns of contraceptive use in teenage and adult women suggested that 15- to 19-year-olds were most likely to report sporadic and ineffective contraceptive use as compared with older women (Glei, 1999).

FACTORS INFLUENCING ADOLESCENT SEXUAL BEHAVIORS

A number of variables have been associated with adolescent sexual behavior. These variables can be grouped into several categories: familial, religious, peer, academic, past abuse, and psychological characteristics.

Family structure, processes, and communication all have a substantial influence on adolescent sexual behavior. Family structure has been consistently associated with adolescent sexual risk taking. For example, Upchurch, Aneshensel, Sucoff, & Levy-Storms (1999) found that girls and boys who live in single-parent or stepparent families have an earlier age of sexual debut than girls and boys who live with both biological parents. Earlier sexual initiation among adolescents from single-parent homes is potentially due to the limited resources available to some single parents to supervise their adolescents. Studies examining parental monitoring have demonstrated that decreased parental monitoring is associated with sexual risk behaviors (Li et al., 2000; Miller, McCoy, Olsen, & Wallace, 1986).

Family processes have also been associated with adolescent sexual behavior. Consistently, controlling and strict parenting styles have been associated with earlier sexual initiation and greater sexual activity among adolescents (Rodgers, 1999; Miller et al., 1986), whereas parents who are moderately strict with their children are more likely to have adolescents who practice responsible sexual behavior (Miller et al., 1986). Further, boys who perceive higher levels of emotional support from their parents are more likely to delay sexual initiation (Upchurch et al., 1999).

Research examining the relationship between parent–adolescent communication and adolescent sexual attitudes and behavior is equivocal. However, in general, adolescents who report better communication with their parents are more likely to delay sexual initiation than those who report having poor communication with their parents (Brooks-Gunn & Furstenberg, 1989; Karofsky, Zeng, & Kosorok, 2000). The influence of parent–adolescent communication on adolescent sexual behaviors may be mediated by the quality of both the relationship and the communication. Adolescents who report a higher level of relationship satisfaction with their mothers are less likely to engage in sexual intercourse, more likely to use contraception when they do engage in intercourse, and less likely to become pregnant. Relationship satisfaction is also associated with the adolescent's intention to initiate sex within the next year (Miller, Norton, Fan, & Christopherson, 1998). Collectively, these findings highlight the significant impact the parent–adolescent relationship has on adolescent sexual attitudes and behaviors.

Research examining the relationship between religion and adolescent sexual behaviors has produced equivocal findings. For example, Roche and Ramsbay (1993) reported that adolescents who frequently attended religious services were more conservative in their premarital sexual attitudes and behavior, whereas other variables, such as religiosity, residence, age, parents' education, nationality, and religious affiliation, were found to be largely insignificant. However, a study by Holder and colleagues (2000) found that religious attendance did not significantly predict sexual behavior; rather, perceptions of spiritual connectedness with friends predicted sexual behaviors. For adolescents who choose to abstain from sexual intercourse, participation in religious groups may reinforce that choice. In contrast, another study compared adolescents who viewed themselves as very religious with those who viewed themselves as less religious and found that the two groups did not differ in having engaged in sex or in their expectation to engage in intercourse in the next year (Donnelly, Duncan, Goldfarb, & Eadie, 1999). Taken together, these results suggest the need for further research to determine how religious beliefs and spirituality influence teenage sexual behaviors. This field of research would also benefit from more specific definitions and measures of religiosity and spirituality to allow for comparisons across studies.

It is well established that the importance of peer relationships substantially increases during adolescence. As a result, peers have more influence on adolescent behaviors, including sexual behaviors. Adolescent sexual behaviors are also influenced by their perceptions of peer sexual attitudes and behaviors. For example, greater peer disapproval of sexual activity was associated with sexual abstinence among adolescents (Beal, Ausiello, & Perrin, 2001). Younger adolescents may be especially susceptible to peer influence, as younger girls reported friends having sex as a primary reason for sexual initiation (Rosenthal et al., 2001). Similarly, sixth-grade males who perceived other males as being sexually active were more likely to be sexually active than sixth-grade males who did not (Robinson, Telljohann, & Price, 1999). However, this study did not find the same effect for girls.

Associating with peers who engage in deviant behaviors is also related to adolescent sexual behavior. One study compared adolescents who reported a history of a single sexual partner with those who had multiple partners and found that those with multiple partners were more likely to have friends who had sex, used alcohol, and had been in a jail or a detention center than those with a single partner (Whitaker, Miller, & Clark, 2000). In addition, males with multiple partners were more likely to have a friend who had gotten someone pregnant. These findings suggest that sexual behavior may just be one of a constellation of co-occuring deviant behaviors. Research examining the relationship between educational factors and sexual behavior is relatively limited. The majority of studies have found an association between adolescent sexual behavior and school attitudes and/or performance. In one study decreased educational investment was associated with increased sexual behavior among adolescent girls, but not among boys (Ohannessian & Crockett, 1993). However, boys' sexual behavior predicted later involvement in school activities. The authors concluded that for girls, becoming sexually active may decrease educational aspirations and school achievement, whereas for boys sexual activity may result in missing academic opportunities and may interfere with future career goals. Further, differences in attitudes toward school have also been associated with number of sexual partners. One study found that adolescents who had multiple partners were more likely to have been suspended or held back a grade, liked school less, and expected their achievement to be lower than those with a single partner (Whitaker et al., 2000). Finally, grade point average (GPA) in school has been associated with sexual behaviors and outcomes of sexual behaviors among adolescents. As an example, a longitudinal study found that 8th-grade GPA significantly predicted whether an adolescent experienced a pregnancy before the 12th grade (Scaramella, Conger, Simons, & Whitbeck, 1998). Thus it appears that academic achievement is at least indirectly related to sexual behaviors and risk taking. However, further research is needed to determine the nature and meaning of these relationships.

A history of sexual abuse or coercion has also been associated with the behaviors and outcomes of adolescent sexual risk taking. Unfortunately a large number of female adolescents have experienced unwanted sexual activity, with one national survey reporting that 22% of females who reported first sexual intercourse at age 13 indicated that it was either nonvoluntary or unwanted (Abma et al., 1995). Women who had had at least one experience of sexual coercion were more likely to engage in high-risk sexual behaviors, such as having sex under the influence of alcohol or drugs and having sex with a stranger, than those without a history of abuse or coercion (Biglan, Noell, Ochs, Smolkowski, & Metzler, 1995). Moreover, sexual abuse is associated with negative outcomes of adolescent sexual behavior, such as pregnancy and sexually transmitted diseases (Biglan et al., 1995; Roosa, Tein, Reinholtz, & Angelini, 1997).

Psychological functioning has a considerable influence on adolescent sexual behaviors. Higher levels of distress are consistently associated with greater sexual activity among adolescents (Tubman, Windle, & Windle, 1996). Psychological functioning has also been associated with high-risk sexual behaviors and a history of STDs (Shreir, Harris, et al., 2001). Researchers have also found an association between low self-esteem and inconsistent contraceptive use in adolescent girls (Miller, Forehand, & Kotchick, 2000).

Very few studies have examined how cognitive factors such as decision making, problem-solving skills, and appraisals influence sexual behavior among adolescents. However, one study found that adolescent girls may defer control to their male partners when making decisions regarding STD protection (Rosenthal et al., 1999). These findings suggest the need to promote a sense of control over STD protection and contraception among adolescent girls.

The relationship between adolescent substance use and sexual risk taking is well established. Adolescents who abuse substances are more likely to engage in more high-risk sexual behaviors and experience more negative outcomes related to their sexual behavior than adolescents who do not (Tapert, Aarons, Sedlar, & Brown, 2001). The robust association between substance use and sexual risk taking is hypothesized to be a function of (1) a constellation of common factors that lead to both substance abuse and sexual risk behaviors and (2) the disinhibiting influence of alcohol or other drugs that increase the likelihood of engaging in sexually risky behaviors (Santelli, Robin, Brener, & Lowery, 2001).

PREVENTION OF PREGNANCY AND SEXUALLY TRANSMITTED DISEASES IN ADOLESCENCE

As rates of infection with sexually transmitted diseases (STDs) and pregnancy increased among adolescents in the 1980s and early 1990s, a variety of prevention programs were developed and implemented. As the body of research on these prevention programs increases, it becomes clearer that there is a need for multiple types of interventions, based on the characteristics of participants who are targeted (such as age, relationship status, types of high-risk behaviors engaged in, etc.). It is important to continue to increase the effectiveness and long term impact of prevention programs on participants, as behavioral change remains the only way to reduce the rate of many of the problems associated with risky sexual behavior. Developing and implementing HIV risk-reduction programs is particularly crucial because there are still no medical cures for HIV. Although other forms of bacterial STDs are not commonly fatal because there are available medical treatments, they can have serious associated sequelae, such as infertility and birth defects in developing fetuses. Other viral forms of

STDs (such as herpes, human papilloma virus, and hepatitis B) currently have few, if any, effective treatments. This section reviews the current debate on abstinence-only programs, highlights the types of programs that have been found to be successful or that offer innovative and promising approaches, and highlights specific questions that should be addressed prior to the development of future intervention programs.

Abstinence Programs

Currently, there is a debate over the implementation of programs that present information only on abstinence as compared with those that offer information on both abstinence and contraception. The argument for abstinence-only programs is that giving adolescents information about contraception implies permission to become sexually active. Indeed, some proponents of abstinence-only programs suggest that any other type of sexual education will increase rates of teen sexual activity. Abstinence-only programs are still relatively new, and few well-designed experimental studies have yet been completed. In a recent review of teen pregnancy programs, only three studies met criteria for evaluation, and none of those studies demonstrated efficacy (Kirby, 2001). However, several more rigorous evaluations are currently taking place, and these results should be available in the near future.

One randomized controlled trial has compared the effects of an abstinence-based program with one that stresses how to protect oneself with condoms (Jemmott, Jemmott, & Fong, 1998). This program was conducted with inner-city African American students in sixth and seventh grades. Follow-up assessments were conducted at 3, 6, and 12 months. Results showed that those who participated in the abstinence intervention were less likely to have engaged in sexual intercourse at the 3-month follow-up than those in the comparison group but that differences had disappeared by the 6-month follow-up. Those who participated in the safer-sex intervention reported more consistent condom use at 3 months than those in the comparison condition and reported a higher frequency of condom use at all three follow-ups. For the 25% of participants who reported sexual intercourse at baseline, the safer-sex intervention group reported less sexual intercourse at 6 and 12 months than the comparison or abstinence group.

The age of participants in abstinence-only programs may be important. It is possible that abstinence interventions might be most effective with cohorts of younger children who are not likely to become sexually active in the near future. These programs may prove to be less effective when presented to older adolescents who have already begun to engage in intercourse or those who are developing long-term, stable relationships. Additionally, as more programs are developed, abstinence-based interventions may also increase in their effectiveness.

Clearly, decisions about the implementation of abstinence-only programs should be made based on replicable scientific studies rather than on political considerations. The results from rigorous studies can be used to improve programs to make them increasingly effective. The consequences of early involvement in sexual activity can be myriad (increased risk of unintended pregnancies, consequences to unwanted children, infection with diseases, sexual coercion, and violence, to name a few), and delaying the onset of intercourse could have beneficial effects. However, it is also clear that many adolescents engage in sexual activity, and doing so without protection (both birth control and disease prevention) can lead to many of the same negative consequences; hence the ongoing need for effective education about ways to protect oneself.

Educational Programs

Initially in the 1980s there was societal and governmental support for programs that taught students to "just say no" to sexual intercourse and drugs. Although these programs may have increased students' knowledge and intentions to abstain from intercourse or drug use, they had little effect on students' actual behaviors (Christopher & Roosa, 1990; Huszti, Clopton, & Mason, 1989; Overby, Lo, & Litt, 1989). The failure of simple educational programs to effect long-lasting changes in risky sexual behaviors is not surprising. Although the behaviors necessary to prevent HIV/STD infection or pregnancy can be described briefly and simply, actually putting these behaviors into practice requires changes in a series of complex and essentially private behaviors. One formulation of the broad range of behaviors and skills necessary to implement risk-reduction behaviors includes a long and varied list (Fisher & Fisher, 1992). These skills include: accepting the fact that one is a sexual person; knowing the behaviors necessary to prevent pregnancy or HIV/STD infection; negotiating the use of safer sexual behaviors with a potential sexual partner; leaving the relationship if risk-reduction behaviors are not used consistently; acquiring condoms; performing-AIDS related preventive behaviors; seeking out and receiving pregnancy, STD, or HIV antibody testing, if necessary; continuing to set and follow the limits necessary to engage routinely in risk reduction behaviors; and reinforcing oneself to prevent possible relapse. As can be seen from this list, effective risk reduction requires a number of complicated actions. These skills require the use of formal operational thinking in order to plan ahead and recognize the long-term consequences of one's own behaviors, which can be a particular challenge to adolescents who are just beginning to develop these capabilities.

Adolescents are just beginning to negotiate the complexity of romantic and sexual relationships. It may be unrealistic to ask them to introduce abstinence or condoms into their relationships without helping them to acquire and practice the skills necessary to accomplish this task. Given the complex emotional, interpersonal, and developmental issues surrounding the sexual behavior of adolescents, it is clear that efforts aimed at simply providing basic information about pregnancy, STD, and HIV prevention are inadequate. Unfortunately, most schools that do provide HIV or pregnancy prevention programs do so using simple informational techniques, which are almost assuredly doomed to fail in bringing about the desired behavioral changes.

Community-Based Interventions

With the increasing awareness of the complexity of changing sexual behavior, interventions have increasingly focused on building skills and addressing antecedents to sexual risk taking. These longer programs have been implemented in both school-based and community settings. Many of these skill-based programs follow similar formats and generally differ only on the theoretical underpinnings and how much time is spent on each skill (i.e., some programs may spend more time on communication, others on values clarification; St. Lawrence et al., 1995; Stanton et al., 1996). As an example, one randomized clinical trial evaluated an eight-session (lasting 90 to 120 minutes) community-based program for African American adolescents and demonstrated significant behavioral changes over a 1-year follow-up (St. Lawrence et al., 1995). The skills-based group focused on communication and condom skills, as well as influencing attitudes about safer sex. The intervention had a differential effect on males and females. Males entered the intervention with significantly greater levels of sexual activity than females. Following the skills-based intervention, they showed significant decreases in unprotected sexual activity, decreases that were maintained over the year-long follow-up period, as compared with those in the comparison group. Females who received the skills-based training maintained lower levels of unprotected sexual activity over the follow-up period, whereas females in the comparison group increased their overall level of sexual activity. Condom use in male and female adolescents increased following the skills-based intervention but gradually decreased for males over the 1-year follow-up. Although concerns have been raised that programs that explicitly educate about condom use and/or other contraceptives will increase sexual activity, this study found the opposite effect. Adolescents in the education-only condition were more likely to begin sexual activity (31% of abstinent adolescents at baseline) than were those in the skills-based group (11%).

School-Based Programs

School-based programs have had varied effects on measured behavioral outcomes. Some evaluated programs have had little effect (Kirby, 2001; Kirby, Korpi, Barth, & Cagampang, 1997; Lieberman, Gray, Wier, Fiorentino, & Mahoney, 2000). Several school-based programs have shown positive behavioral findings (Main et al., 1994; Kirby, Barth, Leland, & Fetro, 1991). One program, Get Real About AIDS, presented information about HIV/AIDS over 15 consecutive school days to 9th- through 12th-graders. Activities were presented in classrooms and were reinforced with other school-based activities over those 3 weeks (such as posters displayed around the school; Main et al., 1994). In addition to basic education, the program focused on increasing students' perceived vulnerability to HIV and positive reasons to be abstinent and on skills-building components, including proper condom use and refusal communication skills. This quasi-experimental evaluation found that, at 6-month follow-up, students in the intervention schools were more likely to report having purchased a condom, and sexually active students were more likely to report that they had used a condom more often during sexual intercourse over the past 2 months. A somewhat similar program, the 17-session Reducing the Risk, focused on teaching effective communication skills, as well as increasing perceived vulnerability (Kirby et al., 1991). After 18 months, students in the intervention classes who had not engaged in intercourse were less likely to initiate sexual activity as compared with those in the control classrooms. Students in the intervention conditions who were sexually active were more likely to use contraception. A replication study of this curriculum found similar results (Hubbard, Giese, & Rainey, 1998).

One program offers an intriguing twist on the more traditional programs reviewed here. This program compared two types of interventions designed to prevent a range of adolescent health risks, including pregnancy, in schools in high-crime areas in an urban setting (Hawkins, Catalano, Kosterman, Abbott, & Hill, 1999). The intervention sought to decrease a range of health risks by attempting to increase health-protective factors that are associated with a broad range of problems (delinquency, school failure, drug abuse, teen pregnancy). Differences from previous programs, however, included a focus on younger children (starting in the first grade), support and training offered to parents and teachers, as well as the children, and a focus on increasing participants' bonding to both school and family rather than focusing on one specific health-risk behavior (such as unprotected intercourse). Children were followed until age 18. Children received age-appropriate training in interpersonal problem-solving skills such as communication, decision making, negotiation, conflict resolution, and refusal skills. No further interventions were offered after sixth grade. Significantly fewer of those children who participated in the full intervention repeated a grade, committed a violent delinquent act, used alcohol heavily (drinking 10 or more times in the previous year), engaged in sexual intercourse, had multiple sexual partners, or became or got someone pregnant. Although not all health-related risks were reduced, of interest is the long-term effect, without booster sessions, on some risky health behaviors between the 6th and 12th grades. The authors suggested these long-term effects, in contrast to the other specific health-risk programs, may be due to the early emphasis on helping the child bond with the school and parents, which may provide a protective factor against engaging in high-risk health behaviors. In addition, this intervention, in contrast to others reviewed, offered services to teachers and parents that reinforced the activities provided to the children; the authors suggest that this intervention may have contributed to the long-term effects (Hawkins et al., 1999).

Clinic-Based Programs

Although school-based interventions allow prevention messages to be presented to a large audience of adolescents, they may include many who are not now at high risk. Interventions designed for clinic settings reach fewer adolescents but can target those at high risk (such as those presenting for treatment of STDs or contraceptive services). Individuals seeking health-related services might be likely to perceive themselves to be at increased vulnerability and thus may be more receptive to the messages, particularly if the messages were targeted to the individual's needs and concerns. One approach, using a tailored computer program to help adolescents make choices about contraception, did not demonstrate significant changes at the 12-month follow-up (Chewning et al., 1999). However, the model of a personalized computer program is intriguing and, with further modifications, may be effective.

One recent randomized study examined the use of a motivational interviewing prevention intervention for adolescents presenting to a clinic for treatment of a current STD (Shrier, Ancheta, et al., 2001). Motivational interviewing (MI) focuses on increasing motivation at various points along a continuum of behavior change (Miller & Rollnick, 2002). MI strategies have been developed to deal with the resistance, ambivalence, and lack of objective self-assessment that are common, particularly among those who are beginning the process of behavior change. In the intervention participants received a session tailored to their current intentions to change their behavior. Participants received booster sessions at 1, 3, and 6 months. At the 6-month follow-up, significantly fewer intervention participants reported an increase in sex with a nonprimary partner, but results disappeared at 1 year. These results are encouraging, as some significant changes occurred as the result of a 30-minute initial session. Modifications may need to be made to the use of MI to adapt it for the developmental level of adolescents (who may have more trouble with the concept of long-term future intentions) and to increase long-term behavior change.

HIV Prevention Programs for Special Populations

Several groups of adolescents are at particularly high risk for HIV infection because of the groups' involvement with high-risk sexual and/or drug use behaviors. Adolescents who are engaging in especially high-risk behaviors may benefit from special programs targeted to their type of risk. Among adolescents at high risk are runaways in urban centers, who often engage in unprotected sex and intravenous drug use (Yates, MacKenzie, Pennbridge, & Cohen,1988). In response to the high risk of this population, an innovative HIV risk-reduction program was implemented in a New York City shelter for teenage runaways (Rotheram-Borus, Koopman, Haignere, & Davies, 1991). The intervention was intensive (up to a total of 20 sessions, with a median number of 11 sessions), taught specific coping skills for high-risk situations, and included referrals for health and psychosocial care. Results indicated that abstinence was not significantly affected by the intervention; however, the program did significantly increase the consistent use of condoms at 3- and 6-month follow-ups. Interestingly, attendance at 15 or more sessions appeared to be associated with the greatest changes in behavior.

It is important to remember that by adolescence some individuals have already identified themselves as homosexual or bisexual and engage in homosexual relationships. These adolescents are at particularly high risk for HIV infection because of the riskiness of unprotected anal intercourse, coupled with the secrecy and denial that often accompany adolescent homosexual relationships. One study of more than 34,000 junior and senior high school students in Minnesota found that 10.7% of the population identified themselves as being "unsure" of their sexual orientation, 1.1% described themselves as bisexual or predominantly homosexual, and 1% reported homosexual experiences (Remafedi, Resnick, Blum, & Harris, 1992). These adolescents are in great need of nonjudgmental risk-reduction intervention programs targeted for their unique needs. Several risk-reduction programs have been found to be effective in intervening with adolescents who identify themselves as gay or bisexual. Two such programs are the Youth and AIDS Project (YAP; Remafedi, 1998) and MPOWERMENT in northern California (Kegeles, Hays, Pollack, & Coates, 1999).

FACTORS TO CONSIDER IN DESIGNING EFFECTIVE PREVENTION PROGRAMS

Developmental Considerations

Adolescents are a particularly difficult group to educate about avoidance of pregnancy and prevention of HIV and other STDs (Huszti et al., 1989). In order to design an effective prevention program for adolescents, several developmental characteristics must be taken into account. Because members of this age group are in the process of moving away from the family and seeking their independence, they often experiment with a variety of new behaviors. Experimentation with sex and drug use is common, both of which can increase the risk of pregnancy or contagion with HIV or other STDs. Peers take on an increased importance during adolescence, and peer groups often subtly or blatantly encourage behavioral experimentation. Adding to the difficulty of designing prevention programs is adolescents' perception of personal invulnerability. Many adolescents tend to believe that they are invulnerable to personal harm, a perception supported by the fact that they are unlikely to have experienced negative consequences from sexually risky health behaviors (Elkind, 1967). Therefore strategies to increase adolescents' perceived vulnerability might be particularly important. Some programs cover pregnancy and HIV and STD prevention together to increase the odds that adolescents may know someone who has experienced one of these negative outcomes. Other programs have used speakers who have acquired HIV infection to make these consequences more real to the participants. Others have used experiential activities to increase adolescents' sense of vulnerability.

It is also important to clearly define the recommendations being made. For example, abstinence is often stated to be the only 100% effective way to prevent unintended pregnancies and infection with STDs. However, this is true only when abstinence is defined as avoiding vaginal, anal, and oral intercourse, as well as any activity that would lead to contact with genital fluids (such as mutual masturbation). Although this point may seem clear to some, there is tremendous variation in how adolescents define abstinence. One study asked college students to define whether a variety of behaviors constituted sex or intercourse (Horan, Phillips, & Hagen, 1998). Almost one-fourth of respondents (24%) felt that anal intercourse was not sex, 37% did not define oral intercourse as sex, and 47% did not define anal–oral contact as sex. Although none of these behaviors will lead to pregnancy, they all could lead to infection with a variety of sexually transmitted diseases. It is important to distinguish between monogamy and serial monogamy. Because adolescents tend to engage in a series of monogamous dating relationships, they may not understand that these relationships are risky. For the purposes of reducing the risk of HIV/STD infection, a monogamous relationship should be explicitly defined as "one lifetime sexual relationship."

Combination Prevention Programs

Recently, interest has increased in developing prevention interventions that target unintended pregnancies and HIV and STD prevention in one program. Because the consistent use of condoms can prevent all of these consequences, it makes sense to target all three issues together. However, as primary relationships progress over time, couples generally stop using condoms and begin using other forms of contraception that do not also prevent diseases (Civic, 2000). Those couples who continue to use condoms are most likely to report doing so for pregnancy prevention (Whaley, 1999). Unfortunately, a significant number of individuals remain at risk for sexually transmitted diseases through their primary relationships, although they are often unaware of this risk (Misovich, Fisher, & Fisher, 1997). However, few couples who are invested in a relationship are likely to consider that their partner might put them at risk for diseases. Thus interventions that combine prevention messages, specifically emphasizing that condoms are an effective method of birth control that also prevent disease, may increase the use of condoms in primary relationships and provide the benefit of decreasing both unintended pregnancies and infection with STDs.

It is important to consider several factors related to the prevention of disease when developing a combination prevention program. For adolescents, it is important to help them understand the various consequences of unprotected intercourse. For example, because viral STDs are currently incurable (including HIV, herpes simplex virus [HSV], and human papilloma virus [HPV], which appears to be a primary cause of cervical cancer), it is important to help adolescents understand that the only certain way to avoid infection with STDs is to avoid any activities that involve contact with vaginal or seminal fluid. For those adolescents who choose not to practice abstinence, it is important to clearly define "consistent use" by stressing the need to use latex condoms "each and every time." Programs can recommend a range of reliable forms of contraception to prevent unintended pregnancy; however, to also prevent diseases, the consistent use of condoms is necessary, even if other forms of contraception are used.

Condom Skills and Efficacy

Although most programs recommend the use of male latex condoms, explicit instruction in their use often is not provided. Condom use has increased among adolescents, but unless they are used correctly, there is still a risk of disease transmission. Analyses of the 1995 National Longitudinal Study of Adolescent Health found that, on questions of correct condom use (such as leaving space at the tip, the use of Vaseline as a lubricant, the efficacy of lambskin condoms), as many as 52% of adolescents were unaware of the correct answer (Crosby

& Yarber, 2001). There have been recent concerns about the efficacy of condoms. A recent National Institute of Health (NIH) panel examined the evidence for the efficacy of condoms to prevent a range of STDs (National Institute of Allergy and Infectious Diseases [NIAID], 2001). Overall, studies have consistently shown that latex condoms provide good protection from infection with HIV and gonorrhea (NIAID, 2001). The methodology for evaluating the efficacy of condoms for other STDs was inadequate at this time (Cates, 2001). Contrary to many media reports, this conclusion does not mean that condoms were ineffective, but rather that more methodologically rigorous studies need to be completed to ensure that they are efficacious in preventing a range of other sexually transmitted diseases. Of note, however, is that condoms appear to be less effective in the prevention of HPV and HSV, as these viruses can live on and be transmitted through skin outside of the genital area protected by condoms (NIAID, 2001).

Considerations for Designing Effective Programs

Several authors have suggested elements that appear to be common to programs that demonstrate a behavioral outcome. A recent review of pregnancy prevention programs suggested that there are 10 elements that distinguish effective programs (Kirby, 2001):

1. They focus on at least one sexual behavior that leads to pregnancy.
2. They are based on theoretical principles.
3. They clearly give a message about abstinence or the use of condoms and/or other contraceptives.
4. They provide basic information about the risks of unprotected sex.
5. They provide a way to address social pressures that adolescents experience.
6. They provide examples of and practice with assertive communication to allow adolescents to negotiate condom use or to refuse unsafe sexual activity.
7. They provide experiential learning that allows for personalization of the messages and skills.
8. They focus on behavioral goals and use teaching methods that are appropriate to the age of the participants.
9. They last longer than several hours.
10. They are led by individuals (adults or peers) who believe in the program and have received adequate training to implement the groups.

St. Lawrence and colleagues (1995) also stress the importance of interventions being culturally relevant to the participants.

The length of programs also seems to be important. Most of the successful interventions for adolescents have been 8 and 15 sessions in length. Although the total amount of time may be important, the spacing of the interventions may also be a consideration. One recent study examined the effectiveness of a community-based HIV-prevention intervention for adolescents (Rotheram-Borus, Gwadz, Fernandez, & Srinivasan, 1998). Adolescents were randomly assigned to a seven-session program, a three-session program that was equivalent in total time to the seven-session program, and a no-intervention condition. Results found that over 3 months, participants in the seven-session program had fewer unprotected acts of intercourse and fewer sexual partners as compared with the other two conditions. Interestingly, the only difference between the seven-session and three-session programs was the number of sessions (total time and content were identical). Similar results were found for a prevention program with gay adolescents (Rotheram-Borus, Murphy, Fernandez, & Srinivasan, 1998). In both studies, proposed behavioral mediators (attitudes and perceived vulnerability) changed in both intervention groups, but only the seven-session group demonstrated behavioral change. The authors suggested that consistent with learning theory, individuals may need to have information spaced over time with opportunities to practice skills learned in groups (Rotheram-Borus, Gwadz, et al., 1998). In addition, it is possible that adolescents may have difficulties sustaining attention over a 3½ hour session and thus may have missed more information as well.

Future Directions for Program Development

Although progress has been made in the development of prevention interventions, much work is left to complete. Clearly, one of the biggest challenges for program developers is to design interventions that facilitate long-term behavioral change. Although many of the programs reviewed herein are promising, behavioral change is rarely sustained beyond 1 year, and most occurs for only 3 to 6 months. The addition of booster sessions might help increase the long-term effects of current interventions. The type of booster sessions (i.e., in group formats, via phone, etc.), the length of these sessions, and the most effective timing of the sessions are all critical questions to examine. In addition to increasing the long-term effectiveness of interventions, it is important to identify which elements contained in the programs are most efficacious with adolescents. Future programs need to examine theory-based interventions in order to determine which programmatic elements are most important for different populations of adolescents. Programs for adolescents who are already sexually active should probably contain different elements than programs targeted to adolescents who are not yet sexually active. Although the majority of programs have been developed for early to mid-adolescence, one intriguing program began offering interventions in first grade. The optimal age at which prevention programs should begin in order to engender long-term behavioral change should also be examined. In addition to age differences, adolescents do not constitute a homogeneous group. The factors that motivate one subpopulation to engage in abstinence or to use condoms consistently during sexual intercourse will not necessarily motivate another subgroup. Therefore, developmental research should be undertaken with each targeted group of adolescents prior to the development of any risk-reduction intervention.

Previous research on pregnancy and HIV/STD prevention programs has suggested several programmatic elements that should be considered in developing new programs. Those programs that combine education with specific skill-building exercises are effective in encouraging behavioral changes. These programs appear to need at least 10–12 contact hours to facilitate actual changes in behaviors. These programs appear to be effective in increasing the use of condoms or other contraception but not as successful in encouraging abstinence. Few programs have incorporated parent interventions, but this component may well be an important addition, particularly for younger teens, as parental attitudes and communications appear to influence teens' behavior. Clearly, peer attitudes and behaviors are an important influence on adolescent behavior. As adolescents begin to develop romantic and sexual relationships, it may be helpful to present information and skills-based activities to both members of couples. Little research has been done examining how intervening with both members of a couple may modify risky sexual behaviors. However, given the difficulty of convincing a partner to practice consistently safer sex, providing an intervention simultaneously may help encourage behavior change.

Future programs must also include a systematic evaluation component that is comprehensive, that assesses specific risk-related behaviors, and that provides for long-term follow-up assessments. Previous research has shown that high levels of knowledge, positive attitudes, and positive intentions do not necessarily translate into behavioral changes. If programs do not include a behavioral evaluation component, investigators run the risk of concluding that the programs are successful when they may not necessarily increase the actual desired behaviors. As much as possible, studies should attempt to use reliable and valid instruments to ensure that the results are meaningful. In addition, similar measures or behaviors should be used across studies. Currently, such a wide variation exists among the behaviors being measured and the types of questionnaires utilized that it impossible to compare results across studies.

REFERENCES

Abma, J. C., Chancra, A., Mosher, W. D., Peterson, L. S., & Piccinino, L. J. (1997). Fertility, family planning and women's health: New data from the 1995 national survey of family growth. National Center for Health Statistics. *Vital Health Statistics, 23*(19), 5–9.

Alan Guttmacher Institute. (2000). *Fact sheet: Contraceptive use*. New York: Author.

Alan Guttmacher Institute. (2002). *Teenage sexual and reproductive behavior in developed countries: Can more progress be made?* New York: Author.

Beal, A. C., Ausiello, J., & Perrin, J. M. (2001). Social influences on health-risk behaviors among minority middle school students. *Journal of Adolescent Health, 28*, 474–480.

Biglan, A., Noell, J., Ochs, L., Smolkowski, K., & Metzler, C. (1995). Does sexual coercion play a role in the high-risk sexual behavior of adolescent and young adult women? *Journal of Behavioral Medicine, 18*, 549–568.

Brooks-Gunn, J., & Furstenberg, F., Jr. (1989). Adolescent sexual behavior. *American Psychologist, 44*, 249–257.

Cates, W. (2001). The NIH condom report: The glass is 90% full. *Family Planning Perspectives, 33*, 231–233.

Centers for Disease Control and Prevention. (1993). *HIV/AIDS surveillance report* (Vol. 1, no. 22). Atlanta, GA: Author.

Centers for Disease Control and Prevention. (1996). Youth Risk Behavior Surveillance System—United States. *Morbidity and Mortality Weekly Report, 45*(No. SS-4), 1–86.

Centers for Disease Control and Prevention. (1998). Trends in sexual risk behaviors among high school students—United States, 1991–1997. *Morbidity and Mortality Weekly Report, 47*, 749–752.

Centers for Disease Control and Prevention. (2000). *HIV/AIDS surveillance report*. Atlanta, GA: Author.

Centers for Disease Control and Prevention. (2002). Teenage births in the United States: State trends, 1991–2000, an update. *National Vital Statistics Record, 50*(9), 1120–1124.

Chewning, B., Mosena, P., Wilson, D., Erdman, H., Potthoff, S., Murphy, A., & Kuhnen, K. K. (1999). Evaluation of a computerized contraceptive decision aid for adolescent patients. *Patient Education and Counseling, 38*, 227–239.

Christopher, F. S., & Roosa, M. W. (1990). An evaluation of an adolescent pregnancy prevention program: Is "just say no" enough? *Family Relations, 39*, 68–72.

Civic, D. (2000). College students' reasons for nonuse of condoms within dating relationships. *Journal of Sex and Marital Therapy, 26*, 95–105.

Crosby, R. A., & Yarber, W. L. (2001). Perceived versus actual knowledge about correct condom use among U. S. adolescents: Results from a national study. *Journal of Adolescent Health*, 128, 415–420.

Donnelly, J., Duncan, D. F., Goldfarb, E., & Eadie, C. (1999). Sexuality attitudes and behaviors of self-described very religious urban students in middle school. *Psychological Reports, 85*, 607–610.

Elkind, D. (1967). Egocentrism in adolescence. *Child Development, 38*, 1025–1034.

Fisher, J. D., & Fisher, W. A. (1992). Changing AIDS-risk behavior. Psychological Bulletin, 111, 455–474.

Glei, D. A. (1999). Measuring contraceptive use patterns among teenage and adult women, *Family Planning Perspectives, 31*, 73–80.

Harlap, S., Kost, K., & Forrest, J. D. (1991). *Preventing pregnancy, protecting health: A new look at birth control choices in the United States*. New York: Alan Guttmacher Institute.

Hawkins, J. D., Catalano, R. F., Kosterman, R., Abbott, R., & Hill, K. G. (1999). Preventing adolescent health-risk behaviors by strengthening protection during childhood. *Archives of Pediatrics and Adolescent Medicine, 153*, 226–234.

Holder, D. W., Durant, R. H., Harris, T. L., Daniel, J. H., Obeidallah, D., & Goodman, E. (2000). The association between adolescent spirituality and voluntary sexual activity. *Journal of Adolescent Health, 26,* 295–302.

Horan, P. F., Phillips, J., & Hagan, N. E. (1998). The meaning of abstinence for college students. *Journal of HIV Prevention and Education for Adolescents and Children, 2,* 51–66.

Hubbard, B. M., Giese, M. L., & Rainey, J. (1998). A replication study of Reducing the Risk: A theory-based sexuality curriculum for adolescents. *Journal of School Health, 68,* 243–247.

Huszti, H. C., Clopton, J. R., & Mason, P. J. (1989). Effects of an AIDS educational program on adolescents' knowledge and attitudes. *Pediatrics, 84,* 986–994.

Jemmott, J. B., Jemmott, L. S., & Fong, G. T. (1998). Abstinence and safer sex HIV risk-reduction interventions for African American adolescents: A randomized controlled trial. *Journal of the American Medical Association, 279,* 1529–1536.

Karofsky, P. S., Zeng, L., & Kosorok, M. R. (2000). Relationship between adolescent–parental communication and initiation of first intercourse by adolescents. *Journal of Adolescent Health, 28,* 41–45.

Kegeles, S. M., Hays, R. B., Pollack, L. M., & Coates, T. J. (1999). Mobilizing young gay and bisexual men for HIV prevention: A two-community study. *AIDS, 12,* 1753–1762.

Kirby, D. (2001). *Emerging answers: Research findings on programs to reduce teen pregnancy* [summary]. Washington, DC: National Campaign to Prevent Teen Pregnancy.

Kirby, D., Barth, R. P., Leland, N., & Fetro, J. V. (1991). Reducing the risk: Impact of a new curriculum on sexual risk-taking. *Family Planning Perspectives, 23,* 253–263.

Kirby, D., Korpi, M., Barth, R. P., & Cagampang, H. H. (1997). The impact of postponing sexual involvement curriculum among youths in California. *Family Planning Perspectives, 29,* 100–108.

Koyle, P., Jensen, L., Olsen, J., & Cundick, B. (1989). Comparison of sexual behaviors among adolescents having an early, middle, and late first intercourse experience. *Youth and Society, 20,* 461–475.

Li, X., Stanton, B., Cottrell, L., Burns, J., Pack, R., & Kaljee, L. (2000). Patterns of initiation of sex and drug-related activities among urban low-income African-American adolescents. *Journal of Adolescent Health, 28,* 46–54.

Lieberman, L. D., Gray, H., Wier, M., Fiorentino, R., & Mahoney, P. (2000). Long-term outcomes of an abstinence-based, small-group pregnancy prevention program in New York City schools. *Family Planning Perspectives, 32,* 237–245.

Main, D. S., Iverson, D. C., McGloin, J., Banspach, S. W., Collins, J. L., Rugg, D. L., & Kolbe, L. J. (1994). Preventing HIV infection among adolescents: Evaluation of a school-based education program. *Preventive Medicine, 23,* 409–417.

Miller, B., McCoy, J., Olsen, T., & Wallace, C. (1986). Parental discipline and control attempts in relation to adolescent sexual attitudes and behavior. *Journal of Marriage and the Family, 48,* 503–512.

Miller, B. C., Forehand, R., & Kotchick, B. A. (2000). Adolescent sexual behavior in two ethnic minority samples: A multi-system perspective. *Adolescence, 35,* 313–333.

Miller, B. C., Norton, M. C., Fan, X., & Christopherson, C. R. (1998). Pubertal development, parental communication, and sexual values in relation to adolescent sexual behaviors. *Journal of Early Adolescence, 18,* 27–52.

Miller, W. R., & Rollnick, S. (2002). *Motivational interviewing: Preparing people for change* (2nd ed.). New York: Guilford Press.

Misovich, S. J., Fisher, J. D., & Fisher, W. A. (1997). Close relationships and elevated HIV risk behavior: Evidence and possible underlying psychological processes. *Review of General Psychology, 1,* 72–107.

Moore K. A., Driscoll, A., & Lindberg, L. D. (1998). *A statistical portrait of adolescent sex, contraception, and childbearing,* Washington, DC: National Campaign to Prevent Teen Pregnancy.

National Campaign to Prevent Teen Pregnancy. (2002). *Halfway there: A prescription for progress in preventing teen pregnancy.* Washington, DC: Author.

National Institute of Allergy and Infectious Diseases. (2001). *Workshop summary: Scientific evidence on condom effectiveness for sexually transmitted disease (STD) prevention.* Washington, DC: Author.

Ohannessian, C., & Crockett, L. (1993). A longitudinal investigation of the relationship between educational investment and adolescent sexual activity. *Journal of Adolescent Research, 8,* 167–182.

Overby, K. J., Lo, B., & Litt, I. F. (1989). Knowledge and concerns about acquired immunodeficiency syndrome and their relationship to behaviors among adolescents with hemophilia. *Pediatrics, 83,* 204–210.

Remafedi, G. (1998). The University of Minnesota youth and AIDS projects' adolescent early intervention program: A model to link HIV-seropositive youth with care. *Journal of Adolescent Health, 23,* 115–121.

Remafedi, G., Resnick, M., Blum, R., & Harris, L. (1992). Demography of sexual orientation in adolescents. *Pediatrics, 89,* 714–721.

Robinson, K. L., Telljohann, S. K., & Price, J. H. (1999). Predictors of sixth graders engaging in sexual intercourse. *Journal of School Health, 69*(9), 369–375.

Roche, J. P., & Ramsbay, T. W. (1993). Premarital sexuality: A five-year follow-up of attitudes and behavior by dating stage. *Adolescence, 28,* 67–80.

Rodgers, K. B. (1999). Parenting processes related to sexual risk-taking behaviors of adolescent males and females. *Journal of Marriage and Family Therapy, 61*, 99–109.

Roosa, M. W., Tein, J. Y., Reinholtz, C., & Angelini, P. J. (1997). The relationship of childhood sexual abuse to teenage pregnancy. *Journal of Marriage and the Family, 59*, 119–130.

Rosenthal, S. L., Cohen, S. S., DeVillis, R. F., Biro, F. M., Lewis, L. M., Succop, P. A., & Stanberry, L. R. (1999). Locus of control for general health and STD acquisition among adolescent girls. *Sexually Transmitted Diseases, 26*, 472–475.

Rosenthal, S. L., VonRanson, K. M., Cotton, S., Biro, F. M., Mills, L., Succop, P. A. (2001). Sexual initiation: Predictors and developmental trends. *Sexually Transmitted Disease, 28*, 527–532.

Rotheram-Borus, M. J., Gwadz, M., Fernandez, I., & Srinivasan, S. (1998). Timing of HIV interventions on reductions in sexual risk among adolescents. *American Journal of Community Psychology, 26*, 73–96.

Rotheram-Borus, M. J., Koopman, C., Haignere, C., & Davies, M. (1991). Reducing HIV sexual risk behaviors among runaway adolescents. *Journal of the American Medical Association, 266*, 1237–1241.

Rotheram-Borus, M. J., Murphy, D. A., Fernandez, I., & Srinivasan, S. (1998). A brief intervention for adolescents and young adults. *American Journal of Orthopsychiatry, 68*, 553–564.

St. Lawrence, J. S., Brasfield, T. L., Jefferson, K. W., Alleyne, E., O'Bannon, R. E., & Shirley, A. (1995). Cognitive-behavioral intervention to reduce African-American adolescents' risk for HIV infection. *Journal of Consulting and Clinical Psychology, 63*, 221–237.

Santelli, J. S., Lindberg, L. D., Abma, J., McNeely, C. S., & Resnick, M. (2000). Adolescent sexual behavior: Estimates and trends from four nationally representative surveys. *Family Planning Perspectives, 32*, 156–165, 194.

Santelli, J. S., Robin, L., Brener, N. D., & Lowry, R. (2001). Timing of alcohol and other drug use and sexual risk behaviors among unmarried adolescents and young adults. *Family Planning Perspectives, 33*, 200–205.

Scaramella, L. V., Conger, R. D., Simons, R. L., & Whitbeck, L. B. (1998). Predicting risk for pregnancy by late adolescence: A social contextual perspective. *Developmental Psychology, 34*, 1233–1245.

Shrier, L. A., Ancheta, R., Goodman, E., Chiou, V. M., Lyden, M. R., & Emans, S. J. (2001). Randomized controlled trial of a safer sex intervention for high-risk adolescent girls. *Archives of Pediatrics and Adolescent Medicine, 155*, 73–79.

Shrier, L. A., Harris, S. K., Sternberg, M., & Beardslee, W. R. (2001). Associations of depression, self-esteem and substance use with sexual risk among adolescents. *Preventative Medicine, 33*, 179–189.

Stanton, B. F., Li, X., Ricardo, I., Galbraith, J., Feigelman, S., & Kaljee, L. (1996). A randomized, controlled effectiveness trial of an AIDS prevention program for low-income African-American youths. *Archives of Pediatrics and Adolescent Medicine, 150*, 363–372.

Tapert, S. F., Aarons, G. A., Sedlar, G. R., & Brown, S. A. (2001). Adolescent substance use and sexual risk-taking behavior. *Journal of Adolescent Health, 28*, 181–189.

Tubman, J. G., Windle, M., & Windle, R. C. (1996). Cumulative sexual intercourse patterns among middle adolescents: Problem behavior precursors and concurrent health risk behaviors. *Journal of Adolescent Health, 18*, 182–191.

Upchurch, D. M., Aneshensel, C. S., Sucoff, C. A., & Levy-Storms, L. (1999). Neighborhood and family contexts of adolescent sexual activity. *Journal of Marriage and the Family, 61*, 920–933.

Whaley, A. L. (1999). Preventing the high risk sexual behavior of adolescents: Focus on HIV/AIDS transmission, unintended pregnancy or both? *Journal of Adolescent Health, 24*, 376–382.

Whitaker, D. J., Miller, K. S., & Clark, L. F. (2000). Reconceptualizing adolescent sexual behavior: Beyond did they or didn't they. *Family Planning Perspectives, 32*, 111–117.

Yates, G. L., Mackenzie, R., Pennbridge, J., & Cohen, E. (1988). A risk profile of runaway and non-runaway youth. *American Journal of Public Health, 78*, 820–821.

Part V

EMERGING ISSUES

40

Racial and Ethnic Health Disparity and Access to Care

RONALD T. BROWN
BERNARD FUEMMELER
ESTHER FORTI

Racial and ethnic health disparities refer to the inequality or differences in amount and quality of health care accorded to various racial and ethnic groups. In this chapter we expand the discussion of health disparity to also include demographic shifts in health status, patterns in access to care, health care utilization, differences in disease prevalence, and behaviors related to disease prevention and health promotion among various racial and ethnic groups.

DEMOGRAPHIC SHIFTS IN HEALTH STATUS

Racial and ethnic minorities currently constitute approximately one-fourth of the population in the United States. By the year 2050, this number is expected to increase to nearly 50% (U.S. Bureau of the Census, 2000). A growing body of literature has provided compelling evidence to indicate that racial and ethnic minorities are at greater risk for morbidity and mortality with a number of chronic illnesses, particularly those associated with behavioral and social factors (e.g., cardiovascular disease, cancer; Kaplan, Everson, & Lynch, 2000). This shift in demographics within the nation's population, coupled with the disparities in morbidity and mortality across ethnic groups, constitutes a major challenge in pediatric public health care. Correspondingly, important federal initiatives have been launched to reduce these racial and ethnic disparities in health (U.S. Department of Health and Human Services, 1998a).

ACCESS TO CARE PATTERNS

A number of explanations have been offered for the persisting and increasing racial and ethnic disparities in health. For instance, lower socioeconomic status and the lack of access to quality health care are considered to be primary contributing factors in racial and ethnic disparities (Giachello & Arrom, 1997). Poor education and insufficient economic resources limit access to health insurance, connection to health care systems, and quality medical care, which further limit health promotion and disease prevention. Moreover, for ethnic and racial minorities and vulnerable populations, environmental risks (e.g., crowded living conditions and substandard housing) also may be risk factors for poor health. Notwithstanding these aforementioned risk factors, it is equally likely that the broader social, cultural, and political climate may influence racial and ethnic disparities in health. Societal racism, discrimination, and a dearth of culturally competent care within most of our health care system also contribute to this state of affairs (Giachello & Arrom, 1997).

HEALTH CARE UTILIZATION PATTERNS

Relative to their Caucasian counterparts, individuals from racial and ethnic minority groups generally are reported to have fewer visits to health care providers for ambulatory care, fewer screenings for cancer, fewer immunizations, and a higher frequency of hospitalizations (Health Care Financing Administration, 1995). Of interest are the findings that these individuals also wait longer to seek necessary medical care, present with a greater frequency of acute medical health problems, and tend to use more "home remedies" as a first response to illness. Furthermore, underreporting and denial of discomfort are frequent means of coping behavior for some minority and ethnic groups (Wilson, Rodrigue, & Taylor, 1997).

Racial and ethnic health disparities have only recently been addressed among pediatric populations. Unfortunately, limited epidemiological data are available on the health status and access to care of minority youth populations (Giachello & Arrom, 1997). In fact, children and adolescents have been underrepresented in clinical, biomedical, and health services research (Lohr, Dougherty, & Simpson, 2001). The primary purpose of this chapter is to summarize the extant literature on racial and ethnic disparities in pediatric health conditions and access to health care. Recognition of these disparities will provide direction for future practice, policy, and research within the field of pediatric psychology. The chapter provides an in-depth review of the putative factors associated with racial and ethnic health disparities specific to pediatric populations (e.g., immunizations, asthma, oral health, mental health) and tertiary care settings (e.g., psychiatric disorders). This review is followed by a summary in which we present recommendations for practice, policy, and research in pediatric psychology to eliminate health disparities among children and their families.

FACTORS ASSOCIATED WITH HEALTH DISPARITIES IN PEDIATRIC POPULATIONS

Biological Factors

Although certain diseases are associated with specific ethnic groups (e.g., higher prevalence of sickle cell disease among African Americans), findings from the Human Genome Study have revealed that genetic differences account for only a small percentage of the variance in health outcomes among major racial and ethnic groups (Lewontin, 1982). For some ethnic and racial groups, evidence suggests a higher incidence of certain health conditions, including hypertension and cancer among African Americans, pancreatic and stomach cancers among Hispanic women, and a higher incidence of strokes among Asian Americans (Wingood & Keltner, 1999). Although genetics cannot entirely explain this phenomenon, it appears that many of these conditions are familial among specific racial and ethnic groups. It is likely that social and behavioral pathways also influence these conditions. In support of this notion, some have observed that social and behavioral conditions interact synergistically with biological predispositions, possibly resulting in the occurrence of specific diseases among various ethnic groups (Thompson & Gustafson, 1996).

Socioeconomic Factors

Socioeconomic status represents a cluster of variables including education, occupation, and income, that serve as indicators of an individual's position within a social system (House & Williams, 2000). Socioeconomic and cultural factors have been demonstrated to be salient determinants of health outcome, with health outcome being positively associated with socioeconomic standing (Wingood & Keltner, 1999). Specifically, socioeconomic status affects health care outcomes, as it limits access to preventive health care due to factors such as poor or no insurance coverage, exposure to less optimal environmental conditions (e.g., lead exposure, pollutants, and toxic wastes), and greater occupational hazards (e.g., disadvantaged individuals are more likely to perform manual labor, in which there is greater risk of injury). Furthermore, children from less affluent families have decreased access to quality health care and evidence-based diagnostic and treatment procedures (Wingood & Keltner, 1999). Finally, evidence exists that children from more rural areas have less access to medical care, placing them at greater risk for poor health outcome (Brown, Ojeda, Wynn, & Levan, 2000). Notably, however, a majority of studies that have controlled for socioeconomic status as a predictor of health outcome reveal that these differences between racial and ethnic groups diminish (House & Williams, 2000). Nevertheless, some differences still remain, thereby suggesting that, although social class may account for some of the variance in health outcome, other factors may also have an impact.

Psychosocial Systems

Psychosocial systems include the family and its social network, community norms regarding health behaviors, cultural practices, societal attitudes regarding ethnic and racial diversity, and the health care system. Regarding familial influences on health outcome, it has been demonstrated that families are important to children's adoption of health practices and behaviors (Brown, 2002). For example, the family plays an important role in dietary habits and physical activity. Moreover, when children are confronted with an illness, the family is a critical factor in facilitating adaptation and social support, variables that are crucial to adherence with treatment regimens, adjustment, and quality of life (Kazak, Segal-Andrews, & Johnson, 1995).

The community has been found to be influential in the practice of health behaviors. One example is social marketing practices that are targeted toward specific ethnic communities. Alcohol and tobacco products have been notoriously recognized as being targeted toward communities with a higher percentage of African American and Latino individuals. In one investigation, Moore, Williams, and Qualls (1996) examined whether the targeting of alcohol and tobacco products for advertisement actually increased alcohol and tobacco consumption. Findings revealed that younger African Americans consumed alcohol and tobacco at lower rates than did their Caucasian counterparts, although as the African Americans increased in age, these rates surpassed those of Caucasians. Another microcosm of the community is the school setting, in which health practices among students may be supported, taught, and reinforced. For example, schools that provide messages of smoking prevention in combination with health education are apt to produce behaviors that are compatible with good health (Flay et al., 1995).

Finally, the health care system in this country does not necessarily reflect the diversity of cultures of individuals who are the recipients of health care. Stated more simply, the United States health care system typically reflects white middle-class values (Giachello & Arrom, 1997). Examples of this scenario within health care systems include the failure to provide for bilingual services in most medical centers, the lack of cultural sensitivity among some health care providers, and a shortage of minority providers. Frequently, stereotypes of racial and ethnic groups may impede the relationship among consumers (i.e., the patients) and health care providers.

Health Risk Behaviors

Another major area associated with persisting disparities in health includes those behavioral practices by specific ethnic and racial groups that may result in disease. These behaviors include tobacco use, substance use, dietary practices, and physical inactivity. Although these behaviors place individuals at increased risk for disease morbidity and mortality, they are not necessarily the single contributor to disease. Rather, behaviors interact with other factors, such as lack of access to health care, and ultimately result in poor health and disease.

Tobacco

Use of tobacco is a leading cause of a number of diseases, including cancer and cardiovascular disease (U.S. Department of Health and Human Services, 2000). Specific ethnic and racial groups are at increased risk for morbidity and mortality associated with these diseases. Although the 1970s and 1980s witnessed a decrease in smoking among most adolescents, there has been particular concern regarding the increase in smoking behaviors among adolescents who are African American and Hispanic (U.S. Department of Health and Human Services, 1998b). For example, rates of smoking among African American youths have increased 80% relative to the decrease among Caucasian adolescents, thereby placing African American youths at greater risk for specific types of cancer and cardiovascular disease. Of even greater concern are findings that these smoking behaviors persist into adulthood and that African Americans are less likely to cease smoking during adulthood than their Caucasian counterparts are (Centers for Disease Control and Prevention, 1998).

Alcohol and Substance Use

With regard to alcohol and substance abuse, the corpus of literature generally suggests no racial and ethnic differences with regard to abuse of and dependence on any types of substances. In fact, in a comprehensive review of the literature, Kandel (1995) concluded that Caucasians actually report higher rates of alcohol abuse and dependence than do other racial and ethnic groups. Similar trends have been reported for drug substances (Schumacher

& Milby, 1999). This trend is also found among adolescent populations, with African American youths reporting substantially lower current and binge drinking than Caucasian and Hispanic youths (Centers for Disease Control and Prevention, 2000). Moreover, of those substances previously abused more frequently among more affluent individuals, such as cocaine and opiates, recent data suggest that cocaine use has shifted to include lower socioeconomic groups residing in urban areas, largely due to the easier access more disadvantaged groups now have to these substances (Schumacher & Milby, 1999).

Dietary Practice

National surveys of health and nutrition have revealed that a substantial proportion of the population in this country across all ages are overweight (Centers for Disease Control and Prevention, 2000; National Center for Health Statistics, 1997). Women of minority racial and ethnic groups are at greater risk for being overweight than Caucasian women (52% of African Americans, 50% of Hispanics, and 34% of Caucasians). However, few differences have been found between minority ethnic and racial groups and their Caucasian counterparts in the prevalence of obesity among infants and young children. Thus these data have been interpreted to suggest that racial differences in dietary practices that result in adult obesity occur during preadolescence and adolescent years (Spear & Reinold, 1999). A study by McNutt et al., 1997, found that 9- to 14-year-old schoolgirls who were African American engaged in a greater frequency of dietary practices associated with weight gain (e.g., consuming foods high in fat content and calories) than a comparison group of Caucasian children. It is possible that cultural beliefs about diet and weight shape these health-compromising behaviors. For instance, investigators have demonstrated that African American adolescent females have a higher preferred weight and are more tolerant of obesity in their partners than are young Caucasian females (Kumanyika, Wilson, & Guilford-Davenport, 1993; McNutt et al., 1997).

Physical Activity

Multiple health benefits are associated with physical activity (e.g., prevention of hypertension, Type II diabetes, heart disease, depression, osteoperosis; Harris, Caspersen, DeFriese, & Estes, 1989). Physical inactivity is a significant risk factor in the development of cardiovascular disease and other health problems and is equally comparable to other risk factors, such as smoking, hypertension, and hyperlipidemia. Caspersen and Merritt (1995) have reported that over one-half of the nation's population is physically inactive or does not engage in regular physical activity. Although physical inactivity does not necessarily appear to be a pressing problem among young children, physical activity levels declines during adolescence (Centers for Disease Control and Prevention, 2000). Among adolescents, physical inactivity also has been associated with health-compromising behaviors (Pate, Heath, Dowda, & Trost, 1996). This inactivity is of particular concern during adolescence, as it is likely to persist during the adult years, placing young people at particular risk for later health problems.

Regarding activity practices among specific racial and ethnic groups, epidemiological data indicate that women who are African American are less physically active than their Caucasian counterparts (Sanderson & Taylor, 1999). Similarly, Mexican American men and women have been reported to be less active than whites (Crespo, Keteyian, Heath, & Sempos, 2000). Among adolescents, similar racial and ethnic patterns of inactivity have been noted. In particular, students who are Caucasian are more likely to engage in moderate or vigorous activity than students who are Hispanic and African American (Centers for Disease Control and Prevention, 2000).

Taken together, the data suggest that individuals from ethnic and racial minority groups evidence greater health-compromising behaviors than do individuals who are Caucasian. These behaviors include more smoking, poorer dietary practices, and less physical activity. In pediatric populations, the patterns of health-compromising behaviors are less clear, although they begin to emerge at adolescence. This finding is of particular concern for minority populations.

Economic Influences

A greater number of minorities are apt to have fewer economic resources relative to nonminority individuals (Children's Defense Fund, 1990; Mendoza, 1994). These economic inadequacies coupled with a lack of education regarding health promotion, interact to sufficiently limit the opportunities of minority individuals to attain those health outcomes commensurate with their more affluent Caucasian counterparts. Simply put, insufficient economic resources severely limit insurance coverage and relegate these individuals to either a lower standard of care or health care that is less accessible relative to those from more affluent populations. It has been well documented that individuals from racial and ethnic minorities do not have appropriate insurance coverage relative to nonminority groups (Aguilera, 1992). As Giachello and Arrom (1997) have astutely observed, the lack of health care coverage is one of the most salient difficulties that minority children encounter in the health care arena. Specifically, lack of insurance limits the array of opportunities for both health promotion and delivery of care.

Regular or usual sources of care refer to an established clinical facility that an individual uses on a routine basis, mainly for primary care services (Giachello & Arrom, 1997). Data have revealed that, even when taking into account differences in insurance coverage and income, minority children are less likely to have a usual source of primary care at an identified private practice or clinic setting (Newacheck, Hughs, & Stoddard, 1996). Minority children are also less likely to receive the care of a physician, even when they have symptoms that require the attention of a health care provider.

HEALTH DISPARITIES FOR PRIMARY AND TERTIARY CARE POPULATIONS

In this chapter we choose to discuss four topical areas to illustrate the issues of health disparities among pediatric populations: immunizations, oral health, asthma, and mental health. Our rationale for choosing these specific topical areas is that they are health issues relevant for all children, with the possible exception of asthma, although this is a pervasive childhood chronic illness.

Immunizations

Significant disparities have been demonstrated in immunization patterns among minority children and those from lower-social-class backgrounds. Wood et al. (1995) found that, among low-income children, nearly one-half of African American children and 30% of Latino children had not received all major vaccinations during infancy. More alarming is that by the age of 2 years, 75% of African American children and more than one-half of Latino children were not up-to-date with immunizations (Wood et al., 1995). Similar disparities in both ethnic and racial immunization rates have been revealed in 28 urban areas within this country. Fortunately, however, immunization rates for minority children have been observed to increase, with one investigation documenting that 90% of the children in the survey had received appropriate immunizations (Centers for Disease Control and Prevention, 1997). Further, this study revealed that the disparities in immunization rates among Caucasian, African American, and Hispanic children had significantly narrowed. Some experts (Moore, Fenlon, & Hepworth, 1996; Wood et al., 1995) have concluded that these disparities are due to insurance status and family characteristics rather than race or ethnicity. Not surprisingly, children residing in inner-city urban areas received fewer immunizations relative to their more economically advantaged peers. Clearly, public health programs designed to increase immunization rates among children from lower income backgrounds, in which minorities are overrepresented, have demonstrated significant impact in increasing immunizations (Centers for Disease Control and Prevention, 1997).

Asthma

Asthma has been found to be slightly more prevalent among African American children than among white children (Centers for Disease Control and Prevention, 1994). Additionally, African American children with asthma have greater disease morbidity and more frequent hospitalizations than Caucasian children (Centers for Disease Control and Prevention, 1994; Taylor & Newacheck, 1992). Some experts have attributed these disparities in morbidity to the existence of differential patterns of health care for children who are minorities. For example, nonwhite children show longer clinic waiting times, fewer visits to the doctor, and more utilization of the emergency room for primary care services (Moore & Hepworth, 1994; Wood, Hayward, Corey, Freeman, & Shapiro, 1990). Patterns of care for minority children with asthma echo those patterns observed among African American adults with asthma. That is, similar to adults, children are more likely to make emergency room visits for care and are less apt to receive primary care services for the management of their asthma (Lozano, Connell, & Koepsell, 1995). In further support of this notion, one study revealed that African American children enrolled in the Medicaid program who had been hospitalized for asthma made significantly fewer primary care visits following hospitalization relative to their Caucasian counterparts, even after adjusting for socioeconomic status.

Disparities in asthma morbidity have also been attributed to the higher likelihood of exposure to environmental conditions that may exacerbate asthma symptoms. For instance, smoke, dust, mold, and dander may be very difficult to control or contain in more crowded living environments within the inner city (Creer & Bender, 1995). Additionally, issues such as familial discord and patient nonadherence that contribute to difficulties in managing the disease tend to occur more frequently among lower socioeconomic status families for whom multiple stressors exist (Creer & Bender, 1995).

Oral Health

Oral diseases such as dental decay among pediatric populations remain one of the most prevalent health problems in this country (U.S. Department of Health and Human Services, 1991). Among children from low-income backgrounds, dental decay is frequently untreated, resulting in pain, failure to digest food properly, and poor appearance. For example, among children who are African American and Hispanic, oral caries were more frequent than among their Caucasian counterparts (Kaste et al., 1996). More important, a greater number of minority children, particularly those from less affluent backgrounds, are less likely to receive appropriate dental care for cavities (U.S. Department of Health and Human Services, 1991). Poor dental hygiene, resulting in halitosis and missing teeth, may be associated with a negative self-image that results in diminished self-competence (Cohen & Gift, 1995). This can be particularly critical to children and adolescents, for whom appearance plays an important role in social acceptance.

Unlike some chronic conditions, oral diseases and dysfunction are preventable through comprehensive oral health care delivery systems. Underserved communities comprising children from lower socioeconomic backgrounds frequently lack access to prophylactic oral hygiene and behaviors that are compatible with good oral health care (e.g., adequate mouth care, healthy dietary choices, tobacco use cessation, restriction of heavy alcohol use; U.S. Department of Health and Human Services, 1991). Given the strong association between oral health and general physical well-being and quality of life, the promotion of oral health among children seems a prudent investment in the public health of our nation's children.

Mental Health

Consistent with the literature on other chronic diseases, it is important to understand racial, ethnic, and demographic disparities in the identification and management of psychiatric disorders. The corpus of adult psychiatric literature reveals clear distinctions in diagnosis of specific disorders, inpatient psychiatric admissions, outpatient services, and pharmacotherapies. For example, research has demonstrated that individuals of African American and Asian descent are more likely to receive a diagnosis of psychosis or organic brain dysfunction than are Hispanic or Caucasian individuals (Chung, Mahler, & Kakuma, 1995; Leo, Narayan, Sherry, Michalek, & Pollock, 1997). In addition, an investigation by Chung et al. (1995) reveals that even after controlling for socioeconomic status, African American individuals are more likely than Caucasians to receive a diagnosis of substance abuse disorder, whereas Caucasian individuals are more likely to receive a diagnosis of a personality disorder. With regard to inpatient mental health services, the highest rates of hospitalization have been found among Native Americans and Alaskan natives (Snowden & Cheung, 1990). In addition, an overrepresentation of inpatient admissions has been observed among African Americans compared with Caucasians and Hispanics (Snowden & Cheung, 1990; Strakowski, Shelton, & Kolbrener, 1993). With regard to outpatient mental health services, mixed findings have been reported. Some studies have noted that African American individuals shower greater utilization of outpatient services (Blank, Tetrick, Brinkley, Smith, & Doheny, 1994) than whites, whereas other researchers have indicated that African Americans underutilize services, particularly when they do not have insurance that covers mental health care (Bui & Takeuchi, 1992). Finally, with regard to pharmacotherapy, compelling evidence suggests that African American individuals are more apt to receive neuroleptic drug therapy than are Caucasians (Collazo, Tam, Sraemek, & Herrera, 1996). Caucasians are more apt to be prescribed antidepressant medication (Chung et al., 1995). Thus, with regard to the adult literature, there is evidence of significant disparity in diagnosis, management, and utilization of mental health services among racial and ethnic groups.

Although the data are scant, the few studies available in the pediatric literature are generally consistent with the adult research. Demographic factors have not been found to predict mental health service utilization after controlling for social class (McCabe et al., 1999;

McKay, Pennington, Lynn, & McCadam, 2001). Nonetheless, African American children have been found to be overrepresented in the child psychiatric population primarily due to diagnostic practices (Scott & Morris, 2000). Some of the literature in the area of foster care is of relevance. For children in foster care, ethnic and racial minorities are frequently overrepresented, among whom studies have revealed that minority children are less likely to receive mental health services than are those who are not from minority groups (Garland et al., 2000). A particularly disturbing fact is that this remains the case even after controlling for the severity of emotional and behavioral problems, suggesting that disparities persist even among children who display significant symptoms (Garland et al., 2000). Interestingly, greater frequencies of neglect and physical abuse have been reported for children and adolescents from ethnic and racial minorities (Cappelleri, Eckenrode, & Powers, 1993). Clearly, additional research must be mounted to determine whether the aforementioned disparities emanate from patterns of referral, accessibility to providers, or cultural issues related to mental-health-seeking behaviors.

There has been recent concern about the ever-shrinking mental health resources for pediatric populations (American Academy of Pediatrics, 2000). Brown and Freeman (2002) have recommended providing mental health services within the primary care setting, particularly for children in underserved areas. In part, this recommendation has come in response to a shortage of pediatric mental health providers, especially in rural and disadvantaged communities (American Academy of Pediatrics, 2000; Brown & Freeman, 2002). In fact, in underserved areas, access to mental health care from providers other than primary care physicians is almost nonexistent. Data from the Great Smoky Mountains Study of Youth, an epidemiological investigation of psychopathology and mental health service use among children, suggest that the major system providing mental health services to children is the educational system. In fact, the school system was the sole provider of mental health services for most children, with 70 to 80% of children receiving services in educational settings (Burns et al., 1995). Clearly, the pediatric primary care setting and school health clinics represent critical venues for the delivery of children's mental health care. Nonetheless, Brown and Freeman (2002) have identified several barriers to the appropriate assessment and management of psychopathology in the primary care setting. These barriers include inadequate training of primary care pediatricians, insufficient resources to manage emotional disturbances in their patients, and unfamiliarity with the nature and benefits of psychological services in the community.

Patient barriers in access to mental health care include lack of resources for travel, time demands due to multiple medical appointments, inadequate cultural competence of physicians, and the stigma associated with the receipt of psychological services. Specifically, negative physician attitudes regarding ethnic and racial minorities have been associated with difficulties in the delivery of psychological services (Brown, 2002).

SUMMARY AND FUTURE DIRECTIONS FOR PRACTICE, POLICY, AND RESEARCH

In review, among racial and ethnic minority populations, as compared with Caucasians, researchers have noted the following: (1) certain disease conditions are familial among specific racial and ethnic groups; (2) health behavior is associated with cultural beliefs; (3) insufficient economic resources that severely limit insurance coverage relegate children and adolescents who are minorities to a lower standard of care or less accessible care; and (4) differential patterns of health care utilization are still in existence.

Several federal initiatives have been launched to address the continued disparities in health among ethnic and vulnerable pediatric populations. For example, the Presidential Initiative on Race calls for a commitment to identify and address health disparities in minority and other vulnerable populations (Satcher, 2000). Healthy People 2010's Goal II focuses on the elimination of health disparities based on race and ethnicity (U.S. Department of Health and Human Services, 1998a). One hundred percent access and zero disparities are the objectives and major drive for programs offered by many federal and state agencies. Eliminating these health disparities among minority youth will necessitate special efforts at promoting health, preventing disease, and delivering culturally appropriate care within the local community setting.

Racial and ethnic minorities are at greater risk for morbidity and mortality for a number of chronic diseases, particularly those associated with behavioral and social factors. Moreover, barriers to health care involve language and communication difficulties, encounters with health care providers who lack knowledge of a child's cultural background, and feelings of isolation among parents (Williams, Yu, Jackson, & Anderson, 1997). All of these aforementioned factors constitute a major challenge in pediatric public health care.

When designing programs and treating diseases, providers cannot assume that what works for majority children will also work similarly for minority children. It is, therefore, important for practitioners who work with children and their families to gain a better understanding of health and culture. Understanding culture and its relationship to service delivery is believed to increase access to, as well as utilization of, services to improve quality of life. This understanding mandates training of health care providers and their staffs in culturally appropriate health care. Many training programs concerning culturally appropriate health care delivery are available.

Increased access to and utilization of appropriate health services can reduce many of the disparities seen in racial and minority children. Racial and ethnic minorities are more likely than Caucasians to be uninsured and poor. A lack of adequate health insurance decreases access to and utilization of preventive and medical services, as well as access to a regular source of care.

Several public programs are available to address this problem. Medicaid acts as a safety net for low-income children. The Children's Health Insurance Program (CHIP) implemented by states with federal matching funds increases the number of children who are eligible for coverage by supporting those families whose incomes are low but above Medicaid level as set by the states (Children's Defense Fund, 2000). The Women, Infants, and Children (WIC) program has been in existence for many years and provides needed resources for women and infants. We recommend that health care providers create and maintain linkages with Medicaid, CHIP, and WIC programs through case management strategies for their pediatric patients and families.

Among pediatric populations, health disparities occur frequently in the areas of health care costs, dissemination of educational prevention programs, and issues related to access and treatment adherence. Policymakers are encouraged to continue advocating for public programs to address health disparities by increasing funding streams for school-based services, including oral health and sexual health, community health promotion intervention programs for youth and families, and provision of low-income primary and specialty services for children through agencies such as federally qualified community health centers.

Future research should be undertaken to determine whether health disparities among children emanate from family cultural issues related to health-seeking behaviors, patterns of referral, culturally appropriate care, or accessibility to providers. A major problem that limits our understanding of the relationship between race, ethnicity, and health is the dearth of quality national and state data sets that enable longitudinal comparisons. According to a report by the Commonwealth Fund (2001), it is essential to collect and report data from existing federal programs and new program initiatives, including block grants, on enrollees by ethnicity, race, and primary language to facilitate the process of closing the gaps in health care. Use of ethnographic techniques, as well as surveys, is highly recommended to identify the family's perceptions about a disease condition and subsequent health practice behavior. These data can be used in formulating appropriate intervention strategies.

In summary, to meet the challenge of an increasingly diverse population and to close the gaps in health among ethnic and racial children, society and pediatric psychologists need to: (1) understand culture and its relationship to health practice; (2) provide access to health care for all Americans through federal programs; (3) collect and report data on health status indicators across race and ethnicity for comparison; (4) provide training in culturally appropriate health care for health and social services providers; and (5) develop strategies to increase the minority health care workforce. Working together as a nation, we can meet the national goal of 100% access and zero disparities in pediatric health care and psychological services delivery to all children and adolescents.

REFERENCES

Aguilera, E. (1992). *Hispanics and health insurance: Vol. I. Status*. Washington, DC: National Council of La Raza and Labor Council for Latin American Advancement.

American Academy of Pediatrics. (2000). Clinical practice guideline: Diagnosis and evaluation of the child with attention-deficit disorder. *Pediatrics, 105,* 1158–1170.

Blank, M. B., Tetrick, F. L., Brinkley, D. F., Smith, H. O., & Doheny, V. (1994). Racial matching and service utilization among seriously mentally ill consumers in the rural south. *Community Mental Health Journal, 30,* 271–281.

Brown, E. R., Ojeda, V. D., Wynn, R., & Levan, R. (2000). *Racial and ethnic disparities in access to health insurance and health care*. Retrieved December 23, 2001, from Los Angeles, CA: University of California, Los Angeles, Center for Health Policy Research website: *http://www.healthpolicy.ucla.edu*

Brown, R. T. (2002). Society of Pediatric Psychology presidential address: Toward a social ecology of pediatric psychology. *Journal of Pediatric Psychology, 27,* 191–201.

Brown, R. T., & Freeman, W. S. (2002). Primary care. In D. Marsh & M. Fristad (Eds.), *Handbook of serious emotional disturbance in children and adolescents* (pp. 428–444). New York: Wiley.

Bui, K. V., & Takeuchi, D. T. (1992). Ethnic minority adolescents and the use of community mental health care services. *American Journal of Community Psychology, 20,* 403–417.

Burns, B. J., Costello, E. J., Angold, A., Tweed, D., Stangl, D., Farmer E. M., & Erkanli, A. (1995). Children's mental health service use across service sectors. *Health Affairs, 14,* 147–159.

Cappelleri, J. C., Eckenrode, J., & Powers, J. L. (1993). The epidemiology of child abuse: Findings from the Second National Incidence and Prevalence Study of Child Abuse and Neglect. *American Journal of Public Health, 83,* 1622–1624.

Caspersen, C. J., & Merritt, R. K. (1995). Physical activity trends among 26 states, 1986–1990. *Medicine and Science in Sports and Exercise. 27,* 713–20.

Centers for Disease Control and Prevention. (1994). *Chronic disease in minority populations*. Atlanta, GA: Author.

Centers for Disease Control and Prevention. (1997). Vaccination coverage by race/ethnicity and poverty among children aged 19–35 months, 1996. *Morbidity and Mortality Weekly Report, 46,* 963–968.

Centers for Disease Control and Prevention. (1998). *Tobacco use among U.S. racial/ethnic minority groups—African Americans, American Indians and Alaska Natives, Asian Americans and Pacific Islanders, and Hispanics: A report of the surgeon general*. Atlanta, GA: Author.

Centers for Disease Control and Prevention. (2000). *Youth risk behavior surveillance: United States, 1999*. Atlanta, GA: Author.

Children's Defense Fund. (1990). *A report card, briefing book, and action primer*. Washington, DC: Author.

Children's Defense Fund. (2000). *The state of America's children*. Washington, DC: Author.

Chung, H., Mahler, J. C., & Kakuma, T. (1995). Racial differences in treatment of psychiatric inpatients. *Psychiatric Services, 46,* 586–591.

Cohen, L., & Gift, H. (1995). *Disease prevention and oral health promotion: Socio-dental sciences in action.* Munksgaard, Copenhagen: Federation Dentaire International.

Collazo, Y., Tam, R., Sraemek, J., & Herrera, J. (1996). Neuroleptic dosing in Hispanic and Asian inpatients with schizophrenia. *Mt. Sinai Journal of Medicine, 63,* 310–313.

Commonwealth Fund. (2001, October). *Lack of racial and ethnic health data hinders efforts to close the gaps in health care: New Release.* New York: Author.

Creer, T. L., & Bender, B. G. (1995). Pediatric asthma. In M. C. Roberts (Ed.), *Handbook of pediatric psychology* (2nd ed., pp. 219–240). New York: Guilford Press.

Crespo, C. J., Keteyian, S. J., Heath, G. W., & Sempos, C. T. (2000). Leisure-time physical activity among US adults: Results from the Third National Health and Nutrition Examination Survey. *Archives of Internal Medicine, 156,* 93–98.

Flay, B. R., Miller, T. Q., Hedeker, D., Siddiqui, O., Britton, C. F., Brannon, B. R., Johnson, C. A., et al. (1995). The television, school, and family smoking prevention and cessation project: VIII. Student outcomes and mediating variables. *Preventive Medicine, 24,* 29–40.

Garland, A. F., Hough, R. L., Landsverk, J. A., McCabe, K. M., Yeh, M., Ganger, W. C., & Reynolds, B. J. (2000). Racial and ethnic variations in mental health care utilization among children in foster care. *Children's Services: Social Policy, Research and Practice, 3,* 133–146.

Giachello, A. L., & Arrom, J. O. (1997). Health service access and utilization among adolescent minorities. In D. K. Wilson, J. R. Rodrigue, & W. C. Taylor (Eds.), *Health-promoting and health compromising behaviors among minority adolescents* (pp. 303–320). Washington, DC: American Psychological Association.

Harris, S. S., Caspersen, C. J., DeFriese, G. H., & Estes, E. H., Jr. (1989). Physical activity counseling for healthy adults as a primary preventive intervention in the clinical setting. *Journal of the American Medical Association, 261,* 3588–3598.

Health Care Financing Administration. (1995). *Summary Report to Congress: Monitoring the impact of medicare physician payment reform on utilization and access.* Baltimore, MD: Author.

House, J. S., & Williams, D. R. (2000). Understanding and reducing socioeconomic and racial /ethnic disparities in health. In B. D. Smedley & S. L. Syme (Eds.), *Promoting health: Intervention strategies from social and behavioral research* (pp. 81–124). Washington, DC: National Academy Press.

Kandel, D. B. (1995). Ethnic differences in drug use: Patterns and paradoxes. In G. Botvin, S. Schinke, & M. Orlandi (Eds.), *Drug abuse prevention with multi-ethnic youth* (pp. 81–104). Newbury Park, CA: Sage.

Kaplan, G. A., Everson, S. A., & Lynch, J. W. (2000). The contribution of social and behavioral research to an understanding of the distribution of disease: A multilevel approach. In B. D. Smedley & S. L. Syme (Eds.), *Promoting health: Intervention strategies from social and behavioral research* (pp. 37–80). Washington, DC: National Academy Press.

Kaste, L. M., Selwitz, R. H., Oldakowski, R. J., Brunelle, J. A., Winn, D. M., & Brown, L. J. (1996). Coronal caries in the primary and permanent dentition of children and adolescents 1–17 years of age: United States, 1988–1991. *Journal of Dental Research, 75,* 696–705.

Kazak, A., Segal-Andrews, A. M., & Johnson, K. (1995). Pediatric psychology research and practice: A family systems approach. In M. C. Roberts (Ed.), *Handbook of pediatric psychology* (2nd ed., pp. 84–104). New York: Guilford Press.

Kumanyika, S., Wilson, J. F., & Guilford-Davenport, M. (1993). Weight-related attitudes and behaviors of black women. *Journal of the American Dietetic Association, 93,* 416–422.

Leo, R. J., Narayan, D. A., Sherry, C., Michalek, C., & Pollock, D. (1997). Geopsychiatric consultation for African-American and Caucasian patients. *General Hospital Psychiatry, 19,* 216–222.

Lewontin, R. (1982). *Human diversity.* New York: Scientific American Books.

Lohr, K. N., Dougherty, D., & Simpson, L. (2001). Methodologic challenges in health services research in the pediatric populations. *Ambulatory Pediatrics, 1,* 36–38.

Lozano, P., Connell, F. A., & Koepsell, T. D. (1995). Use of health services by African American children with asthma on Medicaid. *Journal of the American Medical Association, 274,* 469–473.

McCabe, K., Yeh, M., Hough, R. L., Landsverk, J., Hurlburt, M. S., Culver, S. W., & Reynolds, B. (1999). Racial/ethnic representation across five public sectors of care for youth. *Journal of Emotional and Behavioral Disorders, 7,* 72–82.

McKay, M. M., Pennington, J., Lynn, C. J., & McCadam, K. (2001). Understanding urban child mental health service use: Two studies of child, family and environmental correlates. *Journal of Behavioral Health Services Research, 28,* 475–483.

McNutt, S.W., Hu, Y., Schreiber, G. B., Crawford, P. B., Obarzanek, E., & Mellin, L. (1997). A longitudinal study of the dietary practices of black and white girls 9 and 10 years old at enrollment: The NHLBI Growth and Health Study. *Journal of Adolescent Health, 20,* 27–37.

Mendoza, F. S. (1994). The health of Latino children in the United States. *The Future of Children 3,* 43–72.

Moore, D. J., Williams, J. D., & Qualls, J. W. (1996). Target marketing of tobacco and alcohol-related products to ethnic minority groups in the United States. *Ethnicity and Disease, 6,* 83–98.

Moore, P., Fenlon, N., & Hepworth, J. T. (1996). Indicators of differences in immunization rates of Mexican American and white non-Hispanic infants in a Medicaid managed care system. *Public Health Nursing, 13,* 21–30.

Moore, P., & Hepworth, J. T. (1994). Use of prenatal and infant health services by Mexican-American Medicaid enrollees. *Journal of the American Medical Association, 272,* 297–304.

National Center for Health Statistics. (1997). *Health, United States: 1996–1997 Injury Chartbook*. Hyattsville, MD: Author.

Newacheck, P. W., Hughs, D. C., & Stoddard, J. J. (1996). Children's access to primary care: Differences by race, income, and insurance status. *Pediatrics, 97,* 26–32.

Pate, R. R., Heath, G. W., Dowda, M., & Trost, S. G. (1996). Associations between physical activity and other health behaviors in a representative sample of US adolescents. *American Journal of Public Health, 86,* 1577–1581.

Sanderson, B. K., & Taylor, H. A., Jr. (1999). Physical activity. In J. M. Raczynski & R. J. DiClemente (Eds.), *Handbook of health promotion and disease prevention* (pp. 191–206). New York: Kluwer Academic/Plenum.

Satcher, D. (2000). Eliminating racial and ethnic disparities: The role of the ten leading health indicators. *Journal of the National Medical Association,92,* 315–318.

Schumacher, J. E., & Milby, J. B. (1999). Alcohol and drug abuse. In J. M. Raczynski & R. J. DiClemente (Eds.), *Handbook of health promotion and disease prevention* (pp. 207–230). New York: Kluwer Academic/ Plenum.

Scott, J. R., & Morris, T. L. (2000). Diagnosis and classification. In M. Hersen & R. T. Ammerman (Eds.), *Advanced abnormal child psychology* (2nd ed., pp. 15–32). Mahwah, NJ: Erlbaum.

Snowden, L. R., & Cheung, F. K. (1990). Use of inpatient mental health services by members of ethnic minority groups. *American Psychologist, 45,* 347–355.

Spear, B. A., & Reinold, C. (1999). Obesity and nutrition. In J. M. Raczynski & R. J. DiClemente (Eds.), *Handbook of health promotion and disease prevention* (pp. 171–190). New York: Kluwer Academic/Plenum.

Strakowski, S. M., Shelton, R. C., & Kolbrener, M. L. (1993). The effects of race and comorbidity on clinical diagnosis in patients with psychosis. *Journal of Clinical Psychiatry, 54,* 96–102.

Taylor, W. R., & Newacheck, P. W. (1992). Impact of childhood asthma on health. *Pediatrics, 90,* 657–662.

Thompson, R. J., Jr., & Gustafson, K. E. (1996). *Adaptation to chronic childhood illness*. Washington, DC: American Psychological Association.

U.S. Bureau of the Census. (2000). Population projections of the United States by age, sex, race, and Hispanic origin: 1995–2050. *Current Population Reports, 10,* 1125–1130.

U.S. Department of Health and Human Services. (1991). *Healthy People 2000: National health promotion and disease prevention objectives* (DHHS Publication No. PHS 91-50212). Washington, DC: U.S. Government Printing Office.

U.S. Department of Health and Human Services. (1998a). Report on health disparities. *Public Health Reports,* 113, 372–375.

U.S. Department of Health and Human Services. (1998b). *Tobacco use among U.S. racial/ethnic minority groups: A report of the surgeon general.* Atlanta, GA: Centers for Disease Control and Prevention.

U.S. Department of Health and Human Services. (2000). *Reducing tobacco use: A report of the surgeon general.* Atlanta, GA: Centers for Disease Control and Prevention, National Center for Chronic Disease Prevention and Health Promotion, Office on Smoking and Health.

Williams, D. R., Yu, Y., Jackson, J. S., & Anderson, N. B. (1997). Racial differences in physical and mental health: Socioeconomic status, stress and discrimination. *Journal of Health Psychology, 2,* 335–351.

Wilson, D. K., Rodrigue, J. R., & Taylor, W. C. (1997). *Health promotion and health compromising behaviors among minority adolescents*. Washington, DC: American Psychological Association.

Wingood, G. M., & Keltner, B. (1999). Sociocultural factors and prevention programs affecting the health of ethnic minorities. In J. M. Raczynski & R. J. DiClemente (Eds.), *Handbook of health promotion and disease prevention* (pp. 561–577). New York: Kluwer Academic/Plenum.

Wood, D., Donald-Sherbourne, C., Halfon, N., Tucker, M. B., Ortiz, V., Hamlin, J. S., et al. (1995). Factors related to immunization status among inner-city Latino and African-American preschoolers. *Pediatrics, 96*(2), 295–301.

Wood, D. L., Hayward, R. A., Corey, C. R., Freeman, H. E., & Shapiro, M. F. (1990). Access to medical care for children and adolescents in the United States. *Pediatrics, 86,* 666–673.

41

Health-Related Quality of Life in Pediatric Populations

ALEXANDRA L. QUITTNER
MELISSA A. DAVIS
AVANI C. MODI

Over the past two decades, tremendous progress has been made in defining and measuring quality of life and in recognizing its importance as a health outcome. The origins of this movement go back more than 50 years, to the World Health Organization's broadened definition of health as "a state of complete physical, mental, and social well-being, and not merely the absence of disease or infirmity" (World Health Organization [WHO], 1947, p. 29). This statement laid the groundwork for conceptualizing health as multidimensional and focused attention away from the biomedical model, which emphasized physiological indices of health, and toward a biopsychosocial model that considered the patient's ability to function in his or her daily life (Engel, 1977; Schor, Lerner, & Malspeis, 1995). Although health-related quality of life (HRQOL) was initially criticized as vague and difficult to define, a consensus has emerged that HRQOL is multidimensional and should include four core domains: (1) disease state and physical symptoms, (2) functional status, (3) psychological and emotional functioning, and (4) social functioning (Aaronson, 1989). It should also be patient oriented rather than physician oriented, reflecting the individual's subjective evaluation of his or her daily functioning and well-being (Schipper, Clinch, & Olweny, 1996). Furthermore, rigorous standards of measurement development and psychometric analysis have been applied to measures of HRQOL (Aaronson, 1989; Ware & Sherbourne, 1992).

Research on HRQOL has flourished as a result of advances in medical technology and treatment, efforts to reduce health care costs, and the growing prevalence of chronic illnesses in adult and pediatric populations. Efforts to develop reliable and valid measures of HRQOL have been highly successful, particularly in adult populations, and this success has fostered the use of these measures in several different contexts. HRQOL measures are now used for many purposes: (1) as primary or secondary outcomes in clinical trials; (2) to evaluate new pharmaceutical and surgical interventions; (3) to describe the impact of an illness on a patient's psychosocial functioning; (4) to analyze the costs and benefits of medical interventions; and (5) to aid in clinical decision making (Levi & Drotar, 1998). To date, the vast majority of this research has been conducted with adult populations. However, over the past 10 years, interest in HRQOL research with children and its utilization within pediatric populations has grown.

PROGRESS IN MEASUREMENT DEVELOPMENT AND RESEARCH ON PEDIATRIC HRQOL

In order to evaluate the progress made in HRQOL research with pediatric populations, a systematic review of the published literature from 1990 to 2001 was conducted. This is an expansion of a previous review that spanned the years between 1966 and 1995 (Schor, 1998). As can be seen in Figure 41.1, tremendous growth in the pediatric HRQOL literature has occurred from 1990 to 2001, with annual citations increasing from slightly more than 20 in 1990 to more than 110 in 2001. It is also important to note that measurement studies represent less than 20% of published studies from 1990 through 1998, but they represent almost half of the citations in the past few years. This trend is likely to continue given the impetus to utilize HRQOL measures in both research and clinical trials.

The purpose of this chapter is to provide a comprehensive review of HRQOL research with pediatric populations that will serve both as a benchmark of our progress thus far and as a means of stimulating future research. In this chapter, we describe different types of HRQOL measures. Next, we discuss the unique developmental challenges we face in measuring HRQOL in children who vary in their cognitive and emotional maturity, followed by a discus-

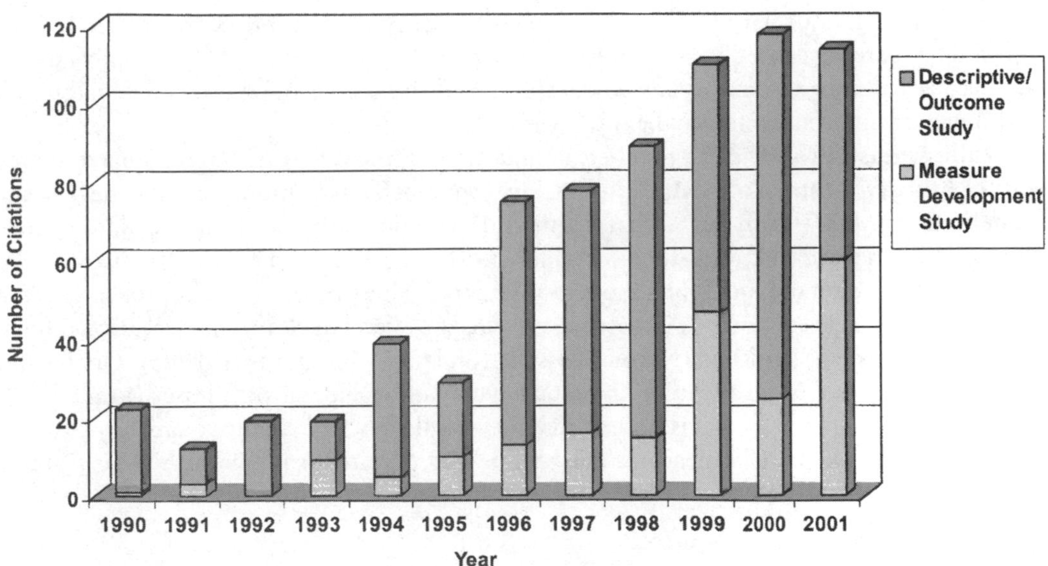

FIGURE 41.1. Review of Medline citations of HRQOL in children and adolescents from 1990 to 2001.

sion of using parent proxy reports to measure children's HRQOL. In the next section, we review cutting-edge methodological issues that affect interpretation of HRQOL scores, such as response shift, that have rarely been addressed in the pediatric literature. Finally, we propose several important directions for future research, including the application of HRQOL measures in clinic settings, development of international HRQOL measures, requirements for pharmaceutical claims, and the need for measures of parental HRQOL.

HRQOL MEASURES

Several different types of instruments have been developed to measure HRQOL, including utility, generic, and disease-specific measures. The decision about which type of measure to use will depend on the purpose of the assessment and the context in which the information will be utilized. The following sections outline the advantages and disadvantages of each type of HRQOL measure.

Utility Measures

Utility measures were derived from economic and decision-making theories and were designed to measure health status in terms of societal preferences for different levels of functioning (Kaplan et al., 1989; Torrance, 1987). The Quality of Well-Being scale (QWB; Kaplan et al., 1989) is the most well known and widely used utility measure. In developing the QWB, adults were asked to order their preferences for particular health states and conditions along a continuum from 0 to 1, weighted for the desirability of these conditions (Kaplan et al., 1989). Utility measures have several advantages: (1) they produce a single number representing the global construct of HRQOL, which is simpler to use in statistical analyses (Juniper, 1997; Kaplan, et al., 1989); (2) they can be used in conjunction with cost and health care utilization data to calculate the cost–benefit ratio of clinical interventions and medical procedures (e.g., comparing the cost–benefit ratios of kidney transplants and long-term dialysis); and (3) they estimate societal values regarding desired health states (Quittner, 1998). This last point is especially important because, although advances in medicine have made it *possible* to treat certain conditions, the human or financial costs may be too great.

Utility measures also have a number of limitations. First, it may not be possible to represent the broader construct of HRQOL with a single number. As mentioned earlier, the consensus definition of HRQOL indicates that it is multidimensional (e.g., physical, social, role functioning; Aaronson, 1989), and studies to date clearly suggest that a particular disease may affect one dimension of functioning more than another. Thus, because this approach yields a single value, it has been shown to be less sensitive to the effects of clinical interventions (Juniper, 1997; Orenstein, Pattishall, Nixon, Ross, & Kaplan, 1990; Quittner, 1998). Finally, the preference weights derived for utility measures were not developed with input from adolescents or younger children, and it is unclear that they would have the cognitive capacity to make such judgments. Thus utility measures may not be appropriate for use with this age group.

Generic Measures

Generic measures assess HRQOL with general items that are applicable to many different medical populations and typically assess functioning in several domains. A number of different generic HRQOL measures have been developed for adults (e.g., Nottingham Health Profile, Hunt McEwen, & McKenna, 1996; Short Form-36, Ware & Sherbourne, 1992) and, more recently, generic HRQOL measures have also been developed for children and parents (Child Health Questionnaire [CHQ]; Landgraf, Abetz, & Ware, 1996; Pediatric Quality of Life Questionnaire (PedsQL; Varni, Seid, & Kurtin, 2001). The major benefit of generic instruments is that scores can be compared across diseases (Guyatt & Jaeschke, 1990; Juniper, 1997; Quittner, 1998). Generic measures, such as the SF-36 and the PedsQL, are quick and easy to administer. In contrast, the child-report version of the CHQ contains more than 80 items and can be quite difficult and time-consuming for children to complete. Although generic measures typically assess a broad range of dimensions that encompass HRQOL, they lack the precision and sensitivity needed to measure these dimensions for a particular illness. Thus generic health profiles may not be responsive to small, but important, changes resulting from therapeutic interventions (Juniper, 1997).

Disease-Specific Measures

In the past decade, interest in developing disease-specific measures of HRQOL has increased. Researchers have recognized the limitations of using generic measures in clinical trials, and this recognition has spurred the development of new, disease-specific HRQOL measures. Disease-specific measures are designed to: (1) assess areas of functioning most likely to be affected by a particular illness (e.g., fatigue, nausea); (2) utilize items that are clinically relevant; and (3) include items that have strong face validity and meaning for children (Quittner, 1998; Spieth & Harris, 1996). In general, disease-specific measures tend to be more responsive to the effects of clinical interventions and are more sensitive to meaningful changes in health status and daily functioning (Juniper, 1997). The primary limitation of these measures is the inability to compare scores across diseases. Examples of disease-specific measures of HRQOL for children include the Paediatric Asthma Quality of Life Questionnaire (PAQLQ; Juniper et al., 1996a), the Cystic Fibrosis Questionnaire (CFQ; Modi & Quittner, in press; Quittner, Buu, Davis, Modi, & Watrous, 2003; Quittner, Buu, Watrous, & Davis, 2000), and the Quality of Life in Epilepsy Inventory—Adolescents—48 (Cramer et al., 1999). Recently, Varni and colleagues (2001) used a modular approach to HRQOL assessment, combining generic items with disease-specific modules (PedsQL™ 4.0; Varni et al., 2001). The PedsQL consists of a core set of generic items designed to assess physical, emotional, social, and school functioning, followed by a set of disease-specific items targeted to pediatric asthma, rheumatology, diabetes, cancer, and cardiac conditions. The benefit of using this approach is that the generic scales allow for cross-condition comparisons, whereas the disease-specific modules enhance sensitivity and responsiveness.

CHALLENGES OF MEASURING HRQOL IN CHILDREN AND ADOLESCENTS

Developmental Issues

Measures of HRQOL for children provide an opportunity to assess the child's unique perspective on how a chronic illness affects his or her daily life. Although this measurement presents several challenges and some skepticism exists about its feasibility, the importance of capturing this perspective should spur pediatric researchers to develop measures of HRQOL that can be reliably completed by very young children (Goodwin, Boggs, & Graham-Pole, 1994; Quittner, Buu, et al., 2000). Self-report methods are the most commonly used; however, specific developmental issues need to be considered when using these measures with children, including: (1) their cognitive ability to understand and respond to the items; (2) the response options that work best for them; (3) their ability to recall information; and (4) the identification of the functional domains that are most developmentally appropriate (Quittner, Buu, et al., 2000; Wallander, Schmitt, & Koot, 2001).

Age is strongly related to cognitive ability, and as children grow older, their perceptions of HRQOL can change (Annett, 2001). For example, younger children (i.e., preschoolers) have a static perception of health that limits their understanding that health can change over time. In addition, they often make incorrect attributions about the causes of illness, conceptualizing them as immanent justice or contagion. These factors can significantly affect a child's ability to accurately report on his or her HRQOL. However, as children enter middle childhood, they have an increased understanding of the causes of disease and are better able to interpret physiological symptoms as indicators of health or illness, suggesting a higher level of cognitive functioning (Burbach & Peterson, 1986). For example, a school-age boy with asthma may experience tightness in his chest and increased wheezing, which he perceives as interfering with his ability to participate in sports and extracurricular activities. Thus he is likely to report an increase in symptoms of asthma and lower HRQOL scores on domains of physical and school functioning. In contrast, a younger child who has the same symptoms may not associate these physical indicators with a decreased ability to play sports and participate in daily activities. Thus his HRQOL scores on these two domains may not be highly correlated (Juniper, 1997). This example illustrates one of many potential interactions between developmental maturity and assessment of children's HRQOL.

Many of these limitations can be addressed by using an interviewer to administer an HRQOL measure to younger children. Interviewers can assess the child's ability to provide reliable responses to a measure by asking practice questions. For example, Quittner, Buu, and colleagues (2000) have included two practice questions in the version of the CFQ that is administered to children ages 6 to 11 (e.g. "If I asked you if you go to the moon *always, often, sometimes,* or *never*, which answer on the card would you choose?"). If the child is unable to understand the practice question and responds inappropriately, it is clear that his or her responses to the measure will be invalid. Interviewers may also recognize biases in the child's responses (i.e., choosing only the end points of the scale) and can prompt them to think through their answers. Although interviewers may be quite helpful in administering HRQOL measures, it is important to provide training in how to ask nonleading questions and elicit unbiased responses. Pictorial representations (e.g., smiley faces) may also help to engage the child's interest, increase understanding of the items, and sustain his or her attention (Eiser & Morse, 2001). Finally, using computers (e.g., touch screens) may also facilitate the assessment of HRQOL in children (Ravens-Sieberer, Theiling, & Bullinger, 1999).

Another issue to consider is the recall interval that is most appropriate for children. HRQOL measures with shorter recall periods are likely to elicit more accurate responses. Friedman (1990) found that children ages 3–4 years have an adequate understanding of time and are able to report the duration of activities they engage in on a day-to-day basis. It may be useful, however, to elicit concrete examples of activities that can anchor the beginning and end of the time period being assessed (Quittner, 1998, 2000).

Parent-Proxy Issues

Historically, HRQOL measures for children have been completed by parents or physicians as proxy informants because of a perception that children lack the cognitive and emotional maturity to accurately report their own HRQOL (Eiser, 1985). A number of researchers have advocated the use of parents as the most valid informants of their child's HRQOL (Theunissen et al., 1998; Verrips, Vogels, den Ouden, Paneth, & Verloove-Vanhorick, 2000); however, it is now recognized that parents may have a limited understanding of their children's internal states (i.e., emotional functioning) and few opportunities to observe their social interactions (Levi & Drotar, 1998). Further, there is growing evidence that children can reliably complete HRQOL measures and that their perspective, although different at times from parents', is equally valid and important (Eiser & Morse, 2001; Quittner, 1998; Quittner, Sweeny, et al., 2000).

A central question regarding the use of proxy measures of HRQOL is the extent to which parents and other informants agree with the child's own view of his or her HRQOL. In general, the evidence regarding convergence between parent and child reports of HRQOL is mixed, with higher correlations reported for domains of functioning that are observable, such as physical functioning and externalizing behaviors (Modi, Pappachan, & Quittner, 2001; Verrips et al., 2000), and lower correlations for areas that are difficult to observe. For example, Quittner and colleagues (2001) found greater convergence between children and their parents on domains such as respiratory and digestive functioning on the CFQ (Modi et al., 2001; Quittner, Davis, Modi, Buu, & Lippstreu, 2001). Conversely, lower agreement between children and their parents has been found on HRQOL scales of emotional and social functioning, presumably because parents are less aware of their child's social behavior with peers (Davis et al., 2001; Verrips et al., 2000). Evidence is also mixed with regard to whether children overestimate or underestimate their level of functioning in relation to their parents. Several studies have found that children rate their physical functioning *lower* than their parents do (le Coq, Boeke, Bezemer, Colland, & van Eijk, 2000; Modi & Quittner, 2002; Theunissen et al., 1998). Parents, on the other hand, generally report lower HRQOL scores than their children do in the domains of self-esteem, competence, and social functioning (Ennet et al., 1991; Theunissen et al., 1998). Although agreement between respondents is not perfect, discrepancies suggest that each has a unique perspective on HRQOL that should be measured.

To date, there is little empirical data on the reasons for differences in parent and child ratings of HRQOL; however, several issues have been considered. First, children may be reluctant to disclose to parents the physical and emotional difficulties they are having. Thus, in an effort to protect their parents, children may present themselves in a more positive light. Second, parents' responses may be influenced by their concerns about how the illness will affect their child's future, leading them to report lower HRQOL scores in some domains. Parental distress related to the impact of caring for a child with a serious, chronic illness or premorbid parental functioning may also affect their ratings of the child's HRQOL (Eiser & Morse, 2001; Quittner, 2000). Finally, there are several domains of functioning (e.g., school, peer relations) about which parents have little firsthand knowledge, and thus their ratings may differ from the child's, which are based on direct experience.

Despite the fact that this difference in perspective leads to lower agreement on some HRQOL scales, the scales may also serve to highlight important clinical issues that the medical team should address. For example, parents may not realize that their child has begun to have difficulty climbing stairs or walking long distances and that fatigue is now affecting his or her performance at school. Having the child's own report of HRQOL provides an opportunity for both parents and health care professionals to address these changes in physical functioning. More research is needed to examine when and under what conditions parent and child ratings of HRQOL are likely to differ in order to determine whether this represents "noise" in the measurement of the construct or meaningful differences in perspective. In the meantime, having both child and parent proxy measures provides additional information that may be viewed as complementary rather than divergent (Eiser & Morse, 2001).

The use of proxy raters of HRQOL may be particularly important in circumstances in which it is the only means of measuring the child's HRQOL. This procedure might include very young children (e.g., below age 4), children who are developmentally delayed, and children who are in the terminal stages of a disease. In these cases, proxy respondents provide a critical window into the child's level of functioning, and research on the reliability and utility of their reports is an important contribution.

METHODOLOGICAL ISSUES AFFECTING INTERPRETATION OF HRQOL DATA

As HRQOL measures are more frequently incorporated into clinical trials as primary or secondary outcomes, knowing how to interpret the clinical significance of observed changes has become critical. In contrast to objective physical indices, such as weight, pulmonary functioning, and blood glucose levels, which have been extensively researched and are relatively easy to interpret, the clinical significance of a half-point change on a HRQOL measure is not immediately apparent. Is an improvement in a drug-versus-placebo arm of a trial worth the cost of the new drug? In comparing the effects of two treatments, what constitutes a meaningful difference in HRQOL scores? Answering these questions requires determination of the minimal clinically important difference (MCID) for a particular HRQOL measure (Wright, 1996). In addition, interpretation of HRQOL scores in longitudinal studies is complicated by naturally occurring changes in disease trajectory and by the psychological shifts individuals may make in their perception of what is valued. This perception change has been termed "response shift."

Determination of the Minimal Clinically Important Difference (MCID)

The MCID has been defined as the "smallest difference in score in the domain of interest which patients perceive as beneficial and which would mandate, in the absence of troublesome side effects and excessive cost, a change in the patient's management" (Jaeschke, Singer, & Guyatt, 1989, p. 408). For physicians, it has been defined as the "smallest effect size that would lead them to recommend therapy to their patients" (Van Walraven, Mahon, Moher, Bohm, & Laupacis, 1999, p. 717). Ascertaining the magnitude of change that corresponds to the MCID has several important applications, such as evaluating the benefits of new treatments, comparing the effects of two different treatments, calculating sample size, and analyzing the cost-effectiveness of alternative treatments. Many variables can influence the MCID, including side effects of the treatment, the importance of the targeted health outcome, and the method used to calculate the MCID (Barber, Santanello, & Epstein, 1996; Van Walraven et al., 1999). Although a number of articles have been written comparing different approaches to determining the MCID in HRQOL research, there is currently no consensus on which approach is best (Hays & Woolley, 2000; Samsa et al., 1999). Two basic approaches for determining the MCID have been developed: (1) anchor-based methods and (2) distribution-based methods. Anchor-based approaches to benchmarking compare the observed differences to an external standard, with the patient typically making the judgment of what the minimal important difference is. Conversely, distribution-based methods rely on statistical procedures to identify the MCID. To date, little research using either approach has been conducted with HRQOL measures for children and adolescents, and, as a first step, it might be helpful to use both methods and then make comparisons.

Response Shift

Another major concern about the interpretation of HRQOL scores is the phenomenon known as response shift. Response shift has been defined as the change in a respondent's internal standards that form the basis of their reports of functioning on a HRQOL measure (Sprangers & Schwartz, 1999). Thus patients faced with a life-threatening or chronic disease may accommodate to their illness over time or shift their values in terms of the activities they consider most valuable. Response shift may serve as a potential threat to the validity of using HRQOL data as a primary or secondary outcome.

The notion of response shift has tremendous relevance for children and adolescents with chronic medical conditions. For example, an adolescent with epilepsy who is experiencing increased problems with fatigue, concentration, and short-term memory (due to seizure medications) may report lower HRQOL scores on physical and school functioning. Because of her medications and increased fatigue, she is not able to drive, but she has learned to ask her friends for rides and reports higher scores on social functioning. This apparent "disconnect" between lower scores in one domain and higher scores in another may indicate a response shift.

Several issues must be considered in examining response shift in pediatric populations. First, it may be very difficult to employ qualitative methods to assess response shifts in children. These methods usually involve asking for retrospective evaluations of changes in HRQOL since the first assessment (the "Then-Test"), which younger children may find difficult. The other methods of assessing response shift may be easier to adapt for use by children and adolescents (e.g., card sort procedures), and certainly qualitative probes and interview questions can be adapted to pediatric populations. Another challenge to consider is the normal shift in functioning that is likely to occur with development. How can these normative, developmental changes (e.g., increasing socialization with age) be distinguished from changes in functioning in response to a chronic illness? Research on response shift is important, particularly when data is collected over time (Bossart, Clay, & Willson, 2002). However, appropriate application of these methods to child and adolescent HRQOL data will require a great deal of additional research.

FUTURE DIRECTIONS FOR HRQOL APPLICATIONS AND MEASUREMENT

As research and clinical applications of HRQOL measures for pediatric populations have grown, exciting new areas for future research have emerged. Although we have noted the need for additional research throughout this chapter, we would like to highlight five directions that will likely shape the field over the next 10 years: (1) the use of HRQOL measures in clinical settings to aid in decision making; (2) the development and use of international HRQOL measures; (3) the use of HRQOL outcomes in drug trials to establish promotional and labeling claims; (4) the application of computerized-adaptive testing methods in HRQOL assessment; and (5) the development of parent measures of HRQOL.

Application of HRQOL Measures in Clinical Settings

One potentially important application of HRQOL measures for children with chronic illnesses is to incorporate them into routine health care. Children with chronic illnesses are typically seen every 3 to 4 months in their subspecialty clinics (e.g., pulmonology, endocrinology), and there is currently no systematic assessment of their psychosocial functioning. HRQOL measures could easily be completed by children and parents during their long waiting times in clinics, either on an annual basis or at each clinic visit. Use of a reliable and valid HRQOL measure that provides information on a variety of domains of functioning (e.g., physical, social, school) could highlight areas of concern that should be addressed by the clinical team and could aid in medical decision making. In order to convince the health care team of the utility of these measures in the clinic, studies documenting positive changes in practice patterns and increased patient and family satisfaction with the clinic visit will be needed.

International HRQOL Measures

Over the past decade, as medical research and health care have become global enterprises, efforts to develop HRQOL measures that can be used internationally have expanded dramatically. There are several reasons for this growing interest in international HRQOL measures. First, HRQOL is now routinely measured as a secondary outcome in clinical trials evaluating new therapeutic interventions. In order to assess the impact of new drugs or medical interventions on HRQOL, it is important to be able to measure the same concepts across several cultures with the same degree of precision (Anderson, Aaronson, Bullinger, & McBee, 1996). Even within the same country, such as the United States, this may necessitate having both an English and Spanish version of the measure. Second, pharmaceutical companies are increasingly multinational, which has been viewed as a cost-saving strategy and has facilitated the implementation of international clinical trials. As these trials have increased, researchers have recognized the need for reliable, valid, and cross-culturally appropriate HRQOL measures. Pooling data increases sample size and power and makes it possible to compare the effects of new medications or interventions across countries (Anderson, Aaronson, Bullinger, & McBee, 1996). Advances in measurement development and statistics have also played a role in this process. Specific guidelines have been established for the translation and validation of HRQOL measures into other languages (Anderson, Aaronson, Leplege, & Wilkin, 1996), and new statistical techniques, such as item response theory (Hui & Traindis, 1985), have made it possible to systematically test the cultural and conceptual equivalence of items translated into different languages (Henry et al., 1998; Henry, Aussage, Grosskopf, & Goehrs, 2003).

Pharmaceutical Claims and Labeling

The use of HRQOL measures in pharmaceutical trials has grown considerably over the past 5 years, particularly since the Federal Drug Administration strongly recommended their use in 1999 (Beans, 1999). There are several reasons for greater use of HRQOL measures in these trials. First, increased prevalence of chronic diseases has highlighted the importance of assessing how an illness and its treatments affect daily functioning (Quittner, 1998). This is a key concern because there are often trade-offs in terms of the side effects of medications, their cost, and the time it takes to adhere to complex treatment regimens. Thus assessing the benefits of new medications or therapies from the patient's perspective is now seen as a critical component of clinical trials.

Second, including an assessment of HRQOL provides information with which to compare different medications and treatments, thus enabling patients and their health care providers to participate actively in the decision-making process. For example, Juniper and colleagues were able to demonstrate that salmeterol showed greater benefits in HRQOL than salbuterol for adult patients with asthma (Juniper et al., 1995). More recently, improvements in HRQOL were found for Tobramyacin Solution for Inhalation (TOBI) over placebo for children and adolescents with cystic fibrosis (CF), based on parent and child reports on one global rating of change question (Quittner & Buu, 2002).

Finally, in 2000, the FDA approved labeling claims for 21 products and promotional claims for 8 different medications as a result of HRQOL data (Burke, 2000). To make labeling or promotional claims based on HRQOL data, rigorous standards must be employed that are consistent with those used to measure safety and clinical efficacy (Revicki et al., 2000). In the future, the field is likely to see increased attention and interest in using HRQOL data to support promotional claims and labeling for new medications and clinical interventions. Currently, however, no HRQOL claims have been approved by the FDA for medications used for pediatric populations. For some pediatric chronic conditions, there are now HRQOL measures that meet the psychometric and clinical standards required for labeling and promotional claims (e.g., asthma, CF, and cancer), and their systematic use needs to be encouraged in future clinical trials. Thus children, parents and health care providers will be provided with the information they need to make informed choices.

Computerized Adaptive Testing and Item Response Theory

The most recent development in administration of HRQOL measures is the use of computers. A major advantage of this mode of administration is that computers can be programmed to reduce both missed responses and multiple responses to the same question (Caro, Caro, Caro, Wouters, & Juniper, 2001). As a result of the increased use of computers, computerized adaptive testing (CAT) has been developed to administer items based on an individual's unique response to each item, with items presented according to their level of difficulty. Thus each respondent receives a different "adapted" version of the measure based on his or her responses to previous items. This provides an efficient way to determine the respondent's "true score." Historically, this technique has been used for educational testing purposes (e.g., Scholastic Aptitude Test; Graduate Record Exam). However, more recently there has been a call for the application of CAT methods to the assessment of HRQOL (McHorney, 1997).

Parental Health-Related Quality of Life

As primary caregivers, parents of children with chronic illnesses are faced with a number of ongoing stressors, including managing daily treatment regimens, coping with the functional limitations imposed by the child's disease, communicating with the health care team, and facilitating the child's functioning at school. More than two decades of research have documented these additional strains and their effects on parental depression, anxiety, and family functioning (see Quittner & DiGirolamo, 1998, for a review). However, the vast majority of these studies have utilized measures designed to identify individual psychopathology (e.g., clinical levels of depression) rather than the alterations in role functioning and increases in role strain associated with caring for a child with a chronic illness (Quittner, Espelage, Opipari, Carter, & Eigen, 1998; Schultz & Quittner, 1998). This "pathologizing" of parental adaptation to childhood illness has had negative effects, including increased stigma and deemphasis on parents' daily functioning (Quittner & DiGirolamo, 1998). More recently, researchers have begun to investigate the usefulness of measuring parent's HRQOL, instead of relying on traditional, but more limited, measures of psychopathology. This approach has tremendous theoretical and practical significance. First, it frames parental adjustment to childhood chronic illness as a *normative* process involving additional daily responsibilities (e.g., treatment regimens), limitations in major life roles (e.g., difficulty working full time, having less time for other children), and increased strains on close relationships (e.g., marital role strain; Quittner et al., 1998).

Second, it acknowledges that these caregiving responsibilities go beyond what is usually asked of parents and, thus, provides a positive connotation for caregiver burden in this context. For example, parents may be reluctant to complete an inventory asking about their depressive symptoms over the previous week but may be willing to reveal information about how their child's illness affects their everyday activities (e.g., "During the past week, how often did you have sleepless nights because of your child's asthma?"; Juniper et al., 1996b). Thus measures of HRQOL may be more acceptable to parents. Completing a depression measure during a visit to their child's asthma or diabetes clinic may raise concerns for parents about why *they* are the focus of the assessment. Examples of parent QOL measures include the Pediatric Asthma Caregiver Quality of Life Questionnaire (Juniper et al., 1996b) and the Parents' Diabetes Quality of Life Questionnaire (Faulkner & Clark, 1998). In sum, the use of HRQOL measures holds tremendous promise for increasing our understanding of how childhood chronic illnesses affect parents and for pinpointing important areas for intervention. The use of HRQOL measures might result in less negative labeling of parents in pathological terms (e.g., "depressed"), less parental "blaming," and greater acceptance of psychological interventions by parents of children with chronic illnesses. This latter benefit could be the most important of all—facilitating inclusion of psychologists as members of the health care team whose primary role is to ensure that children and parents maintain an optimal HRQOL.

SUMMARY

Over the past decade, there has been widespread acceptance of the importance of the biopsychosocial model, particularly for the management of chronic conditions. This is evident in the dramatic increase in the development of HRQOL measures for pediatric populations and their inclusion in pediatric research. As is so often the case, advancements in HRQOL research have been made first in the adult literature and must now be extended downward to adolescents and children. This extension requires an understanding of complex developmental issues and sensitivity to the unique family context in which children with chronic illnesses grow up. In this chapter, we have outlined an ambitious agenda of future research that will require the attention of pediatric psychologists over the next 10 years. Given our progress in the field over the past decade, we are confident that pediatric psychologists can meet the challenge.

ACKNOWLEDGMENTS

Research was supported in part by grants from the National Institutes of Health (HL47064) and the Cystic Fibrosis Foundation. We would like to thank Wendy Hofer for her insightful comments on an earlier version of this chapter.

REFERENCES

Aaronson, N. K. (1989). Quality of life assessment in clinical trials: Methodological issues. *Controlled Clinical Trials, 10*(4), 195S-208S.

Anderson, R. T., Aaronson, N. K., Bullinger, M., & McBee, W. L. (1996). A review of the progress towards developing health-related quality-of-life instruments for international clinical studies and outcome research. *Pharmacoeconomics, 10*(4), 336–355.

Anderson, R. T., Aaronson, N. K., Leplege, A. P., & Wilkin, D. (1996). International use and application of generic health-related quality of life instruments. In B. Spilker (Eds.), *Quality of life and pharmacoeconomics in clinical trials* (2nd ed., pp. 613–633). Philadelphia: Lippincott-Raven.

Annett, R. D. (2001). Assessment of health status and quality of life outcomes for children with asthma. *Journal of Allergy and Clinical Immunology, 107*, S473–481.

Barber, B. L., Santanello, N. C., & Epstein, R. S. (1996). Impact of the global on patient perceivable change in an asthma-specific QOL questionnaire. *Quality of Life Research, 5*(1), 117–122.

Beans, B. (1999). Drug firms rely on psychologists' expertise. [Electronic version]. *American Psychological Association Monitor, 30*(10). Retrieved March 18, 2002, from http://www.apa.org/monitor/nov99/fp2.html.

Bossart, D. F., Clay, D. L., & Willson, V. L. (2002). Methodological and statistical considerations for threats to internal validity in pediatric outcome data: Response shift in self-report outcomes. *Journal of Pediatric Psychology, 27*(1), 97–107.

Burbach, D. J., & Peterson, L. (1986). Children's concepts of physical illness: A review and critique of the cognitive developmental literature. *Health Psychology, 5*, 307–325.

Burke, L. (2000, September). *Regulatory issues in the use of patient reported outcomes in drug labeling and advertising.* Paper presented at the Health-Related Quality of Life Workshop, Center for Drug Evaluation and Research, Food and Drug Administration, Rockville, MD.

Caro, J. J., Caro, I., Caro, H., Wouters, F., & Juniper, E. F. (2001). Does electronic implementation of questionnaire used in asthma alter responses compared to paper implementation? *Quality of Life Research, 10*(8), 683–691.

Cramer, J. A., Westbrook, L. E., Devinsky, O., Perrine, K., Glassman, M. B., & Camfield, C. (1999). Development of the Quality of Life in Epilepsy Inventory for Adolescents: The QOLIE-AD-48. *Epilepsia 40*(8), 1114–1121.

Davis, M. A., Modi, A. C., Quittner, A., Buu, A., Koenig, J., & Accurso, F. (2001, June). *Psychometric analyses of the cystic fibrosis questionnaire for parents of school-age children.* Poster presented at the European Cystic Fibrosis Conference, Vienna, Austria.

Eiser, C. (1985). *The psychology of childhood illness.* New York: Springer-Verlag.

Eiser, C., & Morse, R. (2001). Quality-of-life measures in chronic diseases of childhood. *Health Technology Assessment, 5*(5), 1–125.

Engel, G. L. (1977). The need for a new medical model: A challenge for biomedicine. *Science, 196*, 129–136.

Ennett, S. T., DeVellis, B. M., Earp, J. A., Kredich, D., Warren, R. W., & Wilhelm, C. L. (1991). Disease experience and psychosocial adjustment in children with juvenile rheumatoid arthritis: Children's versus mothers' reports. *Journal of Pediatric Psychology, 16*, 557–568.

Faulkner, M. S., & Clark, F. S. (1998). Quality of life for parents of children and adolescents with Type 1 diabetes. *Diabetes Educator, 24*(6), 721–727.

Friedman, W. J. (1990). Children's representations of the patterns of daily activities. *Child Development, 61*, 1399–1412.

Goodwin, D. A. J., Boggs, S. R., & Graham-Pole, J. (1994). Development and validation of the Pediatric Oncology Quality of Life Scale. *Psychological Assessment, 6*(4), 321–328.

Guyatt, G. H., & Jaeschke, R. (1990). Measurements in clinical trials: Choosing the appropriate approach. In B. Spilker (Ed.), *Quality of life assessments in clinical trials* (pp. 37–46). New York: Raven.

Hays, R. D., & Woolley, J. M. (2000). The concept of clinically meaningful difference in health-related quality-of-life research: How meaningful is it? *Pharmacoeconomics, 18*(5), 419–423.

Henry, B., Aussage, P., Grosskopf, C., & Goehrs, J. M. (2003). Development of the cystic fibrosis Questionnaire (CFQ) for assessing quality of life in pediatric and adult patients. *Quality of Life Research, 12*, 63–76.

Henry, B., Aussage, P., Staab, D., Prados, C., Grosskoph, C., & Goehrs, J. M. (1998). Assessing cross-cultural validity of the Cystic Fibrosis Questionnaire. *Quality of Life Research, 7*(7), 606–607.

Hui, C. H., & Traindis, H. C. (1985). Measurement in cross-cultural psychology: A review and comparison of strategies. *Journal of Cross-Cultural Psychology, 16*(2), 131–152.

Hunt, S., McEwen, J., & McKenna, S. (1996). *Measuring health status*. London: Croom Helm.

Jaeschke, R., Singer, J., & Guyatt, G. H. (1989). Measurement of health status: Ascertaining the minimal clinically important difference. *Controlled Clinical Trials, 10*(4), 407–415.

Juniper, E. F. (1997). How important is quality of life in pediatric asthma? *Pediatric Pulmonology, 15*(Suppl.), 17–21.

Juniper, E. F., Guyatt, G. H., Feeny, D. H., Ferrie, P. J., Griffith, L. E., & Townsend, M. (1996a). Measuring quality of life in children with asthma. *Quality of Life Research, 5*(1), 35–46.

Juniper, E. F., Guyatt, G. H., Feeny, D. H., Ferrie, P. J., Griffith, L. E., & Townsend, M. (1996b). Measuring quality of life in parents of children with asthma. *Quality of Life Research, 5*(1), 27–34.

Juniper, E. F., Johnston, P. R., Borkhoff, C. M., Guyatt, G. H., Boulet, L., & Haukioja, A. (1995). Quality of life asthma clinical trials: Comparison of salmeterol and salbutamol. *American Journal of Respiratory and Critical Care Medicine, 151*(1), 66–70.

Kaplan, R. M., Anderson, J. P., Wu, A. W., Matthews, C., Kozin, F., & Orenstein, D. (1989). The Quality of Well-Being scale. *Medical Care, 27*(Suppl. 3), S27–43.

Landgraf, J. M., Abetz, L., & Ware, J. E. (1996). *Child Health Questionnaire (CHQ): A user's manual* (1st ed.). Boston, MA: New England Medical Center, The Health Institute.

le Coq, E. M., Boeke, A. J., Bezemer, P. D., Colland, V. T., & van Eijk, J. T. (2000). Which source should we use to measure quality of life in children with asthma: The children themselves or their parents? *Quality of Life Research, 9*(6), 625–636.

Levi, R., & Drotar, D. (1998). Critical issues and needs in health-related quality of life assessment of children and adolescents with chronic health conditions. In D. Drotar (Ed.), *Measuring health-related quality of life in children and adolescents: Implications for research and practice* (pp. 3–24). Mahwah, NJ: Erlbaum.

McHorney, C. A. (1997). Generic health measurement: Past accomplishments and a measurement paradigm for the 21st century. *Annals of Internal Medicine, 127*(8), 743–750.

Modi, A. C., Pappachan, S., & Quittner, A. L. (2001, April). *A new measurement tool for health-related quality of life for children with cystic fibrosis*. Poster presented at the Florida Conference on Child Health Psychology, Gainesville, FL.

Modi, A. C., & Quittner, A. L. (in press). Validation of a disease-specific quality of life measure for children with cystic fibrosis. *Journal of Pediatric Psychology.*

Orenstein, D. M., Pattishall, E. N., Nixon, P. A., Ross, E. A., & Kaplan, R. M. (1990). Quality of well-being before and after antibiotic treatment of pulmonary exacerbation in patients with cystic fibrosis. *Chest, 98*, 1081–1084.

Quittner, A. L. (1998). Measurement of quality of life in cystic fibrosis. *Current Opinion in Pulmonary Medicine, 4*, 326–331.

Quittner, A. L. (2000). Improving assessment in child clinical and pediatric psychology: Establishing links to process and functional outcomes. In D. Drotar (Ed.), *Handbook of research methods in pediatric and child clinical psychology* (pp. 119–143). New York: Plenum Press.

Quittner, A. L., & Buu, A. (2002). Effects of tobramycin solution for inhalation on global ratings of quality of life in patients with cystic fibrosis and pseudomonas aeruginosa infection. *Pediatric Pulmonology, 33*, 269–276.

Quittner, A. L., Buu, A., Davis, M. A., Modi, A. C., & Watrous, M. (2003). *Development and national validation of the Cystic Fibrosis Questionnaire (CFQ): A health-related quality of life measure for cystic fibrosis*. Manuscript under review.

Quittner, A. L., Buu, A., Watrous, M., & Davis, M. A. (2000). *The Cystic Fibrosis Questionnaire (CFQ): User's manual.* Washington, DC: Cystic Fibrosis Foundation.

Quittner, A. L., Davis, M. A., Modi, A. C., Buu, A., & Lippstreu, M. (2001, April). *Validation of the Cystic Fibrosis Questionnaire for parents of children with cystic fibrosis (CFQ-Parent)*. Poster presented at the Florida Conference on Child Health Psychology, Gainesville, FL.

Quittner, A. L., & DiGirolamo, A.M. (1998). Family adaptation to childhood disability and illness. In R. T. Ammerman & J. V. Campo (Eds.), *Handbook of pediatric psychology and psychiatry* (pp. 70–102). Boston, MA: Allyn & Bacon.

Quittner, A. L., Espelage, D. L., Opipari, L. C., Carter, B. D., & Eigen, H. (1998). Role strain in couples with and without a chronically ill child: Associations with marital satisfaction, intimacy, and daily mood. *Health Psychology, 17*, 112–124.

Quittner, A. L., Sweeny, S., Watrous, M., Munzenberger, P., Bearss, K., Nitza, A. G., et al. (2000). Translation and linguistic validation of a disease-specific quality of life measure for cystic fibrosis. *Journal of Pediatric Psychology, 25*, 403–414.

Ravens-Sieberer, U., Theiling, S., & Bullinger, M. (1999, September). *Assessing quality of life in chronically ill children: The parents and the parents' view.* Paper presented at the International Congress of the European Society for Child and Adolescent Psychiatry, Congress Centrum, Hamburg, Germany.

Revicki, D.A., Osoba, D., Fairclough, D., Barofsky, I., Berson, R., Leidy, N. K., & Rothman, M. (2000). Recommendation on health-related quality of life research to support labeling and promotional claims in the United States. *Quality of Life Research, 9*(8), 887–900.

Samsa, G., Edelman, D., Rothman, M. G. L., Williams, G. R., Lipscomb, J., & Matchar, D. (1999). Determining clinically important differences in health status measures: A general approach with illustration to the Health Utilities Index Mark II. *Pharmacoeconomics, 15*(2), 141–155.

Schipper, H., Clinch, J. L., & Olweny, L. M. (1996). Quality of life studies: Definitions and conceptual issues. In B. Spilker (Ed.), *Quality of life and pharmacoeconomics in clinical trials* (2nd ed., pp. 11–24). Philadelphia, PA: Lippincott Raven.

Schor, E. L., Lerner, D. J., & Malspeis, S. (1995). Physicians' assessment of functional status and well-being. *Archives of Internal Medicine, 155*, 309–314.

Schulz, R., & Quittner, A. L. (1998). Caregiving across the life-span: Introduction and future directions. *Health Psychology, 17*, 107–111.

Spieth, L. E., & Harris, C. V. (1996). Assessment of health-related quality of life in children and adolescents: An integrative review. *Journal of Pediatric Psychology, 21*, 175–193.

Sprangers, M. A. G., & Schwartz, C. E. (1999). Integrating response shift into health-related quality of life research: A theoretical model. *Social Science and Medicine, 48*, 1507–1515.

Theunissen, N. C., Vogels, T., Koopman, H. M., Verrips, G. H., Zwinderman, K., Verloove-Vanhorick, S. P., & Wit, J. M. (1998). The proxy problem: Child report versus parent report in health-related quality of life research. *Quality of Life, 7*(5), 387–397.

Torrance, G. W. (1987). Utility approach to measuring health-related quality of life. *Journal of Chronic Diseases, 40*(6), 593–603.

Van Walraven, C., Mahon, J. L., Moher, D., Bohm, C., & Laupacis, A. (1999). Surveying physicians to determine the minimal important difference: Implications for sample-size calculation. *Journal of Clinical Epidemiology, 52*(8), 717–723.

Varni, J. W., Seid, M., & Kurtin, P. S. (2001). PedsQL: Reliability and validity of the Pediatric Quality of Life Inventory Version 4.0 generic core scales in healthy and patient populations. *Medical Care, 39*(8), 800–812.

Verrips, G. H. W., Vogels, A. G. C., den Ouden, A. L., Paneth, N., & Verloove-Vanhorick, S. P. (2000). Measuring health-related quality of life in adolescents: Agreement between raters and between methods of administration. *Child: Care, Health and Development, 26*(6), 457–469.

Wallander, J. L., Schmitt, M., & Koot, H. M. (2001). Quality of life measurement in children and adolescents. *Issues, Instruments, and Applications, 57*(4), 571–585.

Ware, J. E., & Sherbourne, C. (1992). The MOS 36–item short-form health survey (SF-36): I. Conceptual framework and item selection. *Medical Care, 30*(6), 473–483.

World Health Organization. (1947). The constitution of the World Health Organization. *WHO Chronicles, 1*, 29.

Wright, J. G. (1996). The minimal important difference: Who's to say what is important? *Journal of Clinical Epidemiology, 49*(11), 1221–1222.

42

Pediatric Psychology and Public Health

Opportunities for Further Integration in the 21st Century

E. WAYNE HOLDEN

As pediatric psychology moves into the 21st century, it is important to consider our relationships with other professions devoted to improving children's health. Pediatric psychology has developed a strong alliance with traditional medicine that emphasizes the prevention, diagnosis, and treatment of disease, primarily at the level of the individual. In addition, pediatric and clinical psychology, as a whole, have mirrored the evolution of medicine with increasing levels of specialization and an overriding focus on psychology as a tertiary care specialty within the world of medicine (Holden & Black, 1999).

This strong alliance has had many advantages for the growth and legitimization of pediatric psychologists working within the tertiary care medical system and the systematic integration of pediatric psychologists into primary care settings (Kelleher, 1999; Schroeder, 1999; Sobel, Roberts, Rayfield, Barnard, & Rapoff, 2001). A significant limitation of this alliance, however, is the constraining influence that it has placed on the integration of public health models into pediatric psychology, with a corresponding emphasis on population-wide health promotion and prevention in training, research, and practice (Holden & Black, 1999; Holden & Nitz, 1995). Within the area of child and adolescent health, some integration has occurred between pediatric psychology and public health, but the absence of a more formal alliance and planned strategies for integrating the two areas has limited the opportunities that could have potentially resulted from more direct interaction. For the most part, the influences instead have been indirect, with a more limited impact on defining the relationship between the two professions.

With significant technological advances and the globalization of health care, many opportunities exist for developing a more sustained and formal public health focus within pediatric psychology. Public health models and perspectives are consistent with the preventive orientation that has been (Kaufman, Holden, & Walker, 1989; Roberts, 1987) and will continue to be an important component of pediatric psychology (Holden & Black, 1999). Public health concepts and methods must be infused into the day-to-day work of pediatric psychologists and a clear understanding must be developed of the public health agenda as it relates to the development and implementation of public policy (Gold, 1999). Collaboration between the two disciplines also stands to benefit public health, as concepts and methods from pediatric psychology can be more directly integrated into the science and practice of public health as it relates to children's concerns.

This brief chapter provides information on public health as it relates to children's health concerns. First, a definition of public health and the components of the public health mission are outlined. Second, important methodological issues regarding the development and dissemination of public health interventions are highlighted. Third, major public health objectives over the next decade are briefly discussed with, specific reference to Healthy People 2010 (U.S. Department of Health and Human Services, 2000). Finally, two examples of newly initiated public health initiatives targeted toward children are provided.

COMPONENTS OF THE PUBLIC HEALTH MISSION

Public health is concerned with the control of disease and health promotion within large segments of the population. Public health specifically focuses on morbidity and mortality associated with patterns of disease, identification of risk factors for the development of disease, and strategies for disease prevention and eradication. Epidemiology is the basic science underlying public health. Its ultimate goal is to describe the distribution and determinants of disease within populations. Using statistical concepts grounded in population-wide parameters, such as prevalence, incidence, and relative risk, epidemiologists attempt to describe the characteristics of disease within populations and to create empirically supported conceptual models that then serve as the basis for developing and implementing broad-scale public health interventions. Once interventions are developed and implemented, epidemiologists are also concerned with the ongoing surveillance of populations to evaluate the impact of interventions on the patterns and burdens associated with disease.

Public health interventions can take many forms that may be unfamiliar to pediatric psychologists, who typically conceptualize and develop interventions from an individual psychological or behavioral standpoint. The delivery of complex, individually based interventions may be too cost- and time-inefficient for implementation on a population-wide basis. Although much of the research from pediatric psychology contributes information for crafting large-scale public health interventions, the eventual content and delivery of these interventions is influenced by other areas that contribute to the public health mission, such as health education and health communication. For example, health communication strategies designed to promote healthy behaviors and to reduce health risks are often utilized within media campaigns to address a targeted population-wide public health concern (Parvanta & Freimuth, 2000; Smith, 2000). These communication strategies are crafted for different audiences and delivered through multiple media channels to maximize their impact on altering the knowledge, attitudes, beliefs, and behaviors of individuals (Robinson, Patrick, Eng, & Gustafson, 1998). These media campaigns capitalize on advanced information technology and consumer activism in the health arena. The dissemination and impact of these interventions are conceptualized within broad theoretical frameworks such as diffusion of innovations (Rogers, 1995), which provides a metatheory for identifying and capitalizing on community-level determinants for the adoption and support of innovative health promotion strategies.

Program implementation, dissemination, and monitoring are also strong components of the public health approach. These components are reflected in an emphasis on effectiveness at the community level once preventive interventions have been tested in efficacy studies. Efficiency, which is primarily determined by cost-effectiveness and benefit–cost analyses, and equity, which reflects appropriate access to public health interventions, are also important factors for determining the effectiveness of programs. Significant resources are typically devoted to monitoring activities through program evaluation in order to understand potential barriers to program implementation and dissemination (Centers for Disease Control and Prevention [CDC], 1999; Cole, Pogostin, Westover, Rios, & Collier, 1995). This information is used to influence public policy decision making regarding the allocation of resources for disseminating preventive interventions to affect the health status of populations. Although pediatric psychologists may receive some training in program evaluation, they typically are not well prepared for the wide range of methods and strategies that are employed, especially in such areas as utilization-focused evaluation (Patton, 1997), in which stakeholders are heavily involved in the design, implementation, and interpretation of evaluation data. The direct involvement of community members is essential to ensuring the successful implementation and sustainability of health interventions in community settings.

HEALTH OBJECTIVES FOR THE NEXT DECADE

Public health is concerned with changes in health parameters for the nation as a whole, although these overall changes are accomplished by the development and dissemination of specific programs that target different groups and policy changes designed to improve the public health infrastructure across the United States. The Centers for Disease Control and Prevention and the broader public health community play a major role in developing health objectives for the nation. Healthy People 2010 is the most recent set of comprehensive health objectives that have been set for the initial decade of the 21st century (U.S. Department of Health and Human Services, 2000). The leading health indicators to be monitored for the population over the next decade include physical activity, obesity, tobacco use, substance abuse, responsible sexual behavior, mental health, injury and violence, environmental quality, immunization, and access to health care.

These overall health indicators have 467 underlying objectives that provide targets for improved health within the United States. Each of these leading health indicators has direct implications for those working with pediatric populations. Behavior-change strategies will play a critical role in determining whether or not the optimistic goals set for each of the objectives underlying these indicators will be met within the next decade. Each area clearly has important implications for the development of preventive and health promotion interventions within pediatric populations. For example, in the area of tobacco use, the Youth Risk Behavior Surveillance system (Everett, Kann, & McReynolds, 1997) documented that 35% of teenagers reported smoking one or more cigarettes in the previous 30 days in 1999 (CDC, 2000). The Healthy People goal for 2010 is to reduce the prevalence of cigarette smoking by more than half, to 16% or less of the adolescent population. Addressing this goal will require comprehensive intervention strategies that are directed to multiple audiences, including teenagers, their families, school personnel, others who work with teens in the community, and policy makers. It is highly likely that prevention, cessation, and displacement strategies will need to be used in tandem to have a discernable impact on lowering the prevalence of adolescent cigarette smoking.

The objectives that have been set in Healthy People 2010 are being tracked by 190 data sources that provide surveillance information on various aspects of the United States population. Two of the most important existing surveillance systems for tracking the health of adolescents are the Monitoring the Future Study (MTF; Johnston, Bachman, & O'Malley, 1998) and the Youth Risk Behavior Surveillance System (YRBSS; CDC, 2000; Everett et al., 1997). The MTF study is sponsored by the National Institute on Drug Abuse and provides self-report drug use data on a yearly basis from approximately 50,000 randomly sampled 8th, 10th, and 12th graders in both public and private school settings (see the MTF home page: *http://www.isr.umich.edu/src/mtf/index.html*). The YRBSS is a self-report measure sponsored by the Centers for Disease Control and Prevention that is administered biennially to students in grades 9 through 12. This broader survey assesses six categories of health risk behaviors, including injury, tobacco use, alcohol and other drug use, sexual behavior, diet and nutrition, and physical activity (YRBSS home page: *http://www.cdc.gov/nccdphp/dash/yrbs/ov.htm*).

Surveillance systems will provide critical information for tracking the progress that is made in achieving health objectives relevant to children and adolescents over the next decade. Making significant progress on achieving these objectives, however, is dependent on the successful development, implementation, and dissemination of community-based health programs designed to decrease health-risk behaviors and increase health-promotion behaviors among children and adolescents.

PROMOTING THE DEVELOPMENT OF HEALTHY BEHAVIORS AMONG YOUTH

With approval from Congress in early 2000 and authorization for up to $125 million over the next decade, the Centers for Disease Control and Prevention was directed to develop a major national media campaign designed to improve the health status of preteens (CDC, 2001). The Youth Media Campaign (YMC) targets children between the ages of 9 and 13 to influence the development and maintenance of positive health behaviors that will offset the opportunity to engage in health-risk behaviors. This multidimensional and comprehensive national media campaign is based on a displacement strategy that provides opportunities to engage in positive goal-directed activities instead of making bad choices that lead to involvement in negative activities. In addition to targeting preteens with positive health messages, the YMC will involve parents, other influential adults, and community organizations to support the goal of improving the foundation for the development of a lifelong healthy lifestyle in our nation's preteens.

The overall goals of the YMC are to encourage preteens to engage in positive, goal-directed activities with a primary focus on increasing physical activity and involving children in other activities that promote the development of self-esteem and a positive health identity. Parents will be provided clear and practical guidance on approaches to influencing their children. Parents and other community members will also be encouraged to increase their physical activity to provide positive role models for preteens. Media, corporate, and other community organization partnerships will be established to directly involve important community stakeholders in the process of creating and sustaining a community-wide initiative. Each audience segment has been carefully evaluated, and multidimensional communication approaches are being developed to capitalize on currently expanded media and information technology infrastructure for reaching preteens, families, and community members.

The YMC relies on the vast accumulated knowledge base about the development of health-risk behaviors and health-promoting behaviors in preteens and adolescents (Blum, 1998; Fors, Crepaz, & Hayes, 1999; Lowry, Kann, Collins, & Kolbe, 1996; Prinstein, Boergers, & Spirito, 2001; Resnick et al., 1997). Much of this literature is a direct product of research conducted by the various psychological specialty areas working directly with children, including pediatric psychology. For example, it has been clearly documented that low levels of perceived parental monitoring, involvement, or guidance are associated with youth participation in several health-risk behaviors (Li, Feigelman, & Stanton, 2000; Svetaz, Ireland, & Blum, 2000). Consequently, a variety of parenting skills, including communication skills, media literacy, and how to teach resistance, refusal, and independence skills to youth, will be targeted through the initiative.

The YMC will use social marketing techniques and a multimedia strategy to present and disseminate information about the campaign and its activities. Youths are one of the largest populations of media consumers. The amount of information portrayed through the media that encourages the development of health-risk behaviors for this age group is overwhelming. Popular media such as television, movies, video games, and the Internet are observational learning mechanisms that can negatively influence youths by encouraging health-risk behaviors (Strasburger, 1990). Social marketing and mass media have the potential to influence the acceptability of positive health behaviors in much the same way, although there are significant barriers to effectively introducing this information into a youth culture that is riddled with negative, health-damaging messages. Formative research conducted for the YMC suggests that most youngsters want to do the right thing and want to define themselves as strong and healthy (CDC, 2001). Adolescents' peer culture, however, plays a critical role in the development and maintenance of health-risk behaviors (La Greca, Prinstein, & Fetter, 2001). Health promotion messages that generally influence and affect this peer culture are a necessary component of any media campaign that is designed to improve the health choices and decision making of preteens.

The YMC is a major adolescent national health initiative that will be unfolding over the course of the next several years. This initiative is built on years of research by pediatric psychologists and other health professionals devoted to promoting the healthy development of youths. The implementation and dissemination phases of the YMC will likely benefit from continued involvement by the pediatric psychology community to promote the highest level of effectiveness of this campaign to achieve health promotion objectives set for the adolescent population in Healthy People 2010.

ASSESSING THE IATROGENIC EFFECTS OF SUCCESSFUL PUBLIC HEALTH INITIATIVES

The development of vaccines and their widespread dissemination has been a significant public health success story, not only in the United States but also worldwide. Over the latter part of the 20th century, immunizations have become a key component of primary health care for both children and adults. Immunizations have substantially reduced the incidence, morbidity, and mortality associated with a number of previously uncontrolled infectious diseases (Chen & Hibbs, 1998).

With the widespread use of immunizations, however, has come an accompanying increase in concerns regarding potential iatrogenic effects. These concerns are magnified when an intrusive preventive intervention such as immunization is administered on a widespread basis within healthy populations. The relative risks of producing adverse consequences from injecting bioactive agents must be balanced carefully against positive benefits in these situations. Furthermore, the heavy weighting of immunizations to the infancy and early-childhood age ranges places special emphasis on clearly understanding and monitoring closely the potential risks to developing organisms from immunizations. A certain level of adverse consequences is associated with any medical intervention, regardless of whether the intervention is preventive or treatment oriented. The underidentification and lack of effective monitoring of adverse events by the public health community can directly result in morbidity and/or mortality that fuels public concern and potentially decreases adherence to what are otherwise effective prevention programs (Duffell, 2001).

Among its various responsibilities, the National Immunization Program (NIP) within the CDC, along with the Food and Drug Administration, has actively developed and promoted surveillance systems that can assist with the monitoring and investigation of adverse consequences from immunizations (Chen et al., 1997; Chen & Hibbs, 1998). The Vaccine Adverse Event Reporting System (VAERS) was developed following enactment of the National Childhood Vaccine Injury Act of 1986, which mandated the reporting of adverse events following immunizations. The CDC also developed the Vaccine Safety Datalink (VSD), which is a large, linked database that combines vaccine and other health-related information across multiple HMOs providing medical services to approximately 2% of the population. This more extensive, prospectively collected database has been in existence since 1990 to investigate both the short- and long-term adverse consequences associated with immunizations. The VSD provides an important opportunity to investigate comprehensively both proximal and distal adverse consequences associated with immunizations and to evaluate the cumulative impact of multiple immunizations on developmental trajectories in children, a concern that has been raised with increasing frequency over the past decade (Chen & Hibbs, 1998).

Thimerosal is a preservative that has been added to multidose vials of vaccines since the 1930s to control bacterial and fungal contamination. Adding this preservative to vaccines has greatly reduced the possibility of opportunistic infection and subsequent death following immunization. Approximately 50% of thimerosal, however, is an organic mercury compound (ethylmercury) that has established neurotoxic and nephrotoxic effects (Magos, 2000). Cumulative exposures to thimerosal through current childhood immunization schedules may present significant health risks, especially to infants and young children. Neurodevelopmental delays, including autism (Bernard, Enayati, Redwood, Roger, & Binstock, 2001), have been at least anecdotally linked to mercury exposure during infancy and early childhood, with thimerosal cited as a potential contributor to exposure levels. Concerns regarding the negative effects of thimerosal exposure through immunizations prompted the release of a joint statement by the American Academy of Pediatrics and the U.S. Public Health Service (1999) that recommended the elimination of thimerosal as an additive in vaccines. A recent comprehensive review article (Ball, Ball, & Pratt, 2001) evaluating thimerosal in childhood vaccines underscored the importance of conducting rigorous, methodologically sophisticated research to more specifically understand the adverse consequences of thimerosal exposure and to establish toxicity levels for multiple negative outcomes, including neurodevelopmental consequences.

A preliminary analysis of the VSD database conducted in the fall of 1999 by CDC revealed a dose–response relationship between thimerosal exposure and neurodevelopmental disorders. A more definitive study, using the VSD as a sampling frame and collecting more reliable and valid neuropsychological data from a cohort of 7- to 9-year-old children, is under way by the CDC. This study will provide direct information on the potential negative consequences of thimerosal that will assist with decision making regarding the development, manufacturing, and use of multidose versus single-dose vaccine vials in the future. Even if a significant dose–response relationship is not established, the conducting and reporting of this research will serve as a response to antivaccine advocates that the long-term iatrogenic effects of immunizations are being monitored adequately and that the safety of this successful public health intervention is being assured. This should assist with reaching Healthy People 2010 objectives to significantly increase the frequency of completed infant immunization schedules. This study will likely serve as a model for future work that utilizes complex, longitudinal surveillance databases to more intensively track and follow up the health status of children who have been exposed to potentially hazardous agents.

CONCLUSIONS

Pediatric psychologists offer a wide range of expertise and knowledge to assist with crafting and implementing public health interventions to improve the health status of children and adolescents. To date, much of this information has focused on the development of conceptual and theoretical models, isolation of the specific determinants of the development of health-risk and health-promotion behaviors, and efficacy trials of interventions to improve health status. Pediatric psychologists have been much less involved in assessing the effectiveness of interventions once they are placed in community settings, determining their cost-effectiveness, evaluating the degree to which the public has equitable access to such interventions, and monitoring their dissemination across time, including the assessment of iatrogenic effects. These latter issues are more directly tied to health policy and the funding of large-scale initiatives designed to improve the health status of the nation as set forth in the objectives of Healthy People 2010.

An even greater degree of formal collaboration between pediatric psychology and public health is possible in the 21st century. This collaboration will require that pediatric psychologists become more cognizant of concepts and constructs in epidemiology and community-based program evaluation. This change can be accomplished from integrating more formally a public health perspective into the training of pediatric psychologists at the graduate and postdoctoral levels. Pediatric psychologists will also need to make a shift into effectiveness research, with its accompanying emphasis on translating and disseminating more basic science, including the results of efficacy trials, into the field. This includes understanding community-based determinants that influence the effectiveness of those interventions that have survived efficacy trials. This is quite consistent with the general move toward defining and understanding evidence-based practice in community settings for children with mental health needs and their families (Holden, Friedman, & Santiago, 2001).

The future success of public health initiatives for children and adolescents in the United States is based on creating and sustaining communities that promote healthy development through multiple sources of support and care (Costello & Angold, 2000). Interwoven and interlaced universal, selected, and indicated public health interventions can potentially have a cascading effect on prevention and health promotion across multiple domains that affect the health of children and their families (Holden & Nabors, 1999). This effect will increase the level of complexity with which society and the health professions approach the implementation, dissemination, and evaluation of community-based public health programs in the future. An emphasis by pediatric psychology on population-based perspectives can only serve to enhance the profession's impact on improving the nation's health as a whole over the next decade.

REFERENCES

American Academy of Pediatrics and the U.S. Public Health Service. (1999). Joint statement of the American Academy of Pediatrics (AAP) and the United States Public Health Service (USPHS). *Pediatrics, 104,* 568–569.

Ball, L. K., Ball, R., & Pratt, R. D. (2001). An assessment of thimerosal use in childhood vaccines. *Pediatrics, 107,*1147–1154.

Bernard, S., Enayati, A., Redwood, L., Roger, H., & Binstock, T. (2001). Autism: A novel form of mercury poisoning. *Medical Hypotheses, 56,* 462–471.

Blum, R. W. (1998). Healthy youth development as a model for youth health promotion: A review. *Journal of Adolescent Health, 22,* 368–375.

Centers for Disease Control and Prevention. (1999). Framework for program evaluation in public health. *Morbidity and Mortality Weekly Report, 48*(No. RR-11), 1–40.

Centers for Disease Control and Prevention. (2000). CDC Surveillance Summaries, June 9, 2000. *Morbidity and Mortality Weekly Report, 49*(No. SS-5), 1–96.

Centers for Disease Control and Prevention. (2001). *Leveraging kids' desire to do the right thing.* Atlanta, GA: Author.

Chen, R. T., Glasser, J. W., Rhodes, P. H., Davis, R. L., Barlow, W. E., Thompson, R. S., et al. (1997). Vaccine Safety Datalink Project: A new tool for improving vaccine safety monitoring in the United States. *Pediatrics, 99,* 765–773.

Chen, R. T., & Hibbs, B. (1998). Vaccine safety: Current and future challenges. *Pediatric Annals, 27,* 445–455.

Cole, G. E., Pogostin, C. L., Westover, B. J., Rios, N. M., & Collier, C. B. (1995). Addressing problems in evaluating health-relevant programs through systematic planning and evaluation. *Risk, Health, Safety and Environment, 37,* 37–58.

Costello, E. J., & Angold, A. (2000). Developmental psychopathology and public health: Past, present and future. *Development and Psychopathology, 12,* 599–618.

Duffell, E. (2001). Attitudes of parents towards measles and immunisation after a measles outbreak in an anthroposophical community. *Journal of Epidemiology and Community Health, 55,* 685–686.

Everett, S. A., Kann, L., & McReynolds, L. (1997). The Youth Risk Behavior Surveillance System: Policy and program applications. *Journal of School Health, 67,* 333–335.

Fors, S. W., Crepaz, N., & Hayes, D. M. (1999). Key factors that protect against health risks in youth: Further evidence. *American Journal of Health Behavior, 23,* 368–380.

Gold, M. (1999). The changing US healthcare system: Challenges for responsible public policy. *Milbank Quarterly, 77,* 3–37.

Holden, E. W., & Black, M. M. (1999). Theory and concepts of prevention science as applied to clinical psychology. *Clinical Psychology Review, 19,* 391–401.

Holden, E. W., Friedman, R. M., & Santiago, R. L. (2001) Overview of the National Evaluation of the Comprehensive Community Mental Health Services for Children and Their Families Program. *Journal of Emotional and Behavioral Disorders, 9,* 4–12.

Holden, E. W., & Nabors, L. N. (1999). The prevention of child neglect. In H. D. Dubowitz (Ed.), *Neglected children: Research, practice and policy* (pp. 174–190). Thousand Oaks, CA: Sage.

Holden, E. W., & Nitz, K. N. (1995). Epidemiology of adolescent health disorders. In J. Wallander & L. Siegel (Eds.), *Advances in pediatric psychology: Vol. II. Adolescent health problems: Behavioral perspectives* (pp. 7–21). New York: Guilford Press.

Johnston, L. D., Bachman, J. G., & O'Malley, P. M. (1998). *The National Survey on Drug Use from the Monitoring the Future Study, 1975–1977.* Rockville, MD: National Institute on Drug Abuse.

Kaufman, K. L., Holden, E. W., & Walker, C. E. (1989). Future directions in pediatric and clinical child psychology. *Professional Psychology: Research & Practice, 20,* 148–152.

Kelleher, K. J. (1999). Pediatric psychologist as investigator in primary care. *Journal of Pediatric Psychology, 24,* 459–462.

La Greca, A. M., Prinstein, M. J., & Fetter, M. D. (2001). Adolescent peer crowd affiliation: Linkages with health-risk behaviors and close friendships. *Journal of Pediatric Psychology, 26*(3), 131–143.

Li, X., Feigelman, S., & Stanton, B. (2000). Impact of perceived parental monitoring on adolescent risk behavior over 4 years. *Journal of Adolescent Health, 27,* 49–56.

Lowry, R., Kann, L., Collins, J. L., & Kolbe, L. J. (1996). The effect of socioeconomic status on chronic disease risk behaviors among US adolescents. *Journal of the American Medical Association, 276,* 792–797.

Magos, L. (2000). Review on the toxicity of ethylmercury, including its presence as a preservative in biological and pharmaceutical products. *Journal of Applied Toxicology, 21,* 1–5.

Parvanta, C. F., & Freimuth, V. (2000). Health communication at the Centers for Disease Control and Prevention. *American Journal of Health Behavior, 24,* 18–25.

Patton, M. Q. (1997). *Utilization-focused evaluation: The new century text* (3rd ed.). Thousand Oaks, CA: Sage.

Prinstein, M. J., Boergers, J., & Spirito, A. (2001). Adolescents' and their friends' health-risk behavior: Factors that alter or add to peer influence. *Journal of Pediatric Psychology, 26,* 287–298.

Resnick, M. D., Bearman, P. S., Blum, R. W., Bauman, K. E., Harris, K. M., Jones, J., et al. (1997). Protecting adolescents from harm: Findings from the National Longitudinal Study on Adolescent Health. *Journal of the American Medical Association, 278,* 823–832.

Roberts, M. C. (1987). Public health and health psychology: Two cats of Kilkenny? *Professional Psychology: Research and Practice, 18,* 145–149.

Robinson, T. N., Patrick, K., Eng, T. R., & Gustafson, D. (1998). An evidence-based approach to interactive health communication: A challenge to medicine in the information age. *Journal of the American Medical Association, 280,* 1264–1269.

Rogers, E. M. (1995). *Diffusion of innovations* (4th ed.). New York: Free Press.

Schroeder, C. S. (1999). A view from the past and a look to the future. *Journal of Pediatric Psychology, 24,* 447–452.

Smith, W. A. (2000). Social marketing: An evolving definition. *American Journal of Health Behavior, 24,* 11–17.

Sobel, A. B., Roberts, M. C., Rayfield, A. D., Barnard, M. U., & Rapoff, M. A. (2001). Evaluating outpatient pediatric psychology services in a primary care setting. *Journal of Pediatric Psychology, 26,* 395–405.

Strasburger, V. C. (1990). Television and adolescents: Sex, drugs, rock 'n roll. *Adolescent Medicine: State of the Art Reviews, 1,* 161–194.

Svetaz, M. V., Ireland, M., & Blum, R. (2000). Adolescents with learning disabilities: Risk and protective factors associated with emotional well-being: Findings from the National Longitudinal Study of Adolescent Health. *Journal of Adolescent Health, 27,* 340–348.

U.S. Department of Health and Human Services. (2000). *Healthy People 2010: Understanding and improving health* (2nd ed.). Washington, DC: U.S. Government Printing Office.

43

Genetic Disorders and Genetic Testing

KENNETH P. TERCYAK

This chapter focuses on genetic disorders and the role of pediatric psychology in genetic testing-related research and patient care. Pediatric genetic disorders can be defined as a heterogeneous group of conditions that are at least partly caused by hereditary factors (Nussbaum, McInnes, & Willard, 2001) and that are present during infancy, childhood, or adolescence. A hallmark of these conditions is the young age of onset, which results in physical, behavioral, and/or psychological challenges to normal development. Among the issues most relevant for pediatric psychology is its understanding of the stress and coping processes of parents and children encountering genetic testing for diagnostic purposes. In addition, pediatric psychology may confront similar issues among families undergoing predictive testing to determine when symptoms of the disorder might first be seen. Ethical, social, psychological, and behavioral issues are key aspects to all genetic testing encounters. These issues include children's and parents' beliefs about the cause of genetic disorders; cognitive interpretations of risk estimates; emotions such as anxiety, sadness, and guilt; the multifaceted process of decision making regarding participation in testing; and adjusting to and accepting the uncertainty or finality of the test results. The assessment of genetic status also carries with it the need to appropriately educate and counsel parents and their children about such issues and the possible implications of information learned from testing for other family members who might also be physically and/or emotionally affected. Thus a wide spectrum of knowledge about pediatric psychology—ranging from principles of child development to relationships between health and psychological functioning to patient education and counseling and to family processes and communication behaviors—is often called on in genetic consultation.

Though in the past the aforementioned activities have primarily been limited to genetic testing for disorders with relatively low incidence in the pediatric population, recent advances in molecular genetics and laboratory technology are expected to produce an explosion of data regarding more well-known disorders that have long been suspected of having a hereditary basis. These disorders include certain forms of childhood cancer, diabetes, and asthma, as well as some psychiatric conditions—all of which occur relatively frequently among children. As many of these disorders already serve as a focus of research and clinical efforts in pediatric psychology, incorporating a genetic perspective will become increasingly important in the coming decades.

Thus, in order to better prepare the field to operate in the era of molecular genetics, this chapter provides an overview of pediatric genetic disorders and major concepts in medical genetics. It also describes the process and content of genetic counseling and the role of pediatric psychology on a medical genetics team. Several examples of genetic testing are given throughout. Finally, this chapter discusses the attendant ethical, social, psychological, and behavioral implications of rapid progress in predictive genetic testing for children, adolescents, and their families and decisions regarding disclosure of genetic test results.

OVERVIEW OF PEDIATRIC GENETIC DISORDERS

It has been estimated that there are more than 15,000 known genetic disorders, affecting upward of 13 million people in the United States (McKusick, 1998). In terms of children, roughly 3–5% are born with some form of a congenital malformation, which accounts for up to 30% of all infant deaths and up to 50% of all deaths postneonatally (Berry, Buehler, Strauss, Hogue, & Smith, 1987; Hoekelman & Pless, 1988). At one time, as many as 11% of all pediatric hospital admissions were related to genetic disorders, and nearly 20% were related to other congenital malformations (Scriver, Neal, Saginur, & Chow, 1973). Recent evidence confirms these earlier estimates, adding that children hospitalized for genetic disorders and congenital malformations are more likely to experience negative health outcomes than are children hospitalized for other reasons (Yoon et al., 1997). Thus pediatric genetic disorders are significant public health concerns.

BIOLOGICAL ASPECTS

In order to appreciate the full impact that genetic disorders and genetic testing may hold for children and families, it is important to have a basic understanding of medical genetics, including: (1) the three main types of genetic disorders (i.e., single-gene disorders, chromosome disorders, and multifactorial disorders) and (2) their primary modes of inheritance (i.e., recessive and dominant; Nussbaum et al., 2001). It is also important to understand how and why genetic tests are used and interpreted, as well as how medicine's ability to effectively prevent or treat the disorder and the age of onset of the disorder itself, play critical roles in determining whether or not children directly participate in the genetic testing process.

Medical Genetics

A gene is a unit of inheritance passed from parent to offspring. More specifically, it is a sequence of chromosomal deoxyribonucleic acid (DNA) that usually contains the information necessary for making a specific protein in the body. Humans are believed to have between 30,000 and 40,000 genes, which combine to form 23 pairs of chromosomes (packages of genes; 46 total). Each parent contributes one chromosome to each pair, so children inherit half of their chromosomes from their mothers and half from their fathers. One's full complement of DNA is called a genotype, and each child of a parent who carries a disease-causing gene has a 50% chance of inheriting that same gene if the condition is dominantly inherited (i.e., almost always results in a specific physical characteristic). By contrast, recessively inherited conditions appear only if children have received two copies of a disease-causing gene, one from each parent.

The expression of genes in the form of an observable trait, characteristic, or the presence or absence of a disorder (phenotype) cannot always be predicted in advance. Some medical disorders are caused by permanent structural alterations (mutations) in DNA, and these are called single-gene disorders. In dominantly inherited single-gene disorders, there is usually a 1:1 genotype:phenotype correspondence, meaning that having the altered gene leads to disease nearly 100% of the time. An example of a dominantly inherited disorder is hypochondroplasia, and an example of a recessively inherited disorder is hemophilia. Other disorders are caused by rearrangements, duplications, or omissions to the whole chromosome (chromosome disorders) that invariably disrupt the genes residing on those chromosomes; whereas still other disorders are caused by a complex interplay of one or more gene mutations interacting with the environment (multifactorial disorders). Examples of chromosome disorders include Down syndrome and Trisomies 18 and 13, and multifactorial disorders include some forms of cancer and diabetes.

Multifactorial disorders are of particular interest to pediatric psychology because genotype:phenotype correspondence is much more variable than it is in dominantly inherited single-gene disorders and because not all carriers go on to become medically affected. As the natural history of a multifactorial disorder is controlled by both genetic and nongenetic (i.e., environmental) influences, the relative contributions of genes and environment differ for each individual. In many cases, it may be important to identify, prior to the onset of symptoms, those who are at risk to develop the disorder so that appropriate steps may be taken to prevent or control the disease. These steps may include alterations in lifestyle and health behaviors, such as diet, physical activity, and tobacco use, along with medical management (e.g., targeted screening). As many of these behaviors are initiated early in life and are influenced by familial and social norms, the field of pediatric psychology should be able to assist children and their family members in reducing some of their risks. However, more research is necessary to prove the long-term effectiveness of initiating such changes in childhood among those who are genetically susceptible.

Genetic Testing

Genetic testing is the clinical tool used to predict the likelihood of disease occurrence, to identify individuals who carry disease-causing mutations, and to establish prenatal and clinical diagnosis or prognosis (Holtzman & Watson, 1998). Genetic testing is presently available for more than 800 disorders, though not all are necessarily detectable in childhood (GeneTests–GeneClinics, 2001). Genetic testing is similar to other kinds of laboratory testing that may be recommended by a physician, though several features make it unique. For example, genetic testing may be used for both medical management and for personal decision making, and its results usually apply not only to the individual undergoing testing but also to other family members (GeneTests–GeneClinics, 2001).

Indications for Pediatric Genetic Testing

In the case of children and adolescents, several points have been raised about when it is appropriate to use genetic testing. The main points to consider prior to initiating testing are:

1. Testing should produce timely medical benefits, which means that steps to prevent or treat the disorder are presently known or that testing provides medical knowledge to promote the patient's current health and well-being.
2. Substantial psychosocial benefits to competent adolescents should be gained from testing (e.g., it should reduce anxiety and uncertainty or influence reproductive, educational, vocational, insurance, or lifestyle decisions).
3. If the benefits of the test are not available until adulthood, then testing should be deferred.

These points were set forth jointly by the American Society of Human Genetics (ASHG) and the American College of Medical Genetics (ACMG) in 1995 and reaffirmed by the American Academy of Pediatrics (AAP, 2000, 2001) and several other national and foreign health organizations. In the case of genetic testing for pediatric disorders that are typically diagnosed around birth, or during childhood or adolescence, the indications for testing are clear. Less clear is the rationale for predictive testing—in which test results are used to estimate the likelihood that the child will experience the disorder at some point during his or her lifetime.

GENETIC COUNSELING AND PSYCHOLOGICAL ASSESSMENT

In families who have experienced chronic illness, especially those predisposed to hereditary disorders, the potential is high that children's psychosocial development will be affected by such events. Fanos (1997) pointed out that many of these children and adolescents, especially those who have had close relatives who have been ill, will likely have experienced multiple losses as a result of these conditions. Psychological research suggests that nearly one-half of children who grow up in families at increased cancer risk report worrying at least a fair amount about their chances of developing cancer in the future, and 50% report considerable worries that cancer might someday affect a member of their family (Tercyak, Peshkin, Streisand, & Lerman, 2001). Data from community samples suggest that children's thoughts about cancer are not infrequent, especially among those who may be at elevated risk (Chin et al., 1998). For example, in a study in the United Kingdom of perceived vulnerability to common diseases, 34% of adolescents and their parents believed that they were more likely to develop cancer than were their peers, and 46% believed they were just as likely as others to be affected by cancer during their lifetimes (Ponder, Lee, Green, & Richards, 1996). Combined with the emotional component of genetic testing, decision making about participation in testing and adjusting to, accepting, and communicating the uncertainty or finality of the test results are topics well deserving of the attention of practitioners trained in health psychology and counseling.

Genetic Counseling

Genetic testing is usually performed in the context of a genetic counseling consultation. The main components of the consultation are: (1) pretest patient education, (2) informed consent to testing, (3) posttest interpretation of test results, and (4) medical and psychosocial follow-up. These sessions are usually led by a medical geneticist, genetic counselor, nurse, or other health care professional with expertise in hereditary risk management (Nussbaum et al., 2001). In traditional genetic counseling, the counselor's (consultant's) interaction with the patient (client/consultand) is characterized by a Rogerian nondirective approach "aimed at promoting the [patient's] autonomy and self-directedness" (Kessler, 1997).

During genetic counseling, an extensive family medical history is taken and the data are usually presented graphically on a pedigree. A pedigree is a simplified diagram of a family's genealogy that shows family members' relationships to each other and which members are affected with a particular disorder or condition. On the pedigree, squares represent male gender, circles represent female gender, and successive generations of family members are displayed in descending order (eldest to most recent), ending with the child or children of interest. The pedigree is annotated with age and other vital facts. A sample pedigree showing an inherited predisposition to familial adenomatous polyposis (FAP; a colon cancer predisposition syndrome in which hundreds to thousands of precancerous colonic polyps develop, beginning at around 16 years; GeneTests–GeneClinics, 2001) is displayed in Figure 43.1.

As can be seen in the three generations of family members shown on the sample pedigree, the eldest son in the second generation (highlighted box) was previously diagnosed and successfully treated for hereditary colon cancer. His three children (two girls and a boy, ranging in age from 10–15 years old) are each at 50% risk to develop the same condition because FAP is dominantly transmitted. The arrow pointing to the middle child (age 13) indicates the presence of early symptoms of FAP, which are an indication for genetic testing. With this visual aid, the genetic counselor is better able to understand and explain disease patterns.

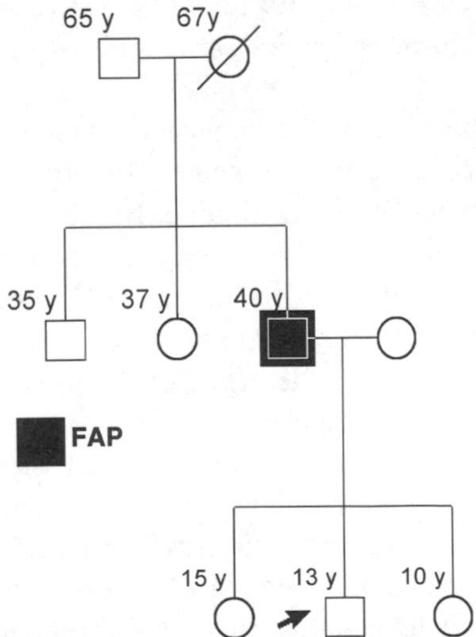

FIGURE 43.1. Pedigree demonstrating familial colon cancer risk.

A genetic counselor's use of a pedigree is not dissimilar to that of a psychologist's use of a genogram to understand a family's history of intergenerational conflict, as suggested in Bowen's family systems theory (Goldenberg & Goldenberg, 1991). In fact, research conducted with adults participating in family cancer-risk assessments suggests that genograms may be quite useful in genetic counseling to highlight family social support structures and communication patterns (Daly et al., 1999).

In addition to similarities in assessment tools used to elicit background information from families, other likenesses between genetic and certain forms of psychological counseling exist. These include the session format (e.g., individual and family sessions) and concepts assessed (i.e., to understand psychological aspects of the disease; Richards, 1996). This overlap, in part, leads to a unification of many of the goals of genetic and psychological counseling and highlights their complementary roles (Weil, 2000).

Role of Pediatric Psychology in Medical Genetics

Though the extent of pediatric psychology's role on a multidisciplinary medical genetics team varies among clinical sites, at least three features most clearly individuate it from that of other team members: (1) expertise in standardized psychological testing, (2) the ability to develop, implement, and modify health recommendations based on behavioral and other lifestyle factors, and (3) the knowledge to conduct child health psychology research and interpret behavioral outcome data.

The formal assessment of cognitive ability, behavior, personality, and academic achievement; structured interviewing; diagnosis and treatment of clinically significant psychological distress; and consulting with schools and other agencies are a unique combination of skills often required in the comprehensive assessment of children suspected of having (and known to already have) genetic disorders. This type of assessment is necessary because many pediatric genetic disorders affect both learning and behavior, particularly the neurobehavioral syndromes. Examples of these disorders include Turner syndrome, fragile-X syndrome, neurofibromatosis, sickle cell disease, Down syndrome, Klinefelter syndrome, phenylketonuria (PKU), Lesch-Nyhan syndrome, Prader-Willi syndrome, and Williams syndrome (see Goldstein & Reynolds, 1999, for review). It is not uncommon to see children with these disorders in a developmental and behavioral pediatrics clinic and for pediatric psychology to provide them with consultations.

In addition, pediatric psychology's role might include measurements of the effectiveness of interventions to prevent or treat pediatric genetic disorders, such as in the case of PKU, which requires dietary restriction of phenylalanine. Most children with PKU will go on to experience severe developmental delays if phenylalanine is not restricted in their diets. Opportunities exist for pediatric psychology to address adherence behaviors among children and adolescents with PKU. For example, Singh, Kable, Guerrero, Sullivan, and Elsas (2000) evaluated the effectiveness of a dietary adherence-promoting intervention delivered at a metabolic camp for adolescent girls with PKU. In addition to providing campers with diet and disease educational information, treatment included discussion groups about attitudes toward dietary adherence; groups were facilitated by experts in nutrition and pediatric psychology. The results of the study suggest short-term improvements in reduced phenylalanine measurements and psychological adjustment, and short- and long-term improvements in campers' diet and disease knowledge. Research by Fehrenbach and Peterson (1989) also highlights the important role that parents' problem-solving skills and stress levels play in children's adherence to the PKU dietary regimen.

PEDIATRIC GENETIC TESTING: A PSYCHOSOCIAL PERSPECTIVE

The past two decades have seen an explosion of adult psychological research on newborn genetic screening, prenatal genetic screening and testing for chromosome disorders, carrier testing for Tay-Sachs disease, sickle cell disease, and cystic fibrosis, and predictive testing for Huntington disease and breast, colon, and other forms of cancer (Hamann & Croyle, 1998; Lerman, Croyle, Tercyak, & Hamann, 2002; Tercyak, Johnson, Roberts, & Cruz, 2001). Many of these studies focused on adults' interests in and motivations for participating in predictive genetic testing, actual test uptake/participation behaviors, and the psychological consequences of learning one's genetic risk status. Largely influenced by a clinical perspective, such works attempted to identify testing participants most likely to experience high levels of psychological distress who might be in need of intervention. Though findings supporting the need for such services depend on the disease in question, a substantial amount of information has been learned about the stress-provoking potential of predictive genetic testing paradigms and characteristic ways in which adults respond to and cope with such news.

Unfortunately, pediatric psychological research has lagged far behind adult research, and many basic issues relating to the psychological experiences of parents, children, adolescents, and their families remain understudied and unknown. As an increasing number of predictive genetic tests become available for commercial use, health care providers and parents alike will be confronted with more and more questions about the appropriateness of these tests for children and adolescents. Further, they will need assistance in discerning what ethical, social, psychological, and behavioral issues are critical to good and poor outcomes when these tests are offered in clinical settings. Limited information is available from predictive testing protocols for Type 1 diabetes and certain forms of hereditary cancer, allowing for preliminary conclusions to be drawn. Nevertheless, remarkable opportunities remain to expand training in pediatric psychology to incorporate genetics into research and clinical practice (Patenaude, 2003).

Although children's direct participation in genetic testing remains a key concern, pediatric psychology must also broaden its focus to recognize the indirect ways that children might be psychologically affected by genetic testing even if children do not participate in testing themselves. One example is communication of parents' genetic test results to their children. In contrast to the substantial amount of information on adult genetic testing participants' communication behaviors toward adult at-risk relatives, there is virtually no information on parents' attitudes, beliefs, intentions, and actual communication behaviors toward children who may be at risk. Furthermore, the outcomes of parents' decisions to disclose or not disclose such information to their children are also unknown and represent a new area of inquiry.

Ethical and Social Issues

Much has been written about the international Human Genome Project (HGP)—a massive research effort designed to construct detailed genetic and physical maps of the entire human genome. With the mapping of the human genome nearly complete (International Human Genome Sequencing Consortium, 2001), information gained from the HGP will have profound implications for individuals, families, and society, including the potential use and misuse of genetic information. To address these issues, the Ethical, Legal, and Social Implications (ELSI) program was established as an integral part of the HGP (Collins et al., 1998). The ELSI program is important to note because it provides a mechanism for scientific research on the implications of human genetics discoveries to be conducted as new information comes to light.

One of the key ethical issues pertaining to children's participation in predictive genetic testing is the adequacy of informed consent (MacDonald & Lessick, 2000). In most states, children under the age of 18 do not have the legal capacity to provide consent for medical procedures, except under unusual circumstances. This responsibility falls to the child's parent(s). There is legitimate concern that parents who pursue predictive genetic testing for their children effectively take away the child's opportunity to choose to do so for him- or herself on reaching the age of majority. Other ethical issues include potential loss of the child's genetic privacy if testing were to be conducted and the possibility of stigmatization and discrimination later on in life if the child were determined to be a carrier of a risk-conferring mutation (AAP 2000, 2001; ASHG/ACMG, 1995; Hanson & Thomson, 2000; Lessick & Faux, 1998; Wertz, Fanos, & Reilly, 1994). In the context of genetic counseling for pediatric genetic disorders, such risks must be carefully weighed against any benefits that might otherwise be received.

Social issues center around the role of the family and the parent-child relationship in decision making about testing and the potential for knowledge gained through genetic test results to alter parent–child relationships and family interaction patterns. Risks to social functioning as a result of learning one's genetic status include impaired or strained relationships with family members and future partners, although these risks cannot necessarily be predicted in advance for any given individual (Michie & Marteau, 1996).

Psychological and Behavioral Issues

Empirical research on psychological and behavioral issues is limited, yet some evidence suggests that children who participate in predictive testing fare satisfactorily. This evidence comes from research-based testing protocols, with its tight controls and extensive monitoring of patient data and safety. Thus the generalizability of these findings to clinical practice is limited, and the information must be interpreted cautiously.

Diabetes

Combined genetic and antibody testing has made it possible to identify infants, children, and adolescents who are at increased risk for developing Type 1 diabetes. The psychological and behavioral impact of predictive testing for this disorder has been investigated in a growing number of studies. Johnson, Riley, Hansen, and Nurick (1990) were among the first to report on such issues in a cohort of 18 children. Immediately following the disclosure of their positive test results (i.e., of being informed that they were at increased risk of developing Type 1 diabetes), children experienced highly elevated anxiety levels. By 4-month follow-up, their distress had remitted to within normal limits. Subsequent work conducted with larger and more diverse samples confirmed these preliminary findings (Galatzer et al., 2001; Johnson & Tercyak, 1995), adding that there is a strong correspondence between parent and child anxiety in predictive testing situations (Johnson & Tercyak, 1995). Other findings indicate that: (1) tested children who are more anxious appear to engage in more coping strategies (Johnson & Carmichael, 2000), including self-initiated lifestyle changes (e.g., modification in diet and exercise patterns) following positive risk notification in an effort to stave off the disease (Johnson & Tercyak, 1995), and (2) mothers who are told that their newborns, children, and adolescents are at risk for developing diabetes are among the most highly anxious (Johnson, 2001; Johnson & Tercyak, 1995). As favorable attitudes toward diabetes screening and prevention exist among those who may be eligible for such services (Lucidarme, Domingues-Muriel, Castro, Czernichow, & Levy-Marchal, 1998; Tercyak, Johnson, & Schatz, 1998), these findings underscore the need to provide appropriate patient education and counseling before and after testing (Roth, 2001).

Cancer

In addition to diabetes, pediatric cancer represents another multifactorial disease for which various predisposition tests currently exist. These include genetic tests that forecast the onset of retinoblastomas, the multiple endocrine neoplasias, Von Hippel–Lindau syndrome, Li-Fraumeni syndrome, and FAP (Nichols, Li, Haber, & Diller, 1998). Several authors have written about the molecular genetics of childhood cancer and its implications for prevention, detection, and treatment (see Israel, 1989, and Knudson, 1993, for reviews). For example, Patenaude (1996) described several reasons that children might be tested for cancer susceptibility, including: (1) clarification of diagnostic information for children with cancer, (2) targeted screening, prevention, or early detection of childhood neoplasias among those determined to be gene carriers or the elimination of aggressive screening among noncarriers, and (3) satisfaction of the parent's or child's desire to learn about the child's genetic risk. Further, many parents of children at risk express an interest in having their children tested for predisposing gene mutations for a variety of cancerous and noncancerous disorders (Benkendorf et al., 1997; Brunger et al., 2000; Hamann et al., 2000; Strong & Marteau; 1995; Tercyak et al., 1998; Tercyak, Peshkin, De Marco, Brogan, & Lerman, 2002). However, parent interest is not sufficient grounds for offering such testing in clinical circumstances without a more complete understanding of the potential pros and cons of that decision. Much remains to be learned about attitudes and interest in genetic testing for cancer in children, about appropriate ways to support these individuals (Grosfeld et al., 1997), and about testing's impact on the family (Rolland, 1999; Tercyak, Streisand, Peshkin, & Lerman, 2000).

One procedure that has been relatively well utilized is predictive testing for FAP—a rare medical condition that, if left untreated, may lead to colon cancer. FAP is inherited in an autosomal dominant fashion. Each child of a parent with FAP has a 50% chance of acquiring the mutation, resulting in a greater than 90% lifetime risk of developing FAP among gene carriers (Lynch & Lynch, 1998). Children are eligible for FAP gene screening because disease symptoms (polyps) may develop during childhood. These polyps are often detected by an annual sigmoidoscopy, and removal of a portion of the affected colon and rectum is recommended to prevent colon cancer from developing (Lynch & Lynch, 1998). Thus one advantage of genetic testing for FAP in childhood is to spare at least some children (i.e., those 50% who are not gene carriers) from continuing frequent and invasive cancer surveillance procedures.

Education and counseling should accompany genetic testing for FAP in all cases, especially when children are involved (Petersen & Brensinger, 1996). This process may help to mitigate the negative psychological outcomes that can be associated with participation in testing and to facilitate healthy patient coping with FAP (Michie, McDonald, & Marteau, 1996). Very little is known about the characteristics of families who choose to have their children undergo screening for FAP gene mutations. Data that are available seem to suggest that, at least in the short term, the process of genetic counseling and testing is agreeable with children and their parents. In one study, children were not found to experience clinically significant increases in their psychological symptoms within 3 months of testing, and neither were their parents (Codori, Petersen, Boyd, Brandt, & Giardiello, 1996). However, children with FAP gene mutations were more likely to experience features of depression if their mothers were affected with FAP; children of affected mothers were also more likely to report greater anxiety after testing. Among parents who were not affected with FAP, follow-up assessments revealed elevations among their general distress scores. A more recent report found anxiety and depression to be within normal limits among children receiving positive test results for up to 1 year following test result receipt (Michie, Bobrow, & Marteau, 2001), further underscoring the relative safety of FAP gene testing for children.

FAMILY COMMUNICATION

Genetic counselors often assess, both before and after testing takes place, the extent to which testing participants are likely to make their test results known to other family members (i.e., disclosure). This assessment helps alert the medical genetics team to potential psychosocial issues that may need to be addressed further, such as family behavioral conflicts that could interfere with important medical information reaching potentially affected individuals (Botkin et al., 1996). Discussing the likelihood, process, content, and potential outcomes of sharing test result information with other family members can also provide some insight into the level of social support participants can be expected to receive and the opportunity for cascade testing to proceed within the family (Bloch, Adam, Wiggins, Huggins, & Hayden, 1992; Daly et al., 1999). In other words, the medical genetics team uses a systems-like approach to consider how the entire family may be affected by the level of communication about one member's genetic testing results. If necessary, psychological interventions to bolster patient coping and communication skills can then be implemented to prepare individuals receiving genetic test results to share this information with other at-risk family members (Daly et al., 2001).

Communication of Parents' Genetic Test Results to Children: A Model

Among the health communication processes that may be of special interest to pediatric psychology are those of parents who must decide if and when to talk with their children about the parents' genetic test results and the potential medical implications of any inherited risks for children. This is an emerging area of inquiry expected to have a substantial impact on clinical practice. Adults often share their knowledge about hereditary disease risk information, including the results of genetic tests, with their adult family members (Lerman, Peshkin, Hughes, & Isaacs, 1998; Ponder & Green, 1996). However, in the case of children, there is usually no immediate medical benefit to the child for the parents to do so, unless medical intervention is available. On the contrary, and in light of the psychological reactions of some parents to learning that they are gene carriers, concerns about psychological risks associated with sharing information about genetic threats to parental health with children have been raised (Tercyak et al., 2000).

Virtually no published studies have tested predictions about how parents might go about making decisions under such circumstances or how children would respond to the news of their parents' illness predisposition (genetic or otherwise). If these data were available, that information could be used to guide and inform parents and clinicians in making decisions related to sharing the results of predictive tests with children. Figure 43.2 presents a hypothetical model of psychological predictors of parental communication of genetic test results to children. The model takes into account social (relationships with family members), cognitive (knowledge, beliefs, and attitudes about testing and the disorder), psychological (stress and coping style), and medical (health care provider behavior and medical benefits and risks) factors—all of which could influence parents' intentions about if and when to share test results with their children. Along with actual test results, these factors are hypothesized to lead to the decision to disclose information about hereditary disease risks to children.

This model also recognizes the four primary stages that make up most health-threat-screening paradigms, which are: (1) pretest counseling, (2) submitting to testing and the waiting period for results to be processed, (3) receipt and interpretation of the result, and (4) outcome and impact. At the pretest counseling stage, factors that are expected to influence parents' intentions to disclose their test results to their children include the advice of health care providers, the level of knowledge parents have about the threat itself and the medical implications for their children, what they think and feel about the threat, the anticipated reaction of the child, and the level of openness in communication among family members. Some of these factors may also exert an influence on one another to produce stronger or weaker intentions toward disclosure, such as parent information-seeking coping style, which could mediate or moderate the relationship between stress and intentions, as well as knowledge, attitudes, and beliefs that might mediate the impact of health care variables. For example, highly distressed parents who vigilantly seek information about the health threat might

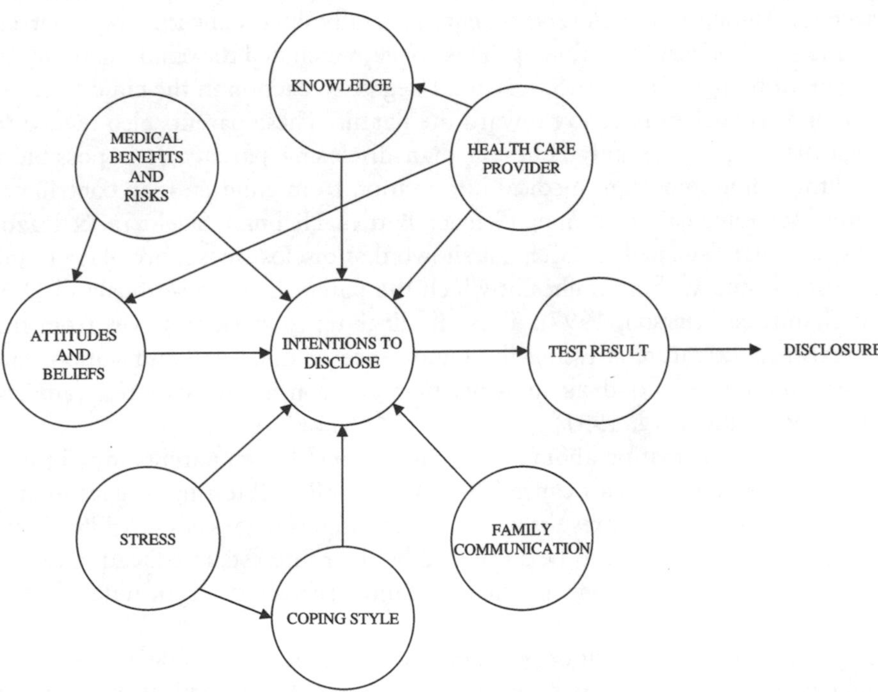

FIGURE 43.2. A hypothetical model of psychological predictors of parental communication of genetic test results to children.

be more likely to want to share this information with their children than distressed parents who prefer to avoid copious amounts of information.

Clearly, parents' intentions to disclose their results are susceptible to change over time, especially as more information about the health threat is acquired and as the information can be reprocessed both emotionally and cognitively. Test results represent an important stage in this model and are expected to interact with parental intentions. For example, it is not uncommon for parents to state early on in testing that they plan to share their results with their children, but only if the results are negative (i.e., the results are "good" news). In the case of predictive testing for adult-onset disorders in which the threat of developing the condition is uncertain, the rationale for immediately disclosing positive or ambiguous results to children might be less clear and more anxiety provoking. Disclosure or nondisclosure of results is but one outcome; others include the emotional and behavioral impact. Following is a summary of research on disclosure of information threatening to parental (and possibly child) health and its impact on well-being.

Factors Associated with Disclosure

Relevant data supporting components of the model come from studies of parents' decision making to share diagnostic medical test results with children—for example, parents who learn that they are HIV-positive and must make decisions about disclosing this information to their children. Wiener and colleagues have found that some, but not all, parents who are infected with the HIV virus tell their children their AIDS risk information (Wiener, Battles, & Heilman, 1998). Reasons given by parents for choosing to tell include not wanting the child to learn the information from someone outside the family and not wanting to keep family secrets. Among nondisclosers, parents generally cited concern over their children's cognitive and psychological functioning. This concern included the child's inability to understand information about HIV/AIDS, fears of a negative reaction in the child (e.g., being sad or scared), and feelings of rejection toward the parent. These parents also tended to report more depression and less family cohesion than disclosing parents. It is possible that the stress of withholding important medical information from children may contribute to parents' poorer psychological functioning (Wiener, Battles, Heilman, Sigelman, & Pizzo, 1996). Other HIV- and AIDS-related research has shown that disclosure is more likely to take place to older children and within families in which the parent is more seriously ill (Armistead, Klein, Forehand, & Wierson, 1997). These findings underscore messages from the family systems treatment literature stressing the importance of open communication patterns to avert crises and resolve conflicts in ways that are consistent with the family's values (Goldenberg & Goldenberg, 1991).

In addition to information about AIDS, data gathered from parents tested for a genetic susceptibility to hereditary breast cancer (BRCA1 and BRCA2 testing) suggest that approximately one-half share their test results with their children (Hughes et al., 1999). Like parents with HIV, these parents appear to be motivated by their interests in educating their children about the illness and in preventing a climate of family secrecy from forming (Tercyak et al., 2002).

The availability of treatment or preventive strategies is likely to be a significant consideration when parents contemplate both genetic testing and communication of risk information. Parents may be more likely to see the benefit of discussing their, or their children's, risk status if there are immediate medical implications, such as altering disease surveillance practices and health behaviors. This situation may be particularly true if the parents have not been seriously ill in the past or are in the presymptomatic phase (Rolland, 1999). Children's abilities to adapt to and understand illness, as well as the factors that cause it (e.g., gene mutations), generally improve with age and maturity through the teen years (Compas, 1998). This gain reflects a fundamental aspect of cognitive development and is consistent with advances in children's thinking capacities (Compas, 1998). Therefore, adolescent children are often told more information about their parents' illnesses than are preadolescent children (Compas et al., 1994; Hilton & Elfert, 1996) and are more involved in the health issues that affect them. Therefore, parents may be more likely to disclose information about predictive test results to adolescents or young adult children than to preadolescent youths (Hughes et al., 1999; Tercyak et al., 2002). The child's gender and premorbid emotional well-being should also be taken into account. There may be compelling reasons that information about the illness is more relevant for one gender than another (e.g., females at risk for hereditary breast or ovarian cancer). Similarly, the parent of a well-adjusted teenager may be more likely to disclose predictive test results to that individual than would the parent of a teen with adjustment difficulties; more positive adjustment and communication have been associated with disclosure (Tercyak et al., 2002).

In addition to the previously noted characteristics of the illness and the child, parent characteristics may be equally important determinants of the disclosure or communication process (Tercyak et al., 2000). For example, it has been shown that parents with higher levels of education (and, therefore, possibly a greater understanding of the genetics of cancer) are less likely to discuss their positive genetic test results for susceptibility to breast cancer with their children (Lerman et al., 1998) and that those with stronger intentions to communicate are more likely to do so (Tercyak et al., 2002). However, parents who experience greater general distress immediately after counseling are somewhat more likely to disclose to children than are parents with less distress (Tercyak, Hughes, et al., 2001). Parent gender may further affect this process. Again, research has found that women may be more likely to share information about having inherited a BRCA1 or BRCA2 mutation with other women than with men (e.g., to their sisters rather than to their brothers), despite the fact that siblings of both genders may be at increased risk (Ponder & Green, 1996). Similarly, Hughes et al. (1999) found that women at high risk for developing breast cancer were more likely to communicate their test results to a sister and to children than were men, which raises issues regarding individual differences in the roles that coping style and social support play.

Decisions about disclosure can lead to several potential outcomes. There are both advantages and disadvantages to disclosing such information to children. Possible advantages of children learning predictive testing results include parent and child emotional relief, better preparedness for the future, and modeling of open communication behaviors (Michie & Marteau, 1996). Disadvantages to testing or disclosure include change in the family's treatment of an affected or at-risk individual, increased worry over health, and decreased self-esteem (Michie & Marteau, 1996). One must also consider the risks and benefits of not sharing such information with youngsters. These include children's anger at not being informed sooner, modeling of family secretiveness, and the belief that no health risks exist when, in fact, they might (which could impede the initiation of more adaptive coping behaviors). Recent data obtained about children of mothers who participate in BRCA1/2 testing suggest that healthy children's thoughts of becoming sick, thoughts about developing cancer, and worries about cancer developing in a family member are moderately related to their symptoms of anxiety, depression, and behavior problems (Tercyak, Peshkin, et al., 2001). However, these symptoms are subclinical and generally remain stable.

Overall, much still remains to be understood about the impact of pediatric genetic testing and the communication of hereditary risk information within families. A child-focused perspective is clearly necessary to solidly advance both research and practice in this area. The importance of the field of pediatric psychology fully embracing these topics is high, particularly for those interested in joining medical genetics teams and cancer centers.

REFERENCES

American Academy of Pediatrics, Committee on Genetics. (2000). Molecular genetic testing in pediatric practice: A subject review. *Pediatrics, 106,* 1494–1497.

American Academy of Pediatrics, Committee on Genetics. (2001). Ethical issues with genetic testing in pediatrics. *Pediatrics, 106,* 1451–1455.

American Society of Human Genetics Board of Directors and American College of Medical Genetics Board of Directors. (1995). Points to consider: Ethical, legal, and psychosocial implications of genetic testing in children and adolescents. *American Journal of Human Genetics, 57,* 1233–1241.

Armistead, L., Klein, K., Forehand, R., & Wierson, M. (1997). Disclosure of parental HIV infection to children in the families of men with hemophilia: Description, outcomes, and the role of family process. *Journal of Family Psychology, 11,* 49–61.

Benkendorf, J. L., Reutenauer, J. E., Hughes, C. A., Eads, N., Willison, J., Powers, M., & Lerman, C. (1997). Patients' attitudes about autonomy and confidentiality in genetic testing for breast–ovarian cancer susceptibility. *American Journal of Medical Genetics, 73,* 296–303.

Berry, R. J., Buehler, J. W., Strauss, L. T., Hogue, C. J., & Smith, J. C. (1987). Birth-weight-specific infant mortality due to congenital anomalies, 1960 and 1980. *Public Health Reports, 102,* 171–181.

Bloch, M., Adam, S., Wiggins, S., Huggins, M., & Hayden, M. R. (1992). Predictive testing for Huntington disease in Canada: The experience of those receiving an increased risk. *American Journal of Medical Genetics, 42,* 499–507.

Botkin, J. R., Croyle, R. T., Smith, K. R., Baty, B. J., Lerman, C., Goldgar, D. E., et al. (1996). A model protocol for evaluating the behavioral and psychosocial effects of BRCA1 testing. *Journal of the National Cancer Institute, 88,* 872–882.

Brunger, J. W., Murray, G. S., O'Riordan, M., Matthews, A. L., Smith, R. J., & Robin, N. H. (2000). Parental attitudes toward genetic testing for pediatric deafness. *American Journal of Human Genetics, 67,* 1621–1625.

Chin, D. G., Schonfeld, D. J., O'Hare, L. L., Mayne, S. T., Salovey, P., Showalter, D. R., & Cicchetti, D. V. (1998). Elementary school-age children's developmental understanding of the causes of cancer. *Journal of Developmental and Behavioral Pediatrics, 19,* 397–403.

Codori, A. M., Petersen, G. M., Boyd, P. A., Brandt, J., & Giardiello, F. M. (1996). Genetic testing for cancer in children: Short-term psychological effect. *Archives of Pediatrics and Adolescent Medicine, 150,* 1131–1138.

Collins, F. S., Patrinos, A., Jordan, E., Chakravarti, A., Gesteland, R., & Walters, L. (1998). New goals for the U.S. Human Genome Project: 1998–2003. *Science, 282,* 682–689.

Compas, B. E. (1998). An agenda for coping research and theory: Basic and applied developmental issues. *International Journal of Behavioral Development,* 22, 231–237.

Compas, B. E., Worsham, N. L., Epping-Jordan, J. E., Grant, K. E., Mireault, G., Howell, D. C., & Malcarne, V. L. (1994). When mom or dad has cancer: Markers of psychological distress in cancer patients, spouses, and children. *Health Psychology, 13,* 507–515.

Daly, M., Farmer, J., Harrop-Stein, C., Montgomery, S., Itzen, M., Costalas, J. W., et al. (1999). Exploring family relationships in cancer risk counseling using the genogram. *Cancer Epidemiology, Biomarkers, and Prevention, 8*(4 Pt 2), 393–398.

Daly, M. B., Barsevick, A., Miller, S. M., Buckman, R., Costalas, J., Montgomery, S., & Bingler, R. (2001). Communicating genetic test results to the family: A six-step, skills-building strategy. *Family and Community Health, 24,* 13–26.

Fanos, J. H. (1997). Developmental tasks of childhood and adolescence: Implications for genetic testing. *American Journal of Medical Genetics, 71,* 22–28.

Fehrenbach, A. M., & Peterson, L. (1989). Parental problem-solving skills, stress, and dietary compliance in phenylketonuria. *Journal of Consulting and Clinical Psychology, 57,* 237–241.

Galatzer, A., Green, E., Ofan, R., Benzaquen, H., Yosefsberg, Z., Weintrob, N., et al. (2001). Psychological impact of islet cell antibody screening. *Journal of Pediatric Endocrinology Metabolism, 14,* 675–679.

GeneTests–GeneClinics (n.d.). Retrieved October 1, 2001, from *http://www.genetests.org*

Goldenberg, I., & Goldenberg, H. (1991). *Family therapy: An overview* (3rd ed.). Pacific Grove, CA: Brooks/Cole.

Goldstein, S., & Reynolds, C. R. (1999). *Handbook of neurodevelopmental and genetic disorders in children.* New York: Guilford Press.

Grosfeld, F. J., Lips, C. J., Beemer, F. A., van Spijker, H. G., Brouwers-Smalbraak, G. J., & ten Kroode, H. F. (1997). Psychological risks of genetically testing children for a hereditary cancer syndrome. *Patient Education and Counseling, 32,* 63–67.

Hamann, H. A., & Croyle, R. T. (1998). Genetic disorders. In A. S. Bellack, M. Hersen, D. W. Johnston, & M. Johnston (Eds.), *Comprehensive clinical psychology* (pp. 409–423). Amsterdam, NY: Pergamon.

Hamann, H. A., Croyle, R. T., Venne, V. L., Baty, B. J., Smith, K. R., & Botkin, J. R. (2000). Attitudes toward the genetic testing of children among adults in a Utah-based kindred tested for a BRCA1 mutation. *American Journal of Medical Genetics, 92,* 25–32.

Hanson, J. W., & Thomson, E. J. (2000). Genetic testing in children: Ethical and social points to consider. *Pediatric Annals, 29,* 285–291.

Hilton, B. A., & Elfert, H. (1996). Children's experiences with mothers' early breast cancer. *Cancer Practice, 4,* 96–104.

Hoekelman, R. A., & Pless, I. B. (1988). Decline in mortality among young Americans during the 20th century: Prospects for reaching national mortality reduction goals for 1990. *Pediatrics, 82,* 582–595.

Holtzman, N. A., & Watson, M. S. (1998). *Promoting safe and effective genetic testing in the United States: Final report of the Task Force on Genetic Testing.* Baltimore: Johns Hopkins University Press.

Hughes, C., Lynch, H., Durham, C., Snyder, C., Lemon, S., Narod, S., et al. (1999). Communication of BRCA1/2 test results in hereditary breast cancer families. *Cancer Research, Therapy and Control, 8,* 51–59.

International Human Genome Sequencing Consortium. (2001). Initial sequencing and analysis of the human genome. *Nature, 409,* 860–921.

Israel, M. A. (1989). Pediatric oncology: Model tumors of unparalleled import. *Journal of the National Cancer Institute, 81,* 404–408.

Johnson, S. B. (2001). Screening programs to identify children at risk for diabetes mellitus: Psychological impact on children and parents. *Journal of Pediatric Endocrinology and Metabolism, 14,* 653–659.

Johnson, S. B., & Carmichael, S. K. (2000). At-risk for diabetes: Coping with the news. *Journal of Clinical Psychology in Medical Settings, 7,* 69–78.

Johnson, S. B., Riley, W. J., Hansen, C. A., & Nurick, M. A. (1990). Psychological impact of islet cell-antibody screening: Preliminary results. *Diabetes Care, 13,* 93–97.

Johnson, S. B., & Tercyak, K. P. (1995). Psychological impact of islet cell antibody screening for IDDM on children, adults and their family members. *Diabetes Care, 18,* 1370–1372.

Kessler, S. (1997). Psychological aspects of genetic counseling: XI. Nondirectiveness revisited. *American Journal of Medical Genetics, 72,* 164–171.

Knudson, A. G., Jr. (1993). Pediatric molecular oncology: Past as prologue to the future. *Cancer, 71,* 3320–3324.

Lerman, C., Croyle, R. T., Tercyak, K. P., & Hamann, H. (2002). Genetic testing: Psychological aspects and implications. *Journal of Consulting and Clinical Psychology, 70,* 784–797.

Lerman, C., Peshkin, B. N., Hughes, C., & Isaacs, C. (1998). Family disclosure in genetic testing for cancer susceptibility: Determinants and consequences. *Journal of Health Care Law and Policy, 1,* 353–372.

Lessick, M., & Faux, S. (1998). Implications of genetic testing of children and adolescents. *Holistic Nursing Practice, 12,* 38–46.

Lucidarme, N., Domingues-Muriel, E., Castro, D., Czernichow, P., & Levy-Marchal, C. (1998). Appraisal and implications of predictive testing for insulin-dependent diabetes mellitus. *Diabetes and Metabolism, 24,* 550–553.

Lynch, H. T., & Lynch, J. F. (1998). Genetics of colonic cancer. *Digestion, 59,* 481–492.

MacDonald, D. J., & Lessick, M. (2000). Hereditary cancers in children and ethical and psychosocial implications. *Journal of Pediatric Nursing, 15,* 217–225.

McKusick, V. A. (1998). *Mendelian inheritance in man: A catalog of human genes and genetic disorders* (12th ed.). Baltimore: Johns Hopkins University Press.

Michie, S., Bobrow, M., & Marteau, T. M. (2001). Predictive genetic testing in children and adults: A study of emotional impact. *Journal of Medical Genetics, 38,* 519–526.

Michie, S., & Marteau, T. M. (1996). Predictive genetic testing in children: The need for psychological research. *British Journal of Health Psychology, 1,* 3–14.

Michie, S., McDonald, V., & Marteau, T. (1996). Understanding responses to predictive genetic testing: A grounded theory approach. *Psychology and Health, 11,* 455–470.

Nichols, K. E., Li, F. P., Haber, D. A., & Diller, L. (1998). Childhood cancer predisposition: Applications of molecular testing and future implications. *Journal of Pediatrics, 132,* 389–397.

Nussbaum, R. L., McInnes, R. R., & Willard, H. F. (2001). *Thompson and Thompson genetics in medicine* (6th ed.). Philadelphia: Saunders.

Patenaude, A. F. (1996). The genetic testing of children for cancer susceptibility: Ethical, legal, and social issues. *Behavioral Sciences and the Law, 14,* 393–410.

Patenaude, A. F. (2003). Pediatric psychology training and genetics: What will twenty-first-century pediatric psychologists need to know? *Journal of Pediatric Psychology, 28,* 135–145.

Petersen, G. M., & Brensinger, J. D. (1996). Genetic testing and counseling in familial adenomatous polyposis. *Oncology (Huntington), 10,* 89–94.

Ponder, M., & Green, J. M. (1996). BRCA1 testing: Some issues in moving from research to service. *Psycho-Oncology, 5,* 223–232.

Ponder, M., Lee, J., Green, J., & Richards, M. (1996). Family history and perceived vulnerability to some common diseases: A study of young people and their parents. *Journal of Medical Genetics, 33,* 485–492.

Richards, M. (1996). Families, kinship and genetics. In T. Marteau & M. Richards (Eds.), *The troubled helix: Social and psychological implications of the new human genetics* (pp. 249–273). New York: Cambridge University Press.

Rolland, J. S. (1999). Families and genetic fate: A millennial challenge. *Families, Systems, and Health, 17,* 123–132.

Roth, R. (2001). Psychological and ethical aspects of prevention trials. *Journal of Pediatric Endocrinology Metabolism, 14,* 669–674.

Scriver, C. R., Neal, J. L., Saginur, R., & Chow, A. (1973). The frequency of genetic disease and congenital malformation among patients in a pediatric hospital. *Canadian Medical Association Journal, 108,* 1111–1115.

Singh, R. H., Kable, J. A., Guerrero, N. V., Sullivan, K. M., & Elsas, L. J., II. (2000). Impact of a camp experience on phenylalanine levels, knowledge, attitudes, and health beliefs relevant to nutrition management of phenylketonuria in adolescent girls. *Journal of the American Dietetic Association, 100,* 797–803.

Strong, L. C., & Marteau, T. (1995). Evaluating children and adolescents for heritable cancer risk. *Journal of the National Cancer Institute Monographs, 17,* 111–113.

Tercyak, K. P., Hughes, C., Main, D., Snyder, C., Lynch, J. F., Lynch, H. T., & Lerman, C. (2001). Parental communication of BRCA1/2 genetic test results to children. *Patient Education and Counseling, 42,* 213–224.

Tercyak, K. P., Johnson, S. B., Roberts, S. F., & Cruz, A. C. (2001). Psychological response to prenatal genetic counseling and amniocentesis. *Patient Education and Counseling, 43,* 73–84.

Tercyak, K. P., Johnson, S. B., & Schatz, D. A. (1998). Patient and family reflections on the use of subcutaneous insulin to prevent diabetes: A retrospective evaluation from a pilot prevention trial. *Journal of Diabetes and Its Complications, 12,* 279–286.

Tercyak, K. P., Peshkin, B. N., DeMarco, T. A., Brogan, B. M., & Lerman, C. (2002). Parent–child factors and their effect on communicating BRCA1/2 test results to children. *Patient Education and Counseling, 47,* 145–153.

Tercyak, K. P., Peshkin, B. N., Streisand, R., & Lerman, C. (2001). Psychological issues among children of hereditary breast cancer gene (BRCA1/2) testing participants. *Psycho-Oncology, 10,* 336–346.

Tercyak, K. P., Streisand, R. M., Peshkin, B. N., & Lerman, C. (2000). Psychosocial impact of predictive testing for illness on children and families: Challenges for a new millennium. *Journal of Clinical Psychology in Medical Settings, 7,* 55–68.

Weil, J. (2000). *Psychosocial genetic counseling.* New York: Oxford University Press.

Wertz, D. C., Fanos, J. H., & Reilly, P. R. (1994). Genetic testing for children and adolescents: Who decides? *Journal of the American Medical Association, 272,* 875–881.

Wiener, L. S., Battles, H. B., & Heilman, N. E. (1998). Factors associated with parents' decision to disclose their HIV diagnosis to their children. *Child Welfare, 77,* 115–135.

Wiener, L. S., Battles, H. B., Heilman, N., Sigelman, C. K., & Pizzo, P. A. (1996). Factors associated with disclosure of diagnosis to children with HIV/AIDS. *Pediatric AIDS and HIV Infection: Fetus to Adolescent, 7,* 310–324.

Yoon, P. W., Olney, R. S., Khoury, M. J., Sappenfield, W. M., Chavez, G. F., & Taylor, D. (1997). Contribution of birth defects and genetic diseases to pediatric hospitalizations: A population-based study. *Archives of Pediatric and Adolescent Medicine, 151,* 1096–1103.

44

Telehealth

DENNIS C. HARPER

In this chapter the focus on telehealth is general and not limiting. Telehealth and telemedicine are often used interchangeably; however, this chapter focuses on a somewhat broader term, "telehealth," which is referred to by the World Health Organization (WHO) as "the integration of telecommunications systems into the practice of protecting and promoting health" (Antezana, 1997, p. 4). Telehealth is generally understood to use advanced telecommunications methods to exchange health information and promote health care across geographic distances and time. Most authors (Darkins & Cary, 2000) use telemedicine as a more restrictive term and focus on "medical" care. In brief, telehealth is *remote* health care. Technology brings the participants together, usually in a visual/auditory format. In the remainder of this chapter this type of remote delivery of health care is referred to as "telehealth."

The following sections highlight several key issues in the history of telehealth, definitions of telehealth and telemedicine, informatics, and the digital convergence of informational strategies in health care, particularly as this new technological application affects pediatric psychology.

BRIEF HISTORY OF TELEHEALTH

The history of telehealth dates to early 1955, when the Nebraska Psychiatric Institute installed a closed circuit two-way microwave video link between the Department of Psychiatry of the Nebraska Medical School in Omaha and a state mental hospital in Norfolk, Nebraska. The system was used for consultations, education, and administration. Success was periodically stalled until the mid-1990s due to high costs, poor image quality, and lack of integration of telehealth into mainstream health care (Darkins & Cary, 2000). Over the next 40 years telehealth moved forward in varying degrees. In the 1970s and 1980s, telehealth became of interest to the National Aeronautics and Space Administration (NASA), the military, and other groups who needed "high tech" consultation systems in very remote and distant settings. This level of technology for the U.S. government facilitated the use of "specialist" consultation combined with high-end technological delivery (i.e., to astronauts and climbers on Mt. Everest).

In the mid- to late 1980s the Internet revolution began, and the public, as well as the professional sector, became interested in fast and highly accessible information technology. Worldwide interest and utilization of telehealth technology was occurring in Scandinavia, New Zealand, and Australia (Darkins & Cary, 2000). Countries that needed remote care delivery systems experimented with cost containment and access to health care across large distances. This form of telemedicine enabled much general consultation (i.e., video conferencing) and specialized in providing short-supply medical consultation in radiology, pathology, dermatology, cardiology, otolaryngology, and, for this discussion, psychiatry. In the mid-1990s the "action" in telecare moved to the United States and was focused on three issues, greater accessibility, better quality through more efficient delivery, and cost reduction in health care delivery (Darkins & Cary, 2000). Three areas surfaced as key foci: prison telemedicine, rural telecare, and home telecare. Prison care and telemedicine emerged as a way to provide much needed health care in a more cost-effective manner and to promote accessibility in a more secure fashion for everyone involved (Bashshur, Sanders, & Shannon, 1997). Rural delivery of specialized care surfaced as another need, especially in providing specialized care in underserved and low-density population areas in which health care specialists are most in short supply. Iowa, Georgia, Missouri, and Texas have been leaders in providing consultations to rural locations with considerable success. In fact, Iowa remains a leader in providing specialized telehealth consultation to children with special health care needs in rural communities (Harper, 2001a). Finally, telecare is currently beginning to move into the home as an adjunct to regular monitoring of chronic health care needs, especially among elderly individuals with diabetes. These systems primarily consist of video phone connections and are becoming cost-effective as essentially a low-end technology system of monitoring health care in the home (Harper, 2001a).

Telehealth trends since 1997 have focused on (1) a general migration of services to the Internet, (2) focus on the home as the site of care, (3) development of noninvasive biosensors, thereby eliminating the role of the physical hospital location, (4) broader involvement of nonmedical practitioners in providing telehealth services, and (5) wireless technology (Darkins & Cary, 2000). The contemporary move to the Internet is largely dependent on the quality of the transmission or bandwidth of the connection, which is related to cost and location. Bandwidth is defined as an agreed-on measure of the capacity of a data channel to exchange information, providing a gauge of a network's capacity to carry data. Larger bandwidths carry more data and enhance the quality of the transmission. The biosensor movement enables practitioners at the off-site location (where the client is) to evaluate and collect physical data remotely. This application will continue to evolve and will likely move into two general directions (Bashshur et al, 1997): (1) higher and more complex technology for superspecialized procedures (remote-computer assisted surgery; noninvasive remote monitoring of physical factors such as heart rate in high-risk infants) and (2) home-focused monitoring of chronic health status, such as diabetes and renal disease. Monitors connected to remote hospital-based computer systems to monitor and remind clients of medications or particular health routines are currently a reality. Low-tech pagers are currently used as "buddy monitors"to monitor and remind people about health routines. Wireless technology, combined with broadband Internet, will enable communication for a variety of remote connections in home or field between provider and client. Laptop video cameras combined with selected biosensors for accessing physical data would enable ease of client participation and facilitate ongoing health consultation without the need to visit special locations. The "virtual clinic" is a technical reality but has to surmount numerous social, professional, cultural, and financial hurdles before becoming widespread (Bashshur et al., 1997). A final trend in telehealth focuses on its utilization and movement toward a broader professional market other than physicians. Nurses, psychologists, and social workers have found that the telehealth venue is becoming an efficient and quality-enhancing tool for regular "consultation and monitoring" of clients (Liss, Glueckauf, & Ecklund-Johnson, 2002).

This brief history illustrates several issues in the evolving status of telehealth. The use of telecommunications in health care was initially precipitated largely by the problem of access and, in some instances, the urgency of particular medical needs. Geography, distance, availability of health care facilities, and limited availability of practitioners for more "complex" care pushed technology to provide some answers to these problems for consumers. Complex technology and remote access issues for the military and NASA combined to generate some interesting inventions and devices. The informational–digital revolution and the Internet provided a pathway for access to more efficient communication between practitioners and consumers (Gilder, 2000). Electronic health care began to evolve; however, acceptance and use of telehealth involves more than lower costs, and the informational access of providers and consumer acceptance are critical and related to a complex interplay of human factors (local politics, personal and professional relationships), costs and reimbursements, technical network design and quality, licensure and statutory regulations for health care, unique liabilities and secure information systems, and the efficacy of the venue for health care distribution.

INFORMATICS AND DIGITAL CONVERGENCE OF INFORMATION

Numerous authors (Gladwell, 2000; Gilder, 2000) have noted that a key aspect of the telehealth movement is in part related to the informational movement or the "information revolution" (Bauer & Ringel, 1999). The information revolution is generally linked to computer development and digitization of all aspects of information. Digitization transforms data into common forms—binary, zero and one. Information, its use, organization, storage, dispersal, availability/access, and complexity are now viewed as a source of power, a commodity for marketing and profit (Davis & Meyer, 1998; Gilder, 2000). Informatics is the applied science of collecting, storing, and retrieving data to support informed decision making (Bauer & Ringel, 1999). There is a complex synergistic relationship between informatics and telehealth systems. Electronic health care and telehealth permit a convergence of information to enable care and complex decision making. The Internet can enable both systems. One example is the electronic medical record (i.e., all aspects of laboratory outcomes, imaging studies, and narrative records; Bashshur et al., 1997).

TELECOMMUNICATION FORMATS AND RELATED ISSUES

There are currently two basic types of telehealth electronic connections. These connections are a function of the particular need of the telehealth consultation and the availability of such connections. Asynchronous connection refers to storage and transmission forward of data or video images. Time is the variable, that is, the video is recorded and then transmitted and displayed at the other end. The amount of delay is dependent on the quality and speed of the particular connection. Synchronous connections usually refer to real-time connections; what is going on between the settings is live at all times. The need for real time is related to the quality of the viewing and speed for visual diagnostic quality.

TELEHEALTH AND RELATIONSHIPS WITH CLIENTS

Telehealth communications raise some issues in the ethical and legal realm. The distance between participants in telehealth alters the context of care and also raises issues in several areas. Is the standard of care changed by telehealth, and does this change affect the quality of care? Do the professionals who consult with distant clients assume obligations consistent with standard therapist/client relationships? Finally, how is confidentiality, privacy, or informed consent assured and maintained in this venue of care?

Licensing issues are of concern primarily due to the potential for cross-state practice and consultation. Licensure to practice given by state statutory systems has long been state specific. In some instances, this regulation has been further reinforced by several states to protect the practice of telehealth and its market integrity (Darkins & Cary, 2000). Another trend is the movement toward a national licensing statute. Such national efforts in medicine have been viewed as unpopular and legally complicated. Cross-state practice implies interstate commerce, which invites federal regulation. Three solutions (Bauer & Ringel, 1999) have been raised: (1) a multistate compact among a group of states, usually contiguous; (2) a model of state practice guidelines that limits practice to only telemedicine; and (3) licensing of particular "Internet practice sites."

Malpractice issues in telehealth have focused on two areas: practice over state lines and whether the "telehealth encounter" actually enables a professional-patient relationship to the point that liability can be assigned. The former point is currently ambiguous, given the jurisdictional confusion over cross-state practice. The relationship issue has found support in case law to the point that the telehealth encounter is consistent with contractual and other professional obligations in client and professional interactions (Viegas & Dunn, 1998).

A related legal issue in the practice of telehealth is standard of care. Standards of care relate to professional requisite skills, training, and expertise to offer or perform a particular service. Presently, no agreed-on standards of care have been offered for telehealth. Numerous suggested voluntary standards have been recently put forth without any statutory approval (American Telemedicine Association, 2002). If the professions are to move forward in the electronic information age, some form of national standards will likely be needed.

Ethical issues for telehealth relate primarily to privacy, confidentiality and security, informed consent, and the professional–client relationship. Privacy and confidentiality are essential to the professional–client relationship and have been problematic at times in the application of telehealth. Internet systems have been violated and will likely continue to have problems. Although any Internet or video conferencing system can be violated, there are some standard safeguards that can and should be applied by all practitioners. Authentication requires a multistep procedure usually consisting of a name and password. Newer devices are commercially available based on retinal scan, voice, or fingerprint. Authorization is a software system configuration that limits access to selected levels of information. Encryption uses an algorithm to scramble information. As telehealth and electronic storage of data become widespread, additional security will be necessary; hopefully, it will be less cumbersome and also more secure (Viegas & Dunn, 1998).

The data on whether the telehealth venue or electronic media (videos, Web chat sites, e-health, e-mail) are sufficient to develop rapport, confidence, and trust receives a very mixed answer generally (Bashshur et al., 1997; Glueckauf, 2002). The existing studies are mostly theoretical and largely descriptive, focusing on both providers' and clients' satisfaction with the medium and utilization rates of telehealth. Data are also available from self-help forums, feedback from research projects, underserved populations with new access to care, and descriptive market surveys of telehealth usage. Stamm (1998) presents a useful and concise review of the data on satisfaction with consultations. For many respondents these data were reported to be as good as those from face-to-face interviews, therapeutic alliance was judged adequate over a series of sessions, and a positive impact on the quality-of-life factors was evident. Glueckauf (2002) continues to raise important questions about efficacy of the entire telehealth technique across different clinical populations. Few studies have provided consistent and useful comparative data between telehealth applications and on-site procedures. Often most studies provide services to resource-limited areas, and respondents are very grateful. Obviously such samples complicate interpretations. Can telehealth as a medium promote confidence, trust, and rapport at a distance? The answer is a qualified yes, but it depends on the quality of the technology, the samples explored, the type of consultation or problem under consideration, and the professionals' overall visual decorum and style.

REIMBURSEMENT

"What is not paid for is not likely to become a viable clinical service"—a statement often made by those working in telehealth. This financial component has been repeated by practitioners in the field of telehealth and telemedicine. Funds for many of these efforts currently represent a combination of grants, private funds, or capitated contractual arrangements for particular populations, most often governmental agencies such as the military or the prison system. Medicare has defined a number of relevant current procedural technology codes (CPT) as applicable for telehealth under the federal budget effective as of January 1, 1999 (Nickelson, 1998). These codes apply to psychological services in certain health provider shortage areas in all 50 U.S. states. Although compensation is limited in amount and breadth of coverage, this action by the federal government signals congressional approval and opens up the market with a precedent for mandated actions for the private sector to note. Capitated payments for telehealth are provided by Medicare. These governmental systems (military/prisons) are high users of telehealth and have developed extensive telecommunications and remote technology in this area, often using dedicated transmission lines for communications. Psychologists should explore these arrangements if they are providing services to such governmental agencies and locations. Home care with Medicare for the elderly is another cost saver and potential area of consultation (McKay, Glasgow, Feil, Boles, & Barrera, 2002). Private carriers are generally reluctant and inconsistent in opening up new markets for payment of telehealth. Nevertheless, in selected states (Illinois, Nebraska, North Dakota, New York, Vermont), some services of physicians, psychologists, and social workers are beginning to be paid.

HIGHLIGHTS FROM THE LITERATURE ON THE CLINICAL APPLICATIONS OF TELEHEALTH

The following sections review selected applications of the literature in telehealth and focus on children with special needs and behavioral telehealth, primarily in the area of mental health and psychiatry. These areas were selected as being relevant to the practice and general role of the pediatric psychologist. The literature in telehealth is expanding rapidly, but to date only preliminary information is available on its general effectiveness in the behavioral, mental health, and rehabilitation areas (Glueckauf, 2002). Considerable literature exists on the medical aspects of telemedicine, usually in the areas of specialized technology applications (e.g., high-tech peripheral biosensors) and general video conferencing for health management. Interested readers can research the extensive literature that is available in these areas (Bashshur et al., 1997; American Telemedicine Association, 2002).

In discussing telehealth applications, it is somewhat important to note the type of transmission in concert with the type of services offered. As noted elsewhere in this chapter, transmission mode does affect the quality of what is being delivered, which in turn may have an impact on the overall outcome and general efficacy of services. The ability to research these issues in telehealth, as noted by Glueckauf (2002), remains one of the central and most pressing issues. The majority of behavioral telehealth applications have been delivered using the store and forward technology over standard phone lines (Stamm, 1998). Video conferencing is also emerging as a communication transaction medium. In fact, Glueckauf (2002) reviews a number of studies in this particular area with promising results. Video conferencing enables the interaction to approach real-time communication. Such connections are usually dedicated (DSL, ISDN) cable lines, which are more efficient, promote higher quality, are usually more secure, and are somewhat more expensive. Use of the Internet for behavioral telehealth has been in the form of specific mental health sites, chat rooms, and online self-help forums (see Telehealth Net: *http://telehealth.net*). Such sites remain controversial because of content, variable professional quality, and ethical issues. Although it is often noted that some help is better than none, this is hardly an endorsement or an assurance of quality. E-mail and text-based sites are also a variation of behavioral health offerings as well. In fact, E-health has become quite popular (Maheu, 2000). With the array of informational telehealth technologies distributed worldwide, it is not surprising that quality and content are highly variable and very difficult to synthesize as to overall effectiveness.

BEHAVIORAL TELEHEALTH

Mental health consultation using a variety of telehealth approaches dates to the late 1950s and early 1960s in the United States. Use of these technologies was and remains related to service shortages of mental health specialists geographically (Bashshur, et al., 1997). Early technology utilized closed circuit television (CCTV) and was the most common mode until the mid-1990s, when computer video conferencing began to be used. Therefore, much of the service provided approached a real-time, reasonable-to-good quality interaction, usually two-way, between participants. Application focused on consultation, assessment, and continuing education (Baer, Elford, & Cukor, 1997; Brown, 1995). These clinical applications utilized diagnostic interviews, medication management, psychotherapy, and general consultation (Brown, 1995; Baer et al., 1997). Clients included adults, outpatients and inpatients, child and family outpatients, adult prisoners, and adults with mental retardation. Diagnostic categories were varied. Baer et al. (1997) reviewed the literature in peer-reviewed journals. Twenty-one studies were reviewed in video conferencing for medical education, clinical psychiatric video conferencing with no controls, clinical psychiatric video conferencing with controls, reliability of psychometric assessment by video, and cost-effectiveness of video consultation. The conclusions were consistent with the variable quality of the studies reported, namely mixed conclusions. A closer inspection of the studies, however, revealed all the problems of most treatment or diagnostic efficacy studies in mental health (e.g., questionable controls, variable interview-based diagnostic procedures, very mixed samples, limited data collection, and brief therapeutic contacts). Even the more well-designed studies often confused or combined the efficacy of mental health outcomes with the satisfaction of the delivery method—telehealth. Several other telehealth studies (Baer et al., 1995; Zarate et al., 1997) with more focused samples and methodology report very high diagnostic rater agreements and reliabilities with clients displaying either obsessive–compulsive disorder or schizophrenia. Higher bandwidth (better clarity of visual images) was associated with higher reliability when comparing telehealth to in-person assessments. Rohland and Flaum (2000), in a small controlled study that utilized telehealth video conferencing in a real-time, two-way system, reported that the results were as "good as face-to-face" consultation, again based on general acceptability ratings of the clients.

Bashshur et al. (1997) and Stamm (1998) provide a balanced summary assessment of behavioral telehealth. Acceptance by providers (psychologists and psychiatrists) and clients was generally positive. Providers were often positively biased in presenting their "own" programs of research or service. Consumers were often "grateful" for receiving hard-to-get services for less travel time and cost. In fact, many programs did not charge for the services. Clearly, outcomes were affected by these factors. Despite increasing usage rates, few projects continue in a self-sustaining mode. Some reasons for this include the following: (1) most programs use telehealth primarily to reduce the distance and access problem; (2) programs were viewed as a peripheral treatment system; and (3) the system was never fully developed, integrated, or maintained in a systemic fashion with the existing health care delivery programs in the treatment setting. As an apparent optional "add-on," sustainability was very difficult. Finally, behavioral telehealth is currently the most frequent "specialty" for consultation in programs in the United States (Stamm, 1998). Consultations in 1997 noted approximately 2,403 contacts based on 27 programs (Stamm, 1998).

TELEHEALTH FOR CHILDREN AND YOUTH WITH SPECIAL HEALTH CARE NEEDS

Children and youth with special needs present a complex array of health care requirements that remain throughout their lifespan. The health care needs referred to in this section include chronic health disabilities (e.g., diabetes, epilepsy, cystic fibrosis), developmental and behavioral disorders (e.g., cerebral palsy, spina bifida, attention-deficit/hyperactivity disorder, mental retardation, autism) and traumatic injuries (e.g., traumatic brain injury, spinal cord injuries). Traditional service models include having the client and family visit multiple individuals in different clinics or teams of professionals in clinics and communicating information in the standard written report whenever it arrives. Much time, energy, travel, costs, and long waits for appointments and late communications characterize these traditional evaluation and treatment service systems. One consumer noted "we are still going through the same thing as parents did 30 years ago . . . there is all this new technology . . . if we had telemedicine none of this would happen" (Wheeler, 1998, p. 16). It is not surprising that telehealth would be considered for providing multispecialty health care services for children and youth with special needs. As early as the 1990s, professionals in rural New York

(Wheeler, 1998) and rural Georgia (Karp et al., 2000) began offering multidisciplinary services to children with special health care needs at remote locations from hospital settings.

These specialized services have utilized store and forward technologies over phone lines and video conferencing over dedicated transmission lines or closed circuit TV. Applications most often included clinical video consultation and were often combined with the work of professionals at the hospital site in consulting, diagnosing, assessing, and managing a client with his or her family and a local professional at the remote site. Variations on these arrangements included a solo professional in a hospital-based location serving a client and family, and multiple professionals in a team in the hospital location consulting with a team in a remote location, either with a client or without a client. These latter video conferencing situations of multiple professionals were often between hospital-based and locally based (medical, educational, social-mental health) individuals. Case conferencing and follow-up is a very frequent purpose of these services.

Dr. Janet Farmer has been a leader at the University of Missouri in Columbia in providing telehealth consultations to special populations. Children and youth are provided telehealth consultations in physical health care, developmental and cognitive review and assessment, behavioral management, and family social concerns. Most frequently, telehealth was used to provide consultation after an initial on-site hospital-based evaluation or treatment. Secondarily, direct evaluation usually consisted of some physical and developmental assessment of a child and discussion of recommendations. Specific applications of problem and diagnosis in special populations have included: consultation on traumatic brain injury (Schopp, 2000), allergy and asthma, neurology, and genetics (Karp et al., 2000), epilepsy (Glueckauf, 2002), orthopedics (Wheeler, 1998), high-risk infants, well-child review, cancer, juvenile onset diabetes, cystic fibrosis, cerebral palsy, mental retardation, autism, behavioral disorders, learning disabilities, attention-deficit/hyperactivity disorder, depression, feeding disorders, postural support design, and augmentative communication (Harper, 2001a). The majority of consultations for special health care contacts involved management and review, as well as follow-up management after earlier on-site evaluations or treatments. Surveys of effectiveness (Karp et al., 2000; Harper, 2001a; J. Farmer, personal communication, January 15, 2002) have shown high acceptance and satisfaction by consumers and some impact on cost reduction of health care, but little data on whether telehealth is an efficacious mode of clinical delivery for chronic health problems or neurodevelopmental disorders commonly treated in multispecialty settings. Glueckauf (2002) raises similar questions and concerns about the applicability of data on telehealth in rehabilitation.

A unique program of health care, "Baby CareLink," has been developed, with some very promising technical and clinical applications. Baby CareLink is a multifaceted telemedicine program located within a hospital neonatal intensive care unit that incorporates video conferencing and World Wide Web technology to permit and enhance regular interactions between families, medical staff, and community providers (Gray et al., 2000).

Baby CareLink provides information to families using both a specially designed WWW-based system and a system of video conferencing from the neonatal intensive care unit. Families are provided with computer equipment on loan during the time their infant is hospitalized. Six major areas of clinical content and resources are present within this system, including a daily clinical report, a message center, a "See Your Infant" section, a family room, a clinical information section, and a section focused on preparation for discharge to the home. Gray and colleagues found that this system significantly improved family satisfaction with inpatient care and significantly lowered costs associated with hospitalization (Gray et al., 2000).

THE IOWA EXPERIENCE

In 1994, the National Library for the Study of Rural Telemedicine was established at the University of Iowa Hospitals and Clinics (UIHC) in Iowa City, Iowa. The UIHC is large 800-bed, high-tech tertiary-care hospital with 4,000 hospital professionals serving Iowa and the midwest. This project was supported by a grant from the National Library of Medicine, and its purpose was to determine health care delivery needs in a rural setting, to develop technical approaches toward their solution, and to test these applications in community settings. This large project lasted 6 years and provided comprehensive telehealth services with a major focus on evaluation. A complete report of this extensive project is available at *http://telemed.medicine.uiowa.edu*. This project became a national model for the research and evaluation of telemedicine.

The National Library of Medicine project developed five major clinical telehealth projects: Pediatric Echo Network, a statewide tele-echocardiographic consultation network; Emergency Department Support for Vascular Ischemia, a Web-based consultation network for rapid diagnosis and treatment of acute cardiac and brain infarction; Telepsychiatry Consultation, a real-time, two-way video conferencing psychiatry service for rural clients; Diabetes Education, a computer, Web-based and Web-TV in-home consultation/management system for rural clients; Specialized Interdisciplinary Consultations, real-time, two-way video conferencing for children and youths with special needs in rural Iowa communities. These projects and their project investigators provided an amazing test bed of clinical applications of telehealth research evaluating a wide range of clinical problems, populations, and technology.

The Specialized Interdisciplinary Consultation telehealth project, under the leadership of Dennis C. Harper (Harper, 2001b), provides a 7-year history of consultation services for children and youth with complex neurodevelomental disorders in rural Iowa communities. The location for the specialized consultation service is the Center for Disabilities and Development (formerly University Hospital School), which is a specialized hospital of the University of Iowa Hospitals and Clinics that provides treatment and evaluation for people with chronic health care concerns and disabilities. A Specialized Interdisciplinary Team, a telehealth consultation service for children and youths with health and developmental disorders was developed and is presently ongoing. This clinical service is unique in that the evaluations are completed by teams of professionals at both sites (hospital and remote), often with parents and children present.

Real-time communication is achieved by using Iowa's Communication Network (ICN), a fiber-optic statewide cable network, linking 99 counties to 800 sites throughout Iowa. This unique fiber-optic transmission system was installed by the state in the mid- to late 1980s. It has been used for long-distance education purposes as well. The Center for Disabilities and Development has a primary telehealth studio, which can connect with the 800 sites and all community hospitals throughout the entire state of Iowa. The telehealth connections for the clinical services consisted of rural hospitals and multicounty public schools.

The following were major highlights of the project: (1) parents became active care managers during their direct participation in telehealth; (2) recommendations for treatment were presented and discussed in "real time," promoting efficiency, coordination, direct practical application, and immediate feedback; (3) follow-up could occur more frequently and in a more timely manner; (4) professional collaboration and rapport increased; (5) major out-of-pocket cost savings were evident for parents; and (6) collaborative and mutual development of clinical telehealth protocols led to the success of the service.

This Specialized Interdisciplinary Consultation project continues on a regular basis at the Center for Disabilities and Development. Its utilization is primarily for follow-up consultation and initial screening of children prior to on-site evaluations and school-based case conferencing for management. It now has a statewide connection with virtually every county and school district throughout the state of Iowa.

CLOSING COMMENTS

The terms "telehealth," "telemedicine," and "telecommunications" only identify a small portion of what is occurring in the field of electronic communications and informational systems. Speed, access, and digital consolidation of information have had and will have a significant impact on human lives, in particular in the health care delivery infrastructure (Davis & Meyer, 1998). Professionals need to understand telehealth and such technology within a number of contexts. Telehealth applications are all about access to service. Access is a key concept in health care delivery. When access is more readily available, many benefits are possible, including reduced morbidity and potentially increased compliance. Secondarily, telehealth becomes sustainable if it assists with community-based infrastructures. Telehealth sets up new professional–client infrastructures of interaction.

The type of equipment, the quality of the transmission, its reliability, and all associated technical aspects can affect the telehealth experience for both providers and consumers. Technology will increase the likelihood of better and faster communications and hopefully less expensive systems. Communication systems are becoming less complicated and ubiquitous. The technical quality of telehealth will continue to improve over time. Is telehealth effective or efficacious as a clinical tool? Telehealth applications have demonstrated that they are able to provide for a variety of diagnostic and treatment services, screening, counseling, psychosocial management, behavioral management, interviewing, and follow-up. Rapport and key aspects of the usual "therapeutic alliance" can be established to some degree. Considerable research needs to focus on identifying the types of clinical problems that are best suited to a telehealth service and whether such services are in fact as good as "face to face." Encouraging results are emerging for helping chronically disabled populations and promoting ongoing health management.

Will telehealth be a reimbursable service? Payment for service will slowly improve, according to a number of experts in the field. Psychologists need to be aware of the national licensing and credentialing requirements in telehealth practice. Most likely, large health care systems will utilize telehealth to provide services for selected "managed" populations such as the military and correctional institutions, as well as to develop contracts with other selected groups.

Does telehealth fit into the clinician's day? Telehealth systems are best offered as a part of a continuum of services within a clinical array as one method for some parts of delivery or health care assistance. Programs that have had continuing success in maintaining telehealth activities after research funds have been depleted have initially integrated them into a variety of aspects of their regular clinical delivery systems. Professionals will note that success of telehealth systems is directly related to how easy they are to use and whether they fit into clinical work patterns and client needs.

Should professionals have training in telehealth? Training in telehealth might be placed in a broader context of training issues related to electronic communications systems, e-mail, Web sites, store and forward technologies, video conferencing, and professional practice of behavioral health assistance, exploring both legal and ethical issues. Psychologists need skills to enhance their marketability with consumers and a competitive edge within the behavioral health care market. Specific training in telehealth in terms of decorum, as well as the technical aspects, would seem to be a reasonable component to expose many students to during their graduate training years.

Are telehealth systems secure? Confidentiality and security remain issues for work in this particular area. Clearly, technology exists to make systems more secure, but we cannot resolve all our problems with technology. This issue will remain and needs to be understood within the ethical, as well as the legal, context of providing these services.

Providing some aspects of health care to people in more convenient locations has clear benefits for their health and quality of life. Economic benefits to consumers of improved access are a compelling reason to continue to explore telehealth services. If assistance is needed, it can be obtained quicker and easier; it is reasonable to do this in some clinical situations. It is not always economical or the best thing to do just because it might be easier. The mental health and medical professionals are not sure about the impact of such services and their overall efficacy on specific health or mental health problems. In order for telecommunications systems to assist with the problems of the underserved, there needs to be better dispersion of specialists and assistance at the right time. The implementation of telehealth will likely continue to be an uphill battle. The least of the difficulties noted by many authors is the technology. Education, support, motivation, and training of providers are critical. A variety of political and social factors often stand in the way of moving toward newer technologies. Pediatric psychologists need to be sensitive to those issues and seek solutions. An overall analysis suggests that telehealth efforts do work in a number of respects. Complex technologies will continue to assist in developing a better quality of life; however, the scientific practitioner's goal is to learn to manage them so that this does in fact happen.

REFERENCES

American Telemedicine Association. (2002, February). Retrieved April, 2002, from *http://www.americantelemed.org.*

Antezana, F. (1997, July). *Telehealth and telemedicine will henceforth be part of the strategy for health for all.* Retrieved December, 2001, from *http://www.who.ch//*

Baer, L., Cukor, P., Jenike, M.A., Leahy, L., O'Laughlen, J., & Coyle, J. T. (1995). Pilot studies of telemedicine for patients with obsessive–compulsive disorder. *American Journal of Psychiatry, 152*(9), 1383–1385.

Baer, L., Elford, R., & Cukor, P. (1997). Telepsychiatry at forty: What have we learned? *Harvard Review of Psychiatry, 5,* 7–17.

Bashshur, R. L., Sanders, J. H., & Shannon, G. (1997). *Telemedicine: Theory and practice.* Springfield, IL: Thomas.

Bauer, J. C., & Ringel, M. A. (1999). *Telemedicine and the reinvention of healthcare: The seventh revolution in medicine.* New York: McGraw-Hill.

Brown, F. W. (1995). A survey of telepsychiatry in the USA. *Journal of Telemedicine and Telecare,* 1, 19–21.

Darkins, A. W., & Cary, M. A. (2000). *Telemedicine and telehealth: Principles, policies, performance, and pitfalls.* New York: Springer.

Davis, S., & Meyer, C. (1998). *BLUR the speed of change in the connected economy.* New York: Warner Books.

Gilder, G. (2000). *Telcosm: How infinite bandwidth will revolutionize our world.* New York: Free Press.

Gladwell, M. (2000). *The tipping point: How little things can make a big difference.* New York: Little, Brown.

Glueckauf, R. L. (2002). Telehealth and chronic disabilities: New frontier for research and development. *Rehabilitation Psychology, 47*(1), 3–7.

Gray, J. E., Safran, C., Davis, R. B., Pompilio-Weitzner, G., Stewart, J. E., Zaccagnini, L., & Pursley, D. (2000). Baby CareLink: Using the Internet and telemedicine to improve care for high-risk infants. *Pediatrics, 106,* 1318–1324.

Harper, D. C. (2001a). *Telemedicine services for children with disabilities in rural Iowa: From research to practice* [CD-ROM]. Bethesda, MD: National Institutes of Health, National Library of Medicine.

Harper, D. C. (2001b). Team-based telemedicine for children with disabilities in rural Iowa. *Telemedicine Journal and e-Health*, *7*, 123.

Karp, W. B., Grigsby, R. K., McSiggan-Hardin, M., Pursley-Crotteau, S., Adams, L. N., Bell, W., et al. (2000). Use of telemedicine for children with special health care needs. *Pediatrics*, *105*, 843–847.

Liss, H., Glueckauf, R. L., & Ecklund-Johnson, E. P. (2002). Research on telehealth and chronic medical conditions: Critical review, key issues, and future directions. *Rehabilitation Psychology*, *47*, 8–30.

Maheu, M. (2000, August). *Telehealth: Delivering behavioral telehealth via the Internet E-health*. Retrieved December, 2001, from *http://telehealth.net/articles/deliver.html*.

McKay, H. G., Glasgow, R. E., Feil, E. G., Boles, S. M., & Barrera, M., Jr. (2002). Internet-based diabetes self-management and support: Initial outcomes from the Diabetes Network Project. *Rehabilitation Psychology*, *47*, 31–48.

Nickelson, D. W. (1998). Telehealth and the evolving health care system: Strategic opportunities for professional psychology. *Professional Psychology: Research and Practice*, *29*, 527–535.

Rohland, B. M., & Flaum, M. (2000, March). *A comparison of telepsychiatry vs. face-to-face care in a rural community mental health setting*. Retrieved December, 2001, from *http://www.nlm/nav-telepsy.html*.

Schopp, L. (2000). Telehealth and traumatic brain injury: Creative community-based care. *Telemedicine Today*, *8*, 4–6, 33.

Stamm, B. H. (1998). Clinical applications of telehealth in mental health care. *Professional Psychology: Research and Practice*, *29*, 536–542.

Viegas, S. F., & Dunn, K. (1998). *Telemedicine: Practicing in the information age*. Philadelphia: Lippincott-Raven.

Wheeler, T. (1998). Telemedicine and special needs children. *Telemedicine Today*, *6*(4), 16–20.

Zarate, C. A., Jr., Weinstock, L., Cukor, P., Morabito, C., Leahy, L., Burns, C., & Baer, L. (1997). Applicability of telemedicine for assessing patients with schizophrenia: Acceptance and reliability. *Journal of Clinical Psychiatry*, *58*, 22–25.

45

International Pediatric Psychology

MAUREEN M. BLACK
AMBIKA KRISHNAKUMAR

International pediatric psychology extends the scientific basis of pediatric psychology across cultures. Global policies in economics, communication, and industry influence our daily lives and contribute to the increasing cultural diversity in many communities. Despite a nearly universal commitment to children through the ratification of the Convention on the Rights of the Child,[1] widespread discrepancies exist in rates of pediatric mortality and morbidity, often related to poverty, sanitary conditions, environmental toxins, infectious agents, and access to health services. Children in many Asian and African countries are much more likely to die before their fifth birthdays or to experience malnutrition and other serious illnesses and disabilities compared with children in Europe, Australia, or the United States (UNICEF, 2001).

Although many common threats to children's health exist across cultures—ranging from biomedical challenges such as infectious diseases, chronic illnesses, and disabilities to psychosocial challenges such as child abuse and neglect—contextual and cultural differences are associated with the meaning that families attribute to children's health and illness. These differences influence choices that families make regarding their care practices, their children's exposure to potential dangers, their requests for assistance, and their response to interventions. This chapter examines three important components of international pediatric psychology: (1) theoretical considerations, (2) methodological considerations, and (3) content areas.

[1]The Convention on the Rights of the Child is an international document that guarantees basic rights of children. It has been ratified by most countries in the world and by the Council of Representatives of the American Psychological Association, but not by the United States.

THEORETICAL CONSIDERATIONS

International pediatric psychology examines the applicability of either adapting existing theories or developing alternative theories to address the behavioral and developmental aspects of children's health and illness across cultures (Black, Eiser, & Krishnakumar, 2000). Beliefs regarding health and illness come from a combination of cultural forces and individual experiences. In many communities, families rely on both Western medicine and indigenous practices (Scrimshaw, 1992), highlighting the importance of recognizing local ethnotheories or beliefs regarding the causes, symptoms, and remedies for illnesses. Harkness and Super (1994) have introduced the concept of a "developmental niche" that includes ethnotheories or beliefs about parenting, the physical and social setting, and the psychological functioning of the child's caregivers. Applied to health and illness, the developmental niche would also include parental ethnotheories of health and illness. Many anthropologists and psychologists advocate adopting an ecological model, which recognizes the importance of cultural, environmental, and social systems on individual behavior (Bronfenbrenner, 1979) and which can be applied to issues related to children's health and illness across cultures.

Parents and community members communicate their understanding of health and illness to their children as they encourage them to adapt to cultural demands and to acquire the health behavioral norms and socialization patterns of their ethnic group (Mindel, Habenstein, & Wright, 1988). Cultural norms and socialization patterns determine how children and families react to health-related situations (e.g., how they define and interpret their symptoms), how they feel about themselves, and how they respond to treatment. In addition, historical experiences of the ethnic group (e.g., racial prejudice) and culturally determined patterns of dealing with issues of health and illness shape families' lives and play a determining role in their behavior, relationships, and socialization practices when faced with health-related situations.

In an example cited by Scrimshaw (2001), in a community in which many children had worms, Guatemalan mothers believed that worms were normal for children unless the worms got agitated and were excreted or coughed up. Agitation often occurred during the rainy season, and mothers reasoned that the worms were frightened by the thunder or lightning. It is likely that the "agitation" was related to the relatively high rates of diarrhea during the rainy season associated with difficulty maintaining hygienic practices. Rather than trying to convince the mothers that their beliefs were wrong, health workers advocated deworming children prior to the rainy season so they would not be bothered by agitated worms. Although this example illustrates the importance of listening to families and trying to understand their beliefs or ethnotheories related to the causes and symptoms of their children's illnesses, it raises questions regarding the responsibility of professionals in educating parents. In addition to recommending deworming prior to the rainy season, if the health workers had linked the problem of worms to community and household hygienic practices, families may have avoided some of the health hazards associated with poor hygienic practices. By incorporating beliefs from children, caregivers, and the community regarding the explanations for children's health and illness, pediatric psychologists can adapt existing theories or develop alternative theories to guide their evaluation and treatment plans.

Ethnotheories regarding children's health and illness vary across cultures. For example, in many Eastern countries, such as India, families may attribute their children's health and illness to spirituality, supernatural powers, and beliefs such as fate, God's will, or karma (the cycle of birth and death in which past deeds determine future life options). Factors that are considered to be central to Western explanations of illness, such as viruses, bacteria, or behavior, are often disregarded (Kohli & Dalal, 1998). In contrast, families in Western countries often rely on individual determinants of children's health and illness. Even when they have exhausted reasonable efforts to identify the etiology of a problem, some families visit multiple practitioners in the search for explanations of their children's illness, either to find a cure or to exonerate themselves from perceived culpability. The attributions that families ascribe to their children's health and illness influence their response to practitioners and their adherence to recommendations. For example, practitioners who focus on individual attributions and recommendations for managing children's illnesses and promoting health may not be well accepted by families who view health and illness from a spiritual or supernatural perspective.

METHODOLOGICAL CONSIDERATIONS

There is a growing demand to develop both global and culturally specific and sensitive measures for evaluating children's health and to determine whether intervention strategies have been effective in reducing the rate of health problems. The necessity to evaluate new treatments involving relatively rare medical and psychological problems, to compare these treatments across cultures, and to monitor the health of diverse cultural and ethnic populations has become of primary concern among health care professionals. To achieve these varied goals, clinicians and researchers often use common measures across cultures. Measures of children's developmental and intellectual capabilities, such as the Bayley Scales of Infant Development and the Wechsler Intelligence Scale for Children, have been translated and used in many cultures. Despite recognition that environmental and nutritional factors influence children's behavior and development (Black, Hess, & Berenson-Howard, 2000), little attention has been paid to the validity of measures of children's behavioral development when used across cultures.

Much caution is warranted when measuring children's behavior, development, and response to health and illness across cultures. Strategies for adapting standardized instruments should extend beyond language translation. Translating the words of a questionnaire or interview does not make the questionnaire valid or reliable for use in another culture. For example, in the translation of the Diagnostic Interview Schedule (DIS) and the Diagnostic Interview Schedule for Children (DISC) from English to Spanish, Canino, Lewis-Fernandez, and Bravo (1997) reported experiencing difficulties in finding equivalent Spanish terms and in formulating questions so that respondents did not under- or overreport specific items. When the McCarthy Scales of Children's Abilities (MSCA) and the Behavioral Style Questionnaire (BSQ) were used with a Jamaican sample, the authors had to make modifications that included the cultural use of certain words and phrases, local pronunciations, and meanings consistent with the country's dialect (Dreher & Hayes, 1993). Decisions about where the instruments are to be administered (home or clinic), whether an interview or questionnaire technique is to be used (differing literacy levels of families), cultural norms concerning expression of illness behaviors, the cultural group's perception of the illness, and the method of help seeking for the illness should be addressed before administration.

In addition, it is not appropriate to assume that questionnaires and techniques validated in one culture can be applied to another culture without examining their cross-cultural equivalence. There are four levels of cross-cultural equivalence (Butcher & Han, 1996; Triandis, Brislin, & Hui, 1988). *Conceptual equivalence* is a comparison between the semantic meaning of the items and constructs in the two languages. *Construct* or *item equiva-*

lence is a measure of whether individuals in different cultural groups respond to the same item in similar ways. *Operational equivalence* refers to the relative performance of the instrument when method of administration varies (e.g., self-report, interview). *Metric equivalence* refers to the ranking of individuals with similar behaviors or symptoms across different cultures. The categories of responses for items within questionnaires should also be considered. Some cultural groups tend to overreport or, in other words, respond to extreme ends of the scale, such as "always" or "never," whereas others are more likely to endorse responses at the middle of the scale. Cultural backgrounds may partially determine how people interpret the rating scales and intervals on a scale. The lack of understanding of what a point on a scale means to members of a particular cultural group can result in the inappropriate interpretation of the responses (Pachter & Harwood, 1996).

Several investigators have provided guidelines for adapting instruments for children across cultures (Bullinger, Anderson, Cella, & Aaronson, 1993; Leung & Van de Vijver, 1996). Rather than merely translating measures, investigators should conduct forward and backward translation and then compare the translated version with the original source, have it reviewed by lay panels and expert committees, and finally conduct psychometric testing of the translated version to examine cross-cultural equivalence, along with reliability and validity.

In addition to concerns about reliability and validity, methodologies that are commonly used in Western societies, such as questionnaires, standardized testing, and observations, are not always appropriate in low- and middle-income countries, where rates of literacy are low and few resources are available for evaluation. Many investigators have called for rapid methods of evaluation that can be used to screen populations (Scrimshaw, 1992). For example, recent evidence has shown that parental concerns regarding specific aspects of their child's development are highly correlated with results from developmental screening tests (Glascoe, 1997), suggesting the importance of relying on parental report. Focusing on parental concerns enables providers to listen to parents and should facilitate the application of culturally consistent interventions (Glascoe, Altemeier, & MacLean, 1989).

CONTENT AREAS

Each year, preventable diseases, including pneumonia, diarrhea, malaria, malnutrition, and measles, claim the lives of more than 10 million children under age 5. Poverty is probably the most prevalent cause of childhood illness and disability (World Health Organization, 1999). Efforts to reduce poverty often require interdisciplinary collaboration with attention to economic and societal reform. However, community, family, and individual-level interventions can all reduce the threat and negative consequences associated with children's illnesses and disabilities. International public health problems, such as the recent epidemic of the human immunodeficiency virus (HIV), have demonstrated the importance of behavioral interventions and collaboration among health professionals from multiple disciplines.

Malnutrition

Millions of young children throughout the world experience malnutrition that is severe enough to stunt their linear growth, with rates exceeding 50% in some low-income countries (UNICEF, 2001). The effects of malnutrition are most severe in the first few years of life, when children's growth is rapid and their nutritional demands are high. The consequences of malnutrition range from the immediate discomfort associated with hunger to long-term deficits in growth and adaptive functioning. There is mounting evidence from Peru (Berkman, Lescano, Gilman, Lopez, & Black, 2002), the Philippines (Mendez & Adair, 1999), Jamaica (Walker, Grantham-McGregor, Powell, & Chang, 2000), and Barbados (Galler, 1984) that stunting associated with malnutrition in the first 2 years of life compromises children's academic performance during school-age years. Unless there are comprehensive interventions that include significant environmental changes, such as adoption (Rutter, 1998; Winick, Meyer, & Harris, 1975), most severely malnourished children experience long-term behavioral and developmental deficits.

An initial response to severe malnutrition was to provide foods high in calories and proteins. Although most food-based interventions limited their evaluations to changes in children's growth, those who examined the impact on children's behavior and development have reported that infants from a rural Mexican village whose diets were supplemented were more active and playful than their peers who were not given supplements, that their behavioral improvements were sustained over time, and that they elicited interactive behavior from their parents (Chavez, Martinez, & Soberanes, 1995). Recent attention has been directed to micronutrient deficiencies, such as iron, zinc, vitamin B-12, and iodine, because these deficiencies are widespread, have negative health consequences, and have been linked to specific behavioral and developmental deficits (Allen, 1994; Black, 1998; Grantham-McGregor, Walker, & Chang, 2000).

Investigators have also begun to recognize the importance of combining nutritional and environmental interventions (Pelto, Dickin, & Engle, 1999). In addition to their growth delays, malnourished children are often wary (Meeks-Gardner, Grantham-McGregor, Chang, Himes, & Powell, 1995), lethargic and inactive and have limited ability to take advantage of environmental opportunities (Grantham-McGregor, 1995). During home observations, mothers of malnourished infants were less sensitive and responsive (Valenzuela, 1997) and more likely to hold or carry their infants rather than play with them (Graves, 1976) than were mothers of healthy infants. Taken together, these observations illustrate the concept of functional isolation that Levitsky and Barnes (1972) described, whereby nutritional deficiencies are partially mediated through caregiving behavior. That is, in addition to the biological consequences of nutritional deprivation, malnourished children are functionally isolated from their surroundings because they do not elicit or use environmental care and enrichment from their families. Interventions that have combined nutrition with environmental stimulation have demonstrated beneficial effects on children's development (Grantham-McGregor, Powell, Walker, & Himes, 1991; Super, Herrera, & Mora, 1990).

Chronic and Infectious Diseases

Epidemiologists estimate that the rates of chronic diseases, such as Type 2 diabetes, will increase dramatically during the early years of the 21st century (Murray & Lopez, 1997). Patterns of family interactions among children with chronic illnesses may vary across cultures, as demonstrated in a recent investigation of Hong Kong youths with Type 2 diabetes (Stewart et al., 2000). Although the children's functioning did not vary by parenting style, even low levels of parent–child conflict were associated with poorer emotional adjustment among the children. Thus, in Hong Kong and perhaps in other countries, families of children with chronic illnesses, such as Type 2 diabetes, may benefit from interventions to promote conflict management.

Infectious diseases, such as HIV and malaria, are prevalent in many low-income countries and are associated with high rates of childhood mortality and morbidity. Children who experience cerebral malaria early in life are at risk for multiple neuropsychological abnormalities that can interfere with cognitive and academic functioning (Boivin, 2002).

Injuries

Injuries are a leading cause of death and disability among children throughout the world. Injuries are classified as intentional (e.g., violence, child abuse) or nonintentional (e.g., poisons, fires, falls, motor vehicles). Injuries of all types are more common in low-income countries than in middle- and high-income countries and are often related to poverty and to the difficulty in protecting children from household and environmental dangers (McQueen, McKenna, & Sleet, 2001). Although little is known about rates of child abuse internationally, investigators in a rural Indian community found that almost half of the parents reported using severe verbal and physical disciplinary techniques (Hunter, Jain, Sadowski, & Sanhueza, 2000). Mothers who reported using severe disciplinary techniques were also more likely to report spousal violence and to have lower levels of education than mothers who did not use severe disciplinary techniques.

Children are often victims in injuries related to war, particularly when land mines have been abandoned in fields (Toole, Waldman, & Zwi, 2001). Motor vehicle accidents are the leading cause of injury-related deaths among people of all ages, particularly in low-income countries in which population rates are increasing, limited attention is paid to automobile or road safety, and access to emergency health care services is limited. Although individual behavioral interventions could be implemented to reduce the likelihood of injuries, there is a need for additional research into community and environmental strategies.

Mental Health

Relatively little attention has been directed to children's mental health in the international arena. High rates of poverty, coupled with limited access to education and health services, increase the likelihood of mental health problems. In addition, children are disproportionately victimized during civil and international conflicts (Toole et al., 2001). There are concerns regarding high rates of posttraumatic stress disorder among children who have experienced major disruptions often associated with war or violence, and intervention strategies are controversial. Some professionals recommend a mental health approach that includes trauma centers and individual therapy, whereas others recommend a community focus that includes reconstruction of community resources and a return to normalcy (Bracken, Giller, & Summerfield, 1995).

To assess the burden of various conditions on health, investigators calculate disability-adjusted life years (DALYs) lost (Murray & Lopez, 1997). Mental health and behavioral problems account for 5 of the 10 leading disorders among individuals in the 15–44 age group in low- and middle-income countries. Depression is the leading cause of mental health disability in this age group. Increasing rates of mental health problems, particularly depression, have led to projections that, by 2020, depression will be second only to cardiovascular disorders in lost DALYs across the world (Murray & Lopez, 1997).

Mothers who are depressed have been described as having intrusive or insensitive interactions with their infants (Cohn, Matias, Tronick, Connell, & Lyons-Ruth, 1986). Infants of depressed mothers are at risk for health and growth problems (Rahman, Harrington, & Bunn, 2002), and children of depressed mothers are at risk for behavioral and developmental problems (Downey & Coyne, 1990), possibly associated with ineffective and inconsistent parenting behavior and lack of attention to the children's physical and emotional needs. The high rates of depression among women throughout the world raise concerns for the health and well-being of their children, particularly because depression often interferes with mothers' ability to benefit from interventions to promote child-rearing practices (Hutcheson et al., 1997).

Environmental Health

Environmental risks can have a disproportionate impact on young children, particularly when they are exposed early in life during periods of rapid growth and development. Lead exposure provides an example of the negative consequences of environmental toxins and the disproportionate burden faced by children in low- and middle-income countries. By studying the blood lead levels of children living near a smelter from ages 2 through 13, investigators demonstrated a clear relationship between increasing levels of lead and decreases in children's cognitive functioning on standardized assessments (Tong, Baghurst, Sawyer, Burns, & McMichael, 1998).

Lead is a heavy metal that has been an important component of industries, especially the automobile industry. High-income countries, such as the United States, Australia, and many European countries, have mandated the use of alternatives, such as lead-free gasoline. However, low-income countries do not have the economic resources to limit lead exposure. Therefore, many children in Africa and Asia are exposed to levels of lead that could damage their cognitive functioning. In addition to the need for strategies to protect children from lead exposure, there are many unanswered questions regarding lead exposure, including dose-related effects, the mechanisms linking exposure to specific deficits, the long-term consequences, and rehabilitation strategies. Many other environmental toxins and contaminants present health challenges to children (McMichael, Kjellstrom, & Smith, 2001). For example, respiratory disease, the leading cause of mortality in children, has been linked to air pollution among infants and young children in Eastern Europe (Bobak & Leon, 1992). In addition to outdoor air pollution, solid fuel used for household cooking in many low-income countries leads to respiratory illnesses and deaths (World Health Organization, 1997). The second leading cause of childhood mortality, diarrhea, has been associated with the lack of basic household services, including safe drinking water and sanitary methods of disposing of excreta.

CONCLUSIONS

Children in low- and middle-income countries are at risk for a wide range of illnesses, often associated with poverty, environmental toxins, unsanitary conditions, limited access to healthy nutrients, and inadequate health care services. Although many illnesses result in behavioral and developmental problems, little is known about effective behavioral interventions. In addition, there is much to be learned about the role of risk and protective factors associated with specific illnesses. With a solid grounding in theories of childhood development, behavioral change, and health; with training in methodologies necessary to develop culturally sensitive, reliable, and valid measures of children's health and illness; and with an understanding of many illnesses confronting children, pediatric psychologists are well positioned to participate in interdisciplinary teams of professionals investigating children's health and illness across international boundaries.

REFERENCES

Allen, L. H. (1994). Vitamin B12 metabolism and status during pregnancy, lactation and infancy. *Advances in Experimental Medicine and Biology, 352*, 173–186.

Berkman, D. S., Lescano, A. G., Gilman, R. H., Lopez, S. C., & Black, M. M. (2002). Effects of stunting, diarrhoeal disease, and parasitic infection during infancy on cognition in late childhood: A follow-up study. *Lancet, 359*, 564–571.

Black, M. M. (1998). Zinc and child development. *American Journal of Clinical Nutrition, 68*, 464S–469S.

Black, M. M., Eiser, C., & Krishnakumar, A. (2000). International research and practice in pediatric psychology: Challenges and new directions. *Journal of Pediatric Psychology, 25*, 363–366.

Black, M. M., Hess, C. R., & Berenson-Howard, J. (2000). Toddlers from low-income families have below normal mental, motor, and behavior scores on the revised Bayley scales. *Journal of Applied Developmental Psychology, 21*, 655–666.

Bobak, M., & Leon, D. A. (1992). Air pollution and infant mortality in the Czech Republic, 1986–1988. *Lancet, 340*, 1010–1014.

Boivin, M. J. (2002). Effects of early cerebral malaria on cognitive ability in Senegalese children. *Journal of Developmental and Behavioral Pediatrics, 23*, 353–364.

Bracken, P. J., Giller, J. E., & Summerfield, D. (1995). Psychological responses to war and atrocity: The limitations of current concepts. *Social Science and Medicine, 40*, 1073–1082.

Bronfenbrenner, U. (1979). *The ecology of human development*. Cambridge, MA: Harvard University Press.

Bullinger, M., Anderson, R., Cella, D., & Aaronson, N. (1993). Developing and evaluating cross-cultural instruments from minimum requirements to optimal models. *Quality of Life Research: An International Journal of Quality of Life Aspects of Treatment, 2*, 451–459.

Butcher, J. N., & Han, K. (1996). Methods of establishing cross-cultural equivalence. In J. N. Butcher (Ed.), *International adaptations of the MMPI-2: Research and clinical applications* (pp. 44–63). Minneapolis, MN: University of Minnesota Press.

Canino, G., Lewis-Fernandez, R., & Bravo, M. (1997). Methodological challenges in cross-cultural mental health research. *Transcultural Psychiatry, 34*, 163–184.

Chavez, A., Martinez, C., & Soberanes, B. (1995). The effect of malnutrition on human development: A 24–year study of well-nourished and malnourished children living in a poor Mexican village. In N. S. Scrimshaw (Ed.), *Community-based longitudinal nutrition and health studies: Classical examples from Guatemala, Haiti, and Mexico* (pp. 302–334). Boston: International Nutrition Foundation for Developing Countries.

Cohn, J., Matias, R., Tronick, E., Connell, D., & Lyons-Ruth, K. (1986). Face-to-face interactions of depressed mothers and their infants. In E. Tronick & T. Field (Eds.), *Maternal depression and infant disturbance* (pp. 31–46). San Francisco: Jossey-Bass.

Dreher, M. C., & Hayes, J. S. (1993). Triangulation in cross-cultural research of child development in Jamaica. *Western Journal of Nursing Research, 15*, 216–229.

Downey, G., & Coyne, J. (1990). Children of depressed parents: An integrative review. *Psychological Bulletin, 108*, 50–76.

Galler, J. (1984). The behavioral consequences of malnutrition in early life. In J. Galler (Ed.), *Nutrition and behavior* (pp. 63–118). New York: Plenum Press.

Glascoe, F. P. (1997). Parents' concerns about children's development: Prescreening technique or screening test? *Pediatrics, 99*, 522–528.

Glascoe, F. P., Altemeier, W. A., & MacLean, W. E. (1989) The importance of parents' concerns about their child's development. *American Journal of Diseases in Childhood, 143*, 955–958.

Grantham-McGregor, S. (1995). A review of studies of the effect of severe malnutrition on mental development. *Journal of Nutrition, 125*, 2233S–2238S.

Grantham-McGregor, S. M., Powell, C. A., Walker, S. P., & Himes, J. H. (1991). Nutritional supplementation, psychosocial stimulation, and mental development of stunted children: The Jamaican study, *Lancet, 338*, 1–5.

Grantham-McGregor, S. M., Walker, S. P., & Chang, S. M., (2000). Nutritional deficiencies and later behavioural development. *Proceedings of the Nutrition Society, 59*, 47–54.

Graves, P. L. (1976). Nutrition, infant behavior, and maternal characteristics: A pilot study in West Bengal, India. *American Journal of Clinical Nutrition, 29*, 305–319.

Harkness, S., & Super, C. M. (1994). The developmental niche: A theoretical framework for analyzing the household production of health. *Social Science and Medicine, 38*, 217–226.

Hunter, W. M., Jain, D., Sadowski, L. S., & Sanhueza, A. I. (2000). Risk factors for severe child discipline in rural India. *Journal of Pediatric Psychology, 25*, 435–448.

Hutcheson, J. J., Black, M. M., Talley, M., Dubowitz, H., Berenson-Howard, J., Starr, R. H., & Thompson, B. S. (1997). Risk status and home intervention among children with failure to thrive: Follow-up at age 4. *Journal of Pediatric Psychology, 22*, 651–668.

Kohli, N., & Dalal, A. K. (1998). Culture as a factor in causal understanding of illness: A study of cancer patients. *Psychology and Developing Societies, 10,* 115–129.

Leung, K., & Van de Vijver, F. (1996). Cross-cultural research methodology. In F. T. L. Leong & J. T. Austin (Eds.), *The psychology research handbook: A guide for graduate students and research assistants* (pp. 351–358). Thousand Oaks, CA: Sage.

Levitsky, D. A., & Barnes, R. H. (1972). Nutritional and environmental interactions in the behavioral development of the rat: Long-term effects. *Science, 176,* 68–73.

McMichael, A. J., Kjellstrom, T., & Smith, K. R. (2001). Environmental health. In M. H. Merson, R. E. Black, & A. J. Mills (Eds.), *International public health* (pp. 379–437). Gaithersburg, MD: Aspen.

McQueen, D. V., McKenna, M. T., & Sleet, D. A. (2001). Chronic diseases and injury. In M. H. Merson, R. E. Black, & A. J. Mills (Eds.), *International public health* (pp. 293–330). Gaithersburg, MD: Aspen.

Meeks-Gardner, J., Grantham-McGregor, S. M., Chang, S. M., Himes, J. H., & Powell, C. A. (1995). Activity and behavioral development in stunted and nonstunted children and response to nutritional supplementation. *Child Development, 66,* 1785–1797.

Mendez, M. A., & Adair, L. S. (1999). Severity and timing of stunting in the first two years of life affect performance on cognitive tests in late childhood. *Journal of Nutrition, 129,* 1555–1562.

Mindel, C. H., Habenstein, R. W., & Wright, R. (1988). *Ethnic families in America: Patterns and variations* (pp. 1–16). Englewood Cliffs, NJ: Prentice-Hall.

Murray, C. J. L., & Lopez, A. D. (1997). Regional patterns of disability-free life expectancy and disability-adjusted life expectancy: Global Burden of Disease Study. *Lancet, 349,* 1347–1352.

Pachter, L. M., & Harwood, R. L. (1996). Culture and child behavior and psychosocial development. *Journal of Developmental and Behavioral Pediatrics, 17,* 191–198.

Pelto, G., Dickin, K., & Engle, P. (1999). *A critical link: Interventions for physical growth and psychological development.* Geneva, Switzerland: World Health Organization.

Rahman, A., Harrington, R., & Bunn, J. (2002). Can maternal depression increase infant risk of illness and growth impairment in developing countries? *Child: Care, Health and Development, 28,* 51–56.

Rutter, M. (1998). Developmental catch-up, and deficit, following adoption after severe global early privation: English and Romanian Adoptees (ERA) Study Team. *Journal of Child Psychology and Psychiatry, 39,* 465–476.

Scrimshaw, S. C. M. (1992). Adaptation of anthropological methodologies to rapid assessment of nutrition and primary health care. In N. S. Scrimshaw & G. R. Gleason (Eds.), *Rapid assessment procedures: Qualitative methodologies for planning and evaluation of health related programmes* (pp. 25–49). Boston: International Nutrition Foundation for Developing Countries.

Scrimshaw, S. C. M. (2001). Culture, behavior, and health. In M. H. Merson, R. E. Black, & A. J. Mills (Eds.), *International public health* (pp. 53–78). Gaithersburg, MD: Aspen.

Stewart, S. M., Lee, P. W. H., Low, L. C. K., Cheng, A., Yeung, W., Huen, K. F., & O'Donnell, D. (2000). Pathways from emotional adjustment to glycemic control in youth with diabetes in Hong Kong. *Journal of Pediatric Psychology, 25,* 393–402.

Super, C. M., Herrera, M. A., & Mora, J. O. (1990). Long-term effects of food supplementation and psychosocial intervention on the physical growth of Columbian infants at risk of malnutrition. *Child Development, 61,* 29–49.

Toole, M. J., Waldman, R. J., & Zwi, A. B. (2001). Complex humanitarian emergencies. In M. H. Merson, R. E. Black, & A. J. Mills (Eds.), *International public health* (pp. 439–514). Gaithersburg, MD: Aspen.

Tong, S., Baghurst, P. A., Sawyer, M. G., Burns, J., & McMichael, A. J. (1998). Declining blood lead levels and cognitive function during childhood: The Port Pirie Cohort Study. *Journal of the American Medical Association, 280,* 1915–1919.

Triandis, H. C., Brislin, R., & Hui, C. H. (1988). Cross-cultural training across the individualism–collectivism divide. *International Journal of Intercultural Relations, 12,* 269–289.

UNICEF (2001). The state of the world children 2001. New York: Author.

Valenzuela, M. (1997). Maternal sensitivity in a developing society: The context of urban poverty and infant chronic undernutrition. *Developmental Psychology, 33,* 845–855.

Walker, S. P., Grantham-McGregor, S. M., Powell, C. A., & Chang, S. M. (2000). Effects of growth restriction in early childhood on growth, IQ, and cognition at age 11 to 12 years and the benefits of nutritional supplementation and psychosocial stimulation. *Journal of Pediatrics, 137,* 36–41.

Winick, M., Meyer, K. K., & Harris, R. C. (1975). Malnutrition and environmental enrichment by early adoption. *Science, 190,* 1173–1175.

World Health Organization. (1997). *Health and environment in sustainable development* (Document WHO/EHG/97.8). Geneva, Switzerland: Author.

World Health Organization. (1999). *The world health report.* Geneva, Switzerland: Author.

Index

B

C

D

F

G

H

I

J

L

M

N

S

T

U

V

W

Y